ORAL CANCER

Edited by

Jatin P Shah MD, MS(Surg), FACS,
Hon FRCS(Edin), Hon FRACS,
Hon FDSRCS(Lond)
Professor of Surgery
Weill Medical College of Cornell University
Chief, Head and Neck Service
EW Strong Chair in Head and Neck Oncology
Memorial Sloan–Kettering Cancer Center
New York, USA

Newell W Johnson PhD, MDSc, FDSRCS,
FRACDS, FRCPath, FFOP(RCPA), ILTM, FMedSci
Professor of Oral and Maxillofacial Medicine and Pathology
WHO Collaborating Centre for Oral Cancer and Precancer
The Guys, Kings and St Thomas' Schools of Medicine,
Dentistry and Biomedical Sciences
Kings College
London, UK

John G Batsakis MD
Professor Emeritus and Former Chairman
Department of Pathology
University of Texas, MD Anderson Cancer Center
Houston, USA

MARTIN DUNITZ

First published in the United Kingdom in 2003
by Martin Dunitz, an imprint of the Taylor & Francis Group,
11 New Fetter Lane, London EC4P 4EE

Tel.: +44 (0) 20 7583 9855
Fax.: +44 (0) 20 7842 2298
E-mail: info.dunitz@tandf.co.uk
Website: http://www.dunitz.co.uk

A CIP record for this book is available from the British Library.

ISBN 1 899066 87 X

Distributed in the United States and Canada by
Thieme New York
333 Seventh Avenue
New York, NY 10001

Distributed in the rest of the world by
Thomson Publishing Services
Cheriton House
North Way
Andover, Hampshire SP10 5BE, UK
Tel.: +44 (0)1264 332424
E-mail: salesorder.tandf@thomsonpublishingservices.co.uk

Composition by Scribe Design, Gillingham, Kent
Printed and bound in Spain by Grafos S.A. Sobre Arte Paple

Contents

Contributors

John G Batsakis
Emeritus Professor and former Chairman
Department of Pathology
University of Texas – MD Anderson Cancer Center
1515 Holcombe Boulevard
Houston, TX 77030, USA

Peter T Blenkinsopp
Honorary Senior Registrar
Eastman Dental Institute – University of London;
Consultant Maxillofacial Surgeon
Queen Mary's University Hospital
Roehampton SW15 5PN, UK

Per Ingvar Brånemark
Director, Institute for Applied Biotechnology
Gothenburg, Sweden;
Visiting Professor
University of Surrey

John F Carew
Assistant Professor
Department of Otorhinolaryngology –
Head and Neck Surgery
Weill Medical College of Cornell University
Assistant Attending Surgeon
Department of Otorhinolaryngology –
Head and Neck Surgery
New York Presbyterian Hospital;
New York, NY 10021, USA

Brian F Conroy
Senior Research Fellow
Department of Biomedical Engineering
University of Surrey;
Eastman Dental Institute – University of London
256 Gray's Inn Road
London WC1X 8LD, UK

Robert Dunlop
Medical Director
St Christopher's Hospice
51–59 Lawrie Park Road
Sydenham
London SE26 6DZ, UK

John Glaholm
Birmingham Oncology Centre
Queen Elizabeth Hospital
Birmingham B15 2TH, UK

Newell W Johnson
Professor of Oral and Maxillofacial Medicine and Pathology
King's College Dental School
Caldecot Road
London SE5 9RW, UK

Snehal G Patel
Clinical Research Associate
Head and Neck Service
Memorial Sloan–Kettering Cancer Center
1275 York Avenue
New York, NY 10021, USA

Jatin P Shah
Professor of Surgery
Weill Medical College of Cornell University;
Chief, Head and Neck Service
EW Strong Chair in Head and Neck Oncology
Memorial Sloan–Kettering Cancer Center
1275 York Avenue
New York, NY 10021, USA

Bhuvanesh Singh
Assistant Professor of Otorhinolaryngology – Head and Neck Surgery
Weill Medical College of Cornell University;
Assistant Attending Surgeon
Head and Neck Service
Memorial Sloan–Kettering Cancer Center
1275 York Avenue
New York, NY 10021, USA

Preface

Oral cancer, the sixth most common cancer worldwide, continues to be the most prevalent cancer related to the consumption of tobacco, alcohol and other carcinogenic products. While the incidence of this cancer remains high in South and Southeast Asia, its traditional highest risk areas, parts of Central and Eastern Europe are seeing alarming increases and now constitute the highest incidence parts of the globe. Encouragingly, however, over the past few years a significant reduction in mortality has occurred in the developed world. This is largely attributed to advances in early diagnosis and implementation of multidisciplinary treatment programs leading to improvement in survivorship and better quality of life. It is also largely a preventable cancer by altering lifestyle: by cessation of tobacco and alcohol abuse and consumption of a healthy diet.

Increasing awareness on the part of the providers of treatment as well as the population in general has led to an increasing proportion of patients presenting with earlier staged disease. Prompt implementation of multidisciplinary treatment with contemporary surgical techniques of reconstructive surgery achieves the goal of preservation or restoration of form and function in an increasing number of patients. Technical advances in free tissue transfer, prosthodontics and implantology have enabled clinicians to achieve an improved quality of life and restoration of esthetics as well as the functions of speech, mastication and swallowing.

The editors and contributors to this work have put together a textbook which provides the state of the art in the management of oral cancer with appropriate details of pathology, epidemiology, surgical techniques, adjuvant therapies, rehabilitation including prosthetics and implantology as well as prevention strategies to cover the broad spectrum of oral cancer management. This textbook should be of significant value to head and neck surgeons, maxillofacial surgeons, otolaryngologists and plastic surgeons involved in oncologic surgery for oral cancer, as well as oral surgeons, dentists and other members of the dental team in providing supportive care to patients with oral cancer. The editors wish to express their appreciation to other contributors who have so generously given their time, expertise and effort in making this a 'complete compendium' for the multidisciplinary management of oral cancer.

Jatin P Shah
Newell Johnson
John Batsakis

I Pathology and Biology

1 Global epidemiology

Newell W Johnson

Definitions of oral cancer

Malignant neoplasms are major causes of fear, morbidity and mortality all over the world. Cancer is one of the five main causes of death in all societies, its relative position varying with age and sex. Fig. 1.1 shows the main causes of death in England and Wales, as a typical example of Western industrialized countries. In developing countries the proportions will differ, infectious being a larger and cardiovascular disease a smaller component. Cancer numbers are important, however. Note how in England and Wales in the past 65 years, infections have declined as a major cause (in spite of the HIV epidemic) so that diseases of the heart and circulatory system now dominate in men, with cancer second; however, cancer dominates in women, especially in the third to sixth decades of life. Globally, 'oral cancer' is the sixth most common cause of cancer-related death, although many people are unaware of its existence.

This text deals with malignant neoplasms affecting the oral cavity, principally the oral mucosa. This disease has much in common with squamous cell carcinomas arising elsewhere in the upper aerodigestive tract, which share common risk factors, so

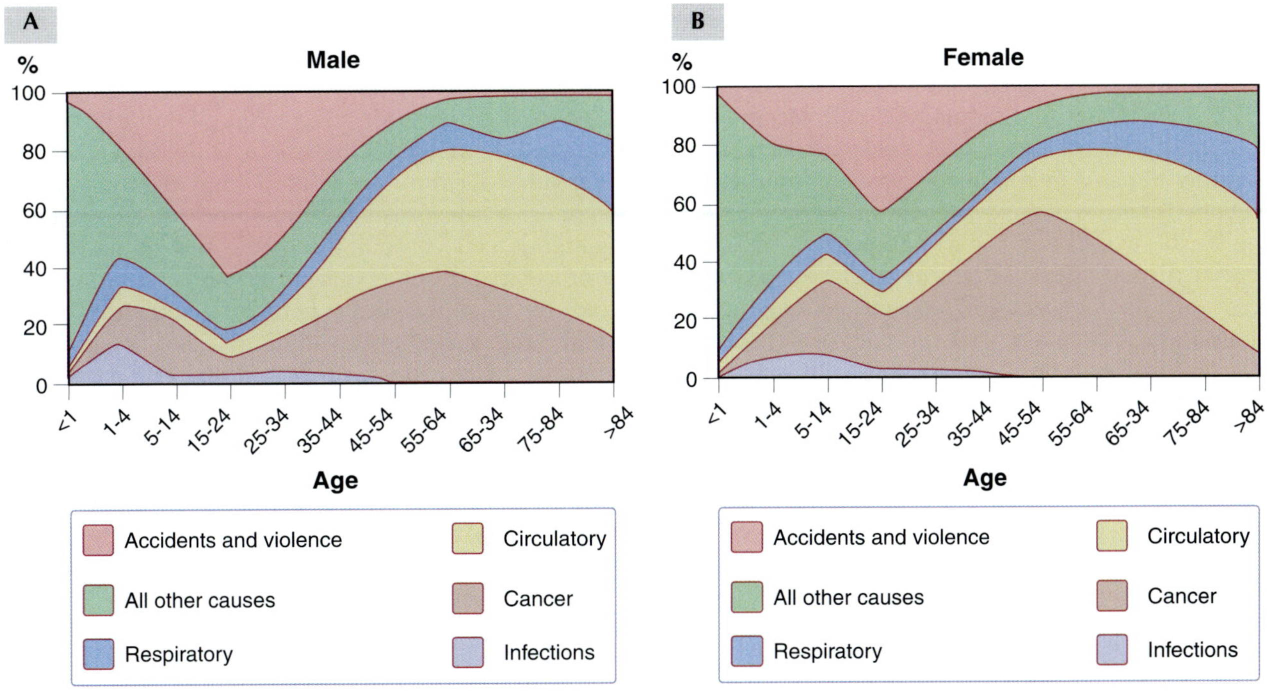

Figure 1.1 Categorization of the major causes of death in England and Wales, in 1996. A: males, B: females. Cancer peaks in childhood and in late middle age. In middle-aged females it is the most common cause of death. (Drawn from data provided by the Office of National Statistics, London, 1997.) There has been a major shift since the 1930s, with infections becoming less common, but cardiovascular diseases remaining the most important.

Table 1.1 Locations as described by the ICD-9

ICD-9 code	Description
140–149	Malignant neoplasms of lip, oral cavity and pharynx
140	Lip
141	Tongue
142	Major salivary gland
143	Gum
144	Floor of mouth
145	Other and unspecified parts of the mouth
146	Oropharynx
147	Nasopharynx
148	Hypopharynx
149	Other and ill-defined sites within lip, oral cavity and pharynx

Table 1.2 Equivalents between ICD revisions 9 and 10

ICD-9 code	Description	ICD-10 code
140–149	Malignant neoplasms of lip, oral cavity and pharynx	C00–C14
140.0–140.9	Lip	C00
141.0	Base of tongue	C01
141.1–141.9	Other and unspecified parts of tongue	C02
143.0–143.9	Gum	C03
144.0–144.9	Floor of mouth	C04
145.2–145.5	Palate	C05
145.0–145.1, 145.6–145.9	Other and unspecified parts of the mouth	C06
142.0	Parotid gland	C07
142.1–142.9	Other and unspecified major salivary glands	C08
146.0–146.2	Tonsil	C09
146.3–146.9	Oropharynx	C10
147.0–147.9	Nasopharynx	C11
148.1	Pyriform sinus	C12
148.0, 148.2–148.9	Hypopharynx	C13
149.0–149.9	Other and ill-defined sites in the lip, oral cavity and pharynx	C14

studies of 'head and neck cancer' are frequently drawn upon when issues relevant to oral cancer are discussed. Reviews of the global epidemiology up to the beginning of the 1990s can be found in references 1 and 2. Of these oral cancers, the vast majority are squamous cell carcinomas arising in the mucous membranes of the mouth and the pharynx. Indeed, of all the oropharyngeal malignancies reported to the SEER (Surveillance, Epidemiology and End Results program of the National Cancer Institute of the United States Public Health Service) registries in the USA between 1973 and 1987, apart from lesions of the salivary glands, gingivae, nasopharynx, nasal cavity and sinuses, more than 95% were squamous cell carcinomas.[3] 'Upper aerodigestive tract alcohol- and tobacco-related oral squamous cell carcinomas' are thus the major head and neck cancers. They constitute a major public health problem worldwide and constitute the major workload of head and neck oncologists worldwide. Our emphasis is thus on mucosal disease. Because cancer at these sites often arises out of long-standing potentially malignant lesions and conditions, so-called premalignant lesions, these are given due consideration; less-extensive coverage is given to other lesions.

Most of the international databases employ the International Classification of Diseases (ICD) coding system of the World Health Organization (WHO), and most of the data currently available are expressed according to the ninth revision of this system (ICD-9): there is, however, a steady trend towards use of the tenth revision (ICD-10). It is particularly important to define these codes and to be clear how many of these precise anatomic sites are included in any particular dataset under study (Table 1.1). The equivalents between revisions 9 and 10 are shown in Table 1.2.

Neoplasms of the major salivary glands clearly have quite distinct natural histories, ill-understood aetiologies and distinct management protocols compared with mucosal cancers. Similarly, nasopharyngeal malignancies are usually Epstein–Barr virus-related carcinomas that differ distinctly from the more widespread alcohol- and tobacco-related squamous cell carcinomas of the rest of the upper aerodigestive tract. Datasets should be examined carefully to determine whether the major salivary glands and nasopharynx are included, as they so often are (ICD codes 140–149 inclusive often being referred to as 'oral' cancers). Some datasets carefully exclude 142 and 147 in order to be consistent about the biological form of neoplasm under consideration. Many datasets make a distinction between lip and intraoral cancer, and we have to be clear whether oral cancer is taken to include oropharynx and hypopharynx in any given dataset.

Incidence rates worldwide

The databases from which these estimates are derived are far from ideal: many parts of the world

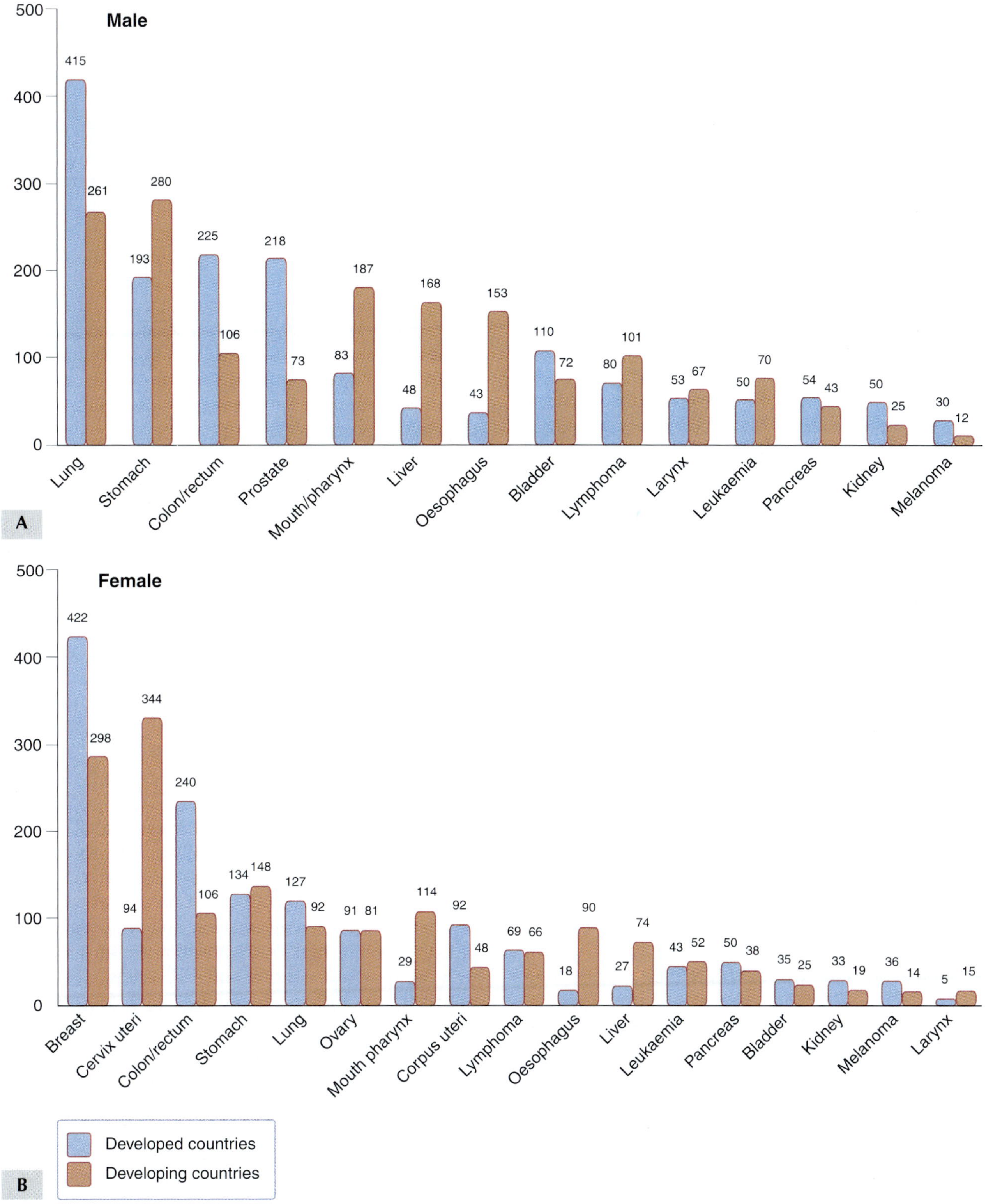

Figure 1.2 Estimated numbers of new cases (thousands) of 14 cancers in men (A), and 17 cancers in women (B), in developed and developing parts of the world. The estimates are for 1985. (Data adapted from Parkin et al.[4])

produce no data at all, in others (often among the most populous), the data may come from localized, atypical regions. Hospital-based cancer registries naturally gather biased information—those cases which present to hospital only; thus, in many developing countries, cases may not come to attention at all, either because of fear or the inability of poor people to access hospital services. This is certainly true of incidence data. Death rates may be even more unreliable because in many developing countries

Table 1.3 Estimated age-standardized incidence rates per 100 000 pa for oral and pharyngeal cancer, in 1985, for 24 world areas. (Data from Parkin et al.[4])

Area	Male	Female
Eastern Africa	14.2	9.5
Middle Africa	15.0	10.0
Northern Africa	15.6	8.7
Southern Africa	13.4	3.4
Western Africa	3.5	2.6
Caribbean	13.3	4.0
Central America	4.6	2.4
South America (temperate)	8.1	2.3
South America (tropical)	18.7	4.9
North America	14.2	5.1
Eastern Asia: China	8.7	6.0
Eastern Asia: Japan	4.5	1.8
Eastern Asia: other	9.3	3.0
South-East Asia	14.5	9.8
Southern Asia	25.1	14.9
Western Asia	9.1	7.5
Eastern Europe	10.7	2.4
Northern Europe	6.5	2.8
Southern Europe	11.4	2.5
Western Europe	16.6	3.2
Australia/New Zealand	15.1	4.8
Melanesia	47.0	25.6
Micronesia/Polynesia	10.0	4.6
USSR	15.7	3.0
All areas	14.0	6.5

follow-up even of treated cases is impossible. Death certification is not always compulsory and there is limited international standardization in the categories of cause of death, let alone calibration of those signing death certificates.

Fig. 1.2[4] plots the estimated numbers of new cases of most common cancers by anatomic site in male and in female patients, comparing so-called developed countries with so-called developing countries. There are striking differences. For both sexes, combined cancer of the mouth and pharynx ICD9 (140–149) ranks sixth overall, behind lung, stomach, breast, colon and rectum and cervix uteri, in that order. In the published data for 1990, oral and pharyngeal sites remain the sixth most common neoplasms within the European Union (EU);[5] however, mouth and pharynx are the third most common site for malignant disease among men in developing countries and the fourth among women. The International Agency for Research on Cancer estimated that in 1985 there were some 413 000 cases worldwide.[4]

The estimated age-standardized rates of the incidence of cancer of the mouth and pharynx (140–149), 1985, by sex and WHO geographic area, are detailed in Table 1.3.[4] Rates range from a low of 1.8/100 000 per annum (for female subjects in Japan) to a high of 47/100 000 per annum (for male subjects in Melanesia). Even given the caveats over precision mentioned above, these figures illustrate the marked global variability in oral cancer incidence. These broad differences are illustrated in the map presented as Fig. 1.3.[6] The highest rates in the world are found in France,[7] the Indian subcontinent, Brazil[8] and Central/Eastern Europe. There are also marked differences between countries in the same geographical region.[9,10]

The ostensibly extremely high rates in the relatively small population of Melanesia have not been researched in detail and may relate to chewing and smoking habits. It has been apparent for decades that the global picture is dominated by the incidence of oral cancer in southern Asia and of oral cavity plus nasopharyngeal cancer in South-East Asia. In India, Bangladesh, Pakistan and Sri Lanka, oral cancer is the most common site and accounts for about one-third of all cancers.[11] Examples of these high rates, age-adjusted to the world population, per 100 000 persons per annum, are listed in Table 1.4 for the six population-based cancer registries in India.[12] Even within the subcontinent there are striking differences in incidence rates. Data relate to 1988–89. More than 100 000 cases of oral cancer occur every year in South and South-East Asia, with poor prospect of survival: about 90% of these cases are attributable to smoking and chewing habits.[13] It is also encouraging that overall rates in India are showing a decreasing trend in successive birth cohorts, particularly among females for intra-oral sites other than tongue (ICD9 143–145), where a mean percentage fall of 16.8% has occurred between 1975 and 1988, although rates remain in the high range of 10–15/100 000 per annum. In Mumbai (Bombay), the incidence of tongue cancer was high: it was 14.9/100 000 per annum (aged 30–74, standardized to the world population) for men and 5.4 for women, but both values showed a fall, of 12.0 and 16.8% respectively, between 1975 and 1988.[14] Unfortunately, it cannot be assumed that these trends apply nationwide and there is growing concern that commercial areca nut and tobacco products will contribute to future rises in the incidence of oral submucous fibrosis and of oral cancer.[15] Furthermore, decreases in the prevalence of traditional pan-chewing habits (see Chapter 2) in the more sophisticated urban areas are more than matched by increases in smoking.

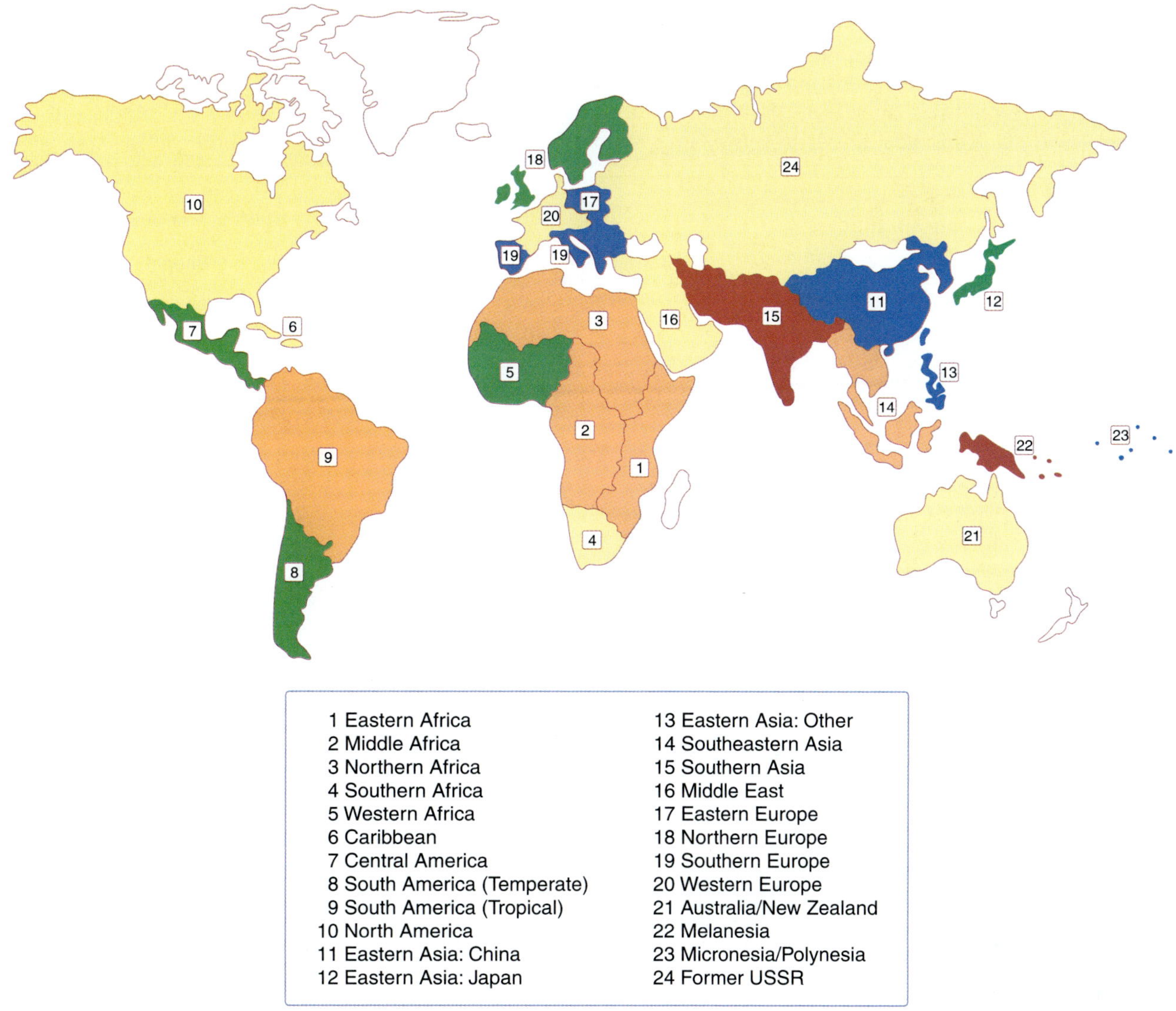

Figure 1.3 Oral cancer rates throughout the world, showing marked geographical variation in incidence. Care is needed in interpretation because some large groupings disguise marked regional variations (Redrawn from Johnson 1997,[6] based on data in Table 1.3.) Cases per 100 000 population per annum (green) 3.05–5.41; (blue) 5.42–7.78; (yellow) 7.79–10.15; (orange) 10.16–12.52; (red) 20–36.3.

Elsewhere in Asia, there is a dramatic increase in mouth cancer incidence (ICD-9 143–149) for both sexes in Japan: it more than doubled between 1973 and 1985 and is still, apparently, rising at 30% or more every 5 years, at least within the Miyagi and Osaka registries.[14] The national data for Japan show this trend to be strongest for men, to be continuing through 1993, and to be strongest for floor of mouth and oropharyngeal cancers. A cohort effect in males born from about 1920 onwards is also apparent.[16] In much of the West, the pattern is completely different: Fig. 1.4 shows the leading sites of new cancer cases and of deaths for the United States of America; these are 1997 estimates.[17] ‘Oral cavity’ cancer in this context includes all ICD 140–149 sites. In males there were 20 900 new cases and 5600 estimated deaths; for females there were 9850 new cases and 2840 deaths (for both sexes 30 750 cases and 8440 deaths). This represents a death-registration ratio of 0.274. In other words, even in an advanced society like the USA, nearly one in three people with oral cancer in time die with, or as a result of, their disease. Elsewhere in North America, notably in the Maritime Provinces of Canada, there is a steep increase in cumulative risk of males developing mouth cancer, increasing in successive birth cohorts, which is reflected in mortality trends.[14] There is also an upward trend for both males and females in Australia and among the non-Maori population in New Zealand. Lip cancer in fair-skinned populations, partly due to ultraviolet light, is a growing problem.[18]

Table 1.4 Incidence rates for oral and pharyngeal cancer (ICD9: 140–149), from the six population-based registries in India, age-adjusted to the world population, per 100 000 persons, in 1988–89. Taken together these represent the most common site group in all of the Indian registries, but there are considerable variations by subsite. Barshi is a rural registry in Maharashtra State; all of the others are urban. (Source: National Cancer Resgistry Programme[12])

A Males

ICD9	Site	Bangalore	Bombay	Madras	Delhi	Bhopal	Barshi
140–149	Lip, oral cavity and pharynx	17.5	26.8	23.6	19.4	38.8	10.8
140	Lip	0.4	0.3	0.6	0.5	0.2	0.0
141	Tongue	4.7	6.5	5.3	7.7	13.2	2.1
142	Salivary glands	0.8	0.4	0.4	0.8	0.5	0.5
143–145	Mouth	3.0	5.8	7.3	3.7	10.4	3.4
146	Oropharynx	1.9	3.2	1.9	3.2	3.8	0.0
147	Nasopharynx	0.6	0.6	0.6	0.6	0.0	0.0
148	Hypopharynx	5.9	8.2	6.5	2.3	8.4	3.5
149	Pharynx, etc.	0.2	1.8	1.0	0.6	2.3	1.3

B Females

ICD9	Site	Bangalore	Bombay	Madras	Delhi	Bhopal	Barshi
140–149	Lip, oral cavity and pharynx	14.9	9.5	14.7	6.4	10.4	1.1
140	Lip	0.1	0.2	0.3	0.3	0.0	0.0
141	Tongue	1.0	1.9	2.1	1.3	1.4	0.0
142	Salivary glands	0.5	0.3	0.2	0.5	0.0	0.0
143–145	Mouth	11.1	3.9	8.2	2.5	6.8	0.6
146	Oropharynx	0.5	0.6	0.4	1.0	0.5	0.0
147	Nasopharynx	0.4	0.2	0.3	0.2	0.5	0.0
148	Hypopharynx	1.2	1.5	2.7	0.6	0.8	0.5
149	Pharynx, etc.	0.1	0.9	0.5	0.0	0.4	0.0

The pattern in Europe, more so than in North America, is cause for great concern. Data from Denmark[19] and from Scotland[20] first drew our attention to dramatically rising trends in oral and pharyngeal cancer incidence, particularly cancer of the tongue, among young adult men. This has now been well documented in many countries, and is reflected in growing mortality rates, as elaborated below. It is most striking in Central and Eastern Europe: in Slovakia, for example, in men aged 35–64 years, oropharyngeal cancer increased from a rate of 6.8/100 000 per annum in 1968–1970 to a staggering 47.9/100 000 in 1987–89.[21]

Age distribution.

The incidence of oral cancer increases with age in all parts of the world. In the West, in 98% of cases the patients are over 40 years of age. This is illustrated in Fig. 1.5 for the UK, for France, and for the EU overall.[22] In the high-prevalence areas of the world, however, in many cases patients are less than 35 years old, owing to heavy abuse of various forms of tobacco. Furthermore, it is now clear that in many Western countries there has been, during the past two or three decades, an alarming rise in the incidence of oral cancer (particularly among younger men), a trend that appears to be continuing.[23] This is reflected in rising mortality rates among younger men (see below).

It is also clear that a number of cases of oral mucosal squamous cell carcinoma occur in both young and old patients, often in the absence of the traditional alcohol and tobacco risk factors, and in which the disease may pursue a particularly aggressive course. These issues are discussed further in Chapter 3.

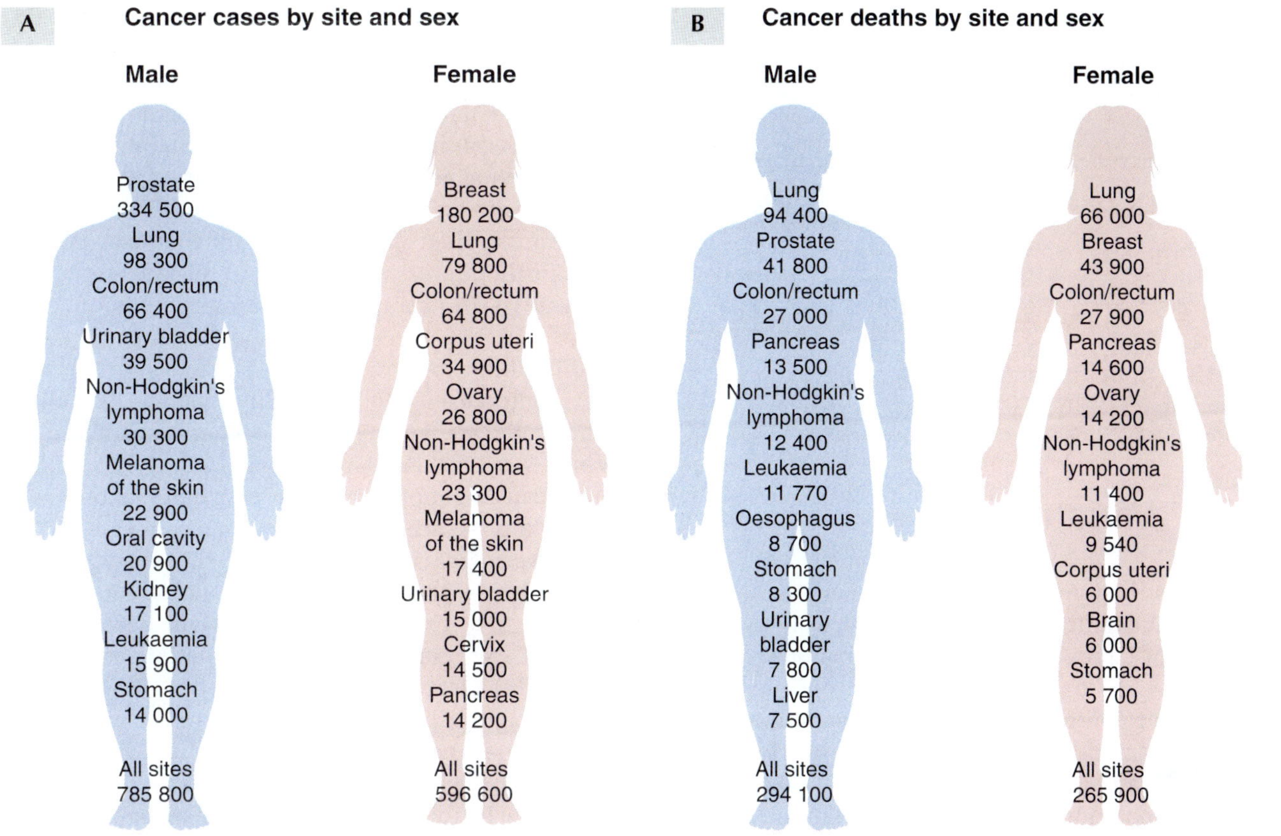

Figure 1.4 Leading sites of new cancer cases (A) and deaths (B) in the USA. Estimates are for 1997 and exclude basal and squamous cell skin cancer and in situ carcinomas, except for bladder. (Data derived from American Cancer Society surveillance research.[17])

Sex distribution

In industrialized countries, men are affected two to three times as often as women, largely because of their greater indulgence in the most important risk factors, such as heavy alcohol and tobacco consumption for intra-oral cancer and sunlight for lip cancer in those who work outdoors. However, the incidence of tongue and other intraoral cancer for women can be greater than or equal to that for men in high-incidence areas such as India, where chewing (and sometimes smoking) are also common amongst women—although this varies considerably from region to region. In the USA, for instance, the death rate per 100 000 population in 1991–93 was 4.4 for males and 1.6 for females (down from 5.9 and 1.9, respectively in 1971–73). Note, however, that because the US population has become larger (22% increase from 1973 to 1993 alone) and because the population over 65 is continuing to become larger and older, actual numbers of deaths have risen steadily over the past 25 years, more so in women (Table 1.5).

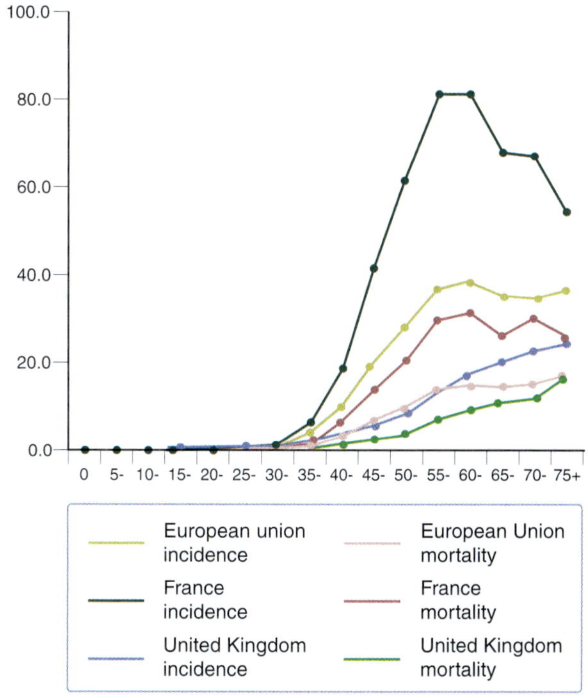

Figure 1.5 Age-specific incidence rates for oral cancer in the UK, in France, where the rates are much higher, and for the European Union overall, as an example of the pattern in the western world. Data refer to the situation in 1990, and for ICD9 sites 140–149. (Source: International Agency for Research against Cancer.[22])

Table 1.5 Actual numbers of deaths from oral and pharyngeal cancer in the USA, by sex, 1973–97. (Source: various tables from American Cancer Society[17])

	1973	1993	1997
Males	5553	5515	5600
Females	2269	2726	2840
Total	7822	8341	8440

Ethnic variations

Ethnicity strongly influences prevalence as a result of social and cultural practices,[24] as well as influencing death rates owing to socioeconomic differences. Where cultural practices represent risk factors, their continuation by immigrants from high-incidence regions to other parts of the world results in comparatively high cancer incidence in immigrant communities. Studies of migrant populations have proved of considerable interest to epidemiologists working in the field of cancer research, in suggesting the extent to which environmental exposures are important in the aetiology of different cancers. For example, it is well established that the high incidence of cancer of the stomach among native Japanese falls over several decades in the immigrant communities to the USA; the high incidence of nasopharyngeal carcinoma in subjects from southern China falls over decades in emigrant communities. Migrant studies relating to oral cancer are meagre. Among Indians living in the Malay Peninsula, for example, the overall incidence of oral cancer has long been considerably higher than that among Malay or Chinese subjects.[25] Similar trends have been noted among Indian migrants from India to Natal in South Africa.[26] Precise estimates of the incidence of oral cancer in ethnic/immigrant subgroups in Europe are not yet available;[27] however, there is an interesting, significant correlation ($r = 0.42$) between the percentage of the population described as Asian and the incidence rate for oral and pharyngeal cancer in the North Thames Region of South-East England.[28] This is also visible in data from the English Midlands.[29] Sverdlow et al.[30] have shown that mortality rates for the 1979–85 period from oral cancer in Indian migrants in England and Wales are increased above rates of those born in England (odds ratio (OR) 2.2; 95% confidence interval (CI) 1.5–3.1); although statistically significant, the study was based on only 30 cases of oral cancer, compared with 4562 other residents. This has been confirmed using incidence data from a total of 7521 cases of upper aerodigestive tract cancer registered in South-East England during the period 1986–91: Asians (i.e. immigrants from India, Pakistan, Bangladesh, Nepal and Sri Lanka: $n = 232$ cases) had significantly higher rates of intra-oral cancer, and residents of Chinese origin ($n = 67$ cases) had significantly higher rates of nasopharyngeal cancer, than the remainder of the local population; furthermore, cancer at these sites presented on average 10–15 years earlier in these groups.[31]

In the United States, as is clear from Fig. 1.6, both the incidence and mortality rates for Black Americans are substantially higher than those for White Americans.[32,33] It is also clear that Black Americans do not appear to be enjoying the same downward trend in mortality rates as are White Americans (see below). Indeed, the incidence for Black men in the USA is so high (20.4/100 000 per annum) that oral/pharyngeal cancer becomes the fourth most common site for malignant disease (Table 1.6). Data on immigrants to the USA of South Asian origin are not available, and oral/pharyngeal cancer does not appear prominently amongst the other recorded racial and ethnic groups, namely Chinese, Filipino, Hawaiian, Japanese, Korean, Vietnamese, Alaska Native, American Indian and Hispanic subjects.

Table 1.6 Incidence rates for the five most commonly diagnosed cancers in males in the USA, 1988–92, for Whites and African Americans. (Source: SEER data, 1996, as quoted in American Cancer Society[17])

African Americans		Whites	
Prostate	180.6	Prostate	134.7
Lung	117.0	Lung	76.0
Colon and rectum	60.7	Colon and rectum	56.3
Oral/pharyngeal	20.4	Urinary bladder	31.7
Stomach	17.9	Non-Hodgkin's lymphoma	18.7

Rates per 100 000 per annum, age-adjusted to the 1970 US standard population.

Mortality rates and trends

As with incidence rates and trends there is much geographical variation. Fig. 1.7[34] plots age-standardized death certification rates for mouth and pharyngeal cancer (ICD9 140–149) in various countries for

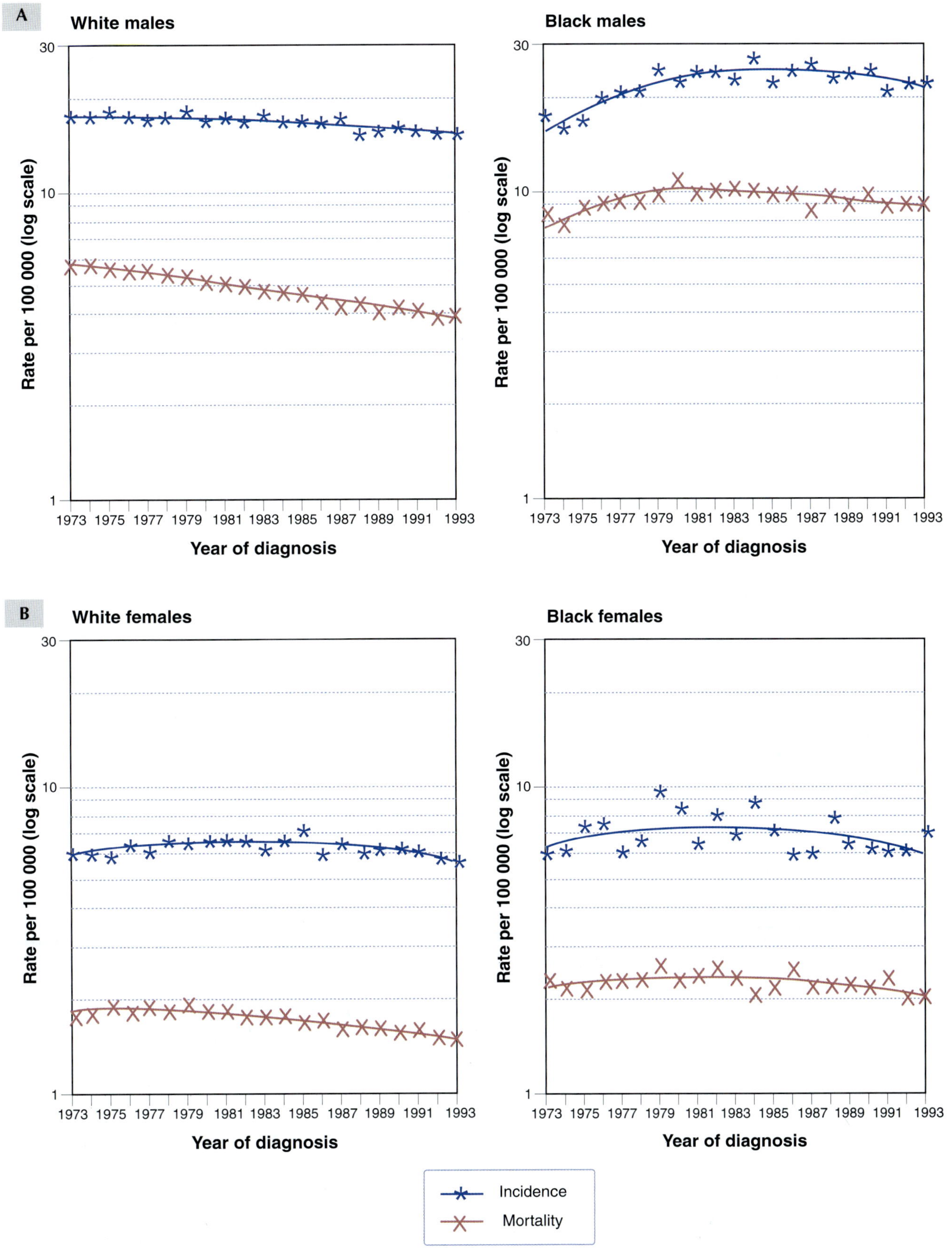

Figure 1.6 Incidence and mortality for oral and pharyngeal cancer in the USA, 1973–1993, for White and Black Americans: A: male, B: female. Incidence rates are derived from the nine standard SEER registries, representing some 14% of the population: mortality rates are from the US National Center for Health Statistics and are total records of all states. SEER is the Surveillance, Epidemiology and End Results Program of the National Cancer Institute, based on data from population-based registries in Connecticut, New Mexico, Utah, Iowa, Hawaii, Atlanta, Detroit, Seattle-Pujet Sound and San Francisco–Oakland. The data may then be extrapolated to the whole US population. Data are published in various print outlets and are available on the World Wide Web at http://www-seer.ims.nci.gov

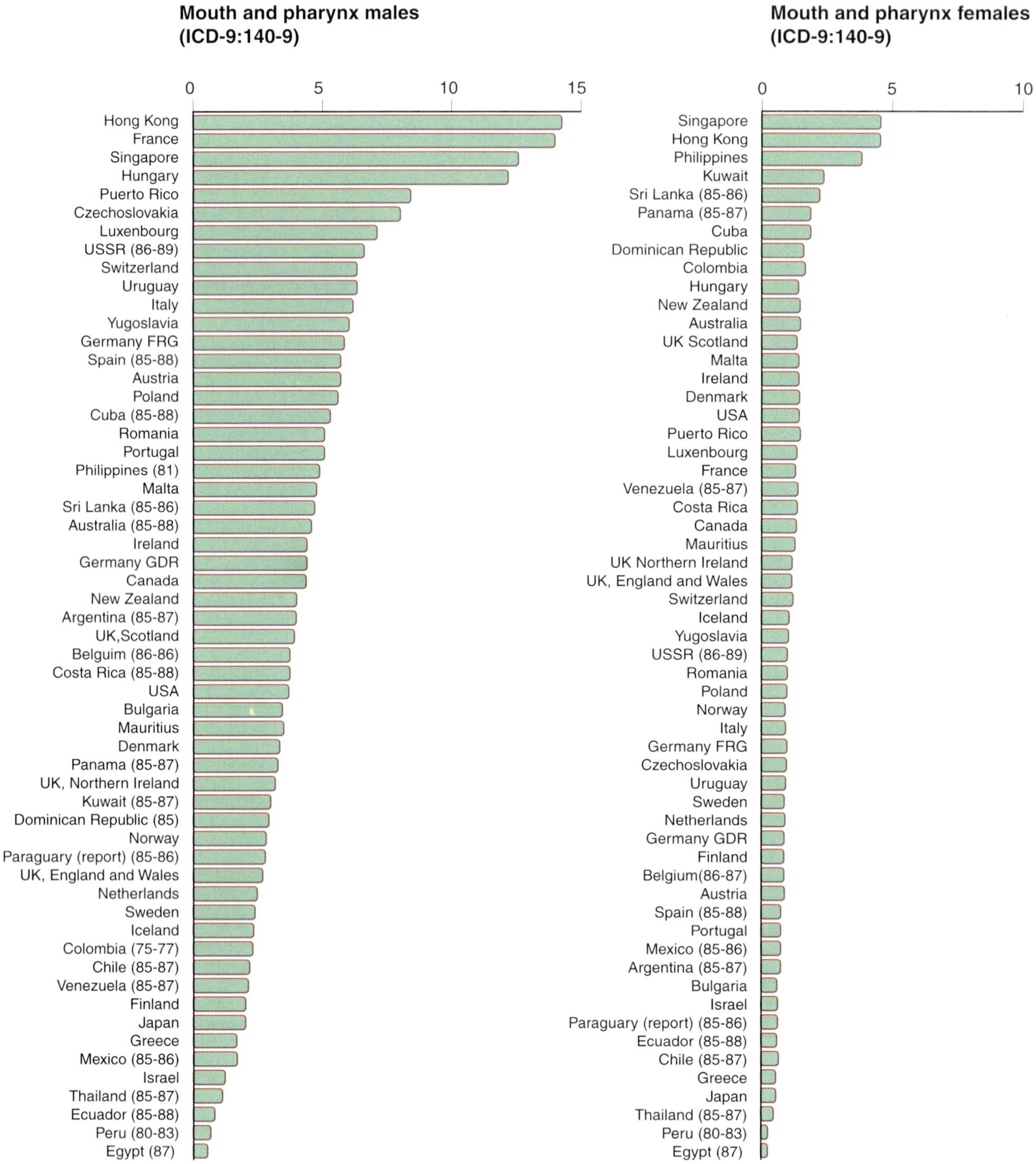

Figure 1.7 Death rates for cancers of the mouth and pharynx (ICD-9: 140–149) in various countries, age standardized to the world population, and derived from death certificate data, for the years 1985–89. See text for further discussion. (Redrawn from Levi et al.[34])

the period 1985–89. These differ by a factor of 24 in male and 15 in female patients. This is, of course, a selected list but the rates for several countries bear comment. Hong Kong and Singapore appear at the top, presumably because of the relatively large contribution of nasopharyngeal carcinoma. Several European countries, namely France, Hungary and Czechoslovakia, also have a high ranking. This is historically linked to heavy alcohol and tobacco use in these communities.

Cancer mortality rates show major changes over time. Fig. 1.8 (A and B for male and female patients, respectively) shows trends between 1930

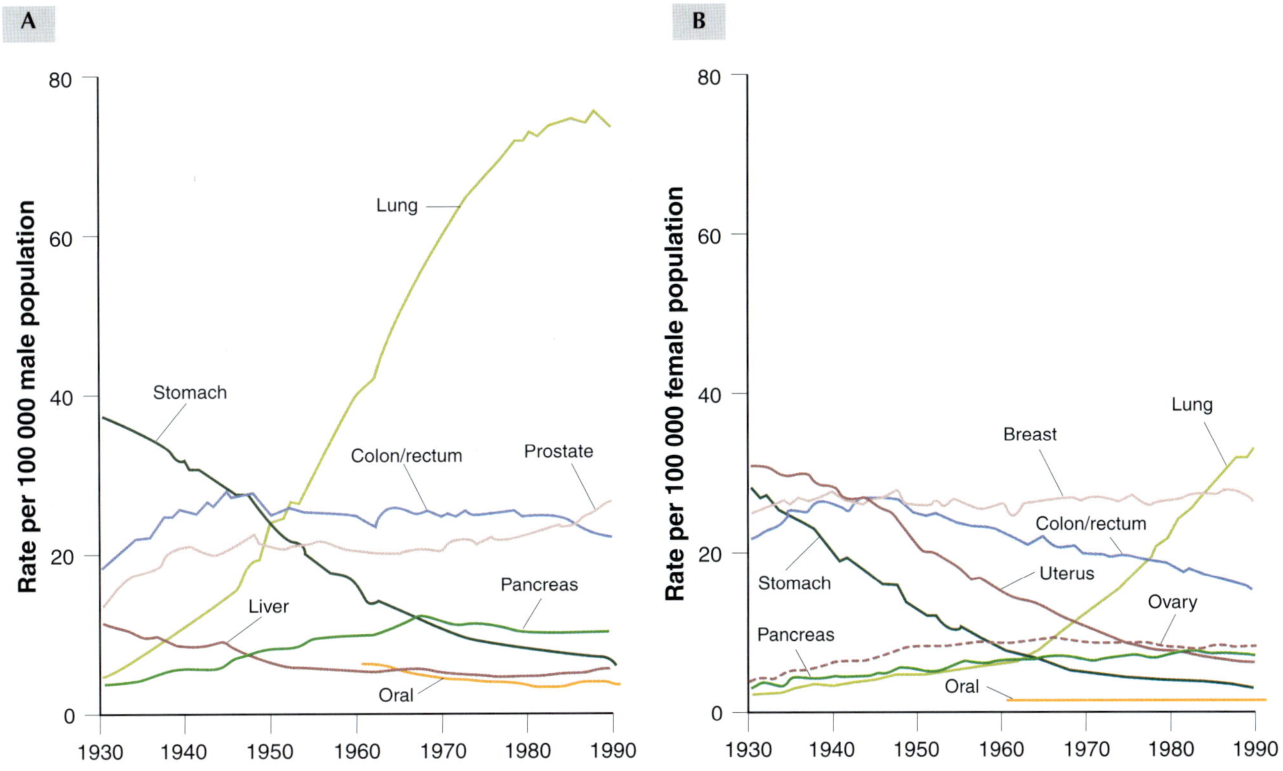

Figure 1.8 Death rates in the USA for six major cancers, compared with those for oral and pharyngeal cancer. Rates are per 100 000 per annum, age adjusted to the 1970 standard population. A: males, B: females. (Redrawn from American Cancer Society.[17])

Table 1.7 Mortality trends for oral and pharyngeal cancer in the USA between 1973 and 1993, by race and sex. (Source SEER Cancer Statistics Review[35])

	All races			Whites			Blacks		
	Total	**Males**	**Females**	**Total**	**Males**	**Females**	**Total**	**Males**	**Females**
All ages									
% change	−22.6	−26.2	−16.3	−26.7	−31.6	−17.5	2.9	10.3	−8.8
Est ann %	−1.4*	−1.7*	−1.0*	−1.7*	−2.1*	−1.1*	−0.1	0.2	−0.3
Under 65									
% change	−26.7	−24.5	−34.0	−33.2	−32.3	−37.5	−1.6	7.3	−21.5
Est ann %	−1.8*	−1.6*	−2.3*	−2.2*	−2.1*	−2.6*	−0.4	0.0	−1.2*
65 and over									
% change	−18.2	−27.8	3.7	−20.4	−31.1	3.4	12.6	16.4	19.1
Est ann %	−1.1*	−1.8*	0.2	−1.3*	−2.1*	0.1	0.6*	0.7*	1.4*

*Indicates that the estimated annual percentage change in rate is statistically significantly different from zero.

and the 1990s for six of the most common cancers in the USA, with oral and pharyngeal cancer added. There have been substantial and significant declines in deaths from stomach cancer in both men and women over the past half century, with truly dramatic rises in deaths from lung cancer due to the smoking epidemic. The female epidemic is some 20 years behind the male epidemic, reflecting societal trends in the incidence of female smoking, and death rates continue to rise in women, although they are now beginning to fall in men. These data show a fall in deaths from oral cancer from 6.0/100 000 per annum in 1962, to 4.5 in 1990–92, in men and a

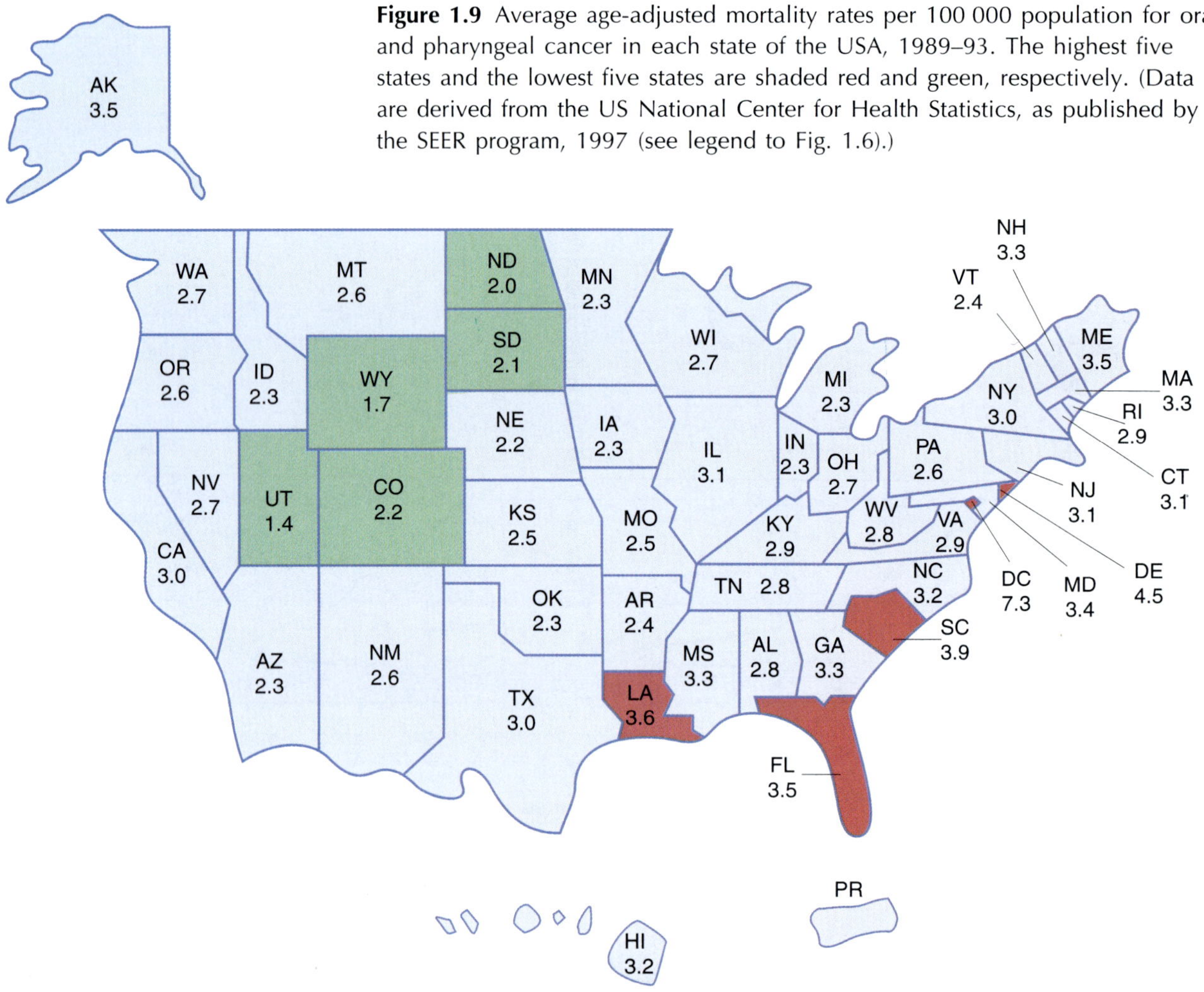

Figure 1.9 Average age-adjusted mortality rates per 100 000 population for oral and pharyngeal cancer in each state of the USA, 1989–93. The highest five states and the lowest five states are shaded red and green, respectively. (Data are derived from the US National Center for Health Statistics, as published by the SEER program, 1997 (see legend to Fig. 1.6).)

steady rate of 1.6/100 000 per annum in women. The SEER program has reported an overall fall in the rate of mortality from oral cancer, between 1973 and 1993, of 22.6% (an estimated annual percentage fall of 1.4). Some of these data are reproduced in Table 1.7, which requires careful interpretation. The table shows a considerable rise (10.3%) in mortality among Black men, even more so in those aged 65 and over (16.4%), an even larger rise in older black women (19.1%) and a smaller but significant rise in mortality among older White women (of 3.4%). Furthermore, for men of all races, the SEER data show a decline in 5-year survival rates from a high of 53.5% in 1974 to 47.5% in 1988 (though there are some fluctuations from year to year).[36] The 5-year survival rates in the SEER registries range from a high of 72.1% for White women in Utah to a low of 24.8% for Black men in metropolitan Atlanta. These striking differences are likely to be explained by a number of factors including socioeconomic condition, age, stage at diagnosis, continued presence or absence of environmental risk factors and access to hospital services. African–American patients have consistently poorer survival outcomes.[37]

Even within the continental United States there is a greater than five-fold regional variation, state by state, in mortality rates (Fig. 1.9):[38] the 'high five' states are clustered in the East and South-East and the 'low five' states in the Midwest. The remaining 40 states have rather similar mortality rates—between 2.3 and 3.4 deaths/100 000 per annum, age-adjusted to the 1970 US standard population. These regional differences are explicable in terms of a combination of ethnic mix, socioeconomic mix and variations in the prevalence and severity of risk factors in these communities, including the use of oral smokeless tobacco in the southern states. Even more striking country-to-country variations are seen within the EU.[39] Figure 1.10 ranks the incidence and mortality rates for oral cancer (ICD 9: 140–149) by country within the EU.[40] There has been approximately a doubling in deaths from oral cancer in the EU between 1970 and 2000, fuelled by younger age groups and therefore continuing well into the 21st

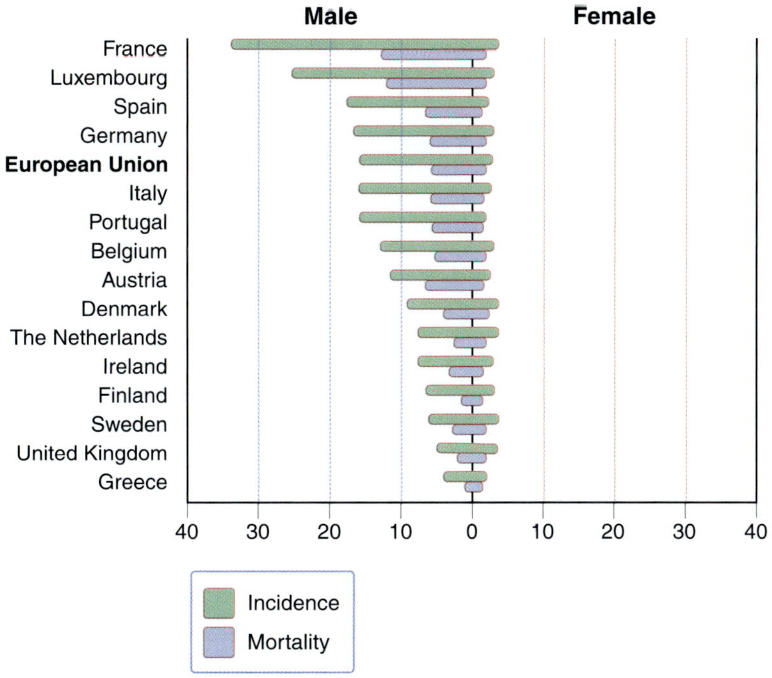

Figure 1.10 The marked variability in incidence and mortality rates for oral and pharyngeal cancer across the European Union.

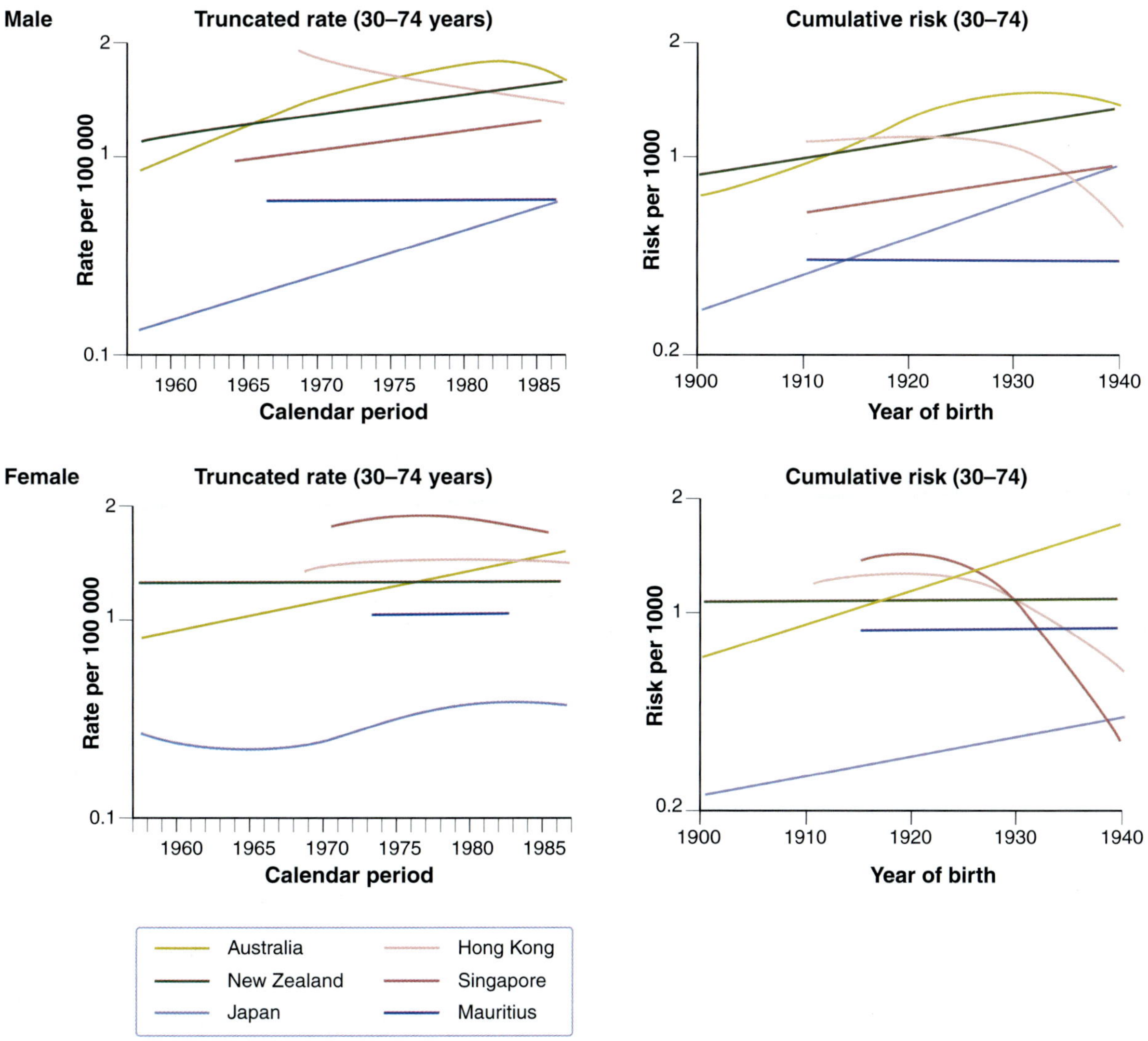

Figure 1.11 Trends in oral and pharyngeal cancer mortality in Oceania.[43]

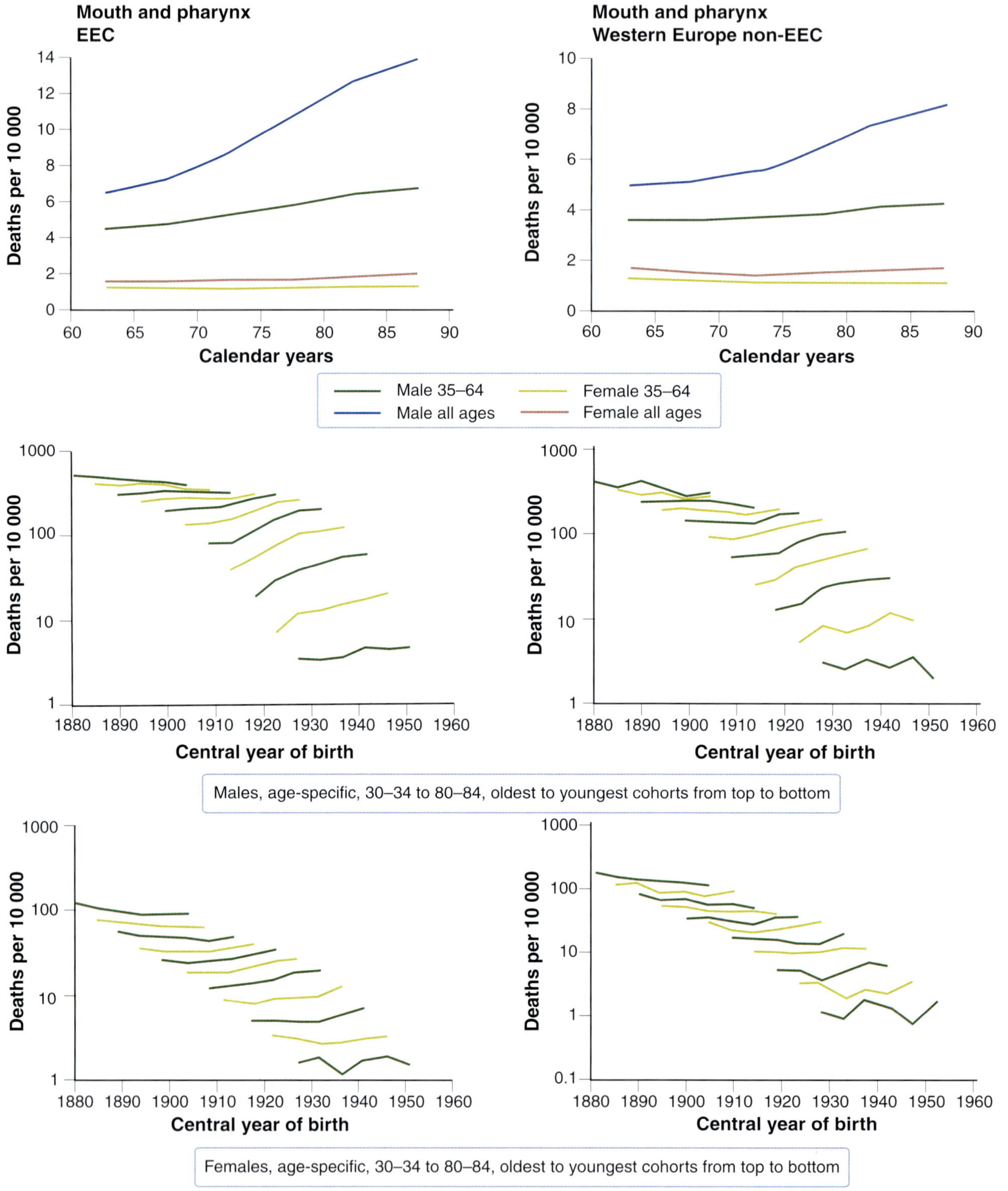

Figure 1.12 Age-standardized death rates of oral and pharyngeal cancer in the countries of the European Economic Community (EEC), 1963–87, showing substantial rises in males, particularly in age cohorts born from about 1915 onwards.[46]

century. The problem is potentially very serious indeed in Central and Eastern Europe, where, as noted above, between threefold and tenfold increases in incidence have been observed within a single generation.[21] Unsurprisingly, in view of their common risk factors, the highest mortality rates in the world for laryngeal cancer in men are found in Hungary, Poland, Slovakia and Romania.[41]

Aside from these important regional and ethnic differences, the overall downward trend in the USA is encouraging. However, much information is now

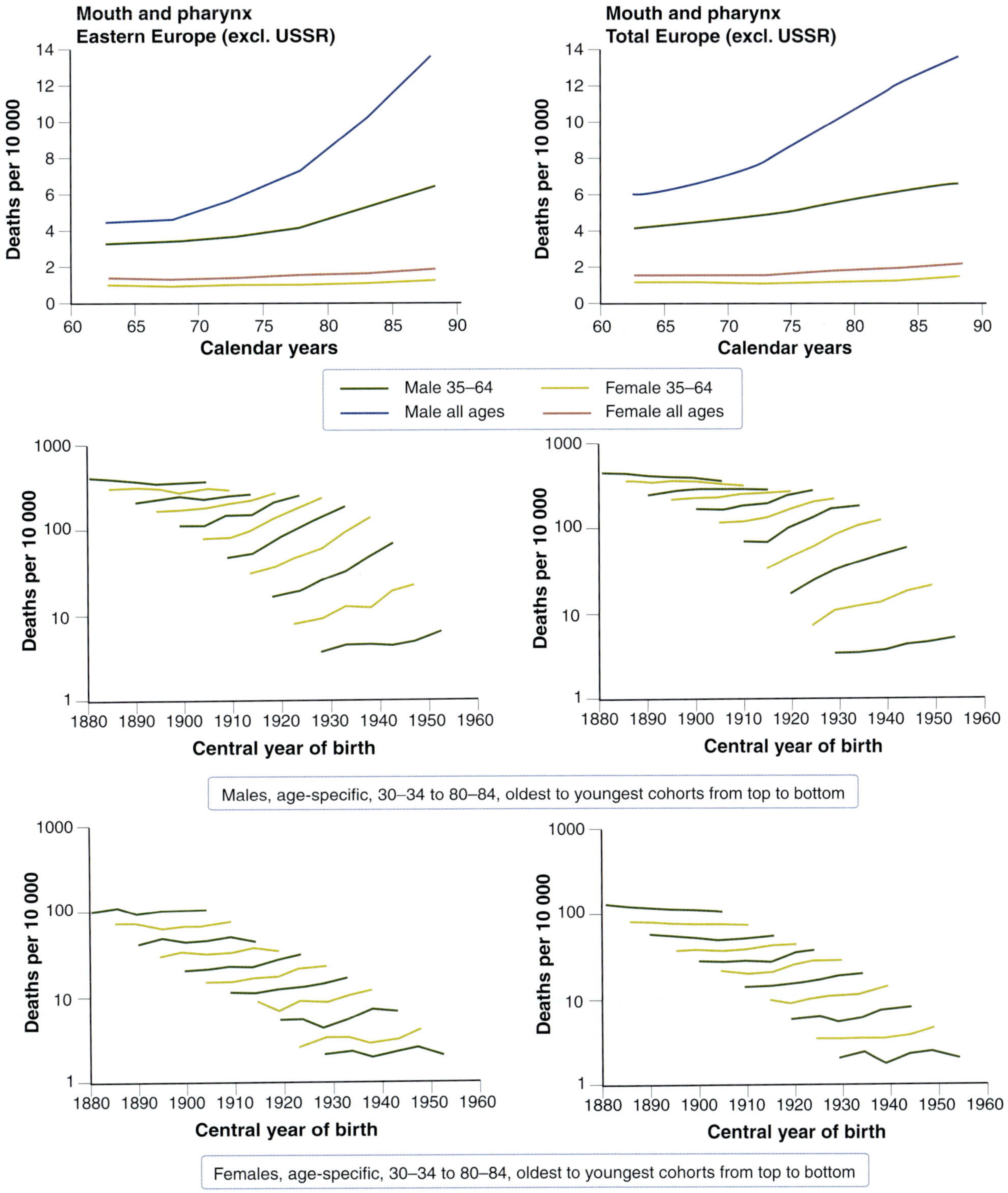

Figure 1.13 Age-standardized death rates for oral and pharyngeal cancer in eastern Europe (outside the EEC), 1963–87. Again there are substantial rises in males with a strong cohort effect.[46]

available to indicate rising trends in both incidence and mortality rates for oral cancer in many other parts of the world.[42] Figure 1.11 reproduces these trends for several major geographical regions, notably in Europe, Australasia and parts of the south American continent.[42] These trends show a strong cohort effect, with individuals born from about the 1920s onwards showing a steady rise in incidence and in mortality rates, albeit from a lower base, than those born in the latter part of the 19th century and the early part of the 20th century.[44,45] For tongue cancer in the USA the change in incidence rates

Table 1.8 Age-period cohort modelling of oral cancer mortality rates in 19 countries with increasing risk. (Source: Macfarlane et al.[42])

Country	Birth cohort with lowest risk	Relative risk for 1940 cohort
Germany	1900	10.12
Hungary	1905	9.32
Czechoslovakia	1905	6.14
Austria	1910	4.80
Spain	1905	3.56
Poland	1910	3.41
Scotland	1915	2.82
Denmark	1910	2.61
Ireland	1915	2.11
Italy	1910	2.09
Switzerland	1910	1.97
England and Wales	1910	1.90
Northern Ireland	1910	1.88
The Netherlands	1905	1.82
Norway	1915	1.62
Canada	1900	1.61
New Zealand	1905	1.47
Portugal	1915	1.46
Australia	1905	1.44

begins with birth cohorts 1938–48.[47] These trends are clearly shown for the European Economic Community (the EU: Fig. 1.12) and even more strongly for Eastern Europe outside the EU (Fig. 1.13).[46] The increases are particularly striking in young and middle-aged men. Table 1.8[42] lists the increase in risk for 19 countries in which increasing risk is consistently demonstrable from the mortality database of the WHO. The relative risk for the cohort born in 1940, and hence now in high-risk age groups, is compared with the birth cohort that shows the lowest risk. The earliest rise in rates appears in the cohort born at the turn of the 20th century in Germany and in Canada; some 15 years later in Scotland, Ireland and Norway. The highest increases are in countries of Central, and then of Western Europe, including parts of Spain;[48] the lowest cohort-based increases have occurred in Norway, Portugal, Canada, Australia and New Zealand. France, which has the highest recorded rates of oral cancer, does not fit this pattern, with rises from 1950–54 to 1980–84, followed by a fall to 1989. There has been little change in overall rates in Sweden and Finland, or in the USA over this period, but subsite analysis for the tongue shows a small rise in Japan with successive cohorts born from 1920, and rises in tongue cancer for young adult men have been reported from the USA.[49] More detailed analysis for England and Wales between 1901 and 1990 is shown in Fig. 1.14[50] for ICD codes 141 and 143–146 (intraoral cancer only) in men. There is a clear rise in both incidence and mortality for the 35–64-year-old group and a striking cohort effect demonstrated in those born from approximately 1915 onwards.

In population terms, survival rates around the world show little evidence of improvement. Cure rates and survival rates have improved with advances in surgical and other techniques in highly specialized, high-volume treatment institutions. Regrettably, such highly expert management is not yet uniformly available and it will be many more decades before these results are reflected in population trends. This is borne out by the Eurocare Study on Survival of Cancer Patients in Europe.[51] Figs 1.15A and B show the relative survival of patients suffering from tongue and oral cavity cancer, respectively, for a number of European countries, in terms of both 1- and 5-year survival rates. Data are presented for Denmark, England, Finland, France, Germany, Italy and Scotland, together with the European average. Overall, these relative survival rates for Europe are 66% at 1 year, 39% at 5 years and 33% at 10 years for the tongue (ICD-9: 141); for the oral cavity (ICD-9: 143–145) they are 71% at 1 year, 46% at 5 years and 38% at 10 years. It is striking that there are no differences in the relative survival rates between the period 1978–80 and the period 1983–85 (Fig. 1.16 A and B). As later data become available it will be of interest to see how the advances in therapeutics and in reconstruction over the last decade have begun to improve these survival rates. Examples of survival curves from one well-documented western industrialized area, the Yorkshire cancer registry in the UK, are shown in Fig. 1.17.[52] There is no significant difference, overall, by age or sex; lip cancer is, biologically, a much less aggressive neoplasm than intraoral cancer and is more readily eradicated. The apparently major differences by treatment modality reflect the fact that smaller and more readily curable lesions will form a proportion of those for whom surgery is the main approach, whereas large (perhaps inoperable) lesions will form a proportion of those treated primarily by radiotherapy. Furthermore these curves do not distinguish the effects of combined modality therapy. The major determinants of survival are discussed in detail in subsequent chapters. They include the following:

- *Patient factors at diagnosis:* Age, sex, socioeconomic status, nutritional status and intercurrent disease,[53] continuing presence of risk factors.[54]
- *Tumour factors:* Site, size, differentiation and biological behaviour of the neoplasm, including

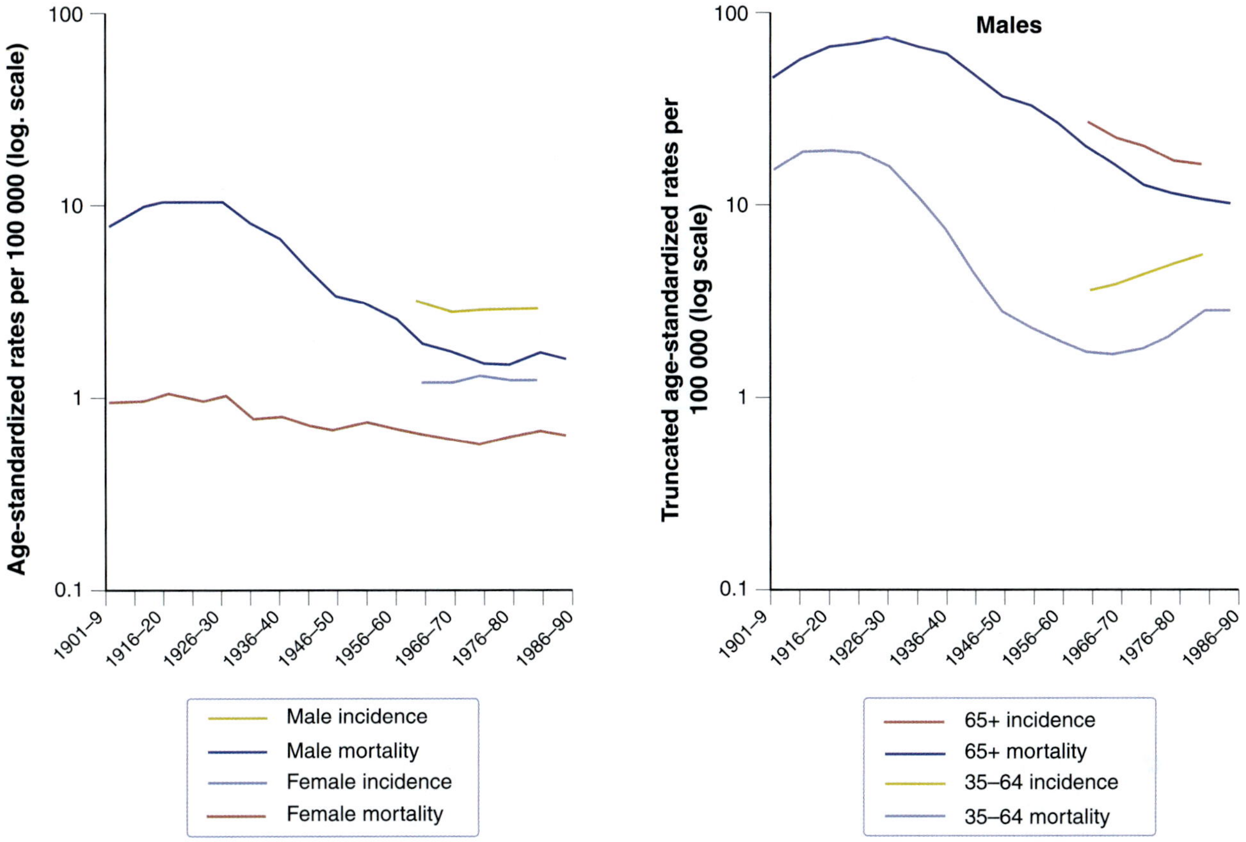

Figure 1.14A Trends in age adjusted intra-oral cancer (ICD9: 141, 143–6) incidence and mortality rates in England and Wales, 1901–90. Note the downward trends last century for older individuals, but rises since the mid 1960s in those aged 35–64, especially in males.[50]

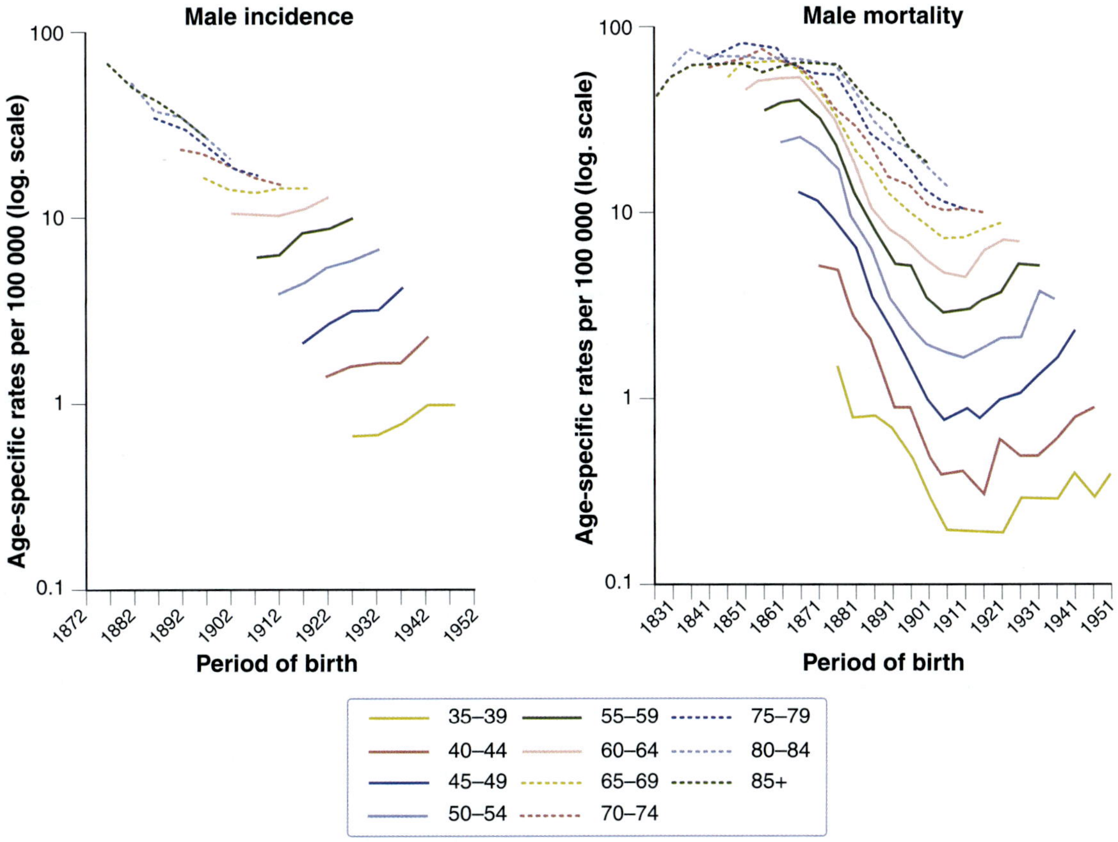

Figure 1.14B The same data as in Fig. 1.14A transformed to birth cohorts, 1872–1951. Note the upturn in the younger cohorts born from approximately 1915 onwards.[50]

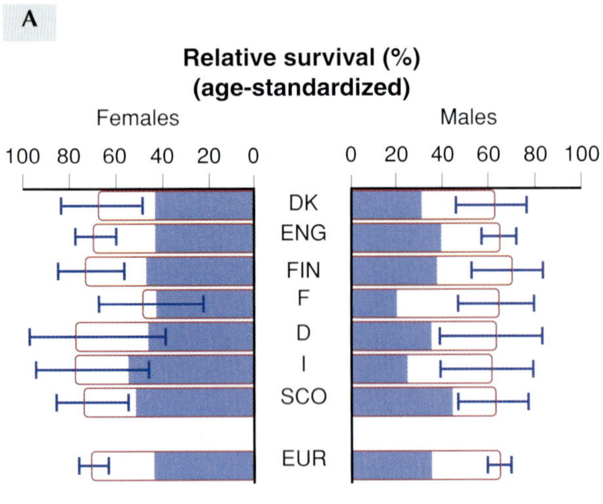

Figure 1.15 Relative 1-year and 5-year survival rates for tongue cancer (A), and for other oral cavity sites (B), in Denmark, England, Finland, France, Germany (D), Italy and Scotland, and for Europe as a whole (age-standardized.)[51]

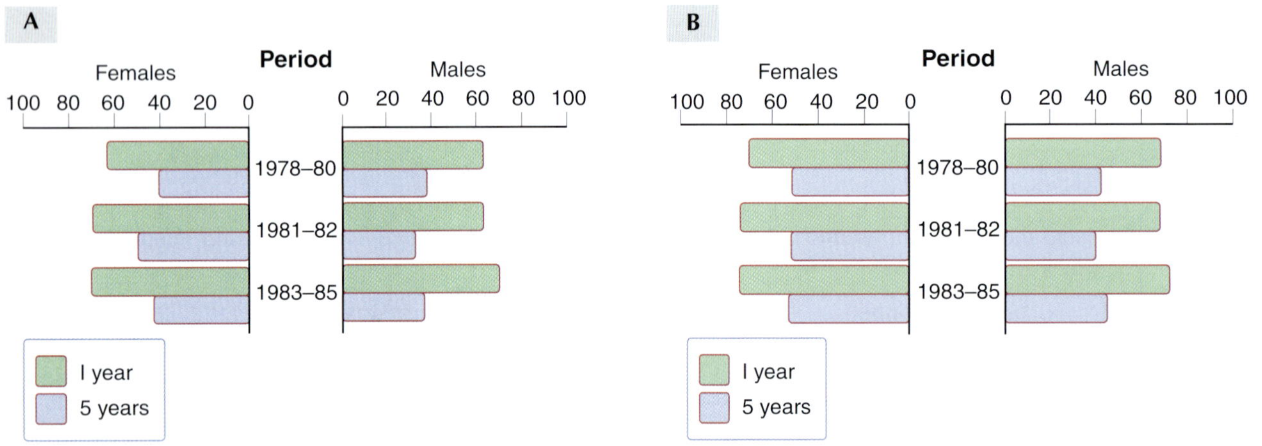

Figure 1.16 Relative survival (%) by time period between 1978 and 1985 in Europe, for tongue (A) and other intra-oral sites (B). No striking trends are apparent.[51]

host immune response, and the extent of regional and distant metastases.

- *Management factors:* Treatment modality and thoroughness, with smaller components derived from the quality and extent of supportive care and aftercare, treatment institution (facilities, including team work; experience, including case load and case mix).

Epidemiology of potentially malignant lesions and conditions

Some definitions

It has already been noted that over 80% of malignant lesions of the mouth and oropharynx are squamous cell carcinomas of the lining mucosae. Although in common use, the term precancerous/premalignant lesion(s) of the upper aerodigestive tract mucosa are unsatisfactory because they imply that perhaps irreversible steps along the multistage process of genetic alterations leading to invasive carcinoma have definitely taken place. However, the risk of a lesion becoming malignant within the life span of the patient is highly unpredictable and relatively low. Furthermore, such lesions may regress. Additionally, in much of the Western world, most of these carcinomas arise without the patient or clinician being aware of a pre-existing lesion.[55] However, in high-incidence areas of the world, notably South Asia, the reverse is the case—tobacco or areca nut chewing habits result in chronic lesions and the majority of oral cancers arise from such lesions (Fig. 1.18D). These carcinomas have a distinctive natural history which is much less

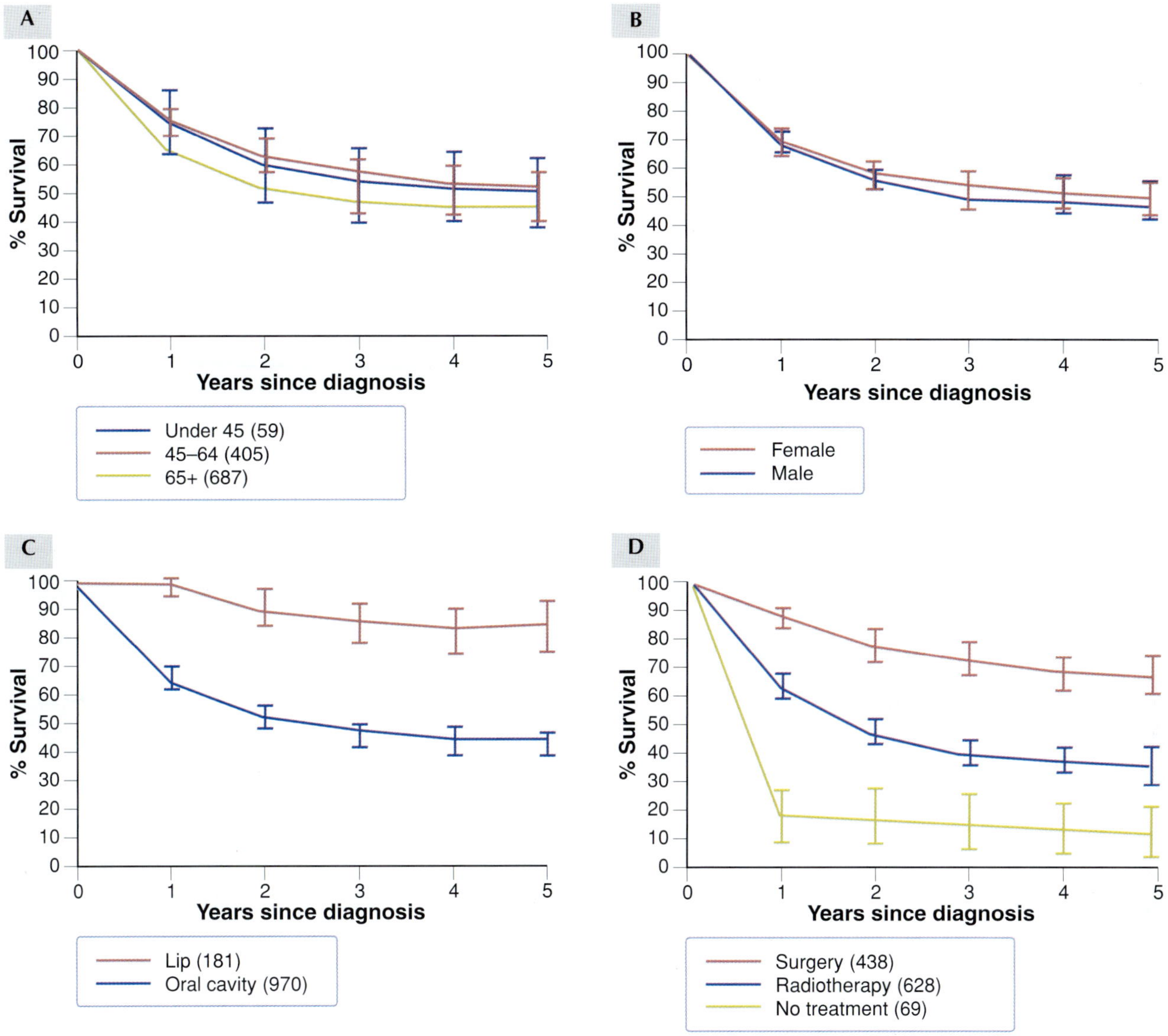

Figure 1.17 Overall survival curves for lip and oral cavity cancer by (A) age, (B) sex, (C) site and (D) major treatment modality, averaged for the years 1979–88, as reported to the Yorkshire Cancer Registry in the UK. See text for further interpretation.[52]

aggressive than carcinomas arising de novo in the West. A preferable term is *potentially malignant lesions and conditions*, among which there is a greater risk of malignant change. This broad group is generally classified under *lesions* and *conditions*, the latter being more generalized and widespread, with significant systemic involvement. They are described in detail subsequently in Chapter 3. These conditions are associated with mucosal atrophy and altered mucosal homeostasis without a discrete lesion being visible clinically. We generally consider the potentially malignant lesions to include leukoplakia and erythroplakia of various clinical presentations (such as homogeneous, verrucous, nodular or speckled) and mixed lesions. Potentially malignant conditions are usually taken to include sideropenic dysphagia (mucosal atrophy associated with chronic iron-deficiency anaemia), erosive lichen planus, oral submucous fibrosis, discoid lupus erythematosis, tertiary syphilis and actinic kerotosis. A range of these lesions is illustrated in Fig. 1.18.

The term leukoplakia has long been rather loosely used by clinicians specializing in oral diseases, in otorhinolaryngology and even in gynaecological medicine. Dentists have tended to follow an old WHO definition describing leukoplakia as 'a white patch which cannot be rubbed off and cannot be characterized clinically or histologically as any other lesion'. We recommend that the term be used only as a clinical descriptor of a white patch or plaque and is never used once histological information is available: this usage is now becoming widely accepted.[56] Biopsy of such lesions is essential to

Figure 1.18 Examples of some potentially malignant lesions and conditions of the oral mucosa.

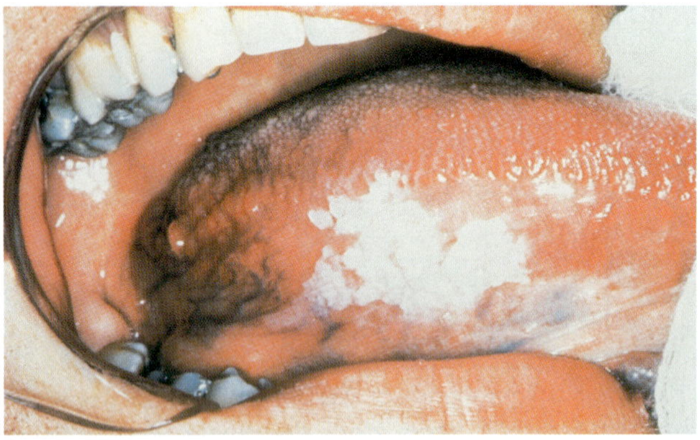

A: Homogeneous white plaque (homogeneous leukoplakia) of the lateral border of the tongue. This appearance is not particularly sinister but this is, in the west, the most common site of intra-oral malignancy, and must be biopsied and followed up.

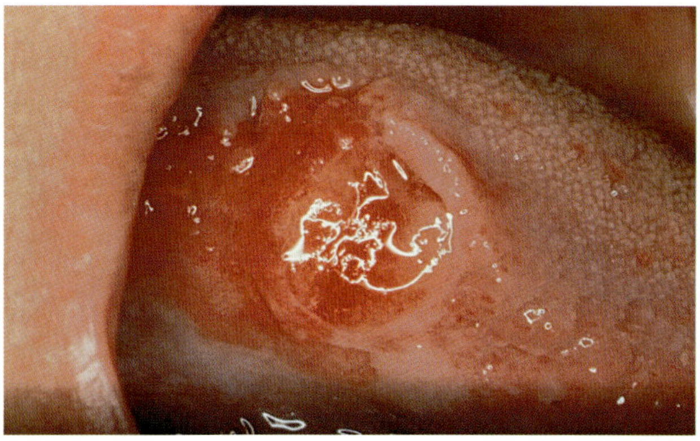

B: Erythroplakia of the lateral border of the tongue. Both the clinical appearance and the site indicate a high risk of this lesion being already an invasive carcinoma, or at high risk of becoming so. It requires immediate definitive treatment. (Courtesy of Professor Paul Bradley, London.)

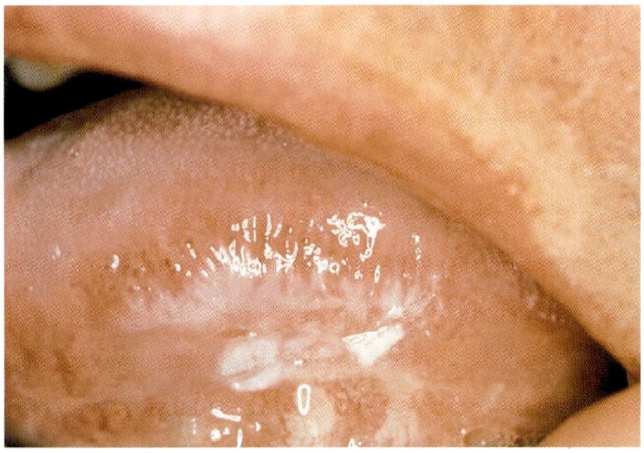

C: A white plaque on the lateral border of the tongue, with a little peripheral erythema. In spite of its relatively innocuous appearance, on biopsy this proved to be an invasive squamous cell carcinoma.

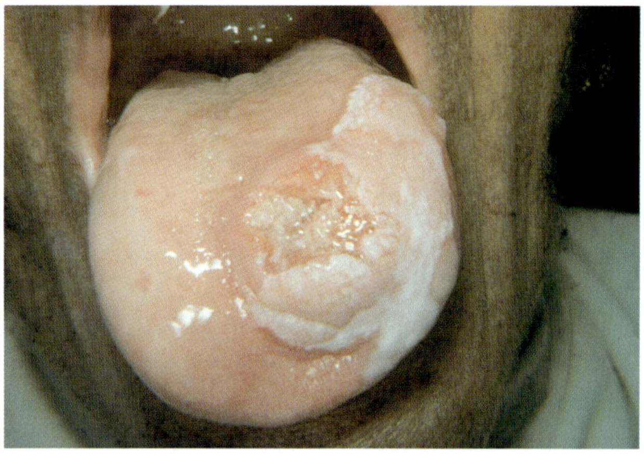

D: A long-standing homogeneous leukoplakia on the dorsum of the tongue, in a south Asian patient, within which a carcinoma has developed. (Courtesy of Prof KAAS Warnakulasuriya, London.)

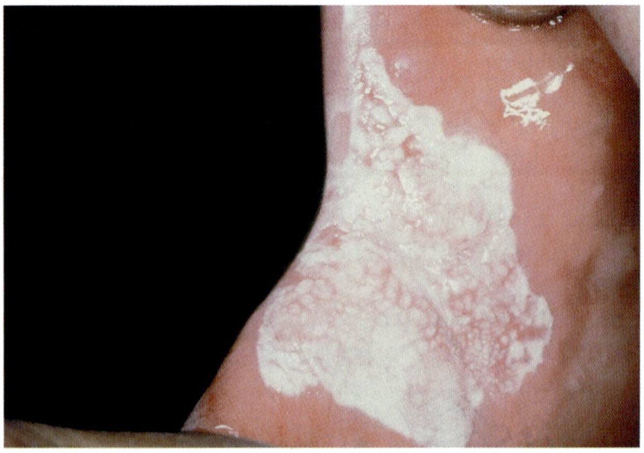

E: Homogeneous leukoplakia at the commissure. Such lesions are often associated with smoking habits, including beedi (see Chapter 2), and may have superficial infestation with candidal hyphae. Although not of a worrying appearance the patient requires thorough investigation, including haematological picture, candidal carriage and biopsy.

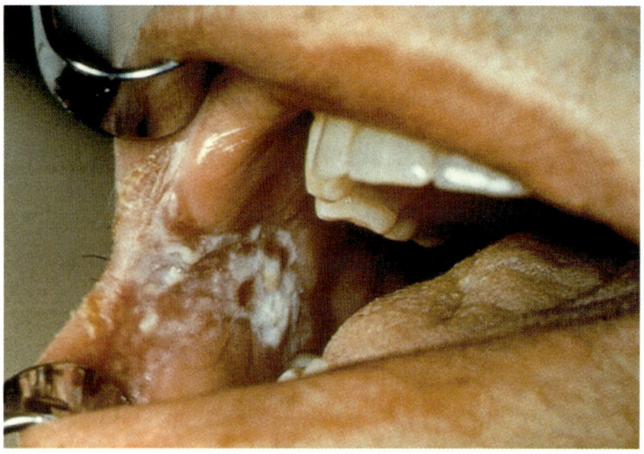

F: This is a more worrying commissural lesion because of the mixed white and red (erythroplakic) areas. These are often described as 'speckled leukoplakia', 'nodular leukoplakia' or erythroleukoplakia. This lesion demands removal with correction of any underlying anaemia and antifungal therapy if organisms are detected.

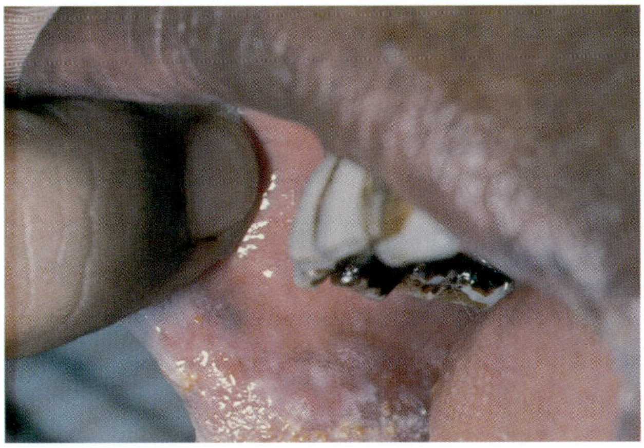

G: Another speckled erythroleukoplakia in a heavy beedi smoker. Candidal infestation was present.

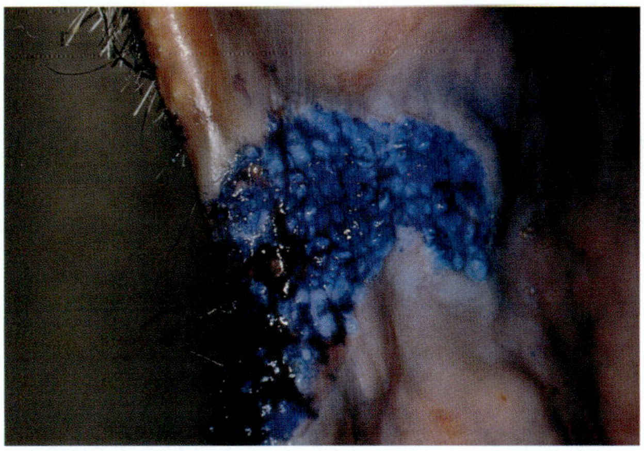

H: This nodular erythroleukoplakia stained heavily with toluidine blue and was severely dysplastic on histological examination.

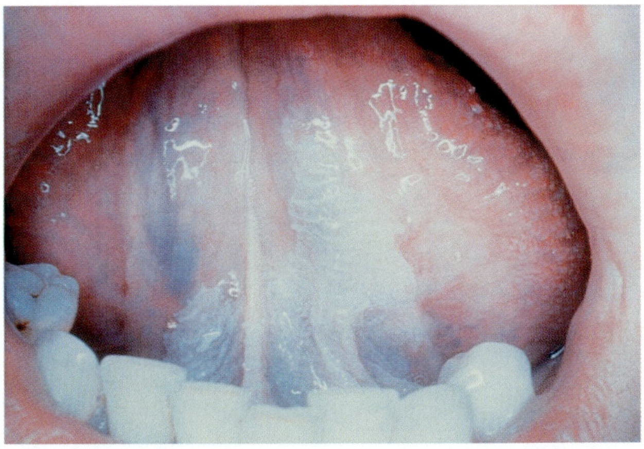

I: Homogeneous leukoplakia on the floor of mouth and ventral tongue. Although not of sinister appearance, some studies have shown this to be a high risk site. One or more biopsies are certainly required as part of treatment planning.

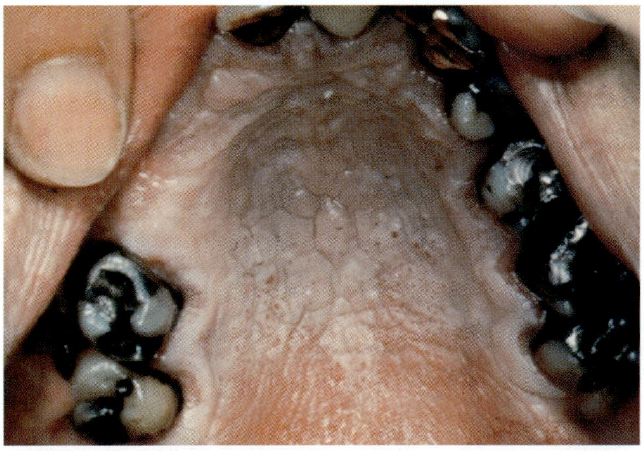

J: Stomatitis nicotina (smoker's palate) in a heavy pipe smoker. Surprisingly, such lesions show a low rate of malignant transformation.

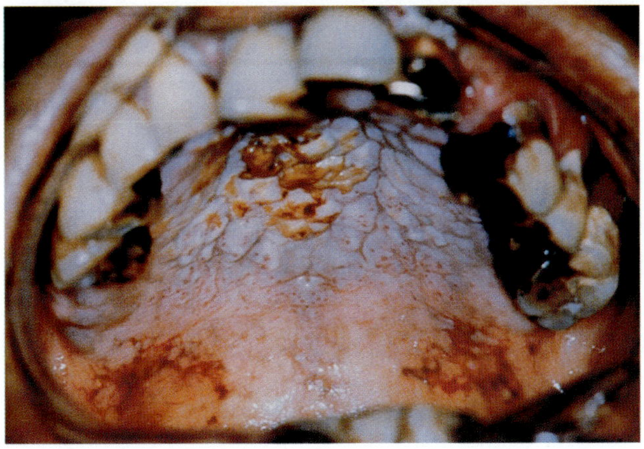

K: Nodular leukoplakia of the hard palate, with erythema of the soft palate, due to reverse smoking (see Chapter 2) in a Filipino woman. The rate of malignant transformation in these lesions in this population is not known, but similar lesions described from parts of India certainly have a relatively high risk. (Courtesy of Dr David Wilson, Adelaide.)

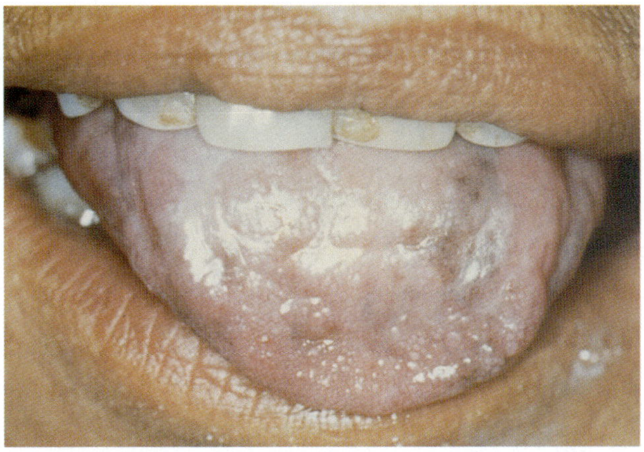

L: A lady with advanced oral submucous fibrosis, showing limited mouth opening, limited tongue protrusion and marked atrophy of lingual mucosa. (Courtesy of Dr Rehana Maher, Karachi.)

continued

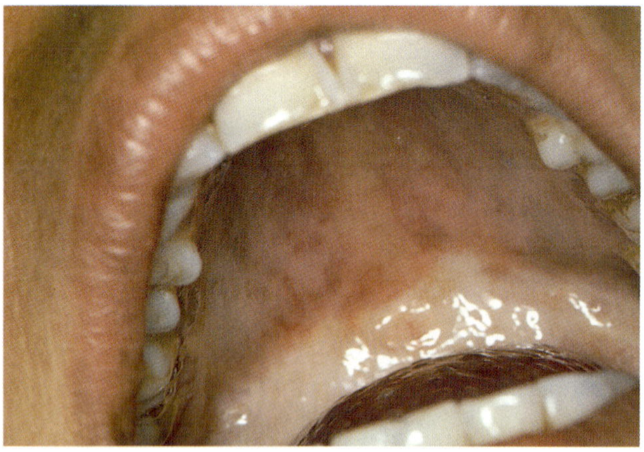

M: Submucous fibrosis. Note the pallor and atrophy of the mucosa of the hard palate and a fibrous band running transversely across, and distorting, the soft palate.

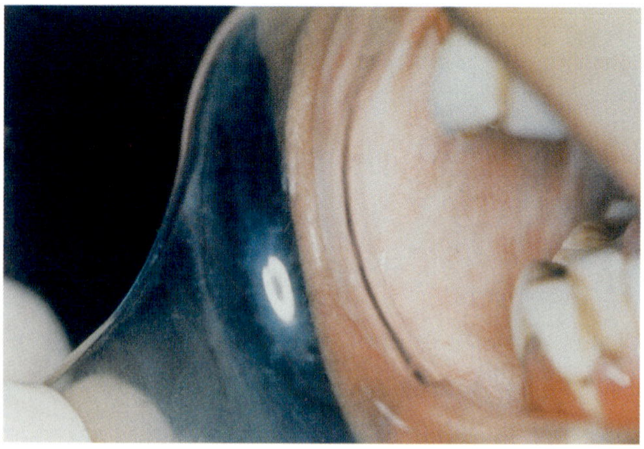

N: Extreme pallor and 'marbling' of the buccal mucosa in oral submucous fibrosis. (Courtesy of Dr Rehana Maher, Karachi.)

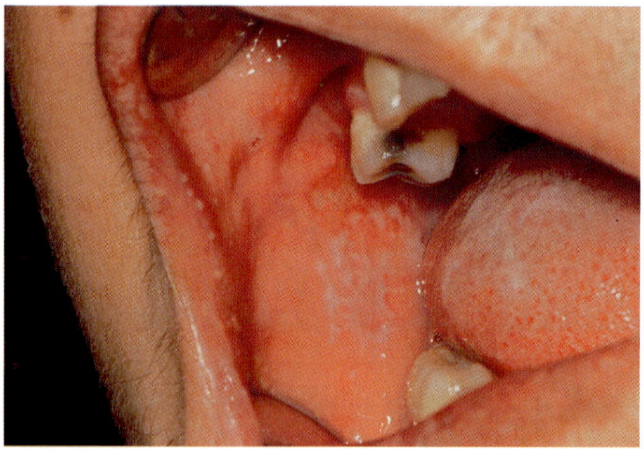

O: Papular and reticular keratin striae of oral lichen planus, on the cheek.

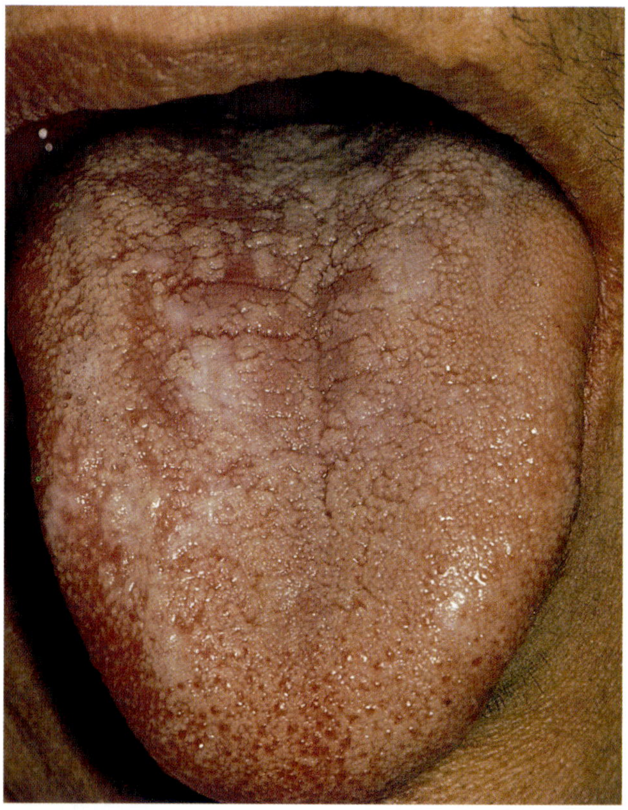

P: The tongue in the same patient as Fig. 1.18O. Note papillary atrophy, erythema and thin blue-white keratin plaques.

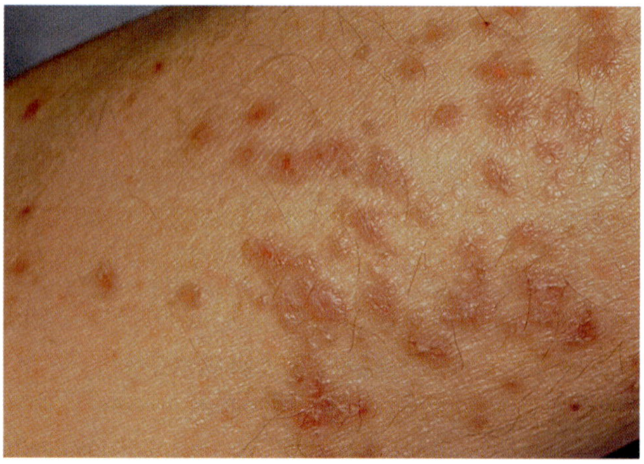

Q: Acute papular eruptions of the skin in the same patient.

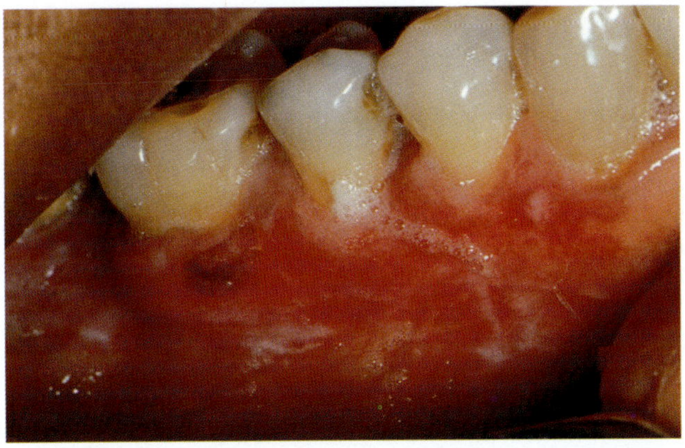

R: Another patient with severe oral lichen planus, showing marked 'desquamative gingivitis' with thinning and erythema of free and attached gingiva, extending to the alveolar mucosa, and covered with reticular keratinized striae.

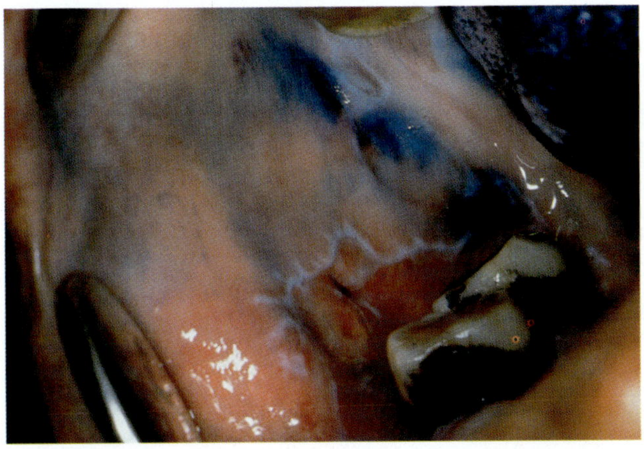

S: Reticular lichen planus of the cheek. The mucosa is very atrophic. Such cases may take up toluidine blue, as shown, and a proportion of these areas may show epithelial dysplasia on histological examination.

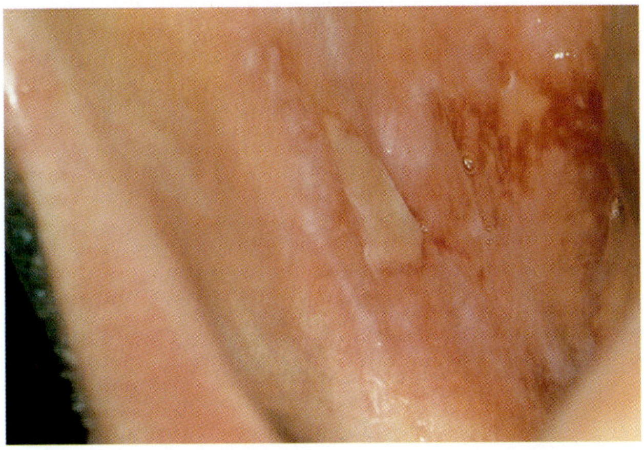

T: Erosive lichen planus of the cheek. It is widely thought that this type of condition has a higher risk of malignant transformation than the more keratinized forms (see text).

establish diagnosis and to estimate the degree of epithelial dysplasia which has value for predicting malignant potential. Biopsy will certainly indicate whether a cancer is already present—provided that the biopsy site or multiple biopsy sites are carefully chosen. Histology may lead to diagnosis of a specific lesion which can present as a white or red plaque, such as lichen planus, chronic candidiasis or lupus erythematosus. Histology helps to characterize tobacco-induced lesions and assists in differentiating these from idiopathic plaques in which no causal factor is evident from history or examination.

The third European Congress on Oral Medicine[57] has recommended that as many as possible of the descriptors given in Table 1.9 be recorded for every lesion and condition.

Diagnostic labels should not be applied until all information is available. White patch not otherwise specified (NOS) is a better term for undiagnosable lesions, which probably represent a considerable, ill-understood spectrum. Keratosis without, or keratosis with, mild/moderate/severe dysplasia are acceptable diagnostic labels for these lesions. Further discussion of the clinicopathologic features of oral white patches is to be found in Chapter 3.

Prevalence and incidence

Because of these unsatisfactory definitions, and the way in which they have changed over time, a very wide range of figures for prevalence and incidence is reported in the literature. This literature is summarized in Table 1.10[58] and further discussed in Chapter 3.

Malignant transformation rates

Data on malignant transformation are limited and difficult to interpret because of variable follow-up, disease definitions, diagnostic criteria and treatment interventions. The literature gives rates of malignant transformation ranging between 0.3 and 17.5% for leukoplakia; a consensus range has been regarded as 3–6%. Schepman and colleagues[59] describe 20/166 (12%) transforming after 6–201 months (median 32 months) in a hospital-based population in The Netherlands; this represents a rate of 2.9% per annum. Women without smoking habits were at significantly higher risk. Importantly, patients who had any form of active treatment did not have a statistically significantly decreased risk of malignant transformation. This latter observation is repeatedly alluded to in the literature and demands extensive

Table 1.9 Descriptors of white, red and related oral mucosal lesions

Clinical markers	Aetiological factors or associations	Histological features
White; red; grey/brown; mixed	Friction; tobacco; restorations; iron and other deficiencies	Epithelial atrophy; hyperplasia; keratinization; dysplasia
Ulcerative; verruciform; nodular	Fungi; viruses: idiopathic	Connective tissue; fibrosis/elastosis; nature and intensity of immune inflammatory infiltrate; vascularity/angiogenesis

Table 1.10 Prevalence of potentially malignant oral lesions and conditions (from Johnson et al.[58])

	Country	No. of persons examined	Prevalence (%)	References
Lesions				
Leukoplakia				
	Guam	2004	0.4	Gerry et al.[60]
	India	4734	3.5	Mehta et al.[61]
	Hungary	5613	3.6	Bruszt[62]
	New Guinea	3996	8.1	Atkinson et al.[63]
	India	30 000	1.6–3.3	Pindborg et al.[64–66]
	India	2004	6.5	Manghi et al.[67]
	India	5000	2.4	Zachariah et al.[68]
	New Guinea	1226	4.6	Pindborg et al.[69]
	India	7286	5.2	Wahi et al.[70]
	India	50 915	0.2–4.9	Mehta et al.[71]
	India	101 761	0.7	Mehta et al.[72]
	India	57 518	11.7	Smith et al.[73]
	India	4559	1.6	Bhonsle et al.[74]
	Sweden	20 333	3.6	Axell[75]
	Germany	4000	2.2	Wilsch et al.[76]
	Burma	6000	1.7	Lay et al.[77]
	Cuba	749	2.1	Rodriguez et al.[78]
	Saudi Arabia	674	1.9	Mani[79]
	USA	23 616	2.9	Bouquot and Gorlin[80]
	USSR	1569	8.0	Zaridze et al.[81]
	Sweden	20 333	0.7–24.8	Axell[82]
	The Netherlands	1000	1.4	Hogewind and Van der Waal[83]
	Thailand/Malaysia	234/233	1.3	Axell et al.[84]
	Hungary	7820	1.3	Banoczy and Rigo[85]
Erythroplakia				
	India	50 915	0.02	Mehta et al.[71]
	Burma	6000	0.1	Lay et al.[77]
Condition				
Oral lichen planus				
	USA	23 616	0.12	Bouquot and Gorlin[80]
	Burma	6000	0.4	Lay et al.[77]
	India	35 000	0.02–0.4	Pindborg et al.[64–66] Zachariah et al.[68]
	India	7639	0.1–1.5	Mehta et al.[71] Pindborg et al.[86]
	Sweden	20 333	1.9	Axell and Rundquist[87]
	Thailand	234	3.8	Axell et al.[84]

Table 1.10 continued

	Country	No. of persons examined	Prevalence (%)	References
	Malaysia	233	2.1	Axell et al.[84]
	Hungary	7820	0.08	Banoczy and Rigo[85]
Oral submucous fibrosis				
	South Africa			
	Pretoria/Johannesburg	1000	0.5	Shear et al.[88]
	Durban	1200	0.6	Dockrat and Shear[89]
	Capetown	—	1.3	Van Wyk et al.[90]
	Durban	2058	3.4	Seedat and Van Wyk[91]
	India			
	Bombay	10 000	0.5	Pindborg et al.[64]
	Lucknow	10 000	0.5	Pindborg et al.[65]
	Bangalore	10 000	0.18	Pindborg et al.[66]
	Trivandrum	5000	1.2	Zachariah et al.[68]
	Ernakulam	10 287	0.4	Pindborg et al.[69]
	Srikakulam	10 169	0.04	Pindborg et al.[69]
	Bhavnagar	10 071	0.2	Pindborg et al.[69]
	Darbhanga	10 340	0.07	Pindborg et al.[69]
	Singhbhum	10 048	0	Pindborg et al.[69]
	Pune	101 761	0.03	Mehta et al.[72]
	Agra	7286	0.6	Wahi et al.[70]
	Goa	5449	0.04	Bhonsle et al.[74]
	Ernakulam	—	0.65	Gupta et al.[92]
	Bhavnagar	—	0.06	Gupta et al.[92]
	Burma	—	0.1	Lay et al.[77]
Precancer				
	Sri Lanka	28 295	4.2	Warnakulasuriya and Nanayakkara[93]

multicentre prospective trials of the efficacy of various treatment modalities.[94]

Interestingly, the rates tend to be on the low side for tobacco-associated lesions such as those common in South Asia, where the incidence of oral cancer is high. In these countries, however, as noted earlier, some 70% of oral cancers develop from such lesions, which thus constitute a substantially increased relative risk of over 50. Idiopathic leukoplakia in Europe and America carries a higher risk. Van der Waal and colleagues[56] give, in arbitrary order, the following features as associated with malignant transformation in oral leukoplakia:

1. Sex; females appear to be at higher risk;
2. Length of duration of the lesion;
3. Lack of obvious risk factors, so-called idiopathic leukoplakia;
4. Location (e.g. floor of mouth or tongue seem to be high-risk sites, but this is influenced by risk habits; in the Amsterdam study[59] the site was not a risk factor;
5. Non-homogeneous types;
6. Colonization by fungi, usually *Candida albicans*;
7. Presence of epithelial dysplasia. In the very informative Northern Ireland cohort, malignant transformation occurred in 15% of dysplasias and 1% of non-dysplasic lesions.[55]

Controversy continues over the malignant transformation rates in oral lichen planus.[95] There are now many reports which describe transformation, ranging from 0 to 5.6% of patients, particularly those with erosive and ulcerative forms (see bibliography in references 82 and 83), but in many of these insufficient evidence is presented to confirm the original diagnosis and there is not always adequate information on smoking and drinking habits. There have always been arguments that the two diseases appeared coincidentally.[96,98] A study from Greece demonstrated the development of squamous cell carcinoma in a mean time of 6.5 years in four of 326 patients followed up from 6 months to 10 years: three had the erosive form, one the papular/atrophic form; none had a family history of cancer, alcohol or tobacco habits or nutritional disturbances.[99] Muzio et al.[100] describe 14/263 (5.32%) of their cases transforming between 3 and 10 years of individual diagnosis of oral lichen planus. Two recent single-case reports of squamous cell carcinoma[101] and of verrucous carcinoma,[102] developing in hepatitis C-related oral lichen planus in the absence of traditional risk factors, add to both our knowledge and confusion. Perhaps a significant factor in the controversy over malignant potential in oral lichen planus is too loose a histological definition of lichen planus: this is discussed further in Chapter 3.

Oral submucous fibrosis clearly has a significant malignant potential, rates as high as 7% over 15 years being reported from the extensive studies in India.[103]

Epidemiology of other oral mucosal neoplasms

Extensive coverage of the clinicopathologic features and natural history of neoplastic and non-neoplastic salivary gland lesions of the oral cavity is given in Chapter 3.

The minor salivary glands of the oral mucosa give rise to neoplasms, in most series from the West representing about 10% of all salivary tumours (5% in the large British series of 1403 patients treated between 1947 and 1992[104]). Most information on site prevalence, however, comes from hospital series and these inevitably demonstrate bias. For example, an early study from Bombay, India, showed 110 of 355 salivary neoplasms seen between 1941 and 1965 to be in the minor glands,[105] and, in Nigeria, 94 of 295 were also intraoral:[106] it is not known whether this reflects real racial or ethnic differences. Importantly, up to 50% of minor gland neoplasms are malignant.[107] Most occur around the junction of the hard and soft palate, followed by the upper lip or cheek, and less commonly the lower lip or tongue (e.g. in a Brazilian series[108] of 164 cases). Tumours of the sublingual gland, which thus present as an oral lesion, are relatively rare and nearly 100% of them are malignant in most of the populations described (e.g. in Israel[109]).

Pleomorphic adenomas are most common, followed by mucoepidermoid carcinomas and adenoid cystic carcinomas (e.g. in the recent series described by Rivera-Bastidas et al.[110]). There may be ethnic/geographical differences in pathological presentation: e.g. in Black South Africans, whereas benign mixed tumours comprised 48% of a case series of 70, polymorphous low-grade adenocarcinoma was the most frequent malignant tumour.[111] With the more overtly malignant tumour types, survival is significantly influenced by clinical stage and histologic grade: 5-, 10- and 15-year survival rates from a large series of cases of malignancy treated at Memorial Hospital, New York, between 1966 and 1991 were 75, 62 and 56%, respectively.[112]

Insufficient evidence exists in the literature to give precise age or sex distributions, but cases are seen between the third and the seventh decades and they tend to present later than do comparable lesions in the major glands, particularly if they are benign and slow growing (e.g. in the African series of Arotiba[113]).

Evidence for risk factors is limited. For tumours of the major glands, exposure to ionizing radiation, even decades earlier, has been implicated,[114] and long-term follow-up of the Nagasaki and Hiroshima survivors show a dose–response effect for both benign and (especially) malignant tumours, most of the effect of which is accounted for by mucoepidermoid carcinoma.[115,116] One study has shown smokers to have eight times the risk of developing Warthin's tumour of the parotid, compared with cases of pleomorphic adenoma,[117] but the former are not minor salivary gland tumours. Given the strong effect of local risk factors for carcinoma arising from the surface epithelium, the permeability of duct epithelium and the closeness of minor salivary glands to the surface, one might suspect tobacco and alcohol to be important in the genesis of minor salivary gland neoplasms. Against this, however, is the low rate of malignant transformation of stomatitis nicotina of the hard palate, a condition with marked reactive change in minor glands.

The majority of malignant melanomata are found on the skin (up to 70% of cases[118]), where exposure to ultraviolet light is the main aetiological agent. Fair-skinned races are more susceptible and episodes of acute sunburn, perhaps decades earlier, are more dangerous than more continuous exposure. Nevertheless, sun-exposed skin is particularly at risk, and the incidence of de novo melanomata, or malignant transformation of naevi, shows a clear association with outdoor occupations and with latitude for fair-skinned races, e.g. on the coast of Queensland, Australia. Melanoma do, nevertheless, develop in mucosae, particularly in the eye, the vulva and vagina, the anus and rectum, the upper respiratory tract and, occasionally, in the oral cavity and lip.[119,120] The non-cutaneous distribution and the features of oral mucosal melanoma are discussed in detail in Chapter 3. The aetiology of oral melanoma remains obscure: it is presumably not related to exposure to ultraviolet light; indeed, Barrett and colleagues have recently argued, on the basis of clinical, histological and immunohistochemical features, that oral melanoma should be regarded as a separate entity and not as a subtype of cutaneous melanoma.[121] A recent review indicates that the mouth may be the primary site for 0.2–8.0% of melanomas.[122] They are always sinister, so that any pigmented patch on the oral mucosa demands full identification, including by biopsy.[123,124] Most present in the fifth to the seventh decades,[125,126] with a male predominance,[127] mostly on the hard palate or maxillary gingivae. They appear to be more common in dark-skinned races[128–130] and in Japanese,[131,132] which raises further questions about predisposing and aetiological factors. Population incidence data are available for oral and nasal melanoma combined from nine cancer registries in the USA, which show an average low rate of 0.041/100 000 per annum, increasing over the period 1973–91.[133] Both sites were equally fatal, with 5-year survival of only 25%.

References

1. Johnson NW. Chapter 1. A global view of the epidemiology of oral cancer. In: Risk markers for oral diseases, Vol 2. Oral cancer: detection of patients and lesions ar risk. Cambridge: Cambridge University Press, 1991
2. Johnson NW. Orofacial neoplasms: global epidemiology, risk factors and recommendations for research. Int Dent J 1991; 41: 365–375
3. Muir C, Welland L. Upper aerodigestive tract cancers. Cancer 1995; 75(Suppl 1): 147–153
4. Parkin DM, Pisani P, Ferlay J. Estimates of the worldwide incidence of eighteen major cancers in 1985. Int J Cancer 1993; 54: 594–606
5. Black RJ, Bray F, Ferlay J, Parkin DM. Cancer incidence and mortality in the European Union. Eur J Cancer 1997; 33: 1075–1107
6. Johnson NW. Oral cancer: a worldwide problem. FDI World 1997; 6(3): 19–21
7. Peng J, Raverdy N, Ganry O, de La Roche-Saint-Andre G, Dubreuil A, Lorriaux A. Descriptive epidemiology of upper aerodigestive tract cancers in the department of Somme. Bull Cancer 2000; 87: 201–206
8. Wunsch-Filho V, de Camargo EA. The burden of mouth cancer in Latin America and the Caribbean: epidemiologic issues. Semin Oncol 2001; 28: 158–168
9. Moore SR, Johnson NW, Pierce AM, Wilson DF. The epidemiology of mouth cancer: a review of global incidence. Oral Dis 2000; 6: 65–74
10. Moore SR, Johnson NW, Pierce AM, Wilson DF. The epidemiology of tongue cancer: a review of global incidence. Oral Dis 2000; 6: 75–84
11. Sankaranarayanan R. Oral cancer in India: a clinical and epidemiological review. Oral Surg Oral Med Oral Pathol 1990; 69: 325–330
12. National Cancer Registry Programme, Indian Council of Medical Research, Ansari Nagar, New Delhi, July 1992
13. World Health Organization. Control of oral cancer in developing countries. Bulle WHO 1984; 62: 817–830
14. Coleman M, Esteve J, Damiecke P, Asland A, Renard H. Trends in cancer incidence and mortality. Lyon: IARC, 1993
15. Gupta PC, Nandarkumar A. Oral cancer scene in India. Oral Dis 1999; 5: 1–2
16. Zheng Y, Kirita T, Kurumatani N, Sugimura M, Yonemasu Y. Trends in oral cancer mortality in Japan: 1950–1993. Oral Dis 1999; 5: 3–9
17. American Cancer Society. Cancer facts and figures. Atlanta: ACS, 1997; 9
18. Moore SR, Allister J, Roder D, Pierce AM, Wilson DF. Lip cancer in South Australia, 1977–1996. Pathology 2001; 33: 167–171
19. Moller H. Changing incidence of cancer of the tongue, oral cavity and pharynx in Denmark. J Oral Pathol Med 1989; 18: 224–229
20. Macfarlane GJ, Boyle P, Scully C. Oral cancer in Scotland: changing incidence and mortality. Br Med J 1992; 305: 1121–1123
21. Plesko I, Macfarlane GJ, Evstifeeva TV, Obsitnikova A, Kramarova E. Oral and pharyngeal cancer incidence in Slovakia 1968–1989. Int J Cancer 1994; 56: 481–486
22. International Agency for Research against Cancer. Cancer in the European Union in 1990. Lyon: IARC, 1996
23. Llewellyn CD, Johnson NW, Warnakulasuriya KA. Risk factors for squamous cell carcinoma of the oral cavity in young people — a comprehensive review. Oral Oncol 2001; 37: 401–418
24. Scully C, Bedi R. Ethnicity and oral cancer. Lancet Oncol 2000; 1: 37–42
25. Ramanathan K, Lakshmi S. Oral cancer in the Chinese male. Asian J Med 1974; 10: 3–7
26. van Wyck CW, Stander I, Padayachee A et al. The areca nut habit and oral squamous cell carcinoma in South African Indians. S Afr Dent J 1992; 83: 425–429
27. Warnakulasuriya KAAS, Johnson NW. Epidemiology and risk factors for oral cancer: rising trends in Europe and possible effects of migration. Int Dent J 1996; 46(Suppl 1): 245–250
28. Thames Cancer Registry. Cancer in South-eastern England. London: 1995
29. Edwards D. Head and neck cancer services in the UK: a study of current management, patient views and factors affecting survival. PhD Thesis, University of London, 1998
30. Sverdlow AJ, Marmot MG, Grunlicj AE, Head J. Cancer mortality in Indian and British ethnic immigrants from the Indian subcontinent to England and Wales. Br J Cancer 1995; 72: 1312–1319

31. Warnakulasuriya KAAS, Johnson NW, Linklater KM, Bell J. Head and neck cancer in Asian and Chinese immigrants resident in Thames Regions. Oral Oncol 1999; 35: 471–475
32. Shiboski CH, Shiboski SC, Silverman S Jr. Trends in oral cancer rates in the United States, 1973–1996. Community Dent Oral Epidemiol 2000; 28: 249–256
33. Skarsgard DP, Groome PA, Mackillop WJ et al. Cancers of the upper aerodigestive tract in Ontario, Canada and the United States. Cancer 2000; 88: 1728–1738
34. Levi F, Lucchini F, La Vecchia C. Worldwide patterns of cancer mortality, 1985–89. Eur J Cancer Prev 1994; 3: 109–143
35. SEER Cancer Statistics Review, 1997, Table IX–1. http://seer.cancer.gov/
36. SEER Cancer Statistics Review, 1997, Table IX–6. http://seer.cancer.gov/
37. Moore RJ, Doherty DA, Do KA, Chamberlain RM, Khuri FR. Racial disparity in survival of patients with squamous cell carcinoma of the oral cavity and pharynx. Ethn Health 2001; 6: 165–177
38. SEER Cancer Statistics Review, 1997, Table IX–9. http://seer.cancer.gov/
39. Smans M, Muir CS, Boyle P. Atlas of cancer mortality in the European Economic Community. IARC Sci Pub No. 107. Lyon: IARC, 1992
40. Atlas of Cancer Mortality in the EU. CD-ROM version, 1997
41. Zatonski W, Smans M, Tyczynski J, Boyle P. Atlas of cancer mortality in Central Europe. IARC Sci Pub No. 134. Lyon: IARC, 1996
42. Macfarlane GJ, Boyle P, Evstifeeva V, Robertson C, Scully C. Rising trends in oral cancer mortality among males worldwide: the return of an old public health problem. Cancer Causes Control 1994; 5: 259–263
43. Coleman MP, Esteve J, Damiecki P, Arslan A, Renard H. Trends in cancer incidence and mortality. IARC Sci Pub No 121. Lyon: IARC, 1993
44. Negri E, La Vecchia C, Levi F, Franceschi S, Serra-Majem L, Boyle P. Comparative descriptive epidemiology of oral and oesophageal cancers in Europe. Eur J Cancer Prev 1996; 5: 267–280
45. La Vecchia C, Tavani A, Franceschi S, Levi F, Corrao G, Negri E. Epidemiology and prevention of oral cancer. Oral Oncol 1997; 33: 302–312
46. Franceschi S, Levi F, La Vecchia C, Lucchini F, Negri E. Comparison of cancer mortality trends in major European areas, 1960–1989. Eur J Cancer Prev 1994; 3: 145–206
47. Schantz SP, Yu GP. Head and neck cancer incidence trends in young Americans, 1973–1997. Arch Otolaryngol Head Neck Surg 2002; 128: 268–274
48. Ruiz Ramos M, Nieto A. Mortality trends from oral cancer in Andalusia, Spain, 1975–1998. Public Health 2001; 115: 338–344
49. Davis S, Severson RK. Increasing incidence of cancer of the tongue in the United States among young adults. Lancet 1987; i: 910–911
50. Hindle I, Downer MC, Speight PM. The epidemiology of oral cancer. Br J Oral Maxillofac Surg 1996; 34: 471–476
51. Berrino F, Sant M, Verdecchia A, Capocaccia R, Hakulinen T, Esteve J. Survival of cancer patients in Europe. IARC Sci Pub No. 132. Lyon: IARC, 1995
52. Joslin C, Rider L, Crellin A. Cancer in Yorkshire; Cancer Registry Special Report Series 2: Head and neck cancer. Leeds: Yorkshire Cancer Organization, 1995
53. Reid BC, Alberg AJ, Klassen AC et al. Comorbidity and survival of elderly head and neck carcinoma patients. Cancer 2001; 92: 2109–2116
54. Macfarlane GJ, Sharp L, Porter S, Franceschi S. Trends in survival from cancers of the oral cavity and pharynx in Scotland: a clue as to why the disease is becoming more common. Br J Cancer 1996; 73: 805–808
55. Cowan CG, Gregg TA, Napier SS, McKenna SM, Kee F. Potentially malignant oral lesions in Northern Ireland: a 20–year population-based perspective of malignant transformation. Oral Dis 2001; 7: 18–24
56. van der Waal I, Schepman KP, van der Meij EH, Smeele LE. Oral leukoplakia: a clinicopathological overview. Oral Oncol 1997; 33: 291–301
57. Johnson NW, van der Waal I, Axell T. Oral leukoplakia. Oral Dis 1997; 3: 47–48
58. Johnson NW, Ranasinghe AW, Warnakulasuriya KAAS. Potentially malignant lesions and conditions of the mouth and oropharynx: natural history—cellular and molecular markers of risk. Eur J Cancer Prev 1993; 2(Suppl 2): 31–51
59. Schepman KP, van der Meij EH, Smeele LE, van der Waal I. Malignant transformation of oral leukoplakia: a follow-up study of a hospital-based population of 166 patients with oral leukoplakia from The Netherlands. Oral Oncol 1998; 34: 270–275
60. Gerry RG, Smith ST, Calton ML. The oral characteristics of Guamanians including the effects of betel chewing on the oral tissues. Oral Surg 1952; 5: 762–781, 884–894, 1004–11
61. Mehta FS, Sanjama MK, Shroff BC, Doctor RH. Incidence of leukoplakia among 'Pan' (betel leaf) chewers and 'bidi' smokers: a study of a sample survey. Indian J Res 1961; 49: 1–7
62. Bruszt P. Stomato-onkologische rehenuntersuchungen in sieben gemeinden sudungars. SSO Schweiz Monatsschr Zahnheilkd 1962; 72: 758–766
63. Atkinson L, Chester JC, Smyth FG, Ten Seldam REJ. Oral cancer in New Guinea: a study in demography and etiology. Cancer 1964; 17: 1288–1289
64. Pindborg JJ, Chawla TN, Misra RK, Nagpaul RK, Gupta VK. Frequency of oral carcinoma, leukokeratosis, leukoedema, submucous fibrosis and lichen planus in 10 000 Indians in Lucknow, uttar Pradesh, India: report. J Dent Res 1965; 44: 615
65. Pindborg JJ, Kalapesi HK, Kala SA, Singh B, Taleyarkhan BN. Frequency of oral and related conditions among 10 000 Bombayites: preliminary report. J India Dent Assoc 1965; 37: 228–229
66. Pindborg JJ, Bhat M, Devanath KR, Naryana HR, Ramachandra S. Frequency of oral white lesions in

10 000 individuals in Bangalore, South India. Preliminary report. Indian J Med Sci 1966; 2: 349–352
67. Manghi SL, Srivastava AN, Saifi AQ. Preliminary study on the epidemiology of Leukoplakia. J India Dent Assoc 1965; 37: 307–309
68. Zachariah J, Mathew B, Varma NAR, Iqbal AM, Pindborg JJ. Frequency of oral mucosal lesions among 5 000 individuals in Trivandrum, South India. J India Dent Assoc 1966; 38: 290–294
69. Pindborg JJ, Barnes D, Roed-Petersen B. Epidemiology and histology of oral leukoplakia and leukoedema among Papuans and New Guineans. Cancer 1968; 22: 379–384
70. Wahi PN, Mital VP, Lahiri B, Luthra UK, Seth RK, Arora GD. Epidemiological study of precancerous lesions of the oral cavity: a preliminary report. Indian J Med Res 1970; 50: 1361–1391
71. Mehta FS, Gupta PC, Pindborg JJ. Chewing and smoking habits in relation to precancer and oral cancer. J Cancer Res Clin Oncol 1981; 99: 35–39
72. Mehta FS, Gupta PC, Daftary DK, Pindborg JJ, Chokso SK. An epidemiologic study of oral cancer and precancerous conditions among 101 761 villagers in Maharashtra, India. Int J Cancer 1972; 10: 134–141
73. Smith LW, Bhargava K, Mani NJ, Malaowalla AM, Silverman S Jr. Oral cancer and precancerous lesions in 57 518 industrial workers of Gujarat, India. Indian J Cancer 1975; 12: 118–123
74. Bhonsle RB, Murti PR, Gupta PC, Mehta FS. Reverse dhumti smoking in Goa: an epidemiologic study of S449 villagers for oral precancerous lesions. Indian J Cancer 1976; 13: 301–305
75. Axell T. A prevalence study of oral mucosal lesions in an adult Swedish population. Odontol Revy 1976; 27: 1–103
76. Wilsch L, Hornstein OP, Bruning H et al. Oral leukoplakia II. Dtsch Zahnarztlz 1978; 33: 132–142
77. Lay KM, Sein K, Hyint A, Ko SK, Pindborg JJ. Epidemiologic study of 6000 villagers of oral precancerous lesions in Bilugyun: preliminary report. Comm Dent Oral Epidemiol 1982; 10: 152–155
78. Rodriguez I, Santana JC, Sanabria J, Banoczy J. Prevalence of oral leukoplakia in Havana city, Cuba. Community Dent Oral Epidemiol 1983; 11: 379–383
79. Mani NJ. Preliminary report on prevalence of oral cancer and precancerous lesions among dental patients in Saudi Arabia. Community Dent Oral Epidemiol 1985; 13: 247–8
80. Bouquot JE, Gorlin RJ. Leukoplakia, lichen planus and other oral keratoses in 23 616 white Americans over the age of 35 years. Oral Surg 1986; 61: 373–381
81. Zaridze DG, Blettner M, Matiakin EG et al. The effect of mass use and smoking on the risk of oral leukoplakia. Cancer Detect Prev 1986; 9: 435–440
82. Axell T. Occurrence of leukoplakia and some other oral white lesions among 20 333 adult Swedish people. Community Dent Oral Epidemiol 1987; 15: 46–51
83. Hogewind WF, van der Waal I. Prevalence study of oral leukoplakia in a selected population of 1000 patients from The Netherlands. Community Dent Oral Epidemiol 1988; 16: 302–305
84. Axell T, Zain RB, Siwamogstham P, Tantiniran D, Thampipit J. Prevalence of oral soft tissue lesions in out-patients at two Malaysian and Thai dental schools. Community Dent Oral Epidemiol 1990; 18: 95–99
85. Banoczy J, Rigo O. Prevalence study of oral precancerous lesions with a complex screening system in Hungary. Community Dent Oral Epidemiol 1991; 19: 265–267
86. Pindborg JJ, Mehta FS, Daftary DK, Gupta PC, Bhonsle RB. Prevalence of oral lichen planus among 7 639 Indian villagers in Kerala, South India. Acta Dermatovenereologica (Stockholm) 1972; 52: 216–220
87. Axell T, Rundquist L. Oral lichen planus—a demographic study. Community Dent Oral Epidemiol 1987; 15: 52–56
88. Shear M, Lemmer J, Dockrat I. Oral submucous fibrosis in South African Indians. S African J Med Sci 1967; 32: 41–46
89. Dockrat I, Shear M. Oral submucous fibrosis in Natal. Proc Int Acad Oral Pathol 1969; 57–63
90. van Wyk CW, Stax J, Farman AG. The prevalence of oral mucosal lesions among a random sample of Asian residents in Cape Town. J Dent Assoc S Afr 1977; 32: 589–592
91. Seedat HA, van Wyk CW. Submucous fibrosis in non-betel nut chewing subjects. J Biol Buccale 1988; 16: 3–6
92. Gupta PC, Mehta FS, Daftary DK et al. Incidence rates of oral cancer and natural history of oral precancerous lesions in a 10-year follow-up study of Indian villagers. Community Dent Oral Epidemiol 1980; 8: 187–333
93. Warnakulasuriya K, Nanayakkara BG. Reproducibility of an oral cancer and precancer detection programme using a primary health care model in Sri Lanka. Cancer Detect Prev 1991; 15: 331–334
94. Marley JJ, Linden GJ, Cowan CG et al. A comparison of the management of potentially malignant oral mucosal lesions by oral medicine practitioners and oral and maxillofacial surgeons in the UK. J Oral Pathol Med 1998; 27: 489–493
95. Barnard NA, Scully C, Eveson JW et al. Oral cancer development in patients with oral lichen planus. J Oral Pathol Med, 1993; 22: 421–424
96. Kovesi G, Banoczy J. Follow up studies in oral lichen planus. Int J Oral Surg 1973; 2: 13–19
97. Fulling HJ. Cancer development in oral lichen planus: a follow up study of 327 patients. Arch Dermatol 1973; 108: 667–669
98. Krutchoff DJ, Cutlert L, Laskowski S. Oral lichen planus: the evidence regarding malignant transformation. J Oral Pathol 1978; 7: 1–7
99. Markopoulos AK, Antoniades D, Papanayotou P, Trogonidis G. Malignant potential of oral lichen planus: a follow-up study of 326 patients. Oral Oncol 1997; 33: 263–269
100. Muzio L, Mignnogna MD, Favia G, Procaccini M, Testa

NF, Bucci E. The possible association between oral lichen planus and oral squamous cell carcinoma: a clinical evaluation on 14 cases and a review of the literature. Oral Oncol 1998; 34: 239–246
101. Porter SR, Lodi G, Chandler K, Kumar N. Development of squamous cell carcinoma in hepatitis C virus-associated lichen planus. Oral Oncol 1997; 33: 58–59
102. Carrozzo M, Carbone M, Gandolfo S, Valente G, Colombatto P, Ghisetti V. An atypical verrucous carcinoma of the tongue arising in a patient with oral lichen planus associated with hepatitis C virus infection. Oral Oncol 1997; 33: 220–225
103. Murti PR, Bhonsle RB, Pindborg JJ, Daftary DK, Gupta PC, Mehta FS. Malignant transformation rate in oral submucous fibrosis over a 17-year period. Community Dent Oral Epidemiol 1985, 13: 340–341
104. Renehan A, Gleave EN, Hancock BD, Smith P, McGurk M. Long-term follow up of over 1000 patients with salivary gland tumours treated in a single centre. Br J Surg 1996; 83: 1750–1754
105. Potdar GG, Paymaster JC. Tumours of minor salivary glands. Oral Surg Oral Med Oral Pathol 1969; 28: 310–319
106. Abiose BO, Oyejide O, Ogunniyi J. Salivary gland tumours in Ibadan, Nigeria: a study of 295 cases. Afr J Med Med Sci 1990; 19: 195–199
107. van der Waal I. Salivary gland neoplasms. In: Prabhu R, Wilson DF, Daftary DK, Johnson NW (eds) Oral diseases in the tropics. Oxford: Oxford University Press, 1991
108. Loyola AM, de Araujo VC, de Sousa SO, de Araujo NS. Minor salivary gland tumours: a retrospective study of 164 cases. Eur J Cancer B Oral Oncol 1995; 31B: 197–201
109. Nagler RM, Laufer D. Tumors of the major and minor salivary glands: a review of 25 years of experience. Anticancer Res 1997; 17: 701–707
110. Rivera-Bastidas H, Ocanto RA, Acevedo AM. Intra-oral salivary gland tumours: a retrospective study of 62 cases in a Venezuelan population. J Oral Pathol Med 1996; 25: 1–4
111. van Heerden WF, Raubenheimer EJ. Intraoral salivary gland neoplasms: a retrospective study of seventy cases in an African population. Oral Surg Oral Med Oral Pathol 1991; 71: 579–582
112. Spiro RH, Thaler HT, Hicks WF, Kher UA, Huvos AH, Strong EW. The importance of clinical staging of minor salivary gland carcinoma. Am J Surg 1991; 162: 330–336
113. Arotiba GT. Salivary gland neoplasms in Lagos, Nigeria. W Afr J Med 1996; 15: 11–17
114. Shore-Freedman E, Abrahams C, Recant W, Schneider AB. Neurilemmomas and salivary gland tumours of the head and neck following childhood irradiation. Cancer 1983; 51: 2159–2163
115. Land CE, Saku T, Hayashi Y, Takahara O, Matsuura H, Tokuoka S. Incidence of salivary gland tumours among atomic bomb survivors. Radiat Res 1996; 146: 28–36
116. Saku T, Hayashi Y, Takahara O et al. Salivary gland tumours among atomic bomb survivors, 1950–1987. Cancer 1997; 79: 1465–1475
117. Kotwall CA. Smoking as an aetiologic factor in the development of Warthin's tumour of the parotid gland. Am J Surg 1992; 164: 646–647
118. Eneroth CM. Malignant melanoma of the oral cavity. Int J Oral Surg 1975; 4: 191–197
119. Sampat MB, Sirsat MV. Malignant melanoma of the skin and mucous membranes in Indians. Indian J Cancer 1966; 3: 228–254
120. Tagaki M, Ishikawa G, Mori W. Primary malignant melanoma of the oral cavity in Japan with special reference to mucosal melanosis. Cancer 1974; 34: 358–370
121. Barrett AW, Bennett JH, Speight PM. A clinicopathological and immunohistochemical analysis of primary oral mucosal melanoma. Eur J Cancer B Oral Oncol 1995; 31B: 100–105
122. Bovo R, Farruggio A, Agnoletto M, Galceran M, Polidoro F. Primitive malignant melanoma of the base of the tongue. Acta Otorhinolaryngol Ital 1996; 16: 371–374
123. Eisen D, Voorhees JJ. Oral melanoma and other pigmented lesions of the oral cavity. J Am Acad Dermatol 1991; 24: 527–537
124. Manganaro AM, Hammond HL, Dalton MJ, Williams TP. Oral melanoma; case reports and review of the literature. Oral Surg Oral Med Oral Pathol Oral Radiol Endod 1995; 80: 670–676
125. Soman SC, Sirsat MV. Primary malignant melanoma of the oral cavity in Indians. Oral Surg Oral Med Oral Pathol 1974; 38: 426–434
126. Liversedge RL. Oral malignant melanoma. Br J Oral Surg 1975; 13: 40–55
127. Chaudry AP, Hampel A, Gorlin RJ. Primary malignant melanoma of the oral cavity: a review of 105 cases. Cancer 1958; 11: 923–928
128. Lewis MG, Kiriyabwire JW. Aspects of behavior and natural history of malignant melanoma in Uganda. Cancer 1968; 21: 876–887
129. Reddy CRRM, Rao R, Ramulu C. Primary malignant melanoma of the hard palate. J Oral Surg 1976; 34: 937–939
130. Goubran GF, Adekeye EO, Edwards MB. Melanoma of the face and mouth in Nigeria: A review and comment of three cases. Int J Oral Surg 1978; 7: 453–462
131. Umeda M, Shimada K. Primary malignant melanoma of the oral cavity: its histological classification and treatment. Br J Oral Maxillofac Surg 1994; 32: 39–47
132. Nakahara H, Kitamura R, Shirasuna K. Simultaneous malignant melanoma and squamous cell carcinoma of the oral cavity: a case report. J Oral Maxillofac Surg 1995; 53: 1455–1457
133. Chiu NT, Weinstock MA. Melanoma of oronasal mucosa. Population-based analysis of occurrence and mortality. Arch Otolaryngol Head Neck Surg 1996; 122: 985–988

2 Aetiology and risk factors for oral cancer

Newell W Johnson

Introduction

Some definitions: *Aetiology* (from Greek *aitia* (cause) and *logos* (science) and late Latin) is that part of medical science which deals with the causes of disease. All diseases have predisposing and direct causes, the former setting the scene in which the latter are more likely to have an effect. Predisposition is always, to some extent, inherited; it is often also a complex societal, cultural and environmental amalgam. For example, inheritance of a propensity to alcoholism, coupled with drunkenness at a particular time and the impairment of judgement and manual dexterity which follows, leads to a road traffic accident: trauma is the direct cause of the injuries sustained. Inheritance of the multiple polyposis coli gene increases the risk of colon cancer, but the more proximate causes related to diet are still influential.

The word *pathogenesis* (*pathos*, suffering or disease; *genein*, to produce) production or development of disease, again from the Greek: is used for the mechanisms involved. These are often difficult to separate, and causes and mechanisms are often described together as aetiopathogenesis. Since all diseases are multifactorial, and all mechanistic pathways complex, with perhaps several routes to a critical outcome such as malignant transformation of a clone of cells, care needs to be taken to ascribe proper weight to any factor under consideration.

We need also to be clear about the sense in which we refer to risk. Many terms are used in different senses by different authors. For the purposes of this discussion we define a *risk factor* as an agent, attribute or behaviour that is directly part of the causal chain of the disease. A *risk marker* or *risk indicator* is associated with the disease, and may or may not be causal: it will have power to predict the presence or likely future occurrence of disease, but may not explain the mechanisms. Socioeconomic status is an example of the latter: it is associated with many diseases, certainly with head and neck cancer, but is not of itself causal; the higher prevalence of smoking, alcohol abuse and poorer nutrition are the relevant factors. Social class is therefore described as a confounder in epidemiological studies of aetiopathogenesis.

In this chapter we approach aetiology in terms of risk factors. In order of importance, risk is dominated by tobacco use, alcohol abuse and nutritional insufficiencies, all of which have heavy confounding with socioeconomic, cultural, religious, racial and geographic variables. We discuss the issues in a logical sequence, starting with genetic factors before going on to environmental factors. Most of what follows relates to squamous cell carcinoma and its precursor lesions and conditions, where the risk factors are relatively well understood. We know little about the aetiology of neoplasms of salivary glands, other soft tissues, bone and the odontogenic apparatus.

Familial and genetic predisposition to oral cancer

There is little evidence of a strong effect of familial and genetic predisposition to oral cancer, but more studies are clearly needed. Certainly, there is nothing yet to suggest a strong association, albeit in a minority of those affected, such as is seen with the carriage of *BRCA 1* and/or *2* for familial breast cancer, or of the *APC* gene in familial adenopolyposis coli. Nevertheless, lip cancer is among the sites that show the strongest cancer clustering within families in the genealogical records of the Utah database, the others being leukaemia, lobular breast cancer, early melanoma and adenocarcinomas of the lung in females.[1] Holloway and Sofaer[2] studied surname distributions for 3658 male cancer cases from the Scottish Cancer Registry for the years 1959–85, comparing them with distributions for 32 468 male deaths in Scotland for 1976. For cancer of the lip there is a mild indication of increased isonomy in patients compared with controls, both within and between regions. This might suggest some genetic predisposition, but may also reflect the fact that families tend to have the same occupation—in this case outdoor work such as farming, fishing and forestry, with exposure to ultraviolet light. For cancer of the tongue, there was some evidence of increased isonomy within but not between regions. Although this could result from inherited susceptibility clustering in different regions, a more likely explanation is that environmental risk factors such as tobacco and alcohol will be common to families. For cancer of the salivary glands there was increased isonomy both within and between regions, again suggesting but not proving that genetic factors are involved; this however is consistent with reports of familial occurrence of malignant salivary tumours.[3,4]

Chapter 1 describes how oral cancer rates are higher in Blacks in the USA, and that this is largely explained by social and environmental factors.[5] The same is probably true for the observation that, in Israel, the risk of developing oral cancer is twice as high in Ashkenazic compared with Sephardic and Eastern Jewish ethnic groups. It is interesting that it is the tongue that is the leading site in the Ashkenazi and Sephardi, whereas the lip and alveolar ridges are most affected in the Eastern Jews, perhaps reflecting type of risk habit.

Perhaps of greater relevance are the studies from Kerala, South India. A familial association was seen in 0.94% of the total oral cancers accrued from January to July 1995, consistent with an autosomal mode of inheritance.[6] Further studies of seven familial cases in comparison with 10 patients with sporadic oral cancer and 14 unaffected first-degree relatives showed no constitutional chromosomal abnormalities. There was a significant difference between patients with oral cancer and unaffected relatives in the sensitivity of chromosomes to bleomycin damage; one unaffected member, who showed enhanced bleomycin sensitivity, later went on to develop an oral cancer, raising the possibility of genetic susceptibility.[7] Again, however, a common environmental source of DNA damage is not excluded.

A similar approach in The Netherlands[8] took 617 first-degree relatives of 105 patients with head and neck cancer and found among them 31 cases of cancer of the respiratory and upper digestive tract, compared with 10 cases in the control group composed of first-degree relatives of the index patient's spouses ($n = 617$). This produced a relative risk of 3.5 ($p = 0.0002$) for first degree relatives, and of 14.6 ($p = 0.0001$) for siblings. This group also studied mutagen sensitivity of lymphocytes and found this to be increased in patients with multiple head and neck cancers, in comparison to those with single tumours and controls. There was no relation to smoking and drinking histories, and the authors propose that a constitutional factor exists that reflects the way genotoxic compounds are dealt with.[9]

It is, of course, important to control for environmental factors in all such studies. This was carefully done in a large case-control study of oral and pharyngeal cancer from the National Cancer Institute in the USA.[10] A similar proportion of patients (46%, $n = 487$) and controls (41%, $n = 485$) reported cancer in a parent or sibling; although trends were apparent, most of these were not statistically significant. The strongest elevated risk was of oral/pharyngeal cancer among those whose sisters developed other cancers, but here the odds ratios (ORs) were only 1.6 (95% confidence interval (CI) 1.1–2.2). Slightly higher ORs emerged in a study in Puerto Rico, but shared lifestyle risk factors were not excluded.[11]

There is rapidly expanding literature describing susceptibility related to inherited capacity to metabolise carcinogens or pro-carcinogens, or impaired ability to repair the consequent DNA damage.[12] This especially appears to involve polymorphisms in GST genes,[13–16] CYP genes,[17–20] the cytochrome P-450 system,[21] but not, according to current evidence, in p53 polymorphisms.[22,23] The evidence for involvement of alcohol dehydrogenase genotypes is conflicting.[24–26] We have to conclude, therefore, that a genetic predisposition to oral cancer, if any, is at best small. This does not preclude it being important in a minority of cases, but the effects are swamped by environmental factors on a population basis. Nevertheless, determination of the reality and nature of these genetic factors would have enormous benefit, not only to at-risk family members, who should thus take particular care to avoid other risks, but in unravelling the molecular mechanisms of oral carcinogenesis, opening the way to better prevention and treatment.

Occupation and risk of oral cancer

Apart from the topic of environmental tobacco smoke (ETS or passive smoking), dealt with below, there is a limited literature on occupation and risk of oral cancer. Butchers in Sweden have a small but significantly increased risk (RR 1.6), no doubt partly confounded by lifestyle factors, but possibly involving industrial exposure, e.g. to viruses, nitrosamines and polycyclic aromatic hydrocarbons.[27]

Effects of solar radiation

It is well established that outdoor workers are at greater risk from lip cancer, because of long-term exposure to ultraviolet light. Those with occupations such as farming, fishing, forestry or postal delivery are at risk. Evidence comes from many countries, including those at high latitudes with clean air through which ultraviolet light penetrates easily (albeit for only part of the year), such as Finland[28] or Sweden,[29] and from countries closer to the equator with regular long hours of sunshine such as rural Greece where lip cancer can account for 60% of oral cancers[30] and in India, for example in fishermen.[31] In Finland, the increased rural risk for lip cancer is confounded by smoking and social class whereas that for oral cavity and pharynx is not; at these latter sites, alcohol was a much stronger confounder than tobacco.[32] A study from California shows that risk for women is strongly related to lifetime solar radiation exposure, but that lipstick and other sunscreens are protective.[33] The lesions that develop are usually well-differentiated squamous cell carcinomas (SCCs) and arise out of long-standing premalignant lesions usually termed solar keratoses. Histologically, these are characterized by hyperorthokeratosis of the epithelium of the vermilion border, usually of the lower lip, with epithelial atrophy and increased deposition of disorganized elastic fibres in the lamina propria (solar elastosis). With time, the degree of epithelial dysplasia increases and many pass through a demonstrable microinvasive stage (see Chapter 3). Obviously, lesions at these early stages are readily cured by limited excision.

Recent falls in the incidence of lip cancer in the Swiss canton of Vaud are interpreted as mostly due to reduced occupational exposure to sunlight and to reduced pipe and cigar smoking.[34] Nevertheless, the effects of early life exposure are long standing: for example, New Zealanders have four or more times the relative risk of developing cutaneous melanoma and lip cancer than do residents of England and Wales, and migrants in both directions retain intermediate risks.[35]

Effects of atmospheric pollution

Part of the urban/rural difference in incidence of head and neck cancer has been related to atmospheric pollution. For example mean sulphur dioxide and smoke concentrations in the atmosphere are positively correlated with squamous cancer of the larynx and, to a lesser extent, the pharynx in data collected from the West Midland region of England 1950–90.[36] There is growing concern all over the world about air pollution in cities and the impact on public health. Oxides of sulphur and nitrogen, carbon monoxide and carbon dioxide, and hydrocarbon particulates (notably 'PM 10s'—particulate material less than 10 μm in diameter, predominantly from diesel engine exhausts) are among the substances causing concern. There is growing evidence that the dramatic rise in the incidence and severity of asthma around the world is related to poor air quality in built-up areas, arising from industrial and vehicular sources. Malignancies of the lower respiratory tract may also increase as a result. The impact on cancer of the mouth is likely to be less, but merits careful study. Not only those who work but also those who live in cities and industrial areas will be at increased risk.

A group in Heidelberg, Germany, has been active in this area over the past decade. Blue-collar workers exposed to dust or inhaled organic and inorganic agents are at increased risk for cancers of the mouth, pharynx and larynx.[37] Most citizens spend more of their time at home than at their place of work or travelling; the quality of indoor residential air is therefore of prime importance. This, naturally, reflects the quality of outdoor air in the locality, but is added to by products of combustion of fossil fuels used for heating and cooking. These factors were addressed in 164 cases of carcinoma of the larynx and 656 controls; 105 cases of pharyngeal cancer

Table 2.1 Risk of upper aerodigestive cancer from domestic fuels. (Source: Dietz et al.[38])

	Odds ratio	*p* value	95% CI
Larynx			
Heating with fossil fuel > 40 years	2.0	0.02	1.10–3.46
Cooking with fossil fuel > 40 years	1.4	0.3	0.76–2.41
Pharynx			
Heating with fossil fuel > 40 years	3.3	0.0005	1.43–7.55
Cooking with fossil fuel > 40 years	2.5	0.05	1.03–6.30
Oral cavity			
Heating with fossil fuel > 40 years	2.4	0.008	1.26–4.40
Cooking with fossil fuel > 40 years	1.6	0.1	0.90–2.97

and 420 controls, and 100 cases of oral cancer and 400 controls.[38] In this study, increased risks for air pollution on the job, traffic jams on the way to work, high traffic emissions in residential areas and outdoor air pollution in residential areas were present for all sites but were not statistically significant. However, household heating with fossil-fuel stoves and cooking with fossil fuels produced statistically significant increased risks at all tumour sites. After taking the important step of adjusting for tobacco and alcohol consumption, the data shown in Table 2.1 were obtained. Socioeconomic differences were excluded as confounders.

Emissions considered to be important were respirable particles to which are bound polycyclic aromatic hydrocarbons (PAHs); cadmium and nitrosamines; carbon monoxide; and volatile organic compounds such as benzenes, styrenes and tetrachlorethylenes. Hard-coal products were suggested as the most dangerous sources.

The importance of fossil-fuel combustion in a work setting is confirmed in a large study in four areas in the USA (1114 cases, 1268 controls), with ORs of approximately 2.0 for cancers at pharyngeal sites. Male carpet installers emerged as at risk, with an OR of 7.7 (95% CI = 2.4–24.9; 23 cases, four controls).[39]

Immunosuppression and lip and oral cancer risk

Individuals with HIV/AIDS are at increased risk for a limited number of neoplasms, especially Kaposi's sarcoma, which commonly presents in the mouth[40] and lymphoma, which occasionally presents as an oral mucosal or intrabone lesion in the jaws.[41] SCCs of the mouth or pharynx are not, however, more common in these patients, and the characteristic oral hairy leukoplakia (OHL) of HIV disease does not appear to undergo malignant transformation (see Chapter 3).

Immunosuppressed organ transplant patients are at increased risk of lip cancer, however, which is principally due to the effects of ultraviolet light, although the effects of smoking, if present, continue to have their role.[42,43]

Tobacco use and risk of oral cancer

There is absolutely no doubt that, on a global scale, the use and abuse of tobacco products is the major cause of oral cancer.[44,45] Alcohol use synergizes with tobacco as a risk factor for upper aerodigestive tract SCCs: this synergism is super-multiplicative for the mouth, additive for the larynx and between additive and multiplicative for the oesophagus.[46] Sorting out the independent effects is difficult, however, because these habits usually overlap. Many believe that the rising incidence of oral cancer in Europe and elsewhere in the Western world is largely due to increasing alcohol consumption (see below). In many developing countries, particularly in the Islamic world and in Moslem communities everywhere, accurate data on alcohol consumption are impossible to obtain because of religious and cultural inhibitions. The issue of tobacco use in non-drinkers, and of alcohol, and poor diet in non-smokers[47] is further addressed in Chapter 3.

Taken together, the effects of tobacco use, heavy alcohol consumption and poor diet probably explain over 90% of cases of oral cancer. The preventive approach is, therefore, clear and all health care professionals have excellent opportunities to contribute.

Every 10 seconds another person dies somewhere in the world as a result of tobacco use. In developed countries as a whole, tobacco is responsible for 24% of all male deaths and 7% of female deaths, rising to over 40% for men in some of the former socialist countries and 17% for women in the USA. This has been calculated to represent an average loss of life for all cigarette smokers of 8 years and, for those whose deaths are directly attributed to tobacco, of 16 years. The proportions of cancer deaths attributed to smoking in developing countries as a whole are lower, being about 21% for men and only 4% for women. However, these figures are rising, the fall in global tobacco consumption in the West being matched by growth in developing countries. Indeed, of the vast majority of the estimated 1100 million smokers in the world, some 800 million are in developing countries, 300 million in China alone! Globally, some 3 million deaths a year have been estimated to be attributable to smoking, rising to 10 million a year in 30–40 years' time when some 7 million will be in developing countries.[48,49] When the use of oral smokeless tobacco is added to these figures and the deaths it contributes through oral, pharyngeal and oesophageal cancer, the seriousness of the global epidemic of tobacco-related diseases is even more staggering.[50] We all share a responsibility to help quell this epidemic.

According to Doll and colleagues,[51] using data from the long-term study on male British doctors, about half of all regular smokers will be killed by their habit. The major causes of such deaths are listed in Table 2.2.

Table 2.2 The major causes of smoking-related deaths

- Cancers of the lung, bladder, pancreas, oesophagus, pharynx and larynx
- Chronic obstructive pulmonary and other respiratory diseases
- Vascular diseases, including coronary artery and peripheral arterial diseases
- Peptic ulceration

Among men in industrialized countries, smoking is estimated to be the cause of 40–45% of all cancer deaths, 90–95% of lung cancer deaths, over 85% of oral cancer deaths, 75% of chronic obstructive lung disease deaths and 35% of cardiovascular disease deaths in those aged 35–69 years. Thus, although oral and pharyngeal cancer figure prominently, lung cancer, other pulmonary diseases and cardiovascular diseases should be the starting points for antitobacco counselling.

Types of tobacco use: a global perspective

The smoking of tobacco in the form of factory-made cigarettes, cigars and cheroots, and loose tobacco in pipes or rolled into hand-made cigarettes, is familiar to all. There is great variation in the tar, nicotine and nitrosamine contents, depending on species, curing, additives and method of combustion. Such smoking habits are the predominant form of tobacco use in the West, and in growing millions in developing countries. With government regulation of tobacco advertising, restrictions on smoking in public transport and other public places, and the awarding of damages to individuals and health authorities (particularly in the USA), manufacturers are increasingly targeting developing countries for sales, especially of their higher-tar varieties. The morality of this is, of course, questionable.

Smokeless tobacco

Much of the tobacco in the world is consumed without combustion, by being placed into contact with mucous membranes, through which the nicotine is absorbed to provide the pharmacological 'benefit'. The practice of nasal snuff, popular in the last century, has faded. However, the use of various forms of snuff, either loose or packeted in small portions, placed in the oral vestibule, is common in Scandinavia and the USA. Tobacco is also prepared in blocks or flakes for chewing, North Americans use the term 'oral smokeless tobacco' for these products. In developing countries, however, tobacco is mostly consumed mixed with other ingredients, as summarized in Table 2.3. There is extensive evidence for the carcinogenicity of these mixtures.[52–55]

Toombak, the form used in Sudan, has been extensively studied in the past decade. It contains unusually high levels of tobacco-specific nitrosamines (TSNs), which are found in the saliva of users.[56] A case-control study of 375 patients with SCC of the lip, buccal cavity and floor of mouth and of 271 patients with similar cancers of the tongue, palate and maxillary sinus, compared with 204 patients with non-squamous oral and non-oral malignant neoplasms, and with 2820 disease-free individuals, shows overall adjusted ORs associated with toombak

Table 2.3 Some common forms of oral smokeless tobacco

Habit	Ingredients	Population
Pan/paan/betel quid	Areca nut, betel leaf/inflorescence, slaked lime, catechu, condiments, with or without tobacco	Indian subcontinent, South-east Asia, Papua New Guinea, part of South America
Khaini	Tobacco and lime	Bihar (India)
Mishri	Burned tobacco	Maharashtra (India)
Zarda	Boiled tobacco	India and Arab countries
Gadakhu	Tobacco and molasses	Central India
Mawa	Tobacco, lime and areca	Bhavnagar (India)
Nass	Tobacco, ash, cotton or sesame oil	Central Asia, Iran, Afghanistan, Pakistan
Naswar/niswar	Tobacco, lime, indigo, cardamom, oil, menthol, etc.	Central Asia, Iran, Afghanistan, Pakistan
Shammah	Tobacco and ash and lime	Saudi Arabia
Toombak	Tobacco and sodium bicarbonate	Sudan

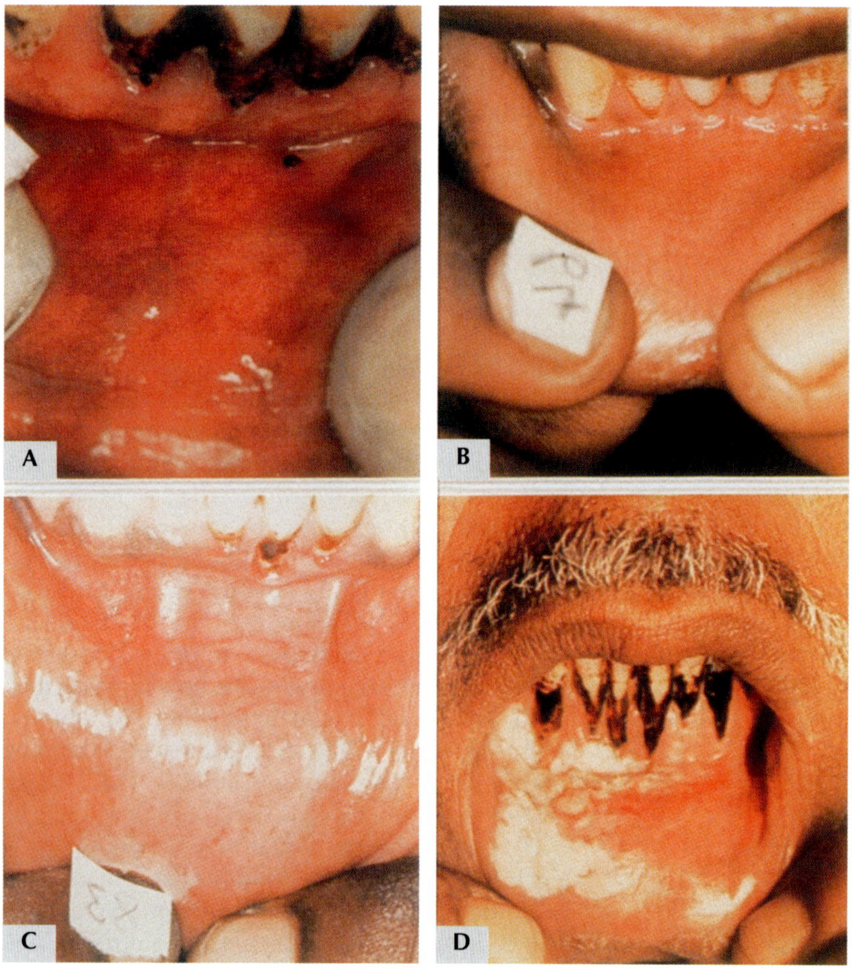

Figure 2.1 Clinical appearance of toombak-associated oral mucosal lesions. A: A superficial lesion with a mild colour change and some wrinkling. B: A superficial white lesion with wrinkling. No obvious thickening or roughness. C: A thickened white or yellowish lesion with furrows and wrinkling. D: A marked, elevated white or yellow/brown lesion with heavy thickening and grooving. Note some reddened furrows are also present. (From Idris et al.[59])

dipping of 7.3 and 3.9, respectively, for the first oral cancer group, compared with hospital and population controls. These effects rise to 11.0 and 4.3, respectively, in long-term users. No significant ORs were found for the second cancer group where the agent is not in direct contact with the cancer site.[57] These toombak-associated carcinomas show a high prevalence of p53 protein aberration/stabilization but a very low prevalence of HPV carriage.[58] Distinctive forms of leukoplakia are common in habitués (Fig. 2.1) but, interestingly, these show a low prevalence of epithelial dysplasia and longitudinal studies are necessary to establish the rate of malignant transformation.[59]

Betel quids (Fig. 2.2)

The recommended terminology is that of the Expert Symposium published in 1997.[60] Betel quids are prepared from areca nut, cured or sun dried, and chopped. These pieces are placed on a leaf of the *Piper betel* vine (in most parts of the world where the habit is indigenous: importantly, this includes emigrant communities), although the inflorescence is used by some, for example in Papua New Guinea (PNG). Slaked lime is an essential ingredient; it lowers the pH dramatically and accelerates the release of alkaloids from both tobacco and nut, with enhanced pharmacological 'lift'. The lime is prepared by baking limestone where available: near coasts this is more often from sea shells or snail shells (such as in Kerala and Sri Lanka) or from coral (as in the Pacific Islands). Customs vary widely. In PNG, for example, areca nut is chewed directly, the lime being smeared on the oral mucosa itself; tobacco is rarely added or chewed, although cigars made from rough local tobacco are commonly smoked[61] and cigarette consumption is now growing. The spread of oral cancer from the coasts to the highlands in PNG has followed the trade in coast-grown areca nuts. The effects of long-term, heavy chewing on the mouth are characteristic and are shown in Fig. 2.3.

The chewing of areca nut in various forms and mixtures is deeply embedded in the social and cultural history of India, Sri Lanka, Pakistan, Bangladesh, Myanmar, Thailand, Cambodia, Malaysia, Singapore, Indonesia, Philippines, New

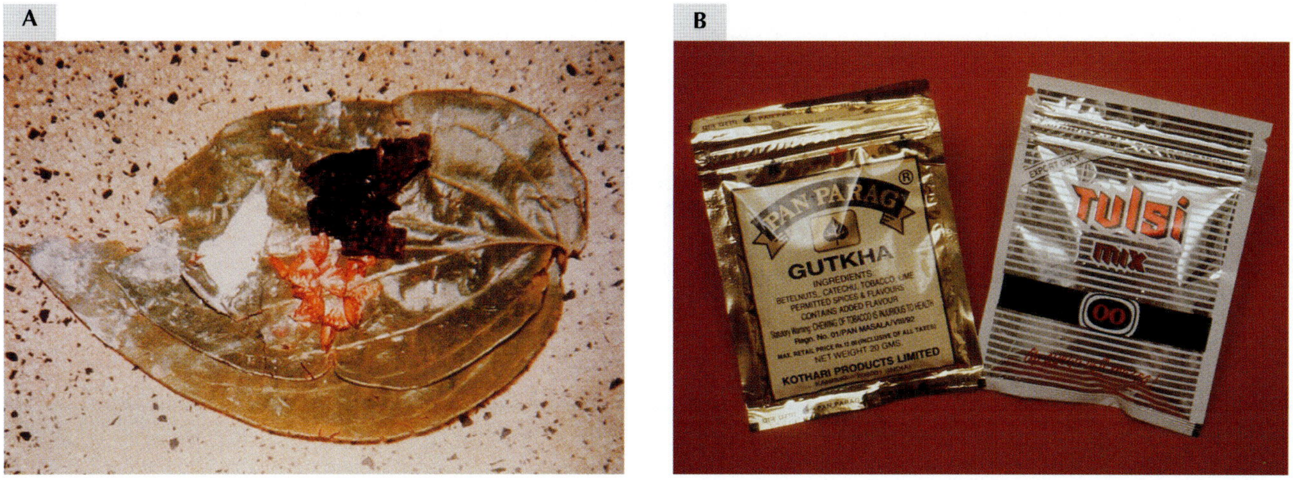

Figure 2.2 A: Ingredients of a traditional betel quid or pan. Chopped areca nut and lime paste are placed on a betel leaf: tobacco and various condiments and sweeteners may be added. B: These days cheap packets of chopped areca nut are widely available. They usually contain other flavourings and frequently include tobacco, in which case they are likely to carry a government health warning. Use of these products may be even more damaging than traditional betel quids, because the leaf of the latter has antioxidant properties.

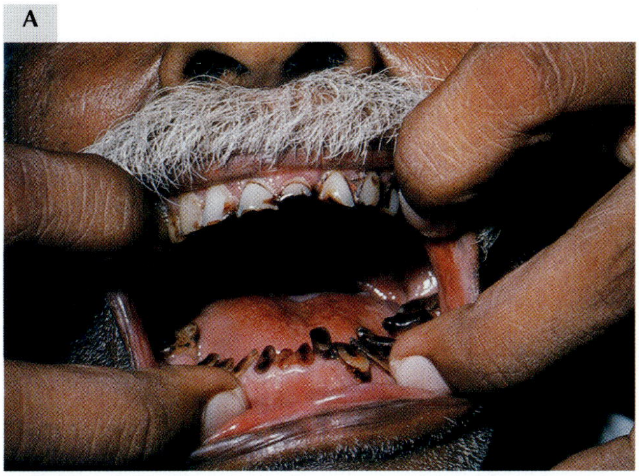

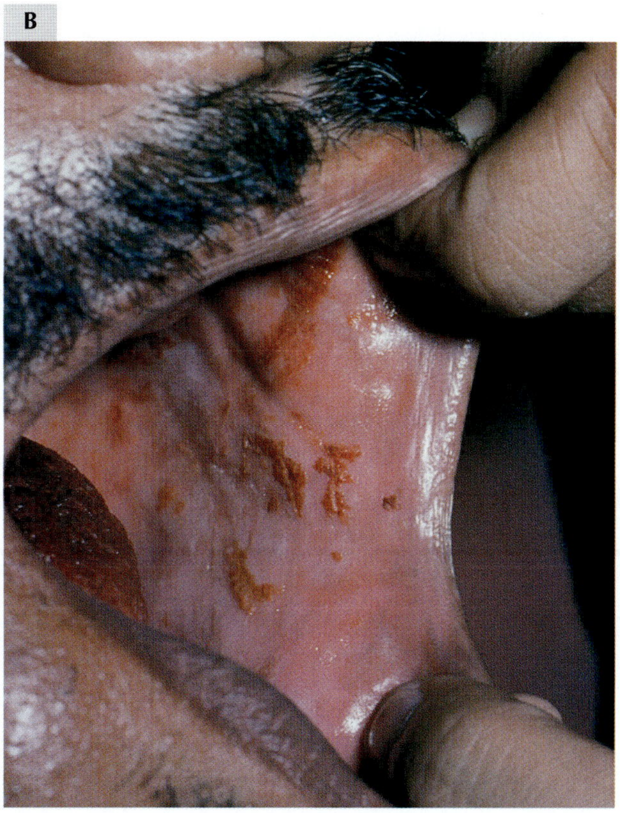

Figure 2.3 A: Severe attrition and tooth staining in a heavy betel quid chewer. B: Atrophic mucosa with superficial plaques of keratin stained by areca extracts.

Guinea, Taiwan and China (Fig. 2.4) and in emigrant communities therefrom. Its use appears in ancient Sanskrit literature. Areca nuts contain potent cholinergic muscarinic alkaloids, notably arecoline and guavacoline, with a wide range of parasympatheticomimetic effects: they promote salivation and the passage of wind through the gut; they raise blood pressure and pulse rate; and they elicit a degree of euphoria by virtue of their GABA receptor-inhibitory properties which contribute to dependence and habituation. There are also bronchoconstrictor effects, and evidence for a role in precipitating and exacerbating asthma and diabetes (reviewed by Boucher[52]). In addition to aspects of oral cancer and precancer, the historical, social and general health aspects of betel quid use are well discussed in the excellent monographs of Bedi and Jones,[63] and of Warnakulasuriya.[64]

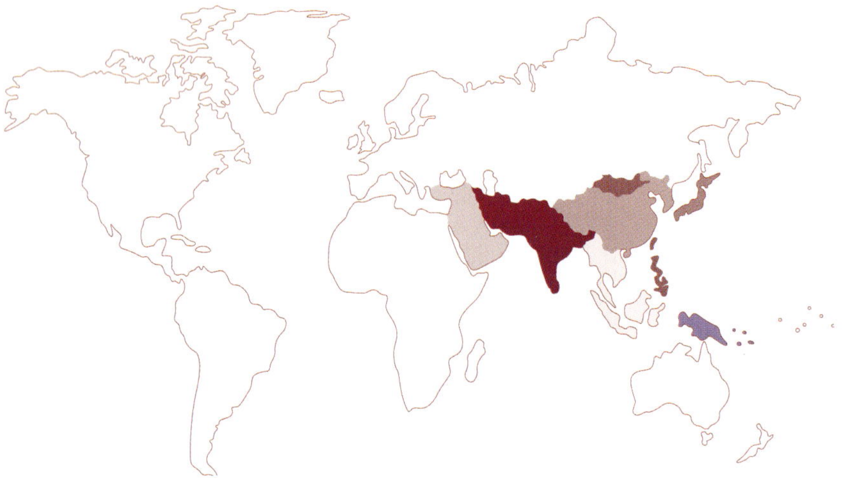

Figure 2.4 Those parts of the globe in which betel quid and other areca nut habits are endemic. These habits are continued amongst emigrants from those parts of the world and are thus found in immigrant communities worldwide.

Daftary et al[53] set out the evidence for the carcinogenicity of betel quid in categories of varying epidemiological weight.

Ecological evidence

It has been known, perhaps for over a century, that there is a high frequency of oral cancer in those parts of the world where areca/tobacco-chewing habits are widespread. The association has a strong ethnic basis and remains in emigrant communities from the Indian subcontinent who continue the habit. Oral submucous fibrosis, for which areca nut itself is the main aetiological agent, is almost exclusively found in those ethnic groups who use pan or areca in other forms, wherever in the world such people reside.

Chewing habits among patients with oral cancer

Descriptive studies in India going back to the 1960s report a high prevalence of oral cancer amongst habitués. For example, in 1962 Paymaster[65] reported that 81% of 4212 oral cancer patients used tobacco: 36% were chewers, 23% were smokers and 22% had both habits. Many similar observations subsequently have been published. There is a strong association between the site of cancer and the site where the quid is habitually placed—again, quite an old observation.[66]

Evidence from cross-sectional studies

Extensive cross-sectional population studies from India, involving over 100 000 individuals, detected 14 oral cancers in chewers of betel quid with tobacco, 24 among other tobacco users and none among non-users of tobacco.[67] In several hospital series in different parts of Thailand, oral cancer ranked second among cancer sites in males in the late 1970s/early 1980s, but by 1990 had dropped to fifth. This has been associated with decreasing use

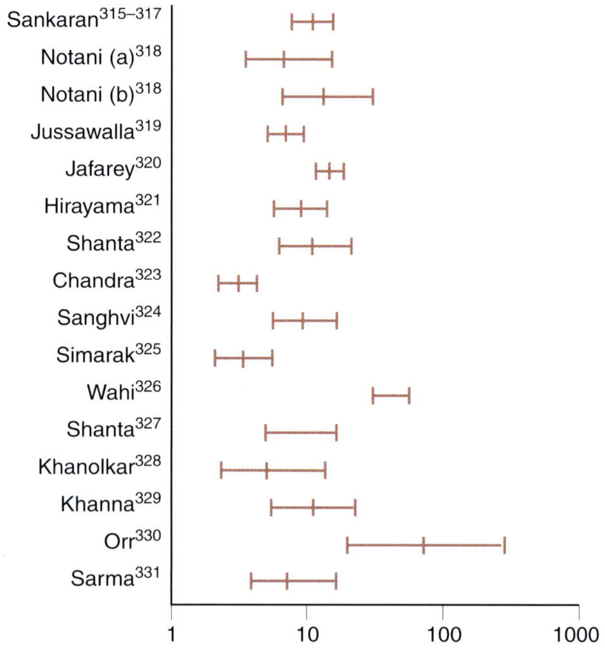

Figure 2.5 Summary of crude odds ratios for the development of oral cancer in populations chewing betel quid in any form, irrespective of smoking habits. (Analysis derived from Thomas and Wilson.[69])

of betel quid, particularly in the cities (reviewed by Reichart[68]); betel quids in Thailand have commonly included tobacco.

Evidence from case-control studies

The carcinogenicity of pan/betel quid mixtures has been clearly established in a meta-analysis of 17 published studies by Thomas and Wilson.[69] These show a range of relative risks (RRs) averaging around 10 (Fig. 2.5). However, as pointed out by Warnakulasuriya,[70] only four studies differentially examine the role of betel quid with and without

Table 2.4 Relative risk (RR) of oral cancer from betel quid with or without tobacco. (Data and cited references from Warnakulasuriya[70])

Reference	Cases/controls	Betel quid with tobacco	Betel quid without tobacco	No chewing habit
Shanta and Krishnamurthi (1959)	Oral cancer	219	33	25
	Controls	35	144	99
	RR	24.8	0.9	1
Chandra (1963)	Oral cancer	138	46	135
	Controls	61	70	256
	RR	4.34*	1.24	1
Hirayama (1966)	Oral cancer	190	35	9
	Controls	215	16	102
	RR	9.1*	1.2	1
Jafarey and Zaidi (1976)	Oral cancer	339	40	88
	Controls	474	216	1690
	RR	13.7*	3.6*	1

*$p < 0.01$

Table 2.5 Effect of cessation of tobacco habits on incidence of lesions in a 10-year follow-up of 12 212 users. (From Gupta et al.[73,315–331])

	Stopped		All others		Incidence ratio
	Incident cases	Incidence/100 000*	Incident cases	Incidence/100 000*	
Leukoplakia					
Men	7	92	183	219	0.42
Women	5	63	54	201	0.31
Lichen planus					
Men	7	107	111	143	0.75
Women	19	396	93	294	1.35

*Age adjusted.

tobacco, and with and without smoking, in cases of oral cancer in South Asian populations (Table 2.4). It is clear that tobacco is the major carcinogen, possibly partly because its presence adds to the compulsion to chew more frequently.

Evidence from prospective studies

Gupta et al.[71] followed up 30 000 individuals over a 10-year period in three areas of India. In Ernakulum the annual age-adjusted incidence of oral cancer was 23/100 000 among betel quid–tobacco chewers compared with zero in smokers and non-habitués: this is the most extensive study of its kind reported.

Evidence from intervention studies

Intensive health education programmes among 36 000 betel quid/tobacco chewers and smokers in India showed a significant regression in precancerous lesions.[72] More significantly, a 10-year follow up of 12 212 users, producing 77 681 person-years of observation in men and 32 544 among women, successfully achieved habit cessation in 6.5% of the men and 14.4% of the women. There was a substantial drop in the incidence of leukoplakia after cessation (incidence ratio 0.31), but not for lichen planus or for several other lesions. As leukoplakia is a potentially malignant lesion in this population, this implies a reduced risk of oral cancer (Table 2.5).[73]

Dose–response relationship
This type of evidence is usually regarded as powerful; unfortunately, few studies exist. However, a dose–response relationship was shown in the classical pioneering studies by Orr in 1933[74] and by Hirayama:[66] the latter showed an RR for oral cancer of 8.4 when the number of quids chewed per day was less than two, rising to 17.6 when the frequency was six times or more per day; individuals who slept with the quid in the mouth had a relative risk of 63.

Areca nut alone as an oral carcinogen

Although the International Agency for Research on Cancer (IARC) concluded in their 1985 publication that 'there was insufficient evidence that the chewing of betel quid without tobacco was carcinogenic to man',[75] we now have to admit this as a probability. Areca nut is certainly the main aetiological agent in oral submucous fibrosis,[76] but in this case-control study 12 of the 14 patients with concurrent oral cancer and submucous fibrosis also used tobacco. Certainly, as seen above from studies in the Indian subcontinent, adding tobacco to betel quids increases their risk. Evidence from elsewhere in the world (e.g. South Africa) is conflicting but now shows that betel quids without tobacco are associated with oral cancer.

In Guam, where areca nut is chewed either alone or with betel leaf only, there is apparently no increase in oral cancer.[77] Conversely, in Taiwan, most heavy chewers of betel quids do not include tobacco, and yet oral cancer is clearly associated with the habit.[78] The risk of malignant transformation of leukoplakia has an OR of 17 (1.94–156.27) for betel nut chewing in Taiwan.[79] In PNG, as already referred to, the predominant chewing habit involves betel vine inflorescence and areca nut, with large quantities of lime applied to the mucosa, but without the addition of tobacco: nevertheless, concurrent cigar smoking is common.[80] Furthermore, the synergistic role of alcohol has not been evaluated in these studies.[81,82] The presence of increased numbers of micronucleated epithelial cells, as a putative intermediate marker of oral cancer risk, has been reported in users of areca nut without tobacco in the Philippines,[83] and in India,[84] in which study chromosomal aberrations and sister chromatid exchanges in phytohaemagglutinin-stimulated peripheral blood lymphocytes were found to be progressively increased in areca nut chewers without disease, through chewers with oral submucous fibrosis, to chewers with oral carcinoma.

Strong evidence that the chewing of areca alone produces oral cancer comes from South Africa: in a study of 143 cases of oral cancer among the Indian immigrant community of the Eastern Cape, 39 of 57 with cheek cancer and 21 of 25 with tongue cancer were nut chewers who did not use tobacco in any form.[85] Finally, a small but well-designed case-control (n = 40:160) study in Taiwan clearly showed a strong carcinogenic effect of the local quids with an OR of 58.4 after adjusting for cigarette smoking and alcohol drinking. Importantly, this showed a strong dose–response relationship, adjusted ORs rising to 275.6 when more than 20 quids were consumed per day, and to 397.5 with more than 40 years of chewing; nevertheless, 18/40 patients drank alcohol and the majority, 32/40, also smoked, so that multiple risk factors are clearly operating in this community.[86] The independent role of areca is confirmed in Pakistan,[87] and reviewed by Trivedy et al.[88]

Animal experiments also support a role: areca nut fibre and cold aqueous extracts of Taiwan betel quids promoted dimethylbenzanthracene (DMBA)-initiated hamster cheek pouch carcinogenesis, in the absence of tobacco products:[89] betel quid alone produced only hyperkeratosis and acanthosis.[90] A number of earlier studies in baboons, monkeys, rats and hamsters are reviewed by Warnakulasuriya.[70] Most of these failed to produce frank neoplasms in the absence of a known artificial/experimental initiator or complete chemical carcinogen. Direct DNA damage has, however, been shown to occur when areca nut extracts are added to human buccal epithelial cells in vitro,[91] and the tannins have been shown to enhance mucosal permeability.[92] The major nitroso compounds formed from areca nut alkaloids are 3-(methylnitrosamino)propionitrile (MNPN), 3-(methylnitrosamino)propionaldehyde (MNPA), *N*-nitrosoguvacoline (NG) and *N*-nitrosoguvacine (NGV), and of these MNPA appears to be the most powerful carcinogen.[93] Jeng et al review the subject comprehensively.[94]

In evaluating the dangers of these complex mixtures it is important to remember that betel leaf itself has been shown to have a protective effect[95] and at least two protective compounds have been identified—β-carotene and hydroxychavicol (an astringent antiseptic). In Taiwan, apparently, over 90% of chewers do not consume rolled betel leaf.[86]

Snuff in Scandinavia and North America

Relevant observations go back decades in the USA. Brown et al.[96] described 'snuff-dipper's cancer' in the southeastern states where the habit of placing snuff in the lower labial sulcus was common: indeed, this was the basis of the classical description of verrucous carcinoma by Ackermann as long ago as 1948[97] and confirmed by McCoy and Waldron much later.[98] Women in the textile industry in this part of the United States have a high prevalence of snuff dipping and elevated death rates from oral

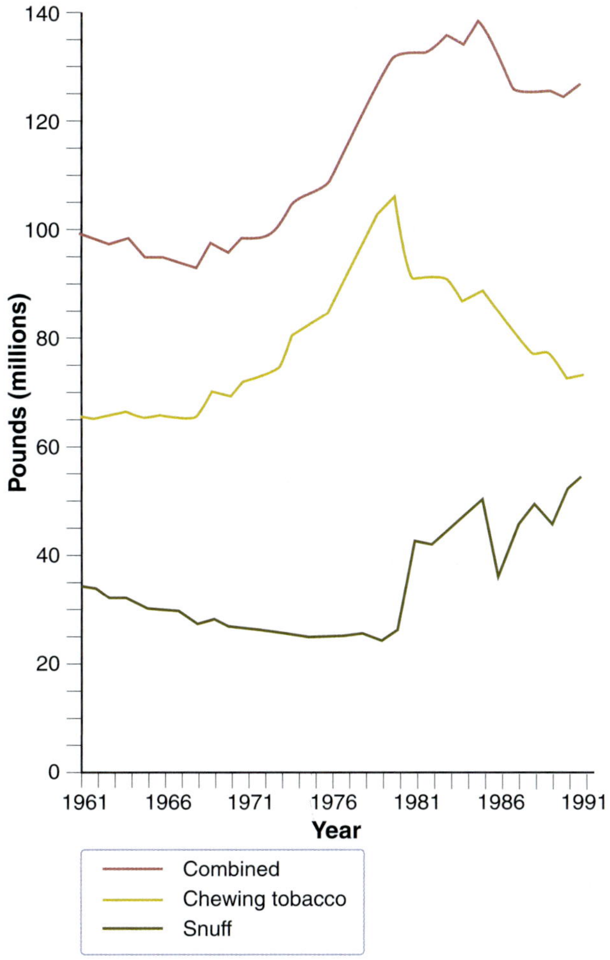

Figure 2.6 Annual consumption of 'spitting' tobacco in the USA, 1961–91.[50]

cancer.[99,100] There is thus evidence that this form of oral smokeless tobacco can be topically carcinogenic.

Concern has been expressed more recently at a growing use of factory-produced portion-packed snuff (Fig. 2.6), and the oral cancers it might cause, particularly among adolescents in the USA.[101] Chewing tobacco and packaged snuff habits are practised by a proportion of prominent sportsmen, particularly baseball players, many of whom are regarded as role models by the young, and there are fears that this habit may be emulated.[102] In 1986 the Surgeon-General of the USA produced a report,[103] which concluded that there was a significant risk to health from oral cancer and other oral lesions, and that it could lead to nicotine addiction and dependence. Congress passed an Act in 1986 which banned the advertising of smokeless tobacco on radio and television and required health warnings on packages and printed advertisements. After some interesting machinations with the law and its interpretation in several European countries, from 1985 onwards, the European Union (EU) banned the sale of portion snuff and loose moist snuff in all of its member states in 1992; when Sweden joined the EU in 1985 it was exempted from the ban on sales, but exports were banned.[104] In the same year the IARC stated that there was sufficient evidence that snuff causes cancer[75] and the Swedish Government required warning labels to be placed on such products.

Table 2.6 Relative risk (RR) and confidence interval (CI) for oral cancer; ICD 9; 140–149; multiplicative model. (From Sterling et al.[107])

	RR	CI
Sex		
Male	1.00	
Female	0.52	0.27–1.00
Race		
White	1.00	
Non-white	2.63	1.31–5.27
Age (years)		
25–44	1.00	
45–64	47.22	6.07–367.19
65–84	84.88	10.71–666.38
85+	206.03	20.00–2122.83
Lifetime smoking (packs)		
0–19 (never)	1.00	
20–11 999	1.07	0.48–2.38
12 000 +	2.85	1.41–5.77
Annual drinking		
0–52 (1 drink/week)	1.00	
53–365 (1 drink/day)	2.75	1.26–5.99
366 +	7.20	3.74–13.88
Occupation		
Professional/managerial/ clerical	1.00	
Blue collar/service/technical	1.06	0.62–1.83
Smokeless tobacco		
0–99 (non-user)	1.00	
100–9999 times	0.92	0.25–3.42
10 000 +	1.21	0.32–4.63

However, the subject remains controversial. Although this habit can produce hyperkeratotic lesions in the area of habitual contact,[105] and there is a notable prevalence even in teenagers in the USA, where 2.9% of males and 0.1% of females from a survey of 17 027 schoolchildren aged 12–17 had lesions associated in a dose-dependent fashion with snuff (particularly) and chewing tobacco,[106] there is as yet limited evidence that malignancies follow; however, judgment must be reserved because there may be a long latent period. Nevertheless, the present evidence does not support the contention that this is a high-risk activity. A study based on combined data of the 1986 US National Mortality Followback Survey (n = 16 598) and the coincident National Health Interview Survey (of 1987), with correction for possible confounders, concluded that the use of smokeless tobacco, either as snuff or chewing tobacco, does not increase the risk of oral cancer or of cancer of the digestive organs. The number of users was, however, small. Alcohol emerged as a major risk factor for oral cancer, with a strong dose–response relationship, as it did to a lesser extent with other digestive cancers. Smoking was associated with risk of oral but not other digestive cancers (Table 2.6).[107] This view of the low cancer risk of smokeless tobacco in the USA has even led to a movement to advocate this practice as a less dangerous alternative to smoking and as an aid to nicotine withdrawal in those addicted to smoking—a suggestion that is highly controversial at present because there are undoubtedly safer forms of nicotine replacement and the cardiovascular effects have not been fully evaluated.[108]

It is clear that the nature of the product varies considerably. Chewing tobaccos differ distinctly from snuff, and snuff as manufactured and used in Europe and North America differs greatly from snuff-like products used in the Middle East, which are made locally in a variety of small-scale industries, by individual vendors, or directly by the users. Products such as toombak, used in the Sudan,[109] and the Shammah of Arabia have, as explained above, exceptionally high tobacco-specific nitrosamine (TSN) contents and are likely to be responsible for the high incidence of oral cancer in those countries.[110] There is, however, a paradox in that the characteristic hyperkeratotic lesions of toombak users show a low prevalence of epithelial dysplasia,[59] as do those described in the USA and Scandinavia. We have opined that, in the case of the Sudan, this might be because those users most susceptible to cancer have already succumbed to their malignancies and do not appear in population studies such as that described here.

In Scandinavia it is now becoming clear that local snuff is not a major risk factor for oral cancer. Two recent case-control studies of oral cancer cases in Sweden have failed to show an association (Table 2.7).[111,112]

Table 2.7 Oral cancer in Swedish snuff users

Reference	No. of pairs	Relative risk	95% Confidence interval
Schildt et al.[84]			
Current users	410	0.6	0.3–1.1
Previous users		1.4	0.7–2.8
Lewin et al.[85]			
Current users	128	1.0	0.7–1.6
Previous users		1.2	0.6–1.9

It is thus a very real argument as to whether snuff might be used to help smokers quit. This approach has been roundly condemned by the anti-tobacco movement in the USA, on the grounds that it, itself, can lead to nicotine addiction, that it ignores the potential role of snuff in other cancers and in cardiovascular diseases, and that other ethically accepted forms of nicotine replacement therapy (such as chewing gums, skin patches and nasal sprays) are widely available. These are real concerns, which require establishment in well-designed studies. It is, therefore, of interest to note two comparatively recent Swedish studies. A case-control study of 585 cases with 10% snuff users and 589 controls with 15% snuff users showed an RR for myocardial infarction of 0.89 (95% CI 0.62–1.29) in snuff users, compared with 1.87 (95% CI 1.40–2.48) in smokers.[113] Another study from health screening of 135 036 construction workers identified 6297 snuff users. The RR for death due to cardiovascular disease was 1.4 (1.2–1.6) for this group, compared with 1.9 (1.7–2.2) for smokers.[114] In addition, no increased risk among snuff users who had never smoked was found among men with the inflammatory bowel diseases, Crohn's disease and ulcerative colitis, in a case-control study.[115] The possibility of increased risk of cancer at other sites has not yet been fully addressed. Nevertheless, on present evidence, it appears that snuff habits as they exist in Scandinavia and, probably, in the USA carry low risks of serious health hazards, including oral cancer. As Axell points out, however, this does not mean that oral snuff use should be encouraged.[116] Absence of evidence of risk does not mean evidence of absence of risk: snuff almost always produces mucosal lesions, and often affects salivary flow and causes gingival recessions.[117] We need to continue to work towards a tobacco-free society.

Smoking and oral cancer

There is overwhelming evidence that active smoking, and growing evidence that passive

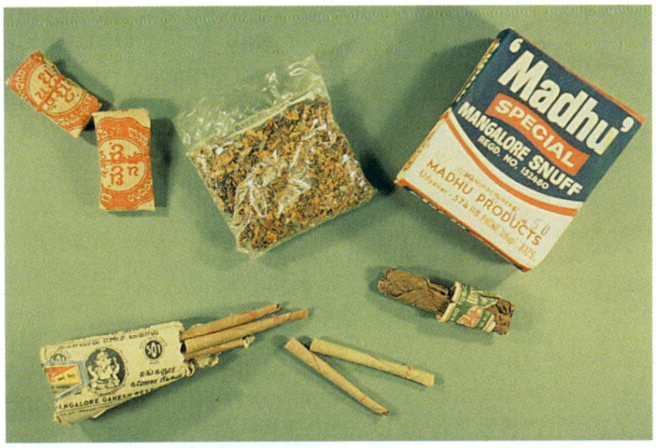

Figure 2.7 Some smoking and smokeless tobacco products common in the Indian subcontinent: packeted snuff, cigars, cut tobacco rolling or pipe, and beedis—cheap tobacco wrapped in a temburni leaf and tied with a cotton thread.

Table 2.8 Cancer deaths due to smoking in the USA, 1985 (US Surgeon-General's report)

Site	% Attributable deaths		Number of deaths pa
	Men	Women	
Lung	90	79	106 000
Lip, oral cavity, pharynx	92	61	7000
Oesophagus	78	75	7000
Bladder	47	37	4000
Kidney	48	12	3000
Larynx	81	87	3000

smoking, are both important in bronchogenic carcinoma. The evidence for active smoking is strong for oral cancer, but other factors are clearly involved, and sorting out their relative contributions remains difficult in spite of continuing research. Discussion in this section relates mostly to studies in the West, avoiding the complications of mixed smoking—often with unusual forms of local tobacco (Fig. 2.7)—and chewing habits discussed above, predominantly in developing countries. These scenarios are helpfully treated separately by Daftary et al.[118] and Binnie.[119] The most comprehensive source of evidence remains the IARC publication of 1986.[120] This evidence is also summarized by the US Surgeon-General's Report of 1989 which lists attributable risk (AR) for cancer at various sites (Table 2.8): the upper aerodigestive sites with which we are here concerned have the highest ARs, in males, of all the many sites for which smoking has been identified as playing a role.

Table 2.9 Alcohol and tobacco habits of 690 consecutive cases of oral cancer in Amsterdam, 1971–91 (Source: Javonovich et al.[127])

Tobacco and alcohol	56%
Tobacco only	14%
Alcohol only	5%
Neither	25%

There is confusion in the literature as to the relative importance of different types of smoking. This partly arises because the lip has not always been separated from intra-oral sites. Ultraviolet light is clearly important for the lip, but not for the mouth. Pipe smoking has long been associated with lip cancer, where consideration has to be given to the nature of the stem and its permeability, and to heat as cofactors. Most of the literature goes back several decades, perhaps because of the decreased popularity of pipe smoking in recent times in the West.[121–124] Some literature suggests that pipe and cigars are less risky for oral cancer than cigarettes,[125] but the very extensive study from North Italy shows higher risks associated with these practices for cancer of the mouth and oesophagus than with cigarettes. Beedi (bidi) smoking, as practised in the Indian sub-continent, is more hazardous than cigarette smoking.[126]

A major difficulty in accurately quantifying smoking risks for oral cancer is the strong synergism of tobacco with alcohol. The importance of tobacco can be inferred from the habits associated with patients with oral cancer in a series of cases from Amsterdam.[127] This series is valuable because it contains a high proportion of cases without either of these major risk factors (Table 2.9). The relative risk for heavy smoking (more than 20 cigarettes per day), adjusted for the effects of alcohol, is highest for the retromolar area, followed by floor of mouth, lower lip, lower alveolus, tongue and lowest for the cheek. For heavy alcohol drinking (more than 4 units per day), adjusted for smoking, the risk is again highest for floor of mouth followed by retromolar area, lower alveolus, tongue, lower lip and again lowest for cheek. The differential by anatomical site is larger for smoking.

A large case-control study from the USA provides good evidence of a dose–response relationship for both tobacco and alcohol[128] (Table 2.10). This is well depicted by the histogram shown in Fig. 2.8.[129]

The relationship between anatomical site of oral cancer and smoking is less clear-cut than with

Table 2.10 Odds ratios for oral and pharyngeal cancer in US males, adjusted for race, age, study location and respondent status. (Source: Blot et al.[128])

Smoking rate	Number of alcoholic drinks per week					
	< 1	1–4	5–14	15–29	30+	Total
Non-smoker	1.0	1.3	1.6	1.4	5.8	1.0
Short duration/former smoker	0.7	2.2	1.4	3.2	6.4	1.1 (0.7–1.7)
1–19/day for 20+ years	1.7	1.5	2.7	5.4	7.9	1.6 (0.9–2.7)
20–39/day for 20+ years	1.9	2.4	4.4	7.2	23.8	2.8 (1.8–4.3)
40+/day for 20+ years	7.4	0.7	4.4	20.2	37.7	4.4 (2.7–7.2)
Pipe and cigar only	0.6	1.0	3.7	4.7	23.0	1.9 (1.1–3.4)
Total	1.0	1.2 (0.7–2.0)	1.7 (1.0–2.7)	3.3 (2.0–5.4)	8.8 (5.4–14.1)	

Ranges are 95% confidence intervals.

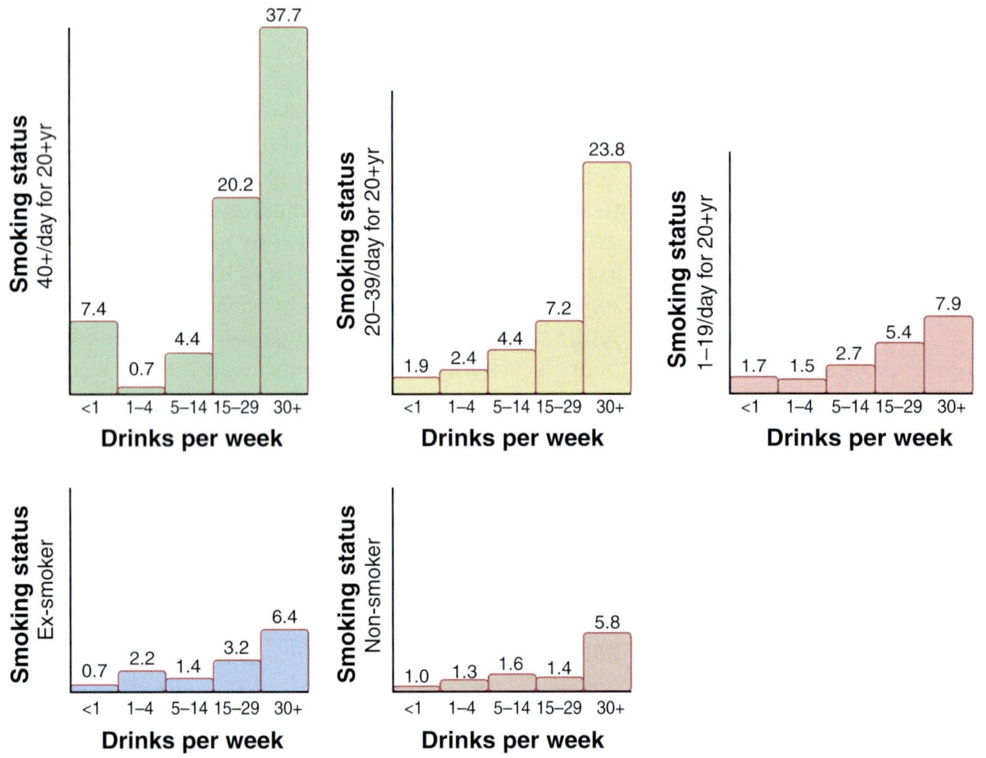

Figure 2.8 Relative risks of oral and pharyngeal cancer in the USA in relation to alcohol and tobacco consumption. (From the Cancer Research Campaign Factsheet 14.14, 1993; after Blot.[129])

smokeless tobacco. It has long been stated that the pooling of carcinogens in saliva gives rise to cancers in the 'gutter' area and thus affects the floor of mouth and the ventral and lateral tongue. Mashberg and Meyers[130] reported in a US population in 1976 that 201 of 207 (97%) asymptomatic, primarily erythroplastic carcinomas were in three locations: floor of mouth, ventral or lateral tongue, and soft palate complex. In the Amsterdam series[127] the floor of mouth and retromolar area were significantly more related to tobacco use than were cancers of the tongue and cheek. However, in another series of 359 cases among male US Veterans, smoking was more strongly associated with soft palate cancers than anterior sites, and alcohol was associated with floor of mouth and tongue lesions.[131] This is interesting because the long-recognized lesions of stomatitis nicotina (syn. smoker's palate) have a low malignant potential (except in reverse smokers; see below). These lesions predominantly affect the hard palate, producing hyperkeratosis without significant epithelial dysplasia, with plugging of the orifices of minor salivary glands and associated congestion and inflammation. Stomatitis nicotina,

Table 2.11 A list of confirmed carcinogens in tobacco smoke. (Source: Davidson et al.[138])

Class	Compound
Aromatic hydrocarbons	
Monocyclic	Benzene
Dicyclic and polycyclic	Benzo(a)anthracene
	Benzo(b)fluoranthene
	Benzo(j)fluoranthene
	Benzo(k)fluoranthene
	Benzo(a)pyrene
	Dibenzo(a,h)anthracene
	Dibenzo(a,e)pyrene
	Dibenzo(a,h)pyrene
	Dibenzo(a,l)pyrene
	Dibenzo(a,l)pyrene
	Ideno(1,2,3-c,d)pyrene
	5-methylchrysene
Aldehydes	Acetaldehyde
	Formaldehyde
Nitrogen compounds	
N-nitroso compounds	4-(methylnitrosamino)-1-(3-pyridyl)-1-butanone (NNK)
	N'-nitrosodimethylamine (NDMA)
	N-nitrodiethylamine
	N-nitroso-*N*-methylethylamine (NEMA)
	N-nitrosonornicotine (NNN)
	N-nitrosopyrrolidine (NPYR)
	N-nitrosopiperidine
	N-nitroso-*n*-butylamine
	N-nitrosodi-*n*-propylamine
Polycyclic aza-arenes	Dibenzo(a,h)acridine
	Dibenzo(a,j)acridine
Miscellaneous nitrogen compounds	4-aminobiphenyl ortho-anisidine
	1,1-dimethylhydrazine
	2-naphthylamine
	2-nitropropane
	Urethane

in the West, is most commonly associated with pipe smoking and both hard and soft palate are relatively uncommon sites of oral cancer.

Reverse smoking, with the lighted end inside the mouth, particularly among females, has been reported for many years from various parts of the world, and a variety of hyperkeratotic and inflammatory changes have been described (see Fig. 1.18K). A high frequency of dysplastic, potentially malignant, lesions and of squamous cell carcinoma (SCC) has been reported among reverse chutta smokers in India along the coastal districts of Visakhapatnam and Srikakulam[132] and in rural Andhra Pradesh.[52,133] Elsewhere in India, in the state of Goa,[134] and in the Caribbean Islands,[135] South America[136] and the Philippines,[137] cancer is not commonly reported.

The mechanisms of tobacco carcinogenesis

There is a vast literature, full coverage of which is outside the scope of this chapter. Over 300 carcinogens have been identified in tobacco smoke or in its water-soluble components which can be expected to leach into saliva.[120] A list of the confirmed carcinogens in tobacco smoke is given in Table 2.11.[138] The major, and most studied of these are the aromatic hydrocarbon benzo(a)pyrene and the tobacco-specific nitrosamines (TSNs), *N*′-nitrosonornicotine (NNN), *N*′-nitrosopyrrolidine (NPYR), *N*′-nitrosodimethylamine (NDMA) and 4–(methylnitrosamino)-1-(3-pyridyl)-1-butanone (NNK).

It has been known since the 1920s that polycyclic aromatic hydrocarbons (PAHs) were the carcinogenic agents present in tars, and this lies behind the tobacco industry's promotion of 'low tar' smoking materials, while continuing to promote 'full strength' brands. Benzo(a)pyrene is a powerful carcinogen and is found in amounts of 20–40 ng per cigarette.[139] The role of *N*-nitrosamines is reviewed by Hoffman and Hecht.[140] The mainstream smoke of a cigarette can contain 310 ng of NNN and 150 ng of NNK.[141] In smoking materials these are generated primarily during pyrolysis, but are also produced endogenously from some forms of smokeless tobacco, quite high levels (a range of 20–890 mg/kg being reported by the IARC) being reached in saliva from, as we have seen, Sudanese toombak, for example.[109] These agents act locally, on keratinocyte stem cells, and are absorbed and act in many other tissues in the body. They produce DNA adducts, principally *O*-6-methylguanine, and these interfere with the accuracy of DNA replication, leading to mutations, which thus contribute to the molecular chain of events leading to malignant transformation of a cell and its clonal derivatives. There is damage to all replicating cells, including those of the immune response (indeed, DNA adducts, or chromosomal instability, resulting from tobacco are most often studied in lymphocytes from peripheral blood).

The metabolism of these carcinogens usually involves oxygenation by p450 enzymes in cytochromes, and then conjugation, in which the enzyme glutathione-*S*-transferase (GST) is involved. Polymorphisms of the p450 and GST genes are currently under active study in the search for genetic markers of susceptibility to head and neck cancer, and indeed to tobacco-related cancers at many other body sites.[142,143] Not all results are consistent, however.[144,145] (See also discussion page 34.)

Marijuana use and head and neck cancer

Although illegal in most countries, recreational use of various extracts of the plant *Cannabis sativa* is widespread. It may be smoked in three ways: as marijuana, which is derived from macerated flowers of the plant mixed with tobacco in a cigarette (under which circumstances the concentration of the active intoxicant, Δ9-tetrahydrocannabinol (THC), is of the order of 1–6% w/v); as hashish, which is dried resin, placed in a pipe (THC 6–10% w/v); or as hash oil (THC 30–60%), which is derived from flowers of the female plant. When burned, the cannabinoids are aromatized and absorbed and a wide range of potential carcinogens is released, including PAHs, benzo(a)pyrene, phenols, phytosterols, acids and terpenes, including nitrosamines at similar levels to those found in tobacco smoke.[146] There are, of course, the products of the tobacco itself.

There are a number of case reports in the English literature of aerodigestive tract cancer in marijuana users and these have been reviewed by Firth.[147] There is also a series of 34 patients aged 20–40 treated in California and reported in the German literature.[148] Firth himself describes oral cancer in 10/70 patients under the age of 45 years in Melbourne. Six of these ten had smoked marijuana at some time, but this is similar to the proportion of users reported in the young Australian population. Although the majority of these cases have been in young patients, adequate details of tobacco and alcohol use are often missing, although some patients, such as the two with tongue cancers described by Caplan and Brigham in 1990, denied use of the latter two risk factors.[149] A study of 173 cases and 176 cancer-free controls at Memorial Sloan–Kettering Cancer Centre in the early 1990s[150] showed ORs for marijuana use, controlling for age, sex, race, education, alcohol and cigarette consumption of 2.6 (1.1–6.6) compared with never users. This rose to OR 3.1 (1.0–9.7) in those aged 55 and under. There was a significant dose–response relationship. Recreational users of marijuana often also enjoy alcohol and tobacco, and tobacco usually forms part of the marijuana smoking mix. It is thus impossible at present to discern an independent risk for the smoking of cannabis products themselves; however, because of their composition, a theoretical risk certainly exists.

Little evidence exists on the risk of marijuana smoking for the development of potentially malignant oral lesions although (as with more conventional tobacco smokers) leukoedema, nicotinic stomatitis, denture-related stomatitis, angular cheilitis and median rhomboid glossitis are more common.[151]

Alcohol and oral cancer

Pure ethanol has never been shown to be carcinogenic in vitro or in animal studies.[152,153] It is presumed to act in concert with other, more direct, carcinogens which may be present in the beverage—so-called congeners—and with other environmental carcinogens, most notably those derived from tobacco. As already discussed, most heavy alcohol consumers also use tobacco so that, from epidemiological data, it is difficult to separate the effects. Nevertheless, some cohort and case-control studies

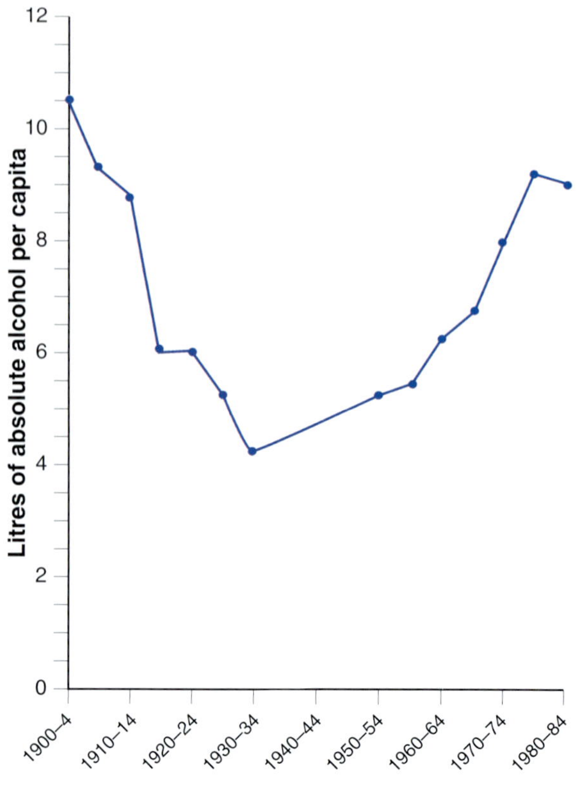

Figure 2.9 Total alcohol consumption in England and Wales, 1900–84; litres of absolute alcohol per capita. (Source: HM Customs and Excise.)

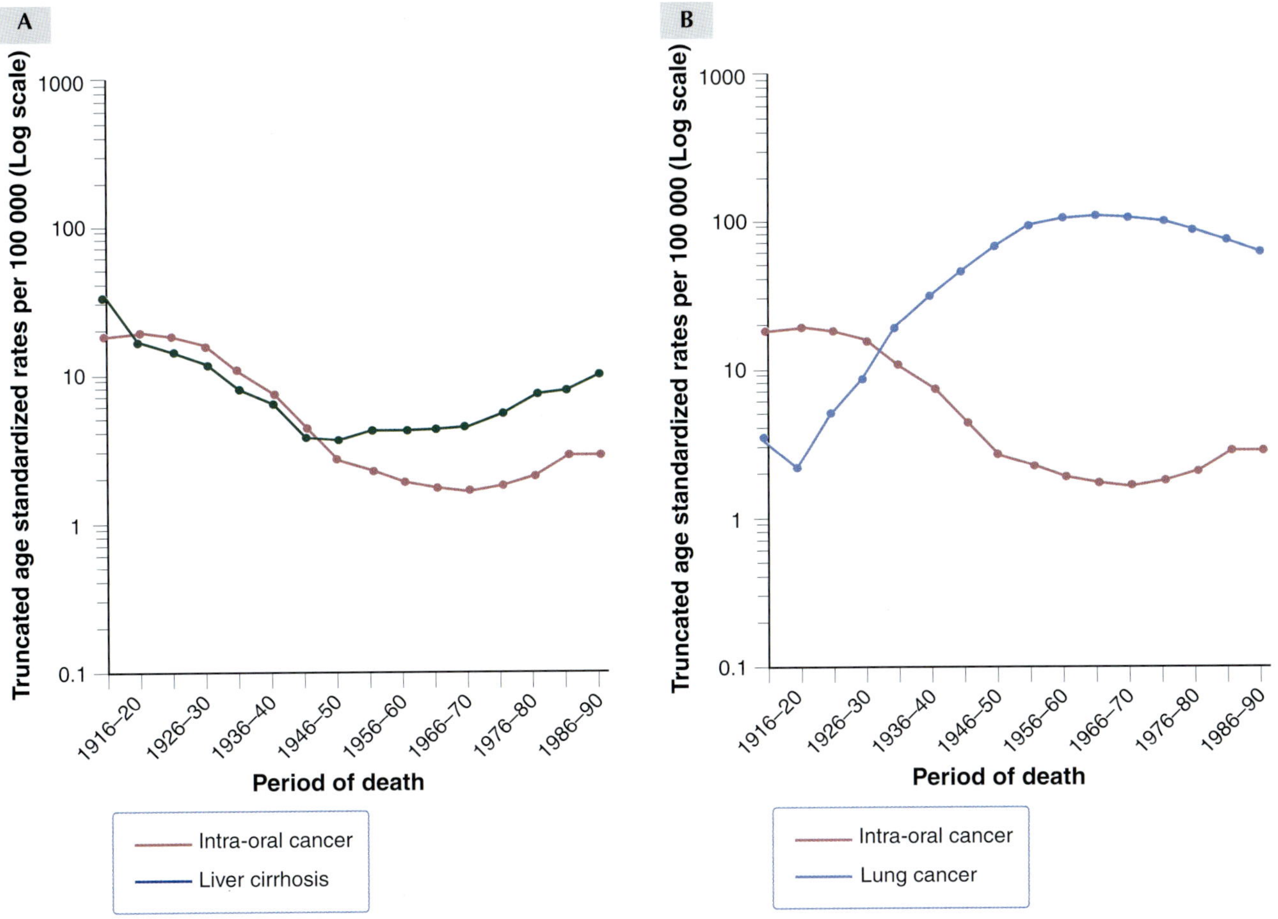

Figure 2.10 A: Trends in the mortality of intra-oral cancer in England and Wales, compared to trends in mortality from liver cirrhosis, 1911–90, for males aged 35–64.[158] B: Trends in the mortality of intra-oral cancer in England and Wales compared to lung cancer mortality, 1911–90, for males aged 35–64.[158]

have found an increased risk of upper aerodigestive tract cancer associated with alcohol drinking in nonsmokers.[154]

The interaction of alcohol use with smokeless tobacco is practically unknown. This is because in most countries where tobacco or pan are used in this way there are either religious or social inhibitions: indeed, in some the use of alcohol is banned by law. This does not mean that alcohol is not consumed, however. Where it is used, it is likely to be produced illicitly, and may as a result contain impurities which add to the risk. In many parts of the Indian subcontinent, for example, local brews distilled from palm juice, 'toddy', are widely available, particularly in rural areas where tobacco habitués may be unable to afford factory made (and therefore quality-controlled) beverages, whether they be of national origin or imported. Recent studies in South India demonstrate a clear role for alcohol.[155,156]

The rise in oral cancer incidence in much of the western world, discussed in Chapter 1, has been related to rising alcohol consumption.[157] In England and Wales, alcohol consumption per capita fell from the beginning of the twentieth century to the 1930s, but has more than doubled since then (Fig. 2.9). Using mortality from liver cirrhosis as a surrogate measure of damage to health from alcohol, Hindle[158] has plotted trends over the twentieth century and shown how they match closely the trends in oral cancer mortality (Fig. 2.10A). Taking deaths from lung cancer as a measure of tobacco damage, it is striking how the trends for oral cancer move, both down and up in the twentieth century, in opposite directions (Fig. 2.10B): this is strong circumstantial evidence that alcohol rather than tobacco is the major factor in the observed trends in oral cancer mortality and, by inference, incidence.

Some of the effect is due to the presence of other carcinogens in the local environment. Apart from those derived from tobacco, beverage congeners include nitrosamines and impurities, the latter particularly in illicit local brews. Brown or dark-coloured drinks may be more dangerous in this

Table 2.12 Odds ratios for oral and pharyngeal cancer in males, according to alcohol habits: Northern Italy, 1984–89. (Source: La Vecchia et al.[171])

	Oral cavity (*n* = 157)	Pharynx (*n* = 134)
Wine (drinks/week)		
≤ 20	1	1
21–34	1.1 (0.5–2.3)	0.7 (0.3–1.6)
35–55	1.9 (0.9–3.7)	1.9 (0.9–3.7)
56–83	4.9 (2.6–9.5)	3.1 (1.6–6.1)
84+	8.5 (3.6–20.2)	10.9 (4.7–25.3)
Beer (drinks/week)		
0	1	1
1–13	1.0 (0.6–1.8)	0.5 (0.3–1.0)
14+	0.8 (0.5–1.4)	0.9 (0.5–1.5)
Spirits (drinks/week)		
0	1	1
1–6	0.7 (0.4–1.3)	0.4 (0.2–0.9)
7+	0.9 (0.6–1.3)	1.2 (0.8–1.8)
Total (drinks/week)		
≤ 19	1	1
20–34	1.1 (0.5–2.5)	0.9 (0.4–2.0)
35–59	3.2 (1.6–6.2)	1.5 (0.8–3.1)
60+	3.4 (1.7–7.1)	3.6 (1.8–7.2)

Ranges are 95% confidence intervals.

Table 2.13 Relative risk of developing upper aerodigestive tract cancer by alcohol and tobacco habits: Paris registry 1975–82. (Source: Brugere et al.[172])

	Tobacco (g/day; adjusted for alcohol)			**Alcohol (g/day[a] adjusted for tobacco)**		
	10–19	**20–29**	**> 30**	**40–99**	**100–159**	**> 160**
Oropharynx	4.0	7.6	15.2	2.6	15.2	70.3
Hypopharynx	7.1	12.6	35.1	3.3	28.6	143.1
Supraglottis	6.1	19.6	48.8	2.6	11.0	42.1
Glottis	3.0	9.5	28.4	0.8#	1.5#	6.1
Epilarynx	1.7#	6.7	14.8	1.9#	18.7	101.4
Lips	4.5	9.7	21.5	1.8#	4.9	10.5
Mouth	3.9	8.6	15.4	2.7	13.1	70.3

[a]15 g alcohol ~ 1 unit.
< 9 g tobacco/day and < 40 g alcohol/day taken as RR of 1, respectively
Confidence limits excluded for clarity, but all except # do not cross unity and are thus significant at the 5% level.

respect and it might be useful, if suitable groups could be adequately matched, to compare the risks in consumers of, say, vodka (which is almost pure ethanol) with those who take predominantly whiskys, which have many congeners.[159] The epidemiological evidence shows that all forms of alcoholic drink are dangerous if heavily consumed.[160] the most dangerous reflecting the predominant habit in the population under study. Thus there is evidence for the role of beer,[128,161–164] wine[165–167] and spirits,[128,163,168,169] which some[169] have taken to implicate ethanol itself. A report from Uruguay, comparing 471 cases of oral and pharyngeal cancer with 471 controls, showed slightly higher ORs for 'pure hard liquor' drinking (3.6; 95% CI 2.1–6.2) than for 'pure wine' drinking (2.1; 1.3–3.3).

Table 2.14 Odds ratios for upper aerodigestive cancer in males according to smoking and drinking habits: northern Italy, 1986–89. (Source: Franceschi et al.[46])

Smoking practice	Alcohol intake (drinks/week)			
	< 35	35–69	60+	Total
Oral cavity/pharynx				
Non-smokers	1	1.6	2.3	1
Light	3.1	5.4	10.9	3.7
Intermediate	10.9	26.6	36.4	14.1
Heavy	17.6	40.2	79.6	25.0
Total	1	2.3	3.4	
Larynx				
Non-smokers	1	1.6	–	1
Light	0.9	5.0	5.4	1.0
Intermediate	4.5	7.1	9.5	5.4
Heavy	6.1	10.4	11.7	6.7
Total	1	1.4	2.8	
Oesophagus				
Non-smokers	1	0.8	7.9	1
Light	1.1	7.9	9.4	2.5
Intermediate	2.7	8.8	16.7	4.0
Heavy	6.4	11.0	17.5	6.6
Total	1	3.1	5.7	

Some of the best evidence for the very significant role of alcohol again comes from the studies in Northern Italy, reviewed by La Vecchia[167,170,171] Table 2.12 extracts data from these studies, deriving estimates from logistic regression adjusted for age, area of residence, years of education, occupation and smoking habits. It is notable from these data that the 95% CIs for ORs for all beverages cross unity until the total alcohol consumption per week is really quite high—above 55 drinks per week. This is consistent with the earlier data from Paris[172] (Table 2.13). Note that, in all of these studies, when the tobacco effect is removed, heavy alcohol consumption itself produces considerable risks, with ORs or RRs of 17, 23, 33, and 70 appearing for oral cancer in the different studies. For these high rates of alcohol use/abuse, the risks are greater than for tobacco, adjusted for alcohol, and of course it is the super-multiplicative synergism already described that is really dangerous. It is also worth observing that self-reported alcohol consumption tends to be underestimated,[153] implying that alcohol may be an even more important factor than the published data indicate. Table 2.14, again from the Italian studies,[46] compares upper aerodigestive sites: the tobacco/alcohol synergism appears to be super-multiplicative for the oral cavity and pharynx, between additive and multiplicative for the oesophagus, and close to additive for the larynx which, simplistically, relates to both agents being present in the mouth, alcohol being present in the oesophagus with smaller amounts of tobacco products, and tobacco products contacting the larynx with fewer constituents of the beverage.

There are several ways in which alcohol is thought to contribute to head and neck cancer, by both local and systemic mechanisms. The IARC Monograph deals comprehensively with the evidence up to the late 1980s.[152] The mechanisms are as follows:

- There is now clear evidence that ethanol increases the permeability of oral mucosa to water itself[173,174] and to many water-soluble molecules, probably including important carcinogens: indeed, increased passage of nitrosonornicotine has been demonstrated in in vitro experiments.[175,176] The effect is greater at 15% than at 5%, but is not further enhanced at 40% ethanol, suggesting the mechanism is related to rearrangement of the epithelial permeability barrier rather than to lipid extraction.[177,178] This means that there will be increased uptake of alcohol itself, and of carcinogens, with enhanced systemic effects. It also implies a solvent action of ethanol on keratinocyte membranes with likely enhanced penetration of carcinogens into proliferating cells where they may exert a direct mutagenic action.[179] A dehydrating effect may contribute.[180] Recent animal experiments in which rats were fed ethanol by stomach tube showed an indirect effect on the permeability of the oral mucosa, because there was decreased synthesis of lipids contributing to the intercellular permeability barrier, perhaps because of liver damage.[181]
- The immediate metabolite of ethanol is acetaldehyde. Some of this may be formed locally and damage cells.[182] Indeed considerable amounts of acetaldehyde can be found in saliva after moderate alcohol consumption, owing to the action of bacterial alcohol dehydrogenases.[183] Production is significantly reduced after three days' use of an antiseptic mouthwash (chlorhexidine), perhaps helping to explain why poor oral hygiene appears to be an independent risk factor for oral cancer in some studies.[184–186] Those genetically predisposed to be more rapid acetylators have been demonstrated to be at increased risk in one recent US study.
- Alcoholic liver disease is common in heavy drinkers and this reduces the detoxification of active carcinogens.[154]
- Alcohol is high in calories, which suppresses appetite in heavy drinkers. Those with a serious

drinking problem become socially fractured, and many choose to spend available cash on drink rather than food. All of this contributes to inadequate diet. Metabolism is further damaged by liver disease. As a result nutritional deficiencies are common,[188] and, as discussed below, these contribute significantly to lowered resistance to cancer.[154]

Unsurprisingly, therefore, alcoholic patients are at especial risk for head and neck cancer, particularly at sites in direct contact with alcohol.[189]

Mouthwash use and risk of oral cancer

As long ago as 1979, concern was expressed about the possibility of high alcohol-containing mouthwashes contributing to oral cancer, when 10 of 11 non-smoking, non-drinking patients with oral cancer (nine female, two male) in the USA were found to be long-term mouthwash users.[190] This was quickly followed up in two case-control studies. The first, among women in North Carolina (206 cases of oral or pharyngeal cancer and 352 controls), found no increased risk when adjusted for snuff-dipping and smoking, although the RR increased to 1.94 (0.8–4.7) among women who did not use tobacco: no consistent dose–response relationship was observed.[191] The second study took 571 cases from the six-city study in the US and matched them with 6047 controls without tobacco-related disease. This showed that daily use of mouthwash was associated with increased risk among females only, whether or not they also used alcoholic beverages and/or tobacco, but the risks were small and showed no dose–response relationship. The study confirmed the strong risks associated with alcohol drinking and tobacco use and, because of confounding by these much more potent factors, these authors concluded that no causal association could be inferred for mouthwash use.[191]

Drawing 866 cases from registries in California, Atlanta and New Jersey, and matching with 1249 controls, Winn and colleagues re-examined the issue some years later.[193] They found increased risks associated with the regular use of mouthwash, of 40% for men and 60% for women, after adjusting for alcohol and tobacco use. Risks generally increased in proportion to frequency and duration of mouthwash use, and were only apparent when the alcohol content of the mouthwash exceeded 25%: the effects were again stronger in women, revealing a maximum OR of 2.4 (1.5–3.9) in those who began regular use before the age of 20 years. This publication raised considerable discussion in several countries (e.g. the UK[194]), many clinicians expressing concern because, in the West at least, smokers may be inclined to use these products heavily to disguise the smell of tobacco. However, in most of the published studies, rarely do ORs exceed 2 with, in most cases 95% CIs spanning unity.

The most recent study, again by Winn and colleagues, with 342 cases and 521 controls in Puerto Rico, showed no increased risk of oral cancer associated with use of mouthwashes containing >25% ethanol.[195] Overall the risk has to be regarded as small, and pales into insignificance compared with those due to tobacco use, heavy alcohol drinking and poor diet. Indeed, critical analysis of all the published literature, including several reviews,[196–198] has led the British, Canadian and American Dental Associations (to name just three) to regard the risks, if any, as insignificant and to endorse certain products of this type for control of dental plaque and gingivitis. It seems prudent, however, to keep the alcohol content as low as possible in formulating the product (alcohol is necessary to dissolve some of the active antimicrobial agents) and certainly to state the composition on the label.

Incidentally, the levels of alcohol in proprietary mouthwashes are unlikely to influence legal proceedings based on exhaled air analyses.[199]

Oral cancer in non-users of tobacco (and/or alcohol)

Because of the overwhelming evidence for the role of tobacco and alcohol, there is great interest in that minority of patients who develop oral cancer in the apparent absence of one or both of these risk factors. Clearly, other factors are operating, as they presumably are in the case of young people who develop these cancers with no exposure, or certainly without the decades of exposure usually associated with high-risk individuals. Lifelong abstainers from both of these prevalent social customs are, in numerical terms, unusual people, and little is known about their wider lifestyle: for example, do they have unusual dietary practices? In addition, we may suspect hereditary, and other environmental factors (including viruses, see below). Thus, we have no understanding of the aetiology, but differences have been described in the natural history of the disease in these cohorts. Rich and Radden[200] found that Australian patients who had never used tobacco or alcohol developed their carcinomas particularly on the buccal mucosa and upper alveolar ridge, and the Amsterdam data[127] were consistent with this. Hodge and colleagues, in a Kentucky population, described 33 of 945 cases (3.4%) of head and neck cancers in non-users of

Table 2.15 Viruses clearly related to human cancers

Virus	Associated neoplasm
DNA viruses	
Epstein–Barr	Burkitt's lymphoma Nasopharyngeal carcinoma Lymphomas in the immunosuppressed
Human herpes virus 8 (KSHV)	Kaposi's sarcoma
Hepatitis B	Hepatocellular carcinoma
Papilloma viruses	Benign papillomas and warts Anogenital (including cervical) cancer Head and neck cancers
RNA viruses	
Human T-cell leukaemia virus (HTLV-1)	Adult T-cell leukaemia
HTLV-2	Hairy cell leukaemia
HTLV-3	Cutaneous T-cell leukaemia

Table 2.16 Proliferative mucosal lesions of the head and neck associated with viruses (as far as possible the order in which the types are listed implies frequency of isolation)

Normal mucosa	HPV-33, 18, 6, 2; EBV; HSV; CMV and many others
Papilloma	HPV-6, 11, 16
Verruca vulgaris	HPV-2, 4, 6, 11
Condyloma acuminatum	HPV-6, 11, 13, 32
Focal epithelial hyperplasia (Heck's disease)	HPV-13 (1, 32, 6, 11)
Keratoacanthoma	?HPV-37
Leukoplakia	HPV-11, 16
Proliferative verrucous carcinoma	HPV-16
Koilocytic dysplasia	HPV-31, 33, 35; 16, 18; 6, 11
Squamous cell carcinoma	HPV-16, 18, 6, 2, 57; ?EBV, ?HSV; ?HHV-6.
Carcinoma of the uterine cervix	HPV-31, 33, 35

Note that for HPVs, currently the most studied family, types 6, 11, 13 and 32 are regarded as 'low risk' and types 16, 18, 31, 33, 35, and 39 as 'high risk'.

tobacco.[201] The non-users of both tobacco *and* alcohol were a definite majority of women, especially older women, and had comparatively few cancers of the floor of the mouth. Other findings in non-user American cohorts are as follows:[202]

- A low incidence of second primaries;
- A higher level of differentiation of the primary lesions;
- A lower frequency of associated oral candidiasis;
- Importantly—*no better overall survival.*

Tan and colleagues have presented a retrospective study of 59 tobacco non-users with squamous cell carcinomas of the head and neck and found that, as with the above studies, significantly more women were involved.[203] Interestingly, this group comprised significantly more patients with tongue cancers and a relatively *high* rate of second primaries in the head and neck. Most importantly, this group had a high exposure to ETS (passive smoking).

None of these studies on the rare cases that occur in non-users of tobacco and/or alcohol dilute the evidence that these substances are far and away the major risk factors. Viral infections and nutritional inadequacies, which are addressed next, are the main hypothetical factors in this group of patients. Much more research is needed in this intriguing area.

Viruses and oral cancer

Understanding of the role of viruses in human carcinogenesis has expanded enormously in the past two or three decades. Although, earlier, there was evidence for viruses being important in the aetiology of malignant disease in animals and in animal model systems (e.g. the Rous sarcoma virus in chickens, the mouse leukaemia viruses), direct evidence for an important role in human cancer was slow to emerge and the molecular mechanisms are only now being elucidated. We now know that viruses contribute to the multistep process of carcinogenesis in many human neoplasms, perhaps to different degrees in different types of cancer or, at least, with different weights of evidence implicating these infectious agents.

Table 2.15 lists those viruses thought to be involved in human cancers. It is now thought that about 15% of all human cancers may have an aetiological relationship to viruses.[204,205] This relationship is, however, difficult to establish because there may be a latent period of one or more decades between the time of initial infection and the appearance of the malignant lesion[206] and because the fingerprint of

Table 2.17 A classification of some viruses important in human disease

Family	Disease
DNA viruses	
Herpesviridae	
(These are icosahedral enveloped particles, ~130 nm in diameter, containing double-stranded linear DNA)	
Human herpes virus 1 (HHV-1) (Herpes simplex virus 1) (HSV-1)	Acute herpetic gingivostomatitis, recurrent herpes labialis
Human herpes virus 2 (HHV-2) (Herpes simplex virus 2) (HSV-2)	Genital herpes, occasionally oral
Human herpes virus 3 (HHV-3) (Varicella zoster virus) (VSV)	Chickenpox, herpes zoster (shingles)
Human herpes virus 4 (HHV-4) (Epstein–Barr Virus) (EBV)	Infectious mononucleosis, nasopharyngeal carcinoma, lymphomas
Human herpes virus 5 (HHV-5) (Cytomegalovirus) (CMV)	Widespread infections of many viscera, including mucosae; severe in the immunocompromised
Human herpes virus 6 (HHV-6)	Not fully determined: febrile illnesses; ?lymphomas in the immunosuppressed
Human herpes virus 7 (HHV-7)	Not fully determined
Human herpes virus 8 (HHV-8) (Kaposi sarcoma herpes virus) (KSHV)	Kaposi's sarcoma, ? primary infusion lymphomas
Poxviridae	
(Brick-shaped enveloped particles, 300 × 240 × 100 nm, also containing double-stranded linear DNA)	
Vaccinia virus	Molluscum contagiosum
Variola virus	Smallpox
Orf	
Parvoviridae	Rashes in children
(Icosahedral enveloped particles, 18–26 nm in diameter, with linear single-stranded DNA)	
Adenoviridae	Pharyngitis, conjunctivitis
(Icosahedral non-enveloped particles, 70–90 nm, containing double-stranded linear DNA)	
Papovaviridae	
(Icosahedral non-enveloped particles, 45–55 nm, containing double-stranded circular DNA)	
Polyoma viruses	Multiple tumours, certainly in the case of mouse polyoma virus and SV40 virus of monkeys. In humans, may be reactivated by immunosuppression
Papilloma viruses	Warts, papillomas, urogenital carcinomas
Hepadnavirus group	Hepatitis B, hepatocellular carcinoma
(Spherical non-enveloped particles, 42 nm diameter, containing circular double-stranded DNA)	
RNA viruses	
Orthomyxoviridae	Influenza
(Spherical, enveloped particles, 80–120 nm, containing single-stranded RNA)	
Paramyxoviridae	
(Spherical, enveloped particles, 100–300 nm, containing single-stranded RNA)	
Para-influenza virus	Para influenza
Mumps virus	Mumps
Measles virus	Measles
Togaviridae	
(Enveloped, single-stranded RNA)	
Rubella virus	Rubella (German measles)

Table 2.17 continued

Retroviridae	
(Spherical, enveloped particles, 80–100 nm, containing single-stranded RNA)	
Human immunodeficiency viruses (HIVs)	AIDS
Human T-lymphotropic viruses (HTLVs: some viruses previously termed HTLVs are now HIVs)	Certain types of leukaemia and lymphomas
Rhabdoviridae	
(Bullet-shaped, enveloped particles, 170 × 70 nm, containing single-stranded RNA)	
Rabies virus	Rabies
Picornaviridae	
(Icosahedral, non-enveloped particles, 20–30 nm, containing single-stranded RNA)	
Rhinoviruses	
Enteroviruses	
Coxsackie	Herpangina; hand, foot and mouth disease; pharyngitis
Echo	Pharyngitis, sialadenitis
Polio	Poliomyelitis

viral infection may have left the affected cells (the so-called 'hit and run' mechanism) or may at least be difficult to detect because large and characteristic or unique parts of the viral genome rarely become integrated into human tissues.

Table 2.16 lists those proliferative mucosal lesions of the head and neck putatively caused by viruses. Current evidence implicates in particular the human papilloma viruses (HPVs), particularly the so-called 'high (oncogenic) risk' genotypes. It used to be thought that herpes simplex virus (HSV) might be involved in oral cancer, and because of the undoubted importance of other herpesviruses, particularly Epstein–Barr virus (EBV) in cancers at other sites (notably nasopharyngeal cancer and lymphomas) and the recently discovered Kaposi's sarcoma-associated herpesvirus (KSHV or HHV8), interest has returned to the study of human herpesviruses (HHVs) in oral squamous cell cancer. Furthermore, because (a) our knowledge of oncogenes in eukaryotic cells is based to a large extent on their identification in viruses, because (b) viral oncogenesis can involve both DNA and RNA viruses, and because (c) disabled viruses (notably adenoviruses) are increasingly used as vectors for gene therapy in cancer, a brief revision of the classification of viruses should be helpful (Table 2.17). A good overview of basic virology and its application to oral diseases can be found in Scully and Samaranayake.[207]

The archetypal DNA oncogenic virus is SV40. Such viruses carry oncogenes which can be directly integrated into the host genome. Retroviruses have relatively simple genomes which encode three genes—GAG, POL and ENV—which produce core proteins, a reverse transcriptase and envelope glycoproteins, respectively. Long terminal repeats (LTRs) are present at each end of the viral genome and these function as promoter and enhancer sequences. The oncogenic retroviruses (sometimes called oncornaviruses) incorporate a fourth gene, an oncogene, by 'hijacking' a host proto-oncogene after integration into host DNA: this can then be

Table 2.18 Retroviral oncogenes

Oncogene	Virus	Tumour
v-*ABL*	Abelson leukaemia virus	Leukaemia
v-*ERB A*	Avian erythroblastosis virus	Helps v-*ERB B*
v-*ERB B*	Avian erythroblastosis virus	Erythroleukaemia
v-*FMS*	Feline sarcoma virus	Sarcoma
v-*H RAS*	Rat sarcoma virus (Harvey strain)	Sarcoma
v-*K RAS*	Rat sarcoma virus (Kirsten strain)	Sarcoma
v-*JUN*	Avian sarcoma virus	Fibrosarcoma
v-*MYB*	Avian myeloblastosis virus	Myeloblastosis
v-*MYC*	Avian myelocytomatosis virus	Leukaemia
v-*SIS*	Simian sarcoma virus	Sarcoma
v-*SRC*	Rous sarcoma virus	Sarcoma

expressed under the influence of viral promoters even though the virus itself may not be capable of replication. Additionally, insertion of a DNA copy of a retrovirus into host genome close to an important proto-oncogene may cause abnormal activity of that gene because of the influence of the viral LTR regions. Even though few retroviruses have so far been convincingly proved to be direct causes of human cancers, their study has led to the identification of the homologous mammalian counterparts, the proto-oncogenes, which may become amplified, mutated or otherwise altered without the direct need for a viral intermediary. For this reason it is instructive to list the best-known viral oncogenes and the animal tumours in which they were first characterized (Table 2.18). This also explains the otherwise potentially confusing terminology and abbreviations used for these mammalian oncogenes.

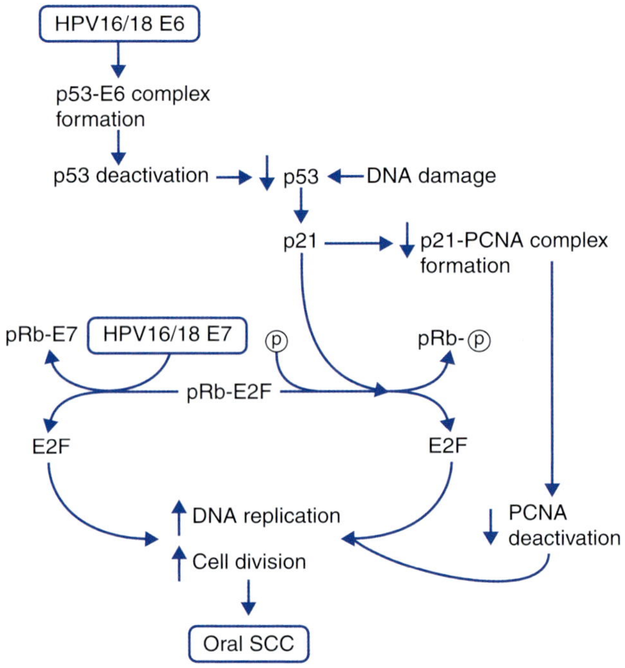

Figure 2.11 An outline of how high-risk HPVs may promote oral carcinogenesis. The E6 protein of these viruses binds to and deactivates p53. When DNA damage occurs, p53 and p21 cannot then be upregulated and hence there is no inhibition of PCNA activity or of pRb phosphorylation: phosphorylated pRb releases activated E2F transcription factors, thus encouraging DNA replication. The E7 protein of HPVs binds directly to pRb with the same effect. (Source: Sugerman and Shillitoe.[215])

The human papilloma virus (HPV)

Papilloma viruses are species and tissue specific. The human papilloma viruses, of which over 75 types have so far been described with some 26 potential new types awaiting classification, are all epitheliotropic, specifically for squamous epithelia, over half being related to skin diseases and the remainder associated with mucosal lesions; mucocutaneous junctions of the anogenital and oral regions are commonly involved. They are DNA viruses with about 7900 base pairs arranged in a double-stranded circular genome encapsulated within an icosahedral protein shell (the capsid), 55 nm in diameter.[208] Viral proteins are encoded by parts of the DNA called open reading frames (ORFs). These sequences are present on only one of the DNA strands, and are divided into early (E) and late (L) regions: E regions (designated E1–E7) are expressed quickly after infection and encode proteins necessary for DNA replication; the L regions (L1 and L2) encode viral capsid proteins later in the process of viral replication. HPVs are typed according to their sequence homology which, currently, is assessed following polymerase chain reaction (PCR) amplification using specific primers. Current convention is that, when there is less than 90% homology of the E6, E7 and L1 ORFs, a new, different type is designated and numbered in order of discovery. Homology above 90% defines a subtype and above 98% a variant.

Papilloma viruses and disorders of epithelial proliferation

There is no doubt that certain types of HPV are highly infectious and directly responsible for lesions associated with epithelial hyperproliferation, notably the common infectious wart or verruca vulgaris and anogenital warts or condylomata (see below). Most of these, however, are benign lesions and the HPVs associated with them have been termed 'low-risk' types.[209] These include HPV types 6, 11, 13 and 32, which have also been described in similar benign lesions of the oral mucosa (i.e. papillomas, condyloma acuminatum, verruca vulgaris and focal epithelial hyperplasia).[210]

Conversely, 'high-risk' HPV types are those associated with premalignant lesions and squamous cell carcinomas—again, most of the evidence coming from anogenital lesions. Among these HPVs 16, 18, 31, 33, 35 and 39 are found most commonly.[209–211] Their viral genomes can become integrated and transcriptionally active in tumours and tumour cell lines, such that the IARC has classified HPV 16 and 18 as carcinogenic in humans (group 1), HPV 31 and 33 as probably carcinogenic in humans (group 2a) and some others as possibly carcinogenic in humans (group 2b); the latest evaluations can be found at the IARC Homepage (http://www.iarc/fr/). Nevertheless, even the high-risk HPVs do not appear to be directly carcinogenic, but seem to require additional modifications of host-cell genes, brought about by physical or chemical carcinogens or other viral infections.[211,212] This is consistent with the multifactorial and multistep nature of human carcinogenesis, in the light of which detection of HPV infection may be a useful risk marker for subsequent malignancy. Indeed, detection and typing of HPV in routine uterine cervical smears is recommended by many; the technology is becoming cheaper and commercial hybridization kits are widely available. Extensive multinational studies are under way to determine the true predictive value of such information and its cost-effectiveness.

The E6 and E7 ORFs of the high-risk HPVs are particularly important because they encode transforming proteins, and can thus be regarded as viral oncogenes. They are thought to act by binding to, and inactivating, the important cell-cycle regulatory tumour suppressor gene proteins p53 and pRb, respectively.[213] They thus act by 'taking the brakes off' the control of cell proliferation, allowing increased DNA synthesis and cell production, and by inhibiting apoptosis. As a result, spontaneous or induced mutations are not eliminated and a transformed state can become established.[214] These mechanisms, particularly in relation to oral cancer, are summarized in a comprehensive review by Sugerman and Shillitoe[215] and illustrated in Fig. 2.11. With in vitro studies using glutathione *S*-transferase-E6 protein, the level of inhibition of site-specific binding of p53 to DNA was, in descending order, HPV 16 E6 > 31 > 18 > 11; furthermore, E7 proteins from high-risk HPV types bind pRb with a higher affinity than do E7 proteins from low-risk types.[216] Mutations conferring higher promoter activity have been found in the long control region (LCR) of genomes of HPVs 16 and 18 isolated from oral cancer cell lines compared with wild-type LCRs.[217] A common polymorphism of the p53 gene may render certain individuals more susceptible to HPV infection and oral carcinogenesis, according to new Indian data.[218]

Table 2.19 Summary of HPV types described in oral SCC and normal oral mucosa with all methodologies combined. (Source: Sugerman and Shillitoe[215])

HPV type	Oral SCC	Normal oral mucosa
1	0/6 (0%)	
2	4/45 (9%)	33/479 (7%)
3	1/28 (4%)	0/33 (0%)
4	1/39 (3%)	
5	0/6 (0%)	
6	62/642 (10%)	90/973 (9%)
7		1/262 (< 1%)
11	68/644 (11%)	30/593 (5%)
13	1/103 (1%)	0/300 (0%)
16	252/1156 (22%)	84/852 (10%)
17	0/6 (0%)	
18	124/881 (14%)	58/535 (11%)
20	0/6 (0%)	
30	0/52 (0%)	
31	0/198 (0%)	8/109 (7%)
32	0/23 (0%)	0/5 (0%)
33	0/231 (0%)	10/67 (15%)
35, 42–44	0/73 (0%)	
45	0/99 (0%)	
51,52,56	0/73 (0%)	
57	1/28 (4%)	0/33 (0%)

Papilloma viruses and oral cancer

HPV 16 is the most common type to be associated with both cervical and oral cancers.[219–221] In vitro studies show that primary human oral epithelial cells can be immortalized by high-risk HPV types;[220,223] however, exposure to tobacco-related chemicals was required for these cells to progress to a fully malignant phenotype.[224,225]

That infection with high-risk HPV, and even demonstrable integration of known viral oncogenes, is neither necessary nor sufficient for the development of oral cancer is supported by our observations that p53 mutations (but not over-expression) correlate with the *absence* of HPV 16 E6.[226] This is consistent with the data from an extensive study by Riethdorf and colleagues,[227] who showed that only about 40% of head and neck squamous carcinomas carrying p53 mutations also carried high-risk HPV, and only about 40% of HPV positive tumours showed p53 mutations. In this study there was no correlation between HPV presence and smoking history and no influence of HPV infection on overall survival rate, either alone or in combination with p53 mutations. In contrast, another study of oral cancer has shown that HPV-negative cases had a poorer prognosis than HPV-positive cases.[228] Much remains to be clarified, therefore, regarding the diagnostic and prognostic value of detecting HPV in oral cancer, especially as the reported prevalences vary so much (see below).

The question of the predictive value of HPV infection in at-risk individuals with or without a detectable potentially malignant lesion is also important. High-risk HPVs have frequently been detected in benign oral lesions and in clinically and histologically normal mucosa.[215,229] Whether detecting them adds to the utility of oral screening is unknown and will require substantial further work. At the time of writing, no longitudinal studies are available and we have to extrapolate from cross-sectional studies on small, selected populations (the IARC is, however, currently coordinating a large international descriptive study of the prevalence of HPV in oral cancer).

Studies of HPV in patients with oral cancer report prevalences varying from 0%[230] to 100%.[231] Possible reasons for such a large variation are the use of different detection methods and differences in the populations studied, not least with respect to prevailing environmental risk factors. One of the major difficulties in the detection of HPV infection in oral cancer is the presence of the virus in only a subpopulation of cells and at low copy number in the infected cells.[232] The methods used in reported studies range from immunocytochemistry (capable of detecting 10 or more copies per cell), through Southern blot hybridization and dot-blot hybridization (1–10 copies per cell), in-situ hybridization (ISH; again more than 10 copies), PCR and in-situ PCR (less than one copy per cell). The literature to 1997 has been extensively and critically reviewed by Sugerman and Shillitoe,[215] whose additive summary is presented as Table 2.19 (individual sources can be ascertained therein). The higher prevalences, unsurprisingly, are reported by studies using the more sensitive techniques. Those using fresh tissue also yield positive results in a higher proportion of cases.

Our own work using a highly sensitive 'nested PCR' method, with two sets of HPV consensus primers to the L1 region, detected HPV DNA in 14/28 (50%) samples of oral SCC and 4/12 (33%) dysplastic mucosae peripheral to the tumours. A novel method based on labelling the PCR products with ^{32}P and the separation of radioactively labelled products on an 8% polyacrylamide gel increased the sensitivity of the detection and allowed identification of the types by subsequent direct sequencing. HPV 16 was found in 13/28 cancers; five of these also harbored HPV 6 and one HPV 6 alone; thus, 14 of the 28 cancers (50%) had no detectable HPV. HPV 16 was the type detected in all four of the 11 potentially malignant tissues (two of which also harboured HPV 6); no other types were found.[233] These results confirm the trend apparent in Table 2.19—namely, that HPV 16, one of the high-risk types of HPV, is that most commonly associated with oral cancer and, possibly, with its immediate precursor stages.

Several important findings emerge from reviewing this considerable, rapidly growing, and often inconsistent literature:

- There appears to be a real trend in the prevalence of HPV infection from normal oral mucosa in healthy patients, through mucosa distant from an oral lesion, through dysplastic or otherwise potentially malignant mucosa, to oral cancer itself.[234,235]
- The detection rate in oral cancer (perhaps 30–50%) is considerably lower than that reported in cervical carcinoma (85–90%), and virus seems less likely to become integrated.
- HPV types 31, 33 and 35, which are commonly associated with cervical cancer, are apparently not found in oral carcinomas, in which HPV 16 and 18 appear to be the most common high-risk types.
- There may be a correlation of high-risk HPV types 16 and 18 with a type of oral mucosal neoplasm, as these seem to be present at lower prevalences in verrucous carcinomas and in keratoses[236] (see above). The literature base is, however, still small and the findings often contradictory. For example, in the now well-recognized entity proliferative verrucous leukoplakia (PVL) (see Chapter 3), the appearance and natural history of which suggest HPV involvement, Palefsky and colleagues[237] found eight of nine lesions from seven patients to contain HPV-16. In UK patients we found only 2/36 samples from seven patients to be positive.[238] Methodological differences cannot, of course, be excluded.
- There may be important geographical differences in HPV infection rates. For example, we have found, using ISH,[239] a surprisingly low prevalence in Sudanese with smokeless tobacco (toombak)-induced oral mucosal lesions, although the use of toombak is known to be associated with a high incidence of oral cancer (see above).
- The finding of these types in normal oral mucosa may suggest that HPV can be latent for long periods before the manifestation of clinical or histological carcinoma. When involved in the carcinogenic process, HPV infection may be an early event.
- There is no apparent relationship between clinical stage and HPV status in SCC of the head and neck. This adds credence to the postulate that HPV involvement is not a late event in the evolution of these cancers.[240–242]
- There may be a predilection of HPV infection for patients with tonsillar carcinoma[242] and elsewhere in Waldeyer's ring.[243]
- There may be a significant association with smoking (see above and reference 244). This has not, however, been found in all studies.[244,245]
- There may be a significant inverse correlation between HPV presence and age: patients more than 60 years of age have a lower prevalence in their tumours.[246] This may impact on the aetiology of oral cancer in younger patients without a typical history of many years' exposure to tobacco and alcohol.

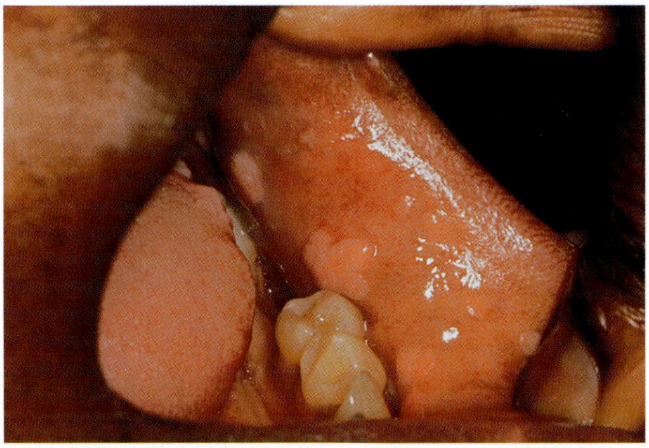

Figure 2.12 Flat papillomas of the buccal mucosa in a patient who had multiple lesions on the lips and elsewhere in the mouth.

- No clear or consistent associations between HPV presence and survival or other behavioural outcomes have been demonstrated.[233,241,247]
- The marked differences described for HPV prevalence rates for SCC of the oesophagus from high- and low-risk geographical areas[248] may apply to oral cancer—hence the importance of the multinational descriptive molecular epidemiological studies currently in progress.
- As technology improves, and methods become ever more sensitive, further variability in rates of HPV infection and integration is emerging.[249]

HPV and benign proliferative lesions of the oral mucosa

The cytological hallmark of HPV infection is the presence of koilocytic atypia of the prickle cell (intermediate) layers of stratified squamous epithelia. This is manifested as ballooning of keratinocytes with densely staining irregular nuclei, often pressed to the side of the cell, surrounded by a perinuclear halo with condensed, amphophilic cytoplasm at its margins. (Distinction should be made between true koilocytosis and vacuolization of cells, such as that seen in white sponge naevus of the oral mucosa, which is not HPV related.) In HPV infection there may also be parakeratinized (dyskeratotic) cells singly or in clusters below the surface layers. Both koilocytotic and dyskeratotic cells may be bi- or multinucleate, and show enlarged nuclei. The association of koilocytosis with the presence of HPV DNA can be confirmed by ISH.

Squamous papilloma and condyloma acuminatum

Benign squamous cell papillomata can be found affecting the oral mucosa in either sex, at any age, particularly in the third to fifth decades. They may be single lesions (usually less than 1 or 2 mm in diameter) or multiple, cohesive lesions. They occur on the soft palate, dorsal or lateral borders of tongue or lower lip (Fig. 2.12). They do not appear to differ from papillomas at other mucosal sites. HPV particles (by electron microscopy), HPV antigens (by immunocytochemistry) and HPV DNA (which identifies mainly HPV 6 and 11) have been found in up to 80% of the lesions studied.[250]

Condyloma acuminatum (venereal wart) of the mouth usually presents as multiple small, white or pink nodules with a verrucous (cauliflower-like) surface. These may proliferate and coalesce to form soft sessile growths up to 1 cm in diameter.[251] Histological distinction from papilloma is difficult and mainly of academic interest, except that this type of lesion more often suggests sexual transmission. Again, HPV particles, HPV structural antigens and HPV DNA 6 and 11 have been found in up to 85% of these lesions.[250]

Verruca vulgaris

The common wart of skin, verruca vulgaris, is relatively rare in the upper aerodigestive tract but is found on the lips, oral mucosa and larynx. It may be difficult to distinguish from papillomata, verrucous hyperplasia and verrucous carcinoma. A true verruca shows, histologically, a prominent granular layer, containing numerous keratohyaline granules just beneath a layer of koilocytes, orthokeratin and thin rete ridges which often curl inwards at the margins of the lesion. Verruca vulgaris of the skin has a clear association with HPV types 2 and 4 and, in keeping with that, designation of oral warts should be limited to lesions with these types.[252] Oral and labial verruca vulgaris are usually associated with HPV type 2, rarely with type 4.

Focal epithelial hyperplasia

Focal epithelial hyperplasia (FEH, or Heck's disease) is a virus-induced benign hyperplasia of the oral mucosa with an ethnic predilection, preponderantly described in Eskimos in Greenland and Alaska (where the prevalence may be as high as 10%), and among Native Americans (prevalence more than 3%); only occasional cases have been described in Caucasians.[253,254]

Clinically, FEH seems to be of two types: (1) circumscribed, sessile, soft, nodular elevations; (2) well-demarcated, soft, slightly elevated papules with a flat surface. Their size ranges between 0.1 and 1.0 cm and both types show an irregular periphery. In the Eskimos some 50% of the lesions may be on the tongue, whereas in American Indians the lip is described as the most common site. Most patients have had lesions for many years and these are not painful.

Histologically, the lesions demonstrate acanthosis, slight parakeratosis and elongation of rete ridges with horizontal anastomoses. Distinctive ballooning of keratinocytes at various levels in the epithelium is described, with mitosis-like aberrations (so-called FEH cells, a form of koilocytosis). Inclusion bodies may be seen in these nuclei and electron microscopy demonstrates HPV-like particles with a diameter of 40–60 nm. HPV types 1, 6, 13, 11 and 32 have been detected.[250,253]

Koilocytic dysplasia

Koilocytic dysplasia (HPV-associated epithelial dysplasia) is believed to be a subtype of oral dysplasia with unique histological features predictive of the presence of HPV DNA.[255] Microscopy shows the simultaneous presence of acanthosis, koilocytosis, keratinocyte multinucleation, nuclear pleomorphism and basal cell hyperplasia. In the cases described there is a striking male predominance (80%) and relatively young age of presentation (39 years); lesions occur mostly on the tongue, lips and buccal mucosa.

It is possible that these lesions will have been classified by others as flat condylomata, Bowen's disease or bowenoid papulosis. HIV seropositivity or risk activities for HIV infection have been found in a quarter of the patients so far described. HPV DNA is detected more often in koilocytic dysplasia than in more conventional oral epithelial dysplasia, either intermediate-risk (31, 33, 35) or high-risk HPV types (16, 18) whether or not they also contain low-risk HPV types (6, 11).

HPV infections in HIV/AIDS patients

As implied above, HPV infections occur in the oral cavity in association with HIV infection and present as verruca vulgaris, condyloma acuminatum and FEH. They have been classified in group II (lesions less commonly associated with HIV infection) by the EC.[256] In the studies reviewed by Schiodt[257] the prevalence ranged from 0 to 5.3%: no cases among HIV-positive or HIV-negative women were found by Shiboski and colleagues,[258] and Lamster and colleagues[259] found cases only among HIV-positive intravenous drug users and not among HIV-positive men who have sex with men.[259] However, unpublished studies in the era of highly active anti-retroviral therapy (HAART) up to early 2002 show a rising incidence in all HIV-positive cohorts on such therapy.

There are insufficient data to conclude that the prevalence of HPV-related oral diseases is higher in HIV/AIDS than in the general population, although it is a clinical impression of the authors that this is the case. As many of these oral infections are sexually transmitted in the population at large it would be surprising if they were not more prevalent in several of the HIV risk groups.

The herpesviruses and oral cancer

Herpes simplex viruses

The epidemiology of cancer of the uterine cervix has long suggested an infective component; for example, this disease is extremely rare in celibates (such as nuns) and shows a relationship to number of sexual partners (not to simple frequency of intercourse). For some time this focused attention on a possible role for HSV type II, as this is a common genital tract viral infection in women, and it is known from studies in vitro that transfection of epithelial cultures with HSV can immortalize such cells. By implication, a role for HSV I (and II, which can be carried in the mouth) was sought in oral carcinogenesis. Evidence in support of this is the clear demonstration from animal studies that HSV can act as a cocarcinogen with tobacco[260] or other chemical carcinogens such as 4-nitroquinoline *N*-oxide (4NQO)[261] and that immunization against HSV can inhibit the cocarcinogenic effect with dimethyl benzanthracene (DMBA).[262]

Several studies in humans have shown that patients with oral cancer have higher antibodies to HSV, but this does not prove a causal relationship.[263] Serum IgA antibodies to HSV I are higher in smokers, and higher again in smokers with oral or other head and neck cancers, suggesting that prolonged exposure to HSV may sensitize the mucosa to tobacco carcinogens. A more likely explanation, however, is that the generalized immunosuppression, particularly of natural killer-cell (NK) activity, which is induced by smoking favours the acquisition or chronicity of HSV infections/carriage, with consequent raised antibody titres.

Stronger, but still circumstantial, evidence comes from a case-control study of 410 pairs drawn from northern Sweden. Univariate analysis showed ORs of 1.9 (0.7–4.5, and therefore not significant) for groups with a clearly stated ('certain') history of HSV-1 infection and 3.3 (1.6–6.5, therefore significant) for groups with a highly suspected ('certain plus probable') HSV-1 infection. Because most reports were of recurrent herpes labialis, lip cancer was analysed separately, revealing ORs of 4.6 (1.7–13) for the highly suspected group. These associations remained in multivariate analysis, which showed HSV infection (OR 3.8; 2.0–7.0), alcohol use (OR 1.5; 1.0–2.3) and current smoking (OR 1.5; 0.9–2.5) to be the major influences.[111]

There is little convincing evidence that HSV gene sequences are present in oral cancer cells, although some studies have claimed to detect HSV antigens.[264] RNA complementary to HSV DNA has been detected by ISH,[265] but there is no evidence for integration. A 'hit and run' hypothesis has long been proposed but is clearly difficult to prove. Currently there is little emphasis placed on HSV in relation to human oral cancer, but the above observations imply a potential role which is worthy of continuing investigation.

Epstein–Barr virus

Because of the very clear relationship of EBV to nasopharyngeal cancer in man,[266] to Burkitt's lymphoma which characteristically affects the jaws (reviewed by Shapira and Peylan-Ramu[267]) and to lymphomata in the immunosuppressed, many have sought evidence for a role in oral squamous cell cancer. Natural infection with EBV occurs worldwide and affects more than 90% of many populations, either subclinically during early childhood or as infectious mononucleosis during teenage years. Spread seems to be mainly by intimate oral contact. The major salivary glands harbour EBV and the virus can be recovered from the saliva of otherwise healthy seropositive individuals. EBV exhibits dual tropism, infecting both B lymphocytes and epithelial cells, particularly those of the nasopharynx. Entry of virus is facilitated by an envelope glycoprotein binding to the C3d receptor on the cell membrane of B cells and to either this or a closely related epitope of the surface of epithelial cells. In oral mucosa this is expressed on cells of the prickle cell layer.[268]

EBV certainly has transforming properties in vitro and many lymphoblastoid cell lines (e.g. Raji) are driven in this way. EBV DNA has been detected in some tonsillar carcinomas, supraglotttic laryngeal carcinoma and some salivary gland carcinomas.[269] However, although we could detect EBV receptors on malignant as well as normal keratinocytes,[268] we could not detect viral DNA in oral cancer by ISH. Although not as sensitive as PCR-based techniques this is an important approach as it allows identification of the cells harbouring virus. Given the high proportion of individuals who will be secreting EBV in saliva, methods which involve wholesale processing of tissue (such as DNA extraction from biopsies) cannot avoid the complication of salivary contamination. Nevertheless, an extensive study from India has reported using PCR to amplify a 239 bp fragment of the *Bam*H1L region of the EBV genome, followed by Southern blot hybridization with EBV oligonucleotide probe, on DNA samples.[270] EBV was detected in 25/103 oral cancer samples (24%), in 13/100 (13%) non-malignant oral lesions (predominantly leukoplakia), in only 3/76 (4%) normal mucosal specimens from the contralateral side of patients with oral lesions and in 10/141 (7%) peripheral blood cells (50 oral cancer patients and 50 with other oral lesions). This is a substantial sample and shows a clear prevalence trend. In a smaller study of Dutch patients using primers for the *Bam*HIW repeat, EBV was found in 100% of the SCC samples ($n = 36$), 78% of premalignant lesions ($n = 9$) and 8% of clinically normal mucosa ($n = 12$). Using primers for the single-copy *BNLF-1* gene, a region of the EBV genome with oncogenic potential, EBV was detected in only 50% of the SCCs and none of the other tissues. These latter authors accept that saliva or infiltrating leukocytes could be the source of the EBV detected, possibly owing to tumour-associated immunosuppression in these patients resulting in increased shedding of EBV. They, and

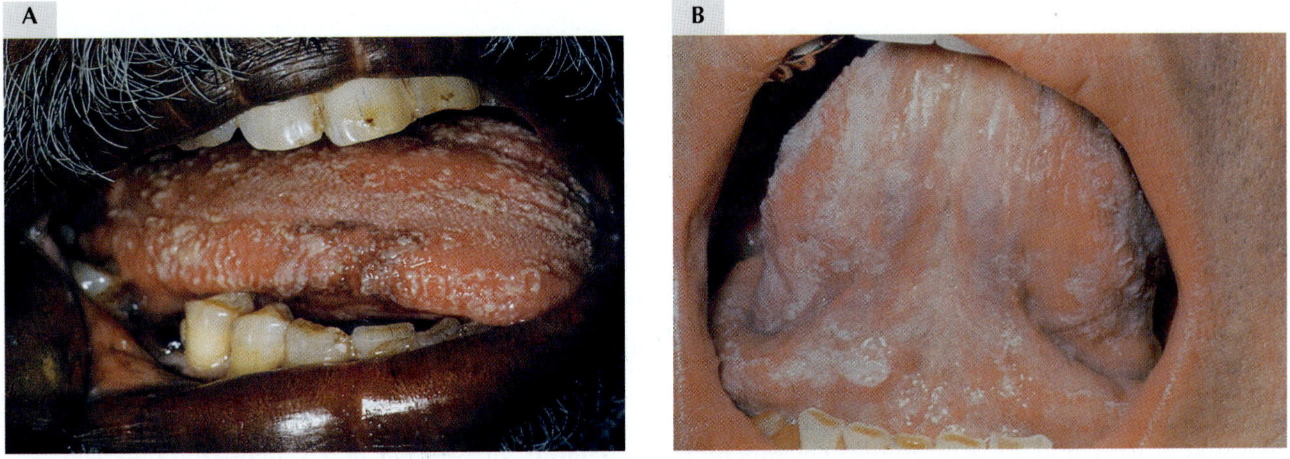

Figure 2.13 A: Oral hairy leukoplakia (Greenspan lesion) on the lateral border of the tongue, mixed with pseudomembranous candidiasis on the dorsum, in an HIV-positive patient. B: A more extensive hairy leukoplakia, affecting lateral and ventral; tongue, and floor of mouth, in an AIDS patient (courtesy Dr Charles Barr, New York).

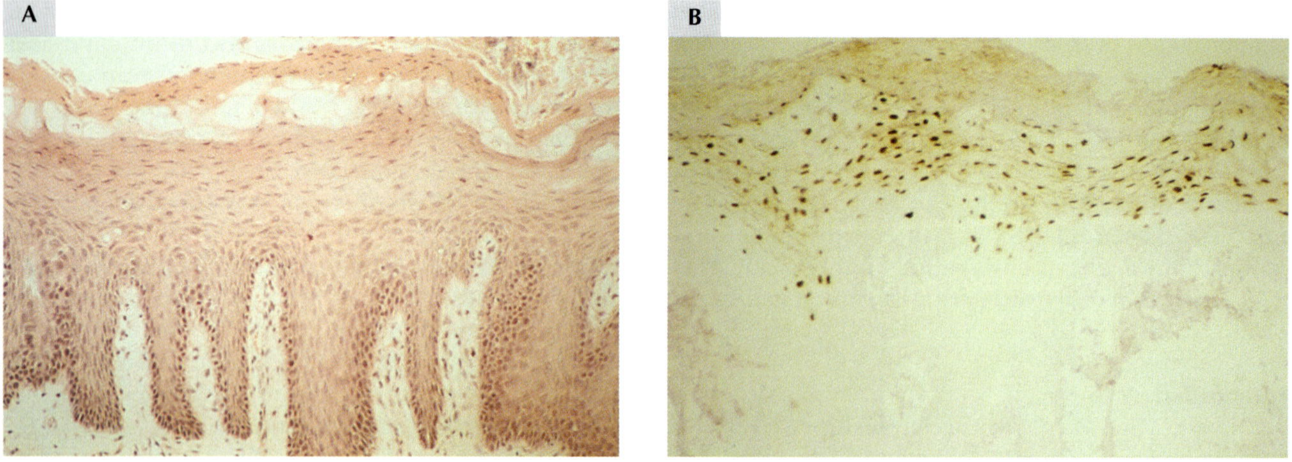

Figure 2.14 A: Histology of oral hairy leukoplakia. Note the modest acanthosis, ballooning of cells in the upper prickle cell layers, a limited hyperparakeratosis, limited rete ridge hyperplasia and absence of an inflammatory infiltrate in the lamina propria. Stained by haematoxylin and eosin. B: An adjacent section to the above, showing EBV in the upper keratinocytes, demonstrated by in situ hybridization.

others, have been unable to demonstrate the clonal presence of EBV in the neoplastic cells of oral SCC. Thus, all of the above is circumstantial evidence but it leaves alive the possibility that EBV may contribute as one of the multiple factors in oral carcinogenesis, at least in a certain proportion of patients. Much is known about the molecular mechanisms of EBV transformation of cell lines in vitro and it remains to be seen whether these are operative in oral epithelia in vivo.

Oral hairy leukoplakia (OHL)

It is now clearly established that OHL, a corrugated plaque-like hyperproliferative lesion of the oral mucosa affecting immunocompromised individuals (Figs 2.13A, B; 2.14A) is EBV driven (Fig. 2.14B) and the molecular mechanisms are known in considerable detail.[269,271–273] However, at the time of writing, no instances of malignant transformation have been reported.

HHV-6

The member of the herpes family designated HHV-6 also has primary tropism for CD4 lymphocytes, but has a productive phase in salivary duct epithelial cells. Primary infection is usually asymptomatic but can cause severe febrile illness in children. Reactivation in later life may be associated with a variety of conditions that show immunological dysfunction. Following a description of the frequent detection of HHV-6 in a small series of patients from India with oral cancers, and elevated levels of anti-HHV-6 antibodies in these patients' sera, one group has now reported a study on Malaysian patients. Up to 80% of oral SCC contained HHV-6 DNA (detected by both PCR: 19/24 cases and ISH: 33/42 cases) or antigen (by ICC: 41/51 cases), with a lower proportion in potentially malignant lesions (leukoplakia and lichen planus): none of seven samples of normal oral tissues were positive by any method.[274] These associations certainly do not establish a role for this virus in oral carcinogenesis, but justify further research.

HHV-8 and Kaposi's sarcoma

Kaposi's sarcoma (KS) and non-Hodgkin's lymphoma (NHL) are common in AIDS patients. EBV is implicated in the cause of up to half of the cases of systemic NHLs and perhaps all of central nervous system lymphomas in these patients. There is growing evidence that another herpes virus, HHV-8 (or KS-associated herpesvirus; KSHV) is implicated in KS. One group has found it at prevalences approaching 100% in KS from all body sites and in all epidemiological groups with KS, including non-HIV-positive 'classical' cases.[275] It has been detected in about half of the oral KS lesions and oral ulcers in HIV-positive patients by others.[276] This is a rapidly moving field. The literature to 1997 has been comprehensively reviewed by Porter and colleagues, who discuss possible pathogenic mechanisms involving the virus producing homologues of human gene products which dysregulate cell cycle arrest and inhibit apoptosis and cell-mediated immune responses.[277]

Hepatitis viruses and oral cancer

Because of the known oncogenic properties of hepatitis B virus in relation to liver cancer, there is

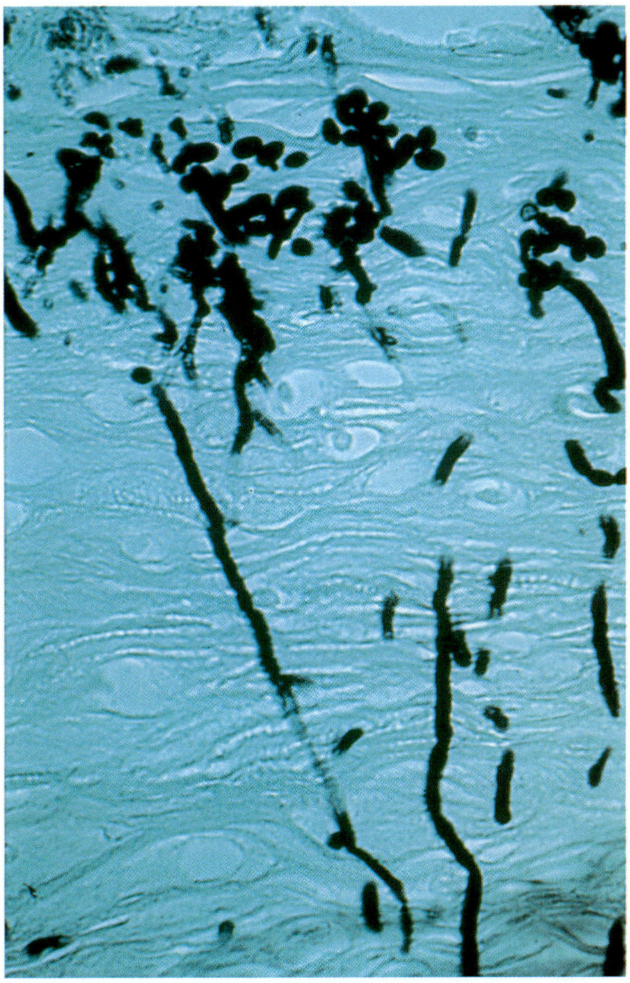

Figure 2.15 Yeasts and hyphae of *Candida albicans*, penetrating the upper layers of the epithelium in a clinical leukoplakia, demonstrated in this section by Grocot's reaction, in which the walls of the organisms are stained black with silver.

speculation as to a possible role for the hepatitis viruses in other epithelial neoplasms. Detection of a high prevalence of hepatitis C antibody in 24/100 oral cancer patients in Japan, and of hepatitis C virus (HCV) RNA in a high proportion of their tumours,[278] poses such a question for oral cancer. There are several case reports of oral cancer arising in lichen planus lesions associated with hepatitis C,[277,279] but the above constitute only early, circumstantial evidence. It has been shown that the NS3 protein of HCV accumulates in nuclei of infected cells and binds to wild-type, but not mutant p53, thus dysregulating the cell cycle.[280] Other theoretical molecular interactions can be speculated upon, but there is as yet no direct evidence in relation to squamous carcinomas. (HBV is a DNA Hepadna virus. HCV is a member of the Flavivirus group and is an enveloped RNA virus.)

Fungal infections

Several species of *Candida*, especially *C. albicans*, are common commensals of the oral cavity. They become opportunistic pathogens when there is immunosuppression, either local (by the use of steroid inhalers) or systemic (e.g. by drugs in transplant patients, or in HIV disease), reduction of competing oral flora (such as in the long-term use of antibiotics), or local changes favouring their proliferation and adherence to oral mucosa: such changes include poor denture hygiene, and the presence of surface roughening or hyperkeratosis, or both. In a proportion of cases of leukoplakia there is superficial invasion by fungal hyphae (Fig. 2.15),[281] particularly those of nodular leukoplakia, and it has been demonstrated that these have a higher risk of malignant transformation. Of 4724 mucosal biopsies accessed by one service in London between 1991 and 1995, periodic acid–Schiff (PAS)-positive fungal hyphae were found in 223 (4.7%), with a significant positive association with moderate or severe dysplasia.[282] There is also a clear association between smoking and the risk of acquiring a candidal infection in the mouth:[283] this also applies to HIV-positive individuals, compounding the risk.[284,285] Patients with iron deficiency, clearly at increased risk for oral cancer (see below), are also more prone to oral candidiasis, indicating an interactive, multifactorial process in oral carcinogenesis, as pointed out by Binnie.[119]

Whether *Candida* spp. invade oral potentially malignant lesions as a secondary event, or are causal in the lesion or the subsequent cancer (or both), remains uncertain. However, a mechanism clearly exists, as these organisms have the enzymes necessary to promote the nitrosation of dietary substrates.[286]

Diet and nutrition in the aetiology of oral cancer

Interest here relates to the roles of iron, of the antioxidant or free-radical scavenging vitamins A, C and E, and to trace elements such as zinc and selenium, for which there is evidence of a protective effect.

The interest in iron goes back to the beginning of the twentieth century, since the recognition (more or less simultaneously in Scandinavia and in England) of a high incidence of upper gastrointestinal tract cancer in middle-aged women suffering from chronic anaemia, with dysphagia and glossitis and atrophy of associated mucosa—the Plummer–Vinson or Patterson–Brown–Kelly syndrome. Both of the

Table 2.20 Odds ratios for oral and pharyngeal cancer according to certain food groups: Pordone, Italy, 1984–89. Includes corrections for age, sex, occupation, smoking and drinking. (From La Vecchia et al.[171])

	Odds ratios for frequency of consumption by tercile[a]	
	Intermediate	High
Pasta or rice	1.1	1.4
Polenta	1.2	1.8
Cheese	1.0	1.7
Eggs	1.4	1.6
Pulses	1.4	1.9
Carrots	0.8	0.7
Fresh tomatoes	0.7	0.5
Green peppers	0.6	0.5

[a]Low consumption is reference category with OR set at 1.

original papers were published in 1919. In animals rendered experimentally iron deficient by venesection and a low-iron diet there is contradictory evidence of the effect on epithelial cell kinetics, with some studies showing increased turnover, theoretically increasing the risk of mutational error[287] and others a decrease.[288] There is agreement, however, that this results in epithelial atrophy[289] and increased cancer risk, clearly shown in such animals when challenged with chemical carcinogens.[290] On the other hand, there is surprisingly little information on the risks of oral cancer associated with anaemia and sideropaenia in human studies: certainly, anaemia of chronic blood loss following hookworm infections and other chronic diseases is common in those parts of south Asia where oral cancer prevails, as is mucosal atrophy—which presumably makes tissues more susceptible to tobacco carcinogens.[291]

There is a large literature on other possible dietary correlates with upper aerodigestive tract cancer, summary reviews of which have been published by La Vecchia and colleagues.[171,292] Studies have looked at broad food groups, specific food items, vitamins and other specific micronutrients and, of course alcohol, which is not discussed further here.

Food groups

Of 13 case-control studies that have examined the association between fruit and vegetable consumption and oral/pharyngeal cancer, 11 report a meaningful inverse association.[292–294] The reduction in risk with fruits, from the highest to the lowest intake, varies from 80% to 20%,[295] and is evident for tongue, mouth and pharynx.[296]

With vegetables the results are less consistent. There is a relationship between total consumption and reduced risk,[297,298] and this is most strongly associated with vegetables rich in carotenes.[166,299] Again, some of the best results come from the northern Italian studies. Table 2.20 summarizes the data from the high-risk area in Northern Italy, based on 302 cases and 699 controls. In this group, high intake of maize revealed two to three times the risk for low intake of maize, possibly because it is less nutritious than other grains and may cause deficiencies of B-group vitamins. In Milan, an area of intermediate risk, high intakes of milk, meat and cheese were associated with reduced risk, somewhat surprisingly in view of the well-established increased risk of these foods for bowel, breast and other cancers; however, these factors probably indicate the better-nourished individuals. Again in Milan, carrots (OR 0.4 for highest vs lowest tercile), green vegetables (OR 0.6) and fresh fruit (OR 0.2) were strongly protective, and the effect is clear when expressed in terms of β-carotene intake. A strong protective effect is evident for carotenoids and vitamin C from vegetables and fruit, and of fibre intake in oral cancer risk in an important study from Beijing, China.[300]

La Vecchia and colleagues[171] estimate that approximately 15% of cases of oral and pharyngeal cancers in Europe can be attributed to dietary deficiencies or imbalances, perhaps accounting for 5000 avoidable deaths per year. Artificial supplementation with micronutrients is discussed in Chapter 18. It should be noted here, however, that obtaining these nutrients from natural foods is more effective than taking dietary supplements. The beneficial effect of high intakes of vegetable and fruits is confirmed, particularly in heavy smokers and alcohol drinkers, in another North-East Italian study.[301]

Dental factors in the aetiology of oral cancer

Clinicians have long noticed an association between poor oral hygiene, poor dental status and oral cancer, and 'dentition' (recorded as number of natural teeth, appliances, sharp or fractured teeth) appears as a correlate in several studies.[302] As these are certain to be confounded by socioeconomic factors, tobacco, alcohol abuse, nutritional and other correlates of cancer risk, it requires carefully designed (and large) case series and case-control studies to evaluate the importance of dental factors. Furthermore, it is well known that, in experimental chemical carcinogenesis experiments in animals, repeated trauma to mucosa localizes the site at which the tumour is likely to appear, increases the yield and reduces the latent period. Many human cases are described of an oral cancer at the site of chronic trauma arising from a broken-down tooth, a denture clasp or an ill-fitting denture flange or excrescence.

Three studies indicate that denture wearing per se is not a risk factor, but that chronic ulceration from an unsatisfactory appliance may promote a neoplasm in the presence of other risk factors. A major study from Brazil, based on 717 cases of cancer of the mouth, pharynx and larynx, and 1434 controls, reports an OR of 2.3 (1.2–4.6) for cancer of the mouth and, interestingly, of 2.7 (1.1–6.2) for cancer of the pharynx with a history of oral sores from ill-fitting dentures.[303] This study also showed that less than daily toothbrushing was associated with an increased risk of tongue neoplasms of 2.1 (1.0–4.3), or of other parts of the mouth of 2.4 (1.0–5.4)—in all cases the logistic regression analyses being carefully controlled for factors such as age, sex, tobacco and alcohol use, ethnicity, income and education. Microorganisms from dental plaque may contribute to chemical carcinogenesis by elaboration of toxins, e.g. nitrosating enzymes: it is also likely that infrequent or inadequate oral hygiene fails to dilute tobacco-derived and other carcinogens present. Data from the study in northern Sweden[111] and from a smaller study in the USA[304] also show no increased risk associated with fillings, dentures or fixed prostheses—nor, importantly, in the Swedish study, with experience of dental radiographic procedures.

Risk factors in young people

The trend of more cases in younger people, described in Chapter 1, has led to several studies of the risk factors involved (reviewed in reference 305). In a study of 116 cases aged 45 years and under,[306] and a comparison with 207 controls who had never had cancer, matched for age, sex and area of residence in South-east England,[307] we have found significant risks associated with tobacco and alcohol use, and poor diet. Importantly, these factors do not explain over a quarter of the cases. There is speculation, as yet unproven, about sexual transmission of disease, related to HPV.[308,309]

Aetiological factors in potentially malignant oral lesions and conditions

The frequent references made earlier in this chapter to aetiological or risk factors for these entities will not be repeated here. In summary (setting aside simple frictional keratoses), leukoplakias—white patches—of several types are strongly associated with tobacco use in all its forms.[310,311] Alcohol has recently been shown to be a significant risk factor for leukoplakia among non-smokers and non-chewers in Kerela, South India, especially among women.[312] In England, alcohol and tobacco act synergistically.[313] Tobacco chewing and alcohol drinking are strong risk factors for erythroplakia in the Indian population, and there is more than multiplacative interaction between alcohol drinking and low fruit and vegetable intake.[314] Paradoxically, although tobacco is undeniably one of the two major aetiological agents for oral cancer, it is not the tobacco-associated lesions that have the highest risk of malignant transformation, but those which appear idiopathic. Oral submucous fibrosis is clearly caused by areca nut chewing in genetically predisposed individuals; malignant transformation is enhanced by tobacco use and nutritional insufficiencies, but can occur without a history of tobacco. The precipitating antigen in the cell-mediated (auto)immune response of lichen planus remains an enigma; transformation is enhanced by traditional risk factors for oral cancer, but can occur in their absence.

References

1. Canon-Albright LA, Thomas A, Goldgar DE, Gholami K, Rowe K, Jacobsen M, McWhorter WP, Skolnick MH. Familiarity of cancer in Utah. Cancer Res 1994; 54: 2378–2385
2. Holloway SM, Sofaer JA. Coefficients of relationship by isonomy among oral cancer registrations in Scottish males. Community Dent Oral Epidemiol 1992; 20: 284–287
3. Newman AN, Calceterra TC, Bhuta S. Familial carcinoma of the submandibular gland. Arch Otolaryngol 1981; 107: 169–171
4. Merrick Y, Albeck H, Nielsen NH, Hansen HS. Familial clustering of salivary gland carcinoma in Greenland. Cancer 1986; 57: 2097–2102
5. Day GL, Blot WJ, Austin DF et al. Racial differences in risk of oral and pharyngeal cancer: alcohol, tobacco and other determinants. J Natl Cancer Inst 1993; 85: 465–473
6. Ankathil R, Mathew A, Joseph F, Nair MK. Is oral cancer susceptibility inherited? Report of five oral

cancer families. Eur J Cancer B Oral Oncol 1996; 32B: 63–67
7. Ankathil R, Bhattathiri NV, Francis JV et al. Mutagen sensitivity as a predisposing factor in familial oral cancer. Int J Cancer 1996; 69: 265–267
8. Copper MP, Jovanovic A, Nauta JJ. Role of genetic factors in the aetiology of squamous cell carcinoma of the head and neck. Arch Otolaryngol Head Neck Surg 1995; 121:157–160
9. Cloos J, Braakhuis BJ, Steen I et al. Increased mutagen sensitivity in head and neck squamous cell carcinoma patients, particularly those with multiple tumours. Int J Cancer 1994; 56: 816–819
10. Goldstein AM, Blot WJ, Greenberg RS et al. Familial risk in oral and pharyngeal cancer. Eur J Cancer B Oral Oncol 1994; 30B: 319–322
11. Brown LM, Gridley G, Diehl SR et al. Family cancer history and susceptibility to oral carcinoma in Puerto Rico. Cancer 2001; 92: 2102–2108
12. Scully C, Field JK, Tanzawa H. Genetic aberrations in oral or head and neck squamous cell carcinoma (SCCHN): 1. Carcinogen metabolism, DNA repair and cell cycle control. Oral Oncol 2000; 36: 256–263
13. Park LY, Muscat JE, Kaur T et al. Comparison of GSTM polymorphisms and risk for oral cancer between African-Americans and Caucasians. Pharmacogenetics 2000; 10: 123–131
14. Gronau S, Konig-Greger D, Rettinger C, Riechelmann H. GSTM1 gene polymorphism in patients with head and neck tumors. Laryngorhinootologie 2000; 79: 341–344
15. Buch SC, Notani PN, Bhisey RA. Polymorphism at GSTM1, GSTM3 and GSTT1 gene loci and susceptibility to oral cancer in an Indian population. Carcinogenesis 2002; 23: 803–807
16. Kietthubthew S, Sriplung H, Au WW. Genetic and environmental interactions on oral cancer in Southern Thailand. Environ Mol Mutagen 2001; 37: 111–116
17. Sreelekha TT, Ramadas K, Pandey M, Thomas G, Nalinakumari KR, Pillai MR. Genetic polymorphism of CYP1A1, GSTM1 and GSTT1 genes in Indian oral cancer. Oral Oncol 2001; 37: 593–598
18. Sato M, Sato T, Izumo T, Amagasa T. Genetically high susceptibility to oral squamous cell carcinoma in terms of combined genotyping of CYP1A1 and GSTM1 genes. Oral Oncol 2000; 236: 267–271
19. Liu S, Park JY, Schantz SP, Stern JC, Lazarus P. Elucidation of CYP2E1 5' regulatory RsaI/PstI allelic variants and their role in risk for oral cancer. Oral Oncol 2001; 37: 437–445
20. Topcu Z, Chiba I, Fujieda M et al. CYP2A6 gene deletion reduces oral cancer risk in betel quid chewers in Sri Lanka. Carcinogenesis 2002; 23: 595–598
21. Bouchardy C, Hirvonen A, Coutelle C, Ward PJ, Dayer P, Benhamou S. Role of alcohol dehydrogenase 3 and cytochrome P-4502E1 genotypes in susceptibility to cancers of the upper aerodigestive tract. Int J Cancer 2000; 87: 734–740
22. Summersgill KF, Smith EM, Kirchner HL, Haugen TH, Turek LP. P53 polymorphism, human papillomavirus infection in the oral cavity, and oral cancer. Oral Surg Oral med Oral Pathol Oral Radiol Endod 2000; 90: 334–339
23. Tandle AT, Sanghvi V, Saranath D. Determination of p53 genotypes in oral cancer patients from India. Br J Cancer 2001; 84: 739–742
24. Nomura T, Noma H, Shibahara T, Yokoyama A, Muramatusu T, Ohmori T. Aldehyde dehydrogenase 2 and glutathione S-transferase M 1 polymorphisms in relation to the risk for oral cancer in Japanese drinkers. Oral Oncol 2000; 36: 42–46
25. Sturgis EM, Dahlstrom KR, Guan Y et al. Alcohol dehydrogenase 3 genotype is not associated with risk of squamous cell carcinoma of the oral cavity and pharynx. Cancer Epidemiol Biomarkers Prev 2001; 10: 273–275
26. Schwartz SM, Doody DR, Fitzgibbons ED, Ricks S, Porter PL, Chen C. Oral squamous cell cancer risk in relation to alcohol consumption and alcohol dehydrogenase-3 genotypes. Cancer Epidemiol Biomarkers Prev 2001; 10: 1137–1144
27. Boffetta P, Gridley G, Gustavsson P et al. Employment as butcher and cancer risk in a record-linkage study from Sweden. Cancer Causes Control 2000; 11: 627–633
28. Pukkala E, Notkola V. Cancer incidence among Finnish farmers, 1979–93. Cancer Causes Control 1997; 8: 25–33
29. Wiklund K, Dich J. Cancer risks among male farmers in Sweden. Eur J Cancer Prev 1995; 4: 81–90
30. Antoniades DZ, Styanidis K, Papanayatou P, Trigonidis G. Squamous cell carcinoma of the lips in a northern Greek population: evaluation of prognostic factors on five year survival rate. Eur J Cancer B Oral Oncol 1995; 31B: 333–339
31. Sankaranarayanan R. Oral cancer in India: an epidemiological and clinical review. Oral Surg Oral Med Oral Pathol 1990; 69: 325–330
32. Pukkala E, Soderholm AL, Lindqvist C. Cancers of the lip and oropharynx in different social and occupational groups in Finland. Eur J Cancer Oral Oncol 1994; 30B: 209–215
33. Pogoda JM, Preston-Martin S. Solar radiation, lip protection, and lip cancer risk in Los Angeles county women. Cancer Causes Control 1996; 7: 458–463
34. Levi F, La Vecchia C, Te VC, Franceschi S. Trends in lip cancer incidence in Vaud, Switzerland. Br J Cancer 1993; 68: 1012–1013
35. Swerdlow AJ, Cooke KR, Skegg DC, Wilkinson J. Cancer incidence in England and Wales and New Zealand and in migrants between the two countries. Br J Cancer 1995; 75: 236–243
36. Wake M. The urban/rural divide in head and neck cancer—the effect of atmospheric pollution. Clin Otolaryngol 1993; 18: 298–302
37. Maier H, de Vries N, Weidauer H. Beruf und Krebs im Bereich von Mundhole, Pharynx und Larynx. HNO 1990; 38: 271–278
38. Dietz A, Senneweld E, Maier H. Indoor air pollution by emissions of fossil fuel single stoves: possibly a

hitherto underrated risk factor in the development of carcinomas in the head and neck. Otolaryngol Head Neck Surg 1995; 112: 308–315
39. Huebner WW, Schoenberg JB, Kelsey JL et al. Oral and pharyngeal cancer and occupation: a case–control study. Epidemiology 1992; 3: 300–309
40. Epstein JB. Management of oral Kaposi's sarcoma and a proposal for clinical staging. Oral Dis 1997; 3(Suppl 1): S124–S128
41. Jordan RCK, Chong L, DiPierdomenico S, Satita F, Main JHP. Oral lymphoma in HIV infection. Oral Dis 1997; 3(Suppl 1): S135–137
42. King GN, Healy CM, Glover MT et al. Increased prevalence of dysplastic and malignant lip lesions in renal transplant recipients. N Engl J Med 1995; 332: 1052–1057
43. de Visscher JG, Bouwes-Bavinck JN, van der Waal I. Squamous cell carcinoma of the lower lip in renal transplant recipients: report of six cases. Int J Oral Maxillofac Surg 1997; 26: 120–123
44. Winn DM. Tobacco use and oral disease. J Dent Educ 2001; 65: 306–312
45. Johnson N. Tobacco use and oral cancer: a global perspective. J Dent Educ 2001; 65: 328–339
46. Franceschi S, Talamani R, Barra S et al. Smoking and drinking in relation to cancers of the oral cavity, pharynx, larynx and esophagus in Northern Italy. Cancer Res 1990; 50: 6502–6507
47. Fioretti F, Bosetti C, Tavani A, Franceschi S, La Vecchia C. Risk factors for oral and pharyngeal cancer in never smokers. Oral Oncol 1999; 35: 375–378
48. Peto R, Lopez AD, Boreham J, Thun M, Heath C Jr, Doll R. Mortality from smoking worldwide. Br Med Bull, 1996; 52: 12–21
49. World Health Organization. Tobacco or health: a global status report. Geneva: WHO, 1997
50. Sullivan LW. Keynote address in: Smokeless tobacco or health. Monograph 2 on Smoking and Tobacco Control. NIH Pub No. 92–3461, Sept 1992: iii–vii
51. Doll R, Peto R, Wheatley K et al. Mortality in relation to smoking: 40 years observations on male British doctors. Br Med J 1994; 309: 901–911
52. Daftary DK, Murti PR, Bhonsle RB, Gupta PC, Mehta FS, Pindborg JJ. Risk factors and risk markers for oral cancer in high incidence areas of the world. In: Johnson NW (ed). Risk markers for oral diseases, vol 2. Oral cancer. Cambridge: Cambridge University Press, 1991: 29–63
53. Daftary DK, Murti PR, Bhonsle RB, Gupta PC, Mehta FS, Pindborg JJ. Oral squamous cell carcinoma. In: Prabhu R, Daftary DK, Wilson DF, Johnson NW (eds) Oral diseases in the tropics. Oxford: Oxford University Press, 1992: 429–448
54. Gupta PC, Hamner JE, Murti PR. Control of tobacco-related cancers and other diseases. Delhi: Oxford University Press, 1992
55. Mehta FS, Hamner JE. Tobacco-related oral mucosal lesions and conditions in India. New Delhi: Jaypee Brothers Medical Publishers, 1993
56. Idris, AM, Nair J, Oshima H, Friesen M, Bronet I, Faustman EM, Bartsch H. Carcinogen specific nitrosamines are present in unusually high levels in the saliva of oral snuff users in Sudan. Carcinogenesis 1992; 13: 1001–1005
57. Idris AM, Ahmed HM, Malik MAO. Toombak dipping and cancer of the oral cavity in the Sudan: a case-control study. Int J Cancer 1995; 63: 477–480
58. Idris AM, Warnakulasuriya KAAS, Johnson NW et al. 1998; personal communication.
59. Idris AM, Warnakulasuriya KAAS, Ibrahim YE, Nilsen R, Cooper D, Johnson NW. Toombak-associated oral mucosal lesions in Sudanese show a low prevalence of epithelial dysplasia. J Oral Pathol Med 1996; 25: 239–244
60. Zain R, Gupta PC, Warnakulasuriya S, Shrestha P, Ikeda N, Axell T. Oral lesions associated with betel quid and tobacco chewing habits. Oral Dis 1997; 3: 204–205
61. MacLennan R, Paissat D, Ring A, Thomas S. Possible aetiology of oral cancer in Papua New Guinea. P N G Med J 1985; 28: 3–8
62. Boucher BJ. Betel quid, smokeless tobacco and general health. In: Bedi R, Jones P (eds). Betel quid and tobacco chewing among the Bangladeshi community in the United Kingdom; usage and health issues. London: Centre for Transcultural Oral Health, 1995: 53–58
63. Bedi R, Jones P (eds). Betel quid and tobacco chewing among the Bangladeshi community in the United Kingdom; usage and health issues. London: Centre for Transcultural Oral Health, 1995: 89
64. Warnakulasuriya S, Peters TJ. Introduction: Biology, medical and socio-economic aspects of areca nut use. Addict Biol 2002; 7: 75–76
65. Paymaster JC. Some observations on oral and pharyngeal carcinomas in the State of Bombay. Cancer 1962; 15: 578–583
66. Hirayama T. An epidemiological study of oral and pharyngeal cancer in central and South East Asia. Bull WHO, 1966; 34: 441–469
67. Mehta FS, Gupta PC, Daftary DK, Pindborg JJ, Choksi SK. An epidemiologic study of oral cancer and precancerous conditions among 101,761 villagers in Maharashtra, India. Int J Cancer 1972; 10: 134–141
68. Reichart P. Oral cancer and precancer related to betel and *miang* chewing in Thailand: a review. J Oral Pathol Med 1995; 24: 241–243
69. Thomas S, Wilson A. A quantitative evaluation of the role of betel quid in oral carcinogenesis. Eur J Cancer Oral Oncol 1993; 29B: 265–271
70. Warnakulasuriya S. The role of betel quid in oral carcinogenesis. In: Bedi R, Jones P (eds). Betel quid and tobacco chewing among the Bangladeshi Community in the United Kingdom. London: Centre for Transcultural Oral Health, 1995: 61–69
71. Gupta PC, Mehta FS, Daftary DK et al. Incidence rates of oral cancer and natural history of oral precancerous lesions in a ten year follow up study of Indian villagers. Community Dent Oral Epidemiol 1980; 8: 287–333

72. Mehta FS. An intervention study of oral cancer and precancer in rural Indian populations: a preliminary report. Bull WHO 1982; 60: 441–446
73. Gupta PC, Murti PR, Bhonsle RB, Mehta FS, Pindborg JJ. Effect of cessation of tobacco use on the incidence of oral mucosal lesions in a ten year follow study of 12,212 users. Oral Dis 1995; 1: 54–58
74. Orr IM. Oral cancer in betel nut chewers in Travancore. Its aetiology, pathology and treatment. Lancet 1933; ii: 575–580
75. International Agency for Research on Cancer. Tobacco habits other than smoking; betel quid and areca nut chewing, and some related nitrosamines. IARC Monographs for the Evaluation of Carcinogenic Risks to Humans. Vol 37. Lyon: IARC, 1985
76. Maher R, Lee AJ, Warnakulasuriya KAAS, Lewis JA, Johnson NW. Role of areca nut in the causation of oral submucous fibrosis: a case-control study in Pakistan. J Oral Pathol Med 1994; 23: 65–69
77. Stich HF, Rosin MP, Brunnemann KD. Oral lesions, genotoxicity and nitrosamines in betel quid chewers with no obvious increase in oral cancer risk. Cancer Lett 1986; 31: 15–25
78. Ko YC, Chiang TA, Chang SJ, Hsieh SF. Prevalence of betel quid chewing habit in Taiwan and related socio-demographic factors. J Oral Pathol Med 1992; 21: 261–264
79. Shiu MN, Chen TH, Chang SH, Hahn LJ. Risk factors for leukoplakia and malignant transformation to oral cancer: a leukoplakia cohort in Taiwan. Br J Cancer; 82: 1871–1874
80. Atkinson L, Purohit R, Reay-Young P, Scott GC. Cancer reporting in Papua-New Guinea; 1958–1970 and 1971–78. National Cancer Institute Monograph No. 62, 1982: 65–71
81. Thomas S, Kearsley J. Betel quid and oral cancer: a review. Oral Oncol Eur J Cancer 1993; 29B: 251–255
82. MacLennan R, Paissat D, Ring A, Thomas S. Possible aetiology of oral cancer in Papua New Guinea. P N G Med J 1985; 28: 3–8
83. Stich HF, Stich W, Parida BB. Elevated frequency of micronucleated cells in the buccal mucosa of individuals at high risk for oral cancer: betel quid chewers. Cancer Lett 1982; 17: 125–134
84. Dave BJ, Trivedi AH, Adhhvaryu SD. Role of areca nut in the cause of oral cancers. Cancer 1992; 70: 1017–1023
85. van Wyk CW, Stander I, Padayachee A, Grobler-Rabie AF. The areca nut chewing habit and oral cancer in South African Indians. S Afr Med J 1992; 83: 425–429
86. Lu CT, Ho YY, Ho CS et al. A case-control study of oral cancer in Changhua County, Taiwan. J Oral Pathol Med 1996; 25: 245–248
87. Merchant A, Husain SS, Hosain M et al. Paan without tobacco: an independent risk factor for oral cancer. Int J Cancer 2000; 86; 128–131
88. Trivedy CR, Craig G, Warnakulasuriya S. The oral health consequences of chewing areca nut. Addict Biol 2002; 7: 115–125
89. Jin Y-T, Tsai S-T, Wong T-Y, Chen F-F, Chen RM-Y. Studies on promoting activity of Taiwan betel quid ingredients in hamster buccal pouch carcinogenesis. Oral Oncol Eur J Cancer 1996; 32B: 343–346
90. Lin LM, Chen YK, Lai DR, Huang YL, Chen HR. Cancer promoting effect of Taiwan betel quid in hamster buccal pouch carcinogenesis. Oral Dis 1997; 3: 232–235
91. Sundqvist K, Grafstrom RC. Effects of areca nut on growth, differentiation and formation of DNA damage in cultured human buccal epithelial cells. Int J Cancer 1992; 52: 305–310
92. van der Bijl P, van Eyk AD. Areca nut extract lowers the permeability of vaginal mucosa to reduced arecoline and arecaidine. J Oral Pathol med 2001; 30: 537–541
93. Sundqvist K, Liu Y, Erhardt P et al. Areca nut toxicity in cultured human buccal epithelial cells. Lyons: IARC Sci Pub 105: 281–285
94. Jeng JH, Chang MC, Hahn LJ. Role of areca nut in betal quid-associated chemical carcinogenesis: current awareness and future perspectives. Oral Oncol 2001; 37: 477–492
95. Nagabhushan M, Amonkar AJ, DeSouza AV, Bhide SV. Nonmutagenicity of betel leaf and its anti mutagenic action against environmental mutagens. Neoplasma 1987 34: 159–168
96. Brown RL, Shu JM, Scarborough JE, Wilkins SA, Smith RR. Snuff dipper's intraoral cancer: clinical characteristics and response to therapy. Cancer 1965; 18: 2–13
97. Ackerman LV. Verrucous carcinoma of the oral cavity. Surgery 1948; 23: 670–678
98. McCoy JM, Waldron CA. Verrucous carcinoma of the oral cavity. Oral Surg Oral Med Oral Pathol 1981; 52: 623–629
99. Blot WJ , Fraumeni JF. Geographic patterns of oral cancer in the United States: aetiologic implications. J Chronic Dis 1977; 30: 745–757
100. Winn DM, Blot W, Shy CM, Pickle LW, Toledo A, Fraumeni JF. Snuff dipping and oral cancer amongst women in the southern United States. New Engl J Med 1981; 304: 749–795
101. Winn DM. Smokeless tobacco and cancer: the epidemiological evidence. CA 1988; 38: 236–243
102. Connolly GN, Orleans CT, Kogan M. Use of smokeless tobacco in major league baseball. New Engl J Med 1998; 318: 1281–1285
103. US Department of Health and Human Services. The health consequences of using smokeless tobacco: a report of the advisory committee to the Surgeon General. Bethesda, Maryland: Public Health Service, National Institutes of Health. NIH Publication No. 86–2874, 1986
104. McCarten B. Smokeless tobacco: the Irish and EU experience. Oral Dis 1998; 4: 56–57
105. Grady D, Greene J, Daniels TE et al. Oral mucosal lesions found in smokeless tobacco users. J Am Dent Assoc 1990; 121: 117–123
106. Tomar SL, Winn DM, Swango PA, Giovino GA, Kleinman DV. Oral smokeless tobacco lesions among adolescents in the United States. J Dent Res 1997; 76: 1277–1286

107. Sterling TD, Rosenbaum WL, Weinkam JJ. Analysis of the relationship between smokeless tobacco and cancer based on data from the National Mortality Followback Survey. J Clin Epidemiol 1992; 42: 223–231
108. Rodu B. For smokers only: how smokeless tobacco can change your life. ISBN 0-945819-77–3. New York: Sulzberger and Graham, 1995
109. Idris AAM, Nair J, Oshima H et al. Unusually high levels of carcinogenic tobacco-specific nitrosamines in the Sudan snuff (toombak). Carcinogenesis 1991; 112: 1115–1118
110. Idris A, Prokopzyk B, Hoffman D et al. Toombak: A major risk factor for cancer of the oral cavity in the Sudan. Prevent Med 1994; 23: 832–839
111. Schildt E-B, Eriksson M, Hardell L, Magnuson A. Oral infections and dental factors in relation to oral cancer: a Swedish case-control study. Eur J Cancer Prev 1998; 7: 201–206
112. Lewin F, Norell SE, Johansson H et al. Smoking tobacco, oral snuff and alcohol in the aetiology of squamous cell carcinoma of the head and neck: a population based case-referent study in Sweden. Cancer 1998, 82: 1367–1375
113. Huhtasaari F, Asplund K, Lundberg V, Stegmyr B, Wester PO. Tobacco and myocardial infarction: is snuff less dangerous than cigarettes? Br Med J 1992; 305: 1252–1256
114. Bolinder G, Alfresson L, Englund A, de Faire U. Smokeless tobacco use and increased cardiovascular mortality. Am J Public Health 1994; 84: 399–404
115. Persson G, Hellers G, Ahlbom A. Use of moist snuff and inflammatory bowel disease. Int J Epidemiol 1993; 22: 1101–1103
116. Axell TE. Smokeless tobacco and oral health: The Swedish experience. Oral Dis 1998; 4: 55–56
117. Axell TE. Oral mucosal changes related to smokeless tobacco usage: research findings in Scandinavia. Eur J Cancer Oral Oncol 1993; 29B: 299–302
118. Daftary DK, Murti PR, Bhonsle RB, Gupta PC, Mehta FS, Pindborg JJ. Risk factors and risk markers for oral cancer in high incidence areas of the world. In: Johnson NW (ed.). Risk markers for oral disease. Vol 2. Oral cancer. Cambridge: Cambridge University Press, 1991: 29–63
119. Binnie WH. Risk factors and risk markers for oral cancer in low incidence parts of the world. In: Johnson NW (ed.). Risk markers for oral disease. Vol 2. Oral cancer. Cambridge: Cambridge University Press, 1991: 64–87
120. International Agency for Research on Cancer. Tobacco smoking. IARC Monographs on the evaluation of carcinogenic risks to humans. Vol 38. Lyon: IARC, 1986
121. Levin ML, Goldstein H, Gerhardt PR. Cancer and tobacco smoking. JAMA 1950; 143: 336–338
122. Wynder EL, Bross IJ, Feldman RM. A study of the aetiological factors in cancer of the mouth. Cancer 1957; 10: 1300–1323
123. Clemmesen J. Statistical studies in the aetiology of malignant neoplasms 1. Review and Results. Acta Pathol Microbiol Scand Suppl 1965; 174.
124. Spitzer WO, Hill GB, Chambers LW, Helliwell BE, Murphy HB. The occupation of fishing as a risk factor for cancer of the lip. New Engl J Med 1975; 293: 419–424
125. Wynder EL, Mushinski MH, Spivah JC. Tobacco and alcohol consumption in relation to the development of multiple primary cancers. Cancer 1977; 40: 1872–1878
126. Dikshit RP, Kanhere S. Tobacco habits and risk of lung, oropharyngeal and oral cavity cancer: a population-based case-control study in Bhopal, India. Int J Epidemiol 2000; 29: 609–614
127. Javonovich A, Schulten EAJM, Kostense PJ, Snow GB, van der Waal I. Tobacco and alcohol related to the anatomic site of oral squamous cell carcinoma. J Oral Pathol Med 1993; 22: 459–462
128. Blot WJ, McLaughlin JK, Winn DM et al. Smoking and drinking in relation to oral and pharyngeal cancer. Cancer Res 1988; 48: 3282–3287
129. Blot WJ. Alcohol and cancer. Cancer Res 1992; Suppl 52: 2119–2123
130. Mashberg A, Meyers H. Anatomical site and size of 222 early asymptomatic oral squamous cell carcinomas: a continuing prospective study of oral cancer II. Cancer 1976; 37: 2149–2157
131. Bofetta P, Mashberg A, Winkelmann R et al. Carcinogenic effect of tobacco smoking and alcohol drinking on anatomic sites of the oral cavity and oropharynx. Int J Cancer 1992; 52: 530–533
132. Gupta PC, Mehta FS, Daftary DK et al. Incidence rates of oral cancer and natural history of oral precancerous lesions in a 10-year follow up study of Indian villagers. Community Dent Oral Epidemiol 1980; 8: 287–333
133. van der Eb MM, Leyton EMS, Gavarasana S et al. Reverse smoking as a risk factor for palatal cancer: a cross sectional study in rural Andhra Pradesh, India. Int J Cancer 1993; 54: 754–758
134. Bhonsle RB, Murti PR, Gupta PC et al. Reverse dhumti smoking in Goa: an epidemiological study of 5449 villagers for oral precancerous lesions. Indian J Cancer 1976; 13: 301–305
135. Quigley LF, Shklar G, Cobb CM. Reverse cigarette smoking in Caribbeans: clinical, histologic and cytologic observations. J Am Dent Assoc 1966; 72: 867–873
136. Morrow RC, Suarez G. Mucosal changes and cancer in intraoral smoking. Laryngoscope 1971; 81: 1020–1031
137. Ortiz GM, Pierce AM, Wilson DF. Palatal changes associated with reverse smoking in Filipino women. Oral Dis 1996; 2: 232–237
138. Davidson BJ, Hsu TC, Schantz SP. The genetics of tobacco-induced malignancy. Arch Otolaryngol Head Neck Surg 1993; 119: 1198–1205
139. Hecht SS, Carmella SG, Murphy SE, Foiles PG, Chung F-L. Carcinogen biomarkers relating to smoking and upper aerodigestive tract cancer. J Cell Biochem 1993; Suppl 17F: 27
140. Hoffmann D, Hecht SS. Nicotine-derived *N*-nitrosamines and tobacco-related cancer: current status and future directions. Cancer Res 1985; 45: 935–944

141. Hoffmann D, Adams JD, Brunnemann KD, Hecht SS. Assessment of tobacco-specific *N*-nitrosamines in tobacco products. Cancer Res 1979; 39: 2505–2509
142. Lafuente A, Maristany M, Arias C et al. Glutathione and glutathione *S*-transferases in human squamous cell carcinomas of the larynx and GSTM1-dependent risk. Anticancer Res 1998; 18: 107–111
143. Hung HC, Chuang J, Chien YC et al. Genetic polymorphisms of CYP2E1, GSTM1 and GSTT1; environmental risk factors and risk of oral cancer. Cancer Epidemiol Biomarkers Prev 1997; 6: 901–905
144. Oude-Ophuis MB, van Leishout EM, Roelofs HM, Peters WH, Manni JJ. Glutathione *S*-transferase M1 and T1 and cytochrome p4501A1 polymorphisms in relation to the risk for benign and malignant head and neck lesions. Cancer 1998; 82: 936–943
145. Veneroni S, Silvistrini R, Costa A, Salvatori P, Faranda A, Molinari R. Biological indicators of survival in patients treated by surgery for squamous cell carcinoma of the oral cavity and oropharynx. Oral Oncol 1997; 33: 408–413
146. Nahas G, Latour C. The human toxicity of marijuana. Med J Aust 1993; 156: 495–497
147. Firth NA. Marijuana use and oral cancer: a review. Oral Oncol 1997; 6: 398–401
148. Wengen DF. Marijuana and malignant tumours of the upper aero-digestive tract in young patients. On the risk assessment of marijuana. Laryngorhinootologie 1993; 72: 264–267
149. Caplan GA, Brigham BA. Marijuana smoking and carcinoma of the tongue. Is there an association? Cancer 1990; 66: 1005–1006
150. Zhang Z-F, Morgenstern H, Spitz MR et al. Marijuana use and increased risk of squamous cell carcinoma of the head and neck. Cancer Epidemiol 1999; 8: 1071–1078
151. Darling MR. Arendorf TM. Effects of cannabis smoking on oral soft tissues. Community Dent Oral Epidemiol 1993; 21: 78–81
152. International Agency for Research on Cancer. Alcohol drinking. IARC monographs on the evaluation of carcinogenic risks to humans. Vol. 44. Lyon: IARC, 1988
153. Tuyns AJ. Alcohol and cancer. Proc Nutr Soc 1990; 49: 145–151
154. Kato I, Nomura AM. Alcohol in the aetiology of upper aero-digestive tract cancer. Eur J Cancer Oral Oncol 1994; 30B: 75–81
155. Balaram P, Sridhar H, Rajkumar T et al. Oral cancer in southern India: the influence of smoking, drinking, paan-chewing and oral hygiene. Int J Cancer 2002; 98: 440–445
156. Iype EM, Pandey M, Mathew A, Thomas G, Sebastian P, Nair MK. Oral cancer among patients under the age of 35 years. J Postgrad Med 2001; 47: 171–176
157. Hindle I, Downer MC, Moles DR, Speight PM. Is alcohol responsible for more intra-oral cancer? Oral Oncol 2000; 36: 328–333
158. Hindle I, Downer MC, Speight PM. The association between intra-oral cancer and surrogate markers of smoking and alcohol consumption. Community Dent Health 2000; 17: 107–113
159. Rothman KJ. The effect of alcohol consumption on risk of cancer of the head and neck. Laryngoscope 1978; 88: 51–55
160. Schecht NF, Pintos J, Kowalski LP, Franco EL. Effect of type of alcoholic beverage on the risks of upper aerodigestive tract cancers in Brazil. Cancer Causes Control 2001; 12: 579–587
161. Bundgaard T, Wildt J, Frydenberg M, Elbrond O, Nielsen JE. Case-control study of squamous cell cancer of the oral cavity in Denmark. Cancer Causes Control 1995; 6: 57–67
162. Merletti F, Boffetta P, Ciccone G, Mashberg A, Terracini B. Role of tobacco and alcoholic beverage in the aetiology of cancer of the oral cavity/oropharynx in Torino, Italy. Cancer Res 1989; 49: 4919–4924
163. Mashberg A, Boffetta P, Winkelmann R, Garfinkel L. Tobacco smoking, alcohol drinking, and cancer of the oral cavity and pharynx among US Veterans. Cancer 1993; 72: 1369–1375
164. Kabat GC, Wynder EL. Type of alcoholic beverage and oral cancer. Int J Cancer 1989; 43: 190–194
165. Andre K, Schraub S, Mercier M, Bontemps P. Role of alcohol and tobacco in the aetiology of head and neck cancer: a case-control study in the Doubs region of France. Eur J Cancer B Oral Oncol 1995; 31: 301–309
166. Franceschi S, Barra S, LaVecchia C, Bidoli E, Negri E, Talimini R. Risk factors for cancer of the tongue and the mouth. A case-control study from northern Italy. Cancer 1992; 70: 2227–2233
167. Barra S, Franceschi S, Negri E, Talamani R, La Vecchia C. Type of alcoholic beverage and cancer of the oral cavity, pharynx and oesophagus in an Italian area with high wine consumption. Int J Cancer 1990; 46: 1017–1020
168. Zheng TZ, Boyle P, Hu HF et al. Tobacco smoking, alcohol consumption, and risk of oral cancer: a case-control study in Beijing, People's Republic of China. Cancer Causes Control 1990; 1: 173–179
169. Boyle P, Macfarlane GJ, Blot WJ et al. European School of Oncology Advisory Report to the European Commission for the Europe Against Cancer Programme: oral carcinogenesis in Europe. Eur J Cancer B Oral Oncol 1995; 31: 75–85
170. Franceschi S, Talamani R, Barra S et al. Smoking and drinking in relation to cancers of the oral cavity, pharynx, larynx, and oesophagus in Northern Italy. Cancer Res 1990; 50: 6502–6507
171. La Vecchia C, Tavani A, Franceschi S, Levi F, Corrago G, Negri E. Epidemiology and prevention of oral cancer. Oral Oncol 1997; 33: 302–312
172. Brugere J, Guenel P, Leclerc A, Rodrigues J. Differential effects of tobacco and alcohol in cancer of the larynx, pharynx and mouth. Cancer 1986; 57: 391–395
173. Lesch CA, Squier CA, Cruchley A et al. The permeability of human oral mucosa and skin to water. J Dent Res 1989; 68: 1345–1349
174. Hsu TC, Furlong C, Spitz MR. Ethyl alcohol as a co-carcinogen with special reference to the aerodigestive

tract: a cytogenetic study. Anticancer Res 1991; 11: 1097–1102

175. Squier CA, Cox P, Hall BK. Enhanced penetration of nitrosonornicotine across oral mucosa in the presence of ethanol. J Oral Pathol 1986; 15: 276–279
176. Du X, Squier CA, Kremer MJ, Wertz PW. Penetration of N-nitrosonornicotine (NNN) across oral mucosa in the presence of ethanol and nicotine. J Oral Pathol Med 2000; 29: 80–85
177. Howie NM, Trigkas TK, Crichley AT, Wertz PW, Squier CA, Williams DM. Short-term exposure to alcohol increases the permeability of human oral mucosa. Oral Dis 2001; 7: 349–354
178. Trigkas TK, Cruchley AT, Williams DM, Wertz P, Squier CA. Human oral mucosal permeability is increased by short term exposure to ethanol. J Dent Res 1993; 72: 694
179. McCoy GD, Wynder EL. Etiological and preventive implications in alcohol carcinogenesis. Cancer Res 1979; 39: 2844–2850
180. Silverman S Jr, Shillitoe EH. Aetiology and predisposing factors. In: Silverman S Jr (ed.) Oral cancer. Atlanta: The American Cancer Society, 1990; 7–39
181. Squier CA, Kremer M, Wertz PW. Ingestion of ethanol increases epithelial permeability in the rat. J Dent Res 1995; 74: 476
182. Enwonwu CO, Meeks VI. Bionutrition and oral cancer in humans. Crit Rev Oral Biol Med 1995; 6: 5–17
183. Homann N, Tillonen J, Meurman JH et al. Increased salivary acetaldehyde levels in heavy drinkers and smokers: a microbiological approach to oral cavity cancer. Carcinogenesis 2000; 21: 663–668
184. Homann N, Tillonen J, Rintamaki H, Salaspuro M, Lindqvist C, Meurman JH. Poor dental status increases acetaldehyde production from ethanol in saliva: a possible link to increased oral cancer risk among heavy drinkers. Oral Oncol 2001; 37: 153–158
185. Moreno-Lopez LA, Esparza-Gomez GC, Gonzalez-Navarro A, Cerero-Lapiedra R, Gonzalez-Hernandez MJ, Dominguez-Rojas V. Risk of oral cancer associated with tobacco-smoking, alcohol consumption and oral hygiene: a case-control study in Madrid, Spain. Oral Oncol 2000; 36: 170–174
186. Homann N, Jousimies-Somer H, Jokelainen K, Heine R, Salaspuro M. High acetaldehyde levels in saliva after ethanol consumption: methodological aspects and pathogenetic implications. Carcinogenesis 1997; 18: 1739–1743
187. Chen C, Ricks S, Doody DR, Fitzgibbons ED, Porter PL, Schwartz SM. N-acetyltransferase 2 polymorphisms, cigarette smoking and alcohol consumption, and oral squamous cell cancer risk. Carcinogenesis 2001; 22: 1993–1999
188. Harris C, Warnakulasuriya KAAS, Gelbier S, Johnson NN, Peters TJ. Oral and dental health in alcohol misusing patients. Alcohol Clin Exp Res 1997; 21: 1707–1709
189. Boffetta P, Ye W, Adami HO, Nucci LA, Nyren O. Risk of cancers of the lung, head and neck in patients hospitalized for alcoholism in Sweden. Br J Cancer 2001; 85: 678–682
190. Weaver A, Fleming SM, Smith DB. Mouthwash and oral cancer: carcinogen or coincidence? J Oral Surg 1979; 37: 250–253
191. Blot W, Winn DM, Fraumeni JF. Oral cancer and mouthwash. J Natl Cancer Inst 1983; 70: 251–253
192. Wynder EL, Kabat G, Rosenberg S, Levenstein M. Oral cancer and mouthwash use. J Natl Cancer Inst 1983; 70: 255–260
193. Winn DM, Blot WJ, McLaughlin JK et al. Mouthwash use and oral conditions in the risk of oral and pharyngeal cancer. Cancer Res 1991; 51: 3044–3047
194. Johnson NW, Warnakulasuriya S. Alcohol in mouthwashes: a health hazard. Br Dent J 1994; 177: 124
195. Winn DM, Diehl SR, Brown LM et al. Mouthwash in the etiology of oral cancer in Puerto Rico. Cancer Causes Control 2001; 12: 419–429
196. Gagari E, Kabani S. Adverse effects of mouthwash use. Oral Surg Oral Med Oral Pathol Oral Radiol Endod 1995; 80: 432–439
197. Elmore JG, Horwitz RI. Oral cancer and mouthwash use: evaluation of the epidemiologic evidence. Otolaryngol Head Neck Surg 1995; 113: 253–261
198. Shapiro S, Castellana JV, Sprafka JM. Alcohol-containing mouthwashes and oropharyngeal cancer: a spurious association due to underascertainment of confounders? Am J Epidemiol 1996; 144: 1091–1095
199. Bhatti SA, Walsh TF, Douglas CWI. Ethanol and pH levels of proprietary mouthwashes. Community Dent Health 1994; 11: 71–74
200. Rich AM, Radden BG. Squamous cell carcinoma of the oral mucosa; a review of 244 cases in Australia. J Oral Pathol 1984; 13: 459–471
201. Hodge KM, Flynn MB, Drury T. Squamous cell carcinoma of the upper aerodigestive tract in nonusers of tobacco. Cancer 1985; 55: 1232–1235
202. Ng SKC, Kabat GC, Wynder EL. Oral cavity cancer in nonusers of tobacco. J Natl Cancer Inst 1993; 85: 743–745
203. Tan E-H, Adelstein DJ, Droughton MLT van Kirk MA, Lavertu P. Squamous cell head and neck cancer in non-smokers. Am J Clin Oncol 1997; 20: 146–150
204. Scully C. Viruses and oral squamous cell carcinoma. Eur J Cancer Oral Oncol 1992; 28B: 57–59
205. Syrjanen S. Viral infections in oral mucosa. Scand J Dent Res 1992; 100: 17–31
206. Vineis P, Brandt-Rauf PW. Mechanisms of carcinogenesis: chemical exposure and molecular changes. Eur J Cancer 1993; 29A: 1344–1347
207. Scully CS, Samaranayake LP. Clinical virology in oral medicine and dentistry. Cambridge: Cambridge University Press, 1992
208. Murphy FA. Virus taxonomy. In: Fields BN, Knipe DM, Howley PM (eds). Fundamental virology, 3rd edn. Philadelphia: Lippincot-Raven, 1996: 15–57
209. zur Hausen H. Human papillomaviruses in the pathogenesis of anogenital cancer. Virology 1991; 184: 9–13
210. Snijders PJF, Scholes AGM, Hart CA. Prevalence of

mucosatropic human papillomaviruses in squamous cell carcinomas of the head and neck. Int J Cancer 1996; 66: 464–469
211. Androphy EJ. Molecular biology of human papilloma virus infection and oncogenesis. J Invest Dermatol 1994; 103: 248–256
212. Eversole LR. Letter to the editor: Papillomaviruses and oral cancer. Oral Surg Oral Med Oral Pathol Oral Radiol Endod 1997; 83: 187–188
213. Bernard H-U, Apt D. Transcriptional control and cell type specificity of HPV gene expression. Arch Dermatol 1994; 130: 210–215
214. Bauer G. Interference of papilloma viruses with p53-dependent and -independent apoptotic pathways. Clues to viral oncogenesis (Review-hypothesis). Oncol Rep 1997; 4: 273–275
215. Sugerman PB, Shillitoe EJ. The high risk human papilloma viruses and oral cancer: evidence for and against a causal relationship. Oral Dis 1997; 3: 130–147
216. Lechner MS, Laimins LA. Inhibition of p53 DNA binding of human papillomavirus, E6 proteins. J Virol 1994; 68: 4262–4273
217. Chen Z, Storthz KA, Shillitoe EJ. Mutations in the long control region of human papillomavirus in oral cancer cells, and their functional consequences. Cancer Res 1997; 57: 1614–1619
218. Nagpal JK, Patnaik S, Das BR. Prevalence of high-risk human papilloma virus types and its association with P53 codon 72 polymorphism in tobacco addicted oral squamous cell carcinoma (OSCC) patients of Eastern India. Int J Cancer 2002; 97: 649–653
219. Woods KV, Shillitoe EJ, Spitz MR, Storthz K. Analysis of human papillomavirus DNA in oral squamous cell carcinomas. J Oral Pathol Med 1993; 22: 101–108
220. Mao EJ. Prevalence of human papillomavirus 16 and nucleolar organiser region counts in oral exfoliated cells from normal and malignant epithelia. Oral Surg Oral Med Oral Pathol 1995; 80: 320–329
221. Yeudall WA. Human papillomavirus and oral neoplasia. Eur J Cancer Oral Oncol 1992; 32B: 61–66
222. Park NH, Min BM, Li SL, Haung MZ, Cherrick HM, Doniger J. Immortalization of normal human oral keratinocytes with type 16 human papillomavirus. Carcinogenesis 1991; 12: 1627–1631
223. Sexton CJ, Proby CM, Banks L et al. Characterization of the factors involved in human papillomavirus type 16-mediated immortalization of oral keratinocytes. J Gen Virol 1993; 74: 755–761
224. Kim MS, Shin KH, Back JH, Cherrick HM, Park NH. HPV-16, tobacco-specific N-nitrosamine, and N-methyl-N-nitro-N-nitrosoguanidine in oral carcinogenesis. Cancer Res 1993; 53: 4811–4816
225. Shin K-H, Tannyhill RJ, Liu X, Park NH. Oncogenic transformation of HPV-immortalized human oral keratinocytes is associated with genetic instability of cells. Oncogene 1996; 12: 1089–1096
226. Penhallow J, Steingrimsdottir H, Elamin F et al. p53 alterations and HPV infections are common in oral SCC: p53 gene mutations correlate with the absence of HPV 16–E6 DNA. Int J Oncol 1998; 12: 59–68
227. Riethdorf S, Friedrich RE, Ostwald C et al. p53 gene mutations and HPV infection in primary head and neck squamous cell carcinomas do not correlate with overall survival: a long-term follow-up study. J Oral Pathol Med 1997; 26: 315–321
228. Chiba I, Shindoh M, Yasuda M et al. Mutations of the p53 gene and human papillomavirus infection as significant prognostic factors in squamous cell carcinomas of the oral cavity. Oncogene 1996; 12: 1663–1668
229. Miller CS, White DK. Human papillomavirus expression in oral mucosa, premalignant conditions, and squamous cell carcinoma. A retrospective review of the literature. Oral Surg Oral Med Oral Pathol Oral Radiol Endod 1996; 82: 57–68
230. Ogura H, Watanabe S, Fukushima K, Masuda Y, Fujiwara T, Yebe Y. Human papillomavirus DNA in squamous cell carcinomas of the respiratory and upper digestive tracts. Jap J Clin Oncol 1993; 23: 221–225
231. Yeudall WA, Paterson IC, Patel V, Prime SS. Presence of human papillomavirus sequence in tumour derived human oral keratinocytes expressing mutant p53. Eur J Cancer Oral Oncol 1995; 2: 136–143
232. Watts SL, Brewer EE, Fry TL. Human papillomavirus DNA types in squamous cell carcinomas of the head and neck. Oral Surg Oral Med Oral Pathol 1991; 71: 701–707
233. Elamin F, Steingrimsdottir H, Warnakulasuriya S, Johnson N, Tavassoli M. Prevalence of human papillomavirus infection in premalignant and malignant lesions of the oral cavity in UK subjects: a novel method of detection. Oral Oncol 1998; 34: 191–197
234. Miller CS, Johnstone BM. Human papillomavirus as a risk factor for oral squamous cell carcinoma: a meta-analysis, 1982–1997. Oral Surg Oral med Oral Pathol Oral Radiol Endod 2001; 91: 622–635
235. Giovanelli L, Campisi G, Lama A et al. Human papillomavirus DNA in oral mucosal lesions. J Infect Dis 2002; 185: 833–836
236. Nielsen H, Norrild B, Vedtofte P, Praetorius F, Reibel J, Holmstrup P. Human papillomavirus in oral premalignant lesions. Eur J Cancer Oral Oncol 1996; 32B: 264–270
237. Palefsky JM, Silverman SS, Abdel-Salaam M, Daniels TE, Greenspan JS. Association between proliferative verrucous leukoplakia and infection with human papillomavirus type 16. J Oral Pathol Med 1995; 24: 193–197
238. Warnakulasuriya S, Speight PM, Tavassoli M, Elamin F, Penhallow J, Johnson NW. Association between proliferative verrucous leukoplakia, p53 protein and HPV infection. Oral Dis 1997; 3(Suppl 1): S28
239. Ibrahim SO, Warnakulasuriya KAAS, Idris AM, Hirsch JM, Johnson NW, Johannessen AC. Expression of keratin 13, 14, and 19 in oral hyperplastic and dysplastic lesions from Sudanese and Swedish snuff-dippers: association with human papilloma virus infection. Anticancer Res 1998; 18: 635–645

240. Mao EJ, Schwartz SM, Daling JR, Oda D, Tickman L, Beckmann AAM. Human papilloma virus and p53 mutations in normal, premalignant and malignant oral epithelia. Int J Cancer (Prev Oncol) 1996; 69: 152–158
241. Haraf DJ, Nodzenski E, Brachman D et al. Human papilloma virus and p53 in head and neck cancer: clinical correlates and survival. Clin Cancer Res 1996; 2: 755–762
242. Snijders PFF, van den Brule AAJC, Meijer CJLM, Walboomers JMM. Papillomaviruses and cancer of the upper digestive and respiratory tracts. Curr Top Microbiol Immunol 1994; 186: 177–198
243. Paz IB, Cook N. Human papillomavirus (HPV) in head and neck cancer. An association of HPV 16 with squamous cell carcinoma of Waldeyer's tonsillar ring. Cancer 1997; 79: 595–604
244. Fouret P, Monceaux G, Temam S, Lacourreye L, St Guily JL. Human papillomavirus in head and neck squamous carcinomas in non-smokers. Arch Otolaryngol Head Neck Surg 1997; 123: S13–S16
245. McKaig RG, Baric RS, Olshan AF. Human papillomavirus and head and neck cancer: epidemiology and molecular biology. Head Neck 1998; 20: 260–265
246. Cruz IBF, Snijders PJF, Steenbergen RDM, Meijer CJCM, Snow GB, Walboomers JMM, van der Waal I. Age-dependence of human papillomavirus DNA presence in oral squamous cell carcinoma. Eur J Cancer Oral Oncol 1996; 32B: 55–62
247. Schwartz SR, Yueh B, McDougall JK, Daling JR, Schwartz SM. Human papillomavirus infection and survival in oral squamous cell cancer: a population-based study. Otolaryngol Head Neck Surg 2001; 125: 1–9
248. Turner JR, Sheen LH, Crum CP, Dean PJ, Odze RD. Low prevalence of human papillomavirus infection in esophageal squamous cell carcinomas from North America. Hum Pathol 1997; 28: 174–178
249. Ha PK, Pai SI, Westra WH et al. Real-time quantitative PCR demonstrates low prevalence of human papillomavirus type 16 in premalignant and malignant lesions of the oral cavity. Clin Cancer Res 2002; 8: 1203–1209
250. Chang F, Syrjanen S, Kellokoski J, Syrjanen K. Human papillomavirus (HPV) infections and their associations with oral disease. J Oral Pathol Med 1991; 20: 305–307
251. Swan RH, McDaniel RK, Dreiman BB, Rome WC. Condyloma acuminatum involving the oral mucosa. Oral Surg Oral Med Oral Pathol 1981; 51: 503–508
252. Adler-Storthz K, Newland JR, Tessin BA, Yeudall WA, Shillitoe EJ. Identification of human papillomavirus types in oral verruca vulgaris. J Oral Pathol 1986; 15: 230–233
253. Lamey P-J, Lewis MAO, Rennie JS, Beattie AD. Heck's disease. Br Dent J 1990; 168: 251–252
254. Pilgard G. Focal epithelial hyperplasia. Report of nine cases from Sweden and review of the literature. Oral Surg Oral Med Oral Pathol 1984; 57: 540–543
255. Fornatora M, Jones AC, Kerpel S, Freedman P. Human papillomavirus-associated oral epithelial dysplasia (koilocytic dysplasia). An entity of unknown biologic potential. Oral Surg Oral Med Oral Pathol Oral Radiol Endod 1996; 82: 47–56
256. EC-Clearing House on oral problems related to HIV infection and WHO Collaborating Centre on oral manifestations of the immunodeficiency virus. Classification and diagnostic criteria for oral lesions in HIV infection. J Oral Pathol Med 1993; 22: 289–291
257. Schiodt M. Less common oral lesions associated with HIV infection: prevalence and classification. Oral Dis 1997; 3: S208–S213
258. Shiboski CH, Hilton JF, Greenspan D et al. HIV-related oral manifestations in two cohorts of women in San Francisco. J Acquir Immune Defic Syndr 1994; 7: 964–971
259. Lamster IB, Begg MD, Mitchell-Lewis D et al. Oral manifestations of HIV infection homosexual men and intravenous drug users. Oral Surg 1994; 78: 163–174
260. Park NH, Sapp JP, Herbosa EG. Oral cancer induced in hamsters with herpes simplex infection and simulated snuff-dipping. Oral Surg Oral Med Oral Pathol 1986; 62: 164–168
261. Larsson PA, Johansson SL, Vahlne A, Hirsch JM. Snuff tumorigenesis: effects of long term snuff administration after initiation with 4-nitroquinoline N-oxide and herpes simplex virus type 1. J Oral Pathol Med 1989; 18: 187–192
262. Park K, Cherrick H, Min B-M, Park NH. Active HSV-1 immunization prevents the co-carcinogenic activity of HSV-1 in the oral cavity of hamsters. Oral Surg Oral Pathol Oral Med 1990; 70: 186–191
263. Larsson PA, Edstrom S, Westin T, Nordkrist A, Hirsch JM, Vahle A. Reactivity against herpes simplex virus in patients with head and neck cancer. Int J Cancer 1991; 49: 14–18
264. Eskinazi DP, Cantin EM. Monoclonal antibodies to HSV-infection-related antigens cross-react with tumour cell lines and tumour tissue sections. Oral Surg Oral Med Oral Pathol 1988; 65: 308–315
265. Eglin RP, Scully C, Lehner T, Ward-Booth P, McGregor IA. Detection of RNA complementary to herpes simplex virus DNA in human oral squamous cell carcinoma. Lancet 1983; ii: 766–768
266. de The G. The Epstein–Barr virus in neoplasms of the head and neck. In: Johnson NW (ed.) Oral cancer: detection of patients and lesions at risk. Cambridge: Cambridge University Press, 1991: 88–95
267. Shapira J, Peylan-Ramu N. Burkitt's lymphoma. Oral Oncol 1998; 34: 15–23
268. Talacko AA, Teo CG, Griffin BE, Johnson NW. Epstein–Barr virus receptors but not viral DNA are present in normal and malignant oral epithelium. J Oral Pathol Med 1991; 20: 20–25
269. Boulter A, Johnson NW, Birnbaum W, Teo CG. Epstein–Barr virus (EBV) associated lesions of the head and neck. Oral Dis 1996; 2: 117–124
270. D'Costa J, Saranath D, Sanghvi V, Mehta AR. Epstein–Barr virus in tobacco-induced oral cancers and oral lesions from India. J Oral Pathol Med 1998; 27: 78–82

271. Cruchley AT, Williams DM, Niedobitek G, Young LS. Epstein–Barr virus: biology and disease. Oral Dis 1997; 3 (Suppl 1): S156–S163
272. Raab-Traub N, Webster-Cyriaque J. Epstein–Barr virus infection and expression in oral lesions. Oral Diseases 1997; 3 (Suppl 1): S164–S170
273. Palefsky JM, Penaranda M-E, Pierik LT et al. Epstein–Barr virus BMRF-2 and BDLF-3 expression in hairy leukoplakia. Oral Dis 1997, 3(Suppl 1): S171–S176
274. Yadav M, Arivanathan M, Chandrashekran A, Tan BS, Hashim BY. Human herpes virus-6 (HHV-6) DNA and virus-encoded antigen in oral lesions. J Oral Pathol Med 1997; 26: 391–401
275. Boshoff C, Whitby D, Talbot S, Weiss RA. Etiology of AIDS-related Kaposi's sarcoma and lymphoma. Oral Dis 1997; 3(Suppl 1): S129–S132
276. Di Alberti L, Porter SR, Speight PM et al. Detection of human herpesvirus-8 DNA in oral ulcer tissues of HIV-infected individuals. Oral Dis 1997; 3(Suppl 1): S133–S144
277. Porter SR, Di Alberti L, Kumar N. Human herpes virus 8 (Kaposi's sarcoma herpesvirus). Oral Oncol 1998; 34: 5–14
278. Nagao Y, Sata M, Tanikawa K, Itoh K, Kameyama T. High prevalence of hepatitis C virus antibody and RNA in patients with oral cancer. J Oral Pathol Med 1995; 24: 354–360
279. Carrozzo M, Carbone M, Gandolfo S et al. An atypical verrucous carcinoma of the tongue arising in a patient with oral lichen planus associated with hepatitis C virus infection. Oral Oncol 1997; 33: 220–225
280. Ishido S, Muramatsu S, Fujita T et al. Wild-type but not mutant-type p53 enhances nuclear accumulation of the NS3 protein of Hepatitis C virus. Biochem Biophys Res Commun 1997; 230: 431–436
281. Rindum JL, Stenderup A, Holmstrup P. Identification of *Candida albicans* types related to healthy and pathological oral mucosa. J Oral Pathol Med 1994; 23: 406–412
282. Barrett AW, Kingsmill VJ, Speight PM. The frequency of fungal infection in biopsies of oral mucosal lesions. Oral Dis 1998; 4: 26–31
283. Arendorf TM, Walker DM. Tobacco smoking and denture wearing as local aetiological factors in median rhomboid glossitis. Int J Oral Surg 1984; 13: 411–415
284. Galai N, Park LP, Wesch J, Visscher B, Riddler S, Margolick JB. Effect of smoking on the clinical progression of HIV-1 infection. J Acquire Immune Def Syndr Hum Retrovirol 1997; 14: 451–458
285. Palmer GD, Robinson PG, Challacombe SJ et al. Aetiological factors for oral manifestations of HIV. Oral Dis 1996; 2: 193–197
286. Krogh P, Hald B, Holmstrup P. Possible mycological aetiology of oral mucosal carcinoma: catalytic potential of infecting Candida albicans and other yeasts in the production of *N*-nitroso-benzylmethylamine. Carcinogenesis 1987; 8: 1543–1548
287. Rennie JS, MacDonald DG. Cell kinetics of hamster ventral tongue epithelium in iron deficiency. Arch Oral Biol 1984; 29: 195–199
288. Ranasinghe AW, Johnson NW, Scragg MA. Iron deficiency depresses cell proliferation in hamster cheek pouch epithelium. Cell Tissue Kinet 1987; 20: 403–412
289. Ranasinghe AW, Johnson NW, Scragg MA, Williams RA. Iron deficiency reduces cytochrome concentrations of mitochondria isolated from hamster cheek pouch epithelium. J Oral Pathol Med 1989; 18: 582–585
290. Prime SS, MacDonald DG, Rennie JS. The effect of iron deficiency on experimental carcinogenesis in the rat. Br J Cancer 1983; 47: 413–418
291. Ranasinghe AW, Warnakulasuriya KAAS, Tennekoon GE, Seneviratne B. Oral mucosal changes in iron deficiency anaemia in a Sri Lankan female population. Oral Surg Oral Med Oral Pathol 1983; 55: 29–32
292. La Vecchia C, Tavani A. Fruit and vegetables and human cancer. Eur J Cancer Prev 1998; 7: 3–8
293. Block G, Patterson B, Subar A. Fruit, vegetables and cancer prevention: a review of the epidemiological evidence. Nutr Cancer 1992; 18: 1–29
294. Potter JD, Steinmetz K. Vegetables, fruit and phytoestrogens as preventive agents. In: Stewart BW, McGregor D, Kleihues O (eds). Principles of Chemo-prevention. IARC Sci Pub No. 139. Lyon, 1992: 61–90
295. Winn DM. Diet and nutrition in the etiology of oral cancer. Am J Clin Nutr 1995; 61: 437S–445S
296. McLaughlin JK, Gridley G, Block G et al. Dietary factors in oral and pharyngeal cancer. J Natl Cancer Inst 1988; 80: 1237–1243
297. Takezaki T, Hirose K, Inoue M et al. Tobacco, alcohol and dietary intake factors associated with the risk of oral cancer among Japanese. Jap J Cancer Res 1996; 87: 555–562
298. Oreggia F, de Stefani E, Correa P, Fierro L. Risk factor for cancer of the tongue in Uruguay. Cancer 1991; 67: 180–183
299. Franco EL, Kowalski LP, Oliveira BV et al. Risk factors for oral cancer in Brazil: a case-control study. Int J Cancer 1989; 43: 992–1000
300. Zheng T, Boyle P, Willett WC et al. A case-control study of oral cancer in Beijing, People's Republic of China. Associations with nutrient intakes, foods and food groups. Eur J Cancer Oral Oncol 1993; 29B: 45–55
301. Tavani A, Gallus S, La Vecchia C et al. Diet and risk of oral and pharyngeal cancer. An Italian case-control study. Eur J Cancer Prev 2001; 10: 191–195
302. Zheng TZ, Boyle P, Hu HF. Dentition, oral hygiene, and risk of oral cancer: a case-control study in Beijing, People's Republic of China. Cancer Causes Control 1990; 1: 235–241
303. Velly AM, Franco EEL, Schlecht N et al. Relationship between dental factors and risk of upper aerodigestive tract cancer. Oral Oncol 1998; 34: 284–291
304. Lockhart PB, Norris CM, Pulliam C. Dental factors in the genesis of squamous carcinoma of the oral cavity. Oral Oncol 1998; 34: 133–139
305. Llewellyn CD, Johnson NW, Warnakulasuriya KA. Risk

factors for squamous cell carcinoma of the oral cavity in young people — a comprehensive review. Oral Oncol 2001; 37: 401–418
306. Llewellyn CD, Linklater K, Bell J, Johnson NW, Warnakulasuriya KAAS. Squamous cell carcinoma of the oral cavity in patients aged 45 years and under: a descriptive analysis of 116 cases diagnosed in the South East of England from 1990–1997. Oral Oncol 2002: in press
307. Llewellyn CD, Linklater K, Bell J, Johnson NW, Warnakulasuriya KAAS. Risk factors for oral cancer in young people: a case-control study of subjects aged under 45 years from southern England. Int J Cancer 2002: submitted
308. Talamini R, Vaccarella S, Barbone F et al. Oral hygiene, dentition, sexual habits and risk of oral cancer. Br J Cancer 2000; 83: 1238–1242
309. Scully C. Oral squamous cell carcinoma; from a hypothesis about a virus, to concern about possible sexual transmission. Oral Oncol 2002; 38: 227–234
310. Banoczy J, Gintner Z, Dombi C. Tobacco use and oral leukoplakia. J Dent Educ 2001; 65: 322–327
311. Schepman KP, Bezemer PD, van der Meij EH, Smeele LE, van der Waal I. Tobacco usage in relation to the anatomical site of oral leukaplakia. Oral Dis 2001; 7: 24–27
312. Hashibe M, Sankaranarayanan R, Thomas G et al. Alcohol drinking, body mass index and the risk of oral leukoplakia in an Indian population. Int J Cancer 2000; 88: 129–134
313. Jaber MA, Porter SR, Gilthorpe MS, Bedi R, Scully C. Risk factors for oral epithelial dysplasia — the role of smoking and alcohol. Oral Oncol 1999; 35: 151–156
314. Hashibe M, Mathew B, Kuruvilla B et al. Chewing tobacco, alcohol and risk of erythroplakia. Cancer Epidemiol Biomarkers Prev 2000; 9: 639–645
315. Sankaranarayanan R, Duffy SW, Day NE, Nair MK, Padmakumary G. A case control investigation of cancer of the oral tongue and the floor of the mouth in Southern India. Int J Cancer 1989; 44: 617–621
316. Sankaranarayanan R, Duffy SW, Padmakumary G, Day NE, Nair MK. Risk factors for cancer of the buccal and labial mucosa in Kerala, southern India. J Epidemiol Community Health 1990; 44: 286–292
317. Sankaranarayanan R, Duffy SW, Padmakumary G, Day NE, Padmanabhan TK. Tobacco chewing, alcohol and nasal snuff in cancer of the gingiva in Kerala, India. Br J Cancer 1989; 60: 638–643
318. Notani PN. Role of alcohol in cancers of the upper alimentary tract, use of models in risk assessment. J Epidemiol Community Health 1988; 42: 187–192
319. Jussawalla DJ, Deshpande VA. Evaluation of the risk in tobacco chewers and smokers, an epidemiologic assessment. Cancer 1971; 28: 244–252
320. Jafarey NH, Zaidi SH. Carcinoma of the oral cavity and oropharynx in Karachi, Pakistan. An appraisal. Trop Doct 1976; 6: 63–67
321. Hirayama T. An epidemiological study of oral and pharyngeal cancer in central and southeast Asia. Bull WHO 166; 34: 41–69
322. Shanta V, Krishnamurti S. Further studies on the aetiology of carcinomas of the upper alimentary tract. Br J Cancer 1963; 17: 8–23
323. Chandra A. Different habits and their relation with cancer of the cheek. Chittaranjan Cancer Hospital Calcutta Natl Cancer Research Centre Bull 1962; 33–36
324. Sanghvi LD, Rao KCM, Khanolkar VR. Smoking and chewing of tobacco in relation to cancer of the upper alimentary tract. Br Med J 1955; 1: 1111–1114
325. Simarak S, de Jong UW, Breslow N et al. Cancer of the oral cavity, pharynx/larynx and lung in North Thailand, case-control study and analysis of cigar smoke. Br J Cancer 1977; 36: 130–140
326. Wahi PN, Kehar U, Lahiri B. Factors influencing and oropharyngeal cancers in India. Br J Cancer 1965; 19: 642–660
327. Shanta V, Krishnamurti S. A study of aetiological factors in oral squamous cell carcinomas. Br J Cancer 1959; 13: 381–388
328. Khanolkar VR. Oral cancer in India. Unio Int Contra Cancrum Acta 1959; 15: 67–77
329. Khanna NN, Pant GC, Tripathi FM, Sanyal B, Gupta S. Some observations on the aetiology of oral cancer. Indian J Cancer 1975; 12: 77–83
330. Orr IM. Oral cancer in betel nut chewers in Travancore, its aetiology, pathology and treatment. Lancet 1933; 2: 575–580
331. Sarma SN. A study into the incidence and aetiology of cancer of the larynx and adjacent parts in Assam. Indian J Med Res 1958; 46: 525–533

3 Clinical pathology of oral cancer

John G Batsakis

Introduction

Of the 52 228 histologically diagnosed cancers of the upper aerodigestive tract reported to the Surveillance, Epidemiology, and End Results (SEER) program of the National Cancer Institute for the years 1973–87, 44.5% were in the oral cavity. Of all other subsites in the aerodigestive tract, only the frequency of occurrence in the larynx exceeded that in oral cavity sites (Table 3.1).[1]

Because of the great numerical dominance of squamous cell carcinoma, the term oral cancer is nearly synonymous with squamous cell carcinoma (Fig. 3.1). In the oral cavity the tongue has been the most common site of origin, followed closely by the floor of the mouth. In an extensive survey of 6181 intra-oral squamous cell carcinomas in Connecticut,

Table 3.1 Cancer of the upper aerodigestive tract: SEER data (1973–1987). (Modified from Muir and Weiland[1])

Anatomic site	Cases (*n*)	Cases (%)
Larynx	14 484	27.7
Tongue	6 745	12.9
Gum/mouth	5 915	11.3
Lip	5 425	10.4
Floor of mouth	4 092	7.8
Hypopharynx	3 432	6.6
Tonsil	3 419	6.5
Major salivary gland	2 913	5.6
Nasopharynx	1 908	3.7
Nose, nasal cavity, middle ear	1 887	3.6
Other oral cavity/pharynx	1 081	2.1
Total	52 228	100.0

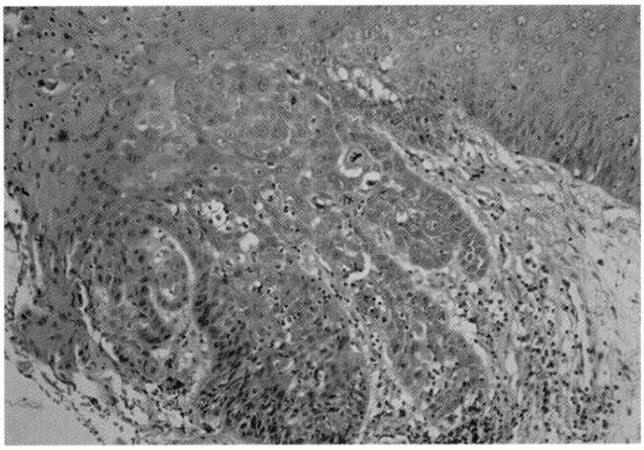

Figure 3.1 Invasive, moderately differentiated squamous cell carcinoma of the buccal mucosa.

moderately differentiated carcinomas were the most common (54.3%), followed by well-differentiated (29.1%) and poorly differentiated carcinomas (16.6%). The oral subsite distribution in the Connecticut study (Table 3.2)[2] is not unlike that

Table 3.2 Intraoral squamous cell carcinoma: Connecticut 1935–85. (Modified from Chen et al.[2])

Intra-oral site	Cases (*n*)	Cases (%)
Tongue	2546	41.2
Floor of mouth	1493	24.2
Palate	682	11.0
Gingiva	572	9.3
Buccal mucosa	375	6.1
Retromolar area	166	2.7
Miscellaneous	347	5.6

Table 3.3 Oral squamous cell carcinoma (n = 740). (Modified from Jovanovic et al.[3])

Site	Male	Female	M/F Ratio
Lower lip	50	6	8.3
Upper lip	1	–	–
Commissure	1	1	1
Tongue	138	108	1.3
Upper alveolar ridge	10	11	0.9
Lower alveolar ridge	31	25	1.2
Floor of mouth	140	59	2.4
Buccal	26	27	1.0
Retromolar	60	20	3.0
Hard palate	8	5	1.6
Multiple (lips and oral cavity)	8	5	1.6
	473	267	1.8

Table 3.4 Oral squamous cell carcinomas: Memorial Sloan–Kettering Cancer Center. (Modified from Shah et al.[4])

Oral site	Carcinomas	
	(n)	(%)
Oral tongue	182	36
Floor of mouth	162	33
Gum	104	21
Retromolar trigone	26	5
Buccal mucosa	26	5
Hard palate	1	
Total	501	100

Table 3.5 Sites of early asymptomatic oral squamous cell carcinomas (n = 222). (Summarized from Mashberg and Meyers[6])

Oral site	Percentage of oral carcinoma
Floor of mouth	45.5
Oral tongue	16.5
Soft palate	13.5
Anterior pillar	10.0
Lip	6.7
Retromolar trigone (lingual aspect)	5.4
Alveolar ridge	1.3
Buccal mucosa	1.0
Hard palate	0.5

published from the Free University Hospital, Amsterdam, The Netherlands (Table 3.3)[3] and Memorial Sloan–Kettering Cancer Center (Table 3.4).[4]

Intra-oral squamous cell carcinoma has a relatively unfavorable prognosis, with an overall 5-year survival rate of 35–50%. The survival rate has, regrettably, remained virtually unchanged over the past three decades and the increase in the incidence of oral cancer accentuates this mortality from the cancer.

The untreated patient with an extensive carcinoma is doomed to an early death. Stell and associates[5] specifically reviewed patients not treated for their squamous cell carcinomas of the head and neck: the commonest reason for not treating the patients was that the carcinoma was too extensive (55%); a further 36% were too old or too infirm to be considered for radical treatment, and 9% of patients refused treatment. The proportion of patients untreated varied according to the site of the primary neoplasm, 25% of pharyngeal tumors being the highest proportional representation. Of 362 patients with oral cavity carcinomas, 54 were in the untreated cohort, with the tongue the leading primary site. The median survival time for all untreated patients was 88 days, but it varied according to the site of the tumor (larynx, 78 days; pharynx, 93 days; oral cavity, 101 days). Untreated patients usually die of complicating respiratory infection. Tumor factors do not significantly affect the survival time in those patients for whom prognosis is predetermined.

The fact that the majority of the untreated patients had too extensive a malignancy is a reflection of late detection, patient neglect and the sometimes asymptomatic character of the carcinomas. Table 3.5 lists the oral subsites of early and asymptomatic squamous cell carcinomas.[6]

With the foregoing serving as preamble to the pathology of oral cancer, a clinicopathologic overview of squamous cell carcinoma at various oral subsites follows. The overview prepares the reader for the appreciation that oral squamous cell carcinoma is not just one disease: there are, besides subsite differences, different precursor lesions and histologic varieties of squamous cell carcinoma (see Chapter 4), each with their own biologic causes and responsiveness to therapy.

The pathology of oral cancer is also not limited to squamous cell carcinomas and their prognostic

Table 3.6 Type of oral mucosa

Type and thickness	Distribution in oral cavity
I. Non-keratinized (lining mucosa) 0.1–0.5 mm	Lips, cheek, vestibular fornix, alveolar mucosa, floor of mouth, ventral tongue, soft palate
II. Ortho/parakeratinized (masticatory mucosa) 0.25 mm	Hard palate, gingiva, filiform papillae of tongue
III. Specialized 0.2–0.9 mm	Dorsal tongue, soft palate; near the palatoglossal folds

factors: it includes lesions with differential diagnostic importance, both mucosal and salivary in origin. These are addressed in the following pages, as is the burgeoning field of molecular pathology (Chapter 5).

Oral squamous cell carcinoma: an overview

Histology of the oral mucosa

The mucosa of the oral cavity is composed of a stratified squamous epithelium and a lamina propria of fibrovascular connective tissue. When the mucosa lies directly on bone, it is called a mucoperiosteum. Elsewhere, there is a submucosa containing fibroadipose tissue and intraoral salivary glands.

In general, masticatory mucosa (attached gingiva and palate) is keratinized; the lining mucosa, which does not overlie bone and has no exceptional functional requirements, is normally not keratinized (Table 3.6). Non-keratinized epithelium has only a basal layer of cells and a stratum spinosum; keratinized epithelium has a stratum corneum of either ortho- or parakeratin. Orthokeratinization is a complete keratinization in which individual keratinocytes are fully keratinized and lose nuclei; parakeratin still retains small, pyknotic nuclei. Orthokeratin is also associated with well-developed keratohyalin granules, the stratum granulosum.

Mitotic activity in the epithelium is found mostly in the basal layer and clustered at the bases of epithelial ridges. Non-keratinized regions of the oral cavity have a higher turnover rate than do parakeratinized or keratinized regions. Approximately 10% of cells in the epithelium are not keratinocytes but are melanocytes, Merkel cells or Langerhans cells. Inflammatory cells also migrate through the epithelium.[7]

Separating the epithelium of the oral mucosa from its subjacent connective tissue is an epithelially derived component, the basal lamina. This consists of lamina lucida and a type IV collagen-containing lamina densa and the lamina reticularis, the collagen network embedded in a glycoprotein matrix produced by connective tissue. The epithelial–connective tissue interface is convoluted, with the degree of convolution a function of the amount of stress to which the mucosa is exposed.[7]

Oral cavity subsites

The lip

The oral labial surface begins at the junction of the vermilion border with the skin and includes only the vermilion surface. The commissures of the oral cavity join the upper and lower lips. The lymphatic drainage of the upper lip may be richer than that of the lower lip. Flow is inferior and frequently bilateral to submental, submandibular, and then to jugulodigastric and other deep jugular nodes.

Carcinoma of the lip is one of the most common malignancies in the head and neck. Excluding non-melanotic skin cancer, carcinoma of the lip accounts for about 12% of all head and neck malignancies, as well as 21.5% of oral cavity cancer.[8] Preponderantly a neoplasm of White men, 50–80 years of age, squamous cell carcinoma of the lips is uncommon in women; less than 15% of patients are younger than 40 years of age.

There is considerable predilection for the lower lip, with 85–95% of all labial carcinomas arising there. The upper lip is the primary site in 2–7% and the commissures in 1–4% of all cases.[9] The exposed vermilion border about halfway between the midline and the commissures is the favored spot in the lower lip; a midline presentation is the preponderant one in the upper lip.

Somewhat less than 50% of the squamous cell carcinomas will have an associated keratotic leukoplakia and/or actinic cheilitis. The great majority (85%) of the carcinomas are well differentiated. The typical squamous cell carcinoma presents as a persistent,

Table 3.7 Cancer of the lips in 1036 patients with 1047 lip cancers. (Modified from data presented by Zitsch et al.[9])

Clinical/pathologic feature	Patients	
	(*n*)	(%)
Sex of patients		
Male	1002	97
Female	34	3
Labial site		
Lower lip	1001	95.6
Upper lip	39	3.7
Commissure	7	0.7
Size of primary		
< 1 cm	312	30
< 2 cm	445	43
< 3 cm	138	12
< 4 cm	49	5
> 4 cm	62	6
Not stated	41	4
Histologic diagnosis		
Squamous cell carcinoma	1001	96
Basal cell carcinoma	11	1
Other	35	3
Level of differentiation of squamous cell carcinoma		
Well	705	70
Moderate	171	17
Poor	24	2
Undifferentiated	45	5
Unknown	56	6

non-healing ulcer or as an exophytic tumor of a relatively short duration, e.g. 6 months. Any mucosal lesion of the lip that does not heal within 2 weeks with appropriate treatment should be biopsied.

At the time of presentation, three-quarters of the carcinomas are less than 2 cm in major dimension. Table 3.7 gives the clinicopathologic characteristics of 1036 lip cancer patients who had a total of 1047 lip cancers.[9]

Extensions from the primary are to the skin of the lip, other areas of the lip mucosa and bone. Only 10–15% or less of patients in the United States have metastases to the cervical lymph nodes at the first presentation to a physician;[8,9] an additional 5–10% will develop this morbid event during the course of the disease.[8] Frequency of nodal metastases correlates with T classification, histologic grade, subsite of involvement and local recurrence. Commissural carcinomas are more aggressive in the USA, with a behavior akin to buccal carcinomas. Recurrences after first excision range from 5% to 20%, with most appearing within 2 years. Infraclavicular dissemination is not common (< 2%).[8,9]

There is an overall 5-year survival of approximately 90%, but cancer of the lip can, and does, kill. Local recurrence has been associated with a determinate survival of 78%, whereas patients having regional recurrences have a survival rate of approximately 50%.[8]

A poor outlook is associated with the following: (1) carcinoma size greater than 2 cm, (2) occurrence on the upper lip or commissures, (3) poor differentiation, (4) perineural invasion, (5) invasion of the mandible, (6) metastasis to cervical lymph nodes, and (7) occurrence in subjects less than 40 years of age.

Mobile tongue (anterior two-thirds)

The anterior two-thirds of the tongue extends from the line of the circumvallate papillae to the undersurface of the tongue at its junction with the floor of mouth. It can be subdivided into tip, lateral borders, dorsum, and ventral surfaces. It is drained primarily by lymphatics coursing inferiorly through the sublingual area and submandibular lymph nodes and posteriorly to the midanterior jugular chain and subdigastric nodes.

Up to 75% of the squamous cell carcinomas of the tongue arise in its mobile part. The carcinomas are no less dangerous than posterior-tongue cancers: that base-of-tongue carcinomas are discovered at a later stage of disease probably is the source of the misconception that base-of-tongue carcinoma is a more lethal disease.[10,11] Although it is found more often in men who are between 50 and 80 years of age, the carcinoma is increasing in frequency in females and younger patients.

The typical carcinoma of the anterior tongue presents as a painless, indurated ulcer on the lateral border. This area is the preponderant site of origin, accounting for three-quarters of the carcinomas. The ventral surface is second in order of frequency with 12–15% of cases, followed by the dorsum (5–7%), and the tip, with 2–3%.[12]

Besides the possibility of overdiagnosis of a granular cell tumor with pseudoepitheliomatous hyperplasia, one has to also consider median rhomboid glossitis in the differential diagnosis of a squamous cell carcinoma of the dorsum of the tongue.[13] This is especially so if biopsy specimens are small or embedded and cut tangentially.

Median rhomboid glossitis is an ovoid-to-rhomboid area on the dorsum of the tongue just in front of the sulcus terminalis. It may be flat or raised, devoid of papillae and slightly purple in color; the surface may be smooth or lumpy; it is usually asymptomatic. The histopathology consists of epithelial parakeratosis and acanthosis with tubular, often branching, ridges. Candidal organisms are often present and the lesion represents a form of chronic candidiasis. There is a subepithelial lymphoid cell infiltration and frequently a supramuscular sclerosis. There have been rare reports of malignant change occurring in median rhomboid glossitis, but the lesion is histologically and clinically benign.

Squamous cell carcinomas of the mobile tongue are most often well- to moderately-well-differentiated. Small localized lesions should be very amenable to cure with either radiation or surgery. Too many stage I and II cancers are, in fact, pathological stage III because of their preoperatively undefined extensions. In about one-quarter of cases there will be extension into adjacent regions, such as the floor of mouth, gingiva, base of tongue, or mandible. There are no substantial microanatomic barriers in the tongue. Crossing the median raphe increases the incidence of contra- or bilateral cervical node metastases. The circumvallate papillae are also not impediments to a spread throughout the tongue.

The incidence of cervical metastasis in squamous cell carcinoma of the oral tongue correlates with the T stage of the primary tumor and appears to be significant even in early stages. Location of the primary on the tongue does not appear to be important with regard to metastasis to the lymph nodes (lesions of the lateral third, 27%; ventral tongue, 24%; tip, 22%; dorsum, 21%).[14] Extension of the carcinoma to the floor of the mouth is, however, associated with an increased frequency of nodal metastases.

Level of differentiation of the carcinoma, separate from size, also seems to have a relationship with the frequency of metastasis to the neck. However, the subjectivity of this factor as well as its inconsistent application hamper judgement on its being an independent factor.

Tumor thickness is a very useful index. Spiro et al.[10] have shown that patients with tongue and floor of mouth carcinomas 2 mm or less in thickness had a treatment failure rate of 1.9% compared with 45.6% for patients whose primary carcinomas were thicker than 2 mm. These data suggest that treatment failure and survival may be dependent more on tumor thickness than on clinical stage (see later).

Recurrences usually occur within the first 24 months, the majority within the first 12 months following primary treatment. Overall survival rates are in the range of 55% 2-year and 34% 5-year survival.[10–12] Uncontrolled disease above the clavicles remains the major source of treatment failure and an approximately 11% second primary rate further thwarts the clinician.

Base of tongue

Although there are clear differences between the incidence, presenting symptoms, and management of carcinomas occurring in the mobile anterior two-thirds of the tongue and the less accessible posterior third (oropharynx), it is important to recognize that these differences are related primarily to site rather than to intrinsic variations in lingual anatomy. Although the circumvallate papillae separate the two tongue areas, there are no barriers to prevent the carcinomas from spreading throughout the tongue. There is also no barrier to crossover into contralateral channels of the tongue's rich lymphatic drainage.

Up to one-third of all squamous cell carcinomas of the tongue arise in the tongue base, an area that extends from the line of the circumvallate papillae to the junction with the base of the epiglottic valleculae and includes the pharyngoepiglottic and glossoepiglottic folds.

As another relatively clinically silent area and not readily visible to self-inspection, carcinomas at the base of the tongue are quite sizable when discovered: 60–90% are T2 or T3.

Typically an ulcerative-infiltrative neoplasm, the base-of-tongue squamous cell carcinoma is moderately well to poorly differentiated and is highly invasive.

The aggressiveness of base-of-tongue squamous cell carcinomas can be appreciated by the fact that (1) 50–75% of patients have clinically positive cervical lymph nodes at diagnosis and 20–30% either have, or will have, contralateral and/or bilateral cervical nodal metastases, (2) almost three-quarters of the carcinomas have extended beyond the base into the anterior tongue, pre-epiglottic space, pharyngeal wall, or mandible; about 20% will invade the larynx.

Floor of mouth

The floor of the mouth is the mucosa covering the anterior and lateral floor of the oral cavity and overlies the mylohyoid and hyoglossus muscles. The lateral and anterior margins are established by the lingual surface of the lower alveolar ridge. The posterior border is formed by the ventral tongue and

Table 3.8 Frequency and sex ratio of floor of mouth carcinoma compared with other oral carcinoma.[5] (From data provided by Barasch et al.,[18] University of Connecticut Oral Biopsy Service 1975–92)

	Floor of mouth	Tongue	Gingiva/ridge	All other sites
Number of cases	176	168	109	122
M/F ratio	2.6	1.1	0.7	1.9

the anterior tonsillar pillars. The lingual frenulum divides the floor of mouth into right and left sides and it is further divided into anterior and posterior zones by the posterior edge of the second molars.

The floor of mouth has a rich lymphatic drainage that is continuous with that of the tongue and gingiva. There is an easy anastomosis between superficial and deep lymphatics and also with opposite sides. Drainage is to the submandibular, submental and deep internal jugular lymph nodes.

Men comprise 70–90% of patients, with an average age at time of diagnosis of 60 years.[15] There has been a recent relatively increased incidence in women. The most common complaint is a sore spot (64%). The mean duration of symptoms to histologic diagnosis is 4 months.[15,16]

An anterolateral location is the origin of predilection but medial extension from the lateral carcinoma is the reason the midline is where most of the carcinomas are noted at diagnosis. If one divides the floor of mouth into thirds, it is seen that 72% of the carcinomas arise in the anterior third, 15% in the mid-third, and 13% in the posterior third.[17]

Table 3.8 gives the frequency and sex ratio of floor-of-mouth carcinomas compared with other oral carcinomas.[18] Table 3.9 from the study by Aygun et al.[17] locates early floor-of-mouth carcinomas and the involved adjacent structures after expansion of the carcinomas.

Squamous cell carcinomas of the floor of the mouth are among the most aggressive and potentially fatal neoplasms of the oral cavity. The difficulty in controlling the carcinomas locally and regionally can be attributed to their proximity to the mandible and also to the intrinsic poor mechanical barrier to spread.

Investigators have noted a relatively high incidence (25–30%) of clinically occult nodal lesions in both T1 and T2 lesions of the floor of mouth, with the positive nodal status increasing with the increase in size of the primary:[8] 40% of patients present with clinical evidence of cervical node involvement.[8,19]

Table 3.9 Carcinoma of the floor of the mouth. (University of Maryland Hospital experience; Aygun et al.[17])

Location in the floor of mouth	**%**
Anterolateral	42
Lateral	22
Multiple or extensive	21
Midline	15
Adjacent structures involved	**%**
Sublingual gland	48
Tongue	25
'Extensive'	21
Gums	6

According to Shafer and Waldron,[20] 21% of leukoplakias and 95% of erythroplasias in the floor of mouth will manifest, on histologic examination, severe dysplasia, carcinoma in situ, or invasive squamous cell carcinoma. A wider range of differentiation is exhibited by floor-of-mouth carcinoma than is seen for lip and tongue carcinomas, but the differentiation subserves size and depth of invasion as far as aggressiveness is concerned.

A retrospective review of 99 patients with squamous cell carcinoma of the floor of mouth who received their primary treatment at Roswell Park Cancer Center from 1971 to 1991 indicated the following:[16]

- 43% of patients had early stage disease (I or II);
- 5-year survival for stages I–IV was 95, 86, 82 and 52%, respectively;
- The incidence of occult cervical metastases for clinical stage I was 21%; clinical stage II, 62%.

The cause of death for patients with floor-of-mouth cancer has been studied by Marks et al.[15] and is presented in Table 3.10.

Table 3.10 Cause of death for patients with floor-of-mouth cancer (n = 94). (Modified from Marks et al.[15])

Cause of death	Percentage of patients
Carcinoma	46
Intercurrent disease	30
Second primary	16
Complications	3
Unknown	5

Hard palate

The oral palate is divided into two parts—an anterior hard palate and a posterior soft palate. The hard palate extends from the inner aspect of the superior alveolar ridge to the posterior edge of the palatine bone; it separates the oral from the nasal cavity. Both palates merge with the maxillary alveolus, sharing a common lymphatic drainage. The lymphatics follow two courses: (a) an anterior and middle pathway through the retromolar region, at times via the submandibular nodes, to the upper internal jugular chain; (b) a posterior route through the posterior tonsillar pillar to the retropharyngeal nodal area and finally into the internal jugular chain.[8]

There is a disproportionate distribution of squamous cell carcinomas between the hard and soft palate in the US population: 75% of these carcinomas occur on the soft palate and 25% on the hard palate.[21] Indeed, the hard palate is the least common site of all intra-oral squamous cell carcinomas in the United States. A comparison of adjacent sites found the alveolar ridge squamous cell carcinomas comprised 9% and the soft and hard palates 4% and 1%, respectively, of all newly diagnosed oral squamous cell carcinomas treated at the Massachusetts General Hospital from 1962 to 1976.[21] This low incidence is to be contrasted with that in South India, where carcinoma of the hard palate is common, especially in young women; reverse chutta smoking is responsible. A relatively high incidence is also noted in Latin America and the Caribbean.

In the United States the carcinoma is most often seen in men between 60 and 70 years of age. The carcinomas are evenly distributed over the palatal surface. In reverse smokers the carcinomas usually develop as a lateral ulcer in the glandular zone of the hard palate. The majority of the carcinomas are well to moderately well differentiated. At the time of diagnosis only about half of the carcinomas are localized to the hard palate: 30% have invaded adjacent structures (underlying bone, floor of the nasal cavity, maxillary sinus, gingiva and soft palate).[21]

Ildstad et al.[21] record an 86% 2-year and 57% 5-year overall survival. Presence or absence of cervical nodal disease is clearly of prognostic significance. Ildstad et al.[21] indicate the dramatic decline in survival in patients who presented at initial clinical-diagnostic staging with evident cervical metastases: they record a 0% 2-year and 5-year survival in this cohort of patients. There is a second primary frequency of 20–30%.

The gingiva (upper and lower alveolar ridges)

The upper alveolar ridge includes the alveolar process of the maxilla and its mucosa extending from the upper gingival buccal gutter to the junction of the hard palate. The posterior margin is the upper end of the pterygopalatine arch. The lower alveolar ridge encompasses the mandibular alveolar process, the mucosa of which extends from its attachment in the buccal gutter to the line of free mucosa of the floor of mouth; posteriorly, it extends to the ascending ramus of the mandible.

Although the mandibular alveolar ridge is anatomically separate from that of the maxilla and is in continuity with the floor of mouth, the two are often combined for data analysis because it is recognized that carcinomas of the ridges exhibit similar clinical behavior.

Alveolar ridge squamous carcinomas comprised 9% of all patients with oral squamous carcinomas reported by Ildstad et al.[21] The carcinomas are neoplasms of the elderly, with the majority of patients in at least their sixth decade of life. Men are more often affected, but there is an impressive increase in the proportion of women with the carcinomas. Like carcinomas of the buccal mucosa, gingival carcinomas are more common in India than in the United States; once again, this is attributable to betel nut and tobacco chewing.

About 70% of the carcinomas arise from the mandibular gingiva, 30% from the maxillary gingiva. The fixed gingiva is more often involved than the free gingiva and edentulous areas more so than areas where dentition is present.

The carcinomas can be insidious in onset and progression. They can be mistaken for persistent gingivitis, periodontal disease or abscess. Focus on these masqueraders can lead to extraction of teeth, with its morbid consequence of an unobstructed neoplastic growth into underlying bone.

Extension of these well to moderately differentiated squamous carcinomas is frequent. From the maxillary gingiva the spread is to the hard palate, maxillary sinus, buccal mucosa, lip, or skin. Carcinomas of the mandibular gingiva can spread to underlying bone, floor of mouth, tongue, retromolar trigone, lip or skin.

Metastases from carcinomas of the lower gingiva have a predilection for levels I and II (submandibular triangle and upper jugular regions). This is especially true for subclinical neck disease, while those patients with clinically positive neck disease are more likely to have involvement of additional nodal levels, particularly level III.[21]

Approximately 13% of the carcinomas are associated with second primaries even though the majority are early stage I–II lesions.[21] Ildstad et al. report a 66% 2-year and 49% 5-year overall survival.[21]

Retromolar trigone (retromolar gingiva)

As its name implies, the retromolar trigone is an approximately triangular mucosal area that covers the ascending ramus of the mandible. The apex of the triangle is next to the maxillary tuberosity behind the last upper molar teeth, and the base is posterior to the last molar tooth. Because of its limited surface area, carcinomas arising in the retromolar trigone have often extended into adjacent structures at the time of discovery. This extension is anteriorly to the gingiva; posteriorly to the anterior tonsillar pillar or fossa; medially to the floor of mouth and posterolateral tongue; laterally to the buccogingival sulcus, buccal mucosa, pterygoid space; or into mandibular bone.

There is an interesting parallel with squamous cell carcinomas of the lower gum. This is not unexpected, as the retromolar trigone is really an extension of the lower gum onto the ascending ramus of the mandible.[22] The biologic behavior of the carcinomas from the two sites is similar in the expression of cervical metastases (39% with carcinomas of the trigone vs 30% of the lower gum).[23] Pathologically proven mandibular bone invasion is not as common for trigone carcinomas as it is in the lower gum (12% vs 36%), but invasion of the maxilla can occur.[22,23]

Carcinomas of the retromolar trigone occur principally in men 50–70 years of age. Delay in discovery is promoted by the false impression of sore throat or dental problems. At the time of discovery, about 60% of the tumors are less than 5 cm and the majority are moderately well differentiated.

There is an incidence of about 30% of second primary neoplasms and this, plus a high incidence of intercurrent disease, accounts for the low 5-year survival of 26%.[22]

Buccal mucosa

The buccal mucosa encompasses the oral mucous membrane of the inner surfaces of the cheeks and lips from the contact line of the opposing lips to the attachment of the mucosa to the alveolar ridges and pterygomandibular raphe.

Squamous cell carcinomas have a predilection for the posterior buccal mucosa, followed by the middle third and, rarely, the anterior third. They arise at the commissures, along the occlusal plane of the teeth, or at the retromolar area. The carcinomas are more common in men (United States), but there is an increasing incidence in women. The carcinomas are uncommon in Blacks and only unusually occur before the age of 40 years. In near-endemic geographic areas such as India and South-East Asia, the incidence in women is equal to (or exceeds) that in men. In the United States, there is a putative association with smokeless tobacco. It is of considerable etiologic interest that buccal squamous cell carcinoma in India is most often on the left side (mid-inferior, posterior-inferior and angle). These sites correspond to the area where the quid is most often placed.

Buccal squamous cell carcinomas are often of the verrucous type or otherwise well differentiated. Exophytic carcinomas are found most often at the level of the buccal commissure; ulceroinfiltrative carcinomas involve the buccinator muscle early and often present a deep, excavating ulcer with diffuse extensions. There is a frequent association with leukoplakia, less so with erythroplasia.

Untreated buccal carcinomas are very destructive, with ulceration through the skin, invasion of bone and the pharyngomaxillary fossa, as well as posterior growth.

The recurrence rate for all types of buccal squamous cell carcinomas is high, and the prognosis for posterior-third buccal carcinomas is very poor. Metastases, most often to regional lymph nodes, will recur in about 56% of cases and approximately 35% of patients present with nodal enlargement. Including patients in whom nodal involvement appeared subsequently, Bloom and Spiro[24] found the incidence of neck metastasis was 39, 56 and 72% of T1, T2 and T3 or T4 lesions, respectively, for an overall incidence of 56%.

Determinate 5-year cure rates, after exclusively surgical treatment, range from 77% and 65% in stage I and II lesions to 27% and 18% in those with stage III and IV lesions, respectively.[24]

Table 3.11 Oral precancerous lesions: a classification. (After Pindborg[27])

Leukoplakia
- Homogeneous
  - Flat
  - Corrugated
  - Pumice-like
  - Wrinkled
- Non-homogeneous
  - Verrucous
  - Proliferative and verrucous
  - Nodular
  - Erythroleukoplakia

Erythroplakia
- Uniformly red
- Red with white nodules

Leukoplakia and related lesions

The requirement for clear definitions for oral white lesions, precancerous lesions, and precancerous conditions has long been recognized. Similar requirements also apply to red lesions or the red component of preponderantly white lesions.

Definition of leukoplakia

In 1978, a World Health Organization (WHO) group defined oral leukoplakia as: 'A white patch or plaque that cannot be characterized, clinically or histopathologically, as any other disease.'[25] The text accompanying the definition indicated that the term leukoplakia does not carry a histologic connotation and should be used only in 'descriptive clinical context'. In a like manner, erythroplakia was defined as a term for bright red patches or plaques that cannot be defined clinically or pathologically as any other condition.

Five years later, at an international seminar, it was decided to avoid the use of the term leukoplakia where there was a known etiologic factor (frictional keratosis, luetic leukoplakia, candidal leukoplakia, etc.), except in those cases where tobacco was believed to be the cause.[26] As a result, the definition of leukoplakia was revised to: 'Leukoplakia is a whitish patch or plaque that cannot be characterized clinically or pathologically as any other disease and it is not associated with any physical or chemical causal agent except the use of tobacco'. The definition of erythroplakia was left unchanged. The seminar also brought forth proposals for an etiologic description for leukoplakia as well as a clinical description. The former considered two categories of leukoplakia: idiopathic (unknown genesis) and those associated with (or thought to result from) the use of tobacco. The clinical description subclassified leukoplakias into a homogeneous type and different types of non-homogeneous leukoplakia. Pindborg[27] elaborated further on these recommendations (Table 3.11).

Dysplasia is rarely seen in homogeneous leukoplakia. Histologic examination reveals either hyperortho- or hyperparakeratosis. Non-homogeneous leukoplakias are rarer than the homogeneous type. The most frequent of the non-homogeneous forms are the nodular leukoplakias and the erythroleukoplakias. The non-homogeneous leukoplakias are almost always the seat of either dysplasia, carcinoma in situ, or squamous cell carcinoma. The malignant potential of nodular leukoplakia and other 'precancerous oral lesions' is seen in Table 3.12.

Table 3.12 Leukoplakia lesions of the oral cavity and their malignant potential. (Modified from Pindborg[27])

Oral lesion	Number of cases	Average follow-up (years)	Number of oral cancers	Relative risk
Nodular leukoplakia	13	2.8	6	3243
Submucous fibrosis	25	6.0	3	8397
Erythematous areas, ulcers	26	2.6	1	303
Ulcerated leukoplakia	105	4.4	1	44
Homogeneous leukoplakia	489	4.8	3	26
Lichen planus	344	3.7	4	16
None of the above	10 145	7.8	4	1

A follow-up international symposium was held in May 1994 to address difficulties in interpretation and application of the proposals of the earlier seminar, published in 1984.[28] The new definitions and guidelines are as follows:

1. *Precancerous lesion*: a morphologically altered tissue in which cancer is more likely to occur than in its apparently normal counterpart. Oral leukoplakia is an example of a precancerous lesion.
2. *Precancerous condition*: a generalized state associated with a significantly increased risk of cancer. Submucous fibrosis is an example of a precancerous condition.
3. *Oral leukoplakia*: a predominantly white lesion of the oral mucosa that cannot be characterized as any other definable lesion; some oral leukoplakias will transform into cancer. A provisional diagnosis of oral leukoplakia is made when a lesion at clinical examination cannot be clearly diagnosed as any other disease of the oral mucosa with a white appearance. A definitive diagnosis of oral leukoplakia is made as a result of the identification and, if possible, elimination of suspected etiologic factors and, in the case of persistent lesions, histopathologic examination. Table 3.13 lists qualifications to be used in the foregoing definitions.
4. *Clinical variants of white and red lesions of the oral mucosa*:
   (a) *Homogeneous leukoplakia*. A predominantly white lesion of uniform flat, thin appearance that may manifest shallow cracks and has a smooth, wrinkled or corrugated surface with a consistent texture throughout.
   (b) *Non-homogeneous leukoplakia*. A predominantly white, or red and white (erythroleukoplakia), lesion that may be irregularly flat, nodular, or exophytic. Nodular lesions have slightly raised, rounded, red and/or white excrescences. Exophytic lesions have irregular blunt or sharp projections.
   (c) *Erythroplakia*. A term used analogously to leukoplakia to designate oral mucosal lesions that present as red areas and cannot be diagnosed as any other definable lesion. The same comments apply to provisional and definitive diagnoses as for oral leukoplakias.
5. *Staging*. Participants of the 1994 international symposium also proposed a staging system for oral leukoplakia. For the provisional diagnosis, size and clinical appearance are coded by the symbols L (size) and C (clinical aspect) as follows:
   - L provisional 1 = < 2 cm, 2 = 2–4 cm, 3 = > 4 cm and x = not specified;
   - C provisional 1 = homogeneous, 2 = non-homogeneous, x = not specified.

Table 3.13 Guidelines for use of definitions of leukoplakia

1. The time for white lesions to regress after elimination of suspected etiologic factors may vary from several weeks to months. A biopsy should be taken when no signs of regression are noted within 2–4 weeks after attempted elimination of suspected factors
2. White lesions for which a local cause can be identified are not to be included among leukoplakias, e.g. frictional lesions, cheek-biting lesions, and lesions associated with dental restorations
3. Various tobacco products and other physical or chemical agents produce a wide range of oral white lesions. These vary also in the risk of malignant transformation. In addition, there is considerable variation in the habits employed with these agents
4. A definitive diagnosis of oral leukoplakia *requires* a biopsy and histopathologic interpretation
5. Histopathologic reports of biopsies of oral leukoplakia should always include a statement on the presence or absence of epithelial dysplasia and, if present, an assessment of the severity. Oral leukoplakias which show epithelial dysplasia carry an increased risk of malignancy
6. If the biopsy specimen of oral leukoplakia shows carcinoma in situ or invasive carcinoma, the provisional diagnosis of oral leukoplakia should be replaced by the histopathologic diagnosis.

For the definitive diagnosis, the symbol P represents pathologic features:

1 = no dysplasia
2 = mild dysplasia
3 = moderate dysplasia
4 = severe dysplasia
x = not specified

Stage grouping is to be used only for oral leukoplakias that have been histologically examined and is three-tiered:

Stage 1 = any L C1 P1 P2
Stage 2 = any L C2 P1 P2
Stage 3 = any L any C P3 P4.

Table 3.14 lists qualifications to be used for the staging system.

The involvement of *Candida albicans* in the etiology or progression of leukoplakic lesions remains controversial. Candida-associated leukoplakia is often ulcerated or of the non-homogeneous type.

Table 3.14 Guidelines for use of classification and staging of leukoplakia

1. Doubt on which L, C, or P category a particular lesion should be allotted, places the lesion in the lower (less advanced) category. This will be reflected in the stage grouping
2. In the case of multiple simultaneous leukoplakias, the one with the highest L category should be classified with the multiplicity of the number of leukoplakia indicated in parentheses, e.g. (L2cm)
3. In the case of the presence of different clinical types, the highest score among the various leukoplakias should be used
4. In the case of multiple biopsies of a single oral leukoplakia, or biopsies taken from multiple leukoplakias, the highest pathologic score of the various biopsies should be used

L, size; C, clinical aspect; P, pathologic features (see text)

Table 3.15 Oral leukoplakia and laryngeal keratosis: a comparison. (From data presented by Bouquot and Gnepp[30] and representing 3857 patients with laryngeal keratosis and 4117 with oral leukoplakia)

Comparative features	Oral leukoplakia	Laryngeal keratosis
Host characteristics		
Age (years)	60	50
Males (%)	60	81
Smokers (%)	66	84
Alcohol abuse (%)	N/A	35
Lesion characteristics		
Average size (cm)	1	1
Average duration at diagnosis (months)	26	7
With erythroplakia at diagnosis (%)	18	16
With carcinoma at diagnosis (%)	7	12
With carcinoma after diagnosis (%)	4	1
Recurrence (%)	18	16
With dysplasia at diagnosis (%)	14	35
With leukoplakia/keratosis adjacent to carcinoma (%)	34	33

The term 'candidal leukoplakia' has been suggested to emphasize the possible participatory or cofactor role in some forms of leukoplakia. Pindborg[29] believed that most, if not all, non-homogeneous forms of leukoplakia are areas of a candidal infection.

Acceptance of the precancerous quality of defined oral leukoplakia preceded, by several decades, a like appreciation of the precancerous nature of laryngeal keratosis. Erythroplakia and erythrokeratosis, long considered high-risk oral mucosal changes, were early ignored in the laryngeal literature because they were often confounded by the inflammatory hyperemia which is almost a constant finding in the larynges of smokers. Table 3.15, based on the studies of Bouquot and Gnepp,[30] compares oral leukoplakia and laryngeal keratosis. The percentage values are the authors' estimates of the most representative and unbiased data.

In most studies, the buccal mucosa and the commissures are the most common sites of involvement by leukoplakia, followed, in Americans, by the floor of the mouth. The gingiva and alveolar ridges are rather uncommon areas of involvement.

Clinical significance

The clinical course of oral leukoplakia is partly dependent on the type of treatment and elimination or persistence of causal factors. The lesions may remain static, decrease or increase in size, or undergo malignant change. Regression is much more likely than malignant transformation. Leukoplakias related to smoking are more likely to persist than those associated with chewing habits. The most common sites for regression to occur are the mucosae of the lips, commissures, and cheeks. Lingual and floor-of-mouth leukoplakia are least likely to regress and are also sites with the highest risk of malignancy.

It is clear that subjects with oral leukoplakia have a higher risk of developing oral cancer than the normal population. In Western countries the rate of malignant transformation is estimated to be between 2 and 6%.[31] The longer the persistence of leukoplakia and, accordingly, the older the patient, the higher the risk of malignancy. Women also appear to be at higher risk than men.[32]

The floor of the mouth and the ventral lingual mucosa have been singled out as special risk sites, regardless of the morphologic type of the leukoplakia. Palatal leukoplakia is usually of the homogeneous type and has a relatively low malignant potential. Probably the most common white patch on the palate is that associated with nicotinic stomatitis (seen predominantly in habitual pipe smokers). There is a diffuse keratosis of the palate's mucosa with chronic inflammation of the palatal glands and plugging of duct orifices with keratin. There is no significant premalignant potential with nicotinic stomatitis.

Erythroplakia (erythroplasia) of the oral cavity is a far more dangerous lesion. There is no apparent gender predilection and the lesions are most frequent in the sixth and seventh decades. In men, the floor of the mouth is the most common site; in women, the alveolar mucosa, gingiva and sulcus mucosa of the mandible are favored. In both sexes, the next most common site is the retromolar region.

In erythroplasia, unlike leukoplakia, a large proportion of cases (40–50%) manifest severe dysplasia or carcinoma. Lumerman and colleagues,[32] in an analysis of 308 cases which included leukoplakia along with erythroplakia and erythroleukoplakia, found a rate of 16% transformation to invasive squamous cell carcinoma within a mean follow-up period of over 33 months.

By means of the clinical appearance and the microscopic severity of dysplasia, observers can predict with a 1.3–17% accuracy which leukoplakic lesions will progress to carcinoma.[33] Cytometric analysis of DNA content has the potential to reduce the subjective quality of prediction. For ploidy data, however, there has been an inconsistency that thwarts their reliability. Whether image cytometry of nuclear features will prove better is as yet unknown. The study by Abdel-Salam et al.[33] is encouraging. The authors developed a model that had a predictive value of 86% in identifying oral white lesions, with or without dysplasia, that will transform to a malignancy. Three variables, related to the nuclear chromatin pattern, exhibited the most discriminating power—mean margination, and standard deviations of clumping and condensation of the chromatin.

Silverman et al.,[31] on the basis of their investigations and those of Lumerman et al.,[32] have given us a contemporary assessment of leukoplakia, dysplasia and malignant transformation:

1. Specific data about correlations between degrees of oral dysplasia, time-related progression, and the influences of cofactors remain unclear.
2. In chronic lesions, the time and occurrence of dysplasia is unknown; an erythematous component in the clinical leukoplakia and discomfort are causes for concern and suspicion.
3. Since there is a risk of malignancy when epithelial dysplasia is found, removal of the lesion is necessary; prospective studies are therefore limited.
4. All subjects with red or white lesions should be carefully followed even though their dysplasias are mild or nil.
5. A high risk for dysplasia and malignant transformation is always associated with proliferative verrucous forms of leukoplakia. Because of this, aggressive treatment is necessary.
6. Of the patients of Silverman et al.,[31] 78% manifested human papilloma virus 16 in their lesional tissue. The high risk may be related to the virus.
7. Development of objective biologic markers is necessary to obviate the subjectivity of definitions of dysplasia.

Table 3.16 Prevalence rates of white oral mucosal lesions. (From the prevalence study by Schepman et al.[34])

Lesion	**Prevalence (%)**
Candidiasis	0.9
Cheek biting	2.3
Frictional lesion	2.5
Geographic tongue	2.3
Dental restoration lesion	0.2
Leukedema	3.0
Nicotinic keratosis	1.0
Leukoplakia	0.6
Lichen planus	0.6
Total	13.4

Schepman et al.[34] tested the revised definitions of oral leukoplakia (provisional and definitive) in a prevalence study of white lesions of the oral mucosa among a selected population of 1000 consecutive subjects from The Netherlands. The investigators deemed the definitions, as well as the classification and staging system, very suitable for epidemiologic studies. The prevalence rates of the target lesions in the 1000 patients studied by Schepman et al.[34] are presented in Table 3.16. The low prevalence rate for leukoplakia may be due to the fact that the majority of the subjects examined were in the 20–29-year-old age group and also to the exclusion of those who were referred for a diagnosis of a white mucosal lesion. Table 3.17 gives an overall impression of the prevalence of oral leukoplakia with a geographic emphasis.[35–44]

Table 3.17 Prevalence of oral leukoplakia

Author and year of study	Country	Number of persons examined	No. of leukoplakias	Prevalence (%)
Pindborg et al. (1965–1966)[35–37]	India	30 000	150–328	1.5–3.3
Gangadarhan and Paymaster (1971)[38]	India	203 249	1422	0.7
Mehta et al. (1972)[39]	India	101 761	685	0.7
Axéll (1976)[40]	Sweden	20 333	717	3.6
Bouquot and Gorlin (1986)[41]	USA	23 616	682	2.9
Hogewind and van der Waal (1988)[42]	The Netherlands	1 000	14	1.4
Banoczy and Rigo (1991)[43]	Hungary	7 820	104	1.3
Ikeda et al. (1991)[44]	Japan	3 131	77	2.5

Proliferative verrucous leukoplakia

Because of the considerable oncologic danger associated with oral proliferative verrucous leukoplakia (PVL), it is singled out for special consideration. Oral PVL is essentially a clinical diagnosis, as the histopathologic features of any lesion along the spectrum of the disease are indistinguishable from non-PVL associated lesions of the same type.

PVL is considered to be a progressive type of oral leukoplakia that is impossible to recognize in its nascent stages.[45] The condition typically begins as non-dysplastic keratosis and develops over time (sometimes 20 or more years) into a confluent, multifocal and widespread oral keratosis with stubborn recurrences and persistences and a high frequency of malignant change.[46–48] The progressive oral mucosal involvement is accompanied by an exophytic and verrucous character of the lesional tissues. Ultimately, many PVLs evolve into invasive carcinoma, with 30% or more of the patients dying of the disease.[47,49]

Although irreversibility is probably intrinsic even in the early flat, non-verrucous form of PVL, it cannot be predicted with a reasonable certainty until the leukoplakia has evolved to the exophytic, verrucous form from which it derives its name. The clinical continuum from hyperkeratosis to carcinoma is also reflected in the spectrum of histologic appearances manifested by PVL. Verrucous carcinoma, conventional well-differentiated squamous cell carcinoma, and histologic verrucous hyperplasia can all exist concurrently within oral PVL. There may also be a progressive dysplasia, but a clinical leukoplakia that shows severe dysplasia at its initial appearance does not qualify.[45]

PVL is most commonly seen in elderly women (age range, 36–90 years; mean, 70.2 years). Patients often indicate a long-time awareness of leukoplakia, sometimes for more than 20 years. Tobacco use history is variable, but abstinence is often claimed.

The buccal mucosa is most often the site of an initial involvement, followed by the hard and soft palate, alveolar mucosa, tongue, floor of mouth, gingiva, and lip, in that order.

In its early form, especially with isolated lesions, the clinical findings of PVL cannot be distinguished from any of the more common types of clinical leukoplakia. These early forms are flat, thickened keratoses. Progression of the disorder is manifested by confluence of lesions, wider mucosal involvement, and an exophytic topography.

The often-noted absence of risk factors ordinarily associated with oral squamous cell carcinoma, the preponderance of women among the patients, and the occurrence at an older age have suggested that the pathogenesis of carcinomas arising in patients with PVL may differ from that of non-PVL-associated carcinoma.[50–52] Palefsky et al.,[50] with a polymerase chain reaction for HPV DNA, studied nine lesions from seven patients with PVL, histologically diagnosed with focal keratosis, papilloma, epithelial dysplasia, and squamous cell carcinoma, and found that eight lesions (89%) were HPV positive, seven for HPV 16. This frequency was higher than the HPV detection rates in non-PVL lesions.

The surgical management of PVL is bedeviled by high recurrence rates and a widespread mucosal involvement that makes total excision often impossible. Only three of the 30 patients studied by Hansen et al.[45] remained free of disease after treatment. Irradiation has not been effective.

Verrucous hyperplasia

We restrict the term verrucous hyperplasia to a histopathologic context only, but include it as one of the evolutionary stages in oral PVL.[47] It need not, however, be part of that peculiar leukoplakia. Outside of the oral cavity, in the sinonasal tract and larynx, verrucous hyperplasia occurs either as an apparently de novo lesion or in association with papillomas. We regard verrucous hyperplasia to be a particularly ominous change in Schneiderian papillomas.[47]

In our opinion, verrucous hyperplasia is an irreversible lesion, often histologically indistinguishable from verrucous carcinoma, i.e. an early form of that neoplasm, although the characteristic feature of a blunted epithelial front pushing into the underlying lamina propria seen in verrucous carcinoma is absent in verrucous hyperplasia.

At any of the mucosal sites, verrucous hyperplasia is a lesion of mature adults. In the oral cavity it is diagnosed most often in patients who are in the sixth through eighth decades. There is a male preponderance. In the oral cavity the gingiva and alveolar mucosa are sites of predilection; the cheeks, tongue, floor of mouth, lip and palate follow. The true and false vocal cords are the laryngeal areas of preference.[47]

Shear and Pindborg[53] have indicated two clinicopathologic patterns in the oral cavity, and we have found the patterns also applicable to sinonasal and laryngeal lesions. The growth patterns are primarily distinguished by the height and degree of keratinization of the verrucous processes. Either a sharp or blunt form may dominate. In the oral cavity and paranasal sinuses the sharp verrucous hyperplasia is most often seen; there is seemingly no particular preference in laryngeal lesions. Combinations of the two forms are also seen.

Prior to the sharp or blunt architecture, verrucous hyperplasia undergoes a sequence of histologic changes that starts with a keratotic, non-dysplastic mucosal thickening (Fig. 3.2) and then progresses through hyperplasia, mucosal clefting, downgrowth, and a verrucous pattern (Figs 3.3, 3.4). Areas of a homogeneous leukoplakia are usually adjacent to (or found elsewhere in) oral verrucous hyperplasia. These are usually absent in the sinonasal lesions, but are found with verrucous hyperplasias of the larynx.

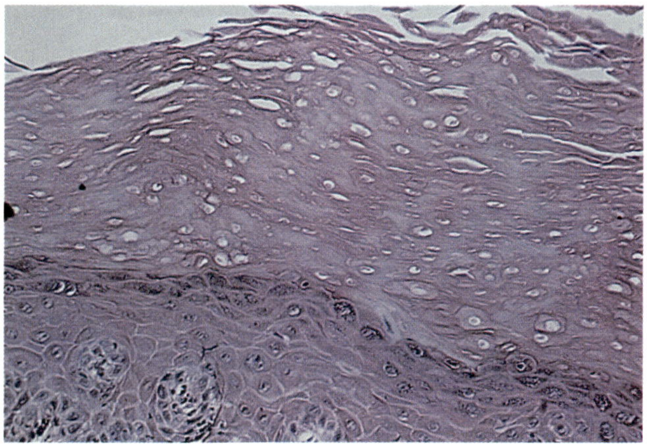

Figure 3.2 A clinical leukoplakia of tongue: marked keratosis without dysplasia.

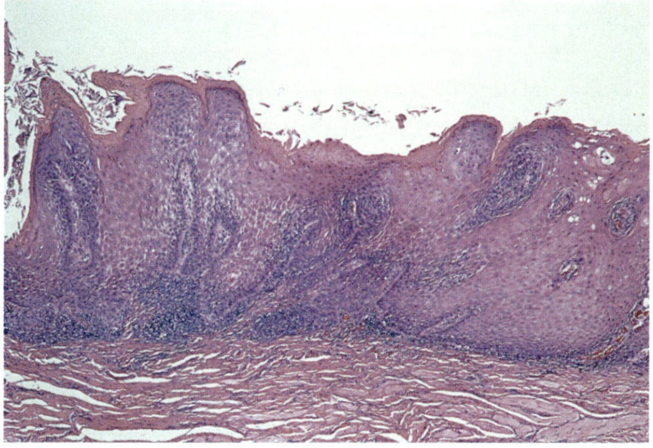

Figure 3.3 Verrucal hyperplasia of the oral cavity.

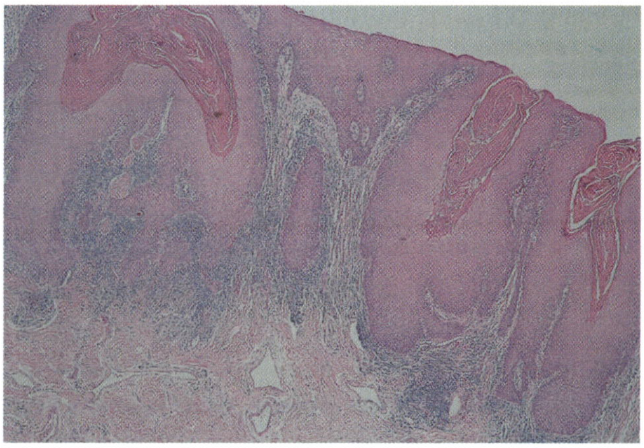

Figure 3.4 Transformation of oral verrucal hyperplasia into early verrucous carcinoma.

Besides the apparent irreversibility of verrucous hyperplasia, the progression to, or the association with, carcinoma is notable. Of 68 patients studied by Shear and Pindborg,[20] seven had coexistent verrucous carcinoma and in seven others there was a conventional squamous cell carcinoma. Slootweg and Müller[49] record similar findings: 37% of their patients had a coexisting or separately occurring

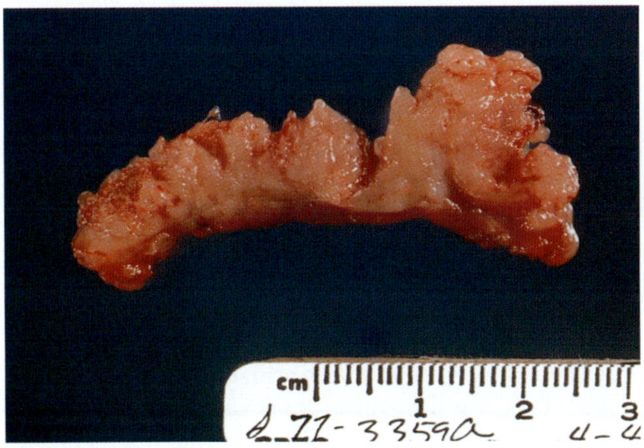

Figure 3.5 Verrucous carcinoma arising in buccal verrucal hyperplasia.

squamous cell carcinoma and in 26% epithelial dysplasia was also present. On the basis of these considerations, together with histologic and clinical data, Slootweg and Müller[49] opine that both verrucous hyperplasia and verrucous carcinoma are only variants of the same disease—verrucous carcinoma (Fig. 3.5).

It is likely that the same principle applies to the lesions of the larynx and Schneiderian mucosa. Schneiderian papillomas are nearly always devoid of a surface keratosis, or even of other areas of cellular keratinization. Keratinization of these papillomas, therefore, has to be regarded as an atypical histologic finding with an ominous portent.[47] In our experience, keratotic Schneiderian papillomas are associated with quick recurrences and an eventual verrucous hyperplasia, with coexistent or subsequent verrucous carcinoma or invasive, conventional squamous cell carcinoma of various degrees of differentiation.

Verrucous hyperplasia in the larynx either is a persistently recurrent lesion or contains a verrucous carcinoma arising from its matrix.

Shear and Pindborg[53] and Slootweg and Müller[49] admit that the lesions of verrucous hyperplasia and verrucous carcinoma may, at times, be indistinguishable. Like these authors, we consider verrucous hyperplasia to be an antecedent stage or early form of verrucous carcinoma and, more important, to have the same biologic potential. For the surgical pathologist, there are guidelines to help distinguish the two lesions but, because of the overlap in histologic features, the guidelines are not criteria. Biopsy specimens at the margins are recommended. With verrucous hyperplasia, the exophytic processes and the majority of the hyperplastic epithelium are entirely superficial to the adjacent normal epithelium. Verrucous carcinoma shows the same superficial exophytic processes, but the retia are broader and extend deeper than the adjacent uninvolved epithelium. As an additional feature, the verrucous processes in verrucous carcinoma often retract a margin of normal epithelium down with them into the underlying stroma.

Human papilloma viruses (HPVs) have been implicated in the genesis of verrucous hyperplasias. Greer et al.[51] have reported that six of 30 verrucous hyperplasias and four of 20 verrucous carcinomas expressed HPV DNA. Shroyer and Greer[52] also found four of an additional 14 verrucous hyperplasias to be HPV DNA positive.

The surgical management of verrucous hyperplasia should be at least like that for verrucous carcinoma. Procrastination, in the hope of reversibility, can lead to possible loss of control and development of overt carcinoma.

To this discussion, we add a 'footnote' expressed by Slootweg and Müller,[49] who eschew the term 'florid oral papillomatosis' and regard lesions so reported as verrucous hyperplasia/verrucous carcinoma.

Hairy leukoplakia

Oral hairy leukoplakia (OHL) is the most recently defined form of leukoplakia. The histopathologic features are distinctive and unlike those of any previously defined oral white lesion.[54–58] They do, however, resemble skin warts and uterine condylomata, both of which are associated with papilloma viruses. Although these lesions were initially thought to be limited to homosexual men, subsequent reports have acknowledged their existence in other populations at risk for AIDS, including those with hemophilia and other transfusion recipients. Some may dispute the adjective 'hairy', but the disorder has become (in nearly all instances) a marker of host immunosuppression, either natural or iatrogenically induced. Nevertheless, examples in immunocompetent subjects have been reported.[57]

The lesion is located mainly on the lateral surface of the tongue and appears as white, slightly raised plaques with a corrugated 'hairy' surface. The plaques range in size from a few millimeters to 3 cm, do not rub off, and are usually not symptomatic. The lesions may also be noted on the buccal or labial mucosa.

Histologically, the free surface is heavily parakeratotic with slender surface projections and corrugations and acanthosis (Table 3.18). Beneath the parakeratotic layer is a band of large, pale staining

Table 3.18 Histopathologic features of hairy leukoplakia of tongue. (From data presented by Schiodt et al.[55])

Features observed	Frequency (%)
In epithelium	
Hyperparakeratosis	100
Hyperplasia/Acanthosis	80
Keratin 'hairs' (hair-like projections)	80
Koilocytosis	98
Bacterial colonies on surface	52
Candidal hyphae in epithelium	43
Inflammation associated with candidal hyphae or leukocytic infiltration of epithelium	0
In connective tissue	
No inflammation	78
Mild inflammation in lamina propria	22

(balloon) cells that form the superior portion of the spinous layer, which is generally thickened. There is a characteristic nuclear chromatin change exemplified by a peripheral condensation of chromatin along the nuclear membrane. Central to this altered chromatin pattern is an amphophilic homogeneous deposit which consists of viral aggregates consistent with Epstein–Barr virus (EBV). Electron microscopy of the balloon cells reveals numerous virions typical of EBV;[58] HPVs are also found.[58] There is no evidence of dysplasia, nor is there any reported association with malignant transformation of this form of leukoplakia over time. Candidal organisms are frequently found on the surface and, in fact, hairy leukoplakia was initially thought to be a severe form of oral thrush.

The differential diagnoses include leukoplakias with atypia, candidiasis, white sponge nevus, oral lichen planus and geographic tongue. The parakeratosis and koilocytosis of hairy leukoplakia and the presence of EBV and HPV help to confirm the diagnosis.

The importance of a correct diagnosis is less that of a confusion with malignancy, but more because OHL seems to be a precursor of AIDS, and can serve as a reasonably reliable marker for the presence of the HIV virus.

Management of OHL is generally unsatisfactory but is usually not necessary beyond routine observation unless esthetics dictate otherwise. Some lesions recede with antifungal therapy, presumably owing to the eradication of candidal organisms. There is, however, never a complete resolution and a return occurs following cessation of treatment.

The significance of a mixed viral (EBV and HPV) infection is unresolved. It may be that a papilloma virus facilitates entry and subsequent replication of EBV in infected cells.

Hairy tongue

So-called 'hairy tongue' is unrelated to hairy leukoplakia. It is the term used to describe an extraordinary elongation of the filiform papillae resulting in a superficial resemblance of hairiness. The affected papillae are generally situated on the medial aspect of the dorsum of the tongue, but extensive involvement may encompass much of the dorsal surface of the anterior two-thirds of the tongue. The color of the involved tongue varies from yellow to black. Pigmentation, when present, is possibly due to medicaments, foodstuffs, tobacco, or products of chromogenic microorganisms.

Hairy tongue has been known for at least several centuries and is an acquired rather than developmental anomaly. Identical lesions have been induced in sheep by feeding them a zinc-deficient diet.

Local factors associated with hairy tongue include smoking, topical antibiotics, astringent mouthwashes and a local pH of 6 or less. It is said to develop also in subjects who have had radiotherapy to the head and neck.[59]

In contrast to a low incidence generally found in healthy subjects, hairy tongue appears to be much more common in patients with advanced cancer. Farman[59] has recorded a 22% incidence in such patients. General ill health is also a factor. Although infection with *Candida* species has been implicated as a factor, hairy tongue is not generally associated with vegetative *Candida* species.

Tylosis

A relationship between tylosis (palmoplantar keratoderma) and carcinoma of the esophagus has been known since 1954.[60] Subsequently, abnormal oral lesions were described in tylotic patients (age range 4–59 years).[60] The oral lesions that presented in childhood were called 'preleukoplakia' and had clinical as well as histologic characteristics similar to those seen in other epithelial disorders such as white sponge nevus and pachyonchia congenita. The adult oral lesions were called leukoplakia but they also had associated areas of abnormal mucosa, resembling those seen in affected children.

The lesions designated preleukoplakia are clinically reminiscent of those seen in leukedema with a gray-white, opalescent appearance, particularly affecting the buccal mucosa. Histologically, there are similarities to leukedema, morsicatio mucosae oris (cheek biting) and white sponge nevus.

There is no inflammatory cell reaction in the lamina propria. The adult form, originally described as 'leukoplakia', is clinically non-specific—in other words, a benign keratosis without special features.

Although it is now recognized that the association of palmoplantar keratoderma with oral mucosal changes is an important clinical sign in the diagnosis of different patterns of focal palmoplantar keratoderma, the relationship to oral cancer is unknown, since epidemiologic factors such as smoking and alcohol drinking are nearly always present.

Because of the problems with the confusing earlier nomenclature, Field et al.[60] recommend use of the term 'leukokeratosis' for the spectrum of diffuse oral lesions seen in the group of tylotic patients and also for the other clinical patterns of focal palmoplantar keratoderma.

Epithelial hyperplasia; dysplasia; carcinoma in situ

The nomenclature applied to histologic epithelial abnormalities of the oral cavity, other than invasive carcinoma, encompasses the terms hyperplasia, dysplasia, and carcinoma in situ. For each, there is the inevitable problem of subjectivity on the part of the surgical pathologist. In addition, there has been too long the assumption that one can transfer criteria for the lesions, from those used to define uterine cervical lesions, to lesions of the head and neck mucosa.

Prior to discussion of the lesions, it should be also appreciated that there are always varying degrees of histologic overlap. Indeed, pseudoepitheliomatous hyperplasia, an exaggerated response to injury, can be one of the most difficult differential diagnoses in oral pathology.

Hyperplasia

A reactive proliferative hyperplasia of the squamous mucosa of the oral cavity is its most common response to injury. A keratotic surface is a usual, but not inevitable, accompaniment. The reactive hyperplasia is characterized by epithelial thickening with a resulting readily identified and intact basal layer. Cellular maturation with a manifest orderly progression is typical. Cytologic atypia is minimal or absent. Division figures are normally found only adjacent to the basal layer of the epithelium. This form of hyperplasia is reversible and should be readily distinguishable from forms of dysplasia (mild, moderate, severe).

Dysplasia

Two histologic signs serve to separate dysplastic growth patterns from benign hyperplasias. Loss of an orderly nuclear mosaic pattern in dysplastic epithelium, manifested by a decreased nuclear/cytoplastic ratio and an irregular random nuclear placement, signals abnormal maturation; usually, the nuclei are more deeply staining and pleomorphic in size and shape. Dyskeratosis is the second sign: not only is keratin almost always found on the surface, there is an abnormal expression of keratin production in the lower parts of the epithelium; this takes the form of either single-cell keratinization or keratin pearl formation. Alterations of nuclear cytomorphology usually accompany the abnormal distribution of keratin.

As indicated above, the oral mucosa (and for the most part, the mucosa of the upper aerodigestive tract) has a proclivity to become hyperplastic and develop keratin as a protective response to any form of injury, including carcinogenic influences. Surface keratinization is rare in dysplasias of the uterine cervix, but is a common occurrence in the upper aerodigestive tract (Fig. 3.6). Here again, the application of histologic criteria for intraepithelial alterations in a non-keratinizing mucosa such as the cervix to the keratinizing oral mucosa has resulted in considerable nosologic confusion.[61,62]

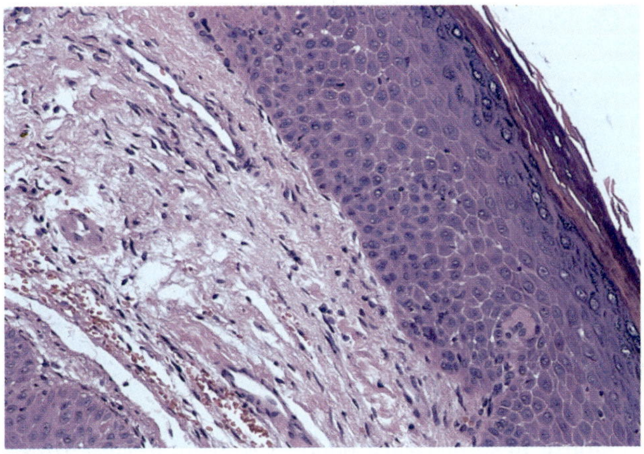

Figure 3.6 Mild dysplasia of basilar layers; this (likely reversible) lesion also shows a modest degree of surface mucosal keratinization.

Table 3.19 Histopathologic features of oral dysplasia

1. 'Drop'-shaped rete processes (wider at their deeper parts than superficially)
2. Altered cellular polarity (changes in the normally long axis parallel to the mucosal surface)
3. Nuclear changes (hyperchromatism, increased nuclear/cytoplasmic ratio and prominent nucleoli)
4. Basal cell hyperplasia with disturbance of the maturational sequence; crowding of cells; increased mitotic activity with abnormal division figures
5. Extensive surface keratinization or, more important, abnormal keratinization of individual groups of cells or single cells in the deeper parts of the epithelium

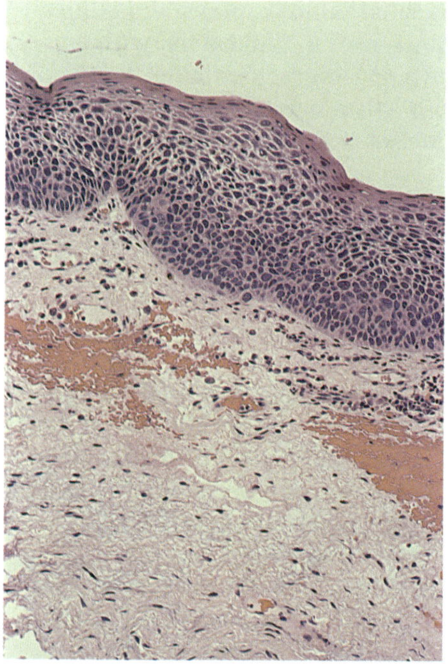

Figure 3.7 Mild dysplasia of oral mucosa.

Table 3.19 lists the general features of dysplasia in the oral cavity. Histologic grading of the degree of the abnormality of the epithelial maturation defines the degree of atypia as mild, moderate or severe (Table 3.20).

Grades I and II are reversible, provided that the provocative stimulus is removed (Figs 3.7, 3.8). Grade III is usually not reversible and in the upper aerodigestive tract is biologically equivalent to carcinoma in situ and microinvasive squamous cell carcinoma (Figs 3.9, 3.10). In many instances, grade III dysplasia lies adjacent to an invasive squamous cell carcinoma. Table 3.21 presents the incidence of dysplastic lesions and carcinomas and their association with the gross mucosal appearance in the oral cavity.[20,62–64]

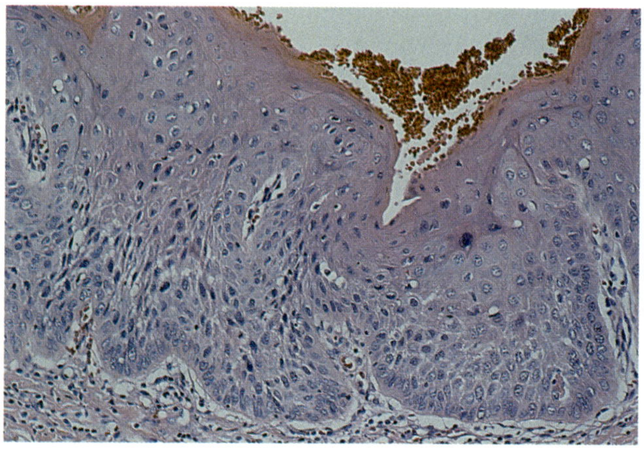

Figure 3.8 Moderately severe dysplasia of oral mucosa.

Table 3.20 Histologic grades of dysplasia

	Grade of dysplasia	Appearance	Significance
I.	Slight or mild	Normal, slightly thinned, or thickened epithelium with some surface keratosis and basal cell hyperplasia; normal mitoses	Evidence of injury, usually reversible if injury cause eliminated
II.	Moderate	Usually thickened and keratotic epithelium; some cellular and nuclear atypia; basal cell hyperplasia with usually normal mitotic activity; abnormal maturation with dyskeratosis	Mucosal change capable of progression or recurrence yet still reversible
III.	Severe keratinizing or nonkeratinizing	Thickened epithelium with prominent keratosis, with or without parakeratosis; abnormal maturation with some basal cell hyperplasia, keratinized cells at all levels; numerous mitoses, many abnormal	Mucosal change with high frequency of progression to invasive squamous cell carcinoma; biologically equivalent to carcinoma in situ

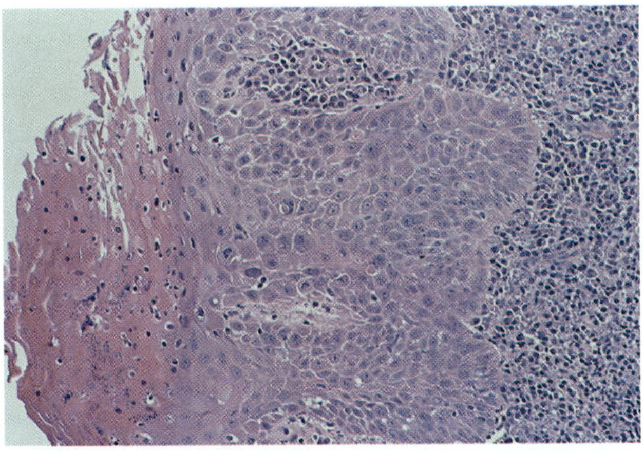

Figure 3.9 Severe keratotic dysplasia of oral mucosa.

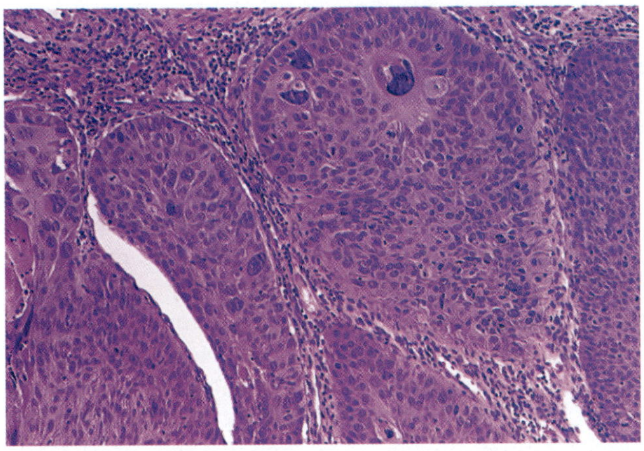

Figure 3.10 Severe keratotic dysplasia of oral mucosa.

Carcinoma in situ

The classic definition of carcinoma in situ is derived from gynecologic pathology. It appears as a top-to-bottom proliferation of basal-like cells, with little or no evidence of epithelial maturation, in a usually thin mucosa. Mitoses are common but keratosis is not.

The classic form is (a) uncommon to rare in the oral cavity, (b) nearly always associated with erythroplakia, (c) rarely an isolated lesion and (d) likely to have a lower frequency of progression to invasive carcinoma than the keratinizing grade III dysplasia.

There are few epidemiologic analyses of upper aerodigestive tract carcinoma in situ; this may be attributed to a lack of definition of the lesion and the inappropriate use of the uterine cervix model for carcinoma in situ. There also is a sampling bias, as in-situ carcinoma may not be especially considered in cases of invasive carcinomas. Singular exceptions to the foregoing are the reports by Bouquot and colleagues.[65,66] In one such report, Bouquot and Gnepp[65] analyzed the National Cancer Institute's Surveillance, Epidemiology and End Results (SEER) data. In that report, the authors assumed that some of the cases diagnosed could be appropriately considered as severe dysplasia. We definitely espouse this reasoning, as we regard severe dysplasia, in-situ carcinoma, and microinvasive squamous cell carcinoma as biologically a common entity.

SEER investigations demonstrate that carcinoma in situ is an extremely rare lesion in the upper aerodigestive tract, representing 2.8% of all upper aerodigestive tract malignancies, although this incidence varies considerably between anatomic subsites—only 1.9% of oral/pharyngeal malignancies and 6.5% in the larynx. This is in stark contrast to the uterine cervix, wherein 66% of all malignancies are carcinoma in situ. Different also is the age distribution of patients with carcinoma in situ of the upper aerodigestive tract: that distribution is almost identical to that of patients with invasive carcinoma of this anatomic site.

Throughout the United States, only 1200 upper aerodigestive tract carcinoma in situ lesions are diagnosed annually; the largest series of oral carcinoma in situ includes only 23 examples.[66]

Table 3.21 Clinical appearance of oral mucosal lesions, associated with histologic findings

Reference	Lesion	Dysplasia (%)	Carcinoma (%)
Waldron and Shafer[62]	Leukoplakia	5	3
Mashberg[63]		7	7
Silverman et al.[64]		2	7
Mashberg[63]	Speckled leukoplakia and erythroplasia	10	57
Silverman et al.[64]		16	23
Shafer and Waldron[20]	Erythroplasia	40	51
Mashberg[63]		2	64 (in situ and invasive)

Table 3.22 Average annual incidence (No. of new cases/100 000 person-years: M and F) for carcinoma in situ in US Whites: SEER population vs Rochester, MN population. (Modified from Bouquot et al.[66])

Anatomic site	US SEER	Rochester, MN
Total upper aerodigestive tract	0.5	1.8 (1.0)[a]
Oral and pharynx	0.2	1.4 (0.6)[a]
Larynx	0.3	0.4

[a]Values in parentheses are those with labial vermilion lesions excluded.

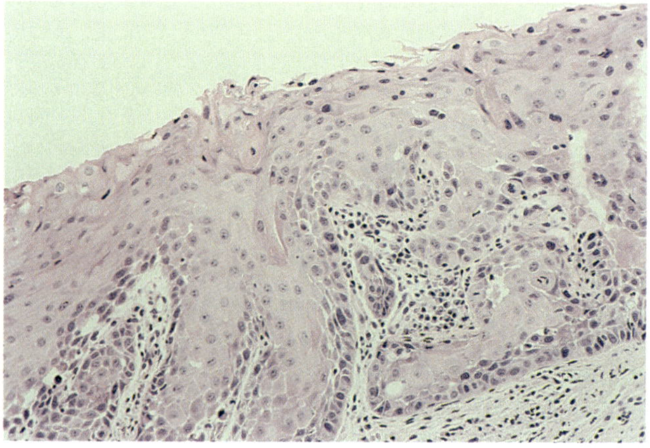

Figure 3.11 Microinvasive squamous cell carcinoma of oral mucosa.

Bouquot's second report was an epidemiologic and clinicopathologic characterization of upper aerodigestive tract in-situ carcinoma in Rochester, Minnesota.[66] Included in this report was a comparison of SEER data and findings in the Rochester, Minnesota population (Table 3.22). As may be seen, there is an excellent correlation between the two studies for carcinoma in situ of the larynx, but a considerably higher rate for oral/pharyngeal carcinoma in situ in the Rochester population (1.4/100 000 person-years vs 0.2 in the SEER population). Much of this difference disappears, however, when vermilion in-situ lesions are excluded from the Rochester data.

For several reasons, the assessment of transformation into invasive squamous cell carcinoma from in-situ carcinoma is difficult, if not impossible. Size of the lesion and, most important, a uniform histopathologic definition must be considered. The low rate of recurrence without invasion (4%) in the Rochester lesions may be related to their relatively small size. Previous investigators have demonstrated a direct correlation between lateral clinical extension and the risk of invasion. Inclusion or exclusion of keratotic or non-keratotic severe dysplasia also confounds data. In the glottis, when 'in-situ carcinoma' and severe dysplasia are both included in follow-up studies, the lesions most closely akin to 'pure' in-situ carcinoma (top-to-bottom dysplasia without keratin) like that seen in the cervix, are least likely to become invasive.[67]

Microinvasive carcinoma

The definition of microinvasive squamous cell carcinoma is fairly consistent, regardless of the anatomical site. Kleinsasser and Glanz[68] define as microinvasive carcinoma of the vocal cords only those carcinomas that have not as yet infiltrated the muscle body of the cords, a depth of invasion of about 3 mm. Microinvasion of the uterine cervix is restricted to a neoplasm infiltrating no more than 2–3 mm from the basal lamina. For the oral cavity, 1.5–2.0 mm has been proposed for microinvasion.[62] At each site, the invasion is further defined as one with an irregular, infiltrative border often accompanied by a reactive desmoplasia and not by the pushing-type expansion of hyperplastic epithelium (Fig. 3.11). If the microinvasive carcinoma is unaccompanied by a more deeply invading carcinoma, it has a low risk (or no risk), for regional metastatic spread. This behavior justifies its inclusion in the biologic triumvirate of grade III or severe dyskeratotic dysplasia, in-situ carcinoma and microinvasive carcinoma.[62,67]

Any discussion of microinvasion must consider the role of the basal lamina of the epithelium. This structure is composed of a number of components, notably type IV collagen and laminin. In general, there is an inconsistent expression of the basal lamina between the epithelium and underlying submucosa as an epithelial lesion progresses through the grades of dysplasia, in-situ carcinoma and invasive carcinoma. Whether this is due to a defect in production or more rapid turnover, including digestion of the basal lamina by carcinoma-excreted proteolytic enzymes, is unclear.[62]

The basal lamina expression in invasive squamous cell carcinoma is also paradoxical. In many instances, cords or cohesive aggregates of carcinoma in the submucosa and lower often express continuous or focal areas of basal lamina. Less apt to express this phenomena are carcinomas that invade as single cells or small, irregular cords. These

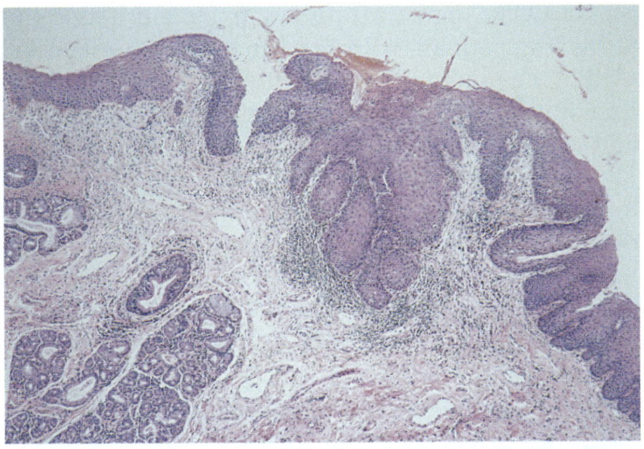

Figure 3.12 Microcarcinoma of buccal mucosa.

findings again serve notice that the distribution of basal lamina cannot distinguish an intraepithelial alteration from invasive carcinoma.

Although there is an acknowledged progression of the precursor lesions to invasive squamous cell carcinoma, it is by no means obligatory. Even the classic carcinoma in situ, a 'restrained carcinoma', does not inevitably give rise to invasive carcinoma. Finally, squamous cell carcinoma of the oral cavity can develop within a completely differentiated, only slightly hyperplastic (or even atrophic) epithelium, in an absence of atypical cells or dysplasia. This type of carcinoma develops directly from the basal cells with the upper layers manifesting some premature keratinization.

Microcarcinoma

A microcarcinoma differs from a microinvasive carcinoma in that it shows further invasive growth and has a macroscopic visibility (a three-dimensional volume of 500 mm^3 at its upper limit of size).[68] Microcarcinomas, thus defined, are rare in the oral cavity and are preponderantly laryngeal neoplasms (Fig. 3.12).

Superficial spreading carcinoma

There is a rarely encountered carcinoma of the upper aerodigestive tract that combines the histologic features of classic in-situ carcinoma with microinvasion. It is clearly not a microcarcinoma because of its usually extensive, lateral growth (superficial spreading, carpet-like) limited to the epithelium except for a few microscopic foci of invasion.[69] Cytologically, the cells are deeply hyperchromatic and basaloid with a full-thickness epithelial involvement. Mitotic activity may be paradoxically low. The esophagus, hypopharynx and larynx have been acknowledged sites of involvement. We have also seen it in the sinonasal tract and oropharynx. There are too few cases to allow any statements on prognosis. In our experience, clear (negative) margins are difficult to achieve, ultimately leading to loss of local control or an evolution to invasive carcinomas.

Oral cancer in the young and old

Patients who have none of the known risk factors for head and neck squamous cell carcinoma are at polar ends of the age span of patients with oral squamous cell carcinoma. Constantinides et al.[70] reported on the elder group, who were preponderantly women: all were over 59 years of age, gave no history of cigarette smoking or alcohol abuse, had no prior irradiation, and no previous treatment for a head and neck carcinoma. Six of the 10 carcinomas involved the oral cavity: six denture wearers had primary carcinomas of the oral cavity, but in only one did the denture abut the primary site. Of especial note, this group of elderly patients with carcinomas had their survival dependent primarily on the number of second primaries and of local recurrences, rather than on the initial stage of the lesion.

Besides denture wearing with an attendant impaired oral hygiene, malignant transformation may also be related to the following: (1) decreased cell immunity from lower levels of lymphokines and decreased T-cell function; (2) relative malnutrition; (3) changes in characteristics of saliva with increased age; (4) impaired repair of cellular breakdown.

The incidence of oral cancer in a young population (under 40 years of age) in the West varies between 0.4 and 5% of total oral cancer; in an Indian series, the incidence was 1.3%.[71] Worldwide, there is a slight preponderance of females. These young patients, especially patients with carcinoma of the tongue, usually do not have a history of obvious etiologic factors.

Table 3.23 compares the frequency of upper aerodigestive tract carcinomas in young adults (under 40 years) and older subjects.[72] There is no coherent information available on oral cancer in children, other than that most pediatric malignancies belong to the sarcoma groups. Writing in 1988, Karja et al.[73] found only 16 case reports of squamous cell carcinoma of the tongue in children aged 0–14 years in the world literature.

Table 3.23 Upper aerodigestive tract carcinomas in young adults and adults. (Modified from Lefebvre et al.[72])

	Younger than 40 years		Older than 40 years	
Site of carcinoma	***(n)***	(%)	***(n)***	(%)
Oropharynx	33	33	776	33
Oral cavity	22	22	404	17
Hypopharynx	20	20	476	21
Endolarynx	9	9	386	17
Nasopharynx	6	6	31	1
Sinonasal tract	1	1	61	3
Other	9	9	183	8

The oral squamous cell carcinomas in the young show no significant histologic difference from counterparts in older patients, other than that there seems to be a greater tendency for carcinomas in the young to be more deeply invasive. Staging of the carcinomas has shown an almost even distribution in both age groups. Carcinomas in the younger age group, however, metastasize early irrespective of tumor size.

Review of the literature indicates conflicting reports of survival rates in younger age groups with oral squamous cell carcinoma. Overall, however, the data indicate a more aggressive behavior of the carcinomas in the young. Although they are possibly not representative of all oral sites, squamous cell carcinomas of the tongue illustrate the aggressiveness of oral cancer in the young.

Less than 4% of squamous cell carcinomas of the tongue present in patients younger than 40 years of age, but they are associated with an overall poor outcome. The available data concerning young patients with squamous cell carcinoma of the tongue point to the high locoregional recurrence rate and a high disease-specific mortality.

Data of locoregional control and survival for the older population with squamous cell carcinoma of the tongue appear to be consistently superior to the results compiled in reviews for the younger population. The poor treatment results in the young are particularly impressive in the light of stage distribution, with 64% of young patients presenting with early I and II stage disease. Sarkaria and Harari,[74] after review of the literature concerning 152 patients younger than 40 years, found a 57% locoregional failure and a 47% mortality rate.

The basis for the poor ultimate treatment outlook in the young patients with the carcinoma is unknown. Unlike the older patients, many young patients have a relatively short or non-existent history of tobacco and alcohol exposure. The Kerala, India experience highlights the multifactorial background that needs to be explored in these patients.[75] In Kerala, oral cancer is the most common cancer in males (perhaps the highest incidence in the world), with age-adjusted rates of 24.2/100 000, and up to 28% of the patients with squamous cell carcinoma of the tongue are younger than 40 years. In a review of 197 consecutive patients treated for tongue cancer in Kerala, 20 of 22 (91%) patients less than 30 years of age did not have a chewing habit, compared with 29 of 175 (17%) of patients older than 30 years.

Examination of *p53* gene mutations in squamous cell carcinomas of the tongue in non-smoking and non-drinking patients under 40 years reveals a marked paucity of mutations;[76] in contrast, young smokers have a mutation incidence of approximately 40%. This difference suggests as-yet unidentified tumor susceptibility genes in the young patients with limited or no exposure to tobacco-related carcinogens.

Multiple primaries, lymph nodes and distant metastasis

Clinicopathologic factors apart from those related to the primary oral neoplasm include (1) second primary carcinomas, (2) status of regional lymph nodes, and (3) distant metastases. The pathologic aspects of each of these factors are described below.

Second primary carcinomas and field cancerization

The development of a multiple (a second) primary tumor in the upper aerodigestive tract and the lung is the main cause of mortality for patients with early-stage carcinoma of the head and neck. The theory of field cancerization assumes that, once a carcinoma is present, the entire mucosa is at risk for the development of other primary carcinomas, and provides an explanation for multiple primaries. Within the field theory reside two hypotheses with respect to the origin of second or multiple primaries: (1) the tumors are genetically unrelated and (2) single-cell transformation is followed by migration of daughter cells and genetically related tumors—a monoclonal vs polyclonal origin.[77]

In truth, neither theory contradicts the field cancerization theory. With the monoclonal hypothesis, malignant cells migrate from the primary carcinoma

Table 3.24 Location and incidence of second primary tumors in patients with squamous cell carcinoma of the oral cavity and lips. (Modified from Jovanovic et al.[80])

Sites of second primary	No. of cases	Incidence/1000 person-years of follow-up
Oral cavity	26	9.9
Lung	19	7.2
Pharynx	13	4.9
Esophagus	8	3.0
Larynx	5	1.9
Lip	3	1.1

and form foci with the potential to form a second carcinoma.[77] Polyclonality assumes that the independent second foci develop at mucosal sites where the field cancerization is most severe.

It is also probable that the distance between the index and second carcinoma is important. Favoring an independent clone of origin are those carcinomas separated by a considerable measure. Related to distance is the primary site. The behavior of laryngeal carcinomas seems to differ from that of oral carcinomas in that the former have a greater likelihood of being followed by a pulmonary cancer.[78]

The reported percentage of multiple primary neoplasms following discovery of an oral squamous cell carcinoma varies from 10 to 27%.[79,80] The majority of these second primaries are found in the oral cavity and pharynx. Although patients have an increased risk of developing cancer of the lung and larynx, the risks are less than those of developing cancer of the upper digestive tract (oral cavity, pharynx, esophagus).

The study by Jovanovic et al.[80] confirms the foregoing (Tables 3.24, 3.25). These investigators studied 727 patients with squamous cell carcinoma of the lip and oral cavity and determined the frequency of second primaries. Of the 727 patients, 96 developed a total of 114 multiple tumors during 2860.2 person-years of follow-up. Of the second primaries, 80% arose in the upper aerodigestive tract, 13% of them synchronous rather than metachronous. In women, the second primary was located mainly in the oral cavity (68%), whereas in men, there was no such predilection. Second primaries of the larynx and esophagus were mainly seen among patients with an index squamous cell carcinoma in the lower part of the mouth (lower alveolar process, floor of mouth and the retromolar region). Compared with the general population, patients with a primary squamous cell carcinoma of the lip and oral cavity had a significantly higher risk of developing an additional cancer in the oral cavity or pharynx, or both. The same cohort did not manifest an increased risk for an additional tumor outside the upper aerodigestive tract. The Jovanovic study[80] indicated that patients with a primary squamous cell carcinoma of the lip and oral cavity have, compared with the general population, a significantly increased risk of developing an additional cancer of the oral cavity and/or pharynx, the risk being 74.7-fold for men and 190.4-fold for women. A 24.6 and 45.3 times higher risk of an additional esophageal tumor was found in men and women, respectively. No increased risk for organs outside the respiratory and upper digestive tracts has been established.

Reasons for the demonstrated regional susceptibility reside in the carcinogenic effects of the use of tobacco and alcohol and in the predisposing quality of oral leukoplakia. With respect to the latter, it has been noted that patients with carcinoma of the tongue together with leukoplakia have a five-fold greater frequency of second primaries than do patients without leukoplakia.[81]

Table 3.25 Second primary tumors in patients with oral squamous cell carcinoma. (Modified from Jovanovic et al.[80])

	Total	Synchronous	Metachronous	Incidence per 1000 person-years follow-up
Total no. of second primaries	114	16	98	39.8
Second primary in the upper aerodigestive tract	91	12	79	31.8
Second primary outside the upper aerodigestive tract	23	4	19	8.0

Table 3.26 Impact of second primary carcinomas on survival. (From data presented by Gluckman and Crissman[83])

(a) Multiple cancers ($n = 548$)

Site	Synchro-nous (%)	Metachro-nous (%)	5-year survival (%)
Oral cavity	20	10.5	15.2
Lip	50	26.8	38.4
Oropharynx	23.8	21.0	22.4
Hypopharynx	8.3	10.9	9.1
Larynx	36.5	16.8	26.7
Overall	27.7	17.0	22.3

(b) Primary (single) cancers ($n = 3793$)

Site	5-year survival (%)
Oral cavity	26.9
Lip	64.6
Oropharynx	27.0
Hypopharynx	13.0
Larynx	43.3
Overall	35.0

Table 3.27 Second primary carcinomas and 5-year survival from time of diagnosis of index carcinoma. (Modified from Jones et al.[84])

Site in the head and neck	No. of patients	Second primary rate (actuarial %)	5-year survival (%)
Oral cavity	715	12.6	47
Oropharynx	494	10.5	40
Hypopharynx	627	5.6	25
Larynx	1245	10.6	64
All sites	3436	9.1	48

Data from the meta-analysis of 40 287 patients by Haughey et al.[82] and a study of a cohort of 5180 patients with head-and-neck cancer by Deleyiannis and Thomas[78] further support the thesis that the site of the primary head-and-neck cancer correlates with the development of a second malignancy. The second set of investigators found that lung cancer developed in 356 (6.9%) of 5180 patients within 15 years of the diagnosis of the index carcinoma.[78] The risk of lung cancer significantly increased with increasing age at diagnosis of the index neoplasm. Men had a significantly higher risk of lung cancer than women. Risk of lung cancer was highest for patients with cancer of the extrinsic larynx, followed in descending order of risk by patients with cancer of the hypopharynx, oropharynx, intrinsic larynx, oral cavity and lip. The stage and grade of the index neoplasm were not significantly related to the development of lung cancer.

Compared with the risk for patients with oral cancer (relative risk = 1.00), the adjusted relative risk of lung cancer developing by site was 0.69 for lip, 1.04 for intrinsic larynx, 2.14 for oropharynx, 1.70 for hypopharynx, and 2.75 for extrinsic larynx. The adjusted cumulative probability of lung cancer developing within 15 years from a diagnosis of head-and-neck cancer by site was 10% for lip, 16% for oral cavity, 18% for intrinsic larynx, 28% for oropharynx, 30% for hypopharynx, and 37% for extrinsic larynx.

The probability of surviving 3 years after the diagnosis of the lung cancer was 15.8% and of surviving 5 years, 8.6%. Tables 3.26 and 3.27 give an overview of the impact of second carcinomas on survival.[83,84]

Status of regional lymph nodes

The involvement of cervical lymph nodes is an essential element of prognosis in head-and-neck cancer (Fig. 3.13). The rate of recurrence in the neck in patients without metastatic lymph nodes is significantly lower than that in patients with positive lymph nodes. The rate does not change significantly in patients free of carcinoma at the primary site, but is affected by other factors such as size, site and stage of the primary carcinoma, as well as the type of neck dissection. In most series, the rate of recur-

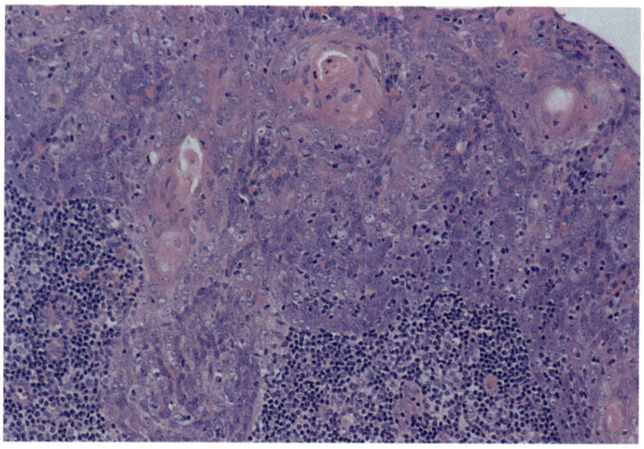

Figure 3.13 Cervical lymph node with metastatic squamous cell carcinoma.

Table 3.28 Frequency of histologically positive lymph nodes in N0 necks. (Modified from Jones et al.[88])

Site of primary	No. of cases	Patients with positive nodes (*n*)	(%)	No. of patients with extracapsular extension
Oral cavity	31	9	29	2
Oropharynx	16	4	25	2
Hypopharynx	32	16	50	6
Larynx	38	8	21	0
Total	117	37	32	10

rence following elective surgery is much lower than in those patients who undergo therapeutic or secondary neck dissection.

It is almost certain that the much worse outlook for patients with stage groupings III and IV compared with I and II is mainly due to an increased lymph node involvement. In general, patients presenting with neck node metastases do half as well as do patients who present with a primary tumor only. It is also considered that the node level affects survival. Spiro and associates[85] suggested five levels of lymph nodes: level I is the submandibular region; levels II, III and IV are upper, middle, and lower deep cervical; and level V is the posterior triangle/ supraclavicular fossa nodes. In the employment of these levels, Spiro et al.[85] found that the 5-year survival fell from 45% for level I to 18% for level IV. No patient with positive level V lymph nodes survived for 5 years. Other clinical studies have confirmed this trend.

Jones et al.[86] performed uni- and multivariate analyses of a number of tumor factors and prognosis in oral cancer. When their data from 524 patients were analyzed by Cox's multivariate regression, only T stage and N stage were found to be significant: both were highly significant predictors of survival, with survival falling with increase in stage. Earlier, Stell[87] had shown that the only relationship between host factors was the one between age and performance status: men with stage III and IV tumors generally were also in poor general health. Concerning survival, he found that, when adjusted survival was studied on treated patients, none of the host factors had an effect.

A number of pathologic findings in the lymph node metastases have been proclaimed as providing additional prognostic information to supplement clinical examination. The findings have been addressed in numerous reports, some presenting contrary data. Overall, however, there is general agreement on several factors that have an appreciable correlation with the rate of cervical recurrence: these are (1) number of lymph nodes involved; (2) extracapsular extension; (3) desmoplastic stromal reaction; (4) invasion of soft tissues, including vascular/lymphatic space; (5) adherence to nerves; (6) invasion of the jugular vein. Table 3.28, from the study by Jones et al.,[88] gives the frequency of histologically positive lymph nodes in N0 necks. The frequency of positive nodes in elective vs therapeutic neck dissections is shown in Table 3.29.[89] The effect of pathologic N stage on prognosis is presented in Table 3.30.

Table 3.29 Histologically positive lymph nodes by primary site of carcinoma.[a] (Modified from Shah[89])

Site of primary carcinoma (no. of patients)	Percentage positive nodes (elective neck dissection)	Percentage positive nodes (therapeutic neck dissection)
Oral cavity (501)	34	76
Oropharynx (207)	31	84
Hypopharynx (126)	17	97
Larynx (247)	37	84
Total (1081)	33	82

[a]Data based on study of 1081 patients undergoing 1119 elective and therapeutic radical neck dissections. The majority of metastatic nodes were in levels I, II and III. Level IV was involved in only 20%. Metastases at level V were encountered in only 4% of patients and were restricted to primary sites from floor-of-mouth and the lower gum.

The study of Olsen et al.,[90] dealing with 284 patients with pathologically confirmed metastatic squamous cell carcinoma who underwent neck dissection without adjuvant therapy, is quite representative of

Table 3.30 Pathologic N stage and survival in oral carcinoma. (From data presented by Jones[86])

No. of nodes	Observed 3-year survival (%)
0	49
1	46
2	27
3+	11
p	<0.0001
Extracapsular extension	**Median survival, months (range)**
Positive	10 (7–17)
Negative	19 (13–38)
p	<0.025

the type of retrospective analysis dealing with these several histologic factors. With a p value of 0.05 or less indicating prognostic significance, the histologic characteristics associated with an increased risk of neck recurrence in the study by Olsen et al.[90] were as follows: four or more lymph nodes involved (compared with one to three lymph nodes), extracapsular extension (gross or microscopic), local invasion, adherence to nerves, and a desmoplastic stromal reaction (Table 3.31). The finding of gross as opposed to microscopic extranodal extension was not a significant factor in the authors' final time-dependent adjusted-hazards ratio. Nodal fixation and location of positive lymph nodes were not analyzed but these factors, too, have prognostic significance.

There is agreement that the outlook for a patient with a fixed cervical lymph node is poor, but there have been different interpretations of what constitutes a 'fixed node'. Two definitions have been used: (1) reduced mobility and (2) fixation to anatomic structures such as the mandible, skull base, carotid artery, skin. The distinction is important: for example, the 5-year cure rate for carcinomas of the oral cavity and oropharynx with single lymph nodes of reduced mobility was 40%, whereas fully fixed lymph nodes carried only a 13% cure rate. Stell and associates,[91] using the truly fixed node as their marker, found an incidence of about 7% in 1863 patients with upper aerodigestive tract squamous cell carcinomas. The incidence of fixed nodes differed between different subsites (oral cavity, oropharynx, piriform sinus and lower alveolus at high risk). There was also an increase in incidence with an increase of T stage of the primary neoplasm. The highest incidence (36%) was found in patients with occult primary carcinomas.

Some protocols retain fixation as a feature; however, in general, size has been used, as it has been shown that a lymph node is unlikely to be truly fixed until its diameter is 6 cm or more.

The significance of the number of positive lymph nodes corroborates earlier findings by Shah et al.[92] (Table 3.32), Snow et al.[93] and Kalnins et al.[94] The considerable decline in 5-year survival rate (if there is histologic evidence of extranodal spread) has been repeatedly affirmed, with only occasional disclaimers. Shigaki et al.[95] found cervical recurrence in 80% of patients having extranodal spread; Pinsolle et al.,[96] on the other hand, did not find a difference in outcome associated with transcapsular spread. They indicate that adequate (combined treatment modalities) treatment may erase its adverse local effects; furthermore, an unexpectedly found

Table 3.31 Histologic risk factors for neck recurrence in patients with cervical lymph node metastases. (Prepared from data presented by Olsen et al.[90])

Risk factor	Contrast[a]	*p* value	2-year recurrence-free survival (%)
No. of histologically positive lymph nodes	>4 vs 1 to 3	0.0002	51 vs 79
Extracapsular disease	Gross/microscopic vs none	0.007	54 vs 91
Extracapsular extension	Gross vs microscopic	0.03	41 vs 58
Vascular/lymphatic space invasion	+ vs –	0.003	42 vs 95
Soft tissue invasion	+ vs –	0.0002	50 vs 84
Jugular vein invasion	+ vs –	0.0004	27 vs 75
Adherence to nerves	+ vs –	0.002	50 vs 75
Desmoplastic lymph node reaction	+ vs –	0.0001	32 vs 86

[a] +, positive; –, negative.

Table 3.32 Oral squamous cell carcinoma: pathologic factors and locoregional failure. (From data provided by Shah et al.[92] and based on 704 patients (370 'cures' and 334 failures)

Factor	Number of patients	'Cures'	Failure
Histopathologic grade			
1	20	15	5
2	465	243	222
3	187	87	100
4	10	7	3
Positive margins	54	12	42
No. of positive lymph nodes			
1	61	29	32
2–3	59	31	28
4–6	58	19	39
7–10	48	12	36
>10	56	19	37
Size of lymph nodes			
<2 cm	152	66	86
2–4 cm	95	32	64
>4 cm	34	11	23
Extracapsular extension	92	28	64
Soft tissue extension	69	22	47

transcapsular spread in patients with N0 node involvement certainly differs in significance from transcapsular spread in patients with N3 node involvement.

Transcapsular extension (Fig. 3.14) is to be distinguished from intracapsular invasion.[97] The significance of the latter has yet to be determined and is probably not portentous. A desmoplastic stromal reaction is characterized by a connective tissue (fibroblastic) reaction of the involved node to the metastatic carcinoma. The desmoplasia, however, is rarely confined to the lymph node and is usually found with transcapsular spread. Olsen et al.[90] found the desmoplastic pattern to be associated with a six-fold to seven-fold increased risk of recurrence in all the proportional hazards models studied. It remains to be seen whether transcapsular extension and desmoplastic stromal reaction are independent contributors to neck recurrence.

Other lymph-node responses (e.g. follicular pattern, sinus histiocytosis, etc.) are not important considerations for recurrence in the neck.

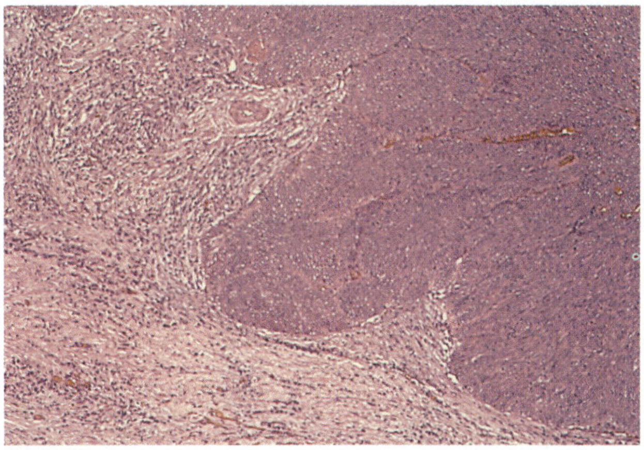

Figure 3.14 Extranodal (transcapsular) extension of a squamous cell carcinoma metastasis to cervical lymph node.

Neither the definition nor the significance of a micrometastasis to the cervical lymph nodes has been established. Moreover, the question of the clinical utility of the extra workload of the complementary multiple sectioning and immunostaining of lymph nodes to detect a micrometastasis remains unanswered. It is undeniable, however, that when a meticulous routine histopathologic examination of cervical lymph nodes is performed, it has been found that the frequency of micrometastasis is high. Data from the study by van den Brekel et al.[98] may be considered typical of the situation. These authors, defining a metastasis measuring 3 mm or smaller as a micrometastasis, found them in 66 lymph nodes in 41 of 92 tumor-positive neck dissection specimens. Detection of these micrometastases influenced postoperative treatment in three of 77 patients with neck node metastases. Sectioning at a deeper level, in 600 originally histopathologically negative lymph nodes from 64 patients, revealed seven additional micrometastases in five patients. Immunohistochemical studies with antikeratin monoclonal antibodies demonstrated four micrometastases in 739 originally histopathologically negative nodes in three of 13 patients.

We agree with the conclusions expressed by van den Brekel et al.,[98] that the additional techniques are best used for studies on the prognostic significance of such metastases and on the accuracy of preoperative staging techniques.

Distant metastases

As local and regional control of head and neck cancer has improved, distant metastases have been increasingly important causes of death. Vikram,[99] for example, noted that, with his population, the overall

Table 3.33 Distant metastases from head-and-neck primary squamous cell carcinoma. (After data presented by Calhoun et al.[101])

	Characteristic	Comment
1.	Percentage of patients with clinical evidence of distant spread	5–25%
2.	Percentage of patients with necropsy evidence of distant spread	≤50%
3.	Size of primary	More commonly associated with increasing T classification
4.	Initial stage of neck disease	N0 = 2–8% N1 = 9–29% N2, N3 = 17–51%
5.	Site of primary	Modest influence; hypopharynx more often than tongue; tonsil more than larynx
6.	Histologic grade	Contradictory reports; probably not significant
7.	Treatment of primary	No apparent influence
8.	Time interval between diagnosis of primary and clinically apparent distant metastasis	Most by 2 years following diagnosis
9.	Metastatic sites	Any organ, but lungs, bone and liver most common Lungs = 52–82% Liver = 6% (clinical) and 17–45% (necropsy) Bone = 20–57% (clinical) and 6–44% (necropsy); spine and ribs most common
10.	Survival	85–90% dead by 2 years; mean survival = 4.2 months

rate of distant metastases had remained about 20% over the prior 20 years, but that the incidence of the metastases occurring with locoregional control had changed from 4% (1960–1965) to 56% (1975–1980) of all patients developing the metastases to distant sites. He and co-workers[100] proposed that the development of multimodality therapy during this time, particularly use of adjunctive radiation therapy, although responsible for the better locoregional control, did little to impede distant metastases. Other investigators indicate that 55–90% of patients who develop distant metastases have coexisting clinical evidence of recurrent locoregional disease.[101] Absence of clinical evidence of locoregional failure is also associated with distant metastases and raises the question of eradication as opposed to only a slowing of the appearance of the locoregional recurrence. In any event, patients with distant metastases do not live long: survival for more than a year is unusual and for more than 2 years is very rare. Table 3.33, derived from a literature review by Calhoun et al.,[101] summarizes factors associated with distant metastases.

Locoregional disease, none the less, still continues as an important (if not the most important) factor as

Table 3.34 Locoregional disease compared with distant metastasis in autopsy series of patients with head-and-neck squamous cell carcinoma. (From data provided by Slootweg et al.[102])

Loclregional disease without distant metastasis (%)	Locoregional disease with distant metastasis (%)	Distant metastasis without locoregional disease (%)	No locoregional disease and no distant metastasis (%)
51–33 (40)[a]	52–23 (36)[a]	10–2 (5.4)[a]	25–12 (19.7)[a]

[a]Average percentages in parentheses.

a cause of death. Slootweg et al.,[102] in a report of autopsy findings in patients with head-and-neck squamous cell cancer, conclude that a major proportion of the patients die with locoregional disease as the single tumor manifestation. Locoregional disease was present in 62% of the autopsied patients, 40% of whom were without carcinoma at other body sites outside the head and neck region. Distant metastasis was observed in 24% of patients; in 19% of these it occurred with concomitant locoregional disease. Second primary tumors were observed in 31% of patients (11% in the head and neck region, the lung, 14% and 6% in miscellaneous other sites). Of the autopsy cohort, 17% died of causes other than the carcinoma. Table 3.34 presents the occurrence of locoregional disease in comparison with distant metastasis in five series of autopsied patients with head-and-neck squamous cell carcinoma.[102]

Table 3.35 Oral minor salivary glands

Name	Location and type of secretion
Superior labial	Lip (labial)/mixed
Inferior labial	
Buccal/retromolar	Vestibular/mixed
Posterolateral palatine	Hard palate/mucous
Palatine	Soft palate/mucous
Glossopalatine	Glossopalatine folds/mucous
Blandin–Nuhn (anterior lingual)	Body of tongue/mixed
von Ebner (posterior lingual)	Base of tongue/serous
Tonsil, lingual (posterior lingual)	Base of tongue/mucous
Intrinsic sublingual	Floor of mouth/mixed

Neoplastic and non-neoplastic salivary gland lesions of the oral cavity

Lesions of oral cavity salivary tissues enter into the differential diagnosis of the much more preponderant squamous cell carcinomas. Some, like necrotizing sialometaplasia, may be particularly challenging in both gross and microscopic respects.

The salivary lesions may be solid or cystic and, with the exception of necrotizing sialometaplasia, are usually non-ulcerated unless subject to trauma. Nearly every class of salivary neoplasm is represented, some with a predilection for the oral cavity (e.g. terminal duct adenocarcinoma, sialoadenoma papilliferum).

Distribution of oral salivary tissue

All regions of the oral cavity contain salivary gland tissue except the gingivae, dorsum of the tongue (anterior two-thirds) and anterior segments of the hard palate, including the raphe. With the exception of those associated with the posterior tongue—the von Ebner's glands—all are pure or predominantly mucus secretors (Table 3.35). For the most part, intercalated ducts are not well developed, striated ducts are lacking, and excretory ducts empty directly into the oral cavity. Capsules are absent and septal compartmentalizations of endpieces are poorly defined and occasionally absent; this is particularly true for the vestibular and palatal glands.

The vestibular glands consist of three contiguous groups—labial, buccal, and retromolar. The vestibular glands are numerous near the midline of the lip but become sparse near the cheek. In the cheek, the number and size of the glands increase more posteriorly.

The palatine glands also consist of three contiguous groups—hard palatine (posterolateral regions of the hard palate), soft palatine (soft palate and uvula), and glossopalatine (near the fauces or palatoglossal folds).

The lingual salivary glands are distributed over the body of the tongue as the Blandin–Nuhn or anterior lingual glands, over the root as the von Ebner or posterior lingual glands, and over the faucial area as the tonsillar or deep posterior glands; within the lingual sulcus is a sublingual group. The glands of Blandin–Nuhn are located on the underside of the tip of the tongue, immediately lateral to the midline. These glands may extend for 25 mm posteriorly. Secretions from the glands are carried to five excretory ducts opening into the sulcus in the region of the frenulum.

The minor salivary glands of the oral cavity are found in the subepithelial connective tissue. These glands secrete in a continuous fashion, and account for approximately 5% of the total daily salivary output of 1 liter. Most of the glands produce a mixed type of secretion, although the glands of von Ebner produce a serous secretion.

Table 3.36 Oral salivary gland tumors: sites of origin. (From data presented by Goldblatt and Ellis[103])

Oral subsite	No.	(%)
Benign		
Palate	686	(60.3)
Buccal mucosa	102	(9.0)
Lip		
Upper	201	(17.7)
Lower	17	(1.5)
Not specified	70	(6.2)
Tongue	23	(2.0)
Floor of mouth	7	(0.1)
Others	31	(2.7)
Malignant		
Palate	449	(53.6)
Buccal mucosa	124	(14.8)
Tongue	90	(10.8)
Floor of mouth	54	(6.5)
Lip		
Upper	11	(1.3)
Lower	4	(0.5)
Not specified	54	(6.5)
Others	51	(6.1)

Table 3.37 Oral salivary gland tumors: histopathologic types. (From data presented by Goldblatt and Ellis[103])

Type[a]	No.	(%)
Benign		
Pleomorphic adenoma	1281	(91.8)
Monomorphic adenoma	61	(4.3)
Oncocytoma	6	(0.4)
Others	48	(3.4)
Malignant		
Adenoid cystic	496	(37.2)
Mucoepidermoid	342	(25.6)
Acinic cell	10	(0.7)
Carcinoma ex pleomorphic adenoma	126	(9.4)

[a]Malignant:benign ratio = 1:1.4.

Neoplasms

The malignant to benign ratio of oral salivary gland tumors is 1.1:1, with the majority of the tumors occurring in the palate, buccal mucosa and the upper lip.[103,104] The palate is the most common location, accounting for 50–60% of the tumors in most series. Tables 3.36 and 3.37 present the various oral subsites and histopathologic classifications of the neoplasms.[102]

Clinical signs and symptoms vary with the site and histologic type, but the tumors usually present as a painless mass, less often as a recently enlarging mass with or without pain or ulceration. Spontaneous ulceration is quite unusual and is mostly due to trauma (dentition, instrumentation, etc.). Treatment and prognosis are dependent particularly on clinical stage, less so by histologic type.

The average age for benign salivary gland tumors, at time of diagnosis, is 43 years; for malignant tumors, 51 years. The sex ratio for both benign and malignant tumors is (M/F) 1/1.3.[104]

Tongue

The tongue accounts for only a small percentage of all intra-oral salivary gland tumors—2.0% of the benign and nearly 11% of the malignant. The site of predilection for malignant lingual salivary tumors is clearly the posterior/base part;[105] benign salivary gland tumors favor the middle to anterior portion of the tongue; adenoid cystic and mucoepidermoid carcinomas account for two-thirds of the salivary gland tumors of the tongue.

Local progression of salivary tumors of the base of the tongue invades adjacent structures including the wall of the pharynx and the mandible. Intracranial extension can occur from direct growth through the cranial vault, but more often through perineural spread—particularly along the trigeminal and glossopharyngeal nerves.

Palate

Salivary tissue is seldom found anterior to a line between the first molars. In this area, fibroadipose tissue is substituted. The midline of the hard palate is also devoid of glands and the attached gingivae are only sparsely populated by glands. The number of glandular elements is greatest in the hard palate, about half as numerous in the soft palate, and least abundant in the uvula. Compactness and collective density are, however, greatest near the junction of the hard and soft palates; here, also, the greatest number of serous acini are found.

In accordance with the distribution of glands, a salivary gland tumor of the palate typically presents in the posterior two-thirds, lateral to the midline and medial to the gingiva. The tumor is most often seen at, or near, the junction of the two parts of the palate. The dominance of pleomorphic adenoma

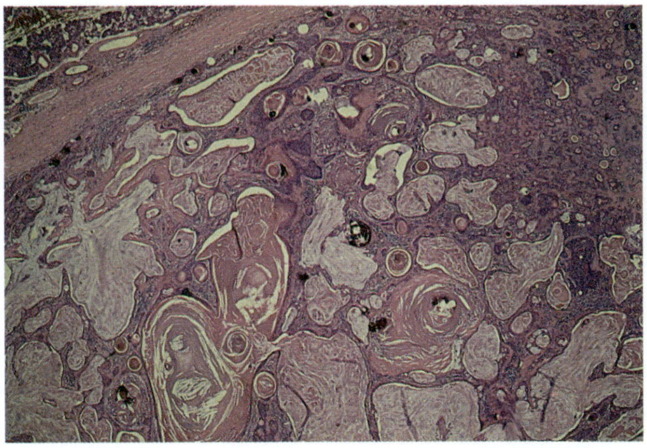

Figure 3.15 Pleomorphic adenoma of the palate.

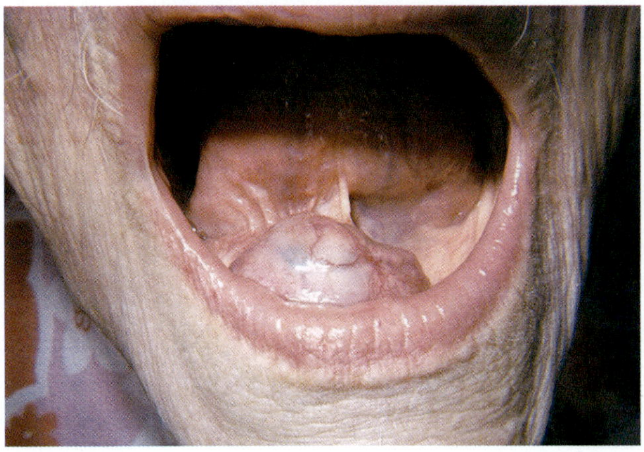

Figure 3.16 Adenoid cystic carcinoma arising in the floor of mouth.

(Fig. 3.15) and adenoid cystic carcinoma as the principal types of salivary neoplasm is seen in Table 3.37.

Two-thirds of pleomorphic adenomas of the palate arise in the posterior third of the hard palate or at the junction of the two palates; one-third of the tumors are found in the soft palate.

Most of the tumors are detected in the third decade of life and women are affected more than men. Tumor size varies from less than 1.0 to over 12 cm. Ulceration of the overlying mucosa is variably reported in up to 10% of cases; in nearly every instance this is not spontaneous.

The frequency of involvement of the underlying palatal bone by pleomorphic adenomas is undefined. In the event, such involvement is one of pressure atrophy or resorption and not infiltration. In rare instances a total rarefaction and even perforation of the hard palate may be seen.

Adenoid cystic carcinoma is not only the most common malignant salivary gland tumor of the palate, it is the most common salivary malignancy of the oral cavity. The notorious neurotropism, local extension, and relatively slow growth of this carcinoma elsewhere apply equally to the oral cavity (Figs 3.16–3.19).

Depending on the published series, the terminal duct adenocarcinoma (Fig. 3.20) or mucoepidermoid carcinoma ranks as the second most common oral salivary gland malignancy. Most of the mucoepidermoid carcinomas are intermediate or low-grade (Figs 3.21–3.24). The terminal duct adenocarcinoma, a biologically low-grade neoplasm, shares a strong neurotropism (small nerves) with the adenoid cystic carcinoma and also a predilection for the palate.[106]

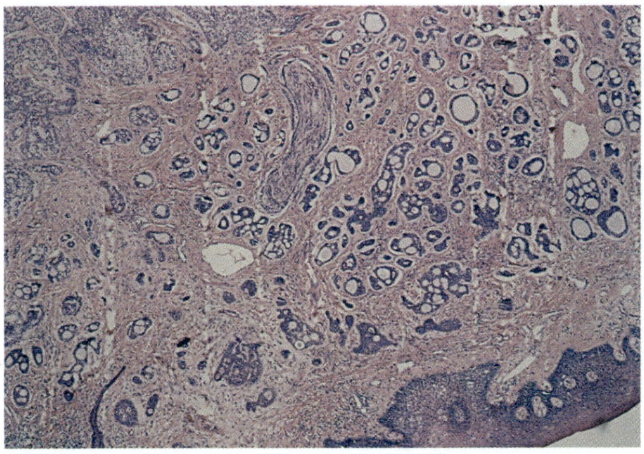

Figure 3.17 Photomicrograph of the adenoid cystic carcinoma depicted in Figure 3.16.

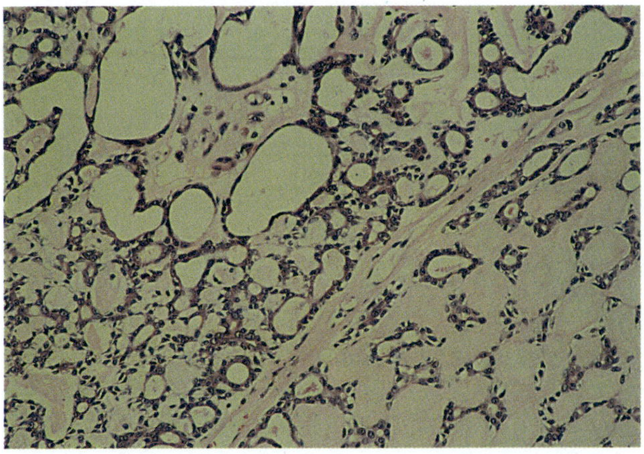

Figure 3.18 Cribriform and cylindromatous patterns of adenoid cystic carcinoma.

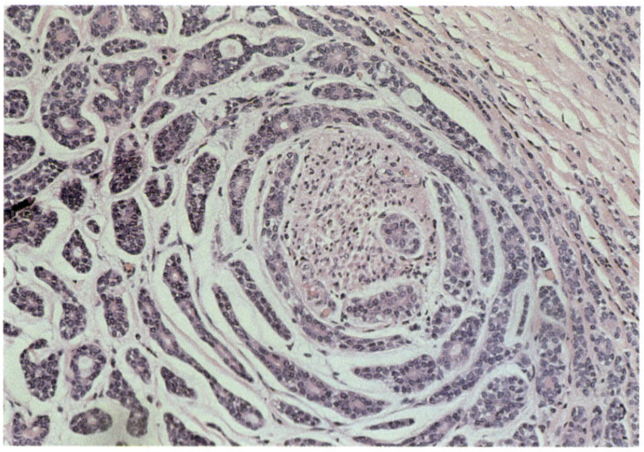

Figure 3.19 Peri- and intraneural invasion by an adenoid cystic carcinoma of the palate.

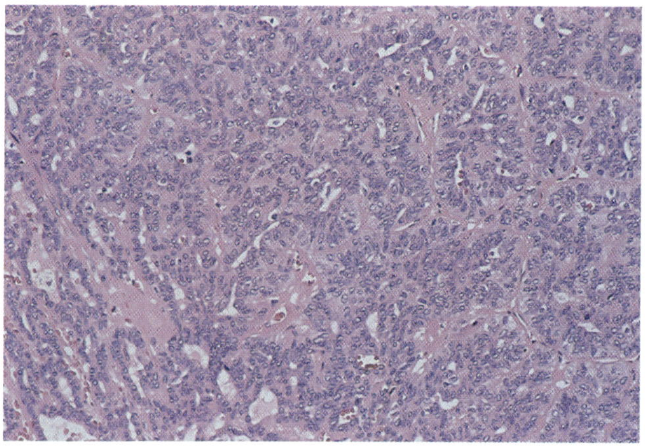

Figure 3.20 Terminal duct (polymorphous low-grade) adenocarcinoma of the palate.

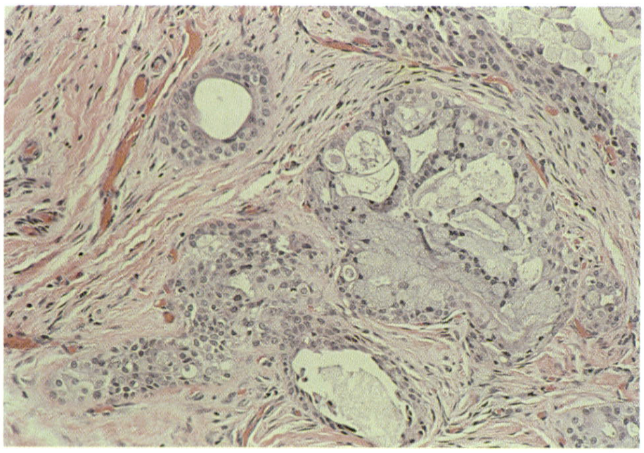

Figure 3.21 Low-grade mucoepidermoid carcinoma of the palate.

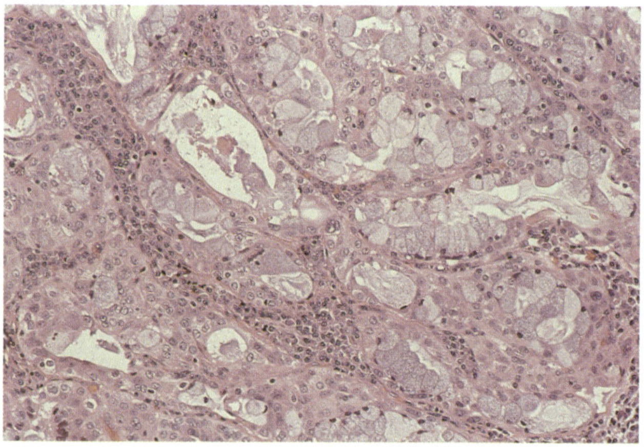

Figure 3.22 Low-grade mucoepidermoid carcinoma of the buccal mucosa showing terminal mucous cell differentiation.

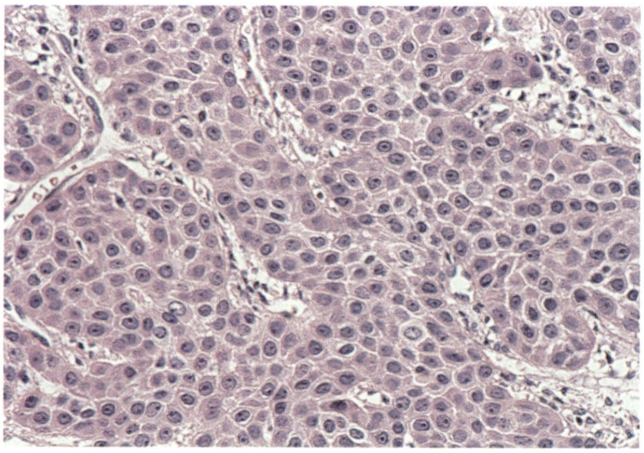

Figure 3.23 Intermediate-grade (II) mucoepidermoid carcinoma composed almost exclusively of intermediate cells.

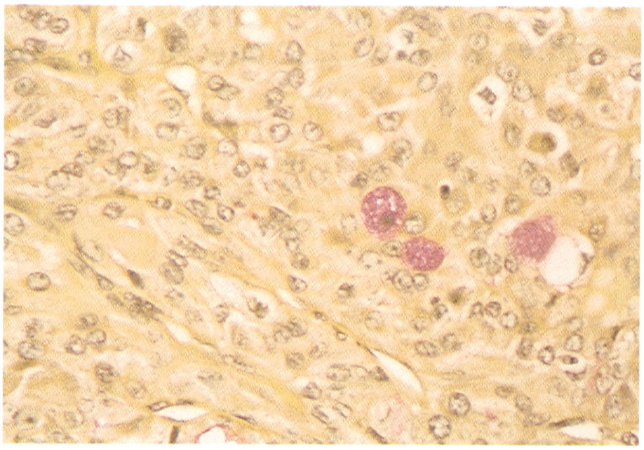

Figure 3.24 Mucicarmine positive cells in a grade II mucoepidermoid carcinoma.

Table 3.38 Salivary gland tumors of the lips (n = 103). (Modified from Neville et al.[107])

Site and type	No. of cases (%)
I. Lip site	
Upper lip	87 (84.5)
Lower lip	16 (15.5)
II. Histologic type of upper lip tumors	
Benign adenomas	
Monomorphic	43 (49.4)
Pleomorphic	37 (42.5)
	80 (92.0)
Malignant tumors	
Adenoid cystic carcinoma	4 (4.6)
Acinic cell carcinoma	2 (2.3)
Adenocarcinoma	1 (1.1)
	7 (8.0)
III. Histologic type of lower lip tumors	
Benign	
Intraductal papilloma	1 (6.2)
Malignant	
Mucoepidermoid carcinoma	13 (81.2)
Acinic cell carcinoma	2 (12.5)
	15 (93.8)

Lips

Four oral pathology laboratories contributed cases of labial salivary gland tumors to the study by Neville et al.[107] (Table 3.38). Of 103 identified tumors, 87 (84.5%) were from the upper lip, whereas 16 (15.5%) were from the lower lip. Of the upper lip tumors, 92% were benign; of the 16 lower lip tumors, 93.8% were malignant. These results confirm findings of earlier investigators, that minor salivary gland tumors are much more common in the upper lip than the lower lip, but that lower lip tumors are more likely to be malignant. Acinic cell carcinomas are rare in anatomic sites other than the parotid gland, and this holds true for intra-oral salivary tissue.

Table 3.39 Inverted ductal papilloma of the oral cavity in 18 patients aged 32–66 years. (From data collected by Hegarty et al.[110])

Oral location	No. of cases
Lower lip	11
Buccal	5
Floor of mouth	1
Soft palate	1
Clinical appearance	1.0–1.5 cm diameter; painless, mucosal punctum
Biologic behavior	Benign; no recurrences, no malignant transformation

Monomorphic adenomas

Monomorphic adenomas can potentially arise from any salivary source but have been reported most often from labial intraoral and parotid salivary glands.[108,109] Those of minor salivary gland origin tend to occur within or adjacent to the upper lip (80%), but the buccal mucosa and palate are not immune (Fig. 3.25). In minor salivary glands, the tumors are usually unencapsulated, firm or cystic, freely movable submucosal nodules. There is a distinct tendency for multicentricity.

Two adenomas, the inverted ductal papilloma[110] and sialoadenoma papilliferum,[111] have either an exclusive or sharp predilection for the oral cavity. Sialoadenoma

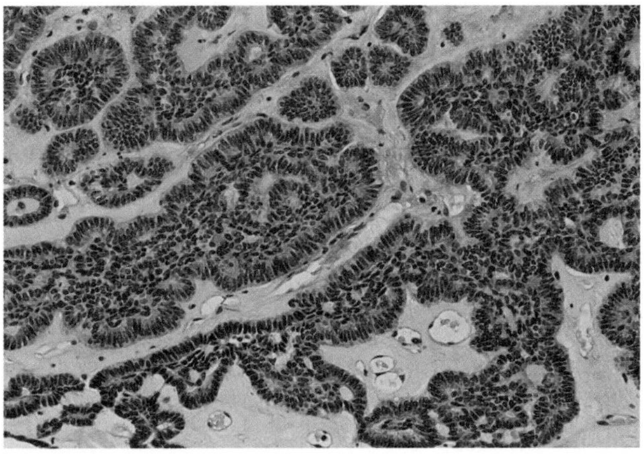

Figure 3.25 Canalicular monomorphic adenoma of the buccal mucosa; this type of monomorphic adenoma is the most common in the oral cavity.

Table 3.40 Benign salivary gland cysts: Hamburg salivary gland register (1965–94). (Modified from Seifert[112])

Classification of cyst	Salivary gland location	No.	(%)
Mucoceles			
Mucous extravasation	Lower lip	1171	(75)
Mucous retention	Lip, cheek, palate, floor of mouth	75	(4.8)
Salivary duct cysts	Parotid	160	(10.25)
Lymphoepithelial cysts	Floor of mouth, parotid	79	(5.1)
Ranula	Sublingual gland	49	(3.1)
Dermoid cysts	Floor of mouth, parotid	24	(1.5)
Polycystic (dysgenetic) disease	Parotid	3	(0.2)

papilliferum, regarded as an analog of the cutaneous syringocystadenoma papilliferum, has a predilection for the palate where it presents as a sessile or pedunculated surface mucosal lesion. The inverted ductal papilloma has a preference for the upper lip and buccal mucosa (Table 3.39). Both adenomas may be mistaken for mucoepidermoid carcinoma.

Non-neoplastic salivary lesions

Salivary cysts

Approximately 6–9% of all salivary gland lesions are various types of benign salivary cysts. The distribution of these cysts is overwhelmingly oral and preponderantly labial and it is the mucocele that dominates all statistics (Table 3.40).[112]

The prevalence of all oral mucoceles is estimated as 2.5/1000 population.[112] The lower lip is most frequently affected, followed by the cheek, palate, floor of mouth and retromolar fossa; the upper lip is rarely affected.

The mucoceles occur most often in children and young adults in an equal sex distribution. Oral mucoceles are usually small, commonly less than 10 mm. Larger mucoceles are prone to occur in the lower lip and the cheek. Histologically, the majority of mucoceles are of the mucous extravasation type; mucous retention cysts account for only a small percentage of the lesions (Figs 3.26, 3.27).

Clinically, the cysts should not pose a diagnostic problem. A low-grade mucoepidermoid carcinoma and cystadenoma are the principal differential diagnoses. Even origin of malignancy from any of the cysts is rare. Seifert[112] found only one example of this, a mucoepidermoid carcinoma arising in a salivary duct cyst, in a series of 1661 salivary gland cysts.

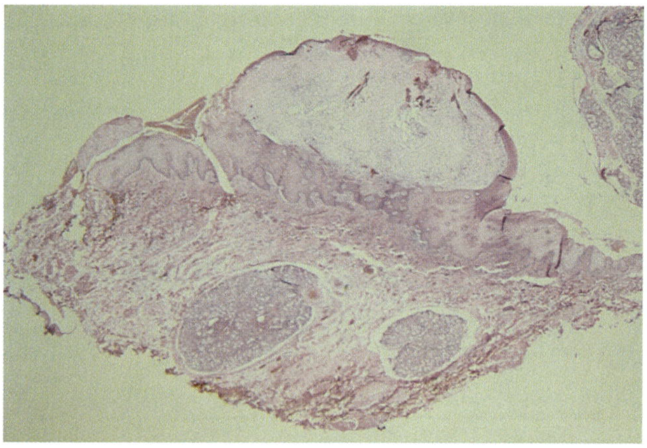

Figure 3.26 Labial mucocele.

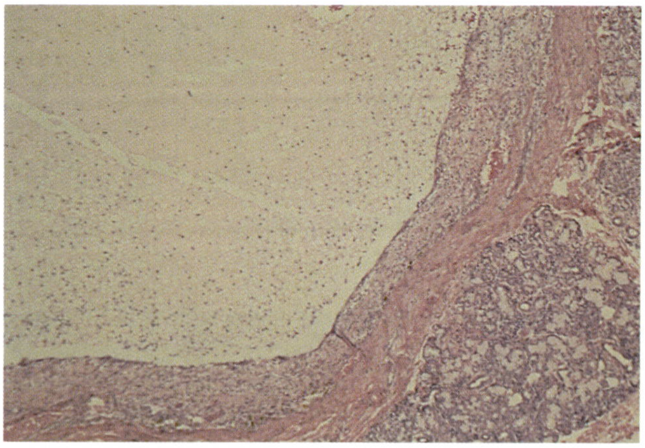

Figure 3.27 Higher magnification of the pseudocystic space in the labial mucocele shown in Figure 3.26.

Adenomatoid hyperplasia

Clinically presenting as a sessile, firm and painless lump in the oral cavity, adenomatoid hyperplasia has been likened to a 'sheep in wolf's clothing'.

Table 3.41 Adenomatoid hyperplasia of minor salivary glands in 58 cases. (Modified from Buchner et al.[113])

Anatomic location	No. of cases	
Hard palate	25	
Soft palate	15	84.5%
Junction of plates	9	
Mandibular retromolar area	4	
Buccal mucosa	2	
Upper lip mucosa	1	
Lower lip mucosa	1	
Ventral tongue	1	

Table 3.41 gives the intra-oral sites of the lesion recorded by Buchner et al.[113] Principal histologic features are hyperplasia and hypertrophy of mucous acini with preservation of lobular patterns.

Necrotizing sialometaplasia

Necrotizing sialometaplasia is a benign, reactive, inflammatory, and usually self-limited disorder of salivary tissues with clinical and histologic features that simulate malignancy, particularly mucoepidermoid and squamous cell carcinomas.[114] Preponderantly a lesion of the minor salivary glands of the palate, necrotizing sialometaplasia can be found in any salivary tissues, including the major salivary glands. In the oral cavity, it has an estimated prevalence of 0.03% of all lesions submitted to biopsy—certainly, an underestimation.[114]

Although squamous metaplasia can be found in several forms of inflammatory and neoplastic disorders of the salivary glands, necrotizing sialometaplasia is a histologically distinctive type with specific diagnostic criteria: these are (1) lobular necrosis of salivary tissue, (2) a time-variable prominence of subsequent granulation tissue and acute and chronic inflammation, (3) squamous metaplasia conforming to duct and/or acinar outlines, and (4) maintenance of the salivary lobular morphology. Adherence to these criteria, especially the last one, excludes other forms of squamous metaplasia, such as that occurring at the periphery of a necrotic cyst (neoplastic or otherwise) and pseudoepitheliomatous hyperplasia extending into ducts (Fig. 3.28).

An ischemic basis for necrotizing sialometaplasia is the most accepted one. This causation is supported not only by experimental evidence but also by clinical and histopathologic observations of the lesions following surgical procedures or radiotherapy at the involved site and an association with thrombosis, Buerger's disease, and emboli. There is also a histologically analogous lesion found adjacent to infarcted areas of the prostate gland.

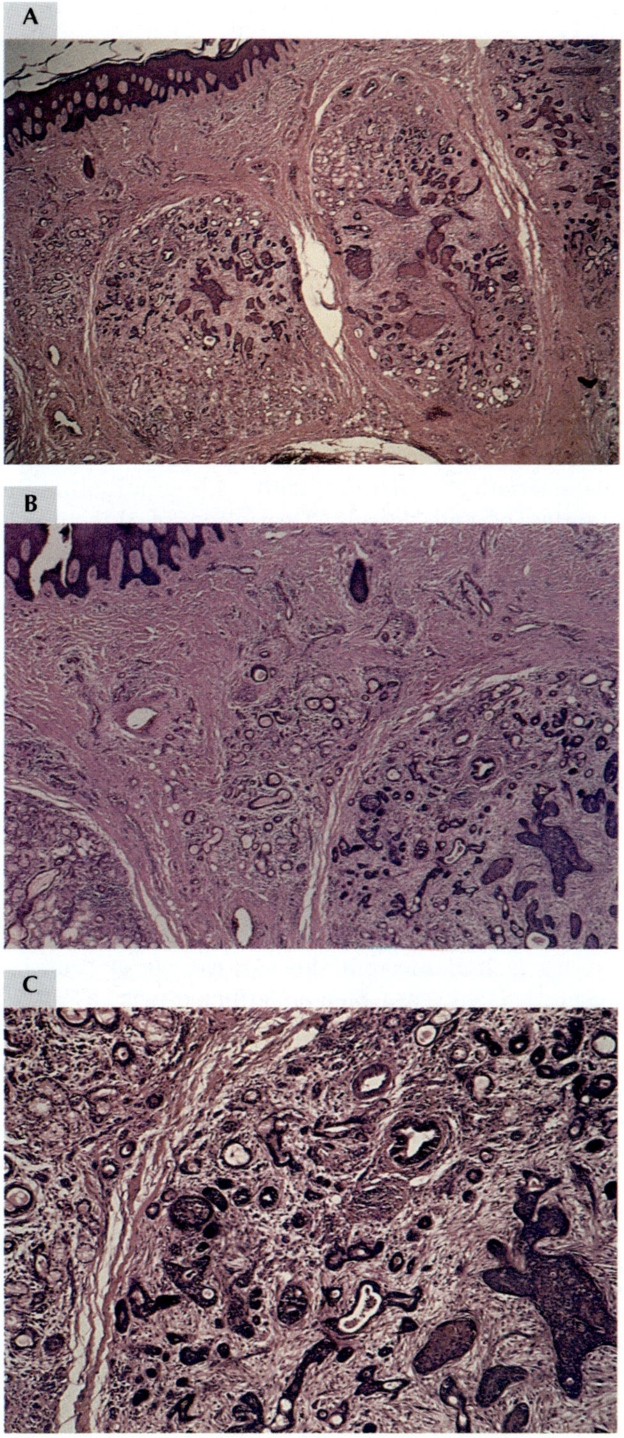

Figure 3.28 A–C Necrotizing sialometaplasia of the palate; note the characteristic preservation of the lobular architecture of the minor salivary gland tissue.

In either minor or major salivary glands, the basic histologic lesion is an infarct of salivary lobules with subsequent repair and metaplasia. The arterial supply of the palate's minor salivary glands is the anterior palatine artery. This vessel enters through the rigid major palatine foramen. The major branches course anterolaterally, with only small branches passing medially to the areas in which necrotizing sialometaplasia has been most often described. The blood supply is vulnerable at the foramen and also distally, where any agent capable of producing compromise or vascular injury can lead to infarct. In the major salivary glands, the arterial vessels follow and accompany subdivisions of the excretory duct system so that each salivary lobule has a separate and distinct blood supply. Even within the lobules, vascular territories are also characteristically distinct, with each culminating in a series of end vessels. Disruption of this blood vasculature after surgical procedures in the major salivary glands is self-evident and accounts for 86% of the reported cases.[114] A similar postoperative sequence is seen in necrotizing sialometaplasia of the upper airway.

Although prior surgery is not often a culprit in necrotizing sialometaplasia of the palate, subtler forms of vascular compromise are still held ultimately responsible. These include dental infections, ill-fitting dentures, and localized mucosal edema.

No age is immune, but the average age at time of diagnosis is 46 years. Men are afflicted twice as often as women and Whites outnumber Blacks by a ratio of 5:1. As Table 3.42 indicates, in the majority of cases the lesion is found on the posterior hard palate, with the junction of hard and soft palates the second most common site.[115] Nearly three-quarters of the palatal lesions are unilateral, and a tenth are bilateral; a lesser number are said to be midline. As salivary tissue is not normally found in the midline of the hard palate, lesions found there are likely to be due to extension or coalescence of unilateral or bilateral lesions. The parotid gland is the major salivary gland most often reported as being involved.

In mucosal sites, necrotizing sialometaplasia most often presents as a deep-seated ulcer, with or without an antecedent swelling or mass. A mass accounts for only about one-third of reported cases, including mucosal and non-mucosal parenchymal sites. Painful lesions are about twice as common as those without symptoms. Paresthesias or anesthesia may also be noted. Bony involvement is not generally described or to be expected, but its presence (rare) does not preclude the diagnosis of necrotizing sialometaplasia.

Different stages of evolution of the lesion often overlap and can occur simultaneously in different areas of the affected salivary tissue. The severity of the infarct also varies. Extensive infarct can lead to a sequestration of necrotic areas and to ulcer formation with the crater-like defects found in some cases of the disorder. The size of the lesions is dependent on the number of affected lobules and the severity of the necrosis. As a result, the diameter of necrotizing sialometaplasia at any salivary site can be less than 1 cm or more than 5 cm. In the series reported by Brannon et al.,[115] the average was 1.8 cm.

The healing process in necrotizing sialometaplasia includes repair of both the ulceration (if present) and of the damaged salivary tissues. Proliferation of surface mucosal cells covers the epithelial defect and often presents as a form of pseudoepitheliomatous hyperplasia. Regeneration of affected ducts and acini is never complete, but the metaplasia of small ducts and acini can be associated with prominent

Table 3.42 Sites of involvement of necrotizing sialometaplasia (n = 184). (From data presented by Brannon et al.[115])

Site	No. of cases	% of total
Palate		
Hard	100	
Soft	10	
Junction	25	
Not specified	7	
Total	142	77.2
Non-palate oral		
Lower lip	7	
Retromolar	5	
Tongue	2	
Buccal	2	
Mucobuccal fold	1	
Tonsillar fossa	1	
Total	18	9.8
Major salivary gland		
Parotid	14	
Sublingual	1	
Submandibular	1	
Total	16	8.7
Other head and neck		
Nasal cavity	5	
Maxillary sinus	1	
Larynx	1	
Incisive canal	1	
Total	8	4.3

nuclei and frequent mitotic figures. It is the combination of an ongoing necrosis and repair that may lead to the mistaken diagnosis of malignancy if the specific criteria are not adhered to.

Necrotizing sialometaplasia generally heals spontaneously, without treatment, within 6–10 weeks. Treatment of symptoms is indicated for patients with painful lesions.[115]

Miscellaneous oral lesions with differential diagnostic import

The differential diagnosis of oral squamous cell carcinomas includes more than salivary benign and malignant lesions: with varying degrees of frequency, other primary or metastatic neoplasms or benign inflammatory lesions enter into diagnostic consideration. Some of these have been presented in the foregoing pages. Other, non-supporting tissue, lesions are now considered.

Pigmented oral lesions

Melanoma

Primary mucosal melanomas are far outnumbered by their cutaneous counterparts in the United States. Table 3.43 presents the frequency of non-cutaneous melanomas by site as derived by Scotto et al.[116] from a study of 432 patients.

Table 3.43 Non-cutaneous melanomas. (Modified from Scotto et al.[116])

Primary site	% of total
Eye	79.0
Vulvovaginal	9.3
Upper respiratory tract and nasopharynx	1.8
Oral cavity and lip	1.6
Others	8.3

Among Caucasians, a fairly constant percentage of all melanomas arises in non-ocular mucous membranes and a fairly constant percentage of these (6–7.5%) takes origin from the oral cavity and upper respiratory tract. There are, however, significant racial differences in the incidence of melanomas at these sites, best exemplified by the incidence of malignant melanomas of the oral cavity in Japanese and melanomas of the nasal cavity in Black Africans. In Japan, the incidence of melanomas among all malignant neoplasms is 0.07%. Oral melanomas make up 7.5% of all melanomas and constitute 34.4% of all mucosal melanomas in the Japanese.

Table 3.44 presents the site distribution of 373 oral malignant melanomas.[117] Nearly 80% of the oral melanomas arise in the mucosa of the upper jaw, with the majority occurring on keratinizing mucosa (Figs 3.29, 3.30).

Table 3.44 Location of 373 oral malignant melanomas. (Modified from Batsakis et al.[117])

Anatomic site	No. of melanomas
Palate	149
Alveolar gingivae	128
Lips	37
Buccal mucosa	25
Gingivopalatine boundary	17
Tongue	12
Floor of mouth	5

Tumor thickness or depth of invasion is one of the most important prognostic factors in cutaneous melanomas. Unfortunately, most reports of oral melanoma have not included this information so a direct comparison between melanoma of the skin and oral mucosa usually cannot be made. Umeda and Shimada,[118] however, did compare the two melanomas (Table 3.45). As can be seen, the great majority of cutaneous melanomas present as stage I

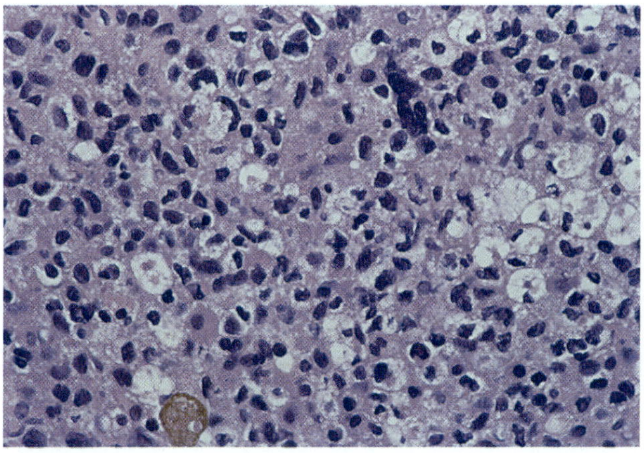

Figure 3.29 Mucosal melanoma of the palate; melanin pigment is sparse.

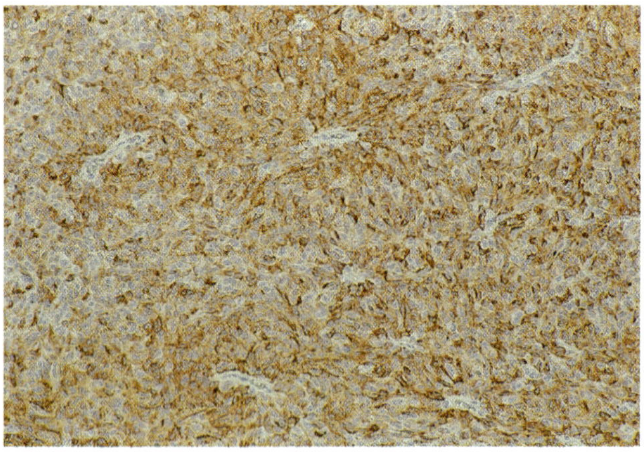

Figure 3.30 Mucosal melanoma: immunohistochemical preparation showing the S-100 protein reactivity of the melanoma cells.

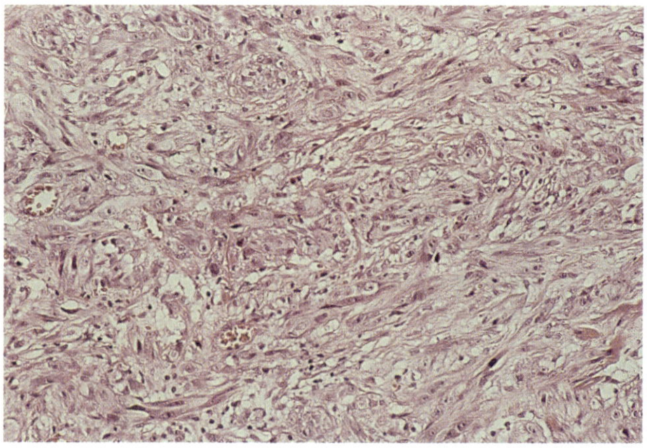

Figure 3.31 Desmoplastic melanoma of the palate: it is this type of melanoma that can be confused with a supporting tissue neoplasm.

lesions, whereas about one-half of oral melanomas have regional metastases (stage II). The greater thickness of oral mucosal melanomas (70% of patients with stage I and 83% of those with stage II oral melanomas have tumor thickness greater than 4.0 mm) indicates that oral melanomas are more advanced at the time of primary treatment. Where there is a tumor thickness greater than 5 mm, lymph nodes are likely to be involved. The most common sites of nodal metastases are the submandibular and upper jugular lymph nodes, which are the same as for oral cavity squamous cell carcinomas. Melanomas of the palate and maxillary gingivae have a high incidence of contralateral neck metastasis.

Umeda and Shimada[118] indicate that there are three growth phases in oral melanomas—a non-elevated, light-brown macular phase, a flat or minimally elevated form that is deeply pigmented, and a nodular phase. The characteristics of oral melanoma with radial growth correspond to those of an oral lentiginous melanoma with a macular, plaque and nodular evolution.

The desmoplastic melanoma is a rare entity within the oral cavity, with a predilection for the maxillary molar gingiva.[119] Like its extra-oral counterpart, it can easily be mistaken for a supporting tissue lesion (Fig. 3.31); immunohistochemistry is essential for correct diagnosis. The lesion is fairly consistently positive for S-100 protein and vimentin but unusually so for HMB-45. The behavior is capricious but the survival rate and prognosis seem better than those for conventional types of melanoma. Long-term follow-up is mandatory because of the supposed low proliferative activity of desmoplastic melanomas.

Oral cavity melanoma has a very poor prognosis.[120,121] Delayed detection partially accounts for this dismal outlook. The median survival rate is low (Table 3.46).

Melanoma metastatic to the oral cavity is rare. An NIH Clinical Center Medical Records database identified 809 patients with metastatic melanoma between 1953 and 1989.[122] Of these 809 patients, 24 (3.0%) had melanoma metastatic to the mucosal or bony structures of the oral cavity. The primary sites

Table 3.45 Tumor thickness in cutaneous vs oral melanomas. (Modified from Umeda and Shimada[118])

Tumor thickness (mm)	Cutaneous melanoma		Oral melanoma	
	Stage I (%) (*n* = 2151)	Stage II (%) (*n* = 290)	Stage I (%) (*n* = 10)	Stage II (%) (*n* = 12)
< 1.5	57	11	0	0
1.5–4.0	33	40	30	17
> 4.0	10	49	70	83

Table 3.46 Survival with oronasal melanoma. (Modified from Chin and Weinstock[121])

Variable	No. of patients	Median survival (months)
A. Location		
Oronasal (all)	182	24
Nasal cavity	80	25
Paranasal sinuses	28	12
Oral cavity	53	25
Gingiva	14	46
Palate	20	22
Nasopharynx	17	27
B. Stage		
Localized	72	39
Regional spread	59	23
Distant spread	26	11

Table 3.47 Amalgam tattoos of the oral cavity. (From data presented by Buchner and Hansen[122])

Location	Cases	
	(*n*)	(%)
Gingiva	76	28.4
Alveolar mucosa	52	19.4
Retromolar area	14	5.2
Mucobuccal fold	21	7.8
Buccal mucosa	61	22.8
Floor of mouth	23	8.6
Tongue	9	3.4
Palate	5	1.8
Labial mucosa	7	2.6
Total	268	100.00

included skin of the trunk, head and neck and limbs, and nasal septal mucosa. The tongue was the most common metastatic site, followed by the buccal mucosa and parotid gland, lip, mandible, submandibular gland and alveolar mucosa. Approximately one-half of the patients with oral metastases also had multiple other sites of involvement. A mean of 4.2 years elapsed between primary tumor and oral metastasis diagnosis. A mean survival of at least 1.7 ± 0.7 years after clinical diagnosis of the oral metastasis was recorded in the NIH series.

Racial pigmentation

The most common clinically apparent melanin deposition in the oral cavity is that related to racial pigmentation and is most readily appreciated in hosts with darker skins, such as Blacks, Orientals and residents of the Mediterranean basin. A lack of circumscription, in contrast to non-racially dependent melanin pigmentation, is characteristic and such pigment can be found on the buccal mucosa, gingivae, hard palate and soft palate, lips and the tongue. Racial pigmentation is increased in smokers.

Amalgam

The most common exogenous and iatrogenic reason for non-melanocytic pigmentation of the oral mucosa is the deposits of dental amalgam.[122] The amalgam tattoo is twice as common as melanotic macules and ten times more common than pigmented nevi of the oral mucosa. The introduction of dental amalgam into oral soft tissues produces the pigmentation. The bluish-black discoloration of the amalgam tattoo is clinically similar to other focal pigmented lesions of the oral mucosa and must be distinguished from pigmented neoplasms, including mucosal melanoma. Radiographically, the presence of opaque particles at the site of pigmentation can establish the diagnosis, but radiographs are negative unless there are gross fragments of amalgam. The location of 268 amalgam tattoos as identified by Buchner and Hansen[122] is shown in Table 3.47.

Nevi

Melanotic macules, nevi, along with racial pigmentation are the three most common benign melanin-pigmented conditions in the oral cavity. The histologic appearance of the oral macule is identical to that of racial pigmentation and is distinguished only by its more discrete nature. To date, melanotic macules of the oral cavity have been benign and without documented evidence of malignant change.

Oral nevi are more common than melanomas of the oral mucosa. Nearly every form of cutaneous nevus can present as an intra-oral lesion, but the intramucosal nevus is the most common. The palate is the most common site for oral nevi, regardless of histologic subtype.

Melanoacanthoma

Despite its ominous-sounding name, melanoacanthoma is a clinically and histologically benign lesion. It is more likely to be reactive than neoplastic. Proposing an alternative nomenclature, to suggest its non-neoplastic nature, Tomich and Zunt[123] suggest the term melanoacanthosis.

The lesion is far more often a cutaneous than an oral cavity disorder. The skin lesions occur preponderantly in Caucasians, tend to develop slowly over a period of years, and present at an average age of 62 years. Intra-oral forms are found almost exclusively in Black women with an average age of 27 years. The oral lesions are typically flat or slightly raised, often appear to expand rapidly and, on occasion, are multifocal. Development of oral lesions has been related to a variety of local physical or chemical trauma and the elimination of such factors contributes to a resolution of the lesion. The oral lesions also have a tendency towards remission after incisional biopsy, as well as a spontaneous regression. This self-limited behavior is in contrast with that of cutaneous melanoacanthomas, indicating that histologic similarity does not distinguish between the reactive oral lesion and the apparent neoplastic character of the skin counterpart.

The histologic features of oral melanoacanthomas are characterized by the presence of benign dendritic melanocytes scattered throughout the layers of the squamous epithelium. There is also an acanthosis, spongiosis, basal layer hyperpigmentation, basal dendritic melanocytes, intra-epithelial melanocytes, dermal melanophages and telangiectasia.

Melanotic neuroectodermal tumor

The melanotic neuroectodermal tumor of infancy is a rare pigmented neoplasm occurring most often in infants during the first year of life.[124–126] There have been 23 synonyms to designate the tumor, underscoring uncertainty over its histogenesis. A neuroectodermal, and probably neural crest, origin is now considered most likely. Molecular biologic studies have also placed the tumor in the peripheral primitive neuroectodermal class or family. Neural crest origin is supported by (1) electron-optic findings of neurosecretory granules, (2) neuroectodermal immunohistochemical reactivity, and (3) the occasional finding of elevated urinary excretion of vanillylmandelic acid (VMA).

In 87% of the reported cases (now over 200), the tumor occurs in the head and neck, the majority in the anterior maxilla (70%). Other sites are the skull (10%), mandible (6–9%), and brain (1–4%).[125] The skin, epididymis, uterus, ovary and mediastinum are infraclavicular sites of reported origin.

There is no gender predilection, but in 82% of cases the tumor is found in patients less than 6 months of age, and 95% occur within the first year of life. The lesion is usually not present at birth.

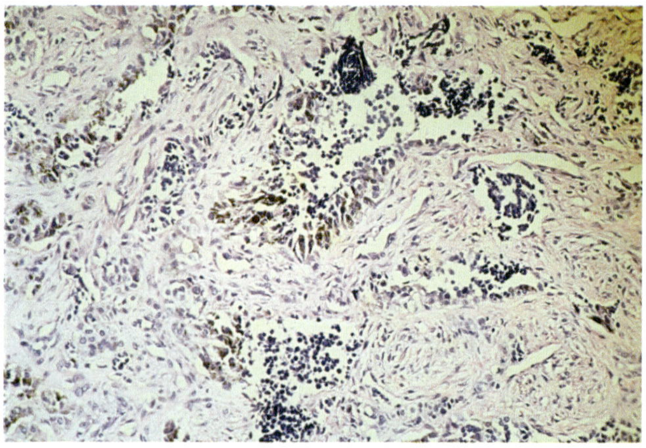

Figure 3.32 Pigmented neuroectodermal tumor of the anterior maxilla; melanin-containing cells are accompanied by smaller neuroblastic cells.

The tumor is a rapidly expanding, non-ulcerated mass appearing most often from the maxilla and which may have an exophytic component on the alveolus. Although it contains melanin, the pigment may not always be clinically evident. Multiple foci are unusual.

The tumor, which is usually only partially encapsulated or is unencapsulated, exhibits cells arranged in clusters or cleft-like spaces within a fibrous stroma. Classically, two cell populations are found: one consists of small, ovoid cells, with little cytoplasm and with hyperchromatic nuclei (Fig. 3.32); the other is an epithelioid cell with more cytoplasm and may contain melanin. By electron microscopy, the duality of the cells is confirmed, with the larger cell type containing melanosomes and the smaller cells displaying neurotubules. The larger cells also show epithelial differentiation, e.g. tonofilaments and immunoreactivity for cytokeratin and epithelial membrane antigen.

Other immunohistochemical findings are a uniform reactivity for neuron-specific enolase, synaptophysin, melanoma associated antigen (HMB 45), and microtubule-associated protein; glial fibrillary acidic protein (GFAP), Leu 7 and S-100 protein have been far less often detected. There may be an occasional myogenic differentiation.

The majority of melanotic neuroectodermal tumors follow a benign course, with a 15% or greater local recurrence rate. The literature indicates a malignancy rate of 6.6%; this may be an overestimate.[126] Four of 13 malignant tumors arose in the maxilla and one other was mandibular; the others were not

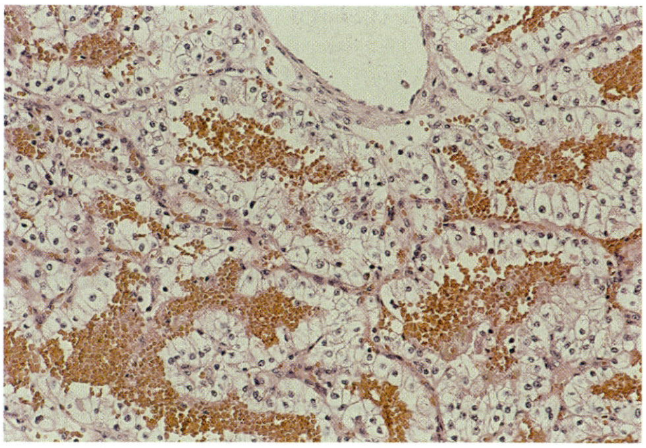

Figure 3.33 Metastatic renal cell carcinoma in the oral cavity; the vascularity and clear cell features are quite characteristic.

Table 3.48 Metastases to oral region. (Modified from Hirshberg and Buchner[127])

Site of primary	Oral mucosa	Jaw bones	Total
Breast	14	85	99
Lungs	42	49	91
Kidneys	22	31	53
Bone	9	29	38
Colorectal	8	26	34
Skin	20	14	34
Neuroblastoma	—	34	34
Female genital tract	10	15	25
Prostate	1	22	23
Liver	7	13	20
Eye	2	17	19
Thyroid gland	—	15	15
Testes	5	10	15
Stomach	6	4	10
Brain	—	8	8
Esophagus	3	4	7
Bladder	1	5	6
Other	7	9	16

from the head-and-neck region. Metastases have been to regional lymph nodes, liver, pleura, bone marrow, pelvis and pelvic organs, bowel and central nervous system (for those arising in the cerebellum). The malignant forms have been composed predominantly of the small non-pigmented cells with histologic similarity to the cells found in neuroblastomas.

Once the tumor has been diagnosed, prompt treatment is necessary to minimize adjacent destruction. The tumor is cured in most instances by a wide local excision with tumor-free margins.

Non-pigmented oral lesions

Non-melanoma metastases

Oral metastatic tumors are uncommon and comprise 1% of malignant oral neoplasms. Almost any malignant neoplasm can colonize in the oral region (Fig. 3.33). Table 3.48 lists the more common primaries.[127] Carcinomas of the breast, lung, kidney, colon and sarcomas of bone head the list; these are also the most common malignancies in general. The primary site differs between genders: in men, the lung, followed by kidney, bone and the colorectum, are the most frequent primary sites; in women, the most common primary site is the breast, followed quite distantly by the genital organs and kidney.

The mandible (particular the molar area) is the most frequently involved bony site in the oral regions. In oral soft tissues, the attached gingiva is the most commonly affected site, followed by the tongue and, with much less frequency, by the other oral soft tissues. The mobile tongue has a slightly higher incidence of metastases than the base and/or posterior border.

Oral metastases are usually evidence of a widespread disease and indicate a grave prognosis: time from detection of the metastasis to death is no more than a few months.

The surprising frequency of reports of metastases of hepatocellular carcinoma to the oral regions deserves comment. Lalikos et al.[128] in 1992 reported the 26th case. Of the 26 cases, 17 (65%) were first diagnosed by discovery of the oral lesion and in seven, metastasis was documented in the absence of pulmonary involvement. Maxillofacial metastases from hepatocellular carcinoma have been recorded almost exclusively in men and in adults. One-third of the metastases are to oral soft tissues; the remainder are to the jaw bones, preponderantly the mandible.

Granular cell tumor

The granular cell tumor, per se, should not enter into diagnostic confusion with squamous cell carcinoma. It is the sometimes present pseudoepitheliomatous hyperplasia associated with the tumor that can be overdiagnosed as a well-differentiated squamous cell carcinoma. The (often histogenetically enigmatic) granular cell tumors have two principal clinicopathologic presentations—an infantile (congenital) epulis form of the gnathic gingiva and a noncongenital aerodigestive and soft-tissue form.[129] The infantile forms only rarely have the aforementioned pseudoepitheliomatous hyperplasia.

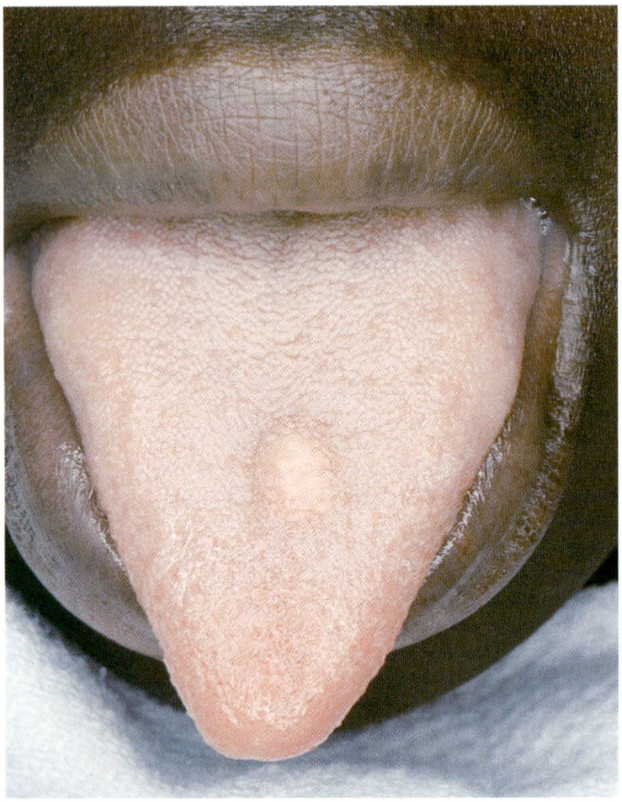

Figure 3.34 Granular cell tumor of the dorsum of the tongue in an 8-year-old boy.

No anatomic site appears resistant to the development of granular cell tumors. Subcutaneous tissues of the head and neck and the oral cavity, especially the tongue, are regions of predilection (Fig. 3.34). They account for about one-third of all granular cell tumors. Why the tongue is so often the site of the tumor is unknown. Trauma is not likely to be a significant factor, as granular cell tumors often occur in relatively non-traumatized areas of the tongue such as the dorsal midline and ventral surfaces. They also present far less often in oral regions that have a relatively high risk of mechanical irritation, such as the lower lip and the buccal mucosa.

The infantile granular cell tumor has a strong predilection for the lateral alveolar ridge of the maxilla, especially the future sites of canine or lateral incisor teeth. Granular cell tumors in older subjects rarely present in this location.

Non-infantile granular cell tumors of the head and neck commonly develop between the third and sixth decades of life, without predilection for either sex. Multifocality at first presentation has been reported to be as high as 16%; usually, it is less than 10%. The tumors are typically not large (< 2 cm), nodular, non-ulcerated, circumscribed, and painless.

There is some degree of squamous hyperplasia of mucosa overlying a granular cell tumor—approximately 50% in overall incidence (Fig. 3.35).[129] A marked degree of this hyperplasia (sufficient to be possibly misdiagnosed as squamous cell carcinoma) is, however, found in about 10% of granular cell tumors. This is a significant factor in granular cell tumors of the larynx, less so in those of the tongue.[129] The finding of an underlying granular cell tumor is fairly strong evidence against the malignant character of the pseudoepitheliomatous hyperplasia and should serve to caution the pathologist. Indeed, only about a dozen reported cases show an actual coexistence of granular cell tumor and squamous cell carcinoma; none of these has been with oral or laryngeal granular cell tumors.

Keratoacanthoma

There is a reservation over including keratoacanthoma in the group of epithelial lesions to be distin-

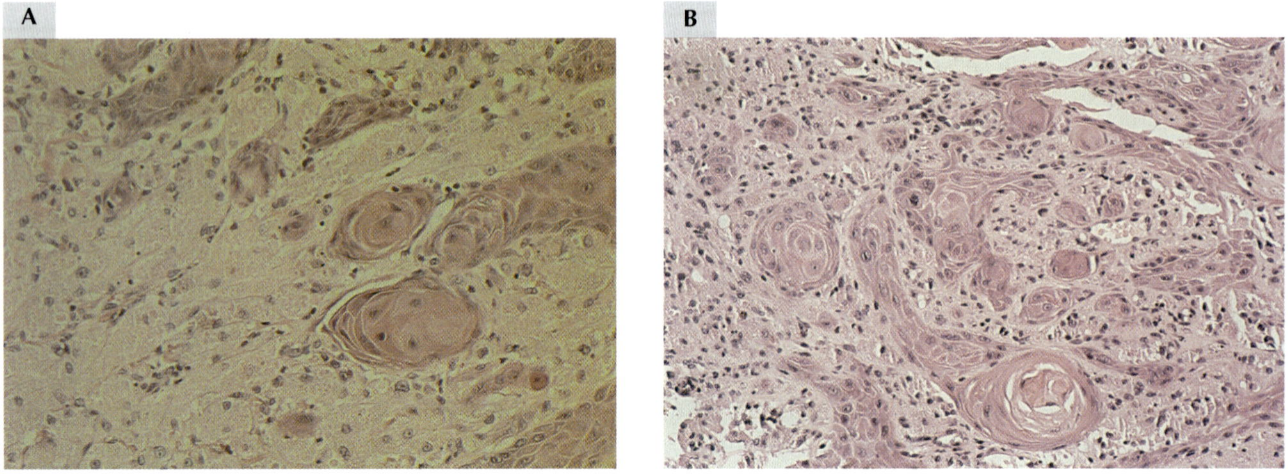

Figure 3.35 A, B Granular cell tumors manifesting varying degrees of a reactive pseudoepitheliomatous hyperplasia.

Table 3.49 Clinical features of oral lichen planus[133]

Form	Features
Reticular	Most common site is buccal mucosa, followed by tongue, gingiva, and lips Many interlacing keratotic lines or stria (Wickham's striae) producing annular or lacy pattern Usually asymptomatic or minimal symptoms
Plaque	Most often over dorsum of tongue and buccal mucosa Multifocal and leukoplakia like May be asymptomatic or have minimal symptoms
Atrophic	Attached gingiva (desquamative gingivitis pattern) is site of predilection; lingual gingiva spared or less involved May coexist with reticular erosive forms Patchy, relatively symmetric, four-quadrant gingival distribution Almost always symptomatic (burning or pain)
Erosive	Changing pattern (weekly) of involvement Erythematous, granular with pseudomembrane or fibrinous layer over erosion; keratotic component at periphery of erosion Usually painful
Bullous	Least common form Predilection for posterior and inferior buccal mucosa, followed by lateral tongue; rarely found on gingiva or lips Bullae or vesicles (up to severel centimeters); ulcers Painful mucosal surface

guished from squamous cell carcinoma. In either its described solitary or eruptive form, intra-oral keratoacanthoma is a very rare lesion. The intra-oral lesion is macroscopically similar to its cutaneous counterpart except that the keratotic core may be lost, leaving an ulcer with rolled and raised margins that may be clinically indistinguishable from those of squamous cell carcinoma. The natural history of an oral keratoacanthoma is unknown, since surgical removal has precluded opportunity for spontaneous regression. Recurrences have not been reported.

So much for the reported examples of intra-oral keratoacanthomas. A clinicopathologic definition of keratoacanthoma is difficult or impossible, and this difficulty is compounded in mucosal rather than cutaneous sites. Definitions run the gamut of a continuous histologic spectrum from lesions that are cytologically benign to those that are cytologically malignant. Others regard the lesion as an abortive squamous carcinoma with the only true test of distinction between keratoacanthoma and squamous cell carcinoma being spontaneous resolution. Schwartz[131] advises that it is sometimes necessary to give, as a diagnosis, 'probable keratoacanthoma; a squamous cell carcinoma cannot be ruled out'. Even perineural invasion and intravascular spread have been regarded as 'alarming but benign phenomena'. Where does this type of arcane pronouncement leave the surgical pathologist? Like Hodak et al.,[132] we regard the solitary keratoacanthoma, cutaneous or mucosal, as a form of squamous cell carcinoma that has a distinctive clinical and histopathologic appearance that may be capable of complete resolution without therapy but requires complete surgical removal.

Lichen planus

Lichen planus is said to afflict 14% of Americans under the age of 75 years. Only 1/100 of these subjects, however, has a severe enough disorder to seek medical attention. The prevalence of oral lichen planus is lower and estimated to be about 1–2%. There may or may not be coexistent cutaneous involvement. Table 3.49 presents the several oral manifestations of lichen planus.[133] Oral lesions are more constant, over time, than those of the skin. Oral lesions are characteristically bilaterally symmetrical; palatal or sublingual involvement is rare; there is frequently an associated oral candidiasis.

Typically, the more common forms of oral lichen planus show hyperparakeratosis and hyperorthokeratosis, with a dense, band-like lymphoid-cell infiltrate at the region of the epithelial basement membrane and superficial stroma. There is a liquefactive degeneration of basal epithelial cells, with obliteration or effacement of the epithelial–stromal junction. A sawtooth configuration of the rete ridges is quite characteristic. A narrow eosinophilic band adjacent to the basement membrane is often noted, as is fibrinogen (demonstrated by direct immunofluorescence). Eosinophilic ovoid (colloid or civette) bodies are necrotic keratinocytes occasionally found at the basal cell level or within the inflammatory infiltrate. A feature stressed by Krutchkoff and Eisenberg[134] is that there must be normal epithelial maturation and cytomorphology.

A chronic lichenoid mucositis due to drugs or foodstuffs serves as a differential diagnosis for oral lichen planus. Plasma cell gingivitis and cinnamon-induced stomatitis are just two examples. The former represents one of three kinds of plasma cellular involvement of the gingiva—neoplastic, idiopathic, and in reaction to allergens present in toothpaste, chewing gum, and flavored mints. The oral mucositis produced by cinnamon contact can be either acute or chronic. The chronic form tends to be keratotic, lichenoid, desquamative, or erythematous. The lesions may be focal and are commonly seen on the buccal mucosa, vestibule, and lateral tongue, or they may be diffuse. The histologic changes are not pathognomonic for cinnamon contact and may be also seen as a contact reaction to other essential oils, fragrances, topical allergens, and other irritants. Most of the contact lesions manifest hyperorthokeratosis and hyperparakeratosis, at times with psoriasiform changes. The stromal changes are lichenoid in distribution, with sawtoothing of rete and obscuration of the basal layer and with a prominent plasma cell constituency. Some patients will show a prominent perivascular chronic inflammatory infiltrate similar to that seen in discoid lupus erythematosus and contact dermatitis.[133]

Whether oral lichen planus may at times undergo malignant change has been debated for almost 80 years. The frequency of this morbid happening has ranged from 0 to 12.5%, depending on the series and also on the criteria used by authors for the definition of lichen planus. In a critical review of 220 cases of reported malignant transformation occurring in oral lichen planus, Krutchkoff et al.[135] found only 15 that satisfied their criteria. There is also a discrepancy in regard to the finding of epithelial dysplasia in oral planus and the rate of development of carcinoma.

In light of the above, it is clear that criteria for lichen planus have not been uniformly applied and that diagnoses have been inaccurate. Despite these deterrents, data from follow-up studies (mean 5.33 years) of 1955 patients with oral lichen planus have shown a fairly consistent overall cancer frequency of 2.8%, although inclusion criteria differed in the four studies reviewed.[136] Validation of a small, yet clinically important, premalignant potential of lichen planus of the oral cavity is offered by Barnard et al.[136] in their careful study of 241 British patients with histologically confirmed oral lichen planus. These authors indicate that nine (3.7%) of the patients developed well-differentiated invasive carcinoma or carcinoma in situ in areas of lichen planus. Most of the carcinomas were in atrophic and/or erosive lesions: six were on the tongue, two on the buccal mucosa, and one on the alveolar ridge. Six of the nine patients were older than 65 years. Voute et al.,[137] in a follow-up of 113 patients with histologically proven oral lichen planus, found three patients (2.7%) who developed squamous cell carcinoma in an average follow-up period of 7 years. In a search for lichen planus in 727 patients admitted for oral cancer, the same authors observed two (0.28%) additional patients with a simultaneous occurrence of oral lichen planus and carcinoma.

It does appear that there is an increased, albeit low, risk for the development of carcinoma in oral lichen planus. This does not apply to cutaneous lesions of lichen planus. Sigurgeirsson and Lindelof,[138] after examining the records of 2071 patients with cutaneous lichen planus, indicated that there was no increased risk of malignant transformation of the skin lesions. They also estimated the risk of developing carcinoma in oral lichen planus to be 0.5–2.6%. The natural history of cutaneous lichen planus differs from that of its oral counterpart: whereas the latter is chronic, skin lesions have a high rate of spontaneous resolution, with almost 90% clearing within 2 years and only a 20% relapse.

Eisenberg and Krutchkoff[139] argue, however, that they remain unconvinced that lichen planus, per se, is premalignant without cofactors of known carcinogens. They stress the importance of clinically and histopathologically distinguishing mucosal epithelial dysplasias that are lichenoid from true lichen planus (Fig. 3.36). The presence of even mild and subtle disturbances of epithelial maturation places a diagnosis of oral lichen planus in a tenuous status. Equally important is their thesis that benign lichenoid conditions (e.g. mucosal and stromal responses to trauma, metals, drugs, foods and microorganisms) can mislead observers clinically and lightoptically.

Perhaps the verdict of Eversole[140] is what we should accept in order to stop the debate: he asks us to acknowledge that (1) there is a small tendency for oral lichen planus to undergo malignant transfor-

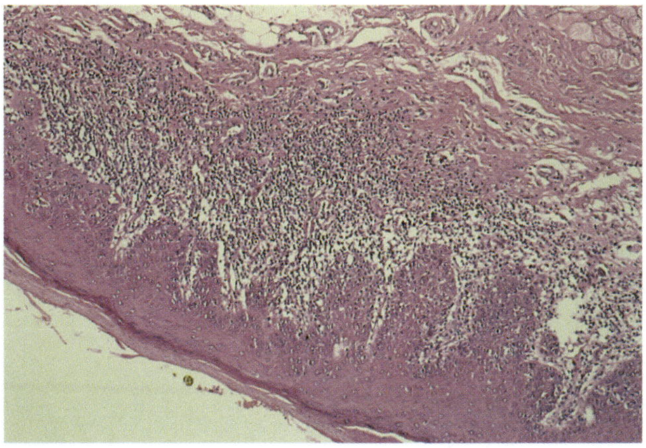

Figure 3.36 Lichenoid dysplasia of oral mucosa.

mation and (2) there is a form of clinical leukoplakia (lichenoid dysplasia) that is precancerous and shares histologic features with lichen planus.

Aphthous ulcer

Aphthous ulcer is a common oral lesion affecting 12–60% of the US population, with the highest rate found in professional school students.[141] Because major aphthous ulcers are uncommon, there are no available studies on their prevalence in the general population. Large aphthous ulcers are, however, more frequent in immunocompromised subjects and at unusual sites like the tonsils and uvula. The floor of the mouth and the tonsillar fossa appear to be areas of predilection.

Despite considerable investigation, the pathogenesis of aphthous ulcers is unknown. During the ulceration phase, there is a decreased CD4/CD8 cell count around the lesion;[141] this ratio reverses to a high level during healing. It is possible that the relative increase in CD8 cytotoxic cells facilitates the ulcerative phase and the relative decrease in CD4 cells delays healing. If allowed to progress, the large aphthous ulcers may be quite destructive locally and clinically mimic a malignancy.

Central odontogenic carcinoma

Although uncommon to rare, squamous cell carcinomas arising in dentigerous cysts can pose problems concerning their tissue of origin (i.e. odontogenic vs oral mucosa). Defined as a cyst surrounding the crown of an impacted or partially erupted tooth and formed from the reduced enamel epithelium, the dentigerous cyst is the second most common odontogenic cyst in the oral cavity.

Malignant transformation in dentigerous cysts is typically a slow process and may take as long as 30 or 40 years. Nearly all of the carcinomas are well differentiated, with the mandible affected twice as often as the maxilla.[142] There is a male preponderance of nearly 3:1 and the average at diagnosis is 64 years. The carcinomas frequently invade marrow spaces and tend to track along the inferior alveolar nerve. It is rare to have metastases to neck nodes.

There is a requirement for hemimandibulectomy or partial maxillectomy, as there is a relatively high recurrence rate after enucleation or en-bloc resection. A 53% 2–6-year survival has been indicated.

Neuroendocrine neoplasms and Merkel cell carcinoma

In extrapulmonary sites, the term 'undifferentiated small cell carcinoma' lacks nosological specificity as a diagnosis. In the oral cavity there are two putative sources for such a neoplasm—oral salivary glands and the oral squamous mucosa. The issue of neuroendocrine features in these carcinomas is a further complicating matter and, at either of the proposed generative sites, there is the complexity of histogenesis, including the Merkel cell.

Koss et al.[143] were the first to propose a salivary tissue origin for small cell carcinomas of minor salivary gland sites in the head and neck. It is not clear whether these authors included tumors that were to be later reclassified as basaloid squamous or high-grade adenoid cystic carcinomas. Allusions were made to possible neuroendocrine origin because the morphology resembled oat cell carcinomas of the lungs, but no histomorphologic investigations were pursued to prove or disprove this thesis.

In any event, small cell carcinomas of salivary glands are rare neoplasms: they account for less than 1% of malignant neoplasms of the major salivary glands and probably a smaller percentage of minor salivary gland carcinomas.[144]

Either a neuroendocrine origin of such neoplasms, or their origin in a stem cell with multidirectional developmental capacity, has been proposed and still is contested.[145] Gnepp and Wick[146] take the assailable position that virtually all salivary-gland small cell carcinomas appear to have neuroendocrine characteristics (as shown by immunohistochemical reactions), even if dense core granules cannot be ultrastructurally demonstrated.

The important question facing the clinician is whether the biologic behavior of the extrapulmonary small cell carcinoma has more similarity to a primary tumor without neuroendocrine differentiation, than to a small cell lung cancer. It does appear

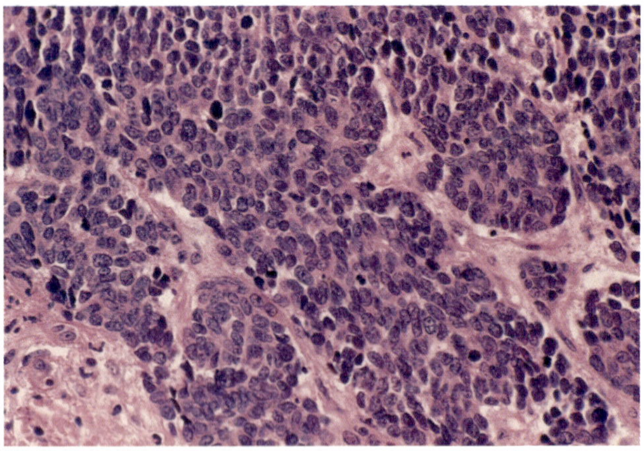

Figure 3.37 Merkel cell carcinoma of the lip.

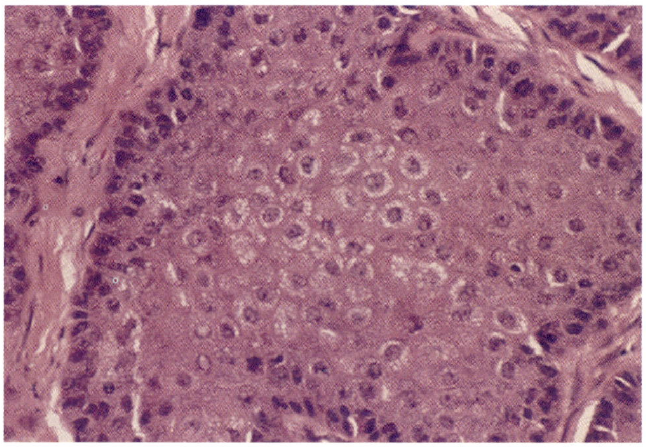

Figure 3.38 Focus of sebaceous cell hyperplasia in the oral cavity.

that the behavior of these small cell carcinomas depends more on their site of origin than on pathologic features. In our experience, neuroendocrine differentiation does not significantly modify the histologic course of extrapulmonary small cell carcinomas. Those occurring in mucosal or salivary gland sites above the larynx, however, appear to be less aggressive than pulmonary and laryngeal forms.

Merkel cells exist ubiquitously in vertebrates from cyclostomes to primates. They are specialized cells in the skin and oral mucosa which participate in the transduction of applied stimuli into neuroelectrical impulses.[147] Neurites arising from subepithelial myelinated fibers terminate within the epithelium in juxtaposition to Merkel cells. In humans, Merkel cell–neurite complexes are found in high numbers in the lip, anterior hard palate and gingiva. The taste buds of lower vertebrates contain Merkel cell-like cells.[147,148]

The head and neck is the major area of predilection for a Merkel cell carcinoma, with the cheeks and eyelids the favorite primary sites. The majority are found on sun-exposed skin, but there have been a few cases involving the oral and nasal cavities (Fig. 3.37).

In the oral cavity, it is likely that Merkel cells arise by a differentiation of basal cells of the surface epithelium. Such an origin would be analogous to the differentiation of chemosensory cells from basal epithelial cells in the nasal and laryngeal mucosa.[149]

Vigneswaran et al.[150] recorded the 12th case of oral/perioral Merkel cell carcinoma in 1992: only two were intra-oral (one, mucobuccal fold and one, buccal); ten of the carcinomas were on the lip mucosa. Like its cutaneous counterpart, an oral Merkel cell carcinoma displays an aggressive clinical course. Eight of the 12 patients manifested regional lymph node and/or distant metastases.

Merkel cell carcinomas manifest a considerable histopathologic heterogeneity. They have been subclassified into trabecular, intermediate and small cell types.[151] In the skin, each type appears to have a degree of prognostic value, the small cell type being associated with the worst outlook.

Immunohistochemistry is very helpful in diagnosis. Three groups of markers are important:

1. Coexpression of two types of intermediate filaments—cytokeratins and neurofilaments;
2. Presence of neuropeptides (e.g. chromogranin, synaptophysin, neuron-specific enolase);
3. Epithelial differentiation markers (e.g. cytokeratins, epithelial membrane antigen and desmoplakins).

Sebaceous lesions

Extracutaneous, extra-ocular sebaceous glands in the head and neck are principally found in the oral cavity and major salivary glands. Sebaceous glands on the lips or buccal mucosa (Fordyce's granules) of humans or higher apes are so common as to be considered the norm rather than exceptional: nearly 80% of adults will show the characteristic yellow-white, single or grouped, pinhead-size granules at these two sites of predilection.[152] Less often they can be found on the retromolar region of the palate, the tongue, frenum, alveolar gingivae, and anterior pillars of the tonsils. The lower lip, especially its central part, is usually devoid of sebaceous glands. It is rare to find sebaceous glands in the oral cavities of subjects younger than 3 years.

Other than an unusual prominence in some individuals, intra-oral sebaceous glands usually are asymptomatic. Tumoral sebaceous lesions are most often hyperplastic–hypertrophic rather than neoplastic (Fig. 3.38). Carcinomas are exceedingly rare.

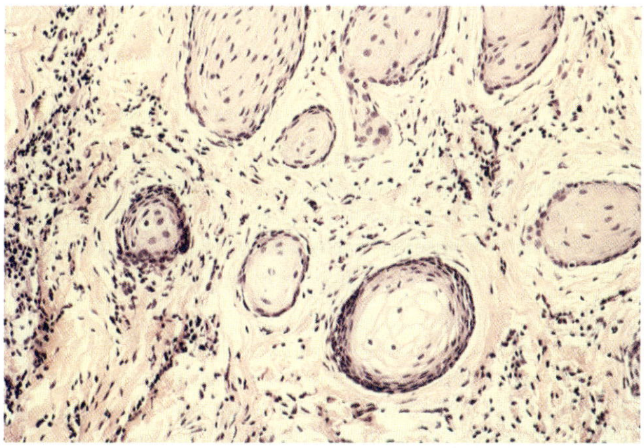

Figure 3.39 Mandibular gingiva with odontogenic epithelial nests.

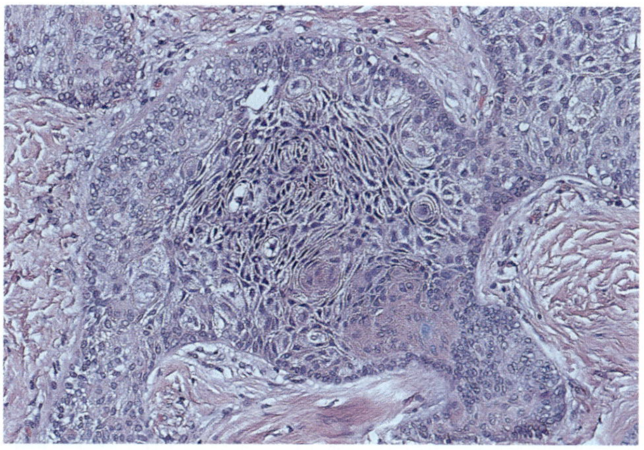

Figure 3.40 Peripheral ameloblastoma of the maxillary oral mucosa.

Microcystic carcinoma

Microcystic adnexal carcinoma is preponderantly a malignancy of the head and neck: of 43 reported examples, 38 arose in the skin of the head and neck; 13 of these were in the upper lip.[130] The neoplasm exhibits a combined eccrine and pilar differentiation. The most characteristic features are keratin cysts, strands of basaloid or squamous cells, sclerotic stroma, areas of ductular differentiation, and the frequent invasion of nerves. Individual cells often have a deceptively bland appearance. Indeed, the cells exhibit few mitotic figures and minimal nuclear atypia. The carcinoma is either poorly circumscribed or uncircumscribed, asymmetric, deeply invasive and horizontally oriented.

As the neoplasm is adnexal, it is only a secondary invader of the oral cavity, particularly those arising in the lips. Nevertheless, it may be confused with an infiltrating squamous carcinoma or salivary carcinoma.

Peripheral epithelial odontogenic tumors

Peripheral epithelial odontogenic tumors are the extra-osseous equivalents of the much more often encountered central gnathic odontogenic tumors. The peripheral tumors arise in the mandibular or maxillary gingiva from the surface mucosa or from dental lamina nests in the submucosa (Fig. 3.39).

A considerable variety of odontogenic tumors take origin in the gingival soft tissues. These include ameloblastoma, adenomatoid odontogenic tumor, calcifying epithelial odontogenic tumor, squamous odontogenic tumor, odontogenic fibroma (gingival epithelial hamartoma, ameloblastic fibrodentinoma), granular cell ameloblastic fibroma, and calcifying odontogenic cyst. The peripheral ameloblastoma is the most frequently encountered (Fig. 3.40). Approximately 5% of all ameloblastomas are considered to be peripheral in origin and approximately 55% of all peripheral epithelial odontogenic tumors are ameloblastomas.[153,154] Table 3.50 presents the clinical aspects of these lesions.

Table 3.50 Clinical aspects of peripheral ameloblastomas (n = 53). (Modified from Nauta et al.[154])

Characteristics	**Findings**	
Age at diagnosis (years)	Range 16–92	Mean 50.2
Gender of patients		
Male	32	60%
Female	19	36%
Not stated	2	4%
Race of patients		
White	31	58%
Black	4	8%
Oriental	8	15%
Not stated	10	19%
Oral site (gingiva)		
Mandible	35	66%
Maxilla	18	34%
Follow-up period	6 months to 8 years	Mean 33 months
Recurrences (gingiva)	8	15%
Mandible	4	
Maxilla	4	
Recurrences after second excision	0	

In keeping with a proposed dual histogenesis, peripheral ameloblastomas without a continuity between tumor and gingival surface mucosa are considered to arise from remnants of the dental lamina. The majority, however, have a continuity with the mucosa and can show multiple connection foci.

The peripheral ameloblastoma is not an aggressive lesion. Invasion of bone is not a feature and 'cure' is usually achieved by conservative excision with adequate margins. There is potential for recurrence, perhaps because of multifocality. A malignant peripheral ameloblastoma is clearly a possibility, but is rare.

The long-standing controversy over whether the peripheral ameloblastoma and basal cell carcinoma are the same or two different lesions has been settled in favor of the former proposal.[153] Still unknown, however, is whether extragingival peripheral ameloblastomas exist. These lesions have been reported in the buccal mucosa and floor of the mouth, and their histogenesis has been attributed to a pluripotentiality of the oral epithelium.

The squamous odontogenic tumor exists in three clinicopathologic forms.[155] The most common arises within gnathic bones and is considered to arise in the periodontium. A so-called mural form develops in association with odontogenic cysts. Completely extra-osseous lesions are rare and are believed to arise from overlying gingival epithelium, much like peripheral ameloblastomas. Malignant change in any of the three types has not been described.

The other histologic types of peripheral epithelial odontogenic tumors are quite rare. The few studies pertaining to them do not allow for complete confidence in predicting biologic behavior, but they appear to have a low recurrence potential and to be nonaggressive lesions.

Cheilitis glandularis, xeroderma pigmentosum, acanthosis nigricans and cancer arising in oral skin grafts

This seemingly odd-fellow collection contains two disorders with primary manifestations in the skin, one that predisposes to labial carcinoma and, the other, a medical curiosity.

Cheilitis glandularis is a chronic suppurative inflammation of the lower lip (rarely of the upper lip) characterized by a swelling of mucosal glands and a mucopurulent discharge through dilated duct openings. The disorder is seen mostly in adult males in whom, with progression of the lesion, there is an increasingly firm enlargement of the lip with eversion.

Between 18 and 35% of cases show a lip squamous cell carcinoma, probably as a result of the eversion and actinic exposure. Most of the carcinomas arise in the deep suppurative type of the cheilitis.

A new cancer developing from grafted skin is a rare event. By the beginning of 1994 there had been eight cases of this development:[156] four arose in oral skin grafts (two buccal and one each on the upper gum and floor of mouth); the esophagus and hypopharynx accounted for the remainder.

An individual with xeroderma pigmentosum is 4800 times more liable to develop a cutaneous squamous or basal cell carcinoma than one not so afflicted: 50% of patients develop a skin malignancy by the eighth year of life.[157]

Xeroderma pigmentosum also predisposes to oral cancer. Patients younger than 20 years of age have an estimated 10 000 times greater frequency of carcinoma of the anterior tongue. Carcinomas of the gingiva and palate also occur with an increased frequency.

Acanthosis nigricans is a mucocutaneous disorder whose early detection of characteristic skin lesions may be crucial to prognosis since the disorder has served as a marker for internal malignancy.[158] More than 90% of these malignancies are intra-abdominal, with gastric carcinoma the type most often associated. Oral lesions of acanthosis nigricans occur in 53% of all cases and they, too, may be markers for the disorder.[158] The discovery of acanthosis nigricans and a malignant tumor is simultaneous in 60% of cases, whereas the mucocutaneous lesion has preceded the carcinoma in about 18% of cases.

The most frequent sites of involvement in the oral cavity by the disorder are the lips (particularly the upper), followed by the tongue, buccal mucosa, and the gingiva. There is no difference between the skin and oral mucosal expression, except that the oral papillary lesions are rarely pigmented. Although there is no predisposition to oral carcinoma, florid papillary oral lesions are most often associated with 'malignant' acanthosis nigricans.[158]

References

1. Muir C, Weiland L. Upper aerodigestive tract cancers. Cancer 1995; 75: 147–153
2. Chen J, Katz RV, Krutchkoff DJ. Intraoral squamous cell carcinoma. Epidemiologic patterns in Connecticut from 1935 to 1985. Cancer 1990; 66: 1288–1296
3. Jovanovic A, Schulten EA, Kostense PJ et al. Squamous cell carcinoma of the lip and oral cavity in The Netherlands; an epidemiological study of 740 patients. J Craniomaxillofac Surg 1993; 21: 149–152

4. Shah JP, Candela FC, Poddar AK. The patterns of cervical lymph node metastases from squamous carcinoma of the oral cavity. Cancer 1990; 66: 109–113
5. Stell PM, Morton RP, Singh SD. Squamous carcinoma of the head and neck: the untreated patient. Clin Otolaryngol 1983; 8: 7–13
6. Mashberg A, Meyers H. Anatomic site and size of 222 early asymptomatic oral squamous cell carcinomas. Cancer 1976; 37: 2146–2153
7. Gartner LP. Oral anatomy and tissue types. Semin Dermatol 1994; 13: 68–73
8. Strong EW, Spiro RH. Cancer of the tongue, lips and oral cavity. In: Pilch YH (ed.). Surgical oncology. New York: McGraw-Hill, 1984: 284–287
9. Zitsch RP, Park CW, Renner GJ et al. Outcome analysis for lip carcinoma. Otolaryngol Head Neck Surg 1995; 113: 589–596
10. Spiro RH, Huvos AG, Wong GY et al. Predictive value of tumor thickness in squamous carcinoma confined to the tongue and mouth floor. Am J Surg 1986; 152: 345–350
11. Ildstad ST, Bigelow ME, Remensnyder JP. Squamous cell carcinoma of the tongue: a comparison of the anterior two thirds of the tongue with its base. Am J Surg 1983; 146: 456–461
12. Ildstad ST, Bigelow ME, Remensnyder JP. Squamous cell carcinoma of the mobile tongue. Clinical behavior and results of current therapeutic modalities. Am J Surg 1983; 145: 443–449
13. Goldenberg D, Ardekian L, Rachmiel A et al. Carcinoma of the dorsum of the tongue. Head Neck 2000; 22: 190–194
14. Silver CE, Moisa II. Elective treatment of the neck in cancer of the oral tongue. Semin Surg Oncol 1991; 7: 14–19
15 Marks JE, Lee F, Smith PG et al. Floor of mouth cancer: patient selection treatment results. Laryngoscope 1983; 93: 475–480
16. Hicks WL, Loree TR, Garcia RI et al. Squamous cell carcinoma of the floor of mouth: a 20 year review. Head Neck 1997; 19: 400–405
17. Aygun C, Salazar OM, Sewchand W et al. Carcinoma of the floor of the mouth: a 20 year experience. Int J Radiat Oncol Biol Phys 1984; 10: 619–626
18. Barasch A, Gofa A, Krutchkoff DJ et al. Squamous cell carcinoma of the gingiva. A case series analysis. Oral Surg Oral Med Oral Pathol Oral Radiol Endod 1995; 80: 183–187
19. Panje WR, Smith B, McCabe BF. Epidermoid carcinoma of the floor of mouth: surgical therapy vs. combined therapy vs. radiation therapy. Otolaryngol Head Neck Surg 1980; 88: 714–720
20. Shafer WG, Waldron CA. Erythroplakia of the oral cavity. Cancer 1975; 36: 1021–1028
21. Ildstad ST, Bigelow ME, Remensnyder JP. Squamous cell carcinoma of the alveolar ridge and palate. A 15-year survey. Ann Surg 1984; 199: 445–453
22. Byers RM, Anderson B, Schwartz EA et al. The treatment of squamous carcinoma of the retromolar trigone. Am J Clin Oncol 1984; 7: 647–652
23. Byers RM, Newman R, Russell N et al. Results of treatment for squamous carcinoma of the lower gum. Cancer 1981; 47: 2236–2238
24. Bloom ND, Spiro RH. Carcinoma of the cheek mucosa. A retrospective analysis. Am J Surg 1980; 140: 556–559
25. World Health Organization Collaborating Centre for Oral Precancerous Lesions. Definitions of leukoplakia and related lesions: an aid to studies on oral precancer. Oral Surg Oral Med Oral Pathol 1978; 46: 518–539
26. Axéll T, Holmstrup P, Kramer IRH et al. International seminar on oral leucoplakia and associated lesions related to tobacco habits. Community Dent Oral Epidemiol 1984; 12: 145–154
27. Pindborg JJ. Clinical relevance of precancerous lesions of oral mucosa. In: Pape H-D, Ganzer U, Schmitt G (eds). Carcinoma of the oral cavity and oropharynx. Berlin: Springer-Verlag, 1994: 9–16
28. Axéll T, Pindborg JJ, Smith CJ et al and an International Collaborative Group on Oral White Lesions. Oral white lesions with special references to precancerous and tobacco-related lesions; conclusions of an international symposium held in Uppsala, Sweden, May 18–21, 1994. J Oral Pathol Med 1996; 25: 49–54
29. Pindborg JJ. Clinical relevance of precancerous lesions of oral mucosa. Recent Results Cancer Res 1994; 134: 9–16
30. Bouquot JE, Gnepp DR. Laryngeal precancer: a review of the literature, commentary, and comparison with oral leukoplakia. Head Neck 1991; 13: 488–497
31. Silverman S Jr, Gorsky M, Kaugars GE. Leukoplakia, dysplasia, and malignant transformation (guest editorial). Oral Surg Oral Med Oral Pathol 1996; 82: 117
32. Lumerman H, Freedman P, Kerpel S. Oral epithelial dysplasia and the development of invasive squamous carcinoma. Oral Surg Oral Med Oral Pathol 1995; 79: 321–329
33. Abdel-Salam M, Mayall BH, Chew K et al. Which oral white lesions will become malignant? An image cytometric study. Oral Surg Oral Med Oral Pathol 1990; 69: 345–350
34. Schepman KP, van der Meij EH, Smeek LE et al. Prevalence study of oral white lesions with special reference to a new definition of oral leucoplakia. Oral Oncol Eur J Cancer 1996; 32B: 416–419
35. Pindborg JJ, Kalapessi HK, Kale SA et al. Frequency of oral leucoplakias and related conditions among 10,000 Bombayites. J All India Dent Assoc 1965; 37: 1–2
36. Pindborg JJ, Chawla TN, Misra RK et al. Frequency of oral carcinoma, leucoplakia, leucoedema, leucokeratosis, submucous fibrosis and lichen planus in 10,000 Indians in Luchnow Uttar Pradesh, India. J Dent Res 1965; 44: 615
37. Pindborg JJ, Bhatt M, Devanath DR et al. Frequency of oral white lesions among 10,000 individuals in Banglore South India. India J Med Sci 1966; 20: 349–352

38. Gangadarhan P, Paymaster JC. Leukoplakia, an epidemiologic study of 1504 cases observed at the Tata Memorial Hospital, Bombay, India. Br J Cancer 1971; 25: 657–668
39. Mehta FS, Gupta PC, Daftary DK. An epidemiologic study of oral cancer and precancerous conditions among 101,761 villagers in Maharashtra, India. Int J Cancer 1972; 10: 134–141
40. Axéll TA. A prevalence study of oral mucosal lesions in an adult Swedish population. Odontol Rev 1976; 27: Suppl 36
41. Bouquot JE, Gorlin RJ. Leukoplakia, lichen planus, and other oral keratoses in 23,616 white Americans over the age of 35 years. Oral Surg Oral Med Oral Pathol 1986; 61: 373–381
42. Hogewind WFC, van der Waal I. Prevalence of oral leucoplakia in a selected population of 1000 patients from The Netherlands. Community Dent Oral Epidemiol 1988; 165: 302–305
43. Banoczy J, Rigo O. Prevalence study of oral precancerous lesions within a complex screening system in Hungary. Community Dent Oral Epidemiol 1991; 19: 265–267
44. Ikeda N, Ishii T, Lida S et al. Epidemiological study of oral leucoplakia based on mass screening for oral mucosal diseases in a selected Japanese population. Community Dent Oral Epidemiol 1991; 19: 160–163
45. Hansen LS, Olson JA, Silverman S. Proliferative verrucous leukoplakia. A long-term study of thirty patients. Oral Surg Oral Med Oral Pathol 1985; 60: 285–298
46. Zakrzewska JM, Lopes V, Speight P et al. Proliferative verrucous leukoplakia. Report of 10 cases. Oral Surg Oral Med Oral Pathol Oral Radiol Endod 1996; 82: 396–401
47. Batsakis JG, Suarez P, El-Naggar AK. Proliferative verrucous leukoplakia and its related lesions. Oral Oncol 1999; 35: 354–359
48. Hall JM, Cohen MA, Moreland AA. Multiple confluent lesions of oral leukoplakia. Arch Dermatol 1991; 127: 887–890
49. Slootweg PJ, Müller H. Verrucous hyperplasia or verrucous carcinoma. An analysis of 27 patients. J Maxillofac Surg 1983; 11: 13–19
50. Palefsky JM, Silverman S, Abdel-Salaam M et al. Association between proliferative verrucous leukoplakia and infection with human papilloma virus type 16. J Oral Pathol Med 1995; 24: 193–197
51. Greer RO, Eversole LR, Crosby LK. Detection of human papilloma virus genomic DNA in oral epithelial dysplasia, oral smokeless tobacco-associated leukoplakias and epithelial malignancies. J Oral Maxillofac Surg 1990; 48: 1201–1205
52. Shroyer KR, Greer RO. Detection of human papilloma virus DNA by in situ DNA hybridization and polymerase chain reaction in premalignant and malignant oral lesions. Oral Surg Oral Med Oral Pathol 1991; 71: 708–713
53. Shear M, Pindborg JJ. Verrucous hyperplasia of the oral mucosa. Cancer 1980; 46: 1855–1862
54. Eversole LR, Jacobsen P, Stone CE et al. Oral condyloma planus (hairy leukoplakia) among homosexual men: a clinicopathologic study of thirty-six cases. Oral Surg Oral Med Oral Pathol 1986; 61: 249–255
55. Schiodt M, Greenspan D, Daniels TE et al. Clinical and histologic spectrum of oral hairy leukoplakia. Oral Surg Oral Med Oral Pathol 1987; 64: 716–720
56. Sciubba J, Brandsma J, Schwartz M et al. Hairy leukoplakia: an AIDS-associated opportunistic infection. Oral Surg Oral Med Oral Pathol 1989; 67: 404–410
57. Eisenberg E, Krutchoff D, Yamase H. Incidental oral hairy leukoplakia in immunocompetent persons: a report of two cases. Oral Surg Oral Med Oral Pathol 1992; 74: 332–333
58. Ficarra G, Gaglioti D, DePietro M et al. Oral hairy leukoplakia: clinical aspects, histologic morphology and differential diagnosis. Head Neck 1991; 13: 514–521
59. Farman AG. Hairy tongue (lingua villosa). J Oral Med 1977; 32: 85–91
60. Field EA, Ellis A, Friedman PS et al. Oral tylosis: a re-appraisal. Oral Oncol 1997; 33: 55–57
61. Crissman JD, Zarbo RJ. Dysplasia, in situ carcinoma and progression to invasive squamous cell carcinoma of the upper aerodigestive tract. Am J Surg Pathol 1989; 13(Suppl 1): 5–16
62. Waldron CA, Shafer WG. Leukoplakia revisited. A clinicopathologic study of 3256 oral leukoplakias. Cancer 1975; 36: 1386–1392
63. Mashberg A, Erythroplasia: the earliest sign of asymptomatic oral cancer. J Am Dent Assoc 1978; 96: 615–620
64. Silverman S, Gorsky M, Lozada F. Oral leukoplakia and malignant transformation. Cancer 1984; 53: 563–568
65. Bouquot JE, Gnepp DR. Epidemiology of carcinoma in situ of the upper aerodigestive tract. Cancer 1988; 61: 1685–1690
66. Bouquot JE, Kurland LT, Weiland LH. Carcinoma in situ of the upper aerodigestive tract. Cancer 1988; 61: 1691–1698
67. Reid BC, Winn DM, Morse DE et al. Head and neck in situ carcinoma: incidence, trends and survival. Oral Oncol 2000; 36: 414–420
68. Kleinsasser O, Glanz H. Microcarcinoma and microinvasive carcinoma of the vocal cords. Clin Oncol 1982; 1: 479–487
69. Carbone A, Volpe R, Barzan L. Superficial extending carcinoma (SEC) of the larynx and hypopharynx. Pathol Res Pract 1992; 188: 729–732
70. Constantinides MS, Rothstein SG, Persky MS. Squamous cell carcinoma in older patients without risk factors. Otolaryngol Head Neck Surg 1992; 106: 275–277
71. Kuriakose M, Sankaranaryanan M, Nair MK et al. Comparison of oral squamous cell carcinoma in younger and older patients in India. Oral Oncol Eur J Cancer 1992; 28B: 113–120

72. Lefebvre JL, Vankemmel B, Adenis L et al. Les carcinomas des voies aerodigestives supérieures avant an (enfants exclus). A propos de 100 cas. Ann Otolaryngol Chir Cervicofac 1987; 104: 89–92
73. Karja T, Syrjanen S, Usenius T et al. Oral cancer in children under 15 years of age. A clinicopathological and virological study. Arch Otolaryngol 1988; 49: 145–149
74. Sarkaria JN, Harari PM. Oral tongue cancer in young adults less than 40 years of age: rationale for aggressive therapy. Head Neck 1994; 16: 107–111
75. Sankaranarayanan R, Nair MK, Mathew B et al. Recent results of oral cancer research in Kerla, India. Head Neck 1992; 14: 107–112
76. Sorensen DM, Lewark TM, Haney JL et al. Absence of p53 mutations in squamous carcinoma of the tongue in nonsmoking and nondrinking patients younger than 40 years. Arch Otolaryngol Head Neck Surg 1997; 123: 503–506
77. Carey TE. Field cancerization: are multiple primary cancers monoclonal or polyclonal? Ann Med 1996; 28: 183–188
78. Deleyiannis FW-B, Thomas DB. Risk of lung cancer among patients with head and neck cancer. Otolaryngol Head Neck Surg 1997; 116: 630–636
79. Jovanovic A, van der Tol IGH, Schulten EA et al. Risk of multiple primary tumors following oral squamous cell carcinoma. Int J Cancer 1994; 56: 320–323
80. Jovanovic A, van der Tol IGH, Kostense PJ et al. Second respiratory and upper digestive tract cancer following oral squamous cell carcinoma. Oral Oncol Eur J Cancer 1994; 30B: 225–229
81. Shibuya H, Amagasa T, Seto K et al. Leukoplakia-associated multiple carcinoma in patients with tongue carcinoma. Cancer 1986; 57: 843–856
82. Haughey BH, Gates GA, Arfken CL et al. Meta-analysis of second malignant tumors in head and neck cancer: the case for endoscopic screening protocol. Ann Otol Rhinol Laryngol 1992; 101: 105–112
83. Gluckman JL, Crissman JD. Survival rates in 548 patients with multiple neoplasms of the upper aerodigestive tract. Laryngoscope 1983; 93: 71–74
84. Jones AS, Morar P, Phillips DE et al. Second primary tumors in patients with head and neck squamous cell carcinoma. Cancer 1995; 75: 1343–1352
85. Spiro RH, Alfonso AE, Farr EW et al. Cervical node metastases from epidermoid carcinoma of the oral cavity or oropharynx: a critical assessment of current staging. Am J Surg 1974; 128: 562–567
86. Jones AS. Prognosis in mouth cancer: tumour factors. Oral Oncol Eur J Cancer 1994; 30B: 8–15
87. Stell PM. Prognosis in mouth cancer: host factors. J Laryngol Otol 1992; 106: 399–402
88. Jones AS, Phillips DE, Helliwell TR et al. Occult metastases in head and neck squamous carcinoma. Eur Arch Otorhinolaryngol 1993; 250: 446–449
89. Shah JR. Patterns of cervical lymph node metastasis from squamous carcinomas of the upper aerodigestive tract. Am J Surg 1990; 160: 405–409
90. Olsen KD, Caruso M, Foote RL et al. Primary head and neck cancer. Histopathologic predictors of recurrence after neck dissection in patients with lymph node involvement. Arch Otolaryngol Head Neck Surg 1994; 120: 1370–1374
91. Stell PM, Dalby JE, Singh D et al. The fixed cervical lymph node. Cancer 1984; 53: 336–341
92. Shah JP, Cendon RA, Farr HW et al. Carcinoma of the oral cavity. Factors affecting treatment failure at the primary site and neck. Am J Surg 1976; 132: 504–507
93. Snow GB, Annyas AA, van Slooten EA et al. Prognostic factors of neck node metastasis. Clin Otolaryngol 1982; 7: 185–192
94. Kalnins IK, Leonard AG, Sako K et al. Correlation between prognosis and degree of lymph node involvement in carcinoma of the oral cavity. Am J Surg 1977; 134: 450–454
95. Shigaki S, Saito R, Kawasaki T et al. Recurrence of carcinoma of the oral cavity, oropharynx and maxillary sinus after radical neck dissection. J Maxillofac Surg 1985; 13: 231–235
96. Pinsolle J, Pinsolle V, Majoufre C et al. Prognostic value of histologic findings in neck dissections for squamous cell carcinoma. Arch Otolaryngol Head Neck Surg 1997; 123: 145–148
97. Johnson JT, Myers EN, Bedetti CD et al. Cervical lymph node metastases: incidence and implications of extracapsular carcinoma. Arch Otolaryngol Head Neck Surg 1985; 111: 534–537
98. van den Brekel MWM, Stel HV, van der Valk P et al. Micrometastases from squamous cell carcinoma in neck dissection specimens. Eur Arch Otolaryngol 1992; 249: 349–353
99. Vikram B. Changing patterns of failure in advanced head and neck cancer. Arch Otolaryngol 1984; 110: 564–565
100. Vikram B, Strong EW, Shah JP et al. Failure at the primary site following multimodality treatment in advanced head and neck cancer. Head Neck Surg 1984; 6: 720–723
101. Calhoun KH, Fulmer P, Weiss R et al. Distant metastases from head and neck squamous cell carcinomas. Laryngoscope 1994; 104: 1199–1205
102. Slootweg PJ, Hordijk GJ, Koole R. Autopsy findings in patients with head and neck squamous cell cancer and their therapeutic relevance. Oral Oncol Eur J Cancer 1996; 32B: 413–415
103. Goldblatt LI, Ellis GL. Salivary gland tumors of the tongue. Analysis of 55 new cases and review of the literature. Cancer 1987; 60: 74–81
104. Waldron CA, El-Mofty SK, Gnepp DR. Tumors of the intraoral minor salivary glands: a demographic and histologic study of 426 cases. Oral Surg Oral Med Oral Pathol 1988; 66: 323–333
105. Roper PR, Wolf PF, Luna MA et al. Malignant salivary gland tumors of the base of tongue. South Med J 1987; 80: 605–608
106. Batsakis JG, El-Naggar AK. Terminal duct adenocarcinomas of salivary tissues. Ann Otol Rhinol Laryngol 1991; 100: 251–253

107. Neville BW, Damm DD, Weir JC et al. Labial salivary gland tumors. Cancer 1988; 61: 2113–2116
108. Batsakis JG. Oral monomorphic adenomas. Ann Otol Rhinol Laryngol 1991; 100: 348–350
109. Batsakis JG, Luna MA, El-Naggar AK. Basoloid monomorphic adenomas. Ann Otol Rhinol Laryngol 1991; 100: 687–690
110. Brannon RB, Sciubba JJ, Giulani M. Ductal papillomas of salivary gland origin: a report of 19 cases and a review of the literature. Oral Surg Oral Med Oral Pathol Oral Radiol Endod 2001; 92: 68–77
111. Cleary KR, Batsakis JG. Sialadenoma papilliferum. Ann Otol Rhinol Laryngol 1990; 99: 756–758
112. Siefert G. Mucoepidermoid carcinoma in a salivary duct cyst of the parotid gland. Contribution to the development of tumours in salivary gland cysts. Pathol Res Pract 1996; 192: 1211–1217
113. Buchner A, Merrell PW, Carpenter WM. Adenomatoid hyperplasia of minor salivary glands. Oral Surg Oral Med Oral Pathol 1991; 71: 583–587
114. Edelman M, Pritchett D. Necrotizing sialometaplasia. Pathology Case Reviews 2000; 5: 221–226
115. Brannon RB, Fowler CB, Hartman KS. Necrotizing sialometaplasia. A clinicopathologic study of sixty-nine cases and review of the literature. Oral Surg Oral Med Oral Pathol 1991; 72: 317–325
116. Scotto J, Fraumeni JF, Lee JAH. Melanomas of the eye and other noncutaneous sites: epidemiologic aspects. JNCI 1976; 564: 489–491
117. Batsakis JG, Regezi JA, Solomon AR et al. The pathology of head and neck tumors; mucosal melanomas, part B. Head Neck Surgery 1982; 4: 404–418
118. Umeda M, Shimada K. Primary malignant melanoma of the oral cavity—its histological classification and treatment. Br J Oral Maxillofac Surg 1994; 32: 39–47
119. Ueta E, Miki T, Osaki T et al. Desmoplastic malignant melanoma of the gingiva; case report and review of the literature. Oral Oncol Eur J Cancer 1996; 32B: 423–427
120. Batsakis JG, Suarez P. Mucosal melanomas. A review. Adv Anat Pathol 2000; 7: 167–180
121. Chin NT, Weinstock MA. Melanoma of oronasal mucosa. Population-based analysis of occurrence and mortality. Arch Otolaryngol Head Neck Surg 1996; 122: 985–988
122. Buchner A, Hansen LS. Amalgam pigmentation (amalgam tattoo) of the oral mucosa. A clinicopathologic study of 268 cases. Oral Surg Oral Med Oral Pathol 1980; 49: 139–147
123. Tomich CE, Zunt SL. Melanoacanthosis (melanoacanthoma) of the oral mucosa. J Dermatol Surg Oncol 1990; 16: 231–236
124. Carpenter BF, Jimenez C, Robb IA. Melanotic neuroectodermal tumor of infancy. Pediatr Pathol 1985; 3: 227–244
125. Stirling RW, Powell G, Fletcher CDM. Pigmented neuroectodermal tumour of infancy: an immunohistochemical study. Histopathology 1988; 12: 425–435
126. Pettinato G, Manivel JC, D'Amore ESG et al. Melanotic neuroectodermal tumor of infancy. A reexamination of a histogenetic problem based on immunohistochemical, flow cytometric, and ultrastructural study of 10 cases. Am J Surg Pathol 1991; 15: 233–245
127. Hirshberg A, Buchner A. Metastatic tumors to the oral region. An overview. Oral Oncol Eur J Cancer 1995; 31B: 355–360
128. Lalikos JF, Sotereanos GC, Nawrocki JS et al. Isolated mandibular metastasis of hepatocellular carcinoma. J Oral Maxillofac Surg 1992; 50: 754–759
129. Kershisnik M, Batsakis JG, Mackay B. Granular cell tumors. Ann Otol Rhinol Laryngol 1994; 103: 416–419
130. Batsakis JG, El-Naggar AK, Weber RS. Two perplexing skin tumors: microcystic adnexal carcinoma and keratoacanthoma. Ann Otol Rhinol Laryngol 1994; 103: 829–832
131. Schwartz RA. Keratoacanthoma. J Am Acad Dermatol 1994; 30: 1–19
132. Hodak E, Jones RE, Ackerman AB. Solitary kerato-acanthoma is a squamous-cell carcinoma: three examples with metastases. Am J Dermatopathol 1993; 15: 332–342
133. Batsakis JG, Cleary KR, Cho K-J. Lichen planus and lichenoid lesions of the oral cavity. Ann Otol Rhinol Laryngol 1994; 103: 495–497
134. Krutchkoff DJ, Eisenberg E. Lichenoid dysplasia: a distinct histopathologic entity. Oral Surg Oral Med Oral Pathol 1985; 60: 308–315
135. Krutchkoff DJ, Cutter L, Laskowski S. Oral lichen planus: the evidence regarding potential malignant transformation. J Oral Pathol 1978; 7: 1–7
136. Barnard NA, Scully C, Eveson JW et al. Oral cancer development in patients with oral lichen planus. J Oral Pathol Med 1993; 22: 421–424
137. Voute ABE, deJong WFB, Schulten EAJM et al. Possible premalignant character of oral lichen planus: the Amsterdam experience. J Oral Pathol Med 1992; 21: 326–329
138. Sigurgeirsson B, Lindelof B. Lichen planus and malignancy. An epidemiologic study of 2071 patients and a review of the literature. Arch Dermatol 1991; 127: 1684–1689
139. Eisenberg E, Krutchkoff DJ. Lichenoid lesions of oral mucosa. Diagnostic criteria and their importance in the alleged relationship to oral cancer. Oral Surg Oral Med Oral Pathol 1992; 73: 699–704
140. Eversole LR. Editorial. Oral Surg Oral Med Oral Pathol 1992; 72: 707
141. Phelan JA, Eisig S, Freedman PD et al. Major aphthous like ulcers in patients with AIDS. Oral Surg Oral Med Oral Pathol 1991; 71: 68–72
142. Gardner A. A survey of odontogenic cysts and their relationship to squamous cell carcinoma. J Can Dent Assoc 1975; 49: 161–166
143. Koss LC, Spiro HR, Hajdu S. Small cell (oat cell) carcinoma of minor salivary gland origin. Cancer 1972; 30: 737–741

144. Batsakis JG, Luna MA. Undifferentiated carcinoma of salivary glands. Ann Otol Rhinol Laryngol 1991; 100: 82–84
145. Hayashi Y, Nagamine S, Yanagawa T et al. Small cell undifferentiated carcinoma of the minor salivary gland containing exocrine, neuroendocrine, and squamous cells. Cancer 1987; 60: 1582–1588
146. Gnepp DR, Wick MR. Small cell carcinoma of the major salivary glands. An immunohistochemical study. Cancer 1990; 66: 185–192
147. Ness KH, Morton TH, Dale BA. Identification of Merkel cells in oral epithelium using antikeratin and antineuroendocrine monoclonal antibodies. J Dent Res 1987; 66: 1154–1158
148. Longo F, Califano L, Mangone GM et al. Neuroendocrine (Merkel cell) carcinoma of the oral mucosa: report of a case with immunohistochemical study and review of the literature. J Oral Pathol Med 1999; 28: 88–89
149. Tachibana T. The Merkel cell: recent findings and unresolved problems. Arch Histol Cytol 1995; 58: 379–396
150. Vigneswaran N, Müller S, Lense E et al. Merkel cell carcinoma of the labial mucosa. An immunohistochemical and ultrastructural study with a review of the literature on oral Merkel cell carcinomas. Oral Surg Oral Med Oral Pathol 1992; 74: 193–200
151. Inoue T, Shimono M, Takano N et al. Merkel cell carcinoma of the palatal mucosa in a young adult. Immunohistochemical and ultrastructural features. Oral Oncol 1997; 33: 226–229
152. Batsakis JG, El-Naggar AK. Sebaceous lesions of salivary glands and oral cavity. Ann Otol Rhinol Laryngol 1990; 99: 416–418
153. Batsakis JG, Hicks MJ, Flaitz CM. Peripheral epithelial odontogenic tumors. Ann Otol Rhinol Laryngol 1993; 102: 322–324
154. Nauta JM, Pander AK, Schoots CJ et al. Peripheral ameloblastoma. A case report and review of the literature. Int J Oral Maxillofac Surg 1992; 21: 40–44
155. Batsakis JG, Cleary KR. Squamous odontogenic tumor. Ann Otol Rhinol Laryngol 1993; 102: 823–824
156. Sado B, Nakamura N, Higuchi Y et al. Squamous cell carcinoma of the oral cavity derived from a skin graft: a case report. Head Neck 1994; 16: 79–82
157. Patton LL, Valdez IH. Xeroderma pigmentosum: Review and report of a case. Oral Surg Oral Med Oral Pathol 1991; 71: 297–300
158. Tyler MT, Ficarra G, Silverman S Jr et al. Malignant acanthosis nigricans with florid papillary oral lesions. Oral Surg Oral Med Oral Pathol Oral Radiol Endodont 1996; 81: 445–449

4 The histology of oral cancer

John G Batsakis

Histopathologic variants of squamous cell carcinoma

Despite being the most common carcinoma in the head and neck, the histopathologic diagnosis of squamous cell carcinoma continues to be the most challenging and difficult of any neoplasm in that anatomic region. The subjective quality of the diagnosis is the basis for the difficulty. Compounding the problem is the number of variants (Table 4.1), each of which has its own criteria, site predilection, and biologic outlook.

Table 4.1 Variants of squamous cell carcinoma of the upper aerodigestive tracts

Conventional squamous cell carcinoma with varying levels of differentiation
Verrucous squamous cell carcinoma and hybrid verrucous squamous cell carcinoma
Basaloid squamous cell carcinoma
Sarcomatoid (metaplastic) squamous cell carcinoma
Adenosquamous carcinoma
Adenoid squamous cell carcinoma and acantholytic squamous cell carcinoma
Papillary squamous cell carcinoma
Lymphoepithelial (nasopharyngeal-type) carcinoma

Verrucous carcinoma

Although verrucous squamous cell carcinoma can be defined in clinical, histomorphologic, and cytokinetic terms as a unique form of squamous cell carcinoma, our knowledge of the lesion has been gained in a more or less heuristic manner. The lesion's biologic activity places it between conventional (non-verrucous) carcinomas (Fig. 4.1) and non-autochthonous hyperplasias of squamous epithelium.[1]

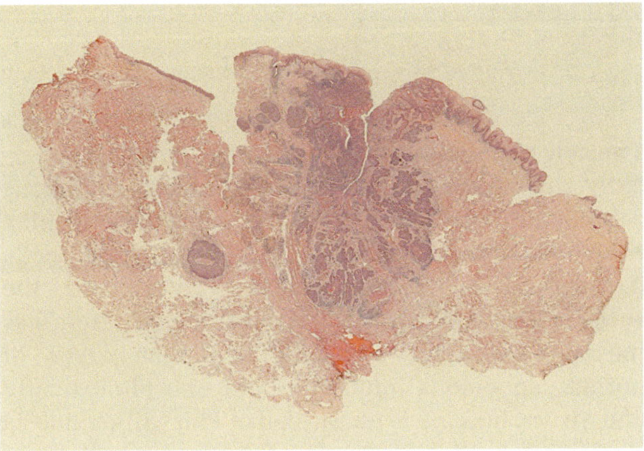

Figure 4.1 Invasive squamous cell carcinoma of the anterior (mobile) tongue.

Predominantly a squamous mucosal lesion, verrucous carcinoma may also be found on cutaneous surfaces, especially in the anogenital region and lower extremities. Whether the carcinomas occur in the upper aerodigestive tract (verrucous carcinoma), on the genitalia (giant condyloma acuminatum), or on the extremities (carcinoma cuniculatum), they are essentially the same.

The mucous membranes of the head and neck are sites of predilection, with the oral cavity and larynx areas especially at risk.

In its early stages, verrucous carcinoma undoubtedly goes unrecognized or unchallenged as just another mucosal or cutaneous verruciform growth. The carcinoma may be both persistent and progressive with a clinical phase that lasts several years. In some patients, however, the lesion appears suddenly or a period of slow growth is followed by rapid enlargement. A clinical leukoplakia often, but not invariably, characterizes the mucosa from which the neoplasm has its origin.[2] The leukoplakia may be diffuse or focal.

Table 4.2 Location of verrucous carcinoma of the oral cavity. (From data presented by Batsakis et al.[1] and Medina et al.[2])

Oral location	No. of cases
Buccal mucosa	147
Gingiva-alveolar	64
Tongue	19
Palate	14
Floor of mouth	12
Lip	5
Retromolar trigone	2
Too diffuse to localize	13

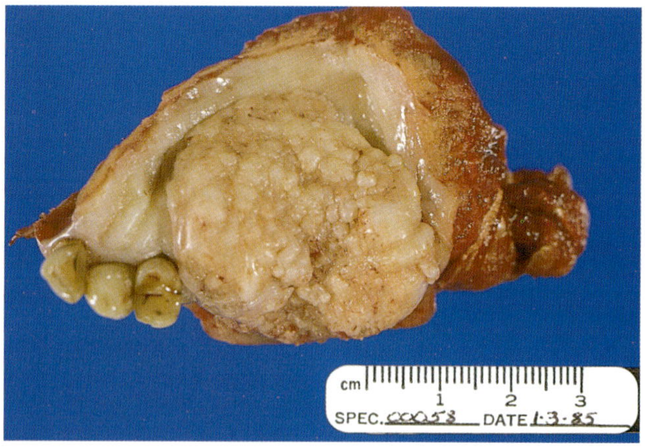

Figure 4.2 Verrucous squamous cell carcinoma of the palate.

The cell kinetics of verrucous carcinomas are apparently distinctive, if not singular, among squamous cell carcinomas. Verrucous carcinomas have a thick zone of non-proliferating, non-keratinized cells between the basal germinative layers and the surface. This non-proliferating cell region resembles the suprabasal or stratum malpighian layer of normal squamous mucosa, both morphologically and in its lack of S-phase cells. This difference is significant in that conventional squamous cell carcinomas manifest S-phase cell distribution throughout all non-keratinized zones.[3] It is unknown, however, whether all verrucous carcinomas are composed of a homogeneous cell population.

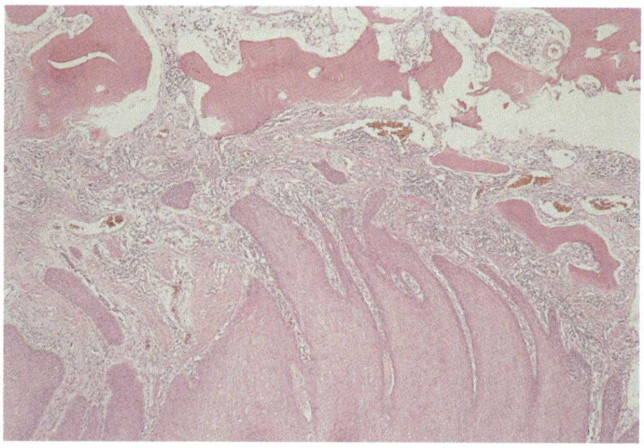

Figure 4.3 Verrucous squamous cell carcinoma invading periosteum of mandible.

In the two main sites of involvement in the head and neck, the oral cavity and the larynx, verrucous carcinoma is a disease of males who are between the ages of 50 and 80 years. At either site, the carcinoma is unusual in a patient younger than 35 years. In the oral cavity, the incidence among all forms of squamous cell carcinoma is between 2% and 4.5%.[2] Table 4.2 presents the site distribution of 276 oral cavity verrucous carcinomas and indicates the buccal mucosa accounts for over one half of the cases.[2]

The gross appearance of the verrucous carcinoma is dependent on several factors: duration of the lesion, degree of keratinization, and accompanying changes in the adjacent mucosa. The oral tumors often arise in clinical leukoplakia and are first relatively soft and circumscribed, becoming firmer and more irregular with time. The fully developed carcinoma is an exophytic gray to gray-red bulky lesion presenting as a rough, shaggy, fungating mass with a papillomatous character (Fig. 4.2).

Contiguous structures may be involved as the tumor's growth continues. When the carcinoma arises in the buccal mucosa or extends into the buccal sulcus, it can grow into the soft tissues overlying the mandible and become fixed to the periosteum. With continued growth it can gradually destroy the periosteum and directly invade and destroy a considerable part of the mandible (Fig. 4.3).

Microscopically, the verrucous carcinoma is broadly based and locally invasive, with papillary frons (Figs 4.4, 4.5). It is composed of highly differentiated squamous epithelial cells that lack the usual cytologic criteria of malignancy (Figs 4.6, 4.7). Mitoses are rare to absent. The surface of the lesion is usually covered by a prominent keratin layer arranged in compressed invaginating folds. The continuity of the surface is maintained by filiform or broader processes of well-differentiated squamous cells. These processes can be likened to a series of church spires (Fig. 4.8). The diagnosis of malignancy is made on the invasive quality of the deep parts of

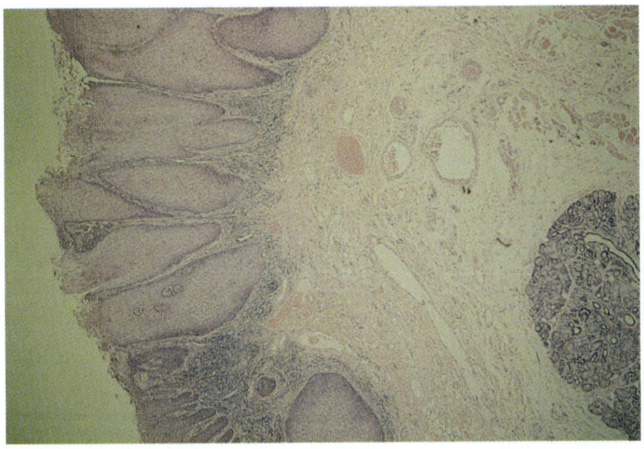

Figure 4.4 Verrucous squamous cell carcinoma of buccal mucosa.

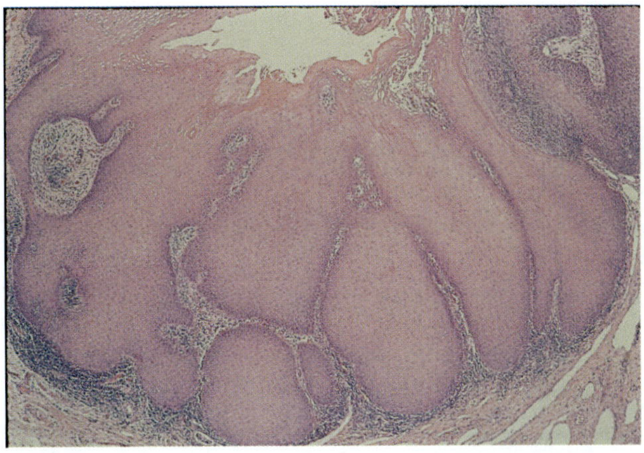

Figure 4.5 Verrucous squamous cell carcinoma of anterior (mobile) tongue.

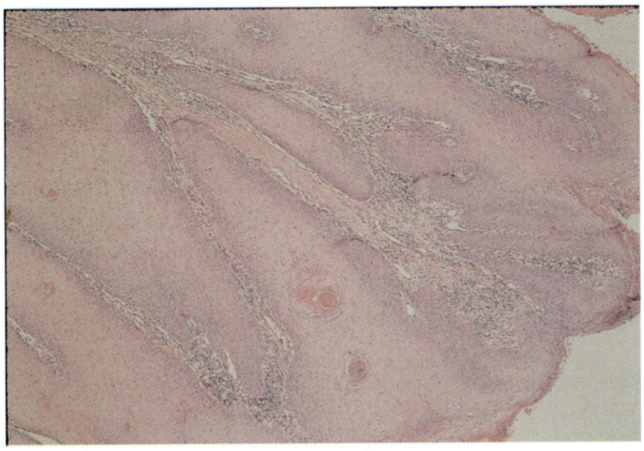

Figure 4.6 Typical verrucous squamous cell carcinoma with blunt invasive and bulbous downgrowth.

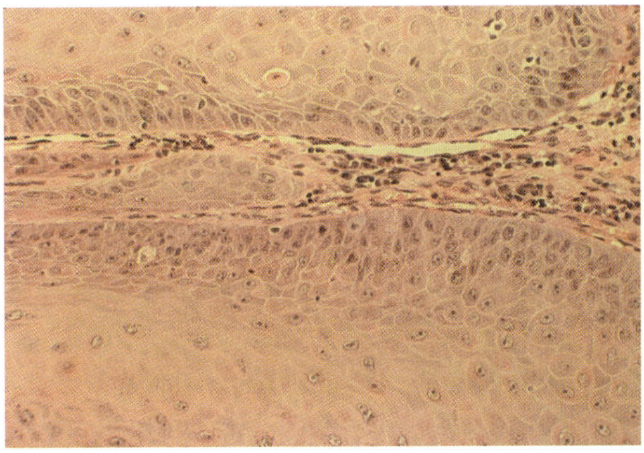

Figure 4.7 Deceptively benign bulbous downgrowth of a verrucous squamous carcinoma.

the tumor. This infiltrative margin is invariably a blunt 'pushing' one with usually a good circumscription. Often the invading tumors grow from a plane that resembles basement membrane. This seems to be a point of confusion for some pathologists who claim they are unable to define invasion. A verrucous squamous cell carcinoma is, by definition, invasive! Typically, but not invariably, there is an associated inflammatory reaction in the stroma. This consists preponderantly of lymphocytes. The inflammatory layer gives the impression of trying to delimit the carcinoma. Intraneoplastic and stromal reactions to keratin or other cellular debris can be found.

Because of the deceptively benign appearance of the neoplastic cells, an accurate surgical pathologic diagnosis requires a biopsy specimen that shows the invasive depth of the lesion. A full-thickness biopsy plus an appropriate clinical description, or, preferably, a personal inspection of the in-vivo lesion should permit a pathologist to distinguish a verrucous carcinoma from benign hyperplasia or other forms of squamous cell carcinoma. The presence of

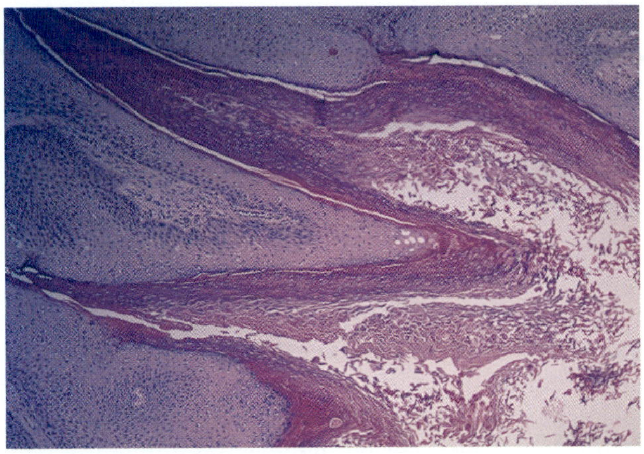

Figure 4.8 Keratotic 'church spire' surface of a verrucous squamous carcinoma.

Table 4.3 Clinicopathologic features of verrucous carcinoma of the oral cavity

Feature	Finding
Site of predilection	Buccal mucosa
Age and sex of patients	Predilection for males older than 50 years
Habits	Tobacco users, poor oral hygiene
Related mucosal changes	Leukoplakia; metachronous or synchronous squamous cell neoplasms
Gross appearance	Exophytic or fungating, usually keratinizing
Differentiation of cells	High degree, uniform; low-grade
Cytologic features of malignancy or severe dysplasia	Rare to absent
Mode of invasion	Pushing or blunt and bulbous
Cellular (host) reaction	Usually prominent
Hybrid forms	20% of oral tumors
Metastatic ability	None in bona fide cases

a regional lymphadenopathy is not an assistance in differential diagnosis and may be misleading. Bona fide and unperturbed verrucous carcinomas do not metastasize, but can be associated with benign lymph node enlargements secondary to the inflammatory reaction associated with the carcinoma. Table 4.3 summarizes the clinicopathologic features of verrucous carcinoma.

The phenomenon of 'anaplastic transformation' following radiation therapy of a verrucous carcinoma has been a factor of contention in the treatment of the neoplasm.[1] It is our consideration that verrucous carcinomas, at any site, are preferably treated with surgical excision. Even at radiation therapy centers the results of local control and survival have not surpassed those obtainable with surgery.[4] It should also be noted that when combination therapy has been used, such management has rarely been a planned program, but one in which surgical salvage followed the failure of radiotherapy.[5]

Selection of surgery over radiotherapy should be predicated on the effectiveness of the modality rather than on the so-called anaplastic transformation. The frequency of the event is clearly overestimated (10–30%).[1] Unknown incidence aside, there are several other disturbing features about the anaplastic transformation phenomenon. The time interval, or latent period, between radiotherapy and the advent of a much more biologically aggressive tumor is short; in fact it must be uniquely so. In five separate reports, the average time interval was 5.4 months.[1] Why this seeming transformation occurs only with this carcinoma and a few others is also not known. It is difficult for us to accept that 'dedifferentiation' of such a phenotypically well-developed lesion as verrucous carcinoma can take place, let alone within the observed limited time span. The term 'anaplastic' also has been used indiscriminately and, unfortunately, perpetuated in the reports of these lesions. Certainly neither the scant microscopic descriptions nor the surprisingly meager light-optic documentation of the tumors in the literature warrant such a classification. Where it has been possible to conclude anything based on either descriptions or photomicrographs, the neoplasms in question have ranged from minimally or nonkeratinizing squamous cell carcinomas to others, best classified as sarcomatoid or metaplastic carcinomas.

Questions can also be raised over the initial diagnosis of verrucous carcinoma. Some are clearly not by contemporary criteria, but are conventional, well-differentiated squamous cell carcinomas. The often large size of the carcinomas lends itself to sampling deficiencies and possible misclassification. It therefore can be seen that both size of the lesion with possible sampling errors and histologic misclassification can play a significant role in the so-called 'transformation process'.

There is certainly the possibility that routine sections may miss areas of less well-differentiated carcinoma within the excised lesional tissue. In that light, the hybrid verrucous carcinoma must be considered (Fig. 4.9). A hybrid verrucous carcinoma is defined as a neoplasm in which there is histologically diagnostic verrucous carcinoma and a non-verrucous squamous cell carcinoma arising synchronously from the same maternal field.[1,2] The non-verrucous carcinoma can be a conventional, well-differentiated squamous cell carcinoma or range to poorly differentiated and non-keratinized.

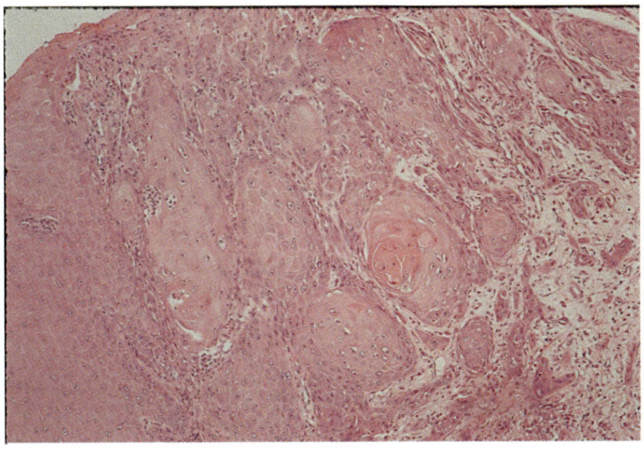

Figure 4.9 Hybrid verrucous squamous cell carcinoma. Conventional invasive squamous cell carcinoma on right with verrucous squamous cell carcinoma in same microscopic field on left.

In an M.D. Anderson series, 20% of oral verrucous carcinomas manifested this hybrid association.[2] This presence could, by clonal stimulation of partially differentiated cells, account for possible 'anaplastic' transformation.

Basaloid squamous cell carcinoma

Basaloid squamous cell carcinoma is an aggressive, histologically distinctive variant of squamous cell carcinoma that has a predilection for the upper aerodigestive tract. Other sites, including the anus (cloacogenic carcinoma), esophagus and uterine cervix may also be involved.

The clinicopathologic features of 90 cases of basaloid squamous cell carcinoma are presented in Table 4.4.[6] These include an occurrence in an elderly population with a mean age of 63 years; a male preponderance (82%); predilection for the base of tongue, pyriform sinus, and supraglottic larynx; and an aggressive clinical behavior with a high incidence of metastases to cervical lymph nodes (64%); distant spread (44%) to lungs, liver, bone, brain, and skin; and death because of the neoplasm (38% lethality at 17 months' median follow-up).

As its name connotes, the carcinoma is distinguished by at least two cytomorphologic components. In addition, the carcinoma manifests both deep and lateral invasion at the time of diagnosis. Since basaloid squamous carcinoma is a variably differentiated squamous cell carcinoma, the recognizable phenotype is, or should be, present. A sampling deficiency of biopsy may not provide a specimen with both components of the carcinoma. Without the squamous cell carcinoma features, a submucosal salivary gland neoplasm, pertinently a high-grade adenoid cystic carcinoma or even a neuroendocrine carcinoma, can be suggested.

Table 4.4 Basaloid squamous cell carcinoma: clinicopathologic features (*n* = 90). (Adapted from Raslan et al.[6])

Age of patients (years)	
Average	63
Range	27–88
Sex of patients	Males (82%)
Anatomic site	%
Base of tongue	24
Piriform sinus	20
Larynx	13
Floor of mouth	9
Larynx–piriform sinus	7
Tonsil	7
Wall of pharynx	6
Base of tongue–larynx	4
Nasal cavity/nasopharynx	3
Hard palate	1
Buccal mucosa	1
Piriform sinus–esophagus	1
Not otherwise specified	3
Size of tumor (cm)	
Average	3.3
Range	1–6
	%
Metastasis to neck nodes	64
Distant metastases	44
Local recurrence	14
Outcome (average follow-up, 21 months; range 1–67 months)	
Dead of disease	38
Alive with disease	18
Alive, no disease	30
Dead of other causes	7
Uncertain or lost to follow-up	8

The carcinomas, even when small, are usually hard and centrally ulcerated with submucosal infiltration. The ulceration can obscure an origin from the surface mucosa, further confusing the diagnosis, especially if the squamous component is lost or obscured.

The squamous carcinoma is usually well to moderately well differentiated and invasive. In-situ carcinoma and/or severe squamous dysplasia are also findings. A multifocal origin over a broad area of affected mucosa has been noted.[7,8] It is, however, the basaloid malignancy that sets this carcinoma apart

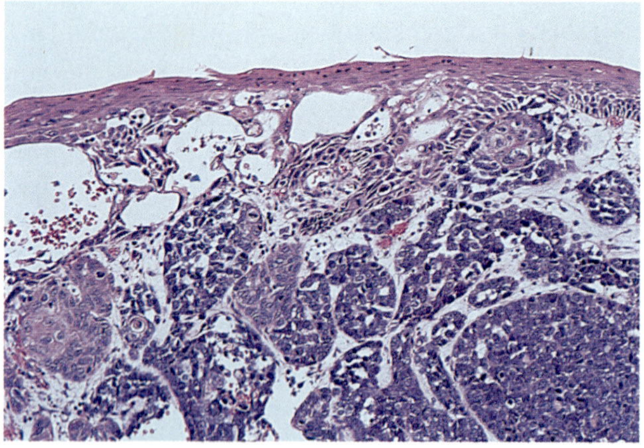

Figure 4.10 Basaloid squamous cell carcinoma showing origin of the basaloid component from an attenuated surface mucosa.

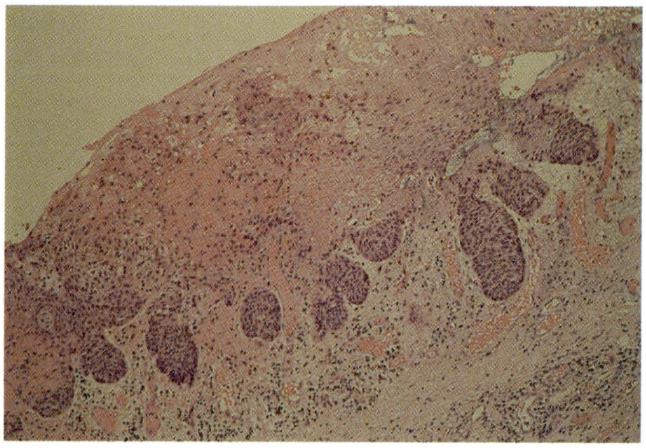

Figure 4.11 Basaloid squamous cell carcinoma with obliteration of surface by necrosis.

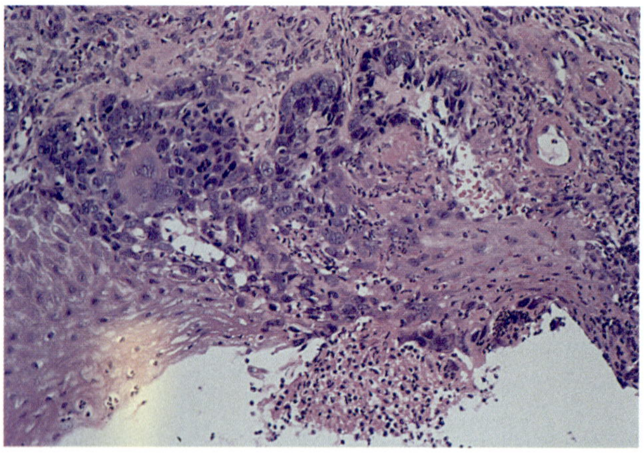

Figure 4.12 Basaloid squamous cell carcinoma showing surface necrosis and biphasic squamous cell and basaloid components.

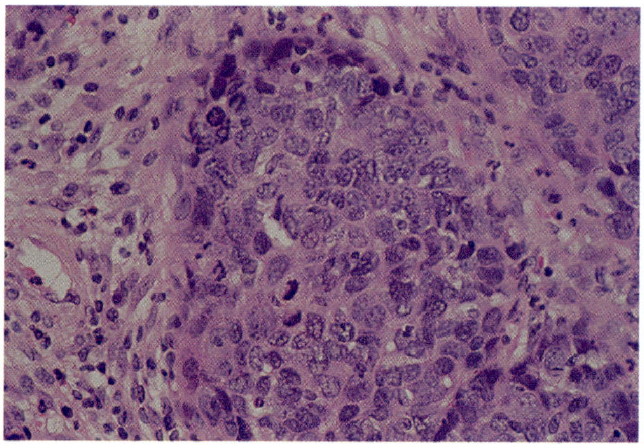

Figure 4.13 Basaloid squamous cell carcinoma (basaloid component) with atypical mitotic figures.

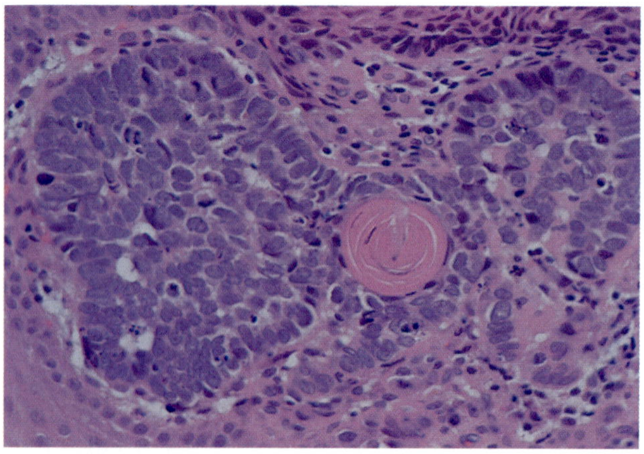

Figure 4.14 Basaloid squamous cell carcinoma. Abrupt keratin formation in a basaloid island.

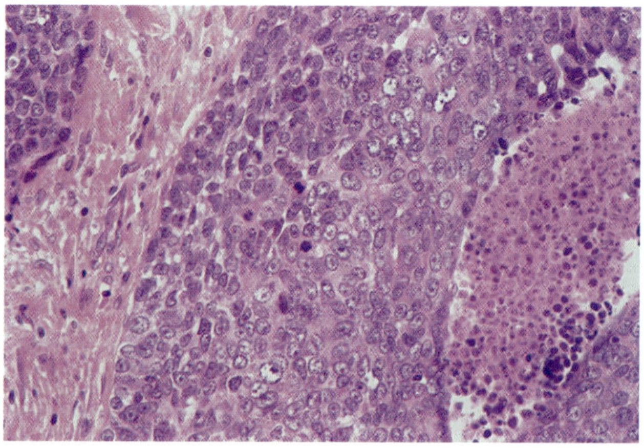

Figure 4.15 Comedo necrosis in basaloid squamous cell carcinoma.

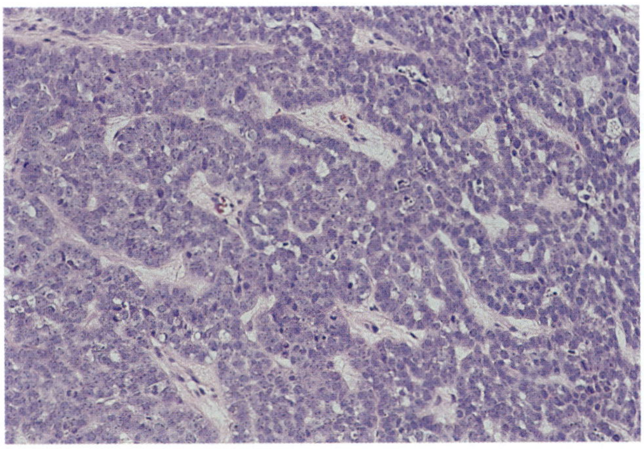

Figure 4.16 Pseudoglandular architecture in a basaloid squamous cell carcinoma.

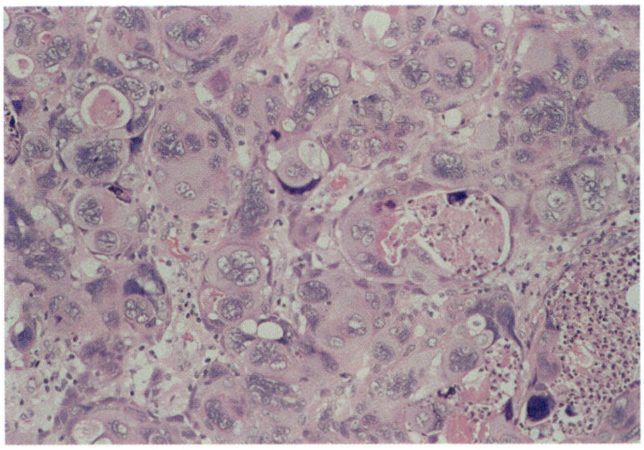

Figure 4.17 Extreme pleomorphism in a basaloid squamous cell carcinoma.

as a distinctive variant of squamous cell carcinoma (Figs 4.10–4.17). The growth pattern of the basaloid cells is often lobular, but can also be in cords or trabeculae. There is a prominent mitotic activity with many atypical or bizarre mitoses. The bulk of the basaloid component may not have a unity with either the squamous carcinoma component or the surface (because of necrosis), but where this is present, it is unequivocal.

The immunochemical profile is one of an epithelial malignancy.[9] Electron-optic findings in the basaloid cells consist of desmosomes, rare tonofilaments, free ribosomes, but no neurosecretory granules, myofilaments, or secretory granules.

Studies of oncogene expression suggest that basaloid squamous cell carcinoma is a distinct variant of squamous cell carcinoma with a poorly differentiated cell population. DNA ploidy studies do not add prognostic information over that by light-optic examination.

The two neoplasms that are most important in the differential diagnosis are adenoid cystic carcinoma and small cell undifferentiated carcinoma with neuroendocrine differentiation.

Adenoid cystic carcinoma does not show foci of squamous cell carcinoma. There is also no significant dysplasia or in situ carcinoma in the overlying mucosa. Mitosis, nuclear pleomorphism, and necrosis are also more conspicuous in basaloid squamous cell carcinoma. Basaloid squamous cell carcinoma is often associated with positive cervical lymph nodes at diagnosis, while adenoid cystic carcinoma is not.

Aside from the rarity of neuroendocrine carcinoma in the oral cavity, they can be distinguished from basaloid squamous cell carcinoma by their prominent nuclear molding and the absence of hyalinosis and mucinous-myxoid changes in the stroma. Paranuclear globular staining for keratin is also a feature not found in basaloid squamous cell carcinoma. The neuroendocrine nature is manifested by immunopositivity for chromogranin, synaptophysin and Leu-7. These are negative in basaloid squamous cell carcinoma.

Table 4.4 certainly indicates the lethality of this variant of squamous cell carcinoma. There is, however, a question whether anatomical location of the primary plays a role. Luna et al.,[8] dealing with basaloid squamous cell carcinomas of the hypopharynx, found no difference in biologic behavior (stage for stage) between conventional squamous cell carcinoma and basaloid squamous cell carcinoma. Basaloid squamous cell carcinomas of the floor of mouth, on the other hand, have a higher recurrence rate and a worse prognosis than matched groups of conventional squamous cell carcinomas, regardless of the grade of the latter.[10] It is possible, although unconfirmed, that there is a correlation between the percentage of basaloid component and prognosis; carcinomas with more than 50% basaloid cells have a poorer prognosis.[10]

Sarcomatoid carcinoma

Reflective of the different theories of histogenesis, sarcomatoid carcinomas have gone by various other designations: carcinosarcoma, spindle cell carcinoma, pleomorphic carcinoma, metaplastic carcinoma, polypoid carcinoma, and pseudosarcomatous carcinoma. Like Wick and Swanson,[11] we believe the continued use of carcinosarcoma as a diagnosis, particularly in the head and neck, is indefensible.

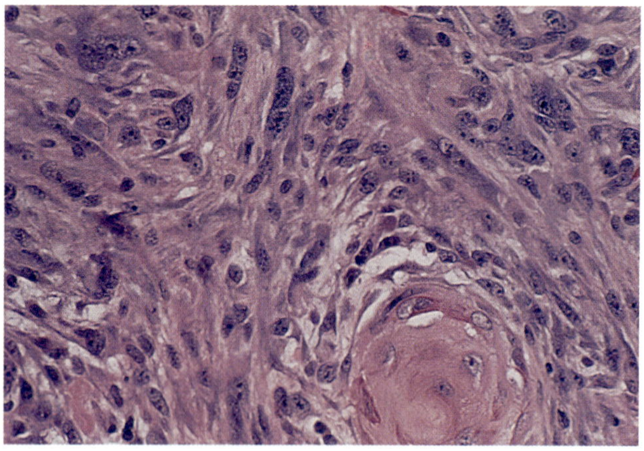

Figure 4.18 Sarcomatoid carcinoma showing a well-differentiated island of squamous cells surrounded by pleomorphic spindle cells.

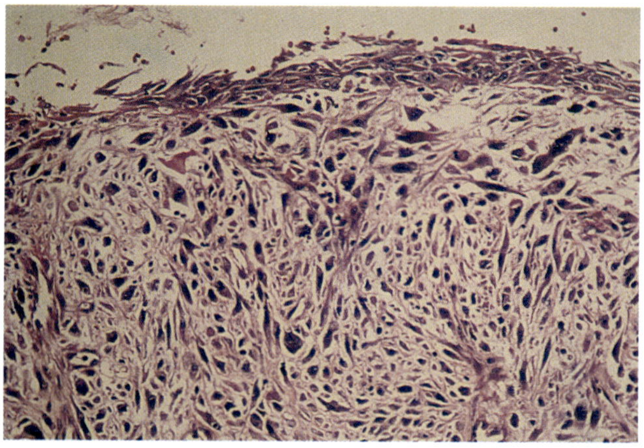

Figure 4.19 Sarcomatoid carcinoma. Highly atypical spindle cells infiltrate beneath an attenuated surface.

This stance is supported by the findings of a monoclonal origin.[12] That said, all malignant neoplasms manifesting an apparent mix of carcinomatous and sarcomatous phenotypes, regardless of whether they are homologous or heterologous, are sarcomatoid carcinomas, albeit with varying degrees of divergent differentiation.

With few exceptions, the definable epithelial malignancy in sarcomatoid carcinoma is a squamous cell carcinoma and the most accepted origin of the usually biphasic histomorphology of a sarcomatoid carcinoma is that the malignant pleomorphic spindle cells derive from a sarcomatous metaplasia of the malignant epithelial cells. Several observations support this view: (1) transitions between the biphasic elements; (2) immunoreactive cytokeratins in the spindle cells; (3) electron-optic features (desmosomes and tonofibrils) of epithelial cells in spindle cells; (4) dual expression of epithelial and mesenchymal differentiation in some of the neoplastic cells; (5) the preponderance of carcinomas rather than sarcomas in locations where sarcomatoid carcinomas occur; and (6) metastases from a sarcomatoid carcinoma may be epithelial only, sarcomatous only, or retain the duality of the primary.[13,14]

Uncommon in absolute terms, sarcomatoid carcinomas are, nevertheless, the most common 'spindle-cell malignancies' of the upper airway and also probably of the upper digestive tract.[11] In the mucosa of the head and neck, the larynx and oral cavity are the sites of predilection, but the tumors also occur in the sinonasal tract, pharynx, and esophagus.[15]

The only assured means of diagnosing a sarcomatoid carcinoma is to require identification of malignant epithelial elements in company with a malignant spindle cell (sarcomatous) population (Fig. 4.18). The identifiable squamous cell carcinoma can be invasive, in-situ, verrucous and variably differentiated. Severe dysplasia, rather than overt carcinoma, may be the only epithelial aberration. Carcinoma may not be demonstrable in all cases, in fact, 28% of the tumors reported by Zarbo et al.[16] were devoid of squamous cell carcinoma (Fig. 4.19).

The morphologic cell type of the spindle cells in a sarcomatoid carcinoma cannot be reliably predicted by routine light-optic examination.[17] At least two additional studies are necessary: (1) electron microscopy (Fig. 4.20) and (2) immunohistochemistry (Fig. 4.21). Assuming there is no sampling bias, the spindle cells in some tumors will show a pure epithelial differentiation, whereas those in other tumors will exhibit only a mesenchymal differentiation. In still others, some of the spindle cells have epithelial markers, others mesenchymal markers, and in some cells there will be features of both lineages. In one series, immunoreactive coexpression was found in 25% of the tumors; epithelial markers in 50% of the tumors.[18] The percentage of cells colored by cytokeratin antigen–antibody reactions varies from 10% or less to more than 90%.

The immunoreactivity of sarcomatoid carcinomas does not always correlate with the ultrastructural findings. Whether this is a reflection of the varying sensitivity and specificity of immunohistochemical markers is not clear. The most reliable epithelial marker is cytokeratin, but staining for epithelial membrane antigen and carcinoembryonic antigen can also be useful. As noted above, none, by themselves, will decorate all the spindle cells in a sarcomatoid carcinoma.

The cytokeratins constitute a family of proteins; at least 19 different human cytokeratin polypeptides

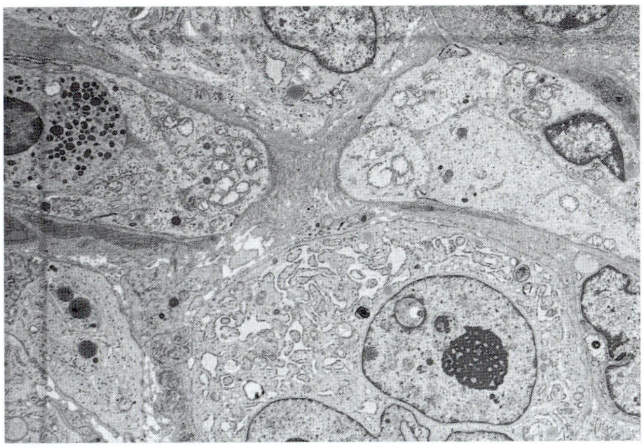

Figure 4.20 Electron micrograph of sarcomatoid carcinoma of tongue illustrating the metaplastic transformation of the squamous cell carcinoma.

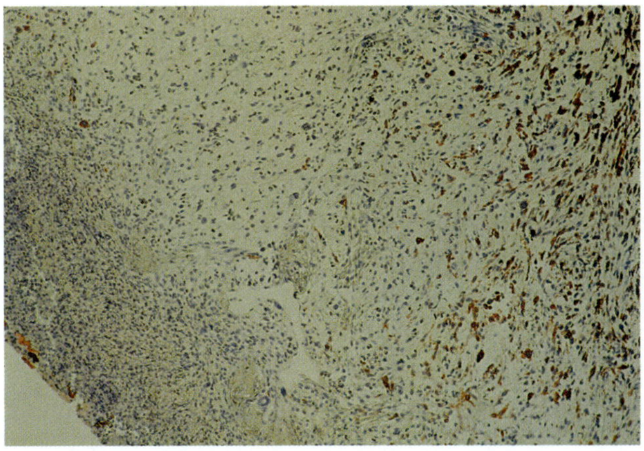

Figure 4.21 Immunohistochemical preparation of a sarcomatoid carcinoma. Keratin positive cells lie deep to the surface (right).

have been distinguished. Different epithelial cells and their carcinomas express different combinations of cytokeratin proteins and it is unlikely that even polyclonal, wide-spectrum antibodies to keratin will be able to detect all of the possible variants of keratin in neoplastic cells. Ogawa et al.,[19] dealing with sarcomatoid carcinomas of diverse sites, found a positivity rate of 59% with anti-high molecular weight cytokeratin antibody alone, 79% with anti-low molecular weight cytokeratin antibody alone, and 88% when both antibodies were used. Reports of sarcomatoid carcinomas of the upper aerodigestive tract indicate keratin expression rates of 50% to 75% (average 58%).[20,21] When possible, electron-optic study should complement the immunohistochemical findings.

Sarcomatoid carcinomas are usually pedunculated or polypoid masses; less often sessile or ulcero-infiltrative lesions. Their size varies from 0.5 to 6.0 cm. If large, they can produce life-threatening obstruction. The carcinoma's surface is nearly always extensively ulcerated and covered by a fibrinonecrotic exudate of varying thickness. There is often a friable quality of the upper part (granulation tissue) of the tumors. Such friability is held responsible for the coughing up of fragments of tumor by some patients.

Demonstrable squamous cell carcinoma or dysplasia may be a minor component (or not detectable), with the sarcomatous elements dominating the microscopic appearance.[22,23] Diligence and the necessity of multiple sections to find an elusive carcinoma are often necessary. It is most reliably found at the base or the margins of the spindle cell proliferation. In most cases, the carcinoma is demarcated and does not exhibit an intermingling with the spindle cell component.

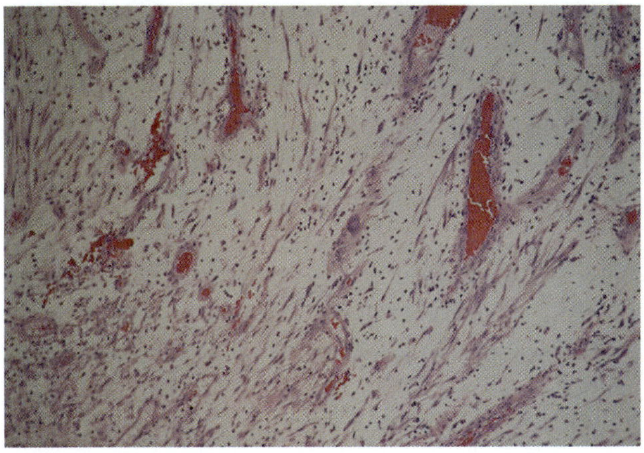

Figure 4.22 Deceptively benign (nodular fasciitis-like) sarcomatoid carcinoma.

The sarcomatous elements can mimic fibrosarcoma, synovial sarcoma, leiomyosarcoma, malignant fibrous histiocytoma or even benign stromal lesions such as a cellular nodular fasciitis and other myofibroblastic proliferations (Figs 4.22–4.24). The spindle cells can be arranged in a fasciculated, myxomatous, or streaming growth pattern, with the fascicular form the most common (Fig. 4.25). One pattern is often dominant in a given tumor, but most of the tumors manifest a combination. Cellular density is variable and so, too, is the pleomorphism shown by cells and their nuclei. Multinucleate giant cells of either foreign body type or bizarre neoplastic form are common (Fig. 4.26). These may be accompanied by metaplastic or malignant osteocartilaginous foci. The latter are frequently associated with prior ionizing radiation to the site of the tumor. The carcinomas may be richly mitotic (often with bizarre division figures) or sparsely population with mitoses.

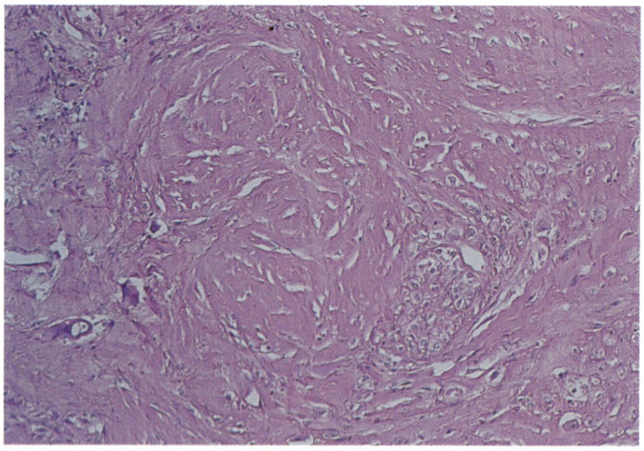

Figure 4.23 Hyalinized matrix of a sarcomatoid carcinoma in a hematoxylin and eosin preparation.

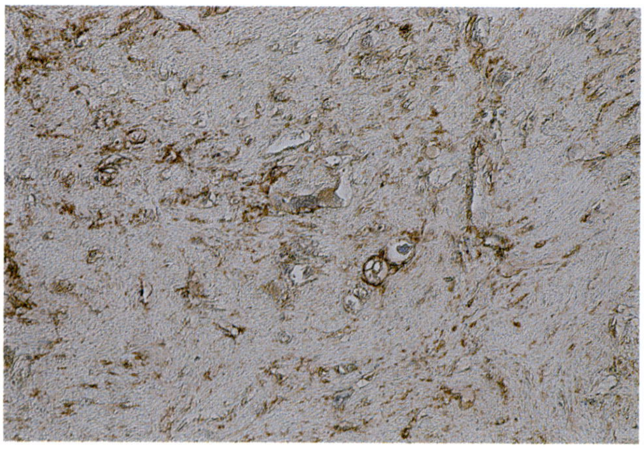

Figure 4.24 Immunohistochemical (keratin) preparation of the tumor shown in Fig. 4.35. Note keratin positive neoplastic cells.

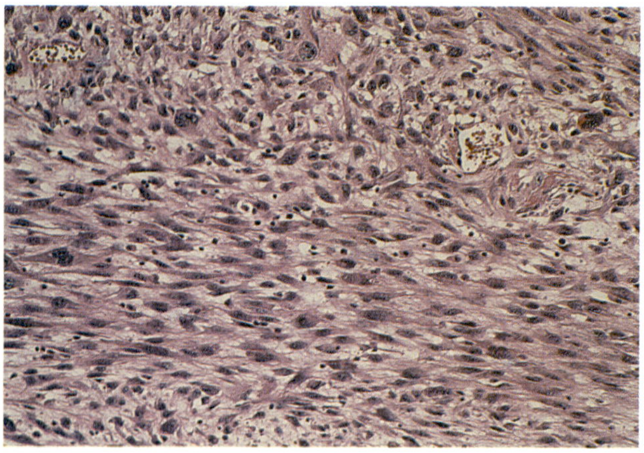

Figure 4.25 Sarcomatoid carcinoma with a fascicular pattern of growth mimicking a supporting tissue malignancy.

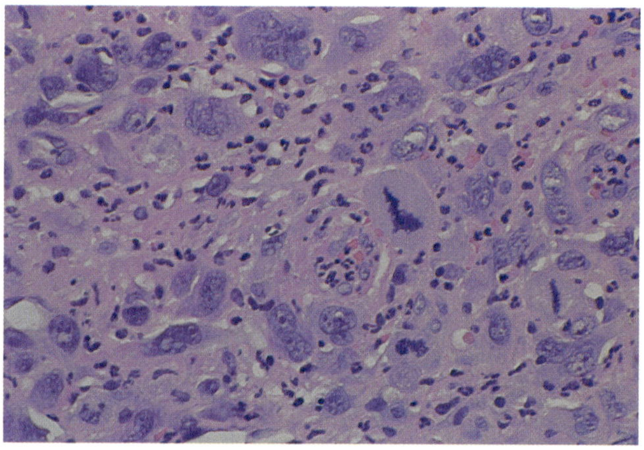

Figure 4.26 Extreme anaplasia of cells in a sarcomatoid carcinoma with abnormal mitoses.

In general, immunohistochemistry and electron microscopy can provide a reasonable direction for defining lines of differentiation in sarcomatoid carcinomas. As noted, however, the complex phenotype exhibited by these tumors may not yield to the demonstration of epithelial features. Compounding the issue is the fact that cytokeratin expression has been also shown in non-epithelial tumors such as leiomyosarcomas, synovial sarcomas, angiosarcomas, melanomas, and other neoplasms. Moreover, the putative mesenchymal marker, vimentin, is expressed in many epithelial tumors and its ubiquitous distribution precludes attaching much significance to it as a cell lineage marker. Even more problematic is the finding of smooth muscle differentiation (electron-optic and immunohistochemical), either alone or co-expressed with cytokeratin in a significant number of sarcomatoid carcinomas. This myogenic profile is interpreted as a manifestation of myofibroblastic differentiation.

Is the fact that not all candidate lesions for a diagnosis of sarcomatoid carcinoma demonstrate a detectable epithelial differentiation in the sarcomatous component a contraindication to the diagnosis? Not if elements of a squamous cell carcinoma are found and the spindle cell elements exhibit cytomorphologic evidence of malignancy, regardless of absent epithelial markers. Possible explanations for the lack of the markers include (1) sampling errors; (2) lack of sensitivity of detection methods, including fixation and processing variables; and (3) the progressive loss of identifiable epithelial markers. Guarino[24] has outlined the rationale for the

Table 4.5 Sarcomatoid carcinoma and related lesions: a classification

Sarcomatoid carcinoma	A biphasic (divergent differentiation) epithelial malignancy. Definable carcinoma with a metaplastic, cytokeratin positive spindle cell component. Metastases can be uniphasic or mixed
Carcinoma with pseudosarcomatous stroma	(a) A uniphasic epithelial malignancy associated with a benign, often atypical, cytokeratin negative, stromal proliferation. Stromal cells exhibit only mesenchymal markers. Metastases are cacinomatous only (b) An epithelial malignancy with postradiation stromal atypia. No cytokeratin reactivity in stromal cells. Metastases are carcinomatous only
Inflammatory myofibroblastic tumor (so-called 'inflammatory pseudotumor')	Part of a spectrum of heterogeneous non-neoplastic or possibly neoplastic histologically benign lesions with mesenchymal (smooth muscle) markers. Potential for recurrence exists

latter in his description of phenotypic conversion from a carcinomatous to sarcomatous appearance as a continuous spectrum of changes.

Unanswered, and probably unanswerable at this time, is whether the stromal cells in a sarcomatoid carcinoma are always part of the spectrum of a mesenchymal differentiation by the carcinoma, or whether there are some instances in which they are literally pseudosarcomatous, reactive cells.[15,22] The problem is heightened when only mesenchymal differentiation is demonstrated in the spindle cells (with or without an accompanying squamous cell carcinoma). In the absence of carcinoma a myofibroblastic tumor (see later) becomes a diagnostic consideration and, in the presence of a carcinoma, the possibility of a reactive fibro-myofibroblastic proliferation to the carcinoma cannot be completely excluded. Batsakis et al.[15] have defended the possibility that various histogenetic mechanisms may be operational and this stance is perpetuated in the current World Health Organization classification of laryngeal tumors.[25]

A classification of sarcomatoid carcinoma and related lesions, based on the foregoing, can be constructed (Table 4.5). The classification stratifies the lesions principally on the basis of evidence of epithelial differentiation of the stromal spindle cells and consequently has an intrinsic weakness. It is offered as a guide, not a listing of diagnostic criteria.

The behavior of a sarcomatoid carcinoma is biologically like that of a conventional squamous cell carcinoma. Once defined as a sarcomatoid carcinoma, the entire lesion should be treated as an epithelial malignancy and managed by surgery, as the primary mode of treatment, as any squamous cell carcinoma of similar stage, location and size. Early stage (T1, T2) lesions have a better overall survival, disease-free interval, and local control. In a review of 154 cases, Batsakis et al.[15] reported a lethality of 42% for all aerodigestive tract tumor sites, but significant differences by specific sites: 34% for laryngeal sarcomatoid carcinomas and 60% and 70%, respectively, for those of the oral cavity and sinonasal tract. The more favorable outlook for tumors of the larynx is attributed to their often glottic location and also to a relative preponderance of exophytic growth. In general, endophytic sarcomatoid carcinomas fare worse. This may be related to a greater depth of invasion and its association with a higher frequency of nodal metastases. Prior radiation therapy has also been associated with a poorer prognosis.[15]

Very little has been done to determine the prognostic impact of the carcinoma's cytomorphology and keratin immunoreactive status. Olsen et al.[21] found the survival rate among patients with negative results of polyclonal keratin stains to be significantly greater than that of patients with positive results of stains ($p < 0.001$ and $p = 0.04$). Ploidy analysis has shown the spindle cells to be non-diploid in most laryngeal tumors studied and their DNA profile to be similar to the co-existent squamous cell carcinoma.[20] As yet, however, the number of cases is too small to judge prognostic significance of the ploidy.

Table 4.6 presents the intraoral sites and outcome of 59 sarcomatoid carcinomas studied by Ellis and Corio.[13] The oral carcinomas exhibited a 2:1 male preference, a preponderance of White subjects and an age range at the time of diagnosis of 29–93 years (mean, 56.6 years). The neoplasms were nearly equally represented in polypoid, exophytic growth

Table 4.6 Sarcomatoid carcinoma of the oral cavity. (Modified from Ellis and Corio[13])

Oral location	No. of cases	Dead of disease
Lower lip	25	10
Tongue	12	4
Alveolar ridge/gingiva	11	3
Floor of mouth	3	2
Maxillary antrum	2	2
Tonsillar pillar/retromolar	2	2
Buccal mucosa	2	0
Upper lip	1	1
Hard palate	1	1

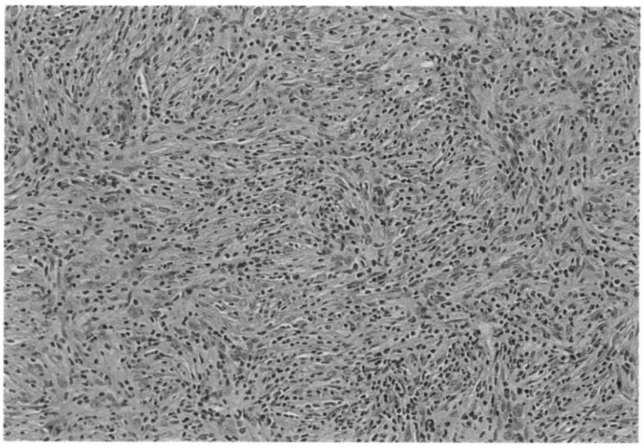

Figure 4.27 Inflammatory (myofibroblastic) pseudotumor. An important differential diagnosis for sarcomatoid carcinoma.

against an endophytic sessile and nodular appearance. Tumor size varied from 0.5 to 5.0 cm (mean, 2.1 cm).

Forty-five of the 59 patients had follow-up information. Of these, 59% were dead of their disease and only 31% were alive without residual or recurrent carcinomas. The mean survival time of patients dead of disease was 1.9 years. Recurrences were noted in 12 patients and metastases in 16. The cervical lymph nodes were the most frequent site of metastasis, 11 or 24%. This is to be compared to sarcomatoid carcinomas arising in the glottis (15%), supraglottis (30%), and hypopharynx (60%). Distant spread occurred in nine patients.

While the outlook is not good for any oral sarcomatoid carcinoma, those of the lower lip have the best survival rate. Mortality in the Ellis and Corio[13] series was not influenced by size of tumor, gross configuration, history of prior radiation, or any histomorphologic characteristic. Surgical resection, with or without neck dissection, resulted in a better survival rate than radiation alone, or the combination of radiation and surgery.

Inflammatory pseudotumor

The 'inflammatory pseudotumor' has become one of the major differential diagnoses in considering sarcomatoid carcinoma (Fig. 4.27). Like sarcomatoid carcinoma, the nomenclature surrounding lesions under the rubric of 'inflammatory pseudotumor' has been bedeviled by an often confusing variety of terms.[26] Moreover, because the term 'pseudotumor' reflects the clinicoradiologic presence of a space-occupying non-neoplastic lesion, it has been used for any mass lesion mimicking a neoplasm.[27] The varied terminology not only points to the use of different diagnostic histologic criteria, but more importantly to the fact the lesion is a heterogeneous entity. A listing of some of the terms used by authors speaks to this point: inflammatory myofibroblastic lesion, inflammatory myofibrohistiocytic proliferation, inflammatory fibromyxoid tumor, xanthomatous pseudotumor, post-inflammatory pseudotumor, plasma cell/histiocytoma complex, and inflammatory fibrosarcoma.

Further compounding the confusion engendered by the nosology is the fact that the tumors have been reported to occur in practically every conceivable site in the body and they can be multifocal. In general, the lesions can be divided into pulmonary and extrapulmonary types, with signs and symptoms related to the mass lesion.

In the head and neck the lesions have been reported in the sinonasal tract, nasopharynx, orbit, oral cavity, larynx, trachea, pharynx, thyroid gland, and salivary glands.

Chan[28] has written the most definitive evaluation of 'inflammatory pseudotumors'. In addition to underscoring the heterogeneity, he also gives a superb clinicopathologic assessment: (1) pulmonary lesions almost invariably have a benign course (recurrence rate, < 5%); (2) lower urogenital tract lesions also pursue a benign clinical course; (3) extrapulmonic and tumors originating outside of the lower urogenital tract, in particular the intra-abdominal masses, are more likely to manifest an aggressive behavior, e.g., local invasion, recurrences and metastasis (rarely); (4) extrapulmonic and extra-urogenital tumors have a reported overall recurrence/persistence rate of approximately 25%, but this varies according to site; (5) the tumors may be histologically misdiagnosed as some form of sarcoma (rhabdo-, leio-, malignant fibrous histiocytoma), lymphoma, plasmacytomas, or anaplastic carcinoma, including sarcomatoid carcinoma, and vice versa.

The unifying feature for this group of lesions is that of a mass comprising a highly variable admixture of bland-looking spindle cells, chronic inflammatory cells, and collagen fibers. Spindle cells may be the major population in some tumors, while plasma cells may be preponderant in others. Most of the tumors contain a combination of these elements. The spindle cells are a mixture of myofibroblasts, fibroblasts, and histiocytes. These are loosely disposed or arranged in a fasicular or storiform growth pattern. Degrees of atypia are seen and that, combined with a prominent fascicular growth pattern, may portend an increased risk of recurrence.

It is almost certain that some so-called inflammatory pseudotumors are genuine neoplasms (especially those with a fasicular growth pattern) and some authors regard all inflammatory pseudotumors as myofibroblastic neoplasms inflammatory myofibroblastic tumors. It is, however, premature to assign an oncogenic basis for all 'inflammatory pseudotumors'. Nonetheless, in the spectrum dominated by apparently non-neoplastic mesenchymal proliferations, the inflammatory myofibroblastic tumor seems to be a neoplasm of limited, but unpredictable biologic potential and a risk for recurrences.

Clonal cytogenetic aberrations have been demonstrated in a few of the tumors, providing further support for a neoplastic process.[28]

There is no current consensus about the inflammatory myofibroblastic tumor's capacity for recurrence and metastases, in part this is due to the uncertainty whether lesions involving multiple sites are multifocal or metastatic. One subgroup, involving the mesentery and retroperiosteum, has been called inflammatory fibrosarcoma (recurrence rate of 37% and metastatic rate of 11%).[29] To date, none of the extra-abdominal tumors have manifested what has been called metastasis.

In summary, benign, non-metastasizing myofibroblastic lesions (probably neoplasms) and inflammatory fibrosarcomas are only two of several types of lesions currently listed under 'inflammatory pseudotumors', which also include reparative, infective and purely inflammatory lesions. The majority of the myofibroblastic tumors behave as indolent, non-metastasizing, occasionally locally recurrent or multifocal lesions.

Squamous cell carcinoma with glandular features

Squamous cell carcinomas of the mucous membranes and skin that display either a real or pseudoglandular architecture have been called adenoid squamous, adenosquamous, acantholytic squamous, pseudoglandular squamous carcinomas and even adenoacanthoma. A consistent misdiagnosis has been mucoepidermoid carcinoma.

The debate over histogenesis has centered on whether the eccrine ducts in the skin and excretory salivary ducts in the mucosa or the basilar cells of the epidermis/mucosa are progenitors. The presence or absence of intracellular mucin, the diagnostic power of which is lamentably weak, is often used as a pivotal feature.

Of far more importance is the prognostic significance of these variants, and since most of these carcinomas occur in the skin and mucous membranes of the head and neck, this is especially pertinent to the head and neck surgeon.[30,31]

Adenosquamous carcinoma

Adenosquamous carcinoma is defined by the World Health Organization as 'a malignant tumor with histological features of both adenocarcinoma and squamous cell carcinoma. The glandular and squamous components occur in close proximity, but are generally distinct'.[25] This unusual neoplasm has been reported in many body sites, including gastrointestinal and upper and lower respiratory and genitourinary tracts as well as skin. In the head and neck, most examples occur in the oral cavity, larynx and paranasal sinuses.

In the oral cavity, 85% of cases arise in the tongue, floor of mouth, and tonsillar–palatine region.[32,33] Patients have an age range from 40 to 75 years (average 57 years). The carcinoma is undeniably an aggressive neoplasm with a high mortality rate after regional or distant metastases. The determinate 5-year survival rate is only 25%.[33,34]

The carcinoma is histologically characterized by an association of an adenocarcinoma and squamous cell carcinoma growing in separate or mixed patterns. In most cases, transition zones are found and intracellular mucin can be detected in the glandular component. There are three basic cell types: basaloid, squamous, and undifferentiated. The glandular carcinoma presents with tubular, alveolar, or ductal structures which are lined by cuboidal, mucous-containing, or poorly differentiated cells (Figs 4.28–4.30).

Mucoepidermoid carcinoma is said to be a difficult differential diagnosis. This should not be if careful

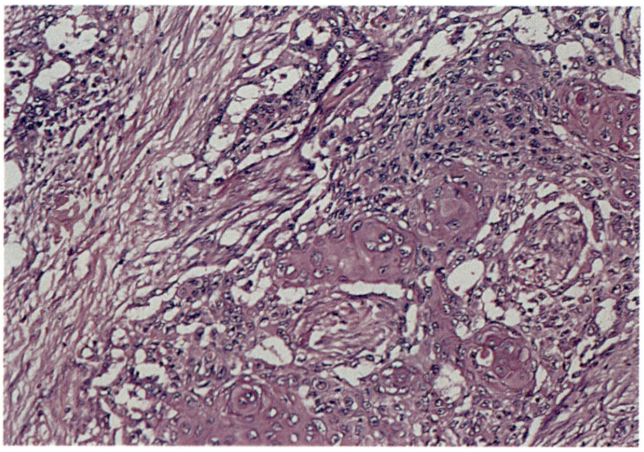

Figure 4.28 Adenosquamous cell carcinoma of oral mucosa with admixture of squamous and glandular elements.

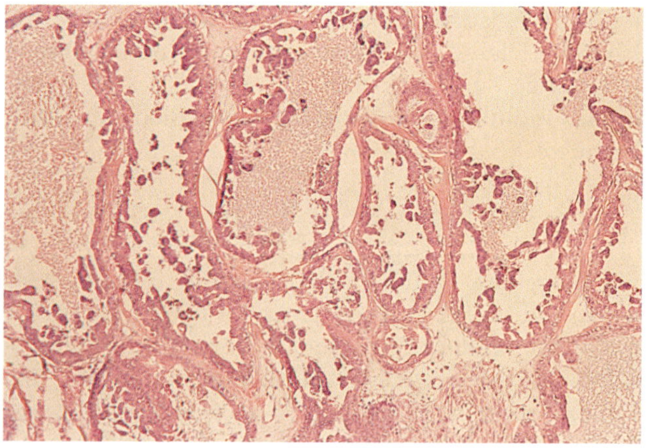

Figure 4.29 Adenosquamous cell carcinoma of the alveolar ridge with marked glandular formations.

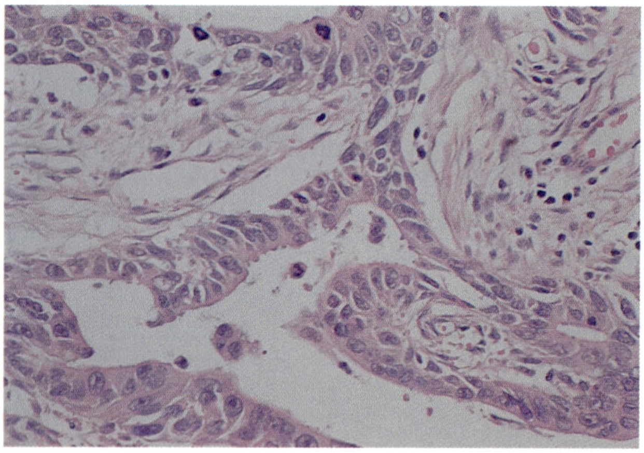

Figure 4.30 Adenosquamous cell carcinoma. This field features the ductal cells of the carcinoma.

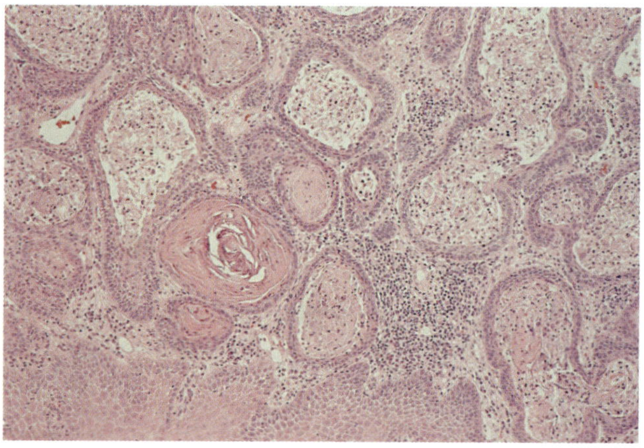

Figure 4.31 Adenoid squamous cell carcinoma with the pseudoglandular spaces created by acantholysis.

attention to cytoarchitecture is followed. The growth pattern of the two neoplasms is quite different. Mucoepidermoid carcinoma rarely has readily recognizable squamous features, except in some high-grade forms. It almost never has demonstrable keratinizing elements. In that respect, the 'epidermoid' in mucoepidermoid carcinoma is adjectival and refers to squamous-like. Unlike mucoepidermoid carcinoma, adenosquamous carcinoma tends to spread throughout the duct system in a vertical and horizontal fashion and often has a prominent mucosal component.[30]

Adenoid squamous carcinoma

Adenoid squamous cell carcinoma is preponderantly a neoplasm of the skin, and especially of the sun-exposed areas of the head and neck.[31] Irrefutable examples also occur in mucosal sites. These include the vermilion borders of the lips, the tongue, other oral mucosa, nasopharynx, sinonasal tract and larynx.[35–37]

Adenoid, pseudoglandular features usually dominate the histologic appearance (Figs. 4.31–4.33). These are usually found deep or deceptively free of the overlying mucosa/epidermis beneath their surfaces. The squamous cell carcinoma is nearly always well differentiated. In some instances, the squamous elements may appear to be only hyperplastic. In the majority of these carcinomas the adenoid feature is initiated in the basal layer of the squamous epithelium. Here it is manifested by a suprabasal clefting and acantholysis followed by a downward rather than upward progression (Figs 4.34–4.35). The end result is a seemingly biphasic carcinoma. A third cytomorphologic component may also be seen.

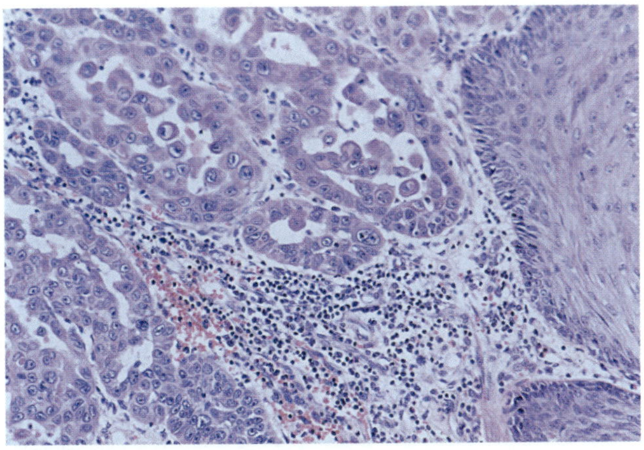

Figure 4.32 Acantholytic adenoid squamous cell carcinoma of the buccal mucosa.

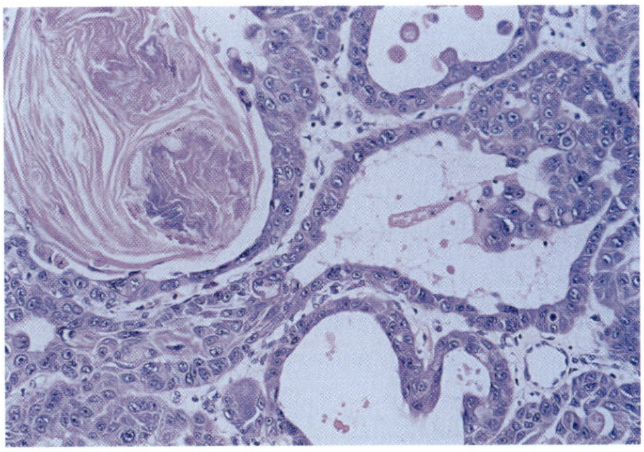

Figure 4.33 Adenoid squamous cell carcinoma of ventral tongue.

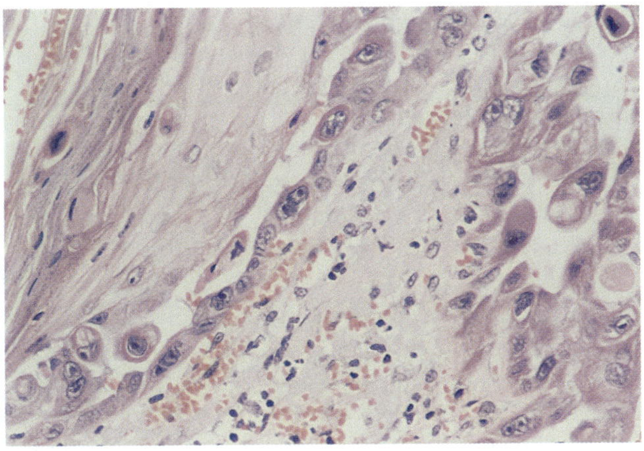

Figure 4.34 Micrograph illustrating the acantholysis forming the adenoid areas of an adenoid squamous cell carcinoma.

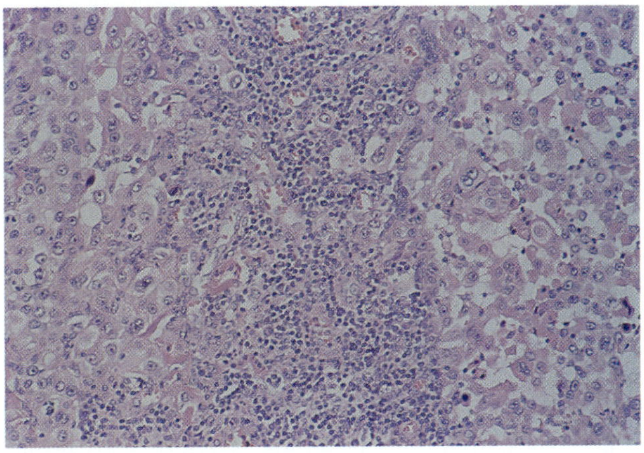

Figure 4.35 Metastatic adenoid squamous cell carcinoma of cervical lymph node.

This one is much less differentiated and can be sarcomatoid, spindled, or clear cell in appearance. A desmoplastic reaction may be an accessory finding.

In instances where the adenoid acantholysis is marked and accompanied by a sarcomatoid element, the squamous derivation can be so obscured that angiosarcoma is a consideration (see later).

It has been our experience that a mucosal head and neck squamous cell carcinoma that demonstrates prominent adenoid features is a carcinoma that has a worse prognosis than conventional squamous cell carcinomas. Less clear is the prognostic impact of adenoid features in the cutaneous counterpart. The differences may be unrelated to the histologic appearances, with depth of invasion and the clinical stage being the determinant factors.

Nasopharyngeal type carcinoma

Undifferentiated carcinoma of the nasopharyngeal type, undifferentiated carcinoma with lymphoid stroma, lymphoepithelioma, lymphoepithelial-like carcinoma, and lymphoepithelial carcinoma are all names applied to a distinctive non-keratinizing carcinoma that is histologically like the undifferentiated forms of carcinoma of the nasopharynx (Fig. 4.36). While morphologically similar, the non-nasopharyngeal lymphoepithelial carcinoma of the upper aerodigestive tracts is less likely to harbor EBV.[38–40]

Besides major salivary gland origin, sites of origin in the head and neck for this carcinoma include tonsil, tongue, soft palate and uvula, floor of mouth, sinonasal tract, larynx, trachea, hypopharynx. Locations outside the head and neck from which the

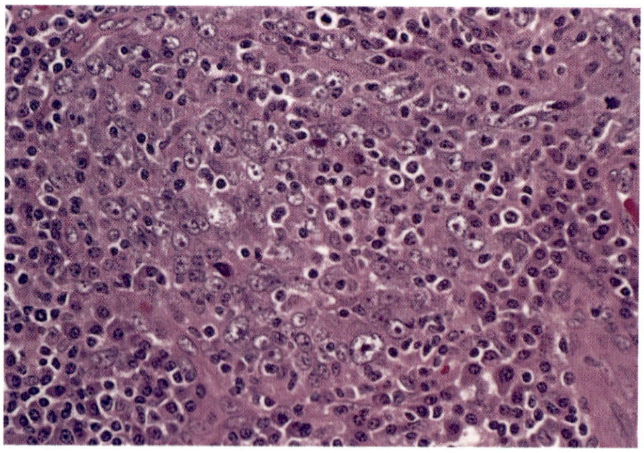

Figure 4.36 Lymphoepithelial carcinoma (nasopharyngeal type) of posterior tongue.

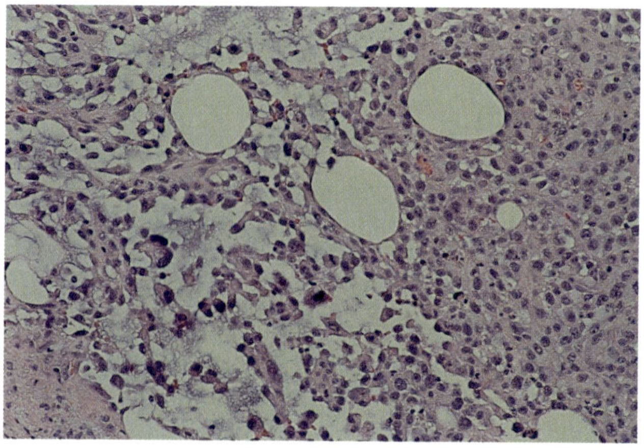

Figure 4.37 Pseudoangiosarcomatous focus in a squamous cell carcinoma.

carcinoma has been reported are the lungs, thymus, stomach, skin, breast, uterine cervix, vagina, and urinary bladder.

Lymphoepithelial carcinoma may present in two equally common histologic forms: a solely undifferentiated carcinoma and a form in which a conventional squamous cell carcinoma is in company with the undifferentiated component. A similar distribution is also seen in the metastases.

The gross appearance of the carcinoma varies from deeply ulcerated to primarily submucosal masses. Microscopically the carcinoma is composed, either partially or totally, of cells with large, round vesicular, sometimes clear nuclei. Each nucleus usually has a single, large, basophilic to deep red nucleolus. Cell cytoplasm is poorly defined, often, therefore, imparting a syncytial growth pattern to the neoplasm. The stroma is composed of small, mature lymphoid cells and occasionally plasma cells that surround and extend into the syncytial aggregates.

Because extant studies have all been retrospective and deal with different sites of involvement and with the rarity of the carcinoma, it is not possible to compare, stage for stage, the prognosis of these lymphoepithelial carcinomas with conventional squamous cell carcinoma. It does appear, however, that the carcinoma is more aggressive with a greater tendency for cervical lymph node involvement and, perhaps, also for distant metastases. In a review of 13 cases, arising in the tonsils and base of the tongue, Bansberg et al.[40] found the carcinomas presenting in an advanced stage, with an 84% distant and regional metastatic rate. Similarity to their nasopharyngeal counterparts was evident in the carcinomas' radiosensitivity and frequent clinical presentation as cervical metastases.

Exaggerated histologic variations

On occasion some of the variants listed in Table 4.1 manifest such exaggerated or unusual features that they simulate other benign or malignant lesions. Pseudoangiosarcomatous[41] and desmoplastic squamous cell carcinomas[42] and extramammary Paget's disease[43] are examples.

Angiosarcoma-like areas in sarcomatoid or anaplastic carcinomas have been well documented, mainly in carcinomas of the breast and thyroid gland, but also in squamous cell carcinomas of the skin and lung. The potential for this deceptive histologic alteration exists in the entire mucosa of the upper aerodigestive tract. We have seen two such lesions, both in recurrent and post-irradiated squamous cell carcinomas of the hypopharynx. Pathogenetically, these pseudoangiosarcomatous carcinomas appear to be markedly exaggerated variants of acantholytic (adenoid) squamous cell carcinoma, with an accumulation of hyaluronic acid in the stroma bringing about a complex of anastomosing channels or spaces lined by neoplastic cells (Fig. 4.37). The cells exhibit a cytokeratin positivity, but are negative with endothelial cell markers.

Desmoplastic squamous cell carcinoma is herein included because there is a small group of oral, particularly lingual, carcinomas that provoke such a pronounced desmoplastic reaction that they may simulate benign pseudosarcomatous lesions such as proliferative myositis or nodular fasciitis. Another distinguishing feature is an apparently unique de novo submucosal evolution.

The carcinoma, as described, is a rapidly growing, diffusely infiltrating lesion of the tongue's musculature. The origin of this peculiar and aggressive carcinoma is unclear. It has been tentatively postulated to be from ducts of minor salivary glands or basal layers of the mucosal epithelium.

Extramammary Paget's disease of oral mucosa, displaying a combination of invasive, intraductal, and intramucosal carcinoma, is a very rare lesion. It does, however, enter into the differential diagnosis of erythroplakic mucosal lesions.

Papillary squamous carcinoma

There is an absence of diagnostic definition for papillary squamous carcinomas of the mucosa of the head and neck. For example, Ishiyama et al.[44] regard the carcinoma as temporally related to proliferative verrucous leukoplakia and posit the neoplasm presents in two morphologic patterns: (1) verrucoid with acroform to polypoid configurations and abundant keratin, cryptic invaginations and large bulbous rete ridges; (2) a more papillary, exophytic carcinoma with epithelial fronds surrounding fibrovascular cores. Neither the photomicrographic depictions nor the clinical course of the first type are those that we consider to be papillary squamous carcinomas. Ishiyama et al.[44] also found a high rate of synchronous or metachronous carcinomas. Stage T3 and T4 carcinomas were associated with a high rate of neck metastases. These are all the findings associated with conventional, albeit exophytic, invasive squamous cell carcinomas arising in a 'soil' of proliferative verrucous leukoplakia.

We are much more restrictive in the definition of papillary squamous carcinoma.[45] The characteristics of a papillary carcinoma are:

- An exophytic squamous proliferation with the overall architecture of a papilloma but with malignant epithelial changes (Fig. 4.38);
- A predilection for the posterior oral cavity, but even more so for the oropharynx, hypopharynx and larynx, and origin not in a leukoplakic background, but rather from a hyperplastic, papillary mucosa, often with increasing dysplasia;
- Often solitary with a prominent fibrovascular core and bearing a strong resemblance to HPV-associated papillomas;
- Most often non-keratinizing or only minimally so;
- Stromal invasion may be absent, difficult to define, or microinvasive in several foci.

Little is known about the biologic course of papillary squamous carcinoma of the oral cavity. If the course is like that of the papillary squamous cell carcinomas of the upper airway the carcinoma should be readily managed, especially if solitary. Because of the putative association with HPV, recurrence or persistence is always a concern.

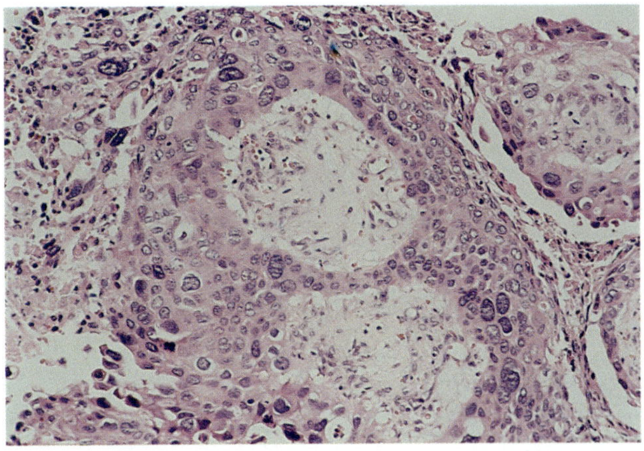

Figure 4.38 Papillary squamous cell carcinoma. There is some retention of papilloma features.

Histopathologic prognostic factors

Over the years, surgical pathologists and clinicians have sought reliable and reproducible histopathologic factors with possible prognostic implication. Some of these have been found wanting while others continue and undergo periodic refinement. Table 4.7 lists the most important current factors.

Histologic grading

There are numerous reports in the literature on the histologic grading of oral squamous cell carcinoma and its value in predicting outcomes and metastasis

Table 4.7 Histopathologic factors with potential prognostic significance

Margins of surgical excision
Angiogenesis density score
Perineural invasion
Histopathologic classification of the carcinoma
Histopathologic grading and scoring systems
Tumor thickness
Tumor depth
Lymphatic/vascular invasion

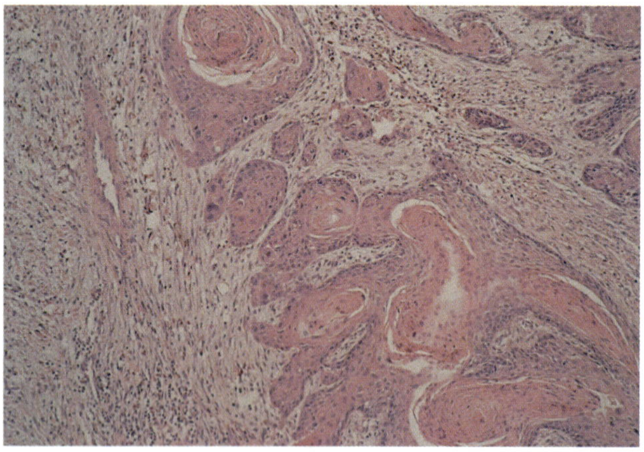

Figure 4.39 Well-differentiated, keratinizing squamous cell carcinoma.

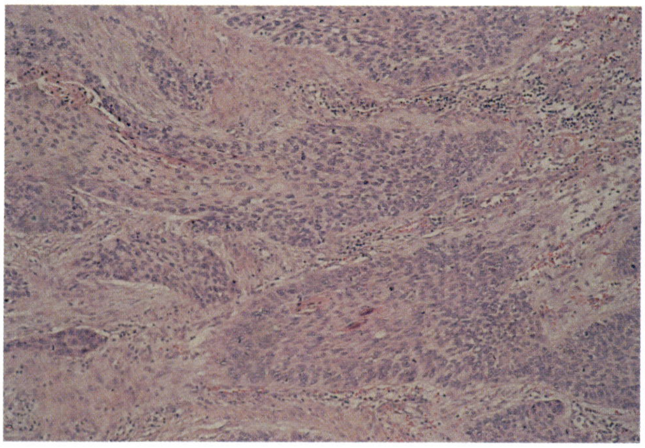

Figure 4.40 Moderately differentiated squamous cell carcinoma.

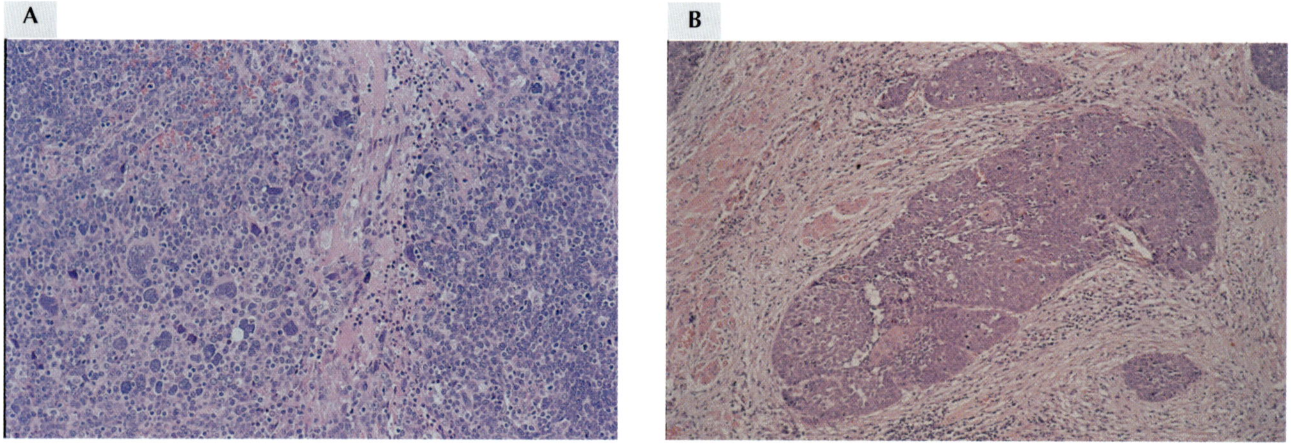

Figure 4.41 A, B Poorly differentiated squamous cell carcinoma.

Table 4.8 Histologic malignancy grading system and point-scoring criteria. (Modified from Woolgar and Scott[48])

	Point score			
Histologic feature	**1**	**2**	**3**	**4**
Degree of keratinization	High, pearl formation	Moderate	Poor, single cells	None
Nuclear polymorphism	Minimal	Moderate	Numerous	Extreme
Mitotic activity (No./10 HPF)	0–15	16–35	36–55	>55
Invasion pattern	Pushing	Bands	Cord or islands	Single cells, cords/islands, < 15 cells
Stage of invasion	Borderline	Into lamina propria	Into submucosa	Into muscle
Stromal lymphoplasmacytic infiltrate	Continuous rim	Moderate, large patches	Minimal, small patches	Absent

Table 4.9 Histologic grading in neoplasms with and without metastasis. (Modified from data presented by Woolgar and Scott[48])

Histologic factor	Chi-squared test statistic (*p* value)
Degree of keratinization	14.17 (0.003)
Polymorphism of nuclei	3.07 (0.38)
Mitotic frequency	11.20 (0.01)
Invasive pattern	25.00 (0.00002)
Invasion stage	8.35 (0.004)
Stromal infiltrate	7.06 (0.7)

to lymph nodes (Figs 4.39–4.41). The relative significance, however, remains uncertain.[46] Grading schemes have evolved over the years with a general acceptance of the one proposed by Anneroth et al.[47] and further modified by Woolgar and Scott (Table 4.8).[48] And it is Woolgar and Scott[48] who give us the most pertinent contemporary perspective on histologic grading.

Of the several histologic features (Table 4.9), the two with independent value in predicting metastasis are the pattern of invasion and degree of keratinization (Figs 4.42–4.44). Both are easily observed, readily reproduced by different observers and for pattern of invasion, show a correlation with in vitro markers of malignancy such as loss of contact inhibition, tumor cell mobility, and secretion of proteolytic enzyme. There is, in addition, a positive correlation between pattern of invasion and the presence of both vascular and perineural invasion.

Woolgar and Scott[48] wisely reject uncertain and difficult to reproduce features such as nuclear polymorphism and lymphoplasmacytic host reaction.

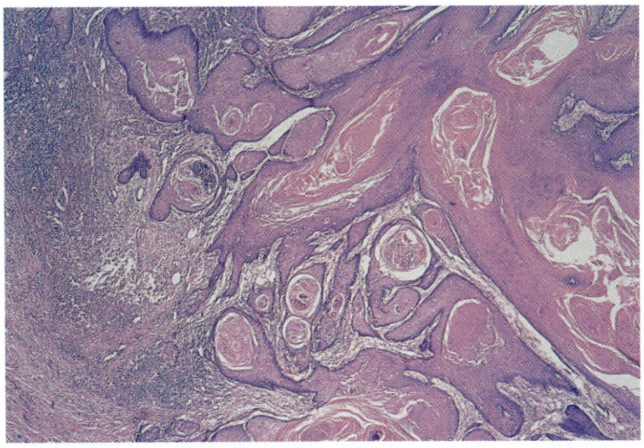

Figure 4.42 Well-differentiated squamous cell carcinoma with easily identifiable keratinization.

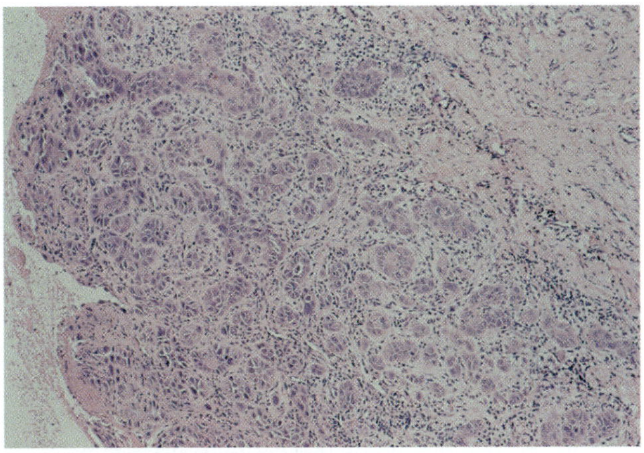

Figure 4.43 Fragmented mode of invasion by a moderately differentiated squamous cell carcinoma.

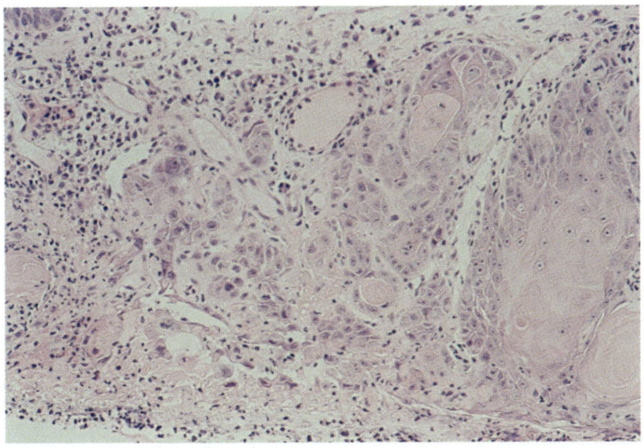

Figure 4.44 Microinvasive squamous cell carcinoma.

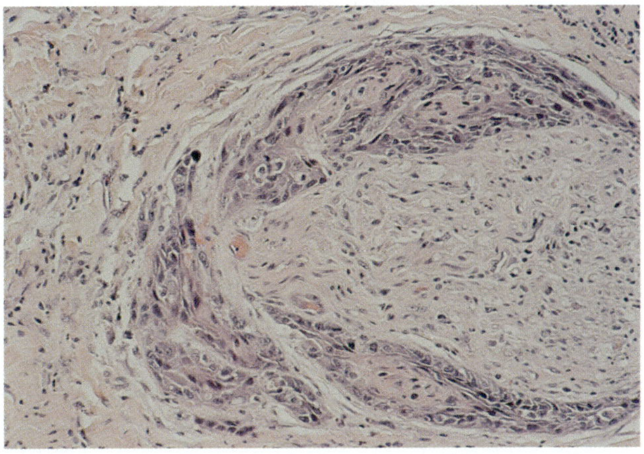

Figure 4.45 Perineural invasion by squamous cell carcinoma.

Table 4.10 Incidence of perineural spread in squamous carcinoma of the head and neck. (Modified from Carter et al.[49])

Primary site of carcinoma	Total no.	Carcinomas with perineural spread	
		At primary	In cervical nodal metastasis
Mobile tongue, floor of mouth	23	6	1
Base of tongue, tonsil, soft palate	8	2	1
Retromolar trigone/alveolus	9	3	6
Pyriform fossa, upper third of esophagus	6	0	6
Larynx	16	2	1
Sinonasal tract	3	1	0
Nasopharynx	1	0	0
Unknown primary	1	0	0
Lips, cheek	3	0	0

It is likely that histologically based grading schemes have run their course, not only because they are being replaced by more objective and reproducible factors, but also because, by and large, they lack independent prognostic significance.

Perineural invasion

Perineural invasion (Fig. 4.45) by squamous cell carcinoma is considered an ominous prognostic sign and has been shown to correlate with an increased incidence of local recurrence, regional lymph node metastasis and a decreased survival.[49–51] Once the carcinoma enters a perineural space, it is possible for it to spread proximally or distally. Extension along the nerve can be for long distances, but Carter et al.,[49,50] in necropsy studies, have indicated that the tumor tends to remain localized to the terminal 1 or 2 cm of the nerve. In a clinicopathologic study of perineural spread in squamous cell carcinoma of the head and neck, Carter and his associates[50,51] demonstrated spread in 24% of an unselected series of 70 patients treated by surgery. Slightly more than half of this group of patients had oral cavity primary carcinomas, particularly from the tongue and floor of the mouth (Table 4.10). The trigeminal nerve, in particular its mandibular division, was most commonly affected. The perineural invasion was more likely with large carcinomas, moderately or poorly differentiated and also showing lymphatic/vascular invasion.

Similar data have been obtained in a study of neurotropic cutaneous tumors.[52] Of 7852 patients who had undergone micrographically controlled excisions of basal cell and squamous cell carcinomas, 37 (0.47%) manifested perineural extension of their carcinomas. Skip areas were uncommon (two of 34) and, if present, a margin of at least 5 mm of uninvolved nerves would likely suffice. In the series, the range of perineural extensions from gross tumors was 3 mm to 9 cm.

As it is with the host of histopathologic factors relating to prognosis, the status of perineural invasion as an independent prognosticator is unclear. Involvement of named nerves and their branches is definitely an adverse factor in any statistical setting. Far less is known about small and no-name nerves.

Lesions mimicking invasion of nerves

Remnants of vestigial or rudimentary epithelial structures that persist are common in the oral region (mucosal and osseous) and include those of both odontogenic and non-odontogenic origins.[53–55] These benign structures can be juxtaneural, perineural and intraneural (Fig. 4.46) and are often incidental

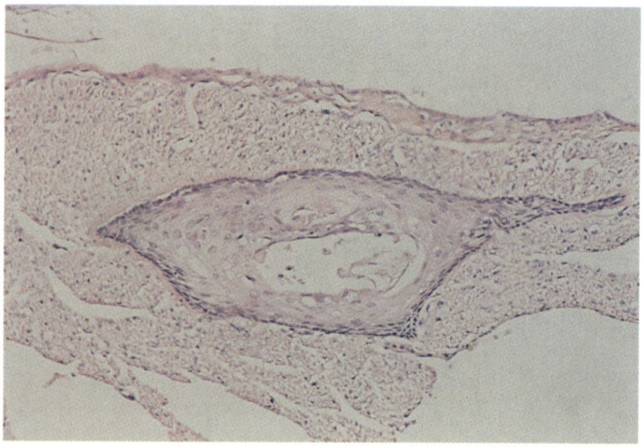

Figure 4.46 Benign epithelial inclusion within nerve.

findings in the microscopic study of other lesions.[53] The juxtaoral organ of Chievitz[56] and the neuroepithelial hamartoma of the oral cavity[57] are two examples.

The anatomic location of the organ of Chievitz is quite consistent. It occurs deep to the medial pterygoid muscle, at the level of the pterygomandibular raphe, and is associated with the long buccal nerve. It is not normally palpable and measures from 0.5 to 2 mm, except when hyperplastic. Histologically it is characterized by squamous epithelial islands and duct-like structures set in a fibrous connective tissue stroma that contains numerous myelinated and non-myelinated nerves in close association with the epithelial elements. The function of the organ remains unknown, although it is thought to have both a neuroreceptor and a secretory function.

The neuroepithelial hamartoma is a gingival lesion composed of round to oval and irregular squamous islands within a collagenized stroma. Small bundles of non-myelinated nerves either collide with the epithelial islands or surround them. The peripheral squamous odontogenic tumor and neurofollicular hamartoma are the principal benign differential diagnosis.

Microvascular invasion

The finding of squamous cell carcinoma within capillaries and/or venules in the immediate vicinity of primary carcinomas of the head and neck has been linked to regional lymph node metastasis.[58–60] Close and associates[58] have rather convincingly demonstrated this relationship. Dealing with 43 primary (T2 or greater) carcinomas, most of which were oral, they found vascular invasion in 35 (81%). Of these, 27 (77%) were found to have nodal metastases. Vascular invasion was absent in eight (19%) of the 43 primary tumor specimens; only two of the eight had histologically confirmed cervical metastases. A 'dose dependency' appears to be at play. Vascular involvement confined to a single vessel has a decreased potential for metastasis.

Neoplastic extension into large vessels is an extremely poor prognostic indicator. In a review of 4300 radical neck dissections, Djalilian et al.[61] found invasion of the jugular vein in 48 cases (1.1%). Forty-four of the patients died (72%) within the first 2 years of the neck dissection. Of these, 13 had metastases to the lungs.

Angiogenesis

Angiogenesis is a fundamental, yet complex physiologic activity. It is central to normal embryonic development, the healing of wounds, and corpus luteum formation. It is now applied to all physiological and pathological forms of neovascularization except vasculogenesis.[62,63] Vasculogenesis is the de novo generation of blood vessels.

The induction of angiogenesis is also required for most tumors to grow beyond 1 to 2 mm in diameter, the limit of simple diffusion of oxygen and nutrients. This correlation between tumor growth and vessel concentration (tumor angiogenesis) has been shown to have a significant relationship with recurrence and prognosis in several types of solid neoplasms.[62] Furthermore, in transgenic mice models, expression of an angiogenic phenotype coincides with, or immediately precedes, frank neoplasia. Angiogenesis also permits metastases. In animal models, onset of angiogenesis is seen to coincide with neoplastic cells in efferent tumor circulation and with metastasis. Conversely, impaired angiogenesis is accompanied by a reduced metastatic rate.

Angiogenesis is controlled by various angiogenic factors which regulate the coordinated extracellular matrix remodeling endothelial cell proliferation, capillary differentiation, and anastomosis necessary to establish a blood supply.[64] The factors can be secreted by neoplastic cells, inflammatory cells and stromal cells. In tumor angiogenesis, these factors and their receptors are important angiogenic molecules. Among the most important of these is vascular endothelial growth factor (VEGF).[65] This dimeric multi-functional glycoprotein mediates its many effects on endothelial cells via two high-affinity tyrosine kinase receptors and is a specific mitogen for endothelium, increases vascular permeability, and induces proteolytic enzymes necessary for vascular remodeling.

While there are other important angiogenic molecules, little is known currently about their place in human tumor angiogenesis. Furthermore, identification of several naturally occurring negative regulators of angiogenesis has led to the appreciation that angiogenesis is balanced between negative and positive stimuli.

Various authors have demonstrated relationships between measures of tumor angiogenesis and prognosis.[66–68] The assessment of tumor angiogenesis by histologic means is by observing and quantifying neovascularization using immunostaining of endothelium. Endothelial cells express a number of markers including factor VIII related antigen, ABH blood group antigens, CD31, CD34, and CD36 and a lectin, Ulex europaeus agglutinin I (UEA-I). The specificity and sensitivity, however, is variable amongst the group of antibodies used to detect the antigens. Quantification is by manual or automated techniques. Choosing the most vascular regions of the tumor or 'hot spots' is another variable for microvessel quantification.

Three studies of head and neck squamous cell carcinomas are illustrative of the potential of angiogenesis as a prognostic indicator. Gasparini et al.[67] showed microvessel density to be increased in 50 patients with locoregional metastases compared with 20 patients without nodal disease. Williams et al.[68] addressed the question of whether this was true in carcinomas of the oral cavity before clinical metastases were evident. In their cohort of patients, 90% of patients with >10% immunostaining developed metastasis to cervical lymph nodes within 2 years. Patients with < 10% staining had no recurrences during the same time period. Analysis using both tumor depth and vessel concentration proved predictive of recurrence. Of the patients with 4 mm or less of tumor depth and less than 10% of staining for angiogenesis, 98% were correctly predicted as having no recurrence. Of those patients with greater than 10% staining and greater than 4 mm tumor depth, 100% developed regional recurrence.

Williams et al.[68] considered only angiogenesis to be an independent predictor of nodal metastases. By combining angiogenesis and tumor thickness an even stronger predictability could be obtained. Penfold and associates[69] came to the same conclusion in their count of microvessels in 41 primary oral squamous cell carcinomas. Tumor microvessel counts correlated with lymph node metastases ($p < 0.001$). This association was independent of tumor size, volume and type of histologic differentiation. When all variables underwent multivariate analysis only vascular count showed a significant association with lymph node metastasis.

On the other side of the ledger, however, is the study on head and neck squamous cell carcinomas by Carrau et al.[65] These investigators found no statistically significant difference between microvessel counts of tumors that metastasized or recurred locally as compared with tumors that did not. The authors, however, were quite circumspect, pointing out that before a 'test' can be accepted as an independent factor, it is necessary that the test be proven to be reproducible, reliable, and simple to perform. This is axiomatic and will require: (1) avoidance of beta errors due to a small number of cases, (2) avoidance of intrinsic flaws in study design, e.g. multiple sites of origin; only one 'hot spot' count, (3) control of sampling errors, (4) evolution of tumor heterogeneity and staining techniques, and (5) a determination as to whether microvessel counts are different for different sites in the upper aerodigestive tract.

Gleich et al.[70] have also determined that tumor angiogenesis, as currently measured, is not of value in predicting tumor aggressiveness in patients with oral cavity T2–T4 carcinomas. After evaluating only the T1 tumors and finding a lack of significant correlation, the authors have proposed that early oral carcinomas may be independent of angiogenesis and that even large oral tumors may have minimal neovascularization, but still have significant metastatic potential.

The current limitations of pathological quantitative angiogenesis together with the facility to monitor several in vivo angiogenic inhibitors have led investigators to examine other measures of tumor angiogenic activity.[65,69] Serum, urine and cerebrospinal fluid levels of factors such as VEGF and tyrosine kinase receptors have been found to be higher in patients with neoplasms than in controls; increasing levels are also associated with advanced tumor grade and stage. Other possible measures of tumor angiogenesis include use of antibodies to specific tumor-associated endothelial epitopes rather than pan-endothelial markers. Alternatively, assessment of other molecules involved in endothelial remodeling such as cell adhesion molecules and proteolytic enzymes may be utilized. Color Doppler, magnetic resonance imaging and positron emission spectroscopy are also being tested as possible non-invasive measures of tumor angiogenesis.

Fox[64] has summarized the current status of the value of the various methods to evaluate tumor angiogenesis. He indicates that the complexity of tumor angiogenesis and the likelihood that different factors at different stages are at play make it unlikely that an accurate assessment of angiogenic activity will be obtained by measuring only one aspect of angiogenesis. None of the current techniques has been validated enough to use in clinical settings. Nevertheless, continued investigations to find an angiogenic index are clearly warranted.

There are important lessons in the study of angiogenesis, particularly as it relates to the metastatic cascade. One lesson is that correlations between molecular factors and what they regulate are not universal. Certain factors may only be transiently expressed or seem to have relevance to a particular type of neoplasm. Equally important is another lesson and that is it is *overall balance* between positive and inhibitor factors which is ultimately the determining event. A prime example of this balance is that between angiogenic and anti-angiogenic factors participating in the angiogenic cascade. The factors can be secreted by tumor cells, tumor-associated macrophages, and even from components of the extracellular matrix. It is the *balance* that is critical in dictating the angiogenic phenotype tumors.

Table 4.11 Cutaneous involvement by upper aerodigestive tract squamous cell carcinomas. (Modified from Cole and McGuirt[71])

Location of primary	No. of patients	Median survival (months)
Oral cavity	19	6
Oropharynx	2	12
Hypopharynx	3	3
Larynx	1	2
Maxillary sinus	1	6

Skin involvement

As might be expected, skin involvement from mucosal squamous cell carcinomas of the head and neck is an extremely poor prognostic factor. Cole and McGuirt,[71] in the largest study to date, found that while direct involvement of skin is a portent of a poor prognostic outcome, it is somewhat less ominous than intradermal lymphatic spread. Patients with a direct involvement had a 7-month median survival; those with lymphatic spread had a 3-month median survival. Table 4.11 indicates only a 6-month median survival for patients with oral cavity primaries.

Surgical margins in squamous cell carcinomas

One of the putative indicators of completeness of the surgical removal is the margin of uninvolved tissue around the excised neoplasm. How generous the margin should be has not, and likely cannot, be defined for all forms of cancer, or for that matter, selected classes of malignancy. Tumor sites, anatomic restrictions, presumed biologic characteristics of the cancer, and the respective advantages of conservation and extended surgery are just some of the factors in the predetermination of adequate margins of resection.[72] There is little doubt, however, that gross residual cancer will yield local persistence and nearly always an increased mortality.

For squamous cell carcinomas of the upper aerodigestive tract, there is a site dependency, not only in the ability of the surgeon to obtain tumor-free margins, but also in the biologic significance of involved or uninvolved limits of excision.[72,73] This variation relates more to the biologic and epidemiologic environment, microanatomic and macroanatomic, of the sites than to any intrinsic histologic differences in the squamous cell carcinomas themselves. These factors also strongly imply that one cannot extrapolate margin significances from carcinomas of the glottis to carcinomas of the oral cavity and pharynx.

It has been claimed that microscopic accuracy of an adequate surgical margin is at least 50%, at least as judged by local recurrences.[72] In part, this rather low assessment is due to pathologic and clinical (surgical) difficulties coincident with the evaluation of preoperatively irradiated tissues and submucosal extension or skip areas. In part, also, must be the contributing factor of lack of close cooperation between surgeon and pathologist.

The definition of positive and negative surgical margins lacks standardization and certainly precision. Irrefutable microscopic evidence is the presence or absence of invasive carcinomas at the line of resection. Intra-epithelial carcinoma at the margins has also been considered as positive. The effects of closeness to a margin and of severe dysplasia at the margin on recurrences and prognosis have not been systematically evaluated. Indeed, neither of these factors is easy to assess. Severe dysplasia remains a highly subjective pathologic impression and as such is capable of being overdiagnosed or underdiagnosed. Measurement is more objective, but its reliability varies with the conditions of measurement. Postremoval and postfixation shrinkage renders these measurements inferior to an in situ, frozen section monitored estimation of distance from the carcinoma. Using excised uterine cervical tissue, Boonstra et al.[74] have indicated that a formalin-fixed, embedded, and sectioned specimen has a total shrinkage of about 15% of the fresh tissue. Formalin fixation produces an overall mean shrinkage of 2.7%, and the dehydration, clearing, and paraffin embedding account for about 12.5%. The actual sectioning of the tissue block and mounting do not increase shrinkage.

A comparable study was carried out by Beaumont et al.[75] on anterior oral squamous cell carcinomas. Significant changes were noted in the longitudinal diameter of the whole specimen between the in situ and the fresh state ($p < 0.004$), and again between the fresh and the fixed state ($p < 0.0002$). The most significant alteration was in the measured diameter of the tumor, with a mean shrinkage of 4.82 mm from the fresh to the fixed state. Of surgical significance were the changes in the surgical margin. The minimal measured surgical margin in situ was 10 mm and, following fixation, this became an average of 5.8 mm. When examined microscopically, the average clearance of tumor was 5.4 mm. There was, therefore, a reduction of 46% from the planned surgical margin before resection to the assessed measurement of microscopic clearance in the surgical pathology laboratory. Table 4.12, prepared from

Table 4.12 Mucosal margin shrinkage. (Modified from Johnson et al.[76])

Time of measurement of margins	Mean length ± SD/% shrinkage	
	Tongue margins	Labiobuccal margins
In situ	12 mm	12 mm
After resection	9.0 ± 0.9 mm/24.8%	7.4 ± 0.8 mm/38.3%
After fixation (formalin)	8.1 ± 1.0 mm/32.5%	6.1 ± 0.9 mm/48.3%
Final prepared histologic slide	8.3 ± 0.8 mm/30.7%	6.3 ± 0.7 mm/47.3%

[a]Data from an experimental canine study. Slide preparation resulted in a slight, statistically non-significant increase in margin size, compared to the formalin-fixed margin.

data in the canine study of oral mucosal margin shrinkages of Johnson et al.,[76] shows strikingly similar conclusions.

Given optimum conditions (surgical and pathologic), what are the prognostic implications of the microscopic determination of the adequacy of local removal of squamous cell carcinomas of the oral cavity and pharynx? It has long been our opinion that histologic grade is subservient to size or T stage of a squamous cell carcinoma as a prognostic indicator. Depending on the skill of the surgeon and the anatomic location of the carcinoma, the T stage may not seriously impair the possibility of securing microscopically free surgical margins. The significance of size, however, bears heavily on local recurrences, and more so on 2- and 5-year survival, even when there are surgically free margins (Table 4.13).[77,78] Furthermore, it is to be accepted that a rather constant number of carcinomas (5–10%) will resist the surgical goal of clear margins, regardless of their apparent T stage.[72]

Based on available information, it appears that lesional tissue within 0.5 cm of a surgical margin, be it severe dysplasia or in situ or invasive carcinoma, places a patient at nearly an equal risk for local recurrence. Failure of local control is not inevitable with such positive margins, but is associated with a nearly 80% incidence of recurrent disease. In the study by Looser et al.,[77] 71% of patients with positive margins manifested recurrence at the primary site, compared with only 32% of patients with negative margins. Byers et al. report similar findings.[78] Extralaryngeal sites with significant recurrence rates after negative margin surgical excision are those in the oral cavity and pharynx (Table 4.14). Looser et al.[77] rank the palate, tonsil, and pharynx, including the pyriform sinuses, the highest, with primary site recurrences of 41.6%, 41.5%, and 37.2%, respectively.

Table 4.13 Free margin status vs (a) clinical stage, (b) T class and local control and survival. (From data presented by Looser et al.[77] (clinical stage) and Byers et al.[78] (T class))

(a) Clinical stage	Local control (%)	5-year survival (%)
I	85.5	61
II	72.6	46
III	64.8	32
IV	47.3	9.3
(b) T class	**Local control (%)**	**2-year survival (%)**
T1	95	86
T2	88	79
T3	86	59
T4	60	25

Table 4.14 Oral squamous cell carcinoma: local recurrences with negative margins. (Modified from Looser et al.[77])

Oral site	No. of carcinomas	No. of recurrences (%)
Tongue	510	166 (32.5)
Gingiva	134	42 (31.3)
Lip	81	7 (8.6)
Palate	137	57 (41.6)
Buccal mucosa	99	33 (33.3)
Floor of mouth	255	67 (26.3)

Table 4.15 Positive margins in relation to primary oral sites. (Modified from Loree and Strong[79])

Oral site	No. of carcinomas	No. of positive margins	(%)
Buccal	12	7	(58)
Maxillary gingiva	19	8	(42)
Mandibular gingiva	57	22	(39)
Hard palate	17	6	(35)
Floor of mouth	137	43	(31)
Tongue	137	37	(27)
Retromolar trigone	25	6	(24)

Table 4.16 Margin histopathology: local recurrence survival. (From data presented by Loree and Strong[79])

Margin	No. of recurrences (%)	5-year survival (%)
Close (within 0.5 cm)	29/83 (35)	51
Dysplasia	3/9 (33)	94
In-situ carcinoma	4/9 (44)	71
Microinvasive carcinoma	10/28 (36)	43

Table 4.17 Margins and local recurrence and survival: oral squamous carcinoma. (Modified from Loree and Strong[79])

Margin	No. of recurrences (%)	5-year survival (%)
Negative	49/269 (18)	60
Positive	46/129 (36)	52

Loree and Strong[79] analyzed the significance of positive margins on survival in a large group of patients (398) with primary oral cavity carcinomas (Table 4.15). The margin was classified as positive according to four criteria: (1) close (within 0.5 cm) margins, (2) 'premalignant' (dysplasia) in the margin, (3) in situ carcinoma of the margin, and (4) invasive carcinoma at the margin (Table 4.16). The incidence of positive margins was directly proportional to the increasing size of the tumor. The overall local recurrence rate in the entire positive margin group was twice the negative margin group, 36% versus 18%, respectively. Positive margins also adversely affected survival; the 5-year survival rates of the positive and negative margin groups were 52.7% and 60%, respectively, a statistically significant difference (Table 4.17). When the impact of postoperative adjuvant therapy was examined, none of the observed differences in survival rates between patients with surgery alone and those with combined therapy was significant. A major finding in the study was that, whereas postoperative radiation therapy to 6000 cGy successfully reduced the local recurrence rate in patients with positive margins, this benefit did not translate to an improved 5-year survival. The patterns of recurrence may change, but the overall risk of failure is increased. Adjuvant postoperative radiation therapy does not appear to decrease the risk of local recurrence in patients with positive margins to a level similar to patients with negative margins not treated with radiation therapy. Tables 4.16 and 4.17 present pertinent data from the study of Loree and Strong.[79]

Scholl et al.[80] evaluated 268 patients with squamous carcinoma of the tongue treated by glossectomy with or without irradiation; of these, 54 (20%) had positive carcinoma margins on the first frozen section evaluation. When the positive margins were subsequently rendered negative the local recurrence rate was worse than if the initial margin was negative (Table 4.18). The employment of immediate postoperative radiation appeared to improve

Table 4.18 Squamous cell carcinoma of the tongue: frozen section margins and local failure after surgery only. (Modified from Scholl et al.[80])

Frozen section margin status	Ty	T1	T2	T3	T4	Total (%)
Negative on first frozen section	2/10	9/72	4/48	5/23	0/4	20/157 (13)
Ultimately negative with additional frozen sections	0/1	3/9	2/8	0/7	1/2	6/27 (22)

Table 4.19 Influence of postoperative radiation on failure at primary site. (From data presented by Vikram et al.[82])

Surgical treatment only (1960–70)		Surgical plus postoperative radiation[a] (1975–80)	
Negative margins	Positive margins	Negative margins	Positive margins
39%	73%	2%	10.5%

[a]Radiation dose of 5000 rad in 5 weeks to 6000 rad in 6 weeks; follow-up for at least 2 years.

Table 4.20 Margin status: results of head and neck intergroup study. (From data presented by Jacobs et al.[84])

	No. of patients (%)	
Site of carcinoma	Positive margins (*n* = 112)	Negative margins (*n* = 575)
Oral cavity	30 (27)	155 (27)
Oropharynx	41 (37)	154 (27)
Hypopharynx	21 (19)	95 (17)
Supraglottis	16 (14)	95 (17)
Glottis	4 (3)	68 (12)
Other	0	8 (1)
Clinical T Stage		
T21	7 (6)	20 (3)
T2	28 (25)	159 (28)
T3	40 (36)	289 (50)
T4	36 (32)	106 (18)
TY	1 (1)	0
Unknown	0	1 (< 1)

local control in this instance. An additional finding in this study was that positive mucosal margins were more often seen in T1 or T2 tumors, whereas positive soft tissue margins were more common in T3 and T4 lesions. The authors indicate that problems with the frozen section technique and its credibility and reliability further add to the impression that when dealing with carcinoma of the tongue, the guiding principle is, and should be, the surgeon's ability to adequately remove all macroscopic disease, and if margins are also microscopically negative without evidence of perineural invasion, the patient probably does not need any additional adjunctive treatment to improve local control. This is echoed by van Es et al.[81] These investigators state that when excision of a small squamous cell carcinoma (T1 and T2) of the mobile tongue or floor of mouth is histologically complete (all margins negative), other histopathologic variables are irrelevant in predicting recurrence at the primary site. The effect of postoperative radiation on failure at the primary site with positive or negative margins as determined by Vikram et al.[82] is shown in Table 4.19.

Dubner and Heller[83] evaluated patterns of recurrence and local control of oral and oropharyngeal carcinomas clinically manifesting invasion of the mandible. They attempted to correlate incidence of recurrence with characteristics of the primary tumor and extent of mandibulectomy. The local recurrence rate was 19% following marginal mandibulectomy and 6% following segmental mandibulectomy. Local recurrence was independent of the size of the carcinoma or extent of metastasis to lymph nodes. Neither invasion of the mandible nor the addition of radiotherapy influenced local recurrence. Ten of 15 patients recurring locally after marginal mandibulectomy were salvaged by further surgery. Most of the local recurrences following segmental mandibulectomy occurred in soft tissues, and not in bone.

From the foregoing the impact of positive margins on survival is clear. The data are institutional experiences, but are comparable to a national experience reported by the Head and Neck Inter-group who found a 16% incidence of positive surgical margins in patients with stage III and IV (operable).[84] Table 4.20 presents the margin status according to the site in the aerodigestive tract and clinical T stage, as reported in the Inter-group study. As expected, patients with positive margins experienced a significantly higher local failure rate (21% versus 9%, $p = 0.003$) and a similar incidence of regional failure relative to the negative margin population. The incidence of distant failure was also significantly higher in the positive margin group (20% versus 12%, $p = 0.42$). The addition of chemotherapy did not change survival. The survival of the patients was approximately one half that of the corresponding negative margin group. With a median survival of only 19 months, the expectation of the positive margin group is not much better than that of the inoperable population.

If the surgical margins are negative, there is certainly no assurance of successful local control (Table 4.21).[77–79,85,86] In fact, clinical T stage may be a more predictable determinant: the smaller the carcinoma with free surgical margins, the higher the local control rate. In like manner, survival of patients with free margins is related almost linearly to the T stage of their carcinomas.[72]

Table 4.21 Published recurrence and survival rates

Reference	Local recurrence (%)		3-year survival (%)	
	+ Margins	− Margins	+ Margins	− Margins
Byers et al.[78]	80	15.8	5	65.8
Looser et al.[77]	71	31.7	30.6	35.9
Chen et al.[85]	55	20	7	39
Loree and Strong[79]	36	18	52	60
Beaumont and Hains[86]	55	35	63	51

Table 4.22 Adenoid cystic carcinoma: margin status and nerve involvement. (Modified from Garden et al.[89])

Gland of origin	No. of patients	+ Margins	Close/uncertain margins	Perineural invasion	Adequate margins and no perineural invasion
Minor salivary glands	122	54	32	74	18
Submandibular/ sublingual	41	11	11	36	4
Parotid	30	15	10	23	1
Lacrimal	5	3	2	3	0

The prognostic implications of a positive microscopic margin also relate to stage of the disease. Stage for stage, there is an increased incidence of recurrences at the primary site—certainly a not unexpected correlation. Survival at 2 and 5 years and longer, however, is more dependent on stage, especially for patients with stage III and IV malignancies.

A significantly lower incidence of local recurrences is reported in patients with primary squamous cell carcinomas of the larynx who have positive surgical margins following conservation laryngeal surgery. In a study by Bauer et al.,[87] 39 of 111 patients undergoing hemilaryngectomy had positive surgical margins (close, gross, and microscopic involvement). Only seven of the 39 developed a local recurrence. Four of the remaining 72 (5.6%) with uninvolved margins developed local recurrence. Inexplicable as these data may seem, they cannot be ignored, and they give support to the notion that site dependency has a significant effect on the results. Patients who are candidates for conservative laryngeal surgery have early-stage carcinomas and hence more favorable prognoses. The disposition of submucosal lymphatic drainage, or lack thereof, in the laryngeal glottis very likely also plays a role in the lower incidence of locoregional recurrences, irrespective of the status of the margins.

Adenoid cystic carcinomas are notorious for invasion into adjacent tissues without well-defined borders and their true extent is often underestimated. As a consequence, the carcinomas are difficult to clear surgically, often resulting in positive margins. In an analysis of outcomes of patients with adenoid cystic carcinomas of the palate, Kuhel et al.[88] reported that 73% of their patients either had disease involving adjacent sites or had carcinoma that appeared to be limited clinically, but showed microscopic extension far beyond the gross margins of the tumor. In addition, adenoid cystic carcinomas have a high rate of perineural invasion. Table 4.22, modified from Garden et al.[89] presents the margin status and nerve involvement of adenoid cystic carcinomas of all salivary sites.

Despite the seemingly random quality of the status of surgical margins, they still provide therapeutic and prognostic guidelines.[90] The advent of perfected molecular technology may add a needed degree of objectivity to the assessment of margins. Brennan et al.[91] have underscored the fallibility of visually inspected margins. They examined the surgical margins and lymph nodes of patients using molecular probes for p53 mutations and found 'molecular-positive margins' in over 50% of patients who were thought to have had completely resected carcinomas. These patients also manifested higher risks for local failure.

Emblematic of the often seen contrary data when studying molecular genetic events is the report by Ogden et al.,[92] who found no statistically significant difference in the rate of second malignant tumors with p53 positive against p53 negative mucosae.

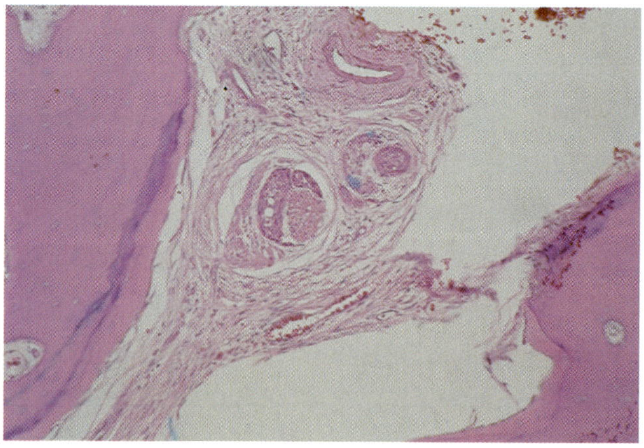

Figure 4.47 Intra-osseous (mandible) perineural invasion by a floor of mouth squamous cell carcinoma.

Oral carcinomas and mandibular margins

Of the various oral carcinoma subsites, the carcinomas related to the mandibular region (alveolar ridge, floor of mouth, lower buccal sulcus, lower retromolar area) are among those with the highest rate of recurrence. Neoplastic invasion of the mandible is one of the factors promoting recurrence. It is therefore critical to determine the presence and extent of bony involvement in the management of patients.[93,94]

Because, too often, the limits of resection of the mandible have been determined by the soft tissue extent of the carcinoma, there is the untoward result of a high percentage of resected mandibles with no evidence of carcinomatous invasion. Clinical examination alone is also misleading. Weisman and Kimmelman[95] have indicated that one-third of histologically proven invasions of the mandible do not show clinical signs of preoperative bone invasion.

The surgeon has several options to evaluate mandibular margins: (1) preoperative radiologic examinations, (2) gross inspection, (3) frozen section and/or imprint evaluation of cancellous bone from the resected mandibular stump, and (4) frozen section of adherent soft tissues. The last is not reliable and provides no information on osseous involvement.

Carcinomatous spread to the mandible is most often in continuity from a primary in the oral cavity. On occasion the invasion is from a contiguous metastasis. Given access to nerves, the carcinomas can utilize them for nerve-related spread (Fig. 4.47). Lymphatic or vascular spread is, however, uncommon.

There are two basic types of involvement of the mandible.[96,97] The first is an erosive form in which the bone recedes before a pushing tumor margin, for example verrucous carcinoma. Here, there is a loss of cortical continuity with a U-shaped or scalloped excavation of medullary bone. Radiologically, there is a well-defined radiolucency with no spicules of bone. The second type is infiltrative, in which there is neoplastic spread into cancellous bone. An ill-defined and irregular lesion is seen on radiographs. A third type, most often seen with adenoid cystic carcinomas, shows a spread through bone marrow without any marked destruction and minimal radiographic changes.

The violated bone surface is rarely, if ever, normal. It shows irregular pitting and various degrees of new bone formation (manifested by spurs and ridges, lined by osteoblasts). The crevices and pits on the bone's surface contain vascular granulation tissue, and it is through these defects that the carcinoma begins its penetration. Perimandibular soft tissues also show various amounts of fibrosis and an active, chronic inflammation, all obscuring periosteal and fascial planes. The obscuration is further compounded by prior radiation.

In the great majority of non-irradiated mandibles, squamous cell carcinomas enter the medullary cavity through the upper borders of the mandible, either through the occlusal ridge alone or in combination with a penetration of either the buccal or lingual plates. This mode amply confirms the importance of cortical bone defects in the edentulous alveolus as a principal route for direct spread into the mandible. Size of the carcinoma does not appear to influence the incidence of bone involvement, but proximity of the tumor to bone does, and carcinomas involving the gingival margins appear to have a particularly high incidence of bone involvement.

Having breached the cortex, the carcinoma can extend vertically and laterally. There may be, at times, a superficial extension beneath a relatively intact cortex and periosteum. Additional spread into the bone is accompanied by a rather consistent and prominent response among bone cells. Carter[98] divides the response into an osteoclast-dependent phase and an osteoclast-independent phase of bone destruction. Each of these responses occurs in advance of the invading carcinoma, and they can coexist. The osteoclastic reaction is always greater than the osteoblastic response and is accentuated with rapidly growing, poorly differentiated carcinomas. Most of the destruction of bone is actually done by the host's cells, particularly osteoclasts. Destruction of bone by the carcinoma itself is a relatively minor, late event. Neither the osteoclastic nor osteoblastic responses are particularly affected by prior irradiation of the bone. New bone formation, mediated by osteoblasts, is most prominent in association with slowly advancing and indolent carcinomas. Periosteal new bone formation is usually seen in front of the neoplastic spread. So, too, is marrow fibrosis.

The presence of dentition significantly influences nerve-related spread. McGregor and MacDonald[99,100] found a four-fold increase of neoplastic spread related to the inferior alveolar nerve edentulous, non-irradiated mandibles as opposed to partially dentate, non-irradiated mandibles. In nearly every instance, however, nerve involvement was also associated with an extensive spread of the carcinoma in the medullary parts of the bone. Skip areas of nerve involvement were unusual. Irradiation did not appear to affect the frequency or extent of nerve involvement.

The difference in nerve-related spread between dentate and non-dentate mandibles is attributable to the difference in vertical height of the occlusal border above the mandibular canal. The progressive resorption of the occlusal surfaces seen in the edentulous mandible brings the alveolar nerve much closer to the mucosa and hence more vulnerable to a direct vertical spread of the carcinoma. The incomplete remodeling of cortical bone and multiple cortical defects associated with alveolar resorption allows direct continuity between the medullary cavity and the overlying mucoperiosteum. Furthermore, the bony changes occasioned by loss of dentition also greatly reduce the distance a floor-of-mouth carcinoma needs to traverse to spread marginally in order to reach the occlusal ridge.

Spread of the carcinoma, erosive or infiltrative, is nearly always through cancellous bone and its marrow spaces. There is little spread deep to an intact overlying mucosa or intact cortex.

Predicting invasion of the mandible is an imperfect exercise. Brown et al.,[101] in a prospective study, concluded that while orthopantomograms (OPGs), bone scans, computed tomography (CT) and magnetic resonance imaging (MRI) were helpful, it was periosteal stripping with direct inspection that was the better predictor of invasion (accurate in all instances in the authors' study). In postirradiated cortical bone, it may not be possible to separate the periosteum, even in the absence of neoplastic invasion, and that can thwart the inspection of the cortex that is the key.

Since cortical bone is usually not amenable to frozen section, it is the cancellous bone of the stump that has been used for determining margins of resection. Touch imprint cytologic preparations or cryostat sections of a curetted sample of the cancellous bone have served as specimens with varying degrees of success and acceptance. Forrest et al.[102] utilized a 1 cm curettage specimen and frozen section and were able to correctly predict adequacy of mandibular resection in 32 (97%) of 33 margins.

It is likely that no single method will suffice in the determination of invasion of the mandible by oral squamous cell carcinomas. A combination of available techniques, tempered by clinical judgement, will produce the best result.

Tumor thickness and depth of invasion

A number of studies have identified tumor thickness as an important prognostic indicator in upper aerodigestive neoplasms, especially as a predictor of regional metastasis.[103–110] Such studies have been postoperative on resected specimens and also preoperative in biopsy specimens.

Distinction needs to be made between depth of neoplastic penetration and tumor thickness. Depth means the extent of growth into tissues beneath an epithelial surface; where epithelium is destroyed, some investigators reconstruct a surface line and measure from this. Penetration can be expressed in millimeters as measured by a micrometer or in terms of a reference to microscopic anatomical deep structures, for example muscle layer, salivary gland layer. Thickness, on the other hand, is a direct micrometer measurement of the vertical bulk of the tumor regardless of the histologic structure of an ulcerative or exophytic form of the tumor's growth.[111] Sites most suitable for thickness measurements are those with some soft tissue beneath the epithelium, i.e., floor of mouth, tongue, buccal mucosa and soft palate. The hard palate and retromolar trigone are less adaptable. Moore et al.[112] found no special advantage to using thickness in laryngeal cancer.

Thickness is perhaps easier to measure, but for carcinomas such as verrucous carcinoma, correlation of outcome is better with depth of invasion.[113]

Ambrosch et al.[114] elected to use depth of invasion as a potential indicator of micrometastasis and found that the depth was the only significant risk factor for metastasis in logistic regression analysis. Contingency table analysis revealed a depth of invasion of 4 mm as the most valuable cut-off point. The risk of metastasizing in oral, oropharyngeal and hypopharyngeal tumors with a depth of invasion greater than 4 mm compared with a depth of invasion of less than 4 mm was more than four-fold ($p = 0.0001$).

Moore et al.[112] found that thickness and depth are both good general indicators of neoplastic aggressiveness. Each manifests good correlation with survival and with regional lymph node metastasis. These investigators agree with Ambrosch and colleagues[114] in indicating that exophytic tumors behave like thin tumors and are best measured from reconstructed mucosal lines.

Using subjective rather than objective measurements of depth of invasion in oral carcinomas, Thompson[113] found that carcinomas confined to the superficial lamina propria seemed to have a better prognosis in relation to the development of cervical metastasis, and this was not influenced by site, size, or degree of differentiation. He used an arbitrary leveling system to assess the depth of invasion. Level 1 indicated a local invasion not beyond one-half the width of the lamina propria. Level 2 lesions involved the deeper half of the lamina propria without infiltration of submucosa or skeletal muscle. Level 3 lesions involved the submucosa when it was present and level 4 carcinomas invaded skeletal muscle. Table 4.23 illustrates the power of depth of invasion compared with other factors.[107]

Table 4.23 Predictive value of factors for cervical lymph node metastasis in carcinoma of tongue. (Modified from Fukano et al.[107])

Factor	All patients[a]
Depth of invasion	0.0003
Mode of invasion	0.0019
T stage	0.0517
Gross appearance (exophytic, endophytic, ulcerative, etc.)	0.4680
Sex of patients	0.4729
Age of patients (≤ 40 years; ≥ 40 years)	0.4984
Level of differentiation of carcinoma (well; other)	0.5453
Location of carcinoma	0.5470

[a]Chi-squared test p value.

Spiro et al.[103] evaluated the predictive value of tumor thickness in squamous cell carcinoma of the oral tongue and floor of mouth. Their retrospective study found a statistically significant association between an increasing thickness of tumor and treatment failure. Tumor thickness greater than 2 mm was noted to have the best correlation with treatment failure and to be a better predictor than T stage (Table 4.24). Failure was most often manifested as regional neck metastases. It was therefore considered that thickness could be used as a guide in the management of the N0 neck. Spiro et al.[103] concluded that patients with primary carcinomas greater than 2 mm thick should be treated with elective therapy to the N0 neck regardless of tumor size.

Table 4.24 Squamous carcinoma of tongue and floor of mouth: tumor thickness and stage. (Modified from Spiro et al.[103])

Tumor thickness	T1	T2	T3
≤2 mm	28	13	2
3–8 mm	18	22	3
≥9 mm	2	14	3
	48	49	8

Mohit-Tabatabai et al.[104] examined the relationship of floor-of-mouth stage I and II cancer to regional metastasis. They too showed a strong correlation between metastasis and tumor thickness. Primary lesions were divided into groups of less than or equal to 1.5 mm, 1.6 to 3.5 mm, and greater than 3.5 mm of tumor thickness. These groups had corresponding regional metastases of 2%, 33%, and 60%, respectively.

The significance of tumor thickness in soft palate carcinomas has been studied by Baredes et al.[115] Their study showed that of 44 patients who had tumor thickness less than or equal to 2.86 mm, 0% had nodal metastases. All patients who had tumor thickness greater than or equal to 3.12 mm had metastases. Furthermore, those patients who had carcinomas of an intermediate depth—greater than 2.86 mm but less than 3.12 mm—had a 60% incidence of nodal disease. These authors also concluded that tumor thickness correlated more directly with nodal disease than did T stage.

Karas et al.[116] examined the relationship between tumor thickness measured in biopsy specimens with the resected specimen in floor-of-mouth carcinoma.

Table 4.25 Tumor depth/thickness and cervical lymph node metastasis

Reference	Oral site	Measurement	Conclusions
Fukano et al.[107]	Tongue	Depth of invasion	Depth greater than 5 mm significantly increased risk of cervical metastases
Ragson et al.[108]	Oral cavity/ oropharynx	Tumor thickness	Thickness greater than 5 mm significantly increased risk of cervical metastases
Brown et al.[109]	Floor of mouth	Tumor thickness	Thickness greater than 2 mm should lead to consideration of elective treatment of neck
Urist et al.[110]	Buccal mucosa	Tumor thickness/ depth of invasion	Poor survival with tumors greater than 6 mm
Mohit-Tabatabai et al.[104]	Floor of mouth	Tumor thickness	Elective neck dissection strongly indicated in N0 lesions more than 1.5 mm thick
Spiro et al.[103]	Tongue/floor of mouth	Tumor thickness	Elective neck therapy appropriate for N0 lesions more than 2 mm thick

A significant overall correlation was found. It was noted that patients whose biopsy specimens exhibited a neoplasm with a thickness less than or equal to 1 mm were likely to have a final tumor thickness of less than 2 mm. On the other hand, all patients with biopsy tumor thickness greater than 2 mm had a final specimen with a thickness greater than 3.5 mm.

Table 4.25 presents six studies relating depth/thickness to nodal metastases.[103,104,107–110]

Ductal invasion

The frequency of involvement into adjacent salivary ducts by oral dysplastic or carcinomatous epithelium is uncommon, but it can be important in the treatment of oral squamous carcinomas. Daley et al.[117] screened routine tissue sections of 1216 cases of oral epithelial dysplasias and squamous cell carcinomas and found 26 (2.14%) that exhibited unequivocal ductal involvement. Floor-of-mouth lesions were especially likely to manifest this finding. So too were severely dysplastic or carcinoma-in-situ lesions. Follow-up on 23 cases indicated that the recurrence rate of pre-invasive lesions with ductal involvement was equal to that of the squamous cell carcinomas. The depth of the ductal dysplasia, however, did not correlate with recurrence rate. Even though uncommon, the involvement of salivary ducts is, nonetheless, significant. Surgical stripping or ablation of such lesions should extend at least 3 mm below the surface to ensure eradication of these reservoirs of dysplastic cells.

Current status and future perspectives of histologic factors

Table 4.7 lists the histopathologic factors considered to be prognostic factors in oral squamous cell carcinomas. For nearly all the factors, one can find a study indicating its significance *vis-à-vis* another. Besides the observation that studies relating to the factors have been mostly retrospective, there are questions to be answered under each category. For margins of excision, the following questions remain: definition of closeness and significance of dysplasia or a carcinoma in situ versus invasive carcinoma. Does more than one positive margin increase risk of recurrence and nodal metastases? Does more than one frozen section of marginal clearance carry a worse outlook? Are 'molecular margins' practical?

Angiogenesis density scoring has a considerable potential, but standardization of scoring is mandatory. Does perineural invasion in mucosal squamous cell carcinoma have as morbid a significance as it does in cutaneous squamous cell carcinomas? What is the significance of size of the involved nerve? Histologic classification by itself may have a bearing, but does size allocation over-ride histologic type? Histologic grade seems not to be a strong factor, but the mode of invasion, for example spider-web, appears to be a useful indicator of aggressiveness.

The three factors with the strongest correlates to metastasis and hence prognosis are tumor thickness, tumor depth, and lymphatic/vascular invasion. For the first two, cut-off points related to anatomic site in the oral cavity need standardization, if possible, and for vascular invasion, establishment as an independent factor is necessary.

Therapy-induced regressive changes in squamous cell carcinoma of the head and neck, while well described, deserve more attention as prognostic factors. Chemotherapy and radiotherapy give rise to regressive changes in squamous cell carcinoma. Histopathologic effects of therapeutic protocols have been mainly concerned with those attributable to chemotherapy alone, but some have also evaluated the findings after preoperative chemoradiotherapy in resected specimens.

The histological characteristics of the carcinomas and associated regressive changes fall into four patterns: (1) complete absence of the carcinoma, (2) foreign body reaction to keratotic material, (3) small foci of residual carcinoma, and (4) extensive persistence of the carcinoma. Associated, non-epithelial alterations include sclerosis, hemorrhage, and atypia of stromal cells.

Except for extensive persistence, the gross appearance is unreliable for conclusions regarding presence or absence of residual neoplasm. In general, the area of the primary neoplasm shows a firm, roughened surface with sclerosis.

Residual carcinoma was absent in the whole specimen in 54% of the cases reported by Valente et al;[118] a lower percentage was reported by Micheau and Richard.[119] Both groups emphasized the possibility that post-therapy regressive changes might mask the carcinoma. These changes are found in all specimens negative for carcinoma and also in instances with minimal as opposed to extensive persistent tumor.

The two most frequent post-therapy changes are stromal sclerosis and keratinized material with a foreign-body-type reaction.[120,121] Whether the keratinized material is the result of extensive destruction of the neoplasm or therapy-induced differentiation has yet to be resolved. The distinction is obviously important. Valente et al.[118] and Micheau and Richard[119] consider the finding to represent a complete absence of carcinoma and this opinion is supported by Kellokumpu-Lehtinen et al.,[120] who did find changes in keratinization patterns in viable tumor after radiation.

References

1. Batsakis JG, Hybels R, Crissman JD et al. The pathology of head and neck tumors: verrucous carcinoma, part 15. Head Neck Surg 1982; 5: 29–38
2. Medina JE, Dichtel W, Luna MA. Verrucous-squamous carcinomas of the oral cavity. A clinicopathologic study of 104 cases. Arch Otolaryngol 1984; 110: 437–440
3. Prioleau PG, Santa Cruz DJ, Meyer JS et al. Verrucous carcinoma. A light and electron microscopic, autoradiographic, and immunofluorescence study. Cancer 1980; 45: 2849–2857
4. Koch BB, Trask DK, Hoffman HT et al. National survey of head and neck verrucous carcinoma. Patterns of presentation, care and outcome. Cancer 2001; 92: 110–120
5. McDonald JS, Crissman JD, Gluckman JL. Verrucous carcinoma of the oral cavity. Head Neck Surg 1982; 5: 22–28
6. Raslan WF, Barnes L, Krause JR et al. Basaloid squamous cell carcinoma of the head and neck: A clinicopathologic and flow cytometric study of 10 new cases with review of the English literature. Am J Otolaryngol 1994; 15: 204–211
7. Wieneke JA, Heffner DK. Basaloid squamous cell carcinoma: an aggressive variant of squamous cell carcinoma of the head and neck region. Pathology Case Reviews 2000; 5: 200–205
8. Luna MA, El-Naggar A, Parichatikanond P et al. Basaloid squamous carcinoma of the upper aerodigestive tract. Cancer 1990; 66: 537–542
9. Banks ER, Frierson HF, Mills SE et al. Basaloid squamous cell carcinoma of the head and neck: a clinicopathologic and immunohistochemical study of 40 cases. Am J Surg Pathol 1992; 16: 939–946
10. Coppola D, Catalano E, Tang C-K et al. Basaloid squamous cell carcinoma of floor of mouth. Cancer 1993; 72: 2299–2305
11. Wick MR, Swanson PE. Carcinosarcomas: current perspectives and an historical review of nosological concepts. Semin Diagn Pathol 1993; 10: 118–127
12. Thompson L, Chang B, Barsky SH. Monoclonal origin of malignant mixed tumors (carcinosarcomas). Evidence for a divergent histogenesis. Am J Surg Pathol 1996; 20: 277–285
13. Ellis GL, Corio RL. Spindle cell carcinoma of the oral cavity. A clinicopathologic assessment of fifty-nine cases. Oral Surg Oral Med Oral Pathol 1980; 50: 523–534
14. Batsakis JG, Suarez P. Sarcomatoid carcinomas of the upper aerodigestive tracts. Adv Anat Pathol 2000; 7: 282–293
15. Batsakis JG, Rice DH, Howard DR. The pathology of head and neck tumors: spindle cell lesions (sarcomatoid carcinomas, nodular fasciitis and fibrosarcoma) of the aerodigestive tracts. Head Neck Surg 1982; 4: 499–513
16. Zarbo RJ, Crissman JD, Venkat H et al. Spindle-cell carcinoma of the upper aerodigestive tract mucosa. Am J Surg Pathol 1986; 10: 741–753
17. Balercia G, Bhan AK, Dickersin GR. Sarcomatoid carcinoma: an ultrastructural study with light microscopic and immunohistochemical correlation of

10 cases from various anatomic sites. Ultrastruct Pathol 1995; 19: 249–263
18. Nakhleh RE, Zarbo RJ, Ewing S et al. Myogenic differentiation in spindle cell (sarcomatoid) carcinomas of the upper aerodigestive tract. Appl Immunohistochem 1993; 1: 58–68
19. Ogawa K, Kim Y-C, Nakashima Y et al. Expression of epithelial markers in sarcomatoid carcinoma: an immunohistochemical study. Histopathology 1987; 11: 511–522
20. Lewis JE, Olsen KD, Sebo TJ. Spindle cell carcinoma of the larynx: review of 26 cases including DNA content and immunohistochemistry. Hum Pathol 1997; 28: 664–673
21. Olsen KD, Lewis JE, Suman VJ. Spindle cell carcinoma of the larynx and hypopharynx. Otolaryngol Head Neck Surg 1997; 116: 47–52
22. Batsakis JG. 'Pseudosarcoma' of the mucous membrane in the head and neck. J Laryngol Otol 1981; 95: 311–316
23. Ellis GL, Langloss JM, Heffner OK et al. Spindle cell carcinoma of the aerodigestive tract: an immunohistochemical analysis of 21 cases. Am J Surg Pathol 1987; 11: 335–342
24. Guarino M. Epithelial-to-mesenchymal change of differentiation; from embryogenetic mechanism to pathological patterns. Histol Histopathol 1995; 10: 171–184
25. Shanmugaratnam K. Histological typing of tumours of the upper respiratory tract and ear. World Health Organization international histological classification of tumors. Berlin: Springer-Verlag, 1991
26. Batsakis JG, Luna MA, El-Naggar AK. 'Inflammatory pseudotumor': what is it? How does it behave? Ann Otol Rhinol Laryngol 1995; 104: 329–331
27. Coffin CM, Watterson J, Priest JR, Dehner LP. Extrapulmonary inflammatory myofibroblastic tumor (inflammatory pseudotumor): a clinicopathologic and immunohistochemical study of 84 cases. Am J Surg Pathol 1995; 19: 859–872
28. Chan JKC. Inflammatory pseudotumor: a family of lesions of diverse nature and etiologies. Adv Anat Pathol 1996; 3: 156–171
29. Meis JM, Enzinger FM. Inflammatory fibrosarcoma of the mesentery and retroperitoneum. Am J Surg Pathol 1991; 15: 1146–1156
30. Batsakis JG, Huser J. Squamous carcinomas with gland-like (adenoid) features. Ann Otol Rhinol Laryngol 1990; 99: 87–88
31. Nappi O, Pettinato G, Wick MR. Adenoid (acantholytic) squamous cell carcinoma of the skin. J Cutan Pathol 1989; 16: 114–121
32. Gerughty RM, Hennigar GR, Brown FM. Adenosquamous carcinoma of the nasal, oral and laryngeal cavities: a clinicopathologic survey of ten cases. Cancer 1968; 22: 1140–1148
33. Napier SS, Gormley JS, Newlands C et al. Adenosquamous carcinoma. A rare neoplasm with an aggressive course. Oral Surg Oral Med Oral Pathol Oral Radiol Endod 1995; 79: 607–611
34. Martinez-Madrigal F, Baden E, Casiraghi O et al. Oral and pharyngeal adenosquamous carcinoma. A report of four cases with immunohistochemical studies. Eur Arch Otorhinolaryngol 1991; 248: 255–258
35. Jones AC, Freedman PD, Kerpel SM. Oral adenoid squamous cell carcinoma: a report of three cases and review of the literature. J Oral Maxillofac Surg 1993; 51: 676–681
36. Takagi M, Sakato Y, Takayama S et al. Adenoid squamous carcinoma of the oral mucosa. Cancer 1977; 40: 2250–2255
37. Ferlito A, Devany KO, Rinaldo A et al. Mucosal adenoid squamous cell carcinoma of the head and neck. Ann Otol Rhinol Laryngol 1996; 105: 409–413
38. MacMillan C, Kapadia SM, Finkelstein SD et al. Lymphoepithelial carcinoma of the larynx and hypopharynx: study of eight cases with relationship to Epstein–Barr virus and p53 gene alterations, and review of the literature. Hum Pathol 1996; 27: 1172–1179
39. Frank DK, Cheron F, Costanzo D et al. Non-nasopharyngeal lymphoepitheliomas (undifferentiated carcinomas) of the upper aerodigestive tract. Ann Otol Rhinol Laryngol 1995; 104: 305–310
40. Bansberg SF, Olsen KD, Gafey TA. Lymphoepithelioma of the oropharynx. Otolaryngol Head Neck Surg 1989; 100: 303–307
41. Banerjee SS, Eyden BP, Wells S et al. Pseudoangiosarcomatous carcinoma: a clinicopathological study of seven cases. Histopathology 1992; 21: 13–23
42. Norris CM Jr, Mustoe RA, Ross JS et al. Desmoplastic squamous cell carcinoma of the tongue simulating myositis or fasciitis. Head Neck Surg 1986; 9: 51–55
43. Theaker JM. Extramammary Paget's disease of the oral mucosa with in situ carcinoma of minor salivary gland ducts. Am J Surg Pathol 1988; 12: 890–895
44. Ishiyama A, Eversole LR, Ross DA et al. Papillary squamous neoplasm of the head and neck. Laryngoscope 1994; 104: 1446–1452
45. Batsakis JG, Suarez P. Papillary squamous carcinoma: will the real one please stand up? Adv Anat Pathol 2000; 7: 2–8
46. Odell EW, Jani P, Sherriff M et al. The prognostic value of individual grading parameters in small lingual squamous cell carcinomas. The importance of the pattern of invasion. Cancer 1994; 74: 789–794
47. Anneroth G, Batsakis JG, Luna MA. Review of the literature and a recommended system of malignancy grading in oral squamous cell carcinomas. Scand J Dent Res 1987; 95: 229–249
48. Woolgar JA, Scott J. Prediction of cervical lymph node metastases in squamous cell carcinoma of the tongue/floor of mouth. Head Neck 1995; 17: 463–472
49. Carter RL, Tanner NSB, Clifford P et al. Perineural spread in squamous cell carcinomas of the head and neck: a clinicopathological study. Clin Otolaryngol 1979; 4: 271–281
50. Carter RL, Pittam MR, Tanner NSB. Pain and dysphagia in patients with squamous carcinomas of

the head and neck: The role of perineural spread. J R Soc Med 1982; 75: 598–600
51. Soo K, Carter RL, O'Brien CJ. Prognostic implications of perineural spread in squamous carcinomas of the head and neck. Laryngoscope 1986; 96: 1145–1148
52. Osguthorpe JD, Abel CG, Lang P et al. Neurotropic cutaneous tumors of the head and neck. Arch Otolaryngol Head Neck Surg 1997; 123: 871–876
53. Dunlap CL, Barker B. Diagnostic problems in oral pathology. Semin Diagn Pathol 1985; 2: 16–30
54. Wysocki GP, Wright BA. Intraneural and perineural epithelial structures. Head Neck Surg 1981; 4: 69–71
55. Lutman GB. Epithelial nests in intraoral sensory nerve endings simulating perineural invasion in patients with oral carcinoma. Am J Clin Pathol 1974; 61: 275–284
56. Miko T, Molnar P. The juxtaoral organ: a pitfall for pathologists. J Pathol 1981; 133: 17–23
57. Mesa M, Baden E, Grodjesk J et al. Neuroepithelial hamartoma of the oral cavity. Oral Surg Oral Med Oral Pathol 1994; 78: 627–630
58. Close LG, Burns DK, Reisch J et al. Microvascular invasion in cancer of the oral cavity and oropharynx. Arch Otolaryngol Head Neck Surg 1987; 113: 1191–1195
59. Poleksic S, Kalwaic HJ. Prognostic value of vascular invasion in squamous cell carcinoma of the head and neck. Plast Reconstr Surg 1978; 61: 234–240
60. Batsakis JG. Invasion of the microcirculation in head and neck cancer. Ann Otol Rhinol Laryngol 1984; 93: 646–647
61. Djalilian M, Weiland LH, Devine KD et al. Significance of jugular vein invasion by metastatic carcinoma in radical neck dissection. Am J Surg 1973; 126: 566–569
62. Folkman J. What is the evidence that tumors are angiogenesis dependent. J Nat Cancer Inst 1990; 82: 4–6
63. Folkman J. Angiogenesis in cancer, vascular, rheumatoid and other diseases. Nature Med 1995; 1: 27–31
64. Fox SB. Tumour angiogenesis and prognosis. Histopathology 1997; 30: 294–301
65. Carrau RL, Barnes EL, Snyderman CH et al. Tumor angiogenesis as a predictor of tumor aggressiveness and metastatic potential in squamous cell carcinoma of the head and neck. Invas Metast 1996; 15: 197–202
66. Craft PS, Harris AL. Clinical prognostic significance of tumour angiogenesis. Ann Oncol 1994; 5: 305–311
67. Yu JL, Rak JW, Carmeliet P et al. Heterogeneous vascular dependence of tumor cell population. Am J Pathol 2001; 158: 1325–1334
68. Williams JK, Carlson GW, Cohen C et al. Tumor angiogenesis as a prognostic factor in oral cavity tumors. Am J Surg 1994; 168: 373–380
69. Penfold CN, Partridge M, Rojas R et al. The role of angiogenesis in the spread of oral squamous cell carcinoma. Br J Oral Maxillofac Surg 1996; 34: 37–41
70. Gleich LL, Biddinger PW, Duperier FD et al. Tumor angiogenesis as a prognostic indicator in T2–T4 oral cavity squamous cell carcinoma: a clinical–pathologic correlation. Head Neck 1997; 19: 276–280
71. Cole RD, McGuirt WF. Prognostic significance of skin involvement for mucosal tumors of the head and neck. Arch Otolaryngol Head Neck Surg 1995; 121: 1246–1248
72. Batsakis JG. Surgical excision margins: a pathologist's perspective. Adv Anat Pathol 1999; 6: 140–148
73. Lee JG. Detection of residual carcinoma of the oral cavity, oropharynx, hypopharynx, and larynx: a study of surgical margins. Trans Am Acad Ophthalmol Otolaryngol 1974; 78: 49–53
74. Boonstra H, Oosterhuis JW, Oosterhuis AM et al. Cervical tissue shrinkage by formaldehyde fixation, paraffin wax embedding, section cutting and mounting. Virch Arch (A) 1983; 402: 195–201
75. Beaumont DG, Hains JD. Changes in surgical margins in vivo following resection and after fixation. Aust J Otolaryngol 1992; 1: 51–52
76. Johnson RE, Sigman JD, Funk GF et al. Quantification of surgical margin shrinkage in the oral cavity. Head Neck 1997; 19: 281–286
77. Looser KG, Shah JP, Strong EW. The significance of 'positive' margins in surgically resected epidermoid carcinomas. Head Neck Surg 1978; 1: 107–111
78. Byers RM, Bland KI, Borlase B et al. Prognostic and therapeutic value of frozen section determinations in the surgical treatment of squamous carcinoma of the head and neck. Am J Surg 1978; 136: 525–528
79. Loree TR, Strong EW. Significance of positive margins in oral cavity squamous carcinoma. Am J Surg 1990; 160: 410–414
80. Scholl P, Byers RM, Batsakis JG et al. Microscopic cut-through of cancer in the surgical treatment of squamous carcinoma of the tongue. Prognostic and therapeutic implications. Am J Surg 1986; 152: 354–360
81. van Es RJJ, Amerongen NN, Slootweg PJ et al. Resection margin as a predictor of recurrence at the primary site for T1 and T2 oral cancers. Evaluation of histopathologic variables. Arch Otolaryngol Head Neck Surg 1996; 122: 521–525
82. Vikram B, Strong EW, Shah JP et al. Failure at the primary site following multimodality treatment in advanced head and neck cancer. Head Neck Surg 1984; 6: 720–723
83. Dubner S, Heller KS. Local control of squamous cell carcinoma following marginal segmented mandibulectomy. Head Neck 1993; 15: 29–32
84. Jacobs JR, Ahmad K, Casiano R et al. Implications of positive surgical margins. Laryngoscope 1993; 103: 64–68
85. Chen TY, Emrich LJ, Driscoll DL. The clinical significance of pathological findings in surgically resected margins of the primary tumor in head and neck carcinoma. Int J Rad Oncol Biol Phys 1987; 13: 833–837
86. Beaumont DG, Hain JD. Surgical margins in oral cavity and oropharyngeal cancer. Aust J Otolaryngol 1992; 1: 47–50
87. Bauer WC, Lesinski SG, Ogura JH. The significance of positive margins in hemilaryngectomy specimens. Laryngoscope 1975; 85: 1–13

88. Kuhel W, Goepfert H, Luna M et al. Adenoid cystic carcinoma of the palate. Arch Otolaryngol Head Neck Surg 1992; 118: 243–247
89. Garden AS, Weber RS, Morrison W et al. The influence of positive margins and nerve invasion in adenoid cystic carcinoma of the head and neck treated with surgery and radiation. Int J Rad Oncol Biol Phys 1995; 32: 619–626
90. Ravasz LA, Slootweg PJ, Hordijk GJ et al. The status of the resection margin as a prognostic factor in the treatment of head and neck carcinoma. J Cranio-Maxillofac Surg 1991; 314–318
91. Brennan JA, Mao L, Hruban RH et al. Molecular assessment of histopathologic staging in squamous cell carcinoma of the head and neck. N Engl J Med 1995; 332: 429–435
92. Ogden GR, Chisholm DM, Morris AM et al. Overexpression of p53 in normal oral mucosa of oral cancer patients does not necessarily predict further malignant disease. J Pathol 1997; 182: 180–184
93. Cleary KR, Batsakis JG. Oral squamous cell carcinoma and the mandible. Ann Otol Rhinol Laryngol 1995; 104: 977–979
94. Haribhakti VV. The dentate adult human mandible: an anatomic basic for surgical decision making. Plast Reconstr Surg 1996; 97: 536–541
95. Weisman RA, Kimmelman CP. Bone scanning in the assessment of mandibular invasion by oral cavity carcinoma. Laryngoscope 1982; 92: 1–4
96. Müller H, Slootweg PJ. Mandibular invasion by oral squamous cell carcinoma. Clinical aspects. J Cranio-Maxillofac Surg 1990; 18: 80–84
97. Slootweg PJ, Müller H. Mandibular invasion by oral squamous cell carcinoma. J Cranio-Maxillofac Surg 1989; 17: 69–74
98. Carter RL. Patterns and mechanisms of localized bone invasion by tumors: studies with squamous carcinomas of the head and neck. Crit Rev Clin Lab Sci 1985; 22: 275–315
99. McGregor AD, MacDonald DG. Routes of entry of squamous cell carcinoma to the mandible. Head Neck Surg 1988; 10: 294–301
100. McGregor AD, MacDonald DG. Patterns of spread of squamous cell carcinoma within the mandible. Head Neck 1989; 11: 457–461
101. Brown JS, Griffith JF, Phelps PD et al. A comparison of different imaging modalities and direct inspection after periosteal stripping in predicting the invasion of the mandible by oral squamous cell carcinoma. Br J Oral Maxillofac Surg 1994; 32: 347–359
102. Forest LA, Schuller DE, Lucas JG et al. Rapid analysis of mandibular margins. Laryngoscope 1995; 105: 475–477
103. Spiro RH, Huvos AG, Wong GY et al. Predictive value of tumor thickness in squamous carcinoma confined to the tongue and floor of mouth. Am J Surg 1986; 152: 345–350
104. Mohit-Tabalabai MA, Sobel HJ, Rush BF et al. Relation of thickness of floor of mouth stage I and II cancers to regional metastasis. Am J Surg 1986; 152: 351–353
105. Jones KR, Lodge-Rigal D, Reddick RL et al. Prognostic factors in recurrence of stage I and II squamous cell cancer of the oral cavity. Arch Otolaryngol Head Neck Surg 1992; 118: 483–485
106. Shah JP, Cendon RA, Farr HW et al. Carcinoma of the oral cavity. Factors affecting treatment failure at the primary site and neck. Am J Surg 1976; 132: 504–507
107. Fukano H, Matsuura H, Hasegawa Y et al. Depth of invasion as a predictive factor for cervical lymph node metastasis in tongue carcinoma. Head Neck 1997; 19: 205–210
108. Ragson B, Cruz R, Hilsinger R. Relation of lymph node metastasis to histopathologic appearance in oral cavity and oropharyngeal carcinoma: a case series and literature review. Laryngoscope 1989; 99: 1103–1110
109. Brown B, Barnes L, Mazariegos J. Prognostic factors in mobile tongue and floor of mouth carcinoma. Cancer 1989; 1195–1202
110. Urist MM, O'Brien CJ, Soong SJ. Squamous cell carcinoma of the buccal mucosa: analysis of prognostic factors. Am J Surg 1987; 154: 411–414
111. Breslow A. Thickness, cross-sectional areas and depth of invasion in the prognosis of cutaneous melanoma. Ann Surg 1970; 172: 902–906
112. Moore C, Kuhns JG, Greenberg RA. Thickness as prognostic aid in upper aerodigestive tract cancer. Arch Surg 1986; 121: 1410–1414
113. Thompson SH. Cervical lymph node metastases in oral carcinoma related to the depth of invasion of the primary lesion. J Surg Oncol 1986; 31: 120–122
114. Ambrosch P, Kron M, Fischer G et al. Micrometastases in carcinoma of the upper aerodigestive tract: detection, risk of metastasizing, and prognostic value of depth of invasion. Head Neck 1995; 17: 473–479
115. Baredes S, Leeman DJ, Chen TS. Significance of tumor thickness in soft palate carcinoma. Laryngoscope 1993; 103: 389–393
116. Karas DE, Baredes S, Chen TS et al. Relationship of biopsy and final specimens in evaluation of tumor thickness in floor of mouth carcinoma. Laryngoscope 1995; 105: 491–493
117. Daley TD, Lovas JGL, Peters E et al. Salivary gland duct involvement in oral epithelial dysplasia and squamous cell carcinoma. Oral Surg Oral Med Oral Pathol Oral Radiol Endod 1996; 81: 186–192
118. Valente G, Vercellino V, Corradi L et al. Histopathological findings after preoperative chemo-radiotherapy in oral and oropharyngeal carcinoma. A study of 28 resected specimens. Oral Oncol Eur J Cancer 1993; 29B: 113–117
119. Micheau C, Richard J. Actins tissulaires de la chimiotherapie intra-arterielle dans les cancers pelv-linguaux el leurs metastases ganglionaires. A propos de 47 cas. Ann Otolaryngol 1975; 92: 499–508
120. Kellokumpu-Lehtinen P, Soderstrom K-O, Kortekangus A et al. Radiation-induced morphological changes and radiocurability in squamous cell carcinoma of the head

and neck region. A preliminary report. Acta Oncol 1990; 29: 517–520
121. Sulfaro S, Frustaci S, Volpe R et al. A pathologic assessment of tumor residue and stromal changes after intraarterial chemotherapy for head and neck carcinomas. A study on serial sections of the whole surgical specimen. Cancer 1984; 64: 944–1001

5 The molecular biology of oral cancer

John G Batsakis

Molecular and genetic aspects

Molecular and genetic studies of squamous cell carcinoma of the head and neck have evolved along two pathways, one pragmatic, the other academic. For the former, it is hoped that by study of the primary carcinoma, a prediction of biologic behavior and prognosis can be made. To date, this is not the case. Many of the so-called prognostic markers have not found a place in routine diagnostic/prognostic strategies. Conflicting data from molecular and genetic studies, expense and technical variability detract from a universal acceptance and application. In addition, the focus of many studies on single markers only ignores the fact that neoplasia and metastasis are multistep processes.

Pursuit of the academic and basic, commendable as it is, too often lacks any translational goal and instead of trying to determine the clinical effect of a genetic aberration, the genetic aberration itself is dissected, leading to further questions. The databanks brought about by such dissection bring to mind T.S. Eliot's rhetorical questions: 'Where is the knowledge that is lost in information? Where is the wisdom that is lost in knowledge?'

In the following we address the information currently available for several genetic and molecular aspects of squamous cell carcinoma of the oral cavity and the metastatic process.

Oncogenes and tumor suppressor genes

Almost all cancer genes (oncogenes and tumor suppressors) have been ascribed some function within the complex pathways of signal generation, receipt and response that regulate cell growth and differentiation. To ensure proper development and homeostasis there are multiple layers of control. Escape from this control requires several mutations to be accumulated within a cell.

Normal genes or cellular protooncogenes can be activated by structural or functional alterations, for example point mutations, truncations, chromosomal rearrangement, gene amplification, proviral insertions. More than 70 of these oncogenes have been identified.[1] In addition to the protooncogenes, several cell cycle regulators, such as certain cyclins and E2F transcription factors, also have tumorigenic potential.

Characterization of protooncogenes and tumor suppressor genes has unveiled the intrinsic interactions and complexities of molecular carcinogenesis and, in the event, diminished the prognostic value of the evaluation of only one such marker. An example is *c-myc*. The *myc* family of protooncogenes currently comprises three members; *c-myc*, *N-myc* and *L-myc*. The best characterized member is *c-myc*. Genetic alterations at the *c-myc* locus and activation of *c-myc* with its protein product disturb the Myc network's central position in the regulation and homeostasis of cell growth.[2] Overexpression can have considerable effects on cell fate, including inhibition of differentiation and promotion of tumor development. The decreased capacity of cells to differentiate is followed by an increased potential to continue cycling and with that the cells become targets for additional somatic mutations.

Tumor suppressor genes encode proteins that may counteract the effect of protooncogenes. In normal cells, these genes modulate growth-promoting signals, transcription, DNA repair, and replication. Like protooncoproteins, their products act at crucial points in the cell cycle to maintain homeostasis. Deletional or mutational loss of function of the tumor suppressor genes also contributes to tumorigenesis.

The concept of the existence of tumor suppressor genes led to the postulate that two independent events were needed to inactivate a given gene.[3] This hypothesis was based on the model of retinoblastoma, in which susceptible individuals with germline mutations of the retinoblastoma (*RB*) gene required inactivation of the remaining allele to develop a malignant phenotype. The family of genes that follow this 'two-hit' model include the *RB* and *p53* genes.[4] The cooperative tumorigenic effect of germline mutations in *p53* and *RB* is seen in heterozygous mice mutant for both genes.[5] These animals have reduced viability and exhibit increased tumor burden and metastatic spread. Several viral and cellular proteins have also been shown to interact with *p53* or *pRB*, altering their functions. Complex formation with these proteins inactivates *pRB* function and leads to cellular immortalization. The loss of one tumor suppressor gene may, however, be compensated by the activity of the other. Without both *pRB* and *p53*, it appears that E2F activation stimulates cell proliferation, allowing tumor formation.[5] High-transformation strains of oncoviruses encode proteins that bind and inactivate both *p53* and *pRB*, indicating the crucial role of these molecules and their close interaction.

Other suppressor genes are being identified. Loss of heterozygosity on chromosome arm 18q in 50–80% of head and neck squamous cell carcinomas has prompted speculation that the 18q arm may contain one or more tumor suppressor genes, including the gene deleted in colorectal carcinomas, the *DCC* gene.[6]

Molecular biology of the cell cycle

The cell division cycle may be viewed as a series of checkpoints or transitions at which certain criteria have to be met before the cell proceeds to the next phase. A simplified approach to these checkpoints is to consider them as downstream effects of signal transduction pathways originating from cellular recognition of DNA damage. When DNA is damaged, a checkpoint is activated to prevent cell cycle progression. This presumably prevents either the cell from replicating the damaged DNA templates in S phase (GI checkpoint) or erroneous chromosomal segregation during mitosis (G2 checkpoint). In higher eukaryotes, cells only divide upon receiving the necessary extracellular stimuli, in the form of circulating hormones or cytokines, or through contact with adjacent cells or substratum. Otherwise, the cells remain in G0, at a state of quiescence.

The molecules that drive cells through the various phases of the cell cycle are called cyclin-dependent kinases. These protein kinases comprise an enzymatic unit and an accessory protein, a cyclin. The kinase remains inactive until bound by its corresponding cyclin, the levels of which vary throughout the cell cycle.[7] The active kinase is therefore a kinase–cyclin complex.

The cyclin-dependent kinases (Cdks) and their regulatory subunits, the cyclins, are key regulators of cell progression, catalyzing transition, both into S phase and into mitosis.[8] Several cyclin/Cdk complexes accumulate as the cycling cells traverse GI phase. In mid to late GI phase, cyclin D/Cdk4 is activated, leading to hyperphosphorylation of the tumor suppressor protein pRb. Phosphorylation of pRb, in turn, disrupts the inhibitory complexes formed between pRb and members of the E2F family of transcription factors, permitting transcription of cyclin E and other genes needed to initiate S phase. With synthesis of cyclin E, cyclin E/Cdk2 is activated, additional substrates are phosphorylated and DNA replication begins. During S and G2 phases, cells accumulate cyclin A/Cdc2 and cyclin B/Cdc2.[8] The activation of these enzyme complexes triggers entry into mitosis (Table 5.1).

As well as the dependence on synthesis of the cyclin, the activity of each cyclin/Cdk complex is also regulated by phosphorylation and dephosphorylation of critical tyrosine and threonine residues, and by the expression of specific inhibitors of the Cdks. Negative regulation is mediated by two groups

Table 5.1 Cyclin-dependent kinases (Cdks) and associated cyclins. (Modified from Gao and Zelenka[8])

Cdk	Cyclin(s)	Presumed function
Cdk 1	Cyclins A, B, B2, B3	G2/M
Cdk 2	Cyclins A, E, D1, D2, D3	G1/S, S
Cdk 3	Not known	G1/S
Cdk 4	Cyclins D1, D2, D3	G1/S
Cdk 5	P35/p25, Cyclins D1, D3	Neuronal differentiation
Cdk 6	Cyclins D1, D2, D3	G1/S
Cdk 7	Cyclin H	Cdk activation kinase transcription regulation
Cdk 8	Cyclin C	Transcription regulation

of proteins: the p21 family, whose members act as broad specificity inhibitors of cyclins D, E, and A complexes, and the p16 family, members of which appear to be specific inhibitors of cdk4 and cdk6.[9]

Only the D cyclins, their kinases, and their inhibitors have been consistently implicated in tumorigenesis. By far the most frequent chromosomal abnormality that affects cyclin D1 is DNA amplification with the amplicon located on chromosome 11q13. Since 1988, a number of studies have addressed the amplification of 11q13 markers in squamous cell carcinomas of the head and neck.[10,11] The proportion of carcinomas with the amplification ranges from 7% to 62%, with an average of 43%.

There is a considerable difference in opinion over the prognostic implications of the amplification. There does seem to be a correlation with more advanced disease (stages III and IV), lymph node involvement, and a reduced overall survival. There is an inconsistent pattern of amplification of cyclin D1 in other cancers and in tumor cell lines. It is very likely that cyclin D1 expression can be affected by other aspects of tumor cell behavior or by genetic abnormalities in other cellular genes as well as being a target of tumor-specific alterations at the DNA level.

The *p53* gene

Mutation, deactivation and disregulated expression of oncogenes and tumor suppressor genes may be key factors in the pathogenesis of oral squamous cell carcinoma.[12] Deactivation of the *p53* tumor-suppressor gene allows cell proliferation and blocks apoptosis of malignant oral keratinocytes. Mutation in the ras oncogene results in persistent mitogenic signaling.[13] Upregulation of c-Myc expression, in the presence of growth factors, provides an additional proliferative signal. Loss of retinoblastoma tumor-suppressor gene (*Rb*) function can contribute to hyperproliferation of oral keratinocytes and simultaneous deactivation of both *p53* and *Rb* is likely necessary for tumorigenesis. Enhanced BcL-2 and reduced Fas expression inhibit tumor cell apoptosis and may convey resistance to cytotoxic drugs and T-cell-mediated cytotoxicity, respectively.[12] Exogenous mutagens such as tobacco, alcohol, and viral oncogenes can cause altered expression of oncogenes and tumor-suppressor genes in some forms of oral squamous cell carcinomas.

The *p53* tumor suppressor gene is found inactivated in a high percentage of tumors of all lineages, usually due to a point mutation in functionally important regions of the gene product.[14] The average percentage of *p53* mutations for squamous cell carcinomas of the head and neck reported in the literature is 37%. This does not include mutations outside exons 5–9. Studies in which sequencing the entire codon of *p53* have been done indicate mutations outside exons 5–8 were least frequent in head and neck malignancies (2%).[15]

Studies of materials from different geographic regions have shown that *p53* exons are unequally affected by mutations.[14] Exon 7 mutation is, in general, the most affected in the USA. The majority of *p53* mutations in head and neck cancer are found in exon 7. In Japan, on the other hand, exons 5 and 8 are the most frequently affected.[14,16]

Accumulating data also suggest that specific patterns of mutations are found in different classes of tumors.[16] G to T transversions are dominant in lung cancer, C to T transitions in skin cancer, and G to A transitions in colorectal cancer. These differences likely reflect the differences in carcinogens, but this is not the sole reason. For example, exposure to cigarette smoke and carcinogens such as benzpyrene is associated with G to T transversions.[16] Although cigarette smoke is an implicated carcinogen in squamous cell carcinoma of the head and neck, G to T transversions are, in general, uncommon in tumors of the oral and nasal cavity, being more frequently found in carcinomas of the larynx and pharynx. The predominant mutation in the head and neck region is a G to A transition.[16]

The *p53* suppressor gene is a single copy gene localized on the short arm of chromosome 17. The gene encodes a nuclear phosphoprotein that functions as a transactivating transcriptional regulator that controls the expression of a set of genes important in the regulation of the cell cycle and in triggering apoptosis after certain types of genomic damage. Upon physical or chemical DNA damage, functional *p53* can either arrest cell cycle progression in late G1 phase, thus allowing repair of the DNA before its duplication, or else induce apoptosis, leading to cell death. Growth arrest is achieved by the transactivational properties of *p53*, which activates a series of genes involved in cell cycle arrest. The apoptotic pathway of *p53* remains incompletely defined.

Mutation of the *p53* suppressor gene is claimed to be the most common genetic alteration associated with human cancer. More than 1000 *p53* mutations have been identified in human neoplasms. The majority of the mutations are found in the central 200 amino acid portion of the protein. Biochemical studies have demonstrated that the core portion of *p53* (residues 102–292) folds into a compact structural domain that contains the sequence-specific DNA binding activity of the protein.

In cells lacking functional *p53*, i.e., neoplastic cells, there is a disruption of normal cell cycle control, inefficient DNA repair, and emergence of genetically unstable cells—all implicating *p53* as a key factor in the control of stability of the genome. The protein encoded by the wild type of *p53* gene is a 53-kD nuclear phosphoprotein, with a half-life of 20 to 30 minutes. Normally, p53 protein is not demonstrable immunohistochemically in normal tissues because of its short half-life. In contrast, the product of the mutated gene has a half-life of 6 to 8 hours, and can be readily visualized by immunochemistry. Although there is some good correlation between immunohistochemical detection of p53 protein and the presence of mutations within the *p53* gene detected by more comprehensive molecular analyses, there are also varying degrees of discordance.[14,17] Reasons for discordance are not only related to techniques and subjective definitions of 'positive', patient selection, and interpretation of data, but also to the fact that missense point mutations are not the only cause of accumulation of the p53 protein. Changes in the half-life of p53 proteins can follow exposure to agents which damage DNA, or deletions, or functional inactivation by the binding of the p53 protein to other viral or cellular proteins. Furthermore, nonsense mutations, deletions and splice site mutations are not associated with a longer half-life of the protein. It should also be noted that immunohistochemical methods can also detect p53 protein stabilization without mutations.

Aside from the foregoing, there are other concerns over the usefulness of the immunohistochemical detection of p53 proteins as a prognostic indicator.[18] The first is the current arbitrary settings of thresholds which distinguish a 'positive' from a negative specimen. Second is the inappropriate drawing of conclusions from only a small number of cases. Third, and maybe the most important, is whether p53 as a prognostic variable, is independent from other, better characterized predictors of neoplastic behavior. There is thus an obvious need for multivariate analysis of data derived from statistically meaningful patient populations. Where this has been done, some studies have shown p53 to be a prognostic factor for overall survival, but not relapse-free survival, or vice versa.[18]

Batsakis and El-Naggar[14] and Dowell and Hall,[18] in well reasoned reviews, point out that the adverse prognostic effect of p53 abnormalities is probably relatively small and that p53 alone cannot assuredly identify a subset of patients with such a low risk of recurrence that treatment would not be indicated.

Not disputed, however, is the importance of p53 in the fundamental understanding of oncogenesis and neoplasia. Although there are many exceptions, there is, in general, an association between abnormal (increased) p53 protein expression and neoplasia, and in many, but not all instances, this is due to mutation. Another critical point is that other indications of increased normal p53 protein expression can represent an objective marker for recent exposure to cellular insults. Studies in the squamous epithelium of the upper aerodigestive tract indicate that these alterations in the expression of p53 protein may precede overt neoplastic changes and may be widespread, often occurring at some distance from any neoplasm, i.e., field change.[19]

The finding of *p53* overexpression and mutation in fields about neoplasms makes the issue of field change more tractable.[20] Immunohistochemical studies indicate overexpression can occur in apparently normal mucosa surrounding a carcinoma, even occasionally when the carcinoma itself is *p53* negative.[19] Smoking, for instance, has been shown to be an inducer of *p53* in otherwise normal mucosa. Non-smoking and non-drinking patients, younger than 40 years, with squamous cell carcinomas of the tongue show infrequent *p53* gene mutations in their carcinomas. Brennan et al.[21] have reported an association between molecular evidence of *p53* gene mutations in normal mucosa and recurrence, with no recurrences in cases where no *p53* mutation was identified.

Immunohistochemical studies on oral cavity and other aerodigestive tract mucosae point to overexpression of p53 as an early event, found in dysplastic lesions before the onset of invasive squamous cell carcinoma. Whether this reflects p53 protein accumulation due to gene mutation, or only a normal p53 response to DNA damage and activity of the carcinogen is not known. It is, however, possible that neoplasia derives from a few mucosal cells carrying a mutation in the *p53* gene, thereby changing its normal form role as a suppressor gene to an oncogene role in its mutant form.

Alteration in the *p53* gene is a gradual process that encompasses several levels of tumor progression, possibly involving at least four different molecular mechanisms: (1) *p53* mutations; (2) deletion of the wild-type allele; (3) increased dosage of the mutant gene by aneuploid increase in chromosome copies, and/or (4) *p53* gene amplification.

The role of the *p53* gene as the 'guardian of the genome' also extends beyond it being one of the keys to unlock oncogenesis. The disruption of programmed cell death (apoptosis) and reduced cell cycle arrest associated with a mutant form of the *p53* gene have been correlated with increased radiation resistance and survival.[22] Introduction, by means of an adenoviral vector, of a functional *p53* gene into a radiation-resistant head and neck squamous cell carcinoma cell line harboring mutant *p53* has restored the G1 block and apoptosis in these cells in vitro. Moreover, the introduced wild-type *p53* sensitized squamous cell carcinoma mouse xenografts to radiotherapy in vivo.[22]

The *mdr-1* gene

Multidrug resistance (MDR) in human cancer is often associated with overexpression of the *mdr*-1 gene which encodes a 170 kDa transmembrane protein, P-glycoprotein (P-gy). Jain and associates[23] used immunohistochemistry and flow cytometry to assess P-gy expression in different stages of oral carcinoma progression. As a summary of the findings:

- A significant increase in the level of P-gy expression ($p < 0.01$) was observed in oral dysplasia as compared with normal oral mucosa, indicating the alterations in the protein may be one of the important early events in oral carcinogenesis.
- A high expression of P-gy was also seen in the oral mucosa adjacent to the tumor in cancer patients as compared with mucosa from cancer-free patients, perhaps a reflection of field cancerization.
- The differential expression of P-gy in normal, dysplastic, and malignant oral tissues points to its association with a more progressed malignant phenotype.
- In the oral cavity, P-gy may play a major role as a xenobiotic transporter in tissue and increased levels likely reflect an innate drug resistance.

The *CD 44* gene

The *CD 44* gene has enjoyed early enthusiasm over its potential for early cancer detection and for analysis of genetic disturbances involved in neoplasia. Reports have indicated altered expression of standard *CD 44* and variant forms of *CD 44* in a wide range of developing epithelial tumors (e.g. gastrointestinal, renal, pulmonary). In most of the cancers studied (notable exceptions are head and neck squamous cell carcinomas and neuroblastomas) there is overexpression of CD 44 protein isoforms in tumor tissue relative to non-neoplastic control tissue.[24] The expression is limited to tumor cells, but is heterogeneous in the tumor.

Noted above is the contrary expression of *CD 44* with squamous cell carcinomas of the head and neck. In normal oral mucosa expression of *CD 44* variant 6 is detected as a membranous protein on the epithelial cell surface. Both basal and spinous layers are strongly stained. There is then a gradual fading into a negative staining of cells in the superficial keratinizing layer. Furthermore, there is a downregulation of the *CD 44* variant in severe dysplasia and oral squamous cell carcinoma. This low expression in oral cancers may indicate a high metastatic potential but, if so, it is clearly different from that in other cancer cells, which nearly all show an increased expression of CD 44 molecules, including variants.[24] This is yet another difference of the squamous mucosa of the upper aerodigestive tract as compared to other epithelia.

Chromosomal imbalances

Genomic abnormalities located on chromosomes 3 and 17 have been implicated in the development and progression of human oral squamous cell carcinoma.[25,26] There are also indications that there is an association between deletion at 3p and aggressive biologic behavior. Numerical gains of chromosomes appear to be more frequent than a significant loss, but the pattern of chromosome aberrations varies considerably from case to case.

Tsuji et al.[26] found polysomy 3 and 17 were significantly increased in oral squamous cell carcinomas when compared to controls. There was, however, no obvious relationship between the degree of polysomies and clinicopathologic factors such as tumor differentiation, stage of disease, DNA ploidy, and clinical outcome.

There is a high rate of loss of heterozygosity (LOH) for tumor suppressor genes in patients with advanced carcinomas of the head and neck. Table 5.2, derived from the study by Gleich et al.,[27] gives the incidence of LOH in 63 subjects with carcinoma of the head and neck. When LOH occurred at both p53 and Rb, there was a demonstrable statistically significant correlation with highly aggressive histologic behavior. Data relating LOH and patient survival are offered in Table 5.3.

Table 5.2 Loss of heterozygosity (LOH) in carcinomas of the head and neck. (From data presented by Gleich et al.[27])

Affected gene	LOH in carcinoma (%)
p53	38
Rb	21
p53 and *Rb*	22

Table 5.3 Loss of heterozygosity (LOH) and patient survival with squamous cell carcinoma of the head and neck. (Modified from Gleich et al.[27])

LOH	No. of patients	DOC	AWC	Alive without cancer	Dead of other causes
p53 and Rb	10	6	1	2	1
p53 alone	9	4	0	4	1
Rb alone	11	2	1	7	1
No LOH	33	5	2	20	3

DOC, died of carcinoma; AWC, alive with carcinoma.

The findings of El-Naggar et al.[28] suggest that genetic alterations correspond to histologic changes and that these alterations are restricted to certain chromosomal regions in early non-invasive squamous lesions and are more widely dispersed in invasive lesions, indicating further acquisition of genetic abnormalities during invasion and progression. A little more than one-quarter of pre-invasive, high-grade dysplasias, studied by El-Naggar et al.,[28] manifested LOH at chromosome 9 loci. Other chromosomal loci showed background alterations that did not exceed 15%. In contrast, invasive carcinoma exhibited a high incidence of alterations at chromosomes 3p, 8p, 9p, and 9q, 11q, and 18q. Chromosome 9p, with 75% alterations, had the highest incidence. Carcinomas with LOH at multiple loci had more aggressive biologic features. The incidence of microsatellite instability was 15% in pre-invasive lesions and 30% in invasive carcinomas. No instability was found in normal squamous epithelium. LOH, but not microsatellite instability, was significantly associated with high grade, high stage, and DNA aneuploidy. This may indicate that instability plays only a minor role in the oncogenesis of the carcinomas.

The *Bcl-2* gene

There is a high frequency of occurrence of abnormalities of *Bcl-2* gene structure or expression in many human neoplasms. The term *Bcl-2* is an acronym for B-cell lymphoma/leukemia-2 gene and the gene is the primary regulator of apoptosis. The gene is essential for the protection of normal cells from apoptosis. Bcl-2 oncoproteins are found in the nuclear envelope, mitochondrial membrane and endoplasmic reticulum, and in a variety of normal tissues. Normally, Bcl-2 proteins are found only in basal or proliferating cells.[29]

The structural abnormality (translocation t [14;18]) of the *Bcl-2* gene is confined to one neoplasm—follicular B-cell lymphoma; the deregulation mechanism in other neoplasms is largely unknown.

The histologic significance of *Bcl-2* overexpression in neoplasms has varied widely in different reports. For squamous cell carcinomas of the head and neck, as a group, poor treatment outcome and shorter overall survival have been associated with *Bcl-2* overexpression in the tumor, irrespective of the treatment modality.[30] That type of neoplasm and anatomic site play a significant role in the prognostic significance of *Bcl-2* overexpression are clearly seen in studies dealing with squamous cell carcinomas of the lung and carcinomas of the head and neck. For each of these carcinomas, overexpression of *Bcl-2* was associated with improved survival.[30]

Once again, genetic complexity dictates that expression of a single gene has to be considered in the context of other related genes and gene products. In the case of *Bcl-2*, these are *Bax*, *Bcl-XL*, *Bcl-XS*, and *Bad*.[30] *Bcl-2* is thought to function largely by antagonizing the cell death inducing effect of *Bax*. Should *Bax* expression be impaired, a cancer cell might be able to escape apoptosis even in the presence of a very low *Bcl-2* expression. The observed variation in the significance of *Bcl-2* overexpression alone could likely be due to differences in the prevalence of abnormalities of related genes.

Before ascribing much importance to *Bcl-2* changes in squamous cell carcinoma of the oral cavity, it is necessary to sort out the interrelationships of related genes, test larger patient sample sizes, and determine variations associated with subsites in the head and neck.

DNA content

There have been numerous studies concerning the prognostic impact of DNA patterns in neoplastic cells. Static as well as flow cytometry has been used for the measurement of the DNA patterns. Each method has certain advantages and limitations. The identification of morphologically irrelevant cells is better achieved by using static cytometry. Results based on a high number of registrations can be obtained by flow cytometry. Flow cytometry also allows a better evaluation of S phase.

According to measuring techniques or type of DNA classification, the frequency of DNA non-diploid tumors among head and neck carcinomas has varied in the literature from 41% to 86%.[31] In like manner, different results have been obtained regarding the inter-relationship between histologic grade and tumor ploidy.[32] In general, non-diploid neoplasms are less differentiated than DNA diploid ones. A higher frequency of metastasis to cervical lymph nodes is also associated with non-diploid carcinomas. Aneuploid neoplasms seem to respond better to preoperative radiotherapy than do diploid carcinomas. Stell[33] reviewed a number of publications involving DNA measurements in cancer of the head and neck using meta-analysis. Survival was better for patients with DNA diploid tumors than for those with non-diploid tumors. The influence of site was evident in that subgroup analyses demonstrated that this was due to carcinomas of the oral cavity. DNA ploidy did not affect outcomes for carcinomas of the larynx. Recurrence after radiotherapy was more often associated with diploid carcinomas.

The independent prognostic significance of proliferative indices such as S phase, proliferating cell nuclear antigen (PCNA), and Ki-67 has also varied between published reports.[34,35] Quantitative studies have shown an increase in PCNA expression from normal mucosa to squamous cell carcinoma. In normal epithelium, Ki-67 antigen is confined to isolated cells adjacent to the basal lamina. In dysplastic and in situ lesions, Ki-67-positive cells can be found throughout the full thickness of the mucosal epithelium. In invasive squamous cell carcinomas, there is a concentration of Ki-67 cells at the periphery. Interestingly, when carcinoma cells mature into keratotic pearls, Ki-67 positivity wanes.

In general, the proliferation markers correlate with T stage and histopathologic grading, again raising the question of independence. Ki-67 is the better immunohistochemical marker. There are far more diverse results with PCNA, explainable, in part, by vulnerability of the antigen in prepared sections.

Ploidy status, including proliferation index, can have possible uses as a predictive factor. The basic difference between a prognostic factor and a predictive factor is that prognostic factors are intended to provide information before treatment; a predictive factor, while it contains prognostic information, can also be used to choose between alternative treatments. In studies of squamous cell carcinoma of the head and neck, the degree of aneuploidy (by flow cytometry) has been found to correlate with the response to induction/adjuvant chemotherapy, as a considerably higher response rate is found in non-diploid subgroups.[36]

Epidermal growth factor receptor

The wide-ranging soluble polypeptide growth factors modulate the growth and differentiation of virtually all cell types, and, by binding to specific cell-surface receptors, they mediate diverse biological effects. Activation of receptors induces an intracellular signaling pathway formed by a chain of messenger proteins. Signal processing ends in the nuclei of cells, where activation or inactivation of transcription factors is responsible for altered gene expression. Growth factors, their receptors, or components of their intracellular signaling system are considered to be key elements for determination of a malignant behavior.[37]

Epidermal growth factor receptor (EGFR), in its physiologic role, controls epithelial cell renewal and also affects the regulation of various non-mitogenic events, for example alterations in cellular metabolism, biosynthesis, differentiation, and angiogenesis.

In humans, the EGFR gene *c-erbB* is found on chromosome 7 and is considered to be a proto-oncogene product found in nearly all adult tissues with the exception of hematopoietic cells. The extracellular domain of EGFR is cysteine-rich and binds ligands, including epidermal growth factor, transforming growth factor (TGF) alpha, heparin-binding epidermal growth factor, and others. The intracellular domain is characterized by its intrinsic protein tyrosine kinase activity.

Many squamous carcinoma cell lines manifest high levels of EGFR. Since the receptor overexpression is often accompanied by an increased production of its ligand TGF alpha, an autocrine pathway likely exists that provides tumor cells with signals that may induce and/or maintain a malignant phenotype.[38]

While there is potential clinical value of EGFR expression in squamous cell carcinomas, there is no demonstrable consistent correlation between EGFR expression and clinical parameters or prognosis of disease.[39]

The present status of EGFR in squamous cell carcinoma of the head and neck can be summarized as follows:

1. The frequent overexpression of EGFR in cell lines may be due to the in vitro culture conditions, to some extent.
2. In vivo, the carcinomas often manifest similar or increased EGFR levels as compared to the basal layer of non-malignant mucosa.
3. The oral mucosa from patients with chronic alcohol and nicotine abuse has an increased expression of EGFR.
4. Overexpression of EGFR is not always related to EGFR gene amplification and/or increased levels of receptor MRNA.
5. EGFR expression does not show a definite correlation with differentiation of the carcinomas.
6. There is an apparent involvement of EGFR expression and the multistep process of head and neck squamous cell carcinogenesis.

Proteinases

The exact role that matrix metalloproteinases and proteinase inhibitors play in neoplastic invasion and metastasis is still largely speculative.[40] While it has been consistently observed that these proteins are increased in a wide range of neoplasms, it is unknown which, if any, are necessary for invasion and metastasis to take place. It is also unclear whether the several matrix metalloproteinases function as independent units or whether they are coordinated by an as yet unknown factor.

In the few studies of patients with head and neck cancer, data have been conflicting on a correlation of specific proteinase expression and metastasis.

Observations that the nuclear matrix undergoes characteristic changes during cell differentiation and that transformation from normal to malignant tissue is associated with distinct nuclear matrix alterations have prompted the examination of nuclear matrix proteins in squamous cell carcinoma of the head and neck. Malignant change from normal oropharyngeal mucosa has been found to be associated with nuclear matrix proteins that are absent in normal mucosa and only found in squamous cell carcinomas. Conversely, several proteins present in the nuclear matrix of normal mucosa are not found in squamous carcinomas.

As for the aforementioned metalloproteinases, however, any disposition on the clinical utility of measuring nuclear matrix protein is premature.[41]

Cell surface carbohydrates

Tumor metastases and invasion may be mediated by cell surface carbohydrates.[42,43] A direct correlation between sialylation and metastatic capacity has been observed in several tumor cell lines and specific glycosylation defects are known to result in a loss of metastatic potential.

The involvement of carbohydrates in metastasis implies that tumor cells with different metastatic potentials possess distinct qualitative or quantitative differences in their glycosylation of membrane glycoconjugates. Correlation between lectin binding and axillary node metastasis in cancer of the breast has been shown, but inconsistently. Studies with oral cancer suggest that cell membrane characteristics, particularly density of sugar residues, may be important in determining the metastatic potential of the cancer.[43]

At the risk of premature judgment, we do not expect important developments from further research on alterations of cell surface carbohydrates and metastasis from squamous cell carcinomas of the oral cavity.

A genetic progression model for head and neck squamous cell carcinoma

The assembling of a torrent of molecular/genetic/biologic information in order to develop a model for the initiation and progression of head and neck squamous cell carcinoma to approximate the colorectal model is bearing fruit. Like colorectal cancer, squamous cell carcinomas are thought to progress through a series of definable clinical and histopathologic stages, all accompanied by a multistep process of accumulated genetic alterations.

In a proposed model of tumor progression in squamous cell carcinoma of the head and neck, deletions of chromosomes 3p, 9p, and 17p have been associated with transitions from normal mucosa to dysplasia, while carcinomas are characterized by additional deletions of 4q, 6p, 8p, 11q, 13q, and 14q.[44] Fragile sites are very vulnerable to carcinogen (virus, tobacco, alcohol) induced breakage. The most common fragile site in humans, FRA3B, is at 3p 14.2 and it has been lost or disrupted in about 85% of squamous cell carcinomas of the head and neck.[44]

Candidate genetic lesions for deletions on chromosome 9p and 13q are mutations of tumor suppressor genes p16 and Rb, located at 9p 21.1 and 13q 14, respectively. The *DPC 4* gene at chromosome band 18q 21.1 is not likely a candidate tumor suppressor gene, since squamous carcinomas of the head and neck only rarely carry mutations of the gene.

It has been shown that deletion of chromosomes 3p, 5q, and 9p is preferentially associated with a high degree of neoplastic differentiation.[44] This is also in accord with the proposed tumor progression model in which allelic losses on 9p and 3p are described in precursor lesions.[44] Comparative genomic hybridization studies by Bockmühl et al.[45] suggest that deletions of chromosomes 4q, 8p, 11q, 13q, 18q, and 21q are associated with tumor progression. Of these, 4q, 11q, and 13q have been described as later events in the progression model.

Table 5.4 Basic steps to achieve metastasis

1. Detachment
2. Invasion and intravasation
3. Circulation
4. Stasis
5. Invasion and extravasation
6. Proliferation

Biology of invasion and metastasis

Brodland[46] has likened the three-step process of carcinogenesis (initiation–promotion–progression) to birthing, i.e., conception, gestation, birth of a malignant lesion. While this may be overly simplistic, it puts our current understanding of the specific molecular mechanisms for degrees of malignancy and development of metastases in a novel perspective. It also serves as a preamble to outlining mechanisms of carcinogenesis and metastasis as articulated by Brodland.[46]

Initiation

Prompted by a variety of carcinogenic agents, for example chemicals, or oncoviruses, initiation produces genetic mutations. For the skin and oral mucosa, initiation is so common that mutational events likely occur many times a day. The mutation may persist and be passed on to the initiated cell's progeny. Most initiated cells, however, never progress beyond the first mutation. A second genetic mutation is necessary for malignant progression. The initiated cell can be histologically indistinguishable from its companion cells.

Promotion

This step is a receptor-mediated process that is reversible. For continued clonal expansion of initiated cells, interaction with a promoter is necessary. Promotion increases the likelihood of progression by increasing the number of initiated cells and thereby proportionally increasing the probability of a second genetic mutation. As for initiation, promotion does not inevitably lead to a malignant lesion, and in some instances is bypassed.

Progression

In this step, the histopathologic changes are readily seen by light-optic examination. Progression can be defined as an irreversible genetic mutation that, with time, usually produces an increasingly malignant pheno- and genotype. The genetic instability in progression leads to increasing growth rates, invasiveness, and adaption by cells to exogenous factors. In Borland's analogy,[46] the birth of a malignant lesion is represented by the progression stage of carcinogenesis.

Following the birth of the malignant neoplasm, the advent of metastasis becomes one of the neoplasm's goals. Table 5.4 lists the six steps to achieve metastasis. An outline of each step follows. The steps are complex, inter-related, and require special adaptations by cells to allow viable metastatic colonies to be established and to survive.

1. Detachment: by this maneuver, the cell becomes independent of its need for cell-to-cell interaction and is prepared for the other cellular adaptations in the metastatic process.
2. Invasion and intravasation: invasion appears to be a three-phase process—cell attachment to the vascular basement membrane, enzymatic degradation of intervening tissue, and migration of the cell into the properly prepared tissue. Tumor cells adept in invasion are richly endowed with receptors that are specific for vascular basement membranes or interstitial cells, e.g., fibronectin receptors. Highly invasive cells also manifest large amounts of proteolytic and hydrolytic enzymes that facilitate the invasion. Chemotaxis or an autocrine mobility factor, or both, are the mechanisms for cellular locomotion and migration of the cells. Intravasation refers to the movement of a tumor cell through vessel walls and into the circulation.
3. Circulation: this may be the most common rate-limiting step of the metastatic process since most of the tumor cells die before achieving stasis. Causative factors for cell death in the circulation include physical (turbulence, shearing forces, collisions) and immunologic factors.
4. Stasis: most metastatic lesions are achieved by passive stasis and lodgment in a capillary bed. Site-specific and non-specific patterns of metastases, however, illustrate the great adaptability

of circulating tumor cells in that the processes do not seem to be dependent on either passive mechanical implantation or site-specific receptors.

5. Invasion and extravasation: tumor stasis does not necessarily yield a viable metastasis. Following stasis, there must be extravasation through the endothelial walls and invasion of the recipient tissues. A requisite is that mechanisms for invasion persist and that physical damage to the cells has not been excessive.
6. Proliferation: often a rate-limiting phase, proliferation of a neoplasm in a foreign environment may not be possible. Production of angiogenic factors by the tumor, autocrine growth factors, responsiveness to local growth hormones, and an insensitivity to local growth inhibitors are all prerequisites for effective proliferation.

Current status

Chromosomal abnormalities are common in oral carcinomas, but a consistent abnormality common to all squamous cell carcinomas has not been identified. The majority of autosomal chromosome arms may be affected, with a recurrent clustering of aberrations on several chromosomal regions. These changes are seen both on short arms (p) and on long arms (q) of the chromosomes. These aberrations may be primary (essential to the malignant process) or secondary (appearing during progression of the carcinoma). The range of characteristic, yet not specific, chromosomal aberrations in oral cancer involves particularly chromosomes 1, 3, 5, 8, 9, 11, 14, 15, and 17. Clustering is especially noted with chromosomes 1, 9, and 4 at positions 1p22, 11q13, 1p36, 9q32, and 11q32.[1]

Allelic loss, considered an early event in oral carcinogenesis, has been especially noted on chromosomes 9p, 3p, and 17p. Chromosome 9 is noteworthy because of the high frequency of allelic loss and the presence of a multiple tumor suppressor gene (MTS-1).[1]

Microsatellite instability is most likely a separate pathogenic mechanism in oral carcinogenesis and has been noted in a number of chromosome sites, including 3p, 6p, 7q, 9p, 11p, and 11q.[1]

Allelotypic analysis is promising since not only does it provide information on accumulated genetic damage, but it may evolve as a useful molecular indication of the behavior of squamous cell carcinoma.

We conclude this section on genetic alterations in squamous cell carcinoma of the head and neck with a comparison of these alterations between English-speaking countries and India and Southeast Asia (Table 5.5).[47] The most striking difference is seen in the prevalence of *p53* mutations, wherein they are infrequent in the Indian subcontinent (7%) but are common in oral carcinomas in England, USA, and Australia (47%). In the West, the *p53* gene in tumors was mutated in a range of codons from exons 4 to 9, with particular 'hot spots' between codons 205 and 248. Multiple genetic abnormalities characterize tumors from India and Southeast Asia, with a preponderance of *H-ras* mutations (35%), LOH of *H-ras* (30%), *N-ras* amplification (28%), and *N-myc* amplification (29%). Interestingly, changes in both *ras* and *myc* are not prevalent in tumors from Europe/USA.[47]

Table 5.5 Genetic alterations in oral squamous cell carcinoma. (Modified from Patterson et al.[47])

Genetic abnormality	Percentage reported: USA, England, Australia	Percentage reported: India, Southeast Asia
1. Mutations		
p53	47.6	7.3
H-ras	6.1	35.0
K-ras	0	6.6
N-ras	0	0
2. Amplifications		
EGF-R	6.2	29.0
C-myc	14.9	20.0
N-myc	0	28.8
L-myc	0	0
H-ras	0	0
K-ras	0	17.3
N-ras	0	28.0
3. LOH *H-ras*	0	30.4

[a]Only gene mutations and amplifications confirmed by DNA sequencing, SSCP or Southern analysis, respectively, are included.

Epigenetic and non-genetic factors

With increasing knowledge of the genetics of cancer has come the appreciation that epigenetic, dysgenetic, and non-genetic factors also play important roles in the process of tumorigenesis. These are, as yet, poorly understood. Whereas genetic events are the consequence of damage to the base sequences, epigenetic events originate from all other alterations affecting DNA and chromosome structures, for example methylation, and a relaxation of genomic imprinting.[48] Such epigenetic changes are effectors of genetic instability via interference with the fidelity of DNA replication and can also lead to a mutator phenotype. Alteration in gene expression leading to genetic instability is the basis of cellular dysgenetics and explains why not all mutations have alterations in chromosomes as the primary cause of the neoplastic progression.

The foregoing non-genetic factors may hold the key to differences in the susceptibility of cells to the development of cancer. Integral to this possibility is tumor promotion, whereby cells enter a program of stress response called activation. Cell activation involves an increase of the replicative life span of the cells and presumably a disturbance of its regulation, leading to genetic instability.

Table 5.6 Causes of chemotherapy and radiotherapy failure. (As proposed by Rew[49])

1. Passive mechanisms
   - structural and genetic heterogeneity of the neoplasm
   - abnormal vascularity and faulty drug perfusion
   - altered physiologic environment (hypoxia, pH)

II. Active mechanisms
   - DNA repair mechanisms
   - expulsion of unwanted drugs (cell membrane-bound pumps)
   - intracellular drug detoxification (e.g. the glutathione system)
   - increased production, genetic up-regulation, and compensation for specific molecular damage
   - proliferation of quiescent clones as compensation for damage and destruction of other cells
   - enhancement of cell survival by downregulation of apoptosis
   - selection and emergence of resistant cell clones (e.g. paradoxical drug resistance) by topoisomerase expression in surviving cells

Therapeutic implications of molecular biology of solid tumors

The ever increasing database on the biology of solid tumors, including oral cancer, has dispelled an earlier mirage of a 'magic bullet' in the non-surgical management of cancer. Every so-called 'breakthrough' and discovery of another 'novel marker' has been followed by an appreciation of the exquisite complexity, subtlety, and indeed, sophistication of the biologic problem. Because of this, treatment gains are likely to be incremental rather than a single, dramatic exposition.[49] As the cellular and molecular biology of cancer advances, authors are shifting their emphasis from diagnostic/prognostic markers to the interruption of regulatory mechanisms of specific aspects of the biology of cancer as prospective therapy. An example is the development of antimetastatic strategies based on the current understanding of the metastatic cascade. Many are predicated on the essential role of matrix-degrading proteases necessary for new vessel formation. Synthetic matrix metalloproteinase(s) inhibitors are known to inhibit human endothelial cell invasion through a reconstituted basement membrane. Other inhibitors of angiogenesis, directed both at cell adhesion molecules and/or proteases, underscore the fundamental comparability between angiogenesis and tumor invasion.[50]

As well as metastasis, nearly every event in the neoplastic process has served as a potential target for new therapeutic strategies. Practically every report of these events concludes with an almost obligatory statement regarding potential therapeutic exploitation. Fortunately, Rew[49] has masterfully summarized many of these efforts and the following is a distillation of his summary. Non-surgical treatment, however, is faced with a host of persistent causes of failure (Table 5.6).

Treatment strategies based on cellular and molecular mechanisms may be divided into conventional or novel categories.[49] An overlap does exist.

Conventional drug treatments have historically been targeted at DNA replication and cellular proliferation, an outcome of the belief that cell production alone was the key to cancer progression.[49] Many of the therapeutic agents in this category may have secondary or alternative modes of action, for example interference with other processes, such as apoptosis. An exploitation of these modes has led to the development of a new range of therapeutic options by combining conventional agents with others such as calcium channel antagonists, for example.

Novel treatments include gene transfer, viral vectors, and immune targeting mechanisms.[49]

Impairment of cell proliferation has been a goal for adjuvant therapy and many drugs can be shown to act selectively in various cell cycle phases. Indeed, the drugs are often defined by their action in

Table 5.7 Characteristics of an effective modulator of neoplastic growth. (As proposed by Rew[49])

1. Reaches all target cells with proliferation potential, particularly neoplastic stem cells
2. Effectively inhibits proliferation or cell division or induces cytostasis or apoptosis
3. Overcomes intrinsic homeostatic and 'drug resistance' mechanisms
4. Overcomes problems imposed by hypoxia, deficient vasculature, abnormal interstitial pressures and pH
5. Possesses an acceptable route, mechanism and frequency of administration
6. Has satisfactory therapeutic ratio, acceptable incidence of side-effects, and produces demonstrable improvement in survival rather than response

relation to DNA synthesis and the cell cycle. Efficacy (therapeutic index) for a drug is based on its greater selectivity for malignant than normal cells.[49] Unfortunately, efforts at disruption of proliferation have not generally been successful and suggest that altered proliferation rates are not a satisfactory explanation of neoplasia. The outcome of therapy based only on cell cycle strategies is bedeviled by the complexity, asynchrony, and heterogeneity of proliferation within the solid tumors; local cell depletion acts as a potent stimulus for reactivation and proliferation of quiescent cells.[49,51]

Increase in cell loss can be as important as a reduction in cell proliferation in determining the clinical progression or arrest of a neoplasm. Many of the cytotoxic drugs which disrupt the cell cycle can also induce apoptosis in neoplastic cells. However, as Rew[49] indicates, there is controversy over the significance and usefulness of apoptosis as a target for drug therapy. Apoptosis may only be a final common pathway for many different initial mechanisms of cell damage.

Another therapeutic strategy is the modulation of tumor growth. Possible targets for cell modulation include cell signaling pathways, enzyme systems, for example protein kinases, oncoproteins, and mechanisms of metastasis. Table 5.7 presents several characteristics of an effective modulating agent as proposed by Rew.[49] A group of drugs which have shown considerable success for a modulating strategy is the hormonally targeted drugs used in breast and prostate cancer.

Novel adjuvant therapies such as immune targeting, antibody-directed therapy, and gene transfer therapy are designed to be extremely selective and specific for target cells. Such features are found in monoclonal antibodies and viruses.

Monoclonal antibodies have been used with success to supplement conventional imaging techniques in the localization of neoplasms. They have the potential for use in therapy, either alone or for targeted delivery of a cytotoxic agent or radioisotope. Problems of antigenicity (systematic or tumor-related) and the risk of anaphylactic and other immunological reactions have not been defined or overcome.[49] Finally, intravenous delivery has with it the likelihood of imperfect diffusion to target cells.

The hope of gene transfer therapy is to introduce corrective genetic signals into abnormal cells. Targets may be somatic or germ cell lines. Various forms of cancer are only a subset of candidate diseases which include metabolic disorders, cystic fibrosis, immune deficiency disorders, and hemoglobinopathies.

Gene transfer techniques which have been employed include immune enhancement, vectoring of biologicals, for example tissue-specific viruses, tissue protection as with bone marrow, selective drug activation by specific genes, and correction of somatic defects.

Any of the gene transfers first require identification of a specific gene and molecular mechanisms in order to achieve a desired cytotoxic or cytostatic effect. Following that, the therapeutic agent must be vectored (for example by a viral agent) into each neoplastic cell, or at least every cancer stem cell.[49] These strategies presuppose knowledge of and identification of stem cells, and the very important existence of a specific tumor antigenicity.

Forms of adoptive immunotherapy also require identification of a tumor antigen in squamous cell carcinoma. Many tumor proteins could potentially function as an antigen to elicit a specific immune response to squamous cell carcinoma tumor cells. That may be the stumbling block—too many antigens and not one that is species rather than individual carcinoma specific. Mutations, of both the *ras* oncogene and the *p53* suppression gene, have been demonstrated to be immunogenic in vitro, but in vivo data are scant.

If antigenic proteins are processed and appropriate conditions are found, binding of the peptides to class I MHC molecules could lead to a CD8+ peptide-specific T cell response, while association of the peptides with class II molecules could yield a CD4T cell response. Both effector arms are potentially useful in modulating tumor growth, mediating cytolysis through either tumor cell apoptosis or by inhibiting angiogenesis. Now to find the candidate antigen!

Other new techniques include genetic pro-drug activation therapy and differential display polymerase chain reaction (for preparation of catalogues of gene expression for individual tumors). Another is immunotherapy using a recombinant vaccine encoding human papilloma virus genes E6 and E7 to generate specific cytotoxic T cells in vivo.[49]

To date, the targeting of the unique physiology of solid tumors for anticancer therapy has not received as much attention as methods based on the cellular and molecular differences between transformed and untransformed cells.

The majority of the differences between the physiology of normal tissues and that of solid tumors stem from differences between the two vasculatures.[52] Research for selective cancer treatment exploiting these differences can be divided into:

1. Hypoxia-selective cytotoxins to take advantage of the unique low oxygen tension in most human solid tumors;
2. Use of the long intravascular half-life of sterically stabilized liposomes to selectively accumulate in the tumors;
3. Inhibition of angiogenesis;
4. Gene therapy activated by the low oxygen environment or necrotic regions of tumors.

Hypoxia-selective cytotoxins The targeting of drug cytotoxicity and/or anticancer drug potentiation to hypoxic cells in solid tumors turns the low oxygen levels in tumors from a disadvantage to an advantage. The killing of hypoxic cells has a greater therapeutic potential than oxygenating the cells or chemically sensitizing them to chemo- or radiotherapy. As Brown and Giaccia[52] point out, the cells killed are the ones resistant to conventional therapy and the hypoxia is more tumor specific. Another significant advantage of hypoxia-selective cytotoxins is their potential to enhance the killing by standard anticancer drugs. Brown and Siim[53] review the clinical activities of these drugs.

Liposomes The leakiness of tumor vessels with their inherent increased permeability has permitted specific targeting of anticancer drugs to tumors using specifically modified liposomes. The attractiveness of allowing high tumor concentrations via liposomes is countered by the fact that the distribution of the liposomes is very heterogeneous and concentrated in perivascular interstitium.[52]

Antiangiogenesis The significance of angiogenesis to neoplastic growth and metastasis has already been presented in this section. Theoretically, antiangiogenesis therapy has some important advantages over standard anticancer treatment.[52]

- It targets a process that is quite tumor specific and hence there is little systemic toxicity.
- With an endothelial cell target, there is a closer proximity to tumor cells.
- The genetic stability of endothelial cells should inhibit development of drug resistance.

While the odds are not insurmountable in developing an effective antiangiogenesis strategy, it must be recalled that different angiogenic molecules regulate distinct steps in the process of angiogenesis. This suggests that any given molecule may be necessary, but is in itself insufficient for the establishment of a viable microvasculature. VEGF and/or its two high-affinity receptors expressed in endothelial cells are the most promising targets. In addition to its specific and potent vascular endothelial mitogenic activity, VEGF also increases vascular permeability.

Gene therapy In this novel approach to anticancer therapy, genetic material is transferred into cells by a variety of techniques with the goal of a selective destruction of cancer cells and sparing of normal cells. Currently, this selective kill is being achieved either by controlling vector delivery and activity or by transgene expression. In exploiting tumor physiology, the hypoxic stress response (the regulation of gene induction by hypoxia) could allow activation of a non-toxic prodrug to a toxic metabolite.[54] However, as with most forms of gene therapy, the targeting of constructs to the tumor remains a significant obstacle.

What does the future hold?

Molecular pathology, and with it molecular-based therapy, is poised to enter the post-genome era. Predicated on the human genome project, with its identification of approximately 19 000 genes, plus tens of thousands of fragments (tentatively identified as partial fragments of genes) termed expressed sequence tags (ESTs), the post-genome era will be driven by high technology, e.g. tissue microarray profiling of cancer specimens and cell lines.[55] The advent of cDNA microarray technology allows effective measurement of the expression of almost every gene in the human genome in a single overnight hybridization experiment. The majority of genes, however, have been only partially characterized and the functions of most are as yet unknown. Because of this, while it may be avant-garde to suggest a 'novel classification of human malignancies based on gene expression' or a 'genetic-based classification',[56,57] it is premature and, unless digested with care, will lead to another decade of superficial exposition.[58–60]

References

1. Scully C, Field JK. Genetic aberrations in squamous cell carcinoma of the head and neck (SCCHB) with reference to oral carcinoma (review). Int J Oncol 1997; 10: 5–21
2. Henriksson M, Lüscher B. Proteins of the Myc network: essential regulators of cell growth and differentiation. Adv Cancer Res 1996; 68: 109–182
3. Knudson AG Jr. Mutation and cancer: statistical study of retinoblastoma. Proc Natl Acad Sci 1971; 68: 820–823
4. Knudson AG Jr. Genetics of tumors of the head and neck. Arch Otolaryngol Head Neck Surg 1993; 119: 735–737
5. Williams BO, Remington L, Albert DM. Cooperative tumorigenic effects of germline mutations in *Rb* and *p53*. Nature Genet 1994; 7: 480–484
6. Jones JW, Raval JR, Beals TF et al. Frequent loss of heterozygosity on chromosome arm 18q in squamous cell carcinomas. Identification of 2 regions of loss—18q 11.1–q12.3 and 18q 21.1–q23. Arch Otolaryngol Head Neck Surg 1997; 123: 610–108
7. Hall M, Peters G. Genetic alterations of cyclins, cyclin-dependent kinases, and Cdk inhibitors in human cancer. Adv Cancer Res 1996; 68: 67–108
8. Gao CY, Zelenka PS. Cyclins, cyclin-dependent kinases and differentiation. Bio-Essays 1997; 19: 307–315
9. Rudoltz MS, Kao G, Blank KR et al. Molecular biology of the cell cycle: potential for therapeutic applications in radiation oncology. Semin Rad Oncol 1996; 6: 284–294
10. Lammie GA, Peters G. Chromosome 11q13 abnormalities in human cancer. Cancer Cells 1991; 3: 413–420
11. Hunter T, Pines J. Cyclins and cancer II: cyclin D and CDK inhibitors come of age. Cell 1994; 4: 573–582
12. Sugarman PB, Joseph BK, Savage NW. Review article: the role of oncogenes, tumour suppressor genes and growth factors in oral squamous cell carcinoma: a case of apoptosis versus proliferation. Oral Dis 1995; 1: 172–188
13. Greenblatt MS, Bennett WP, Holstein M et al. Mutations in the *p53* tumour suppressor gene: clues to cancer etiology and molecular pathogenesis. Cancer Res 1994; 54: 4855–4878
14. Batsakis JG, El-Naggar AE. *p53*: fifteen years after discovery. Adv Anat Pathol 1995; 2: 71–88
15. Ogden GR, Hall PA. Field changes, clonality and early epithelial cancer: possible lessons from *p53*. J Pathol 1997; 181: 127–129
16. Ko LJ, Prives C. *p53*: puzzle and paradigm. Genes Develop 1996; 10: 1054–1072
17. Yandel DW, Thor AD. *p53* analysis in diagnostic pathology. Biologic implications and possible clinical applications. Diagn Mol Pathol 1993; 2: 1–3
18. Dowell SP, Hall PA. The *p53* tumour suppressor gene and tumour prognosis. Is there a relationship? J Pathol 1995; 177: 221–224
19. Crosthwaite N, Teale D, Franklin C et al. *p53* protein expression in malignant, premalignant and non-malignant lesions of the lip. J Clin Pathol 1996; 49: 648–653
20. Boyle JO, Hakim J, Koch W et al. The incidence of *p53* mutations increases with progression of head and neck cancer. Cancer Res 1993; 53: 4477–4480
21. Brennan JA, Mao L, Hruban RH et al. Molecular assessment of histopathologic staging in squamous cell carcinoma of the head and neck. N Engl J Med 1995; 332: 429–435
22. Chang EH, Jang Y-J, Hao Z et al. Restoration of the G1 checkpoint and the apoptotic pathway mediated by wild-type *p53* sensitizes squamous cell carcinoma of the head and neck to radiotherapy. Arch Otolaryngol Head Neck Surg 1997; 123: 507–512
23. Jain V, Das SN, Luthra K et al. Differential expression of multi-drug resistance gene products, p-glycoproteins in normal, dysplastic, and malignant oral mucosa in India. Int J Cancer (Pred Oncol) 1997; 74: 128–133
24. Goodison S, Tarin D. Review: current status of *CD 44* variant isoforms as cancer diagnostic markers. Histopathology 1998; 32: 1–6
25. Roz L, Lee C, Porter S et al. Allelic imbalance on chromosome 3 in squamous cell carcinoma of the oral cavity. Cancer Res 1994; 54: 6481–6488
26. Tsuji T, Mimura Y, Kanekawa A et al. Increased polysomy 3 and 17 detected by fluorescence in situ hybridization (FISH) in oral squamous cell carcinoma. Oncol Rep 1997; 4: 277–280
27. Gleich LL, Biddinger PW, Gartside PS et al. The loss of heterozygosity in retinoblastoma and *p53* suppressor genes as a prognostic indicator for head and neck cancer. Laryngoscope 1996; 106: 1378–1381
28. El-Naggar AK, Goepfert H, Batsakis JG. Molecular genetic analysis of head and neck squamous tumorigenesis by microsatellite markers. In: Werner JA, Lippert BM, Rudert HH (eds). Head and neck cancer—advances in basic research. Amsterdam: Elsevier, 1996: 169–177
29. Pezzella F, Gattu K. What is the value of Bcl-2 protein detection for histopathologists? Histopathology 1995; 26: 89–93
30. Friedman M, Grey P, Venkatesan TK et al. Prognostic significance of *Bcl-2* expression in localized squamous cell carcinoma of the head and neck. Ann Otol Rhinol Laryngol 1997; 106: 445–450
31. Baretton G, Li X, Stoll C et al. Prognostic significance of DNA ploidy in oral squamous cell carcinoma. A retrospective flow and image cytometric study with comparison of DNA ploidy in exisional biopsy specimens and resection specimens, primary tumors and lymph node metastases. Oral Surg Oral Med Oral Pathol Oral Radiol Endod 1995; 79: 68–76
32. Tytor M, Olofsson J, Ledin T et al. Squamous cell carcinoma of the oral cavity. A review of 176 cases with application of malignancy grading and DNA measurements. Clin Otolaryngol 1990; 15: 235–251

33. Stell PM. Ploidy in head and neck cancer: a review and meta-analysis. Clin Otolaryngol 1991; 16: 510–516
34. Störkel S, Reichert T, Reiffen KA et al. EGFR and PCNA expression in oral squamous cell carcinoma—a valuable tool in estimating the patient's prognosis. Oral Oncol Eur J Cancer 1993; 29B: 273–277
35. Slootweg PJ, Koole K, Hordijk GJ. The presence of p53 protein in relation to Ki-67 as cellular proliferation marker in head and neck squamous cell carcinoma in adjacent dysplastic mucosa. Oral Oncol Eur J Cancer 1994; 30B: 138–141
36. Tennvall J, Wennerberg J, Anderson H et al. DNA analysis as a predictor of the outcome of induction chemotherapy in advanced head and neck carcinomas. Arch Otolaryngol Head Neck Surg 1993; 119: 867–870
37. Hsuan JJ. Oncogene regulation by growth factors. Anticancer Res 1993; 13: 2521–2532
38. Christensen ME, Therkildsen MH, Hansen BL et al. Epidermal growth factor receptor expression on oral mucosa dysplastic epithelia and squamous cell carcinoma. Eur Arch Otorhinolaryngol 1992; 249: 243–247
39. Bier H, Hoffman T. Epidermal growth factor receptor in head and neck squamous cell carcinomas. In: Werner JA, Lippert BM, Rudert HH (eds). Head and neck cancer—advances in basic research. Amsterdam: Elsevier, 1996: 225–234
40. Charous SJ, Stricklin GP, Netterville JL et al. Expression of matrix metalloproteinases and tissue inhibitor of metalloproteinases in head and neck squamous cell carcinomas. Ann Otol Rhinol Laryngol 1997; 106: 271–278
41. McCaffery JD, Gagany M, Faust RA et al. Nuclear matrix proteins as malignant markers in squamous cell carcinoma of the head and neck. Arch Otolaryngol Head Neck Surg 1997; 123: 283–288
42. Dennis JW, Laferte S. Tumor cell surface carbohydrate and the metastatic phenotype. Cancer Metast Rev 1987; 5: 185–204
43. Remani P, Bhattahiri VN, Bindu L et al. Correlation of lectin binding with lymph node metastasis in oral cancer. Oral Oncol 1997; 33: 19–22
44. Califano J, van der Rict P, Westra W et al. Genetic progression model for head and neck cancer: implications for field cancerization. Cancer Res 1996; 56: 2488–2492
45. Bockmühl U, Wolf G, Schmidt S et al. Genomic alterations associated with malignancy in head and neck cancer. Head Neck 1998; 20: 145–151
46. Brodland DG. The life of a skin cancer. Mayo Clin Proc 1997; 72: 475–478
47. Patterson IC, Eveson JW, Prime SS. Molecular changes in oral cancer may reflect an etiology and ethnic origin. Oral Oncol Eur J Cancer 1996; 32B: 150–153
48. Simons JWIM. Genetic, epigenetic, dysgenetic, and non-genetic mechanisms in tumorigenesis. Crit Rev Oncogen 1995; 6: 261–273
49. Rew DA. Cell and molecular mechanisms of pathogenesis and treatment of cancer. Postgrad Med J 1998; 74: 77–78
50. Ahmed A, Hart IR. Mechanism of metastasis. Crit Rev Oncol/Hematol 1997; 26: 163–173
51. Rew DA. Heterogeneity, biodiversity and bioperversity in human solid tumours. Eur J Surg Oncol 1996; 22: 469–473
52. Brown JM, Giaccia AJ. The unique physiology of solid tumors: opportunities (and problems) for cancer therapy. Cancer Res 1998; 58: 1408–1416
53. Brown JM, Siim BG. Hypoxia-specific cytotoxins in cancer therapy. Semin Rad Oncol 1996; 6: 22–36
54. Dachs GU, Patterson AV, Firth JD et al. Targeting gene expression to hypoxic tumor cells. Nature Med 1997; 3: 515–520
55. Hoos A, Cordon-Cardo C. Tissue microarray profiling of cancer specimens and cell lines: opportunities and limitations. Lab Invest 2001; 81: 1331–1338
56. Alizadeh AA, Ross DT, Perou CM et al. Towards a novel classification of human malignancies based on gene expression patterns. J Pathol 2001; 195: 41–52
57. Petersen I, Petersen S. Towards a genetic-based classification of human lung cancer. Anal Cellular Pathol 2001; 22: 111–122
58. Jefferies S, Foulkes WD. Genetic mechanisms in squamous cell carcinoma of the head and neck. Oral Oncol 2001; 37: 115–126
59. Baumann M, Bentzen SM, Doerr W et al. The translational research chain: is it delivering the goods? Int J Radiat Oncol Biol Phys 2001; 49: 345–351
60. Grainger DJ. Human gene therapy: are we still expecting too much, too soon? Q J Med 2001; 94: 337–339

II Clinical Management

6 Clinical evaluation and differential diagnosis

John F Carew, Bhuvanesh Singh and Jatin P Shah

The oral cavity is that part of the upper aerodigestive tract which extends from the mucocutaneous junction at the vermilion border of the lips to the anterior surface of the faucial arch. It is lined by squamous epithelium containing interspersed minor salivary glands and it also contains dentoalveolar structures which support the upper and lower dentition. Primary tumors of the oral cavity may arise from the surface epithelium, minor salivary glands or submucous soft tissues, as well as from dental structures, bone or neurovascular tissues.

The oral cavity is the most predominant location in the head and neck region for primary malignant epithelial tumors. Over 30 000 new cases of cancer of the oral cavity are diagnosed in the United States yearly and 90% of these cases are squamous cell carcinomas.[1,2] A majority of patients with cancer in the oral cavity are males, although a rising incidence has been observed in females over the past 50 years (Fig. 6.1).[3] The designated anatomic sites in the oral cavity described by the UICC/AJCC staging system are shown in Fig. 6.2.[4]

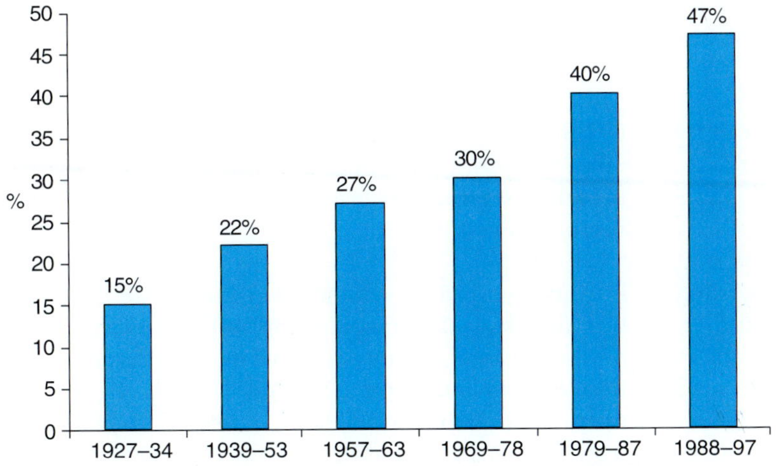

Figure 6.1 Rising incidence of squamous carcinoma of the oral tongue in women as observed at Memorial Sloan-Kettering Cancer Center, New York.

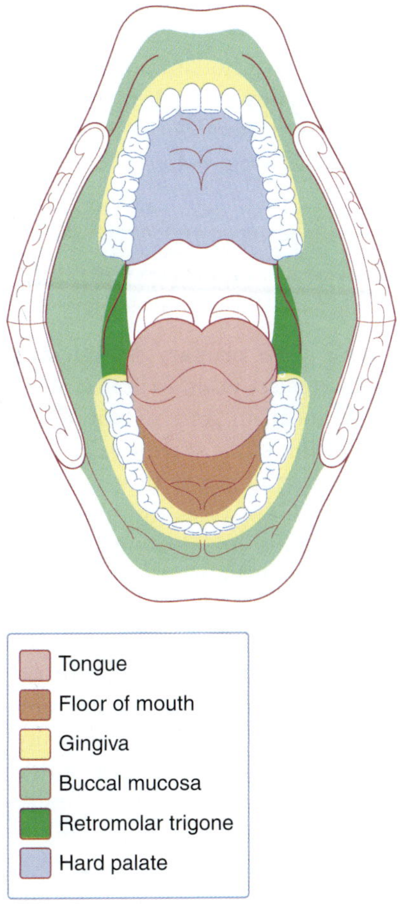

Figure 6.2 Anatomic sites in the oral cavity.

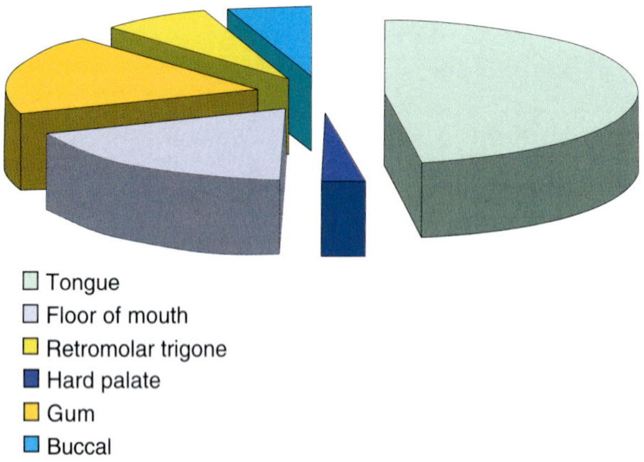

Figure 6.3 Site distribution for squamous carcinomas of the oral cavity at MSKCC (1985–2000).

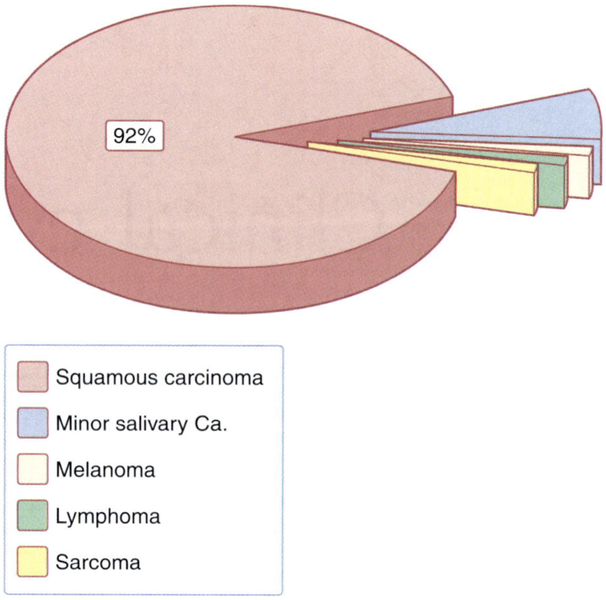

Figure 6.4 Histological distribution for primary malignant tumors of the oral cavity.

The tongue and floor of the mouth are the most common sites of origin for primary squamous cell carcinomas in the oral cavity in the Western world.[1] Retromolar trigone and buccal mucosa are, however, the most frequently encountered primary sites in those parts of the world where tobacco chewing and chewing of betel nuts are most prevalent.[5] The site distribution for primary squamous cancers of the oral cavity in the United States is shown in Fig. 6.3. The frequency of each histologic variant of primary malignant tumors of the oral cavity and oropharynx is shown in Fig. 6.4.

Clinical presentation

Patients with primary malignant tumors in the oral cavity present with a variety of symptoms according to the location and extent of the primary tumor. Superficial, early stage tumors most often present as non-healing ulcers with varying degrees of pain, and occasional episodes of bleeding from the lesion. These tumors are usually present for several weeks to a few months before most patients seek medical attention. Occasionally a suspicious lesion may be identified by the dentist during routine dental examination in asymptomatic patients. Superficial ulcerations and early tumors are often assumed to be non-neoplastic lesions and are treated with oral rinses, topical therapy, or antibiotics. Very early lesions on the gum or the alveolar process can often be mistaken for sepsis around a tooth socket and treated as gingivitis or dental infection. Lack of response to conservative treatment or the presence of a loose tooth, however, should immediately raise suspicion of a malignant process necessitating biopsy to establish tissue diagnosis. The presence of an exophytic lesion with several contiguous loose teeth should raise the index of suspicion for a locally advanced malignant tumor of the gum. A history of a non-healing extraction site should also raise the suspicion of a neoplastic process in a patient who has undergone recent tooth extraction. An ill-fitting denture may be the presenting symptom in some patients with cancer of the gum or palate. In contrast to ulceration, some tumors present as exophyptic growths which may be white to pink in color. Friability and surface bleeding are often a prominent feature. Some white lesions present as papillary growths so characteristic of a verrucous carcinoma.

Further symptoms related to difficulty in mastication and speech often develop with increasing size of the lesion or invasion of the underlying soft tissues and musculature. Very advanced lesions cause significant local pain, referred otalgia, and restriction in the mobility of the tongue. Excessive salivation with reduced mobility of the tongue is an ominous sign and usually suggests a far advanced carcinoma of the oral tongue. Impairment in the oral phase of swallowing with the resultant pooling of saliva and distortion of speech may also result from the continued growth of oral cavity tumors. With further progression and delay of treatment, tumor growth can result in impairment of mastication and deglutition. Oral consumption of food may be restricted to soft foods and patients may lose significant weight. Advanced lesions with invasion of the mandible and the inferior alveolar nerve may produce anesthesia of the skin of the chin. Halitosis secondary to a fungating necrotic tumor is present in some patients with massive lesions. Progressive trismus is a manifestation of local progression of tumor in the masticator space and pterygomaxillary region with invasion of the pterygoid muscles. However, it must be borne in mind that trismus may also be related to chronic submucous fibrosis in patients with a habit of chewing tobacco or betel nuts.[6]

Lesions of the anterior floor of the mouth may cause obstruction of the opening of the Wharton's ducts, leading to obstructive submandibular sialadenitis and a palpable mass in the submandibular region, which may be the presenting symptom.[7] Occasionally, a palpable cervical metastatic lymph node is the presenting symptom of patients with primary cancer in the oral cavity.

The clinical characteristics of the primary tumor arising on the mucosal surface of the oral cavity are variable. The tumor may be ulcerative, exophytic, endophytic, or it may be a superficial proliferative lesion. The visible features of the lesion are usually sufficient to raise the index of suspicion regarding the need for a biopsy to establish tissue diagnosis. Ulcerative lesions are usually accompanied by an irregular edge and induration of the underlying soft tissues. On the other hand, exophytic lesions may present either as a cauliflower-like irregular growth, or they may be flat, pink to pinkish-white proliferative lesions. Occasionally, a red to pink velvety flat lesion is the only manifestation of superficially invasive cancer or carcinoma in situ. Bleeding from the surface of the lesion should raise the suspicion of a neoplasm. Squamous carcinoma with excessive keratin production and verrucous carcinoma present as white, heaped-up lesions with varying degrees of keratin debris on the surface. Papillary projections are often seen in lesions which are accompanied or preceded by a squamous papilloma. Endophytic lesions have a very small surface component but have a substantial amount of soft tissue involvement beneath the surface. Leukoplakia and erythroplakia have a varying incidence of malignancy.[8,9] Speckled leukoplakia has a particularly high incidence of malignant transformation.[10] Multiple primary cancers occur synchronously in approximately 2% of patients with oral cancers.[11] Therefore, a thorough examination of the oral cavity should be performed in every case.

Squamous cell carcinomas, whether exophytic or endophytic, present as lesions arising from, or intimately related to, the surface epithelium. Whenever a lesion is encountered in the oral cavity that is below the epithelium, another differential diagnosis should be considered. These tumors may arise from the structures beneath the mucosa or represent metastatic disease from other sites. Tumors of minor salivary origin present as submucosal masses and most commonly occur where the greatest density of minor salivary glands are found—the hard palate.[12] When these lesions become large, however, the overlying mucosa may ulcerate making it difficult to determine their submucosal origin. Sarcomas may also arise from the soft tissues beneath the mucosa thus presenting as a submucosal mass. Finally, lesions may occasionally involve the epithelium but arise from structures not normally found in the mucosa lining the oral cavity. One example is mucosal melanoma, which may present as a pigmented or non-pigmented lesion of the oral cavity mucosa. Brownish-black pigmented lesions are very characteristic of mucosal melanoma. However, it must be borne in mind that melanosis is quite common in the black population of African descent and those of Asian origin (Figs 6.5–6.65).

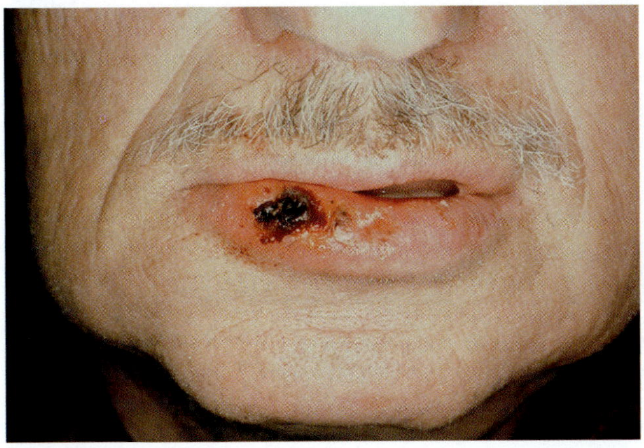

Figure 6.5 Ulcerated superficially invasive squamous cell carcinoma of the lower lip.

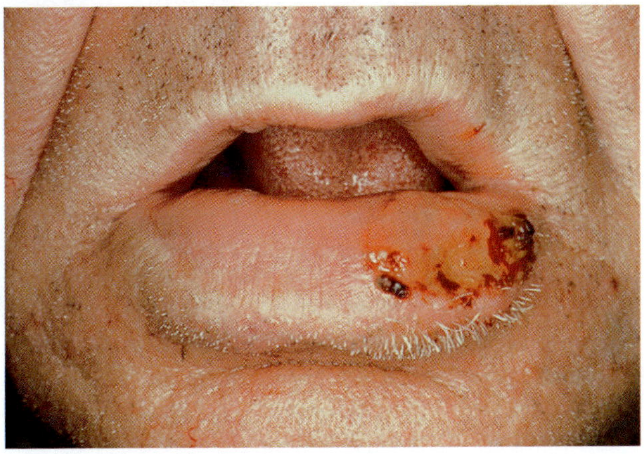

Figure 6.6 Chronic inflammatory ulceration of the vermilion border of the lower lip.

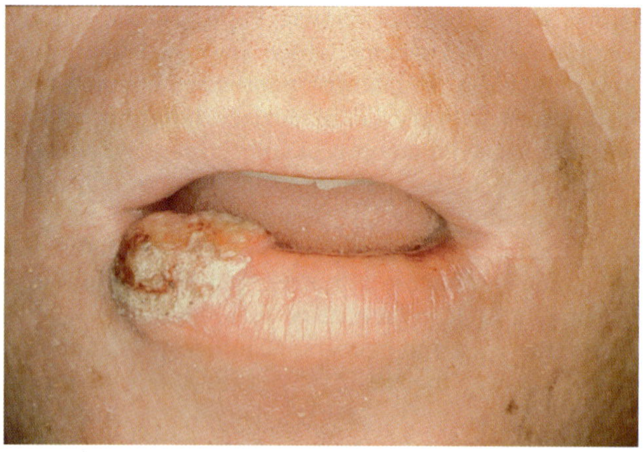

Figure 6.7 Exophytic, well-differentiated, keratinizing squamous cell carcinoma of the lower lip adjacent to the commissure.

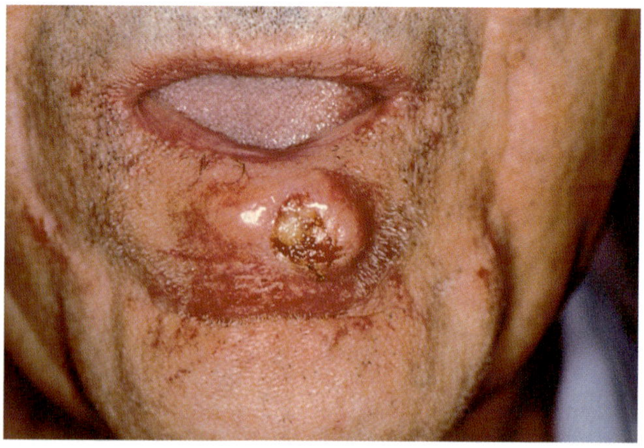

Figure 6.8 Squamous cell carcinoma of the lower lip with invasion of the deep musculature.

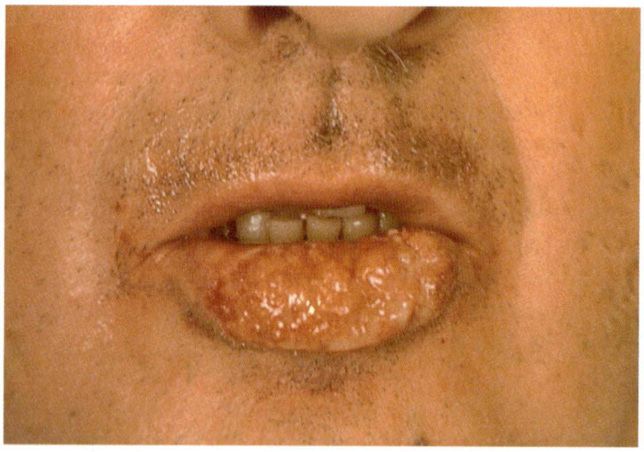

Figure 6.9 Superficial extensive carcinoma of the vermilion border of the lower lip.

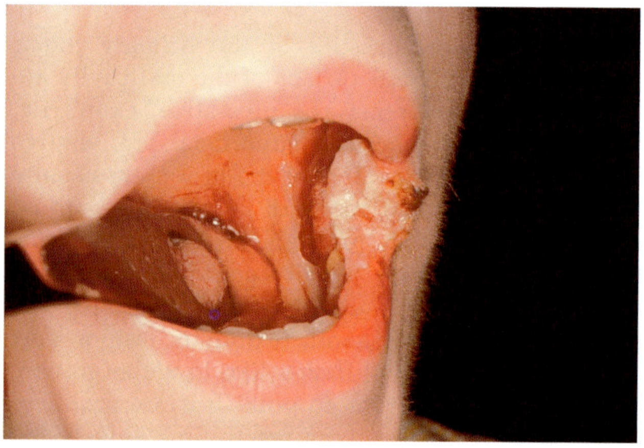

Figure 6.10 Squamous cell carcinoma of the oral commissure extending to the cheek mucosa.

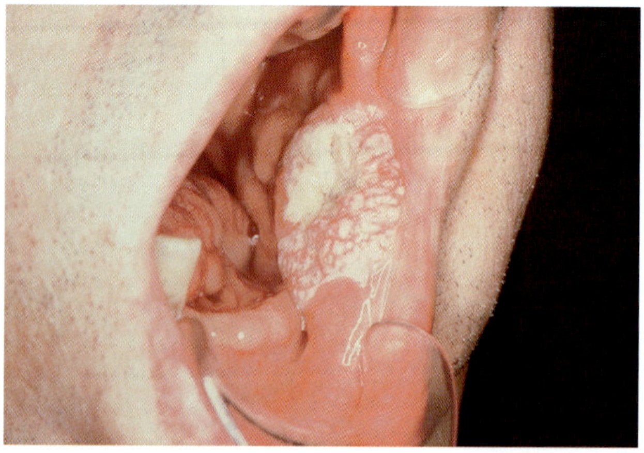

Figure 6.11 Papillary verrucous carcinoma of the oral commissure with extension to the cheek mucosa.

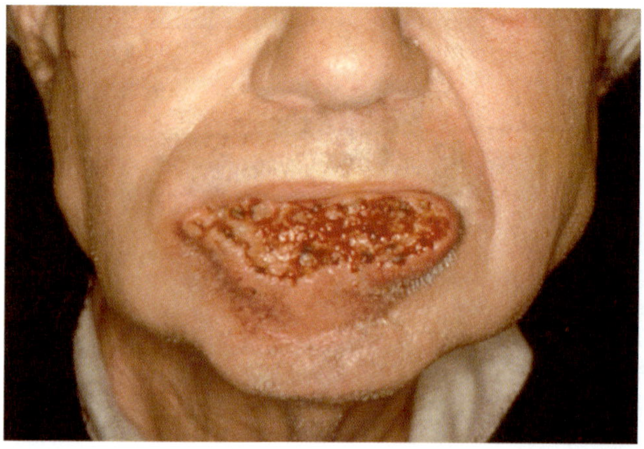

Figure 6.12 Massive carcinoma of the lower lip with invasion of the skin, soft tissues and mandible.

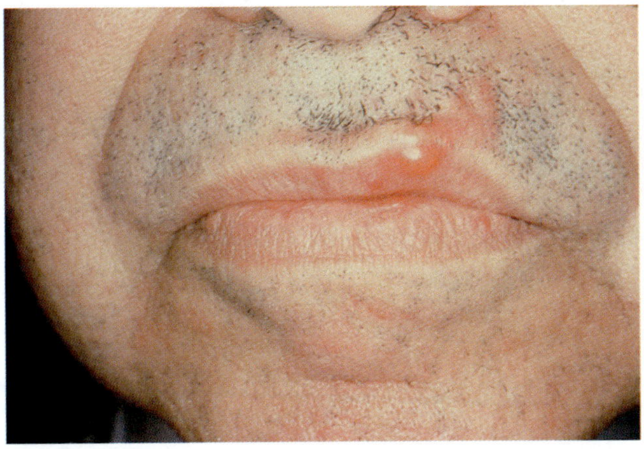

Figure 6.13 Adnexal carcinoma of sweat gland origin involving the vermilion border of the upper lip and adjacent skin.

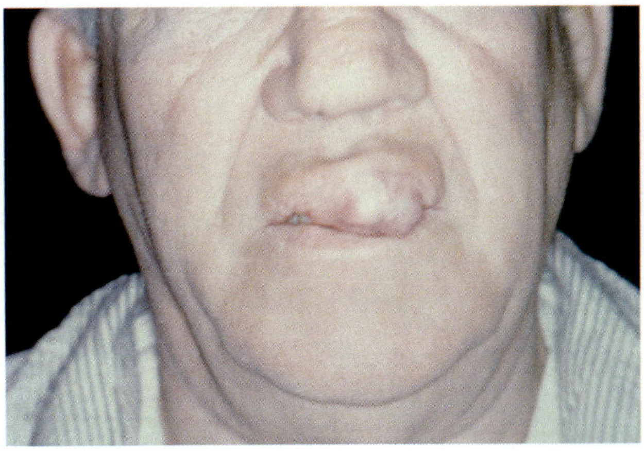

Figure 6.14 Adenoid cystic carcinoma of minor salivary gland origin involving the upper lip.

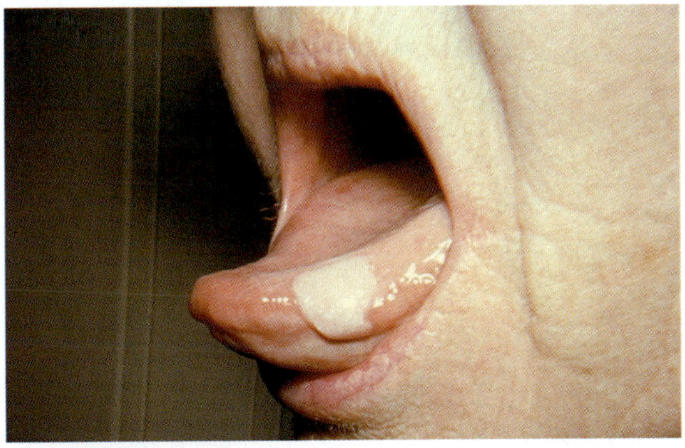

Figure 6.15 Discoid leukoplakia involving the lateral border of the tongue.

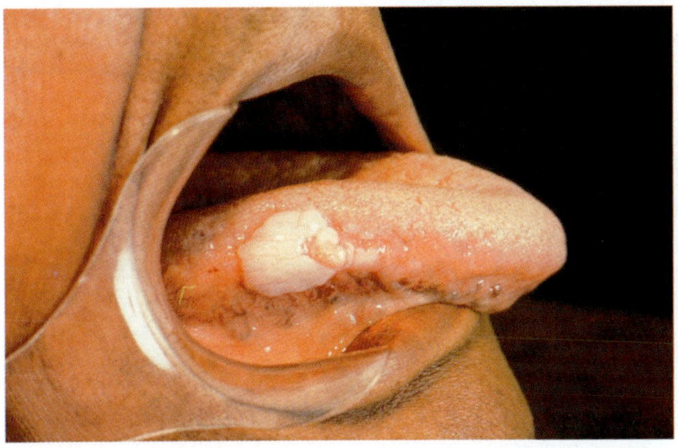

Figure 6.16 Squamous cell carcinoma arising at the periphery of a pre-existing discoid leukoplakia.

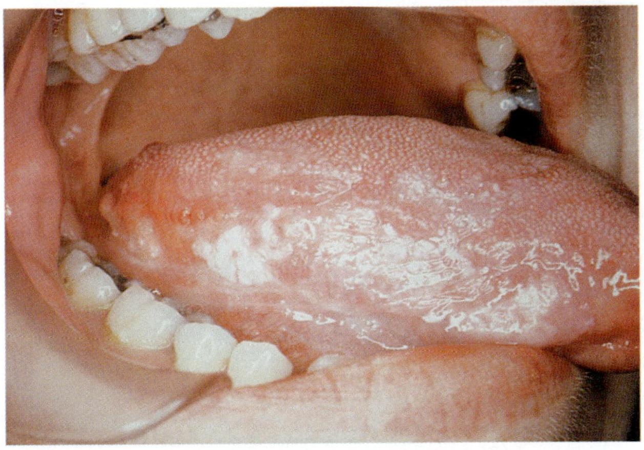

Figure 6.17 Multifocal areas of hyperkeratosis involving the lateral border of the tongue. (Note: no treatment was given to this patient at this juncture.)

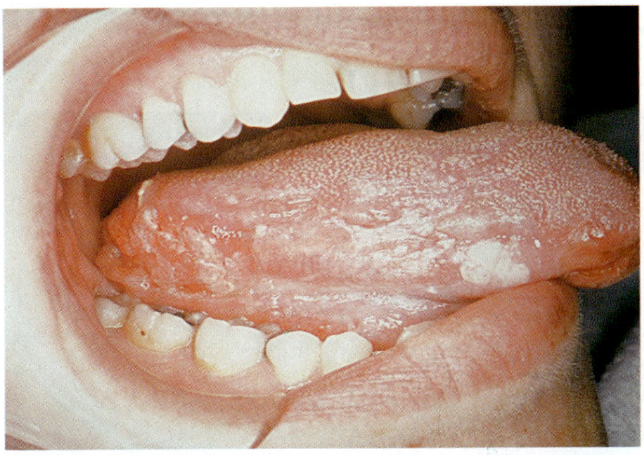

Figure 6.18 Eight months later, the patient shown in Fig. 6.17 has developed two synchronous primary squamous cell carcinomas of the lateral border of the oral tongue involving the junction of the anterior and middle third of the tongue as well as the junction of the middle and posterior third of the tongue on the right-hand side.

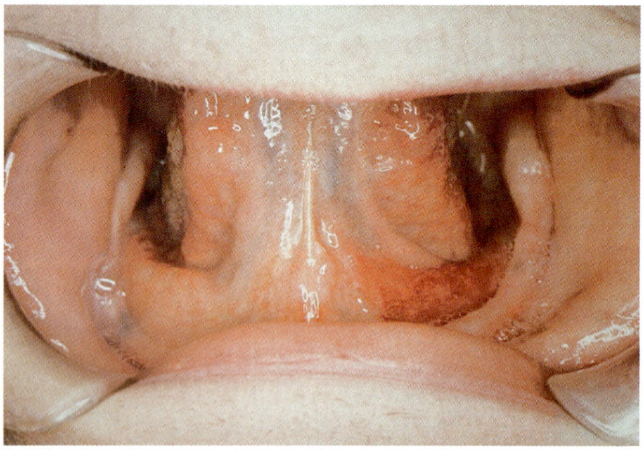

Figure 6.19 Erythroplakia of the anterior floor of the mouth. (Note: no treatment was given to this patient at this juncture.)

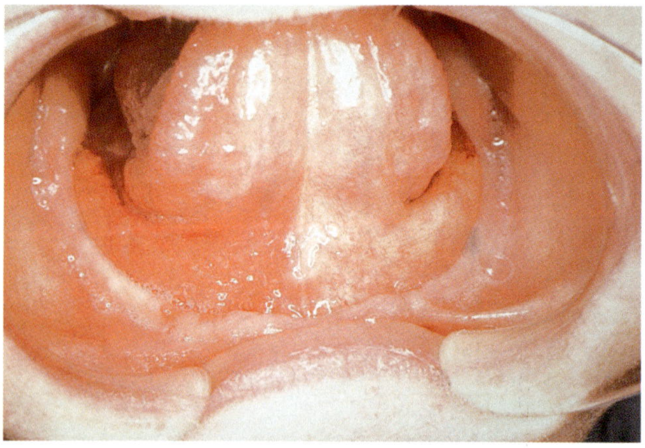

Figure 6.20 Three years later, the patient shown in Fig. 6.17 has superficially invasive squamous cell carcinoma arising in an area of pre-existing erythroplakia.

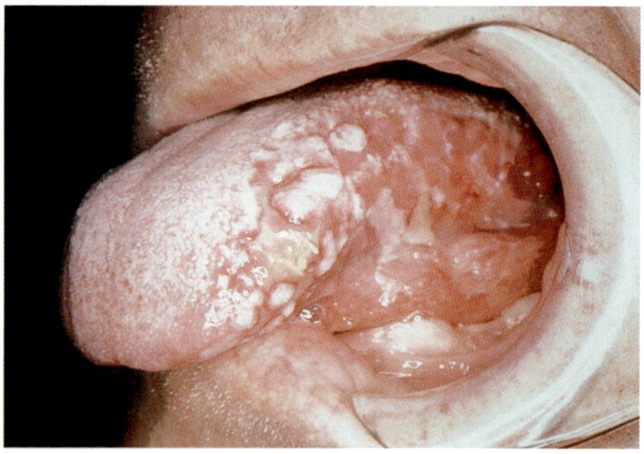

Figure 6.21 Speckled leukoplakia involving the lateral border of the oral tongue.

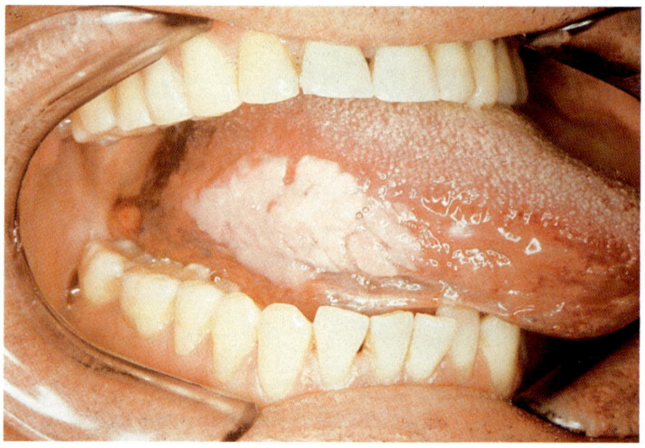

Figure 6.22 Discoid hyperkeratosis involving the lateral border of the oral tongue.

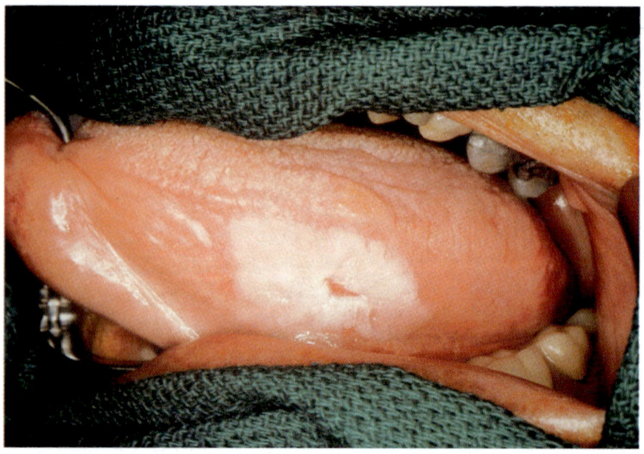

Figure 6.23 Squamous cell carcinoma arising in a pre-existing area of hyperkeratosis.

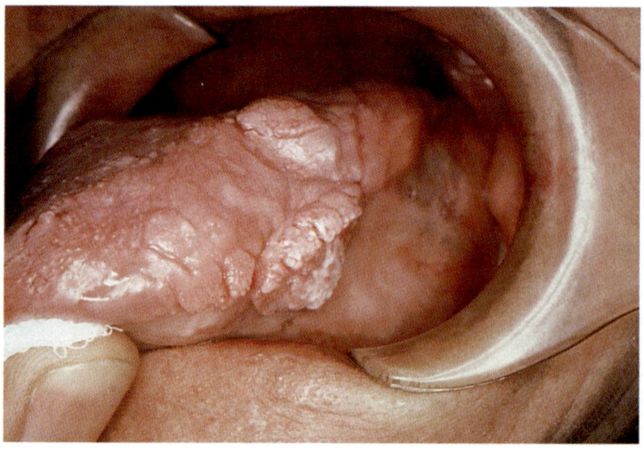

Figure 6.24 Multifocal papillomas of the lateral border of the oral tongue.

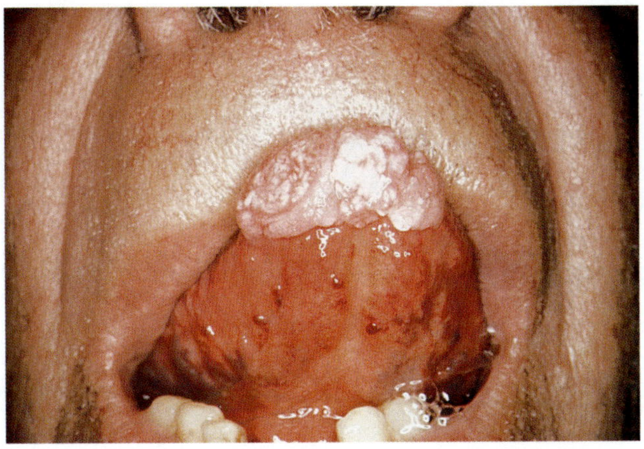

Figure 6.25 Exophytic cauliflower-like squamous cell carcinoma of the tip of the tongue.

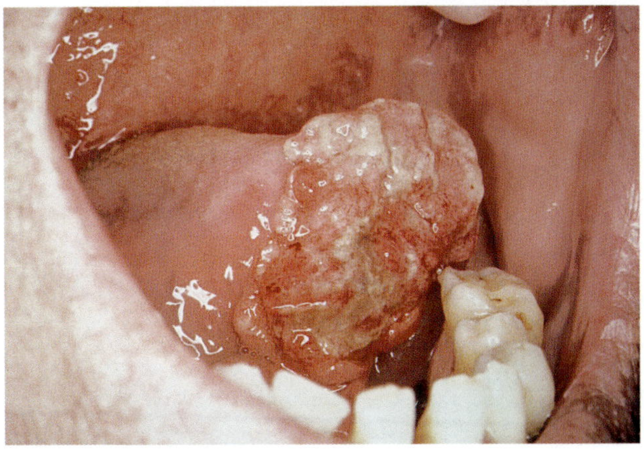

Figure 6.26 Squamous cell carcinoma of the lateral border of the tongue and floor of the mouth.

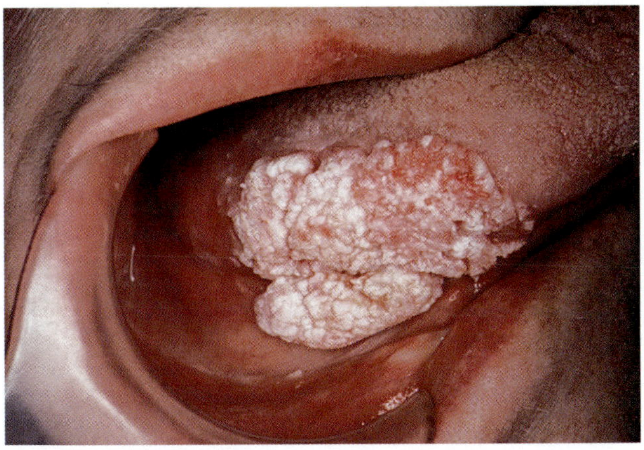

Figure 6.27 Papillary squamous cell carcinoma of the right lateral border of the tongue.

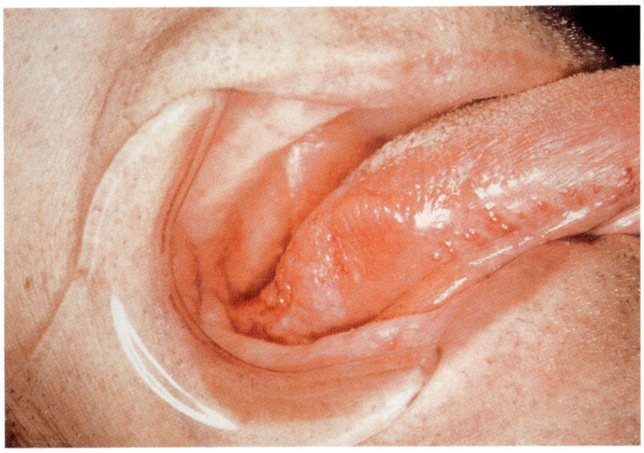

Figure 6.28 Multifocal hyperkeratotic superficially invasive squamous cell carcinoma involving the right lateral border of the tongue.

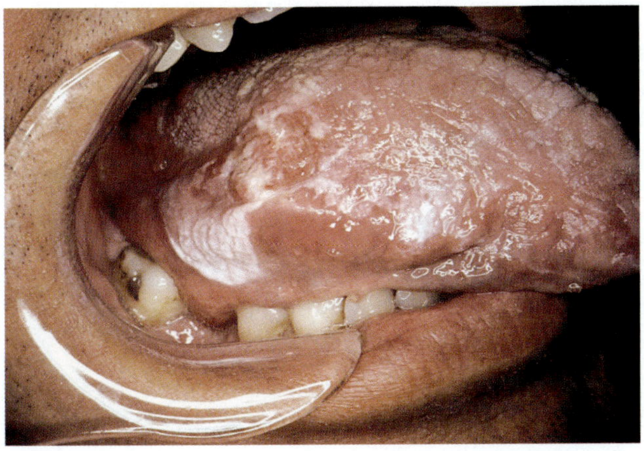

Figure 6.29 Squamous cell carcinoma with adjacent area of hyperkeratosis of the lateral border of the tongue.

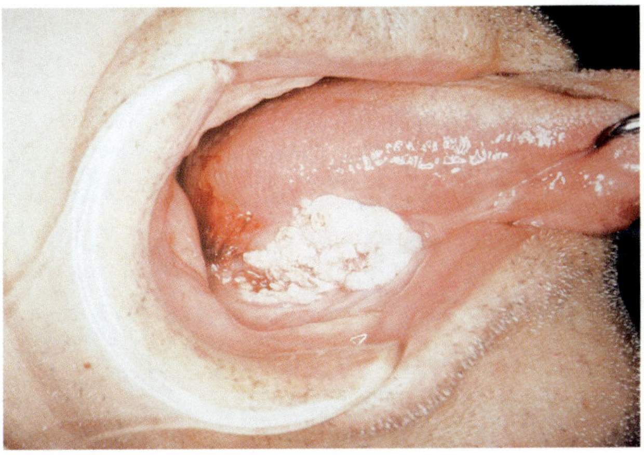

Figure 6.30 Squamous cell carcinoma of the lateral border of the tongue at the periphery of a pre-existing area of hyperkeratosis.

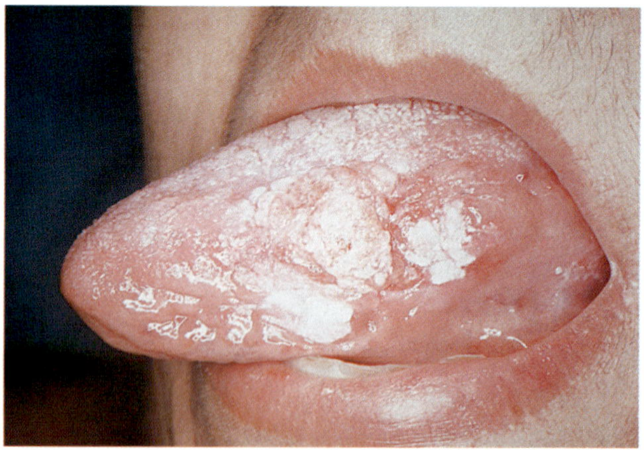

Figure 6.31 Multifocal areas of keratosis with low-grade squamous cell carcinoma of the lateral border of the tongue.

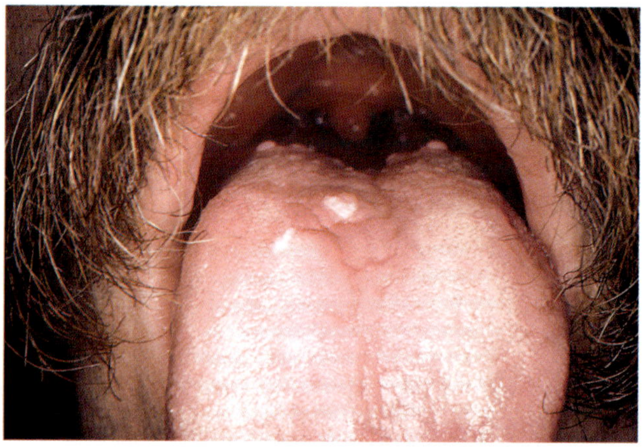

Figure 6.32 Squamous cell carcinoma of the dorsum of the tongue in the mid-line.

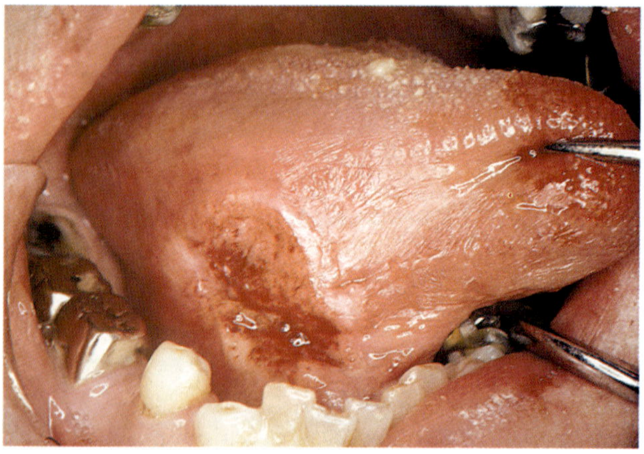

Figure 6.33 Ulcerated endophytic squamous cell carcinoma of the right lateral border of the tongue.

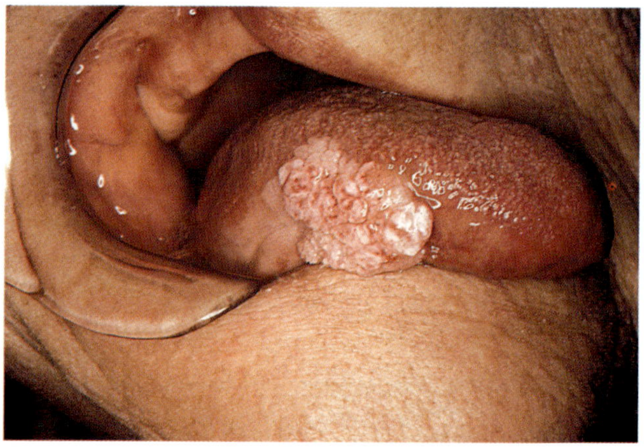

Figure 6.34 Verrucous carcinoma of the lateral border of the tongue.

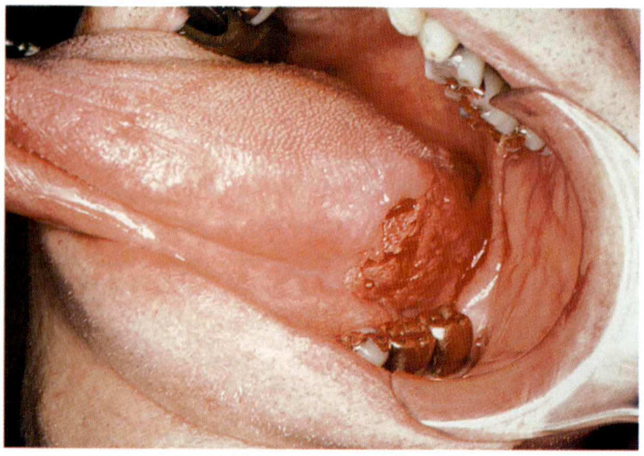

Figure 6.35 Ulcerated endophytic squamous cell carcinoma of the lateral border of the tongue adjacent to the retromolar region.

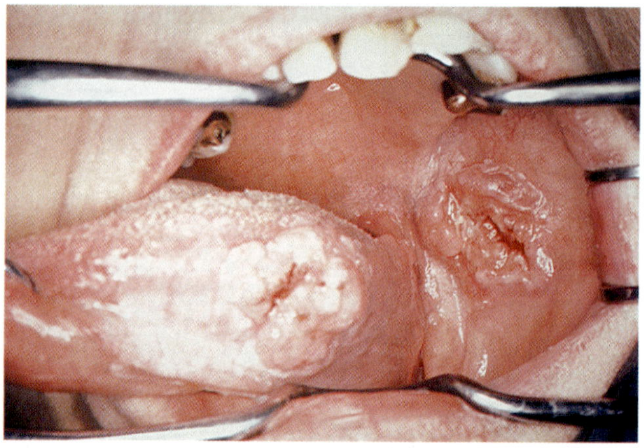

Figure 6.36 Synchronous squamous cell carcinomas of the lateral border of the tongue and buccal mucosa.

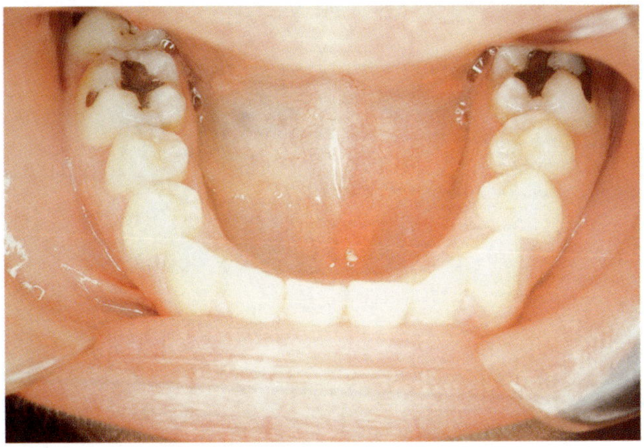

Figure 6.37 Impacted calculus at the opening of left Wharton's duct.

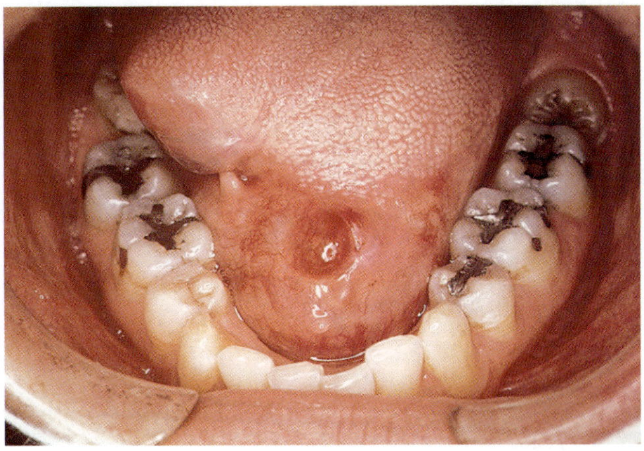

Figure 6.38 Ranula of the floor of the mouth post-previous partial glossectomy.

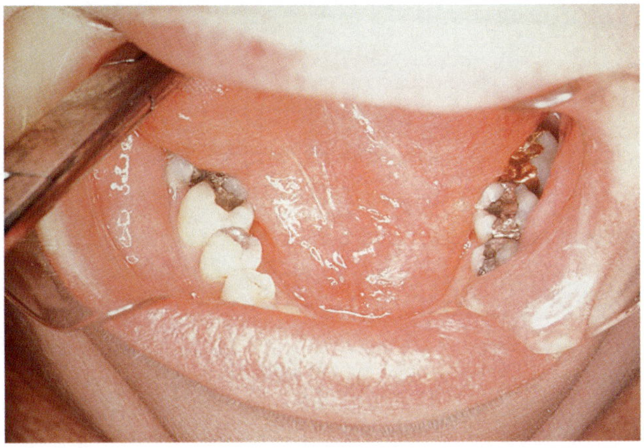

Figure 6.39 Squamous cell carcinoma in a pre-existing area of leukoplakia.

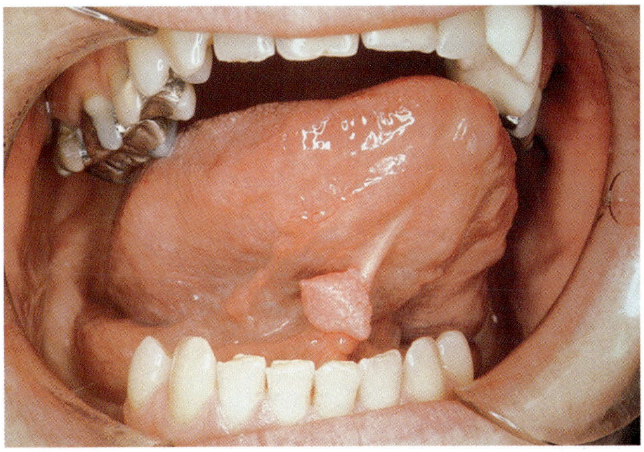

Figure 6.40 Squamous cell papilloma of the anterior floor of the mouth.

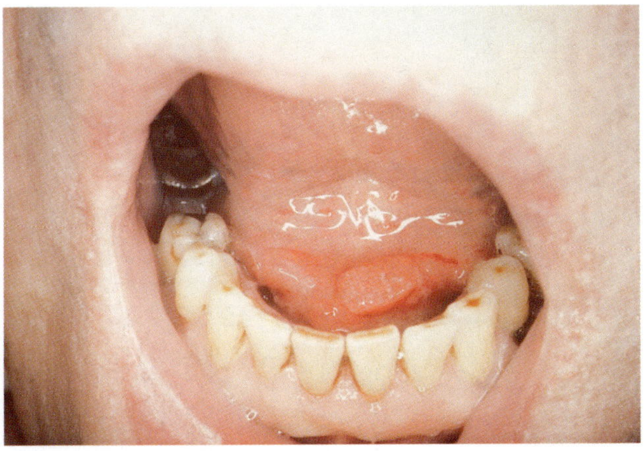

Figure 6.41 Squamous cell carcinoma of the anterior floor of the mouth.

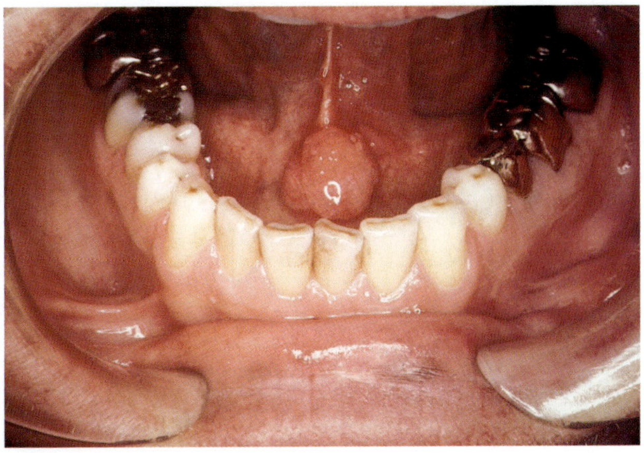

Figure 6.42 Squamous cell carcinoma of the anterior floor of the mouth.

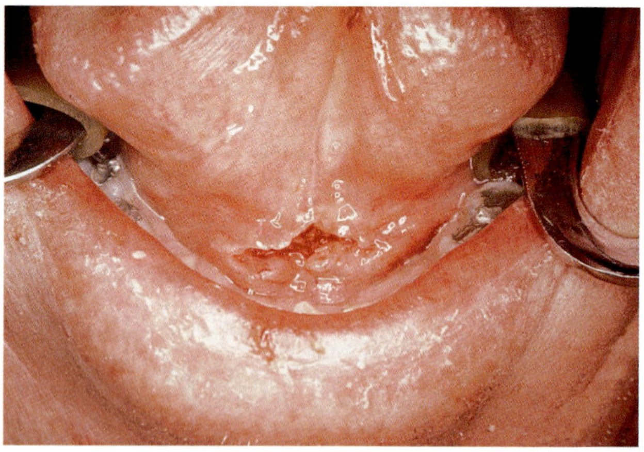

Figure 6.43 Ulcerated infiltrating squamous cell carcinoma of the anterior floor of the mouth.

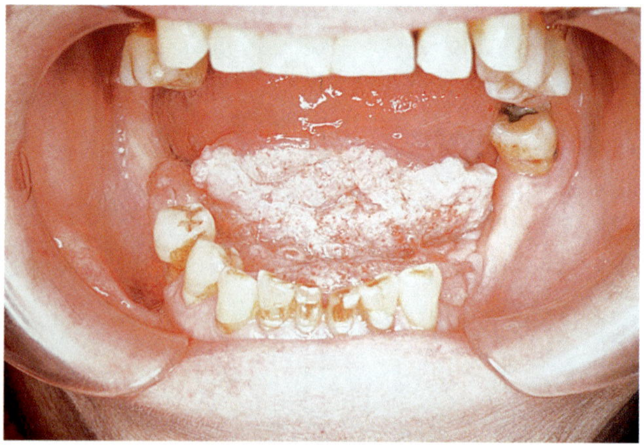

Figure 6.44 Deeply invasive squamous cell carcinoma of the anterior floor of the mouth involving the lingual gingiva.

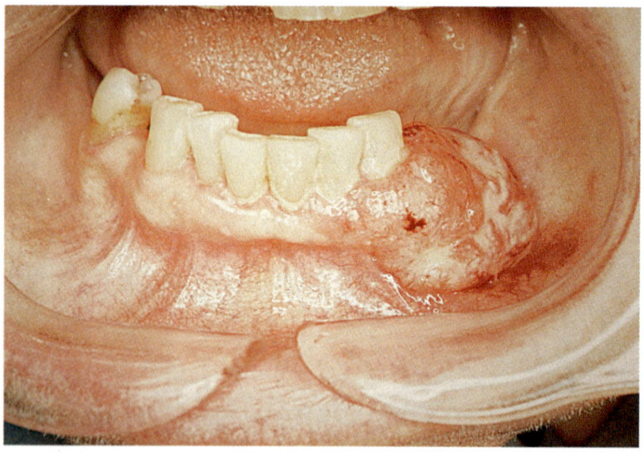

Figure 6.45 Squamous cell carcinoma of the lower gum with invasion of the underlying mandible.

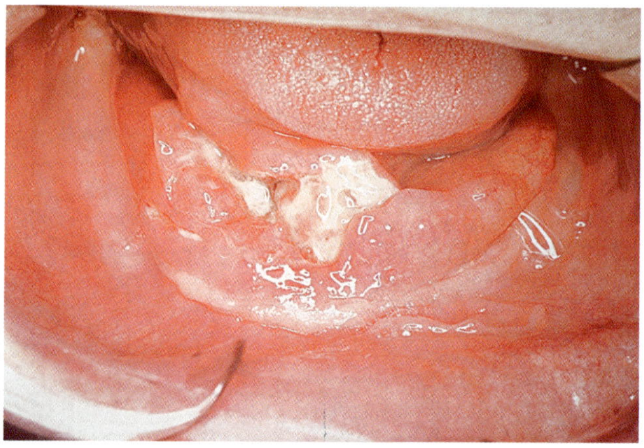

Figure 6.46 Verrucoid deeply invasive squamous cell carcinoma of the anterior floor of the mouth with extension to lower gingiva.

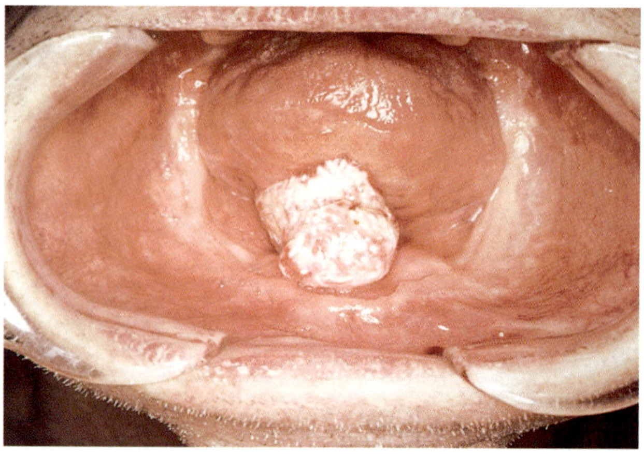

Figure 6.47 Exophytic verrucous carcinoma of the lower gum in the midline extending to the floor of the mouth.

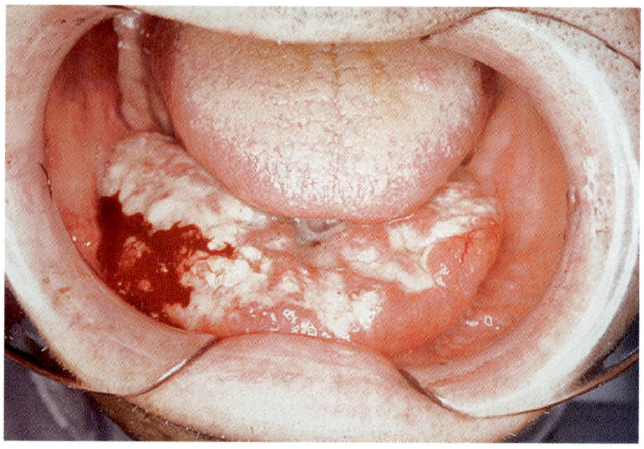

Figure 6.48 Extensive squamous cell carcinoma of the lower gum.

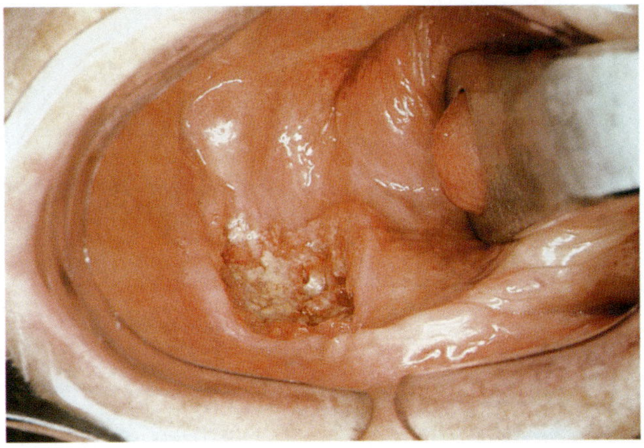

Figure 6.49 Squamous cell carcinoma of the edentulous lower gum with extension to the floor of the mouth.

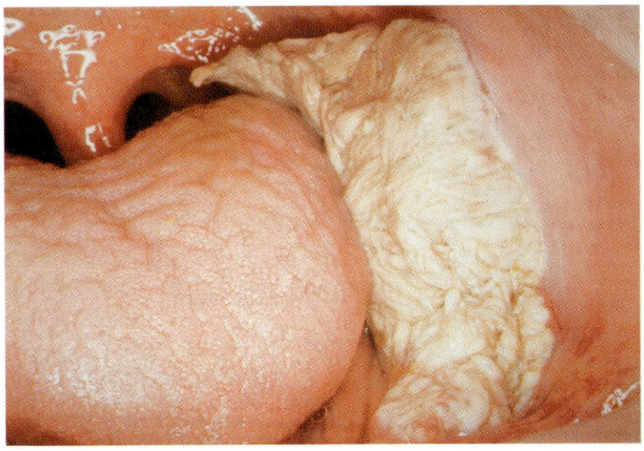

Figure 6.50 Verrucous carcinoma of the left lower gum with extension to the retromolar gingiva.

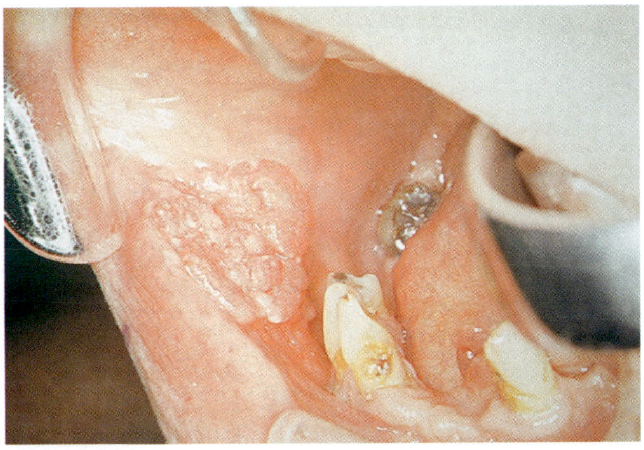

Figure 6.51 Papillary squamous cell carcinoma of the right cheek mucosa.

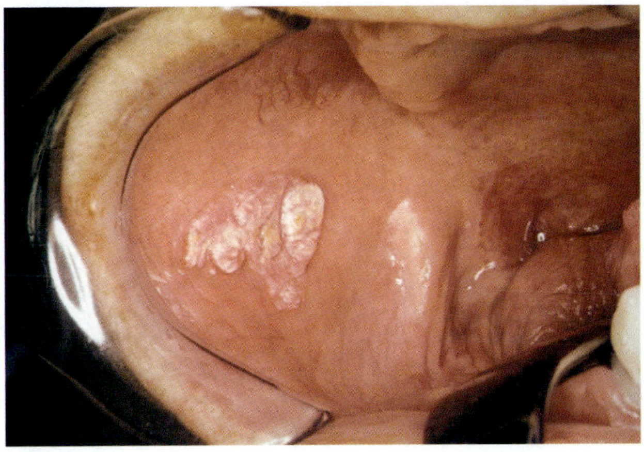

Figure 6.52 Superficially invasive squamous cell carcinoma of the right cheek mucosa.

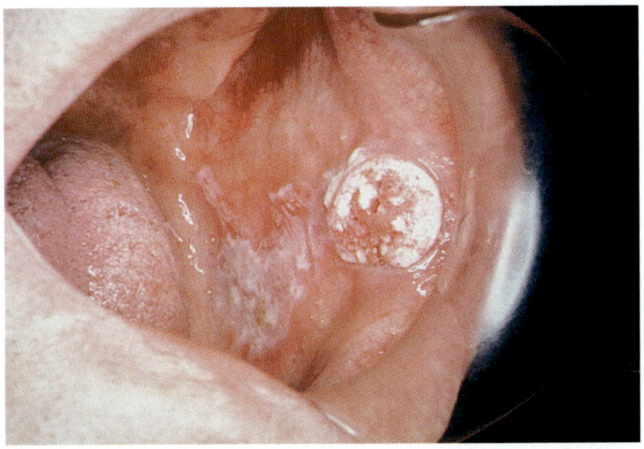

Figure 6.53 Squamous cell carcinoma of the left cheek mucosa with superficial areas of hyperkeratosis.

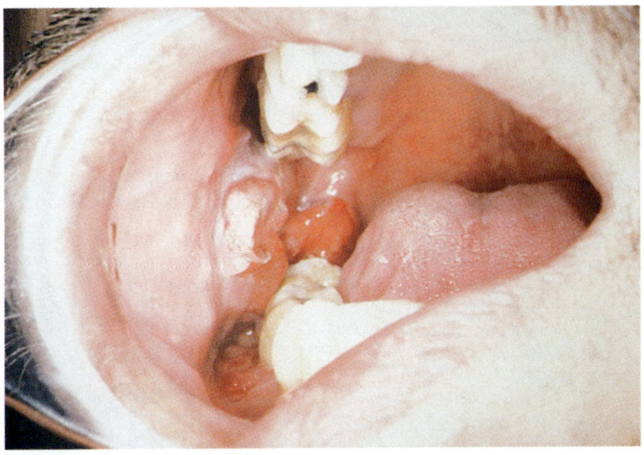

Figure 6.54 Squamous cell carcinoma of the retromolar gingiva.

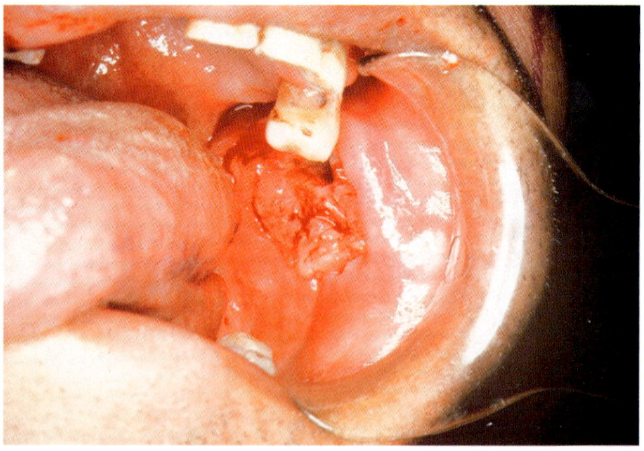

Figure 6.55 Squamous cell carcinoma of the retromolar gingiva with extension to the lower gum and the maxillary tubercle.

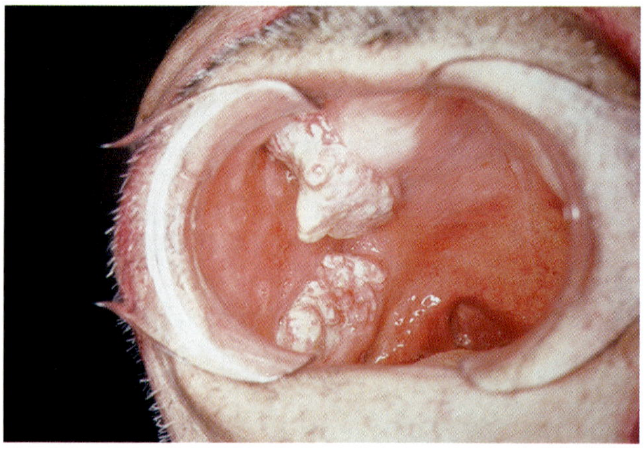

Figure 6.56 Multifocal squamous cell carcinomas involving the lower and upper gum.

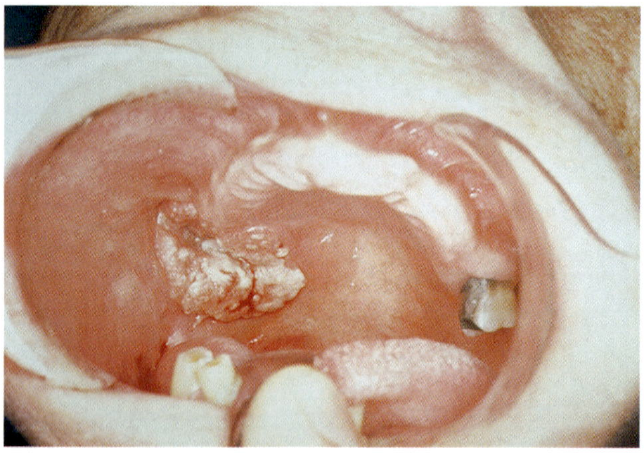

Figure 6.57 Squamous cell carcinoma of the maxillary tubercle and adjacent hard palate.

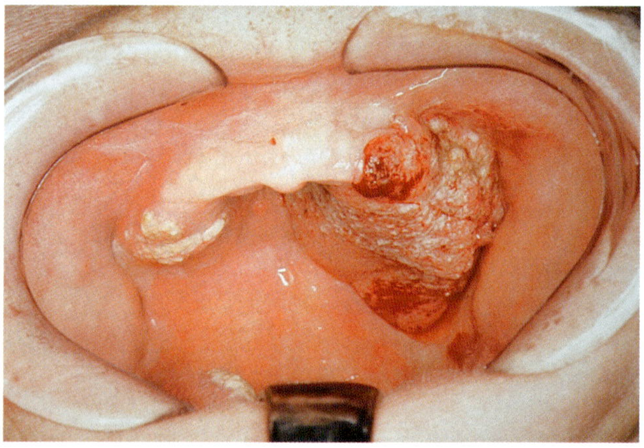

Figure 6.58 Squamous cell carcinoma of the upper gum with extension to the buccal mucosa and hard palate.

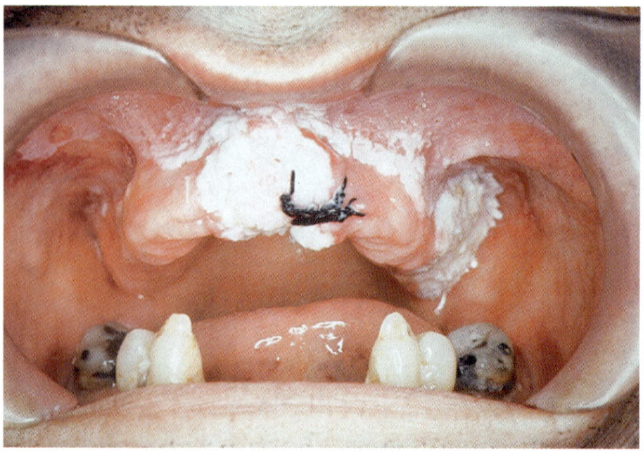

Figure 6.59 Verrucous carcinoma of the upper gum with extensive areas of hyperkeratosis.

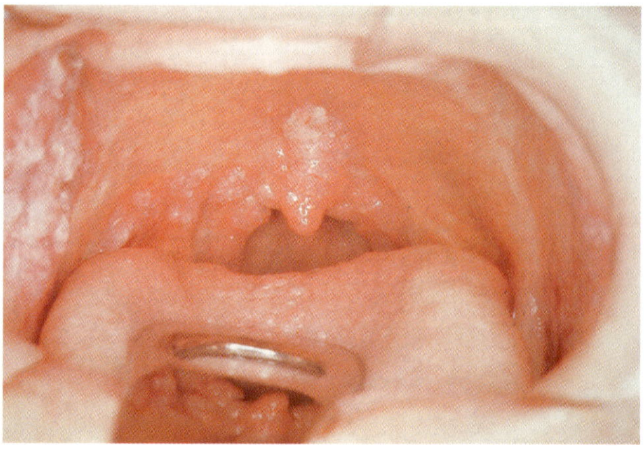

Figure 6.60 Multifocal hyperkeratotic superficially invasive squamous cell carcinoma involving the right cheek mucosa and soft palate.

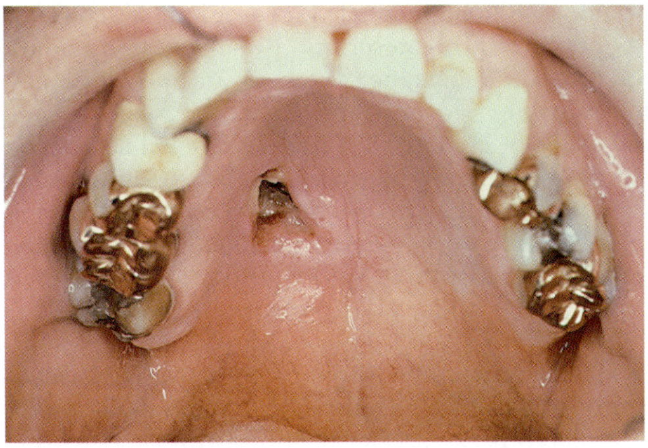

Figure 6.61 Mostly endophytic ulcerated squamous cell carcinoma of the hard palate.

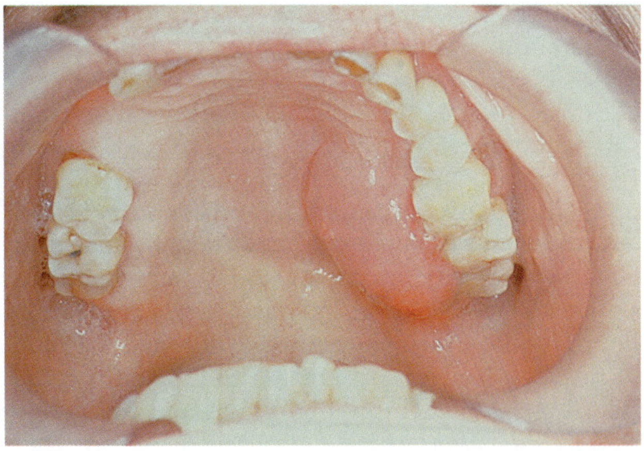

Figure 6.62 Adenoid cystic carcinoma of the hard palate.

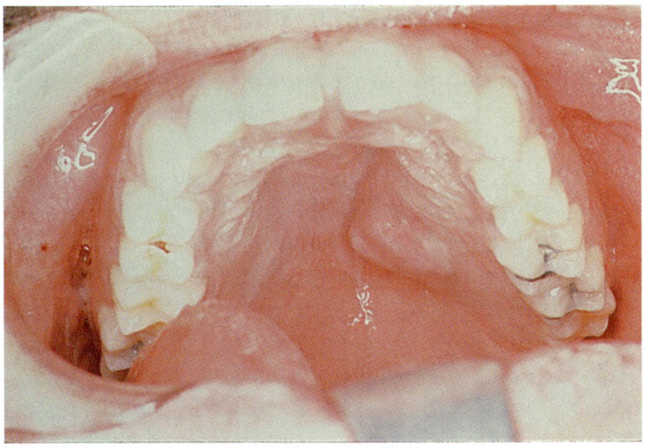

Figure 6.63 Mucoepidermoid carcinoma of the hard palate.

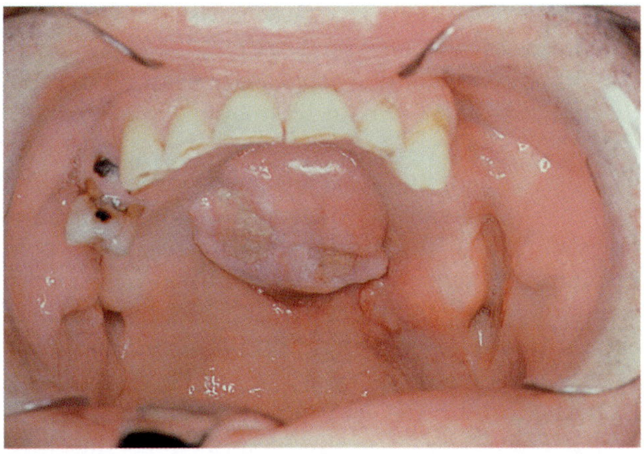

Figure 6.64 Adenocarcinoma of minor salivary gland origin of the hard palate.

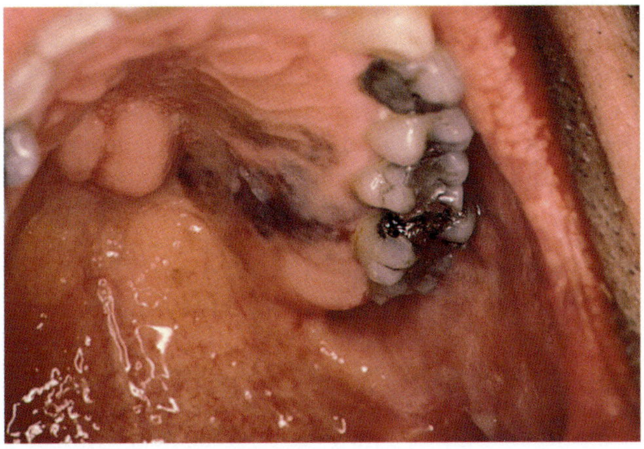

Figure 6.65 Mucosal melanoma involving the hard palate.

A complete examination of the head and neck region should be performed in all patients with tumors of the oral cavity. This examination should include inspection and palpation of the skin of the face and scalp, mucosa of the oral cavity, nasal cavity and nasopharynx, oropharynx, hypopharynx and larynx, cervical lymph nodes, salivary glands, and cranial nerves. An evaluation of sensation of the skin of the cheek, upper lip, chin and lower lip should be performed to assess clinical evidence of perineural involvement. Invasion of the second division of the trigeminal nerve from primary tumors of the upper alveolus and palate may cause anesthesia of the skin of the cheek and upper lip. Similarly, anesthesia of the skin of the chin and lower lip signifies invasion of the inferior alveolar nerve, a branch of the third division of the trigeminal nerve.

The status of regional cervical lymph nodes should be carefully evaluated by systematic palpation of accessible cervical lymph nodes including preauricular, periparotid, submental, prevascular facial, submandibular, deep jugular, and posterior triangle lymph nodes. Nodal levels I, II and III are the ones most commonly involved by regional metastasis from oral cavity cancers.[13–15] Occasionally it is difficult to distinguish an enlarged submandibular salivary gland from an enlarged metastatic level I lymph node. Bimanual palpation through the floor of the mouth may assist in the differential diagnosis. If cervical lymph nodes are enlarged, they should be appropriately described as to their location, size, number, and clinical signs of extranodal spread. Appropriate 'N' staging should be assigned at this time according to the UICC/AJCC staging system.[4]

The major salivary glands (parotid, submandibular, and sublingual) should be carefully examined by bimanual palpation for any masses or lesions. Openings of the Stensen's and Wharton's ducts should be inspected for free flow of saliva. Function of the facial nerve should be documented.

Examination of the nasal cavity with a speculum for any visible or obstructing lesions should be documented. Tumors of the palate or oropharynx may produce secondary nasal obstruction. Similarly, tumors of the nasal cavity or nasopharynx may extend inferiorly to the oral cavity or oropharynx.

Examination of the oral cavity requires careful inspection of the vermilion surface of the lips, labial and buccal mucosa, upper and lower alveolus, as well as mucosa of the gingiva, floor of the mouth, oral tongue, and hard palate. A tongue depressor with satisfactory lighting provides adequate visualization of the accessible sites in the oral cavity. Mobility of the tongue should be evaluated to assess deep infiltration of the musculature of the tongue or invasion of the hypoglossal nerve by tumor. Vitality of the teeth should be checked, particularly in lesions of the lower or upper gum. Palpation of the lesion allows assessment of the third dimension or depth of infiltration of the tumor. Lesions of the floor of the mouth and cheek mucosa should be palpated bimanually. Proximity of the primary tumor to the adjacent bone (mandible or maxilla) should be carefully evaluated and documented to assess the need for bone resection in conjunction with excision of the primary tumor. Numbness of the tongue signifies invasion of the lingual nerve and numbness of the lower teeth and gingiva signifies invasion of the inferior alveolar branch of the third division of the trigeminal nerve. Surface measurements of the tumor are documented for accurate T staging.[4] Accurate clinical description of the lesion should include its appearance, such as ulcerative, fungating, exophytic, or endophytic, as well as the presence of associated features such as leukoplakia or erythroplakia. The presence of multiple primary tumors should be carefully checked. Documentation of the surface characteristics of the mucosa of the oral cavity and oropharynx not involved by tumor is important.

A dental mirror should be used for careful evaluation of the lingual gingivae of the upper and lower alveolar processes. The dental mirror is also used to examine the nasopharynx, hypopharynx, and larynx. The presence of any mucosal lesion should be noted, with accurate description of its visual characteristics. The mucosal surface of the posterior third of the tongue (posterior to the circumvalate papillae) should be carefully scrutinized and the presence of any lesions in the hypopharynx and larynx should be recorded. Adequacy of airway and mobility of the vocal cords should be recorded. Finally, palpation of the base of the tongue is essential to rule out a submucosal tumor mass.

If adequate examination of the hypopharynx and larynx is not feasible with a dental mirror due to poor cooperation from the patient, then a fiberoptic flexible nasolaryngoscope should be used. This may be done without any anesthetic. On the other hand, topical anesthetic may be used in the nasal cavity. The added advantage of using the flexible nasolaryngoscope is that it provides good visual examination of the nasal cavity and nasopharynx and a detailed survey of the hypopharynx and larynx. Video recording or photography may be used to document the findings.

Tissue diagnosis is usually confirmed by a wedge or punch biopsy obtained from the periphery of the lesion, or from the center of the lesion. An adequate volume of viable tissue should be retrieved. Highly keratinizing squamous carcinomas and verrucous carcinomas may not provide satisfactory representative tissue from the surface of the lesion and the diagnosis of invasive carcinoma can be missed from a superficial biopsy. Therefore, where excessive keratin deposit is seen on the surface of an exophytic lesion, the biopsy should be obtained from an adjacent invasive zone or from the depth of the lesion rather than the surface. Similarly, areas of necrotic tumor should be avoided for biopsy. Harvest of viable tissue in a biopsy is generally confirmed if some bleeding occurs at the biopsy site. If a biopsy fails to show carcinoma in a clinically suspicious lesion, then the biopsy should be repeated until the tissue diagnosis is confirmed.

References

1. Landis SH, Murray T, Bolden S, Wingo PA. Cancer statistics, 1998 [published erratum appears in CA Cancer J Clin 1998 May–Jun; 48: 192]. CA Cancer J Clin 1998; 48: 6–29
2. Hoffman HT, Karnell LH, Funk GF, Robinson RA, Menck HR. The National Cancer Data Base report on cancer of the head and neck. Arch Otolaryngol Head Neck Surg 1998; 124: 951–962
3. Ildstad ST, Tollerud DJ, Bigelow ME, Remensnyder JP. Squamous cell carcinoma of the head and neck at the Massachusetts General Hospital: a comparison of biologic characteristics in men and women. Surgery 1986; 99: 7–14
4. Fleming ID, Cooper JS, Henson DE et al (eds). AJCC Cancer Staging Manual, 5th edn. Philadelphia: Lippincott–Raven, 1997
5. Sankaranarayanan R. Oral cancer in India: an epidemiologic and clinical review. Oral Surg Oral Med Oral Pathol 1990; 69: 325–330
6. Norton SA. Betel: consumption and consequences. J Am Acad Dermatol 1998; 38: 81–88
7. Mashberg A, Meyers H. Anatomical site and size of 222 early asymptomatic oral squamous cell carcinomas: a continuing prospective study of oral cancer. II. Cancer 1976; 37: 2149–2157
8. Waldron CA, Shafer WG. Leukoplakia revisited. A clinicopathologic study of 3256 oral leukoplakias. Cancer 1975; 36: 1386–1392
9. Mashberg A. Erythroplasia vs. leukoplasia in the diagnosis of early asymptomatic oral squamous carcinoma [editorial]. N Engl J Med 1977; 297: 109–110
10. Craig RM. Speckled leukoplakia of the floor of the mouth. J Am Dent Assoc 1981; 102: 690–692
11. de Vries N, Van der Waal I, Snow GB. Multiple primary tumours in oral cancer. Int J Oral Maxillofac Surg 1986; 15: 85–87
12. Spiro R. Salivary neoplasms: overview of a 35-year experience with 2,807 patients. Head and Neck Surg 1986; 8: 177–184
13. Shah JP. Patterns of cervical lymph node metastasis from squamous carcinomas of the upper aerodigestive tract. Am J Surg 1990; 160: 405–409.
14. Shaha AR, Spiro RH, Shah JP, Strong EW. Squamous carcinoma of the floor of the mouth. Am J Surg 1984; 148: 455–459.
15. Franceschi D, Gupta R, Spiro RH, Shah JP. Improved survival in the treatment of squamous carcinoma of the oral tongue. Am J Surg 1993; 166: 360–365.

7 Workup and staging

John F Carew, Bhuvanesh Singh and Jatin P Shah

A satisfactory pretreatment work-up for a patient suspected of having cancer of the oral cavity requires a detailed head and neck examination and biopsy to establish tissue diagnosis. The physical examination should document appropriate parameters necessary for clinical staging of the tumor. Further work-up requires assessment of the general medical condition of the patient, nutritional status, dental evaluation and preoperative dental care as well as radiographic evaluation.

A complete physical examination is performed to assess the general physical condition of the patient, predisposing factors related to the development of oral cancer, and associated co-morbid conditions.[1,2] This, in particular, requires assessment of pulmonary function and the status of the cardiovascular system in relation to smoking habit and alcohol consumption. The general nutritional status is evaluated in patients who manifest signs of chronic malnutrition and significant weight loss, since these may have profound effects on wound healing postoperatively.[3]

Radiographic evaluation

Either direct extension of a primary tumor of the oral cavity to the mandible or maxilla or its proximity to bone requires appropriate radiological studies to establish the extent of bone involvement. While the absence of radiographic findings does not rule out bone invasion, bone destruction as seen on radiological studies confirms tumor invasion. Radionucleotide bone scans are often positive prior to radiographic appearance of bone destruction, but they seldom provide accurate information regarding the extent of bone invasion. Bone scans may also be positive in non-neoplastic conditions, such as inflammatory lesions, thus leading to false positive results. In one study, the false positive rate of bone scans in detecting the mandible invasion in oral cavity tumors exceeded 50%.[4]

Plain radiographs of the mandible in anteroposterior and oblique views are not satisfactory as a routine screening procedure to establish or rule out bone destruction. However, a panoramic view of the mandible (orthopantomogram, OPG) is, perhaps, the most important radiographic study to assess the general architecture of the mandible in relation to the dentoalveolar structures and invasion by tumor (Fig. 7.1). It must, however, be appreciated that due to technical reasons the midline of the mandible near the symphysis is not adequately evaluated by a panoramic view. Early invasion of the lingual cortex of the mandible is also not appreciated on a panoramic view. Occlusal films of the body of the mandible and intra-oral dental films are often quite accurate in demonstrating early invasion by tumor (Figs 7.2, 7.3).

Computerized tomograms are generally not optimal for routine evaluation but may be considered in selected circumstances, such as primary tumors of the mandible and those lesions where soft tissue extension from tumors involving the ascending ramus of the mandible is suspected. A CT scan may also be of help in assessing the extent of local

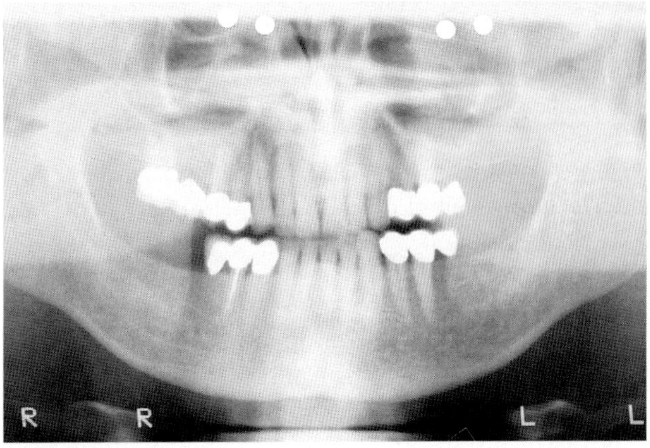

Figure 7.1 Panoramic x-ray (Panorex, orthopan tomogram) of the mandible.

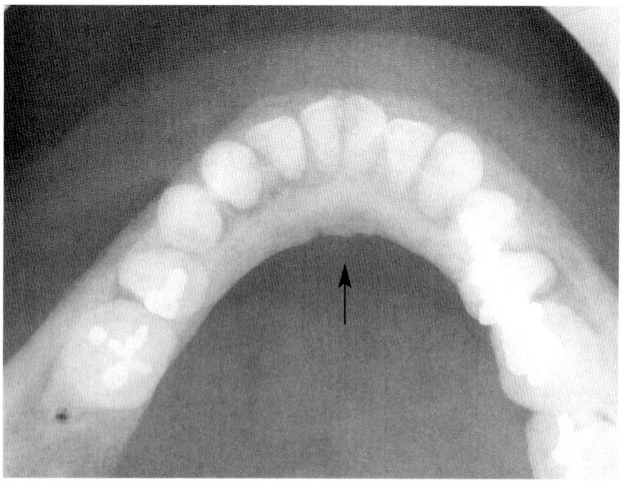

Figure 7.2 Occlusal film of mandibular arch showing early invasion of lingual cortex.

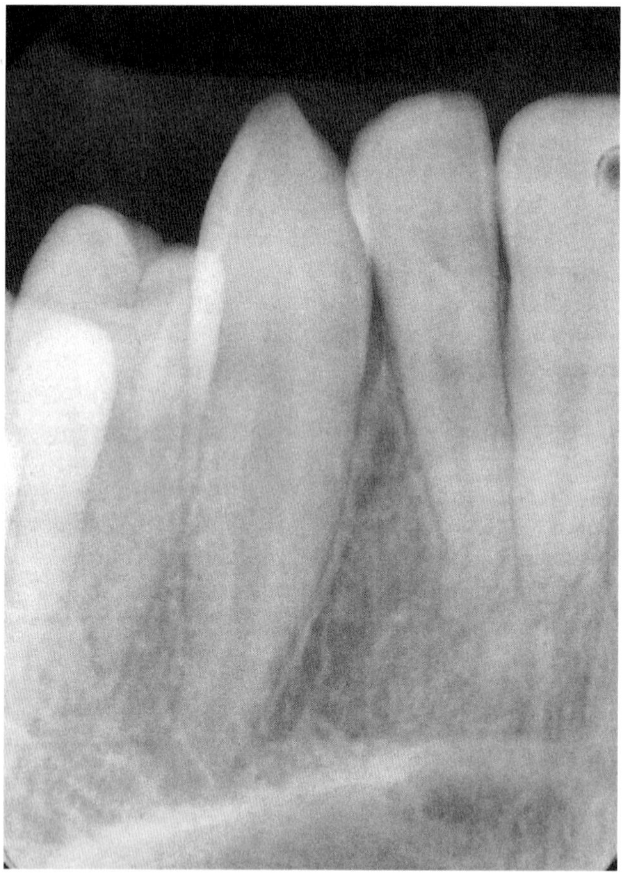

Figure 7.3 Periapical dental film showing fine architectural detail of dental roots.

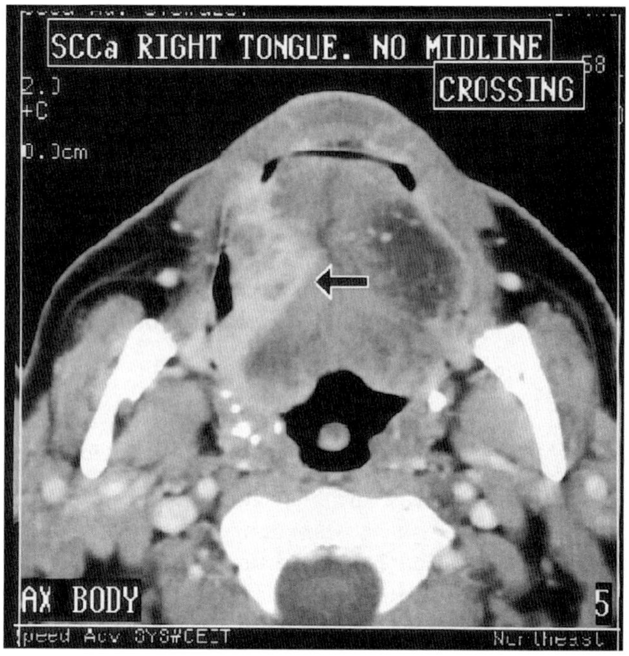

Figure 7.4 Axial view of a CT scan with contrast through the oral cavity of a patient with advanced carcinoma of the tongue.

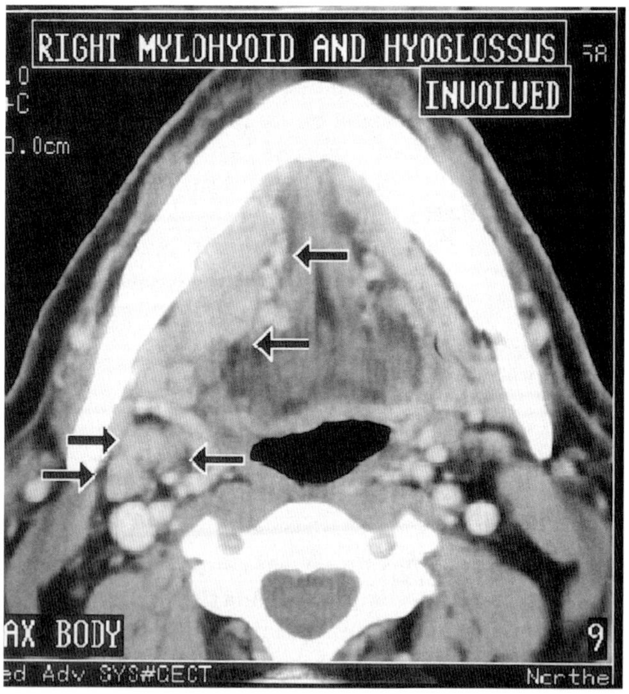

Figure 7.5 CT scan with contrast showing invasion of lingual cortex of the mandible by advanced cancer of the tongue.

invasion by large tumors. Computerized tomography of the oral cavity is optimal when intravenous contrast is used. Soft tissue and bone windows are obtained to demonstrate contrast enhancement due to tumor invasion and bone invasion (Figs 7.4, 7.5). A sophisticated software program for the CT scan called 'Dentascan' provides more accurate details of the mandible and may be considered in appropriate circumstances when dental details are required.[5] (Fig. 7.6) In addition, three-dimensional reconstructions of

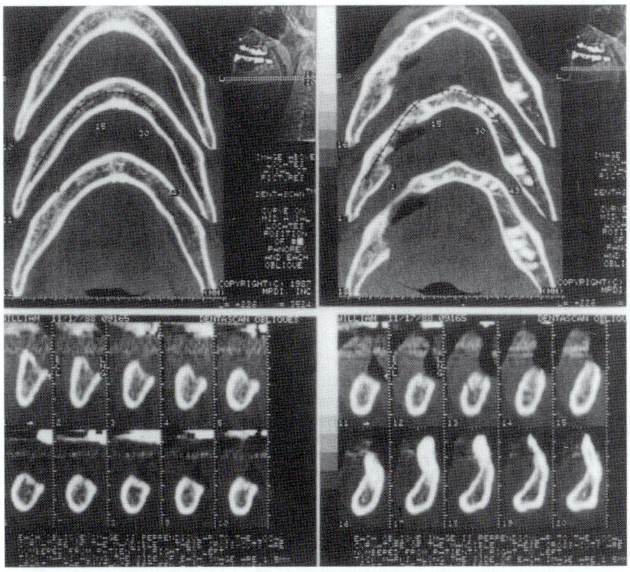

Figure 7.6 Dentascan of the mandible.

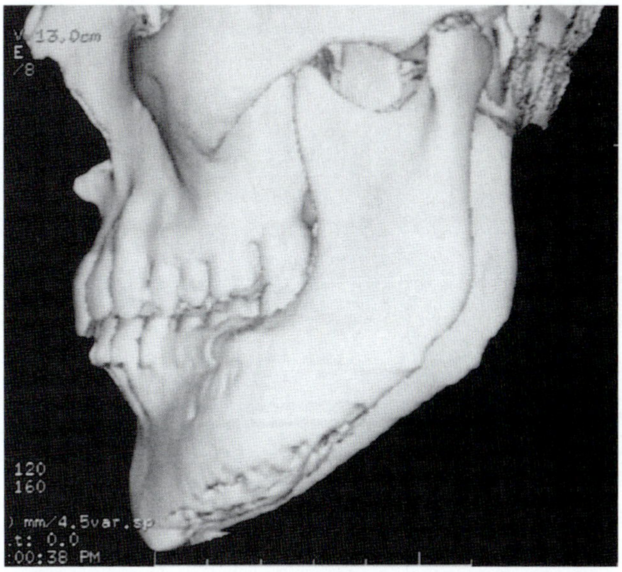

Figure 7.7 Lateral view of 3-D reconstruction of the CT scan of the mandible of a patient with sarcoma.

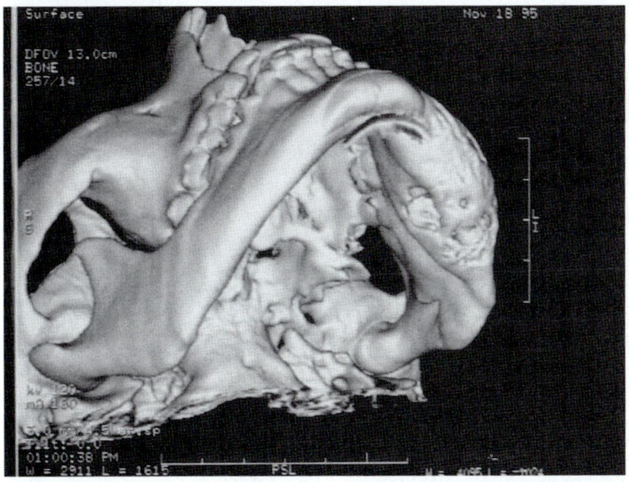

Figure 7.8 Oblique inferior view of 3-D reconstruction of the mandible of the same patient shown in Fig. 7.7.

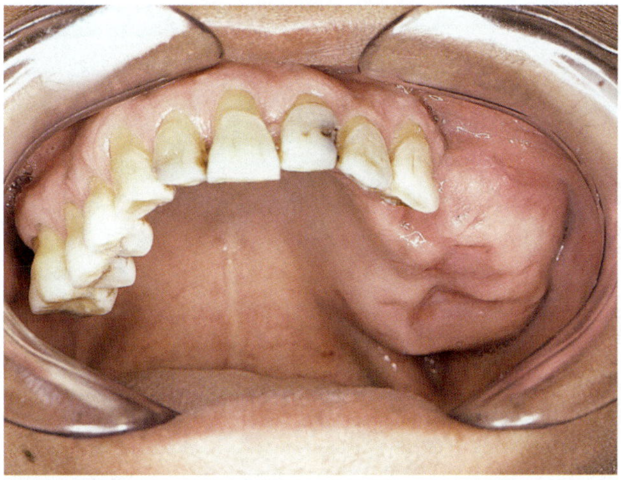

Figure 7.9 Intraoral view of a patient with myxoma of the left maxilla with involvement of the left upper gum.

CT images provide an excellent overview of the mandible or maxilla from any desired angle (Figs 7.7, 7.8). A three-dimensional CT scan and a one-to-one reproduction of the image are of great value to the surgeon for mandible reconstruction with a microvascular free flap. These images are essential in fabricating a graft which matches the resected portion of the mandible.

A CT scan most accurately assesses invasion of the maxilla by primary tumors of the oral cavity such as those arising from the palate or upper alveolus. It is important to obtain coronal cuts with soft tissue and bone windows to adequately assess the extent of tumor involving the hard palate and upper alveolus (Figs 7.9–7.11). Magnetic resonance imaging (MRI) is superior in defining soft tissue details and intracranial extension and allows sagittal images.[6] Axial and sagittal MRI scans of a patient with an exophytic tongue carcinoma vividly demonstrate its third dimension (Figs 7.12, 7.13). Also, in situations when extensive soft tissue invasion in the parapharyngeal space is suspected, an MRI scan is desirable. Bony details are, however, not very clear on MRI, and CT scan is preferred in the assessment of bone involvement. Regardless of the presence or absence of invasion of mandible or maxilla by tumor, if any bone resection or osteotomy is to be undertaken for surgical treatment of a primary tumor of the oral cavity or oropharynx, appropriate radiographic studies of the bone under consideration must be obtained prior to the surgical procedure.

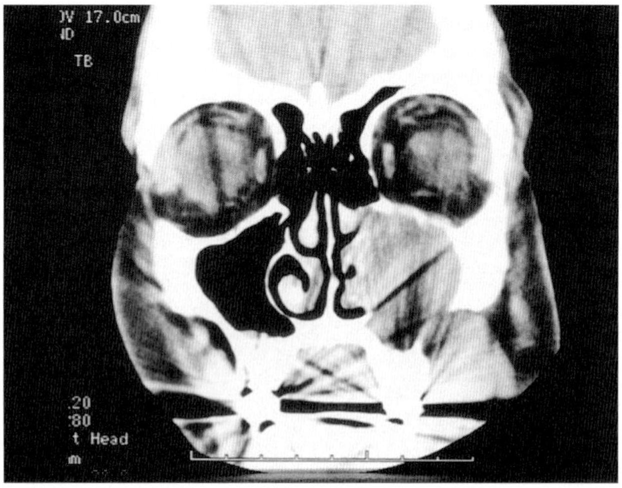

Figure 7.10 Coronal view of the CT scan of the paranasal sinuses with soft tissue window of the patient shown in Fig. 7.9.

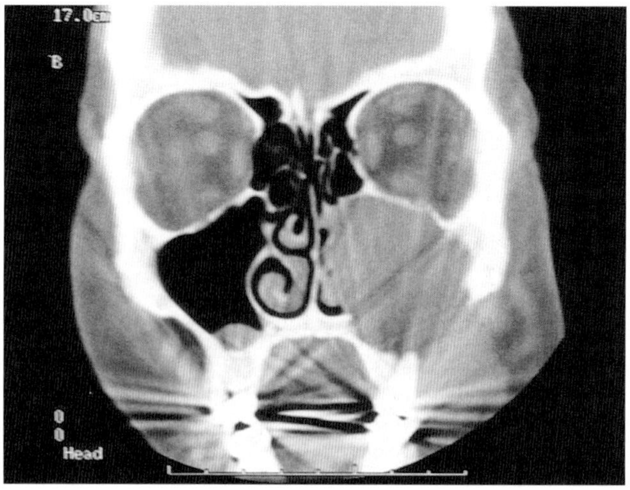

Figure 7.11 Coronal view of the CT scan of the paranasal sinuses with bone window of the patient shown in Fig. 7.9.

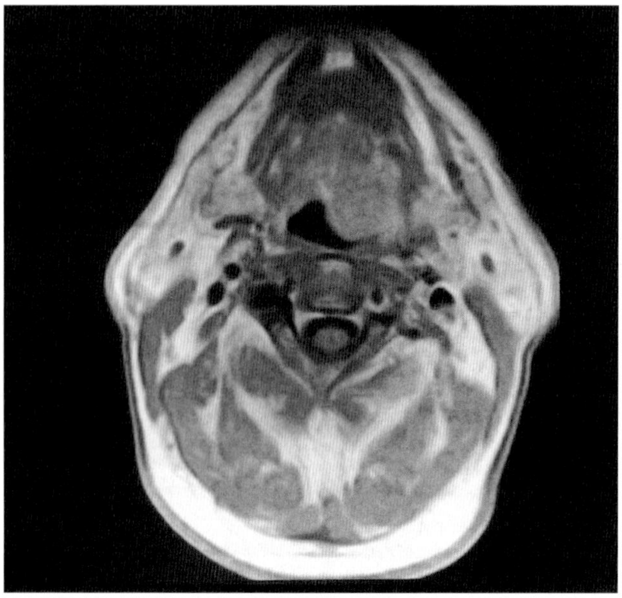

Figure 7.12 Axial view of the MRI scan of a patient with cancer of the base of the tongue.

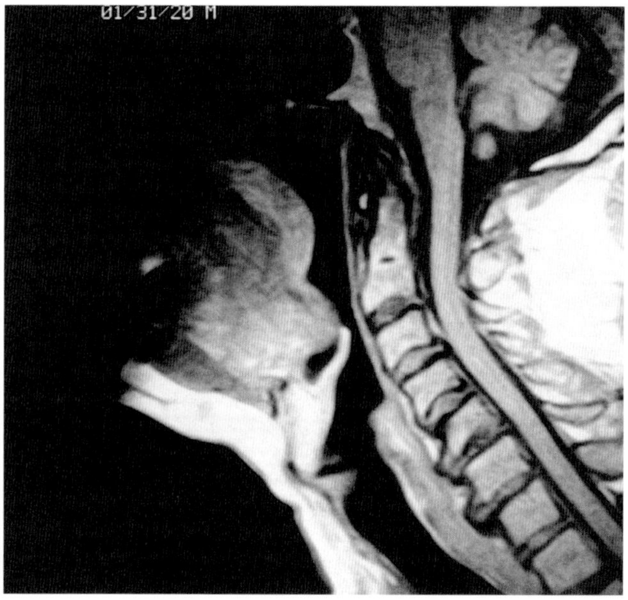

Figure 7.13 Sagittal view of the MRI scan of the same patient showing cancer of the base of the tongue abutting the lingual surface of epiglottis.

Preoperative dental assessment

Many patients with primary carcinomas of the oral cavity have poor oral hygiene.[7] Their dentition is in poor repair and often harbors gross sepsis. It is very important that preoperative dental evaluation and appropriate dental care are provided to achieve an optimal status of hygiene in the oral cavity prior to a surgical procedure.[8] All grossly septic teeth should be adequately assessed for consideration of extraction, either preoperatively or intraoperatively. It is, however, important to emphasize that teeth, whether loose or immobile within the tumor or in its vicinity, should not be extracted prior to the definitive surgical resection. Extraction of teeth near a tumor opens up dental sockets that are vulnerable to implantation of tumor. The efficacy of a satisfactory surgical procedure may be seriously jeopardized under these circumstances.[9]

Deposits of tartar need to be removed and appropriate scaling of the dentition undertaken to avoid dental complications and prevent sepsis in the oral cavity following surgery. Any restorative dental work, however, should be postponed until adequate surgical treatment of the primary oral cancer is completed.

If the contemplated surgical procedure requires resection of any part of the mandible or maxilla, appropriate dental consultation should be obtained for consideration of fabrication of either a mandibular splint or a palatal obturator if required. If a postoperative splint, obturator or dental prosthesis is needed, then it is imperative that dental impressions obtained before surgery are available to allow fabrication of an appropriate prosthesis.

If the patient has received radiation therapy or adjuvant postoperative radiotherapy is anticipated, adequate dental consultation is crucial. It is important that the patient has dental prophylaxis for radiation therapy in terms of extraction and/or treatment of septic teeth, restoration of salvageable teeth and advice regarding fluoride treatment for prevention of caries in remaining viable teeth.

If reconstructive surgery with a ‘free flap’ is anticipated, and if such reconstruction is to be done by a second surgical team, then the choice of free flap should be planned during appropriate preoperative consultation with the reconstructive surgeon. This would entail review of available and applicable free flaps with the patient, including the sequelae and disability at the donor site. Detailed assessment of the circulation of the donor site is essential in patients with peripheral vascular disease and diabetes. Angiograms of the lower extremity may be required in some patients who require fibula free flap reconstruction.

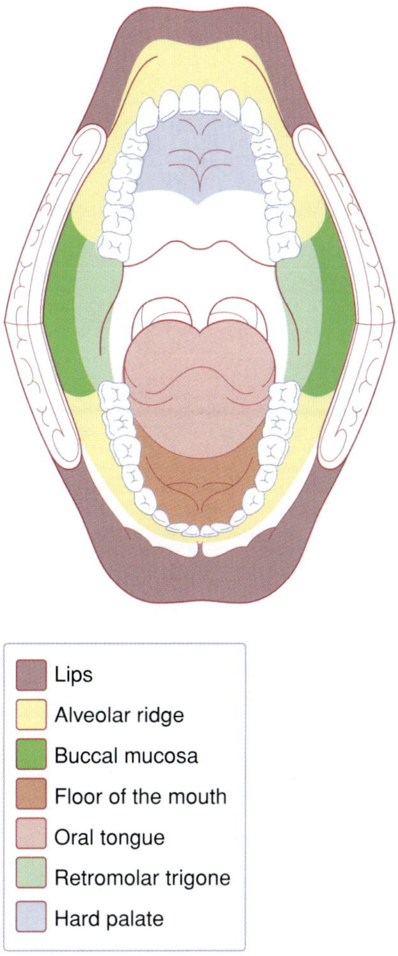

Figure 7.14 Lip and oral cavity: sites and T staging. T_1: < 2 cm; T_2: > 2 cm, < 4 cm; T_3: > 4 cm; T_4: massive tumor which invades adjacent structures.

Preoperative counselling in patients with a history of tobacco and alcohol abuse is vitally important to reduce postoperative morbidity. Cessation of smoking and alcohol also offers long-term benefit by reducing the risk of multiple primary tumors. Alcohol abusers and patients who come for treatment in an inebriated status are at a high risk of alcohol withdrawal symptoms in the postoperative period. They need to be seen preoperatively by psychiatric and rehabilitation specialists to facilitate perioperative management of alcoholism. The presence of these comorbid conditions has a significant impact on postoperative complications as well as prognosis.[1]

Staging for tumors of the oral cavity

Clinical staging for primary tumors of the oral cavity developed by the American Joint Committee on Cancer and the UICC is based on the TNM system.[10] Surface dimensions of the primary tumor are included as the most important parameter for determining primary tumor staging in the oral cavity. One significant deficiency of this staging system, however, is the omission of the third dimension of the lesion since it reflects the depth of infiltration. It is well known that deeply infiltrating but clinically early staged primary tumors of the tongue and floor of the mouth have an increased risk of regional metastasis and death due to disease compared to superficial tumors of the same T stage.[11] Thus, a more aggressive therapeutic approach may have to be considered, including elective treatment of regional lymph nodes for patients with early staged but deeply infiltrating tumors. In contrast, lesions which are at an advanced T stage, but are relatively superficial, have a better prognosis. The primary site staging (T staging) is shown in Table 7.1 (Fig. 7.14).

The N staging system for regional cervical lymph nodes is uniform for all epithelial tumors of the

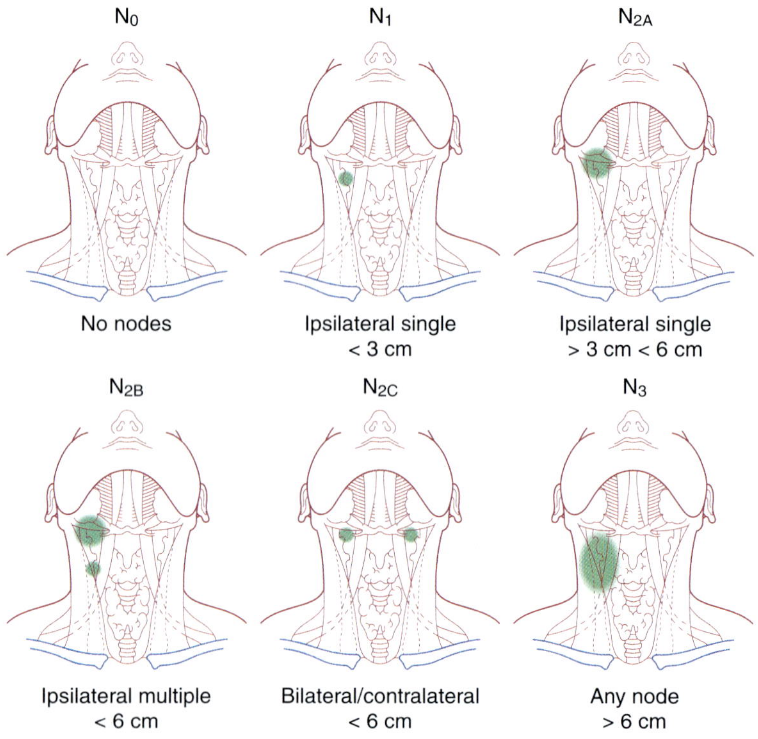

Figure 7.15 Regional lymph nodes: N staging. N_0: no nodes; N_1: ipsilateral, < 3 cm; N_{2A}: ipsilateral, > 3 cm, < 6 cm; N_{2B}: ipsilateral, multiple, < 6 cm; N_{2C}: bilateral/contralateral, < 6 cm; N_3: > 6 cm.

Table 7.1 TNM stage grouping for oral cancer

Stage 0	T_{is}	N_0	M_0
Stage I	T_1	N_0	M_0
Stage II	T_2	N_0	M_0
Stage III	T_3	N_0	M_0
	T_1	N_1	M_0
	T_2	N_1	M_0
	T_3	N_1	M_0
Stage IVA	T_4	N_0	M_0
	T_4	N_1	M_0
	Any T	N_2	M_0
Stage IVB	Any T	N_3	M_0
Stage IVC	Any T	Any N	M_1

upper aerodigestive tract.[10] The nodal staging system takes into account the size and multiplicity as well as the unilateral or bilateral presence of metastatic nodes as the parameters for N staging. The current N staging system is shown in Fig. 7.15. Important prognostic parameters such as the location of the metastatic lymph node as well as the presence of capsular penetration and extranodal spread are not used as parameters in the current N staging system, however. It is well known that the presence of metastatic lymph nodes beyond the first echelon locations and the presence of extranodal soft tissue extensions of metastatic tumor carry a significant negative impact on prognosis.[12,13]

The presence or absence of distant metastasis is documented as M_0 or M_1 by routine work-up that includes a posterior–anterior (PA) and lateral chest radiograph and routine blood chemistries. Specific clinical symptoms or physical findings indicative of distant metastasis require additional investigation such as radiographic studies including a bone scan, radiographs of the skeleton, and CT scans of brain, chest, abdomen, or pelvis. The most frequently involved sites for distant metastasis are lungs, liver and bones.[14] Therefore, a routine chest radiograph and serum chemistries, if normal, are considered sufficient to rule out distant metastasis in the absence of other specific symptoms. The stage groupings for the TNM system classification for oral cancer are shown in Table 7.1.

References

1. Piccirillo JF. Inclusion of comorbidity in a staging system for head and neck cancer. Oncology (Huntingt) 1995; 9: 831–836; discussion 841, 845–848
2. Singh B, Bhaya M, Stern J et al. Validation of the Charlson comorbidity index in patients with head and neck cancer: a multi-institutional study. Laryngoscope 1997; 107 (11 Pt 1): 1469–1475

3. Ondrey FG, Hom DB. Effects of nutrition on wound healing. Otolaryngol Head Neck Surg 1994; 110: 557–559
4. Weisman RA, Kimmelman CP. Bone scanning in the assessment of mandibular invasion by oral cavity carcinomas. Laryngoscope 1982; 92: 1–4
5. King JM, Caldarelli DD, Petasnick JP. DentaScan: a new diagnostic method for evaluating mandibular and maxillary pathology. Laryngoscope 1992; 102: 379–387
6. Crawford SC, Harnsberger HR, Lufkin RB, Hanafee WN. The role of gadolinium-DTPA in the evaluation of extracranial head and neck mass lesions. Radiol Clin North Am 1989; 27: 219–242
7. Maier H, Zoller J, Herrmann A, Kreiss M, Heller WD. Dental status and oral hygiene in patients with head and neck cancer. Otolaryngol Head Neck Surg 1993; 108: 655–661
8. Hurst PS. Dental considerations in management of head and neck cancer. Otolaryngol Clin North Am 1985; 18: 573–603
9. Soo KC, Spiro RH, King W, Harvey W, Strong EW. Squamous carcinoma of the gums. Am J Surg 1988; 156: 281–285
10. Greene FL, Page DL, Fleming ID et al (eds) AJCC Cancer Staging Manual, 6th edn, New York, Springer, 2002
11. Spiro RH, Huvos AG, Wong GY, Spiro JD, Gnecco CA, Strong EW. Predictive value of tumor thickness in squamous carcinoma confined to the tongue and floor of the mouth. Am J Surg 1986; 152: 345–350
12. Spiro RH, Alfonso AE, Farr HW, Strong EW. Cervical node metastasis from epidermoid carcinoma of the oral cavity and oropharynx. A critical assessment of current staging. Am J Surg 1974; 128: 562–567
13. Farr HW, Arthur K. Epidermoid carcinoma of the mouth and pharynx 1960–1964. J Laryngol Otol 1972; 86: 243–253
14. Nishijima W, Takooda S, Tokita N, Takayama S, Sakura M. Analyses of distant metastases in squamous cell carcinoma of the head and neck and lesions above the clavicle at autopsy. Arch Otolaryngol Head Neck Surg 1993; 119: 65–68

8 Factors affecting choice of treatment

John F Carew, Bhuvanesh Singh and Jatin P Shah

The factors that influence choice of initial treatment are related to the characteristics and stage of the primary tumor (tumor factors), to the patient (patient factors), and to the providers of treatment (physician factors). In selecting the optimal treatment, therefore, one should consider these three sets of factors. The ultimate goals in the treatment of cancer of the oral cavity are to:

1. Cure the cancer;
2. Preserve or restore form and function;
3. Minimize the sequelae of treatment, and
4. Prevent multiple primary tumors.

The currently available therapeutic modalities to achieve these goals include surgery, radiotherapy, chemotherapy, combined modality treatments, and primary and secondary prevention strategies including lifestyle changes and chemoprevention.

Tumor factors

Clinical characteristics and histopathological parameters of the tumour listed in Table 8.1 are important factors that influence choice of treatment.

Table 8.1 Tumor factors influencing choice of treatment

Site of the primary tumor
Location in the oral cavity (anterior vs posterior)
Size (T stage)
Proximity to bone (mandible or maxilla)
Status of cervical lymph nodes
Histology (type, grade and depth of invasion)
Previous treatment

Certain primary sites are considered high risk since they have a higher risk for nodal metastasis compared to other sites in the oral cavity. For example, primary tumors of the oral tongue and floor of the mouth have an increased risk of lymph node metastasis compared to similar staged lesions of the hard palate or upper gum.[1–3] Primary tumors located anteriorly in the oral cavity have a lower risk for dissemination to regional lymph nodes compared to similar staged lesions in the posterior part of the oral cavity and oropharynx; for example, primary tumors of the oral tongue versus the base of the tongue.[3,4] Thus, more posteriorly located lesions will require consideration of elective treatment of the clinically negative neck in initial treatment planning.

The size of the primary tumor clearly impacts significantly on the decision regarding choice of initial treatment. Small, superficial primary tumors of the oral cavity are easily accessible for surgical resection through the open mouth. On the other hand, larger tumors will require more extensive surgical approaches for exposure and excision. Additionally, certain primary sites in the oral cavity, such as tumors of the tongue, are easily amenable to initial treatment by radiotherapy, in contrast to those which are situated in proximity to bone such as a lesion of the gum. Similarly, the risk of regional lymph node metastasis increases with increasing size of the primary lesion, necessitating consideration of elective treatment of the clinically negative neck.

The proximity of a primary oral cancer to bone, such as mandible or maxilla, is also an important consideration in treatment selection. Invasion of the alveolar process or lingual cortex of the mandible from tumors of the floor of the mouth, gum or cheek mucosa requires accurate assessment of the underlying bone and appropriate surgical treatment planning to evaluate the need for bone resection. Similarly, a primary tumor of the upper alveolus or the hard palate requires adequate radiological evaluation, appropriate dental consultation for fabrication of a dental prosthesis, and proper treatment planning for satisfactory surgical resection of the primary lesion. Tumors of the hard palate and upper or lower gum, or those that secondarily extend to the mandible or maxilla, are considered suboptimal for definitive treatment by radiotherapy. Not only does proximity of the primary tumor to bone increase the risk of exposure of the involved bone and osteoradionecrosis, but it also reduces the likelihood of a favorable response to ionizing radiation delivered with a curative intent.

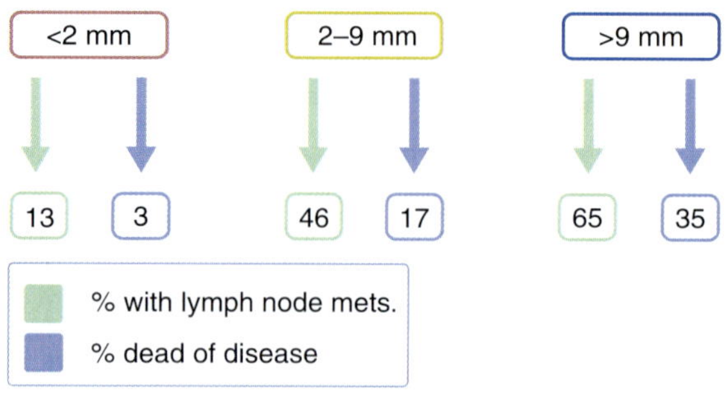

Figure 8.1 Risk of lymph node metastasis and mortality in relation to thickness of primary lesions for T_1 and T_2 squamous carcinoma of the oral tongue and floor of the mouth.

The presence of clinically palpable cervical lymph node metastasis necessitates comprehensive neck dissection as an integral part of surgical treatment planning. The extent of neck dissection, however, will vary upon the extent of nodal metastasis and the location of palpable lymph nodes.

The histology of the primary tumor is an important parameter that influences the selection of initial treatment. While squamous cell carcinomas are radio-responsive, primary carcinomas of minor salivary gland origin and malignant lesions of the somatic soft tissues are considered radio-resistant and are best treated by surgical resection. Most lesions of squamous cell origin have a varying degree of histologic progression from in situ to invasive carcinoma. The histologic grade of the lesion generally reflects the aggressiveness of the tumor. Poorly differentiated carcinomas and undifferentiated carcinomas are predictably more aggressive in comparison to moderately differentiated and well-differentiated carcinomas. However, the most important histologic feature of the primary tumor which impacts on selection of treatment and eventual prognosis is its depth of infiltration. Thin and superficially invasive lesions have a lower risk of regional lymph node metastasis, are highly curable, and offer an excellent prognosis.[5] On the other hand, thicker lesions which are deeply infiltrating have a significantly increased incidence of regional lymph node metastasis, with its adverse impact on prognosis. Similarly, exophytic lesions are considered less aggressive than endophytic lesions of the same site and T stage. The risk of lymph node metastasis and survival in relation to the thickness of the primary lesions for T_1 and T_2 squamous carcinomas of the oral tongue and floor of the mouth are shown in Fig. 8.1. While it would be ideal to know the thickness of the lesion prior to surgical resection, it is clinically impractical to have that information available prior to excision of the primary tumor in many instances. In general, however, thickness of the lesion as appreciated by palpation is a reasonably good indicator of the depth of invasion and therefore its potential for regional lymph node metastasis. Evaluation of the depth of infiltration of the primary lesion is useful in the consideration of whether elective dissection of the regional lymph nodes at risk in the clinically negative neck is necessary.

Previous treatment of another oral cavity tumor will have a significant impact on the selection of treatment for the presenting oral cancer. For example, patients who have previously undergone radiotherapy to the oral cavity for any reason are not considered candidates for any definitive radiotherapy for a second oral cancer. Similarly, patients who may have had significant partial glossectomy in the past may not be considered good candidates for a further glossectomy for a second primary tumor or recurrent tumor due to significant loss of function in relation to speech and deglutition with additional surgery. Alternative treatment programs with brachytherapy or concomitant chemo/radiotherapy should be considered prior to total glossectomy in these patients. Thus, previous treatment clearly influences the selection of therapy for the presenting tumor.

Patients at an advanced stage of disease, that is those presenting with spread to regional cervical lymph nodes or with large primary tumors, i.e. T_3 and T_4, are candidates for combined modality treatment. Currently, surgical resection followed by postoperative radiation therapy is considered standard treatment for patients with stage III and stage IV carcinomas of the oral cavity.

Patient factors

Several factors related to patient characteristics are important in the selection of initial treatment (Table 8.2).

Table 8.2 Patient factors influencing choice of treatment

Age
General medical condition
Tolerance
Occupation
Acceptance and compliance
Lifestyle (smoking/drinking)
Socio-economic considerations

Table 8.3 Physician factors influencing choice of treatment

Surgical skills
Radiotherapy skills
Chemotherapy expertise
Dental and prosthetic services
Rehabilitation services
Support services

In general, older age is not considered to be a contraindication for implementation of appropriate surgical treatment for oral cancer. However, advancing age, intercurrent disease, and debility due to associated cardiopulmonary conditions increase the risk of a major adverse perioperative event. The inability of the patient to tolerate an optimal therapeutic program due to associated co-morbid conditions is thus an important factor which can influence the choice of initial treatment.[6,7] The patient's occupation, and acceptance of and compliance with the proposed treatment are similarly important considerations when the optimal treatment program is designed. The patient's lifestyle, particularly with reference to smoking and drinking, impacts heavily on the selection and tolerance of treatment offered. Unwillingness on the part of the patient to give up these habits causes further complications in therapy and increases the risk of multiple primary tumors. Finally, socio-economic considerations play an increasing role in the selection of treatment. Allocation of resources clearly has to be judged on the basis of outcomes analysis of a particular treatment program.

The geographic location of the patient in relation to the treatment facility and the fiscal impact of the proposed treatment on the patient are also important considerations. In many parts of the world, patients may not have the freedom to choose the treatment facility due to government, insurance, or health care provider regulations. Therefore, when therapeutic decisions regarding the optimal treatment are made, these socio-economic factors must be considered in order to provide the most cost-effective treatment to the patient.

Physician factors

Several physician and health care provider related factors also play an important role in the selection of initial treatment, these are shown in Table 8.3.

Management of cancer of the head and neck requires a multidisciplinary team effort and technical capabilities and support services from various disciplines are essential for a successful outcome. A comprehensive head and neck surgery team consists of a head and neck surgeon, with the availability of other surgical specialists in microsurgery, neurosurgery, vascular surgery, plastic and reconstructive surgery, and dental surgery and prosthetics. Similarly, expertise in radiation oncology including brachytherapy, and integration of combined treatment programs of radio-chemotherapy are essential. A well-qualified team of medical oncologists with expertise in the administration of chemotherapeutic drugs and the management of chemotherapy-related complications is fundamental in the management of patients with advanced disease and recurrent tumors. In addition, physical and psychosocial rehabilitation services are vitally important for long-term restoration of the patient's quality of life. Implicit in such a team is the availability of a psychologist, social worker, and family support groups to provide the patient with all essential services.

Selection of initial treatment

Both surgical resection and radiotherapy are applicable either singly or in combination in the treatment of cancer of the oral cavity. At this time, the role of chemotherapy in the management of oral cancer remains investigational. Small and superficial tumors of the oral cavity are equally amenable for cure by surgical resection or radiotherapy. Therefore, single modality is preferred as definitive treatment in early staged tumors (T_1 and T_2 lesions) of the oral cavity. When the end point of treatment, i.e. cure of cancer, is comparable by either surgery or radiotherapy, other factors must play a role in the selection of the initial treatment. These include complications, cost, convenience, compliance and

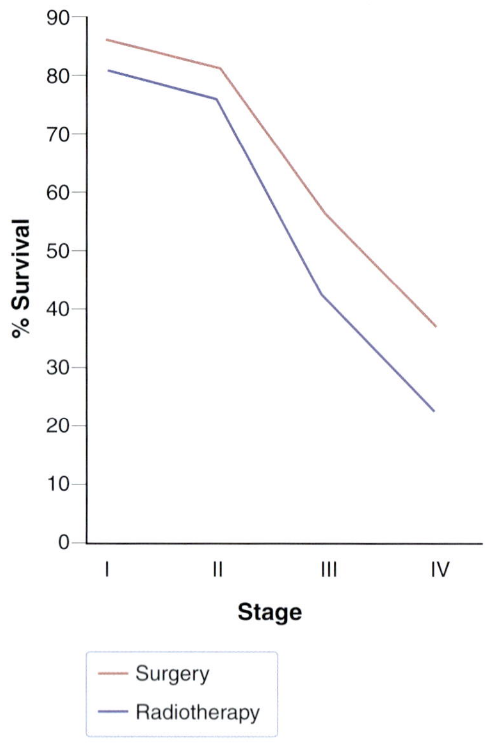

Figure 8.2 The choice of surgery versus radiotherapy: survival with single modality treatment.

long-term sequelae of treatment (Fig. 8.2), as well as site, location, stage, histology, and node status.

In general, primary tumors in the vicinity of bone are not suitable for definitive radiotherapy, due to the fear of exposure of bone with the risk of osteoradionecrosis and its attendant morbidity. Thus, primary tumors of the lower gum, upper gum and hard palate are best treated by surgical resection. On the other hand, primary tumors of the tongue, floor of mouth or cheek mucosa, as well as lips, are readily suitable for radiotherapy as definitive treatment. If radiotherapy is selected as the initial definitive treatment, in most instances a combination of external and interstitial irradiation is required. Small, superficial, selected lesions may be treated by brachytherapy alone. In choosing radiotherapy as definitive treatment, one needs to consider the status of dentition and oral hygiene, since they may significantly impact upon the complications of radiotherapy. The most feared complications of external radiation to the oral cavity are the long-term risks of dental caries and osteoradionecrosis secondary to dental sepsis in the irradiated mandible. Thus, patients with very poor oral hygiene and significant dental sepsis will require total exodontia prior to initiation of radiotherapy. In addition to the above, the long-term sequelae of radiotherapy such as permanent xerostomia and temporary loss of taste are to be considered as important issues in selection of therapy. Other factors such as length of treatment, convenience to the patient, and cost of treatment are also important considerations which will influence selection of initial treatment. If the patient is at a significant risk of developing multiple primary tumors, then radiotherapy may be reserved for its potential use in the future for subsequent primary tumors and may not be the ideal choice of therapy in early staged oral carcinoma.

Initial surgical treatment, on the other hand, provides in a cost-effective manner an expeditious curative treatment for early stage oral cancer with minimal morbidity and essentially no long-term sequelae of treatment. Most early stage primary oral carcinomas can be treated by a relatively simple surgical procedure, usually through the open mouth, with a short hospitalization. The functional sequelae of surgical treatment are minimal and transient. Impairment in the clarity of speech and difficulty with mastication resulting from surgical intervention in the oral cavity are overcome by the patient in a matter of a few weeks. Long-term impairment of speech, mastication, or other debilities are usually not seen. Thus, surgical treatment for early staged oral carcinoma is the therapy of choice in most instances, in the absence of contraindications.

Patients with advanced stage tumors clearly require combined modality treatment for successful outcome. Radiotherapy in combination with surgery can be employed either preoperatively or postoperatively. There are obvious advantages and disadvantages of preoperative radiotherapy when compared to postoperative radiation therapy.

Preoperative radiotherapy delays the implementation of the surgical treatment by several weeks. However, during this time nutrition of the patient can be improved either by nasogastric tube feeding or by supplemental nutrition through a gastrostomy tube. The use of preoperative radiotherapy has been claimed to 'enhance resectability'. However, it must be borne in mind that tumor response with shrinkage of the primary tumor should not influence the extent of surgical resection. It is a well-known fact that tumors do not shrink concentrically and viable islands of tumor cells may still be present in grossly normal appearing tissues adjacent to the residual tumor following preoperative radiotherapy. Therefore, the extent and the margins of surgical resection should be essentially the same as those in the absence of preoperative radiotherapy. In those patients who will require multiple staged reconstruction, preoperative radiotherapy offers an advantage in posing no conflict with such staged reconstructive procedures. However, currently one stage primary reconstruction is considered the state of the art and therefore preoperative radiotherapy is not considered advantageous any more. On the other hand, irradiated tissues may pose a problem with healing of tissue and increase the risk of local wound complications. An additional and important disadvantage of preoperative radiotherapy is dose limitation. It is well known that with increasing dosage of preoperative radiotherapy, the wound complications of surgery increase.

Postoperative radiotherapy, on the other hand, offers significant advantages over preoperative radiotherapy and offers better or comparable local and regional control rates of cancer. There is no delay in implementation of surgical resection and there are no dose limitations with postoperative radiotherapy. Another distinct advantage is the availability of accurate pathologic details of disease following surgery. This information helps in the design of radiation portals and dose as well as in the identification of areas at high risk of recurrence which would benefit from boosting. At present, doses in the range of 6000 cGy to the primary site and neck are recommended, with a boost to areas at increased risk of local recurrence. Postoperative radiotherapy does not influence the extent of surgical resection and healing and wound complications are not an issue since radiotherapy is started after the incisions have healed.

Thus, for patients with advanced disease (stage III and stage IV), a combined treatment program consisting of surgical resection with immediate appropriate reconstruction followed by adjuvant postoperative radiation therapy is currently considered the optimal treatment.

The factors that influence the choice of surgical approach for a primary tumor of the oral cavity or oropharynx are the size of the primary, its depth of infiltration, the site of the primary, anterior versus posterior location, and proximity of the tumor to the mandible or maxilla. Therefore, thorough clinical assessment of the primary tumor is mandatory for selection of the appropriate surgical procedure. Examination under anesthesia is sometimes necessary to decide upon the appropriate surgical approach. The proximity of the tumor to the maxilla or mandible mandates the need for adequate clinical and radiographic assessment to rule out the possibility of bone involvement. If bone resection is required, then the surgical planning should include restoration, reconstruction, or prosthetic rehabilitation of the bony defect.

References

1. Evans JF, Shah JP. Epidermoid carcinoma of the palate. Am J Surg 1981; 142: 451–455
2. Shaha AR, Spiro RH, Shah JP, Strong EW. Squamous carcinoma of the floor of the mouth. Am J Surg 1984; 148: 455–459
3. Franceschi D, Gupta R, Spiro RH, Shah JP. Improved survival in the treatment of squamous carcinoma of the oral tongue. Am J Surg 1993; 166: 360–365
4. Kraus DH, Vastola AP, Huvos AG, Spiro RH. Surgical management of squamous cell carcinoma of the base of the tongue. Am J Surg 1993; 166: 384–388
5. Spiro RH, Huvos AG, Wong GY, Spiro JD, Gnecco CA, Strong EW. Predictive value of tumor thickness in squamous carcinoma confined to the tongue and floor of the mouth. Am J Surg 1986; 152: 345–350
6. Piccirillo JF. Inclusion of comorbidity in a staging system for head and neck cancer. Oncology (Huntingt) 1995; 9: 831–836; discussion 841, 845–848
7. Singh B, Bhaya M, Stern J et al. Validation of the Charlson comorbidity index in patients with head and neck cancer: a multi-institutional study. Laryngoscope 1997; 107(11 Pt 1): 1469–1475

9 Cervical lymph nodes

John F Carew, Bhuvanesh Singh and Jatin P Shah

The single most important factor impacting on the outcome of patients with squamous cell carcinoma of the upper aerodigestive tract is the stage of the disease at the time of initial diagnosis and treatment.[1–21] Patients who present with tumors localized at the primary site without dissemination to regional lymph nodes enjoy an excellent prognosis. On the other hand, once dissemination to regional lymph nodes takes place, the probability of 5-year survivorship, regardless of the treatment rendered, reduces to nearly one half of that seen in early staged patients (Fig. 9.1).[1–3,5,10–12,15,19,21–31]

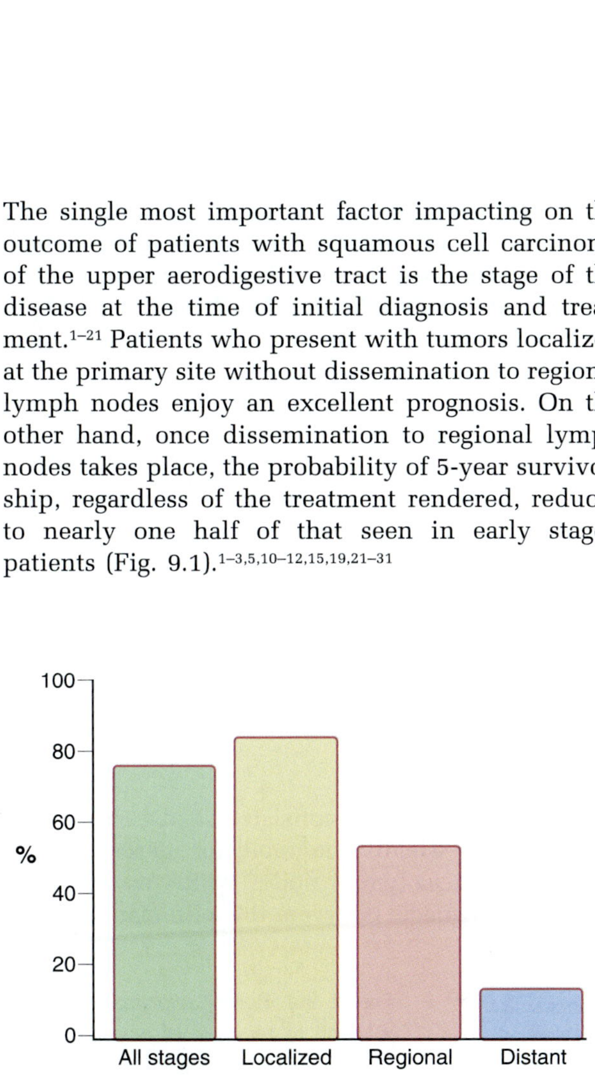

Figure 9.1 Cancer of the oral cavity and pharynx: 5-year survival rates (MSKCC, 1986–95).

In spite of the progress made in the field of early diagnosis by public education and physician awareness in the past few years, still a significant number of patients present with disease at an advanced stage at the time of diagnosis. Reports from the American Cancer Society indicate that over 40% of the patients with squamous carcinomas of the oral cavity and pharynx present with regional dissemination of disease at the time of initial diagnosis (Fig. 9.2).[32] In other parts of the world such as Asia and Latin America, a majority of patients with cancer of the upper aerodigestive tract present with advanced stage disease.[33–41] Thus, management of cervical lymph nodes becomes a vitally important component of the overall treatment strategy for patients with cancers of the head and neck.

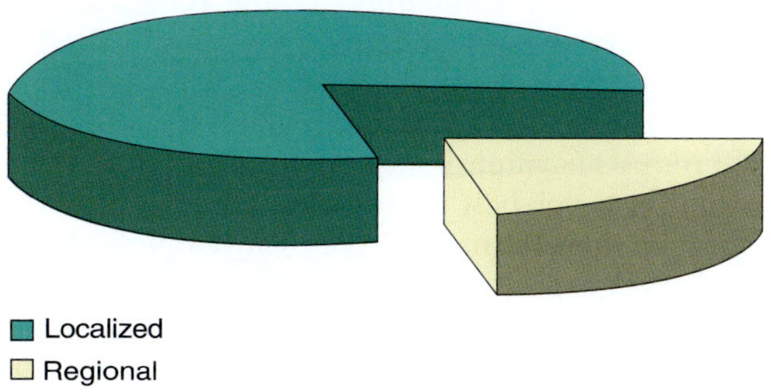

Figure 9.2 Cancer of oral cavity (MSKCC, 1986–95).

Anatomy of regional lymphatics

Regional lymphatic drainage from the scalp and skin of the head and neck region, the mucosa of the upper aerodigestive tract, salivary glands, and the thyroid gland occurs to specific cervical regional lymph node groups. In addition to this, tumor dissemination via regional lymphatics to these lymph node groups occurs in a predictable and sequential fashion.[3,5,24,27,28,42–51] Therefore, specific regional lymph node groups should be appropriately addressed in treatment planning for a given primary site. These include those regional lymph nodes which are accessible for surgical resection and those which are relatively inaccessible for adequate surgical resection.

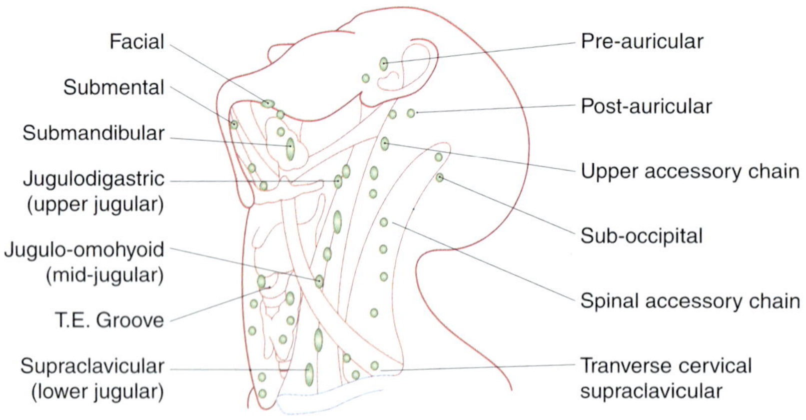

Figure 9.3 Regional cervical lymph nodes. Additional lymph node groups not shown; parapharyngeal, retropharyngeal and superior mediastinal.

The regional lymph nodes of the head and neck region are shown in Fig. 9.3. The preauricular, periparotid and intraparotid lymph nodes are the first echelon lymph nodes for the anterior half of the scalp, the skin of the forehead, and the upper part of the face. The postauricular and suboccipital groups of lymph nodes provide initial drainage to the posterior half of the scalp and the posterior aspect of the external ear. Cervical lymph nodes in the lateral aspect of the neck primarily drain the mucosa of the upper aerodigestive tract. These include the submental, prevascular facial, and submandibular group of lymph nodes located in the submental and submandibular triangles of the neck. Deep jugular lymph nodes include the jugulo-digastric, jugulo-omohyoid, and supraclavicular group of lymph nodes adjacent to the internal jugular vein. Lymph nodes in the posterior triangle of the neck include the accessory chain of lymph nodes located along the spinal accessory nerve and the transverse cervical chain of lymph nodes in the floor of the posterior triangle of the neck. Parapharyngeal and retropharyngeal lymph nodes are at risk of metastatic dissemination from tumors of the pharynx.[52]

The central compartment of the neck includes the delphian lymph node overlying the thyroid cartilage in the midline draining the larynx and perithyroid lymph nodes adjacent to the thyroid gland. Lymph nodes in the tracheo-esophageal groove provide primary drainage to the thyroid gland as well as the hypopharynx, subglottic larynx, and cervical esophagus. Lymph nodes in the anterior superior mediastinum provide drainage to the thyroid gland, the cervical esophagus, and serve as a secondary lymphatic basin for anatomic structures in the central compartment of the neck. Each anatomic subgroup of lymph nodes described above specifically serves as primary echelon lymph nodes draining a specific site in the head and neck region. Thus, location of a palpable metastatic lymph node may often indicate the source of a primary tumor. In Fig. 9.4 the regional lymph node groups draining a specific primary site as first echelon lymph nodes are depicted.

In order to establish a consistent and easily reproducible, user-friendly method for description of regional cervical lymph nodes which establishes a common language between the clinician and the

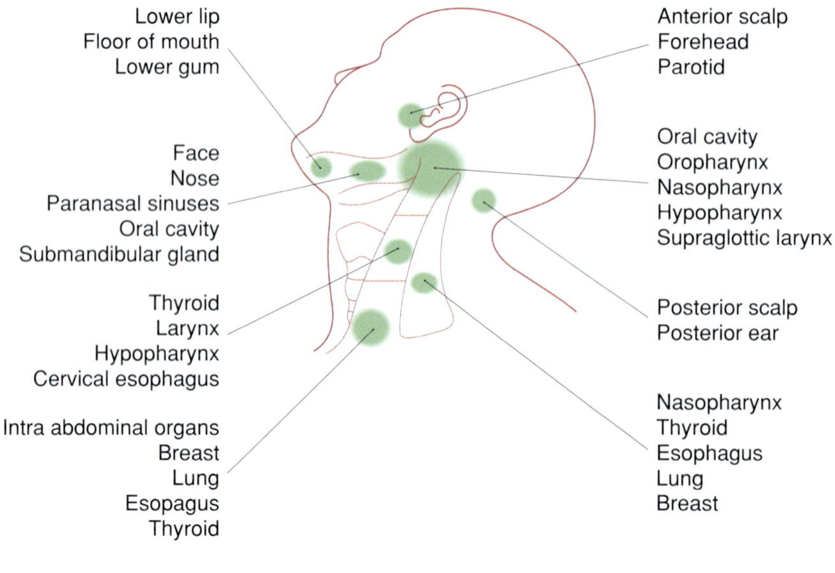

Figure 9.4 Potential primary sites in relation to location of cervical lymph node metastases.

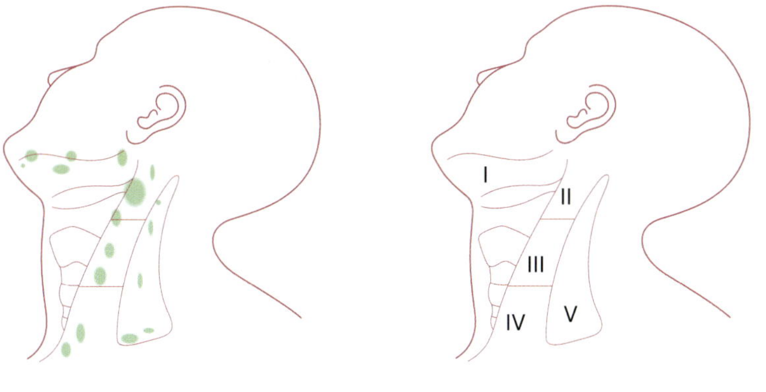

Figure 9.5 Cervical lymph nodes: location and levels.

pathologist, the Head and Neck Service at Memorial Sloan–Kettering Cancer Center in New York has described a leveling system of cervical lymph nodes (Fig. 9.5).[2,3,46] This system divides the lymph nodes in the lateral aspect of the neck into five nodal groups or levels:

Level I Submental group The nodal tissue between the anterior belly of the digastric muscles and cephalad to the hyoid bone.

Submandibular group Nodal tissue in the triangular area bounded by the anterior and posterior bellies of the digastric muscle and the inferior border of the body of the mandible. The lymph nodes adjacent to the submandibular salivary gland and along the facial artery are included in this group.

Level II Upper jugular group Nodal tissue around the upper portion of the internal jugular vein and the upper part of the spinal accessory nerve, extending from the base of the skull up to the bifurcation of the carotid artery or the hyoid bone (clinical landmark). The posterior limit for this level is the posterior border of the sternocleidomastoid muscle and the anterior border is the lateral limit of the sternohyoid muscle.

Level III Mid-jugular group Nodal tissue around the middle third of the internal jugular vein from the inferior border of level II up to the omohyoid muscle or the lower border of the cricoid cartilage (clinical landmark). The anterior and posterior borders are the same as those for level II.

Level IV Lower jugular group Nodal tissue around the lower third of the internal jugular vein from the inferior border of level III up to the clavicle. The anterior and posterior borders are the same as those for levels II and III.

Level V Posterior triangle group Nodal tissue around the lower portion of the spinal accessory nerve and along the transverse cervical vessels. It is bounded by the triangle formed by the clavicle, posterior border of the sternocleidomastoid muscle, and the anterior border of the trapezius muscle.

Level VI Central compartment group Lymph nodes in the tracheoesophageal grooves and perithyroid region, extending from below the hyoid bone up to the suprasternal notch.

Level VII Superior mediastinal group Lymph nodes in the anterior superior mediastinum, extending from the suprasternal notch up to the innominate artery.

Clinical staging of cervical lymph nodes (N staging)

The American Joint Committee on Cancer (AJCC) and the International Union Against Cancer (UICC) has agreed upon a uniform staging system for cervical lymph nodes. This nodal staging system is depicted in Fig. 9.6. The N stages of lymph node metastasis are described in Table 9.1.

This staging system simply reflects the volume of tumor burden in regional lymph nodes which is directly linked to prognosis of the patient. The

Table 9.1 2002 AJCC/UICC staging system for cervical lymph node metastases

N_x	Regional lymph nodes cannot be assessed
N_0	No regional lymph node metastasis
N_1	Metastasis in a single ipsilateral lymph node, < 3 cm in greatest dimension
N_{2A}	Metastasis in single ipsilateral lymph node > 3 cm but < 6 cm in greatest dimension
N_{2B}	Metastasis in multiple ipsilateral lymph nodes, none > 6 cm in greatest dimension
N_{2C}	Metastasis in bilateral or contralateral lymph nodes, none > 6 cm in greatest dimension
N_3	Metastasis in a lymph node > 6 cm in greatest dimension

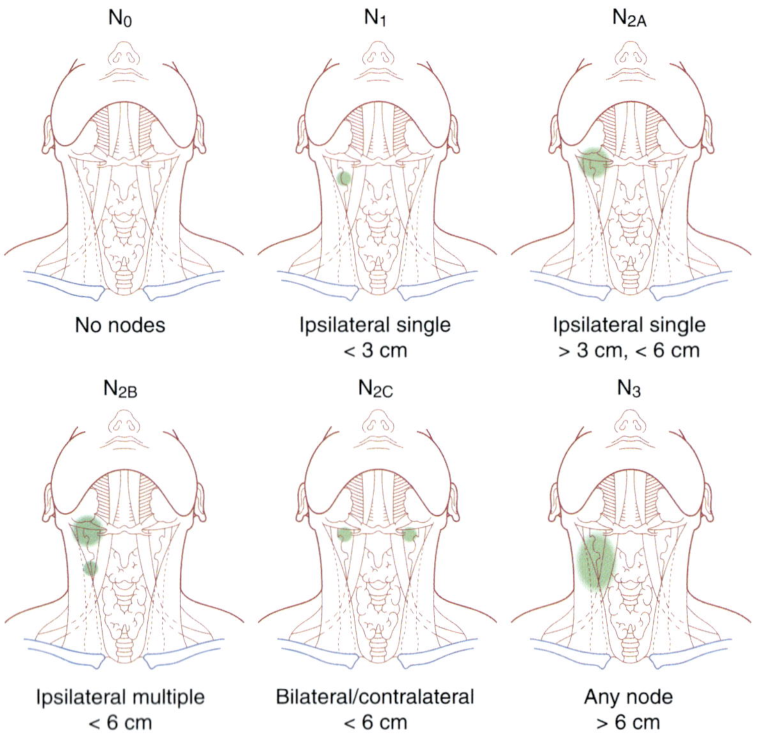

Figure 9.6 AJCC/UICC N staging.

prognosis worsens with increasing N stage. However, there are other prognostic factors pertaining to the lymph nodes which are not included in the current N staging system.

Nodal factors affecting prognosis

Several factors pertaining to the characteristics of the regional lymph node metastasis directly influence prognosis. These include the presence or absence of clinically palpable cervical lymph node metastasis, the size of the metastatic lymph node, the number of lymph nodes involved, and the location of lymph nodes involved by metastatic cancer.[3,5,7,19,21,25,28,52–54] Involvement of lower cervical lymph nodes (level IV) and lower posterior triangle lymph nodes (level V) by metastatic cancer usually implies an ominous prognosis.[7] Thus, involvement of lymph nodes in the lateral neck below the lower border of the cricoid cartilage is of serious prognostic significance. In addition to this, the presence of extranodal spread of metastatic disease by capsular rupture of the lymph node with invasion of the soft tissues clearly impacts on prognosis.[12,14,21,23,55–59] Perivascular and perineural infiltration by tumor as well as the presence of tumor emboli in regional lymphatics also have an adverse impact on prognosis.[5,12,18,53,54,57,60] Therefore, these factors must be considered in developing a treatment strategy for patients in whom regional lymph nodes are involved by metastatic disease, particularly for planning adjuvant therapy and for assessment of prognosis.

Risk of nodal metastasis

Involvement of regional lymphatics by primary squamous cell carcinomas of the upper aerodigestive tract is dependent on various factors related to the primary tumor, including the site, size, T stage, and location of the primary tumor. In addition, histomorphologic features of the primary tumor also influence the risk of nodal metastasis.[3,5,6,8,10,13,22,45,46,51,61–63] The risk of nodal metastasis increases in relation to the location of the primary tumor as one progresses from the anterior to the posterior aspect of the upper aerodigestive tract, i.e. the lips, oral cavity, oropharynx, and hypopharynx (Fig. 9.7).[3,5,45,46,51] For tumors of the larynx and pharynx, the risk of nodal metastasis increases as one progresses from the center of the laryngopharyngeal compartment to the periphery.[3,5,46,51] For example, the risk of regional lymph node metastasis from carcinoma of the true vocal cord is exceedingly small. The risk, however, increases as one progresses from the vocal cords to the false vocal cords, aryepiglottic fold, pyriform sinus, and pharyngeal wall. Nearly two-thirds of patients with primary carcinomas of the hypopharynx present with clinically palpable regional lymph node metastasis.

Within the oral cavity certain primary sites have a significantly increased risk of nodal metastasis compared to the other sites, for example, floor of mouth versus hard palate. In general, the T stage usually reflects tumor burden and therefore the risk of nodal metastasis increases with increasing T stage of the primary tumor at any site.

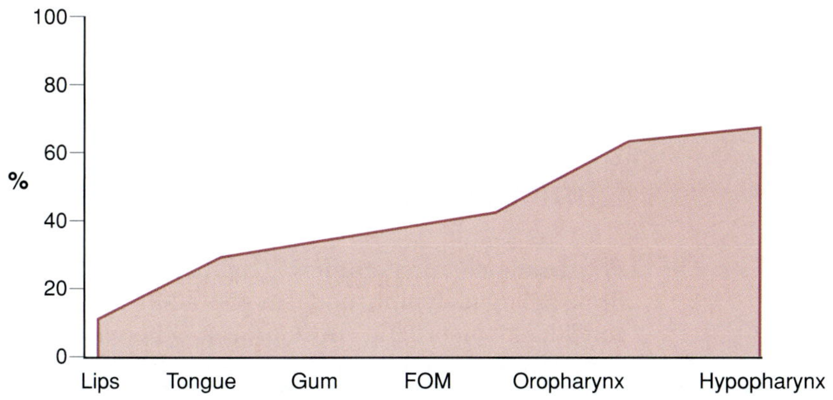

Figure 9.7 Incidence of nodal metastases at presentation in relation to primary site, location.

Certain histomorphological features of the primary tumor also increase the risk of nodal metastasis. Thus endophytic tumors are more inclined to metastasize than exophytic tumors. It has been well documented that for tongue and floor of mouth cancers, tumor thickness is related to the risk of nodal metastases (Fig. 9.8). Poorly differentiated carcinomas have a higher risk of nodal metastases compared to well-differentiated lesions.

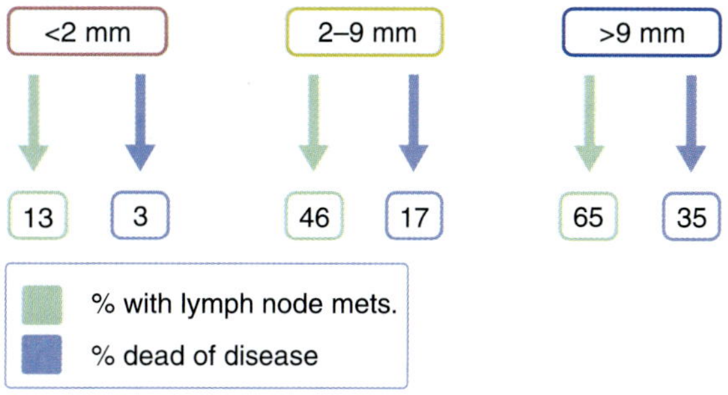

Figure 9.8 Percentage of lymph node metastases and percentage dead of disease, in relation to tumor thickness.

Patterns of neck metastasis

Dissemination of metastatic cancer to regional lymph nodes from primary sites in the upper aerodigestive tract occurs in a predictable and sequential fashion.[3,5,43,45,46,51] Thus, only select regional lymph node groups are at risk of nodal metastases initially from any primary site, in the absence of grossly palpable metastatic lymph nodes. On the other hand, when clinically palpable lymph nodes are present at the time of initial diagnosis, comprehensive clearance of all regional lymph node groups at risk is warranted. Several well-documented studies in the literature have confirmed that select groups of regional lymph nodes are initially at risk for each primary site in the head and neck region. Understanding the sequential patterns of neck metastasis therefore greatly facilitates surgical management of regional lymph nodes in the clinically negative neck where the lymph nodes are at risk of harboring micrometastasis.

For primary tumors in the oral cavity the regional lymph nodes at highest risk for early dissemination by metastatic cancer are limited to levels I, II, and III (Fig. 9.9). Anatomically this translates into regional lymph node groups contained within the supraomohyoid triangle of the neck including the submental, submandibular, prevascular facial, jugulodigastric, upper deep jugular, superior spinal accessory chain of lymph nodes, and mid-jugular

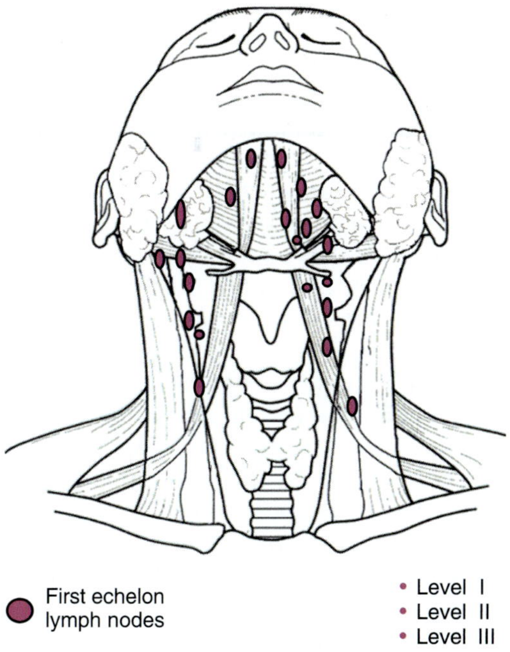

Figure 9.9 Patterns of lymph node metastases for cancer of the oral cavity. First echelon lymph nodes: levels I, II, and III.

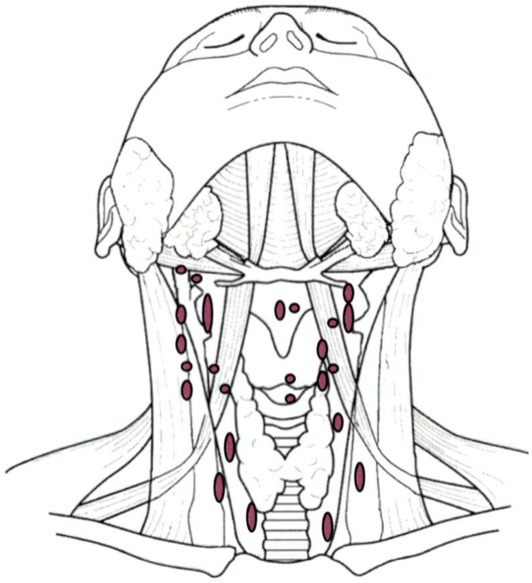

Figure 9.10 Patterns of lymph node metastases for cancer of the larynx and pharynx. First echelon lymph nodes: levels II, III, and IV.

lymph nodes. Skip metastasis to levels IV and V in the absence of metastatic disease at levels I, II, or III occurs in less than 10% of cases.[64] Therefore, if the neck is clinically negative, levels IV and V lymph nodes are generally not considered at risk of harboring micrometastasis from primary squamous carcinomas of the oral cavity.

For tumors on the lateral aspect of the oropharynx, the first echelon lymph nodes at highest risk of harboring micrometastasis in the clinically negative neck are the deep jugular lymph nodes at levels II, III and IV on the ipsilateral side (Fig. 9.10).[27,46,61] The lymph node groups in the deep jugular chain are the jugulo-digastric, highest spinal accessory chain of lymph nodes, mid-jugular lymph nodes, jugulo-omohyoid lymph nodes, and supraclavicular lymph nodes deep to the sternocleidomastoid muscle. Contiguous lymph nodes lateral to the internal jugular vein overlying the cutaneous roots of the cervical plexus are usually considered a component of levels II, III and IV. In patients with primary carcinomas of the oropharynx with a clinically negative neck the risk of micrometastasis to levels I and V is extremely small.[27,46,61,65] Skip metastasis to levels I and V in the absence of disease at levels II, III, or IV is usually not seen. Primary tumors which involve both sides of the midline have a potential of microscopic dissemination of metastatic disease to jugular lymph nodes on both sides of the neck.

Clinical features and diagnosis

The presence of a clinically palpable, unilateral, firm, enlarged lymph node in the adult should be considered metastatic until proven otherwise. The clinically enlarged lymph node may be present at any of the previously described anatomic locations in the head and neck region. The location of a palpable lymph node may point to the potential site of a primary tumor. The important features to note during examination of the neck for cervical lymph nodes are the location, size, consistency, and number of palpable lymph nodes as well as clinical signs of extracapsular spread such as invasion of the overlying skin, fixation to deeper soft tissues, or paralysis of cranial nerves. Histological diagnosis of metastatic carcinoma is usually established by a needle aspiration biopsy and cytological examination of the smears.[2,3,5,24,25,66,67] An enlarged metastatic cervical lymph node may be the only physical finding present in some patients whose primary tumors are either microscopic or occult at the time of presentation. A systematic search for a primary tumor should be undertaken in these patients prior to embarking upon therapy for the metastatic nodes.

Radiographic evaluation

Most patients with palpable cervical lymph node metastasis seldom require radiographic evaluation of the nodes for diagnosis. However, when massive metastatic disease is present, radiographic evaluation by CT scan with intravenous contrast or MRI scan with gadolinium contrast, is desirable to assess the extent of the nodal disease, particularly as it relates to the carotid artery, the skull base, and the parapharyngeal space on the ipsilateral side as well as to evaluate the clinically negative contralateral side.[66,68–72] Several lymph node groups which are not accessible to clinical examination, such as those in the parapharyngeal and retropharyngeal areas, are best assessed by a CT or MRI scan. Similarly, evaluation of lymph nodes in the superior mediastinum is best accomplished with radiographic studies. The radiographic features for diagnosis of a metastatic node are: size, rim enhancement, central necrosis, and extranodal invasion (Fig. 9.11).[68] Ultrasound-guided fine needle aspiration biopsy of a small lymph node often helps to establish accurate tissue diagnosis.[66]

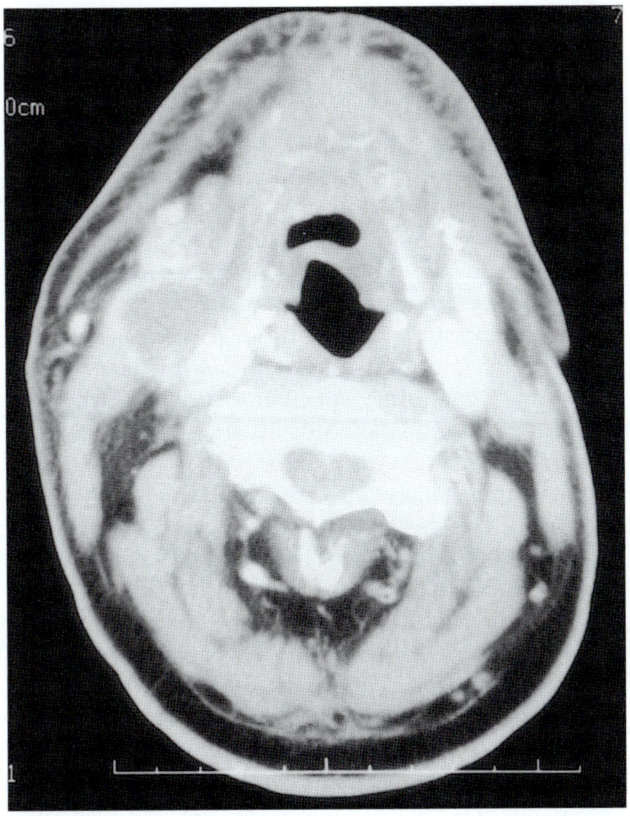

Figure 9.11 CT scan of neck with contrast showing a metastatic lymph node with central necrosis and rim enhancement.

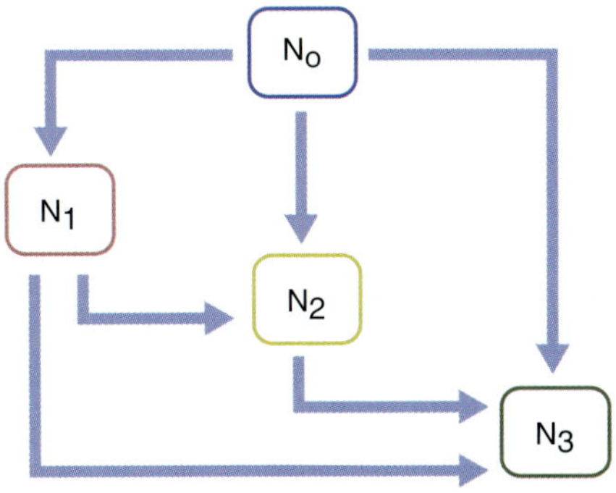

Figure 9.12 Disease progression in untreated N_0 necks.

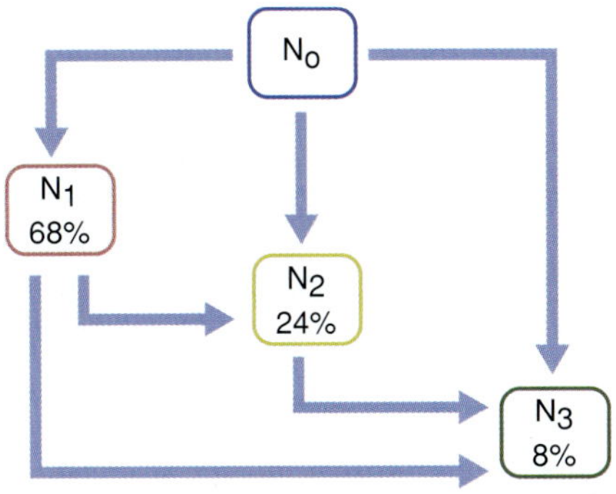

Figure 9.13 Clinical findings at delayed therapeutic neck dissection in untreated N_0 necks.

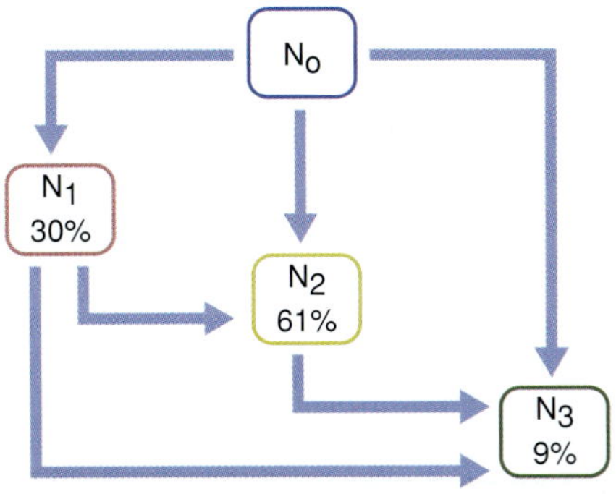

Figure 9.14 Pathologic findings at delayed therapeutic neck dissection in untreated N_0 necks.

Goal of treatment

Clearly the goal of treatment for cervical lymph node metastasis is regional control of disease. Micrometastases and minimal gross metastases may be controlled by radiotherapy alone. However, surgery remains the mainstay of treatment of cervical lymph node metastases since it provides comprehensive clearance of all grossly enlarged lymph nodes and offers accurate histological information on lymph nodes at risk of having micrometastasis in the clinically negative neck.[1,73,74]

While the indications for comprehensive surgical clearance of regional lymph nodes in the neck for clinically palpable metastatic lymph nodes are obvious, the indications for elective treatment of the N_0 neck are less clear.[25,75–78] Statistically, one is unable to document difference in regional control rates or survival between patients undergoing elective neck dissection for micrometastasis or those undergoing therapeutic neck dissection for N_1 disease.[25,66,75,76,78] Unfortunately, however, all patients who are at risk of having micrometastasis do not present for subsequent therapeutic neck dissection with N_1 disease (Fig. 9.12).[56,77] Review of a consecutive series of patients whose N_0 neck was observed initially and who subsequently underwent therapeutic neck dissection shows that a significant number of patients had clinically apparent metastatic disease greater than N_1 (Fig. 9.13).[56,75–77,79–81] Indeed, on pathologic analysis of neck dissection specimens, a majority of the patients had metastatic disease greater than N_1 (Fig. 9.14). It is well known that the prognosis of a patient with metastatic squamous carcinoma to regional cervical lymph nodes is dependent on the extent of nodal disease in the neck. Thus, when a significant risk of micrometastasis to regional lymph nodes is present based on the characteristics of the primary tumor, an elective dissection of regional lymph nodes at risk should be considered.

Table 9.2 Indications for postoperative radiation therapy to the neck

1. Gross residual disease following neck dissection
2. Multiple positive lymph nodes in the neck
3. Extracapsular extension by metastatic disease
4. Perivascular or perineural invasion by tumor
5. Other ominous findings such as tumor emboli in lymphatics, cranial nerve invasion, or extension of disease to the base of the skull

Regional recurrence of metastatic disease in the dissected neck is dependent on the volume of neck metastasis at the time of neck dissection.[53] Regional recurrence following neck dissection for multiple metastatic lymph nodes is prohibitively high.[81,82] Therefore, to enhance regional control rate, postoperative radiation therapy is recommended. The need for adjuvant postoperative radiation therapy, however, depends on the extent of disease in the neck. Regional control of metastatic disease in the neck is significantly enhanced with postoperative radiotherapy.[81–86] Indications for postoperative radiotherapy are listed in Table 9.2.

Selection of initial treatment

The surgical treatment of regional lymph nodes for carcinoma of the oral cavity is based on the understanding of the anatomy of the regional lymphatics, the patterns of regional lymph node metastasis, and the risk of nodal metastasis depending on the characteristics of the primary tumor. When regional metastases are clinically palpable, comprehensive clearance of all regional lymph nodes at risk is mandatory. Classical radical neck dissection remains the gold standard of surgical management of clinically apparent metastatic lymph nodes. However, the morbidity of the operation is significant and therefore it is recommended only under select circumstances. The current indications for classical radical neck dissection are:

1. N_3 disease
2. Multiple gross metastases involving multiple levels
3. Recurrent metastatic disease in a previously irradiated neck
4. Grossly apparent extranodal spread with invasion of the spinal accessory nerve and/or internal jugular vein at the base of the skull
5. Involvement of accessory chain lymph nodes by metastatic disease

On the other hand, when appropriate indications exist, a function-preserving comprehensive neck dissection sparing one or more vital anatomic structures should be considered as long as it does not compromise satisfactory clearance of metastatic disease. Preservation of the spinal accessory nerve alone significantly reduces the morbidity of neck dissection.[87–90] Thus if the spinal accessory nerve is not involved by metastatic cancer, it should be routinely preserved even in patients with clinically palpable metastatic lymph nodes. Such a surgical approach does not adversely impact on local recurrence or long-term survival.[19,43,46,91–93] However, comprehensive clearance of all five cervical lymph node levels must be undertaken when a neck dissection is undertaken for grossly palpable cervical lymph node metastasis. Limited neck dissection for palpable nodal metastasis is considered risky and is not recommended. Preservation of the sternocleidomastoid muscle or internal jugular vein in patients with palpable cervical lymph node metastasis from primary squamous carcinomas of the upper aerodigestive tract is not recommended.

When an elective neck dissection is undertaken to excise cervical lymph nodes at risk of harboring micrometastasis (occult metastasis), it is seldom necessary to perform a comprehensive neck dissection to excise all five levels of lymph nodes. As mentioned earlier, the patterns of cervical lymph node metastasis are predictable and sequential, with involvement of the first echelon lymph nodes initially before dissemination occurs to other lymph node levels. Thus, an elective neck dissection is usually of limited extent, addressing only the lymph node groups at highest risk for a given primary site. Such a limited dissection of lymph nodes is usually considered a 'staging procedure'. The histological information derived from the study of the excised lymph nodes facilitates selection of adjuvant therapy in patients who are at increased risk of neck failure and spares the need for a morbid operation or adjuvant radiotherapy in others who are at reduced risk. Thus, an elective operation for primary tumors of the oral cavity with an N_0 neck requires dissection of lymph nodes at levels I, II, and III.[17,43,50,64,94–98] If the primary tumor crosses the midline, bilateral clearance of levels I, II and III should be undertaken.

Classification of neck dissections

The understanding of the biological progression of metastatic disease from primary sites in the head and neck region to cervical lymph nodes has allowed the development of several modifications of the classical radical neck dissection to reduce morbidity and maintain therapeutic efficacy. In order to standardize the terminology of various types of neck dissections, the following classification scheme is recommended.[43,47–49,97,99]

Comprehensive neck dissection

The term comprehensive neck dissection is applied to all surgical procedures on the lateral neck which comprehensively remove cervical lymph nodes from level I through level V. Under this broad category are included the following operative procedures:

1. *Classical radical neck dissection.*
2. *Extended radical neck dissection* (resection of additional regional lymph nodes or sacrifice of other structures such as cranial nerves, muscles, skin, etc.).
3. *Modified radical neck dissection type I (MRND-I).* This procedure selectively preserves the spinal accessory nerve.
4. *Modified radical neck dissection type II (MRND-II).* This procedure preserves the spinal accessory nerve and the sternocleidomastoid muscle but sacrifices the internal jugular vein.
5. *Modified radical neck dissection type III (MRND-III).* This procedure requires preservation of the spinal accessory nerve, internal jugular vein, and sternocleidomastoid muscle.

Selective neck dissection

These operations selectively remove lymph node groups at designated levels only and do not comprehensively dissect all five levels of lymph nodes. Selective neck dissections are usually employed as staging procedures for the clinically negative neck where the lymph nodes are at risk of harboring micrometastasis. These operations include:

1. *Supraomohyoid neck dissection.* This procedure encompasses dissection of lymph nodes at levels I, II, and III and is recommended as an elective procedure for primary tumors of the oral cavity.
2. *Jugular neck dissection.* This procedure encompasses dissection of lymph nodes at levels II, III and IV.
3. *Anterior triangle neck dissection.* This procedure encompasses lymph nodes removed in supraomohyoid and jugular neck dissections (levels I, II, III, and IV).
4. *Central compartment neck dissection.* This procedure encompasses clearance of lymph nodes in the central compartment of the neck adjacent to the thyroid gland and in the tracheo-esophageal groove (level VI). This operation is recommended for cancers of the thyroid gland.
5. *Posterolateral neck dissection.* This operation encompasses lymph nodes in the occipital triangle, posterior triangle of the neck, and the deep jugular chain of lymph nodes at levels II, III and IV. This operation is recommended for melanomas and squamous carcinomas of the posterior scalp.

Preoperative preparation

No specific preoperative preparation is required for patients undergoing neck dissection other than planning of the incisions for neck dissection, particularly if the primary tumor is to be resected simultaneously. In addition to this, planning of the neck

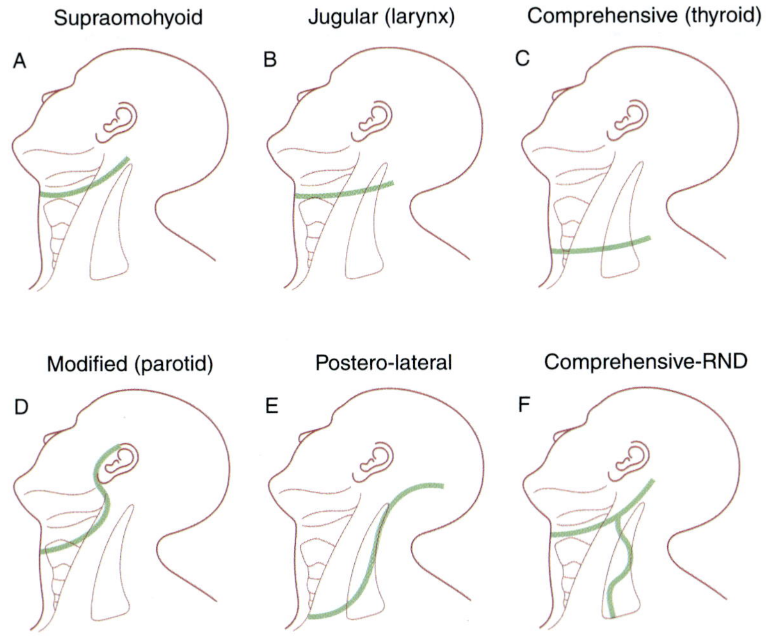

Figure 9.15 Incisions for neck dissections: (A): supraomohyoid; (B): jugular (pharynx); (C): comprehensive (thyroid); (D): modified (parotid); (E): posterolateral; (F): comprehensive—RND.

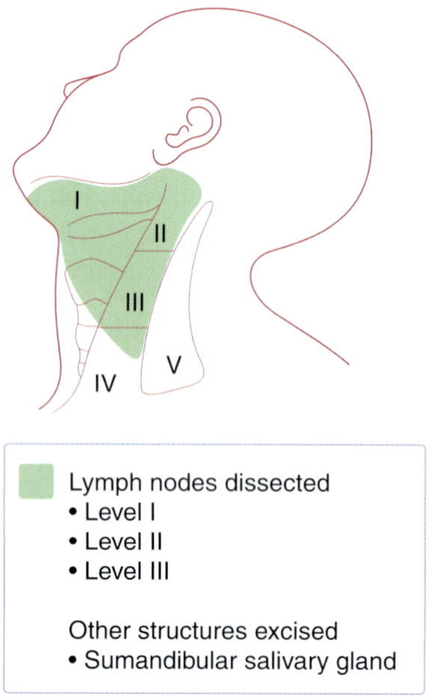

Figure 9.16 Supraomohyoid neck dissection. Lymph nodes dissected: levels I, II and III. Other structures excised: submandibular salivary gland.

dissection incisions must take into consideration any reconstructive effort required to repair the surgical defect created following excision of the primary tumor. The most commonly employed incisions for various types of neck dissections are shown in Fig. 9.15.

Operative techniques

Supraomohyoid neck dissection (SOHND)

This operation may be performed in conjunction with excision of the primary tumor from the oral cavity, either in continuity where the primary tumor and lymph nodes at levels I, II, and III are removed in a monobloc fashion, or as a discontinuous procedure where the primary tumor in the oral cavity may be excised through a peroral approach and the supraomohyoid neck dissection is performed through a separate transverse incision in the upper part of the neck (Fig. 9.16). The incision is placed in an upper neck skin crease extending from the mastoid process towards the hyoid bone up to the midline. If the primary tumor is to be resected perorally, this incision should be satisfactory. On the other hand, if the primary tumor is not accessible through the open mouth or if the primary tumor of the oral cavity is to be excised en bloc with the contents of the supraomohyoid triangle of the neck, then a lower cheek flap approach will be required. The skin incision therefore is extended cephalad in the midline to divide the lower lip.

The skin incision is outlined in Fig. 9.17, with an alternate extension in the midline shown by the dotted line. The patient's neck is extended and rotated to the opposite side to put the skin at the site of surgery under tension.

The skin incision is deepened through the platysma throughout its length (Fig. 9.18). Since the incision is quite low in the neck, the use of electrocautery to divide the platysma has no risk of injury to the mandibular branch of the facial nerve. However, in the posterior aspect of the skin incision attention should be paid to avoid injury to the greater auricular nerve, which can be safely preserved. Similarly, the external jugular vein should be carefully preserved if a microvascular free flap is to be used for reconstructive surgery since it is an excellent recipient vein.

The upper skin flap is elevated first; it remains close to the platysma and the marginal branch of the facial nerve is carefully identified. Posteriorly the greater auricular nerve and the external jugular vein overlying the sternomastoid muscle come into view as elevation of the flap continues. They should be carefully identified and preserved (Fig. 9.19). The nerve is demonstrated here with a hook.

Attention is now focused on careful identification, dissection, and preservation of the mandibular branch of the facial nerve which directly overlies the submandibular salivary gland (Fig. 9.20). This dissection should be performed sharply, either by scalpel or scissors, since use of electrocautery in the vicinity of the mandibular branch can produce temporary paralysis of this nerve. In identifying and preserving the mandibular branch of the nerve, it may become necessary to sacrifice the cervical branch of the facial nerve. Once the nerve is identified and dissected along its course, it is retracted cephalad, along with the upper skin flap, by shifting the nerve with the flap and placing a suture between soft tissues caudad to the nerve and those of the upper cheek flap cephalad to the nerve to form an envelope to protect the nerve. Alternatively, one may elect to identify the posterior facial vein first, as shown in Fig. 9.21. The vein is divided and its stump is suture-ligated at its upper end, with the platysma on the upper skin flap carefully preserving the marginal branch of the facial nerve between the stump of the vein and the platysma muscle. Dissection now proceeds along the lower border of the body of the mandible. The fascial attachments between the sternomastoid muscle and the angle of the mandible are divided. Mobilization of soft tissues along the lower border of the body of the mandible exposes the prevascular facial lymph nodes (Fig. 9.22). These are meticulously dissected and maintained in continuity with the rest of the specimen. The facial artery and its accompanying veins adjacent to these nodes are divided between

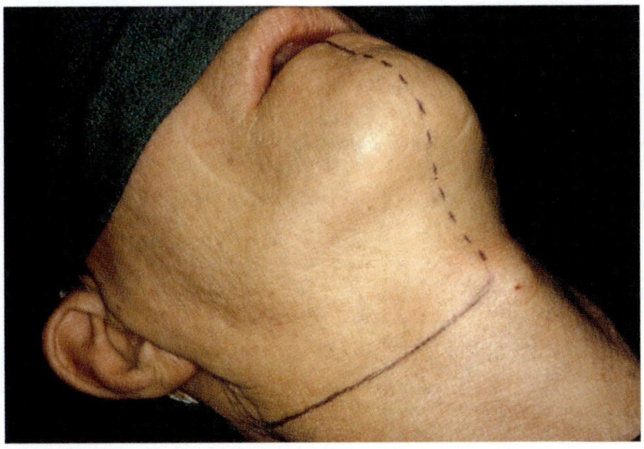

Figure 9.17 Skin incision outlined. Alternate extension for a lower cheek flap is shown with dotted line.

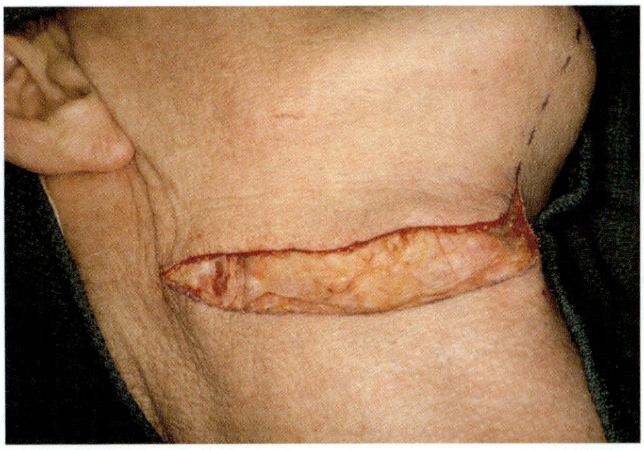

Figure 9.18 Skin incision deepened through platysma.

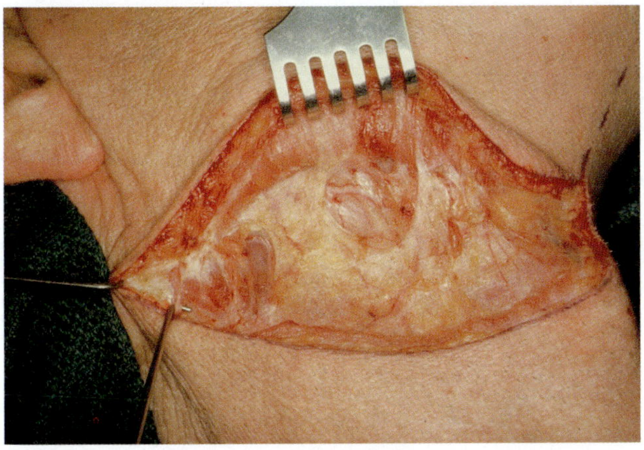

Figure 9.19 Care should be exercised to preserve the greater auricular nerve during elevation of the upper flap.

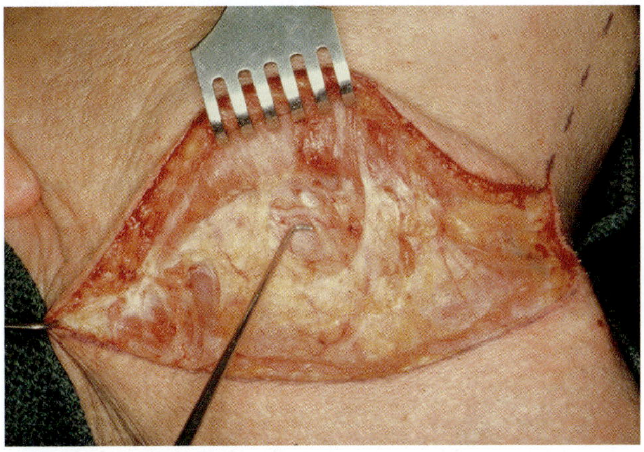

Figure 9.20 The marginal branch of the facial nerve crossing the facial artery and overlying the submandibular salivary gland is preserved.

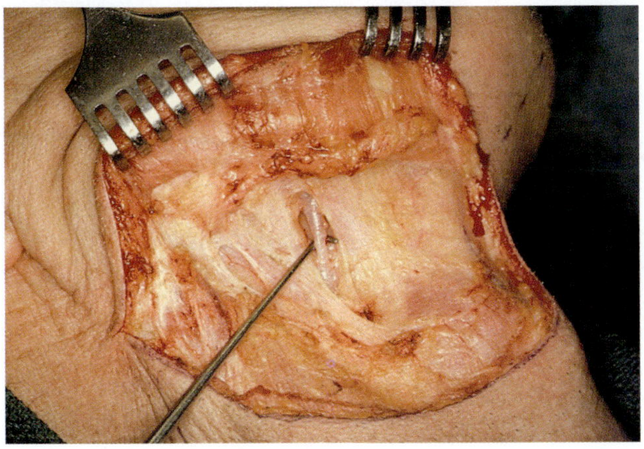

Figure 9.21 Posterior facial vein shown here is divided.

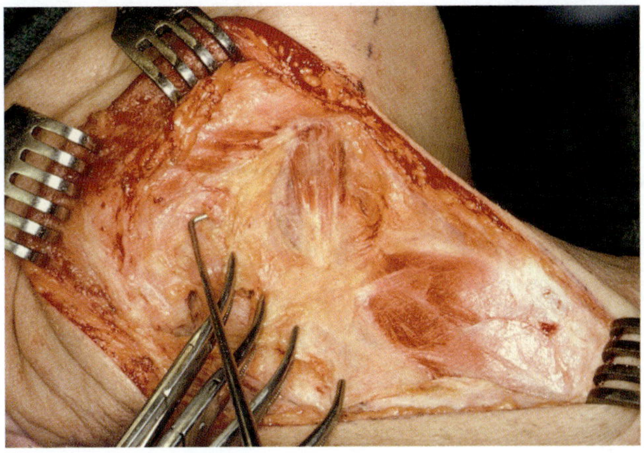

Figure 9.22 The prevascular facial group of lymph nodes adjacent to the body of the mandible are dissected en bloc.

clamps and ligated. Dissection now continues anteriorly along the lower border of the body of the mandible up to the attachment of the anterior belly of the digastric muscle. Soft tissues between the mandible and anterior belly of digastric are separated. At this point, brisk hemorrhage is likely to be encountered from several vessels which provide blood supply to the anterior belly of the digastric muscle and the myelohyoid muscle. The nerve and vessels to the myelohyoid muscle, however, enter parallel to each other in a fascial envelope which is identified, clamped, divided, and ligated (Fig. 9.23). Once all the nerve filaments and vessels along the free border of the myelohyoid

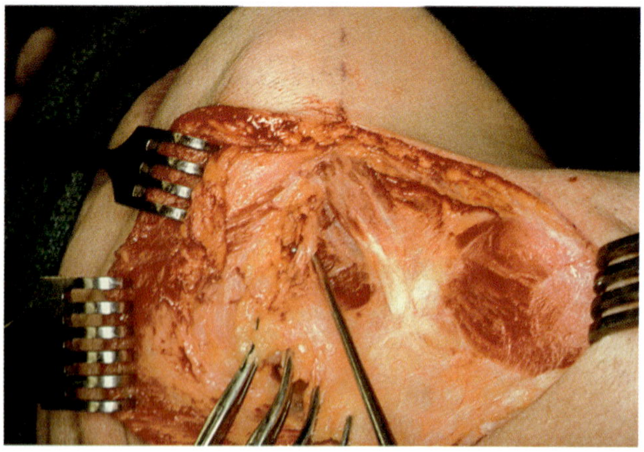

Figure 9.23 The blood vessels to the mylohyoid muscle are divided and ligated.

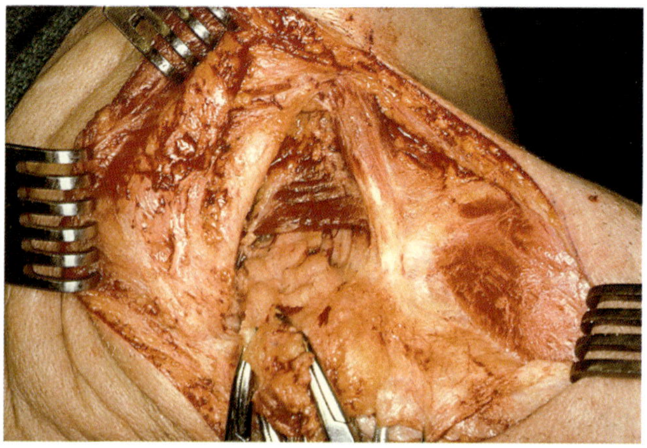

Figure 9.24 The anterior belly of digastric muscle and mylohyoid muscle are exposed.

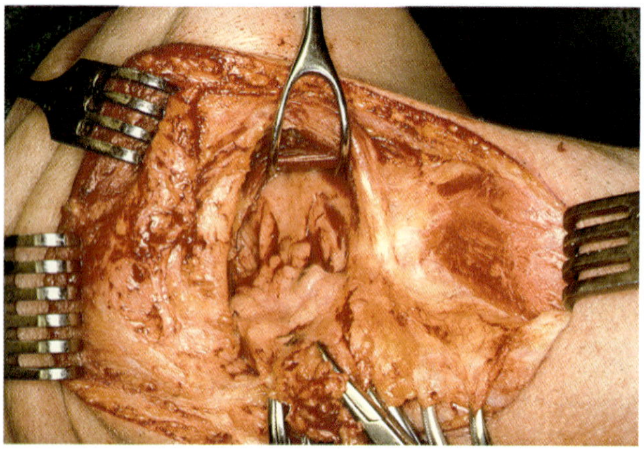

Figure 9.25 The lateral edge of the mylohyoid muscle is retracted medially to expose the Wharton's duct.

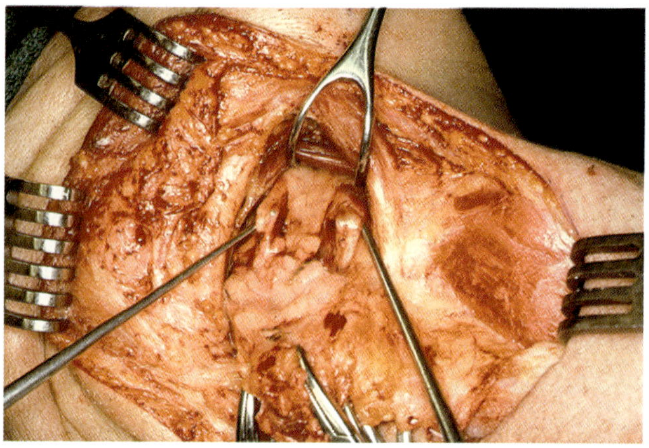

Figure 9.26 The lingual and hypoglossal nerves are identified and protected.

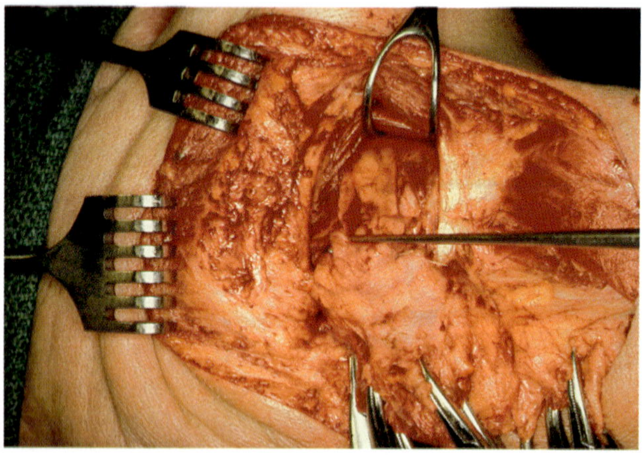

Figure 9.27 The secretomotor fibers to the submandibular salivary gland are divided.

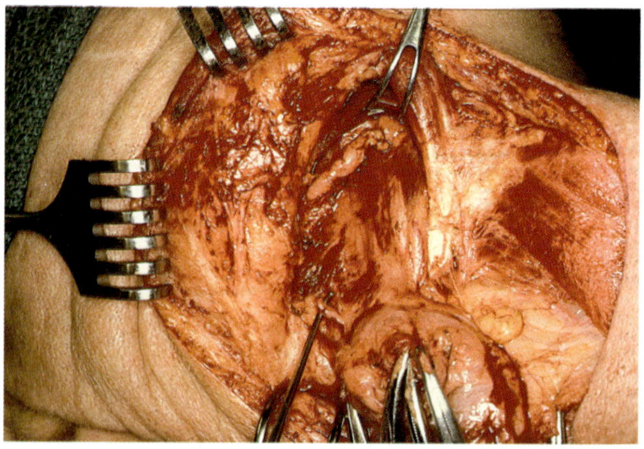

Figure 9.28 The facial artery entering the submandibular salivary gland at its postero-inferior edge is divided and ligated.

muscle are divided, the muscle will come into full view.

Gentle traction on the submandibular salivary gland with several hemostats allows mobilization and delivery of the submandibular gland from its bed (Fig. 9.24). A loop retractor is now placed along the lateral border of the myelohyoid muscle, which is retracted medially towards the chin of the patient (Fig. 9.25). This exposes the undersurface of the

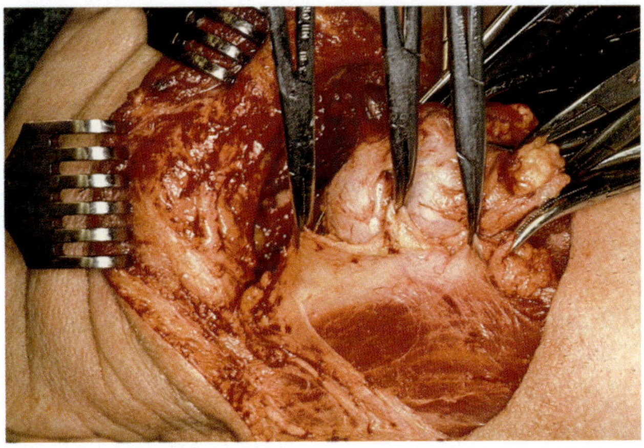

Figure 9.29 The fascia on the anterior border of the sternocleidomastoid muscle is dissected and retracted medially.

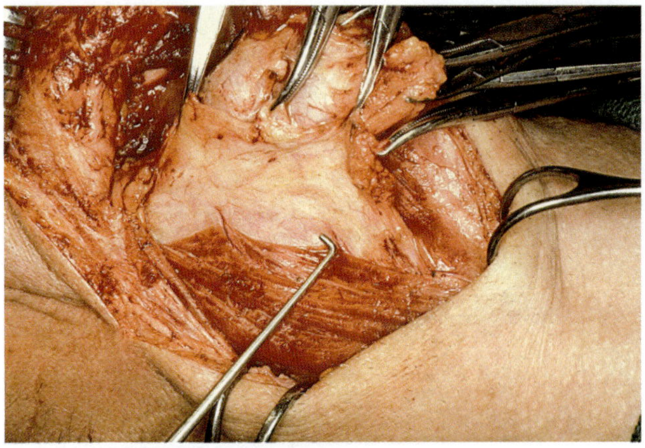

Figure 9.30 Further medial retraction of the fascia provides exposure of the carotid sheath.

floor of the mouth and brings into view the secretomotor fibers to the submandibular salivary gland as they come off the lingual nerve, as well as the Wharton's duct with accessory salivary tissue along the duct. At this juncture, alternate blunt and sharp dissection is necessary to clearly identify the Wharton's duct, and the lingual and hypoglossal nerves in the floor of the mouth as they enter the tongue.

Both the lingual and the hypoglossal nerve are shown in Fig. 9.26, with the Wharton's duct in the middle showing small amounts of salivary gland tissues along its length. Once the lingual nerve is clearly identified, the secretomotor fibers to the submandibular gland are divided. The latter are shown in Fig. 9.27 as they come off the lingual nerve. There is usually a small blood vessel accompanying this nerve so it is divided between clamps and ligated. Similarly, the Wharton's duct is divided between clamps and its distal stump ligated. The entire submandibular gland is now retracted posteroinferiorly, and loose areolar tissue between the salivary gland and the digastric muscle is divided. As one approaches the posterior belly of the digastric muscle, the proximal part of the facial artery as it enters the submandibular salivary gland is exposed (Fig. 9.28). It is divided between clamps and ligated. The entire contents of the submandibular triangle are now dissected off and retracted inferiorly.

Attention is now focused on the region of the tail of the parotid gland and the anterior border of the upper part of the sternomastoid muscle. The fascia along the anterior border of the sternomastoid muscle is grasped with several hemostats and retracted medially to provide traction along its anterior border (Fig. 9.29). Electrocautery is used to clear the fascial attachments from the anterior border of the sternomastoid muscle. Several tiny vessels entering the upper part of the sternomastoid muscle (branches from the occipital and superior thyroid arteries) are divided by electrocautery. Further medial retraction of the specimen exposes the carotid sheath, as shown in Fig. 9.30. The latter is incised and dissection now proceeds cephalad towards the base of the skull.

A hemostat is used to separate the fascia of the carotid sheath, which is divided and retracted medially (Fig. 9.31). This dissection continues cephalad up to the posterior belly of the digastric muscle, which is retracted cephalad to expose the upper end of the jugular vein entering the jugular foramen. Several pharyngeal veins as well as branches of the superior thyroid vein may have to be divided in order to mobilize the specimen.

One of the pharyngeal veins shown in Fig. 9.32 will be divided to facilitate mobilization of the specimen. The sternomastoid muscle is now retracted further posteriorly, exposing the jugular vein in its entirety. The latter is still covered by a fascial envelope containing upper deep jugular and jugulodigastric lymph nodes (Fig. 9.33). The sternomastoid muscle is retracted posteriorly to expose lymph nodes in the accessory chain at the apex of the posterior triangle; these are meticulously dissected out and retracted anteriorly with the rest of the surgical specimen.

While the lymph nodes at the apex of the posterior triangle of the neck are dissected, extreme care should be exercised to identify and carefully preserve the accessory nerve as well as cutaneous and muscular branches of the cervical plexus (Fig.

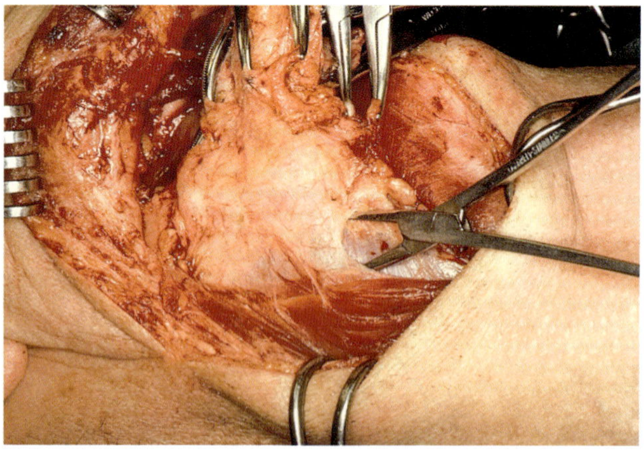

Figure 9.31 The carotid sheath is opened to faciltate its dissection.

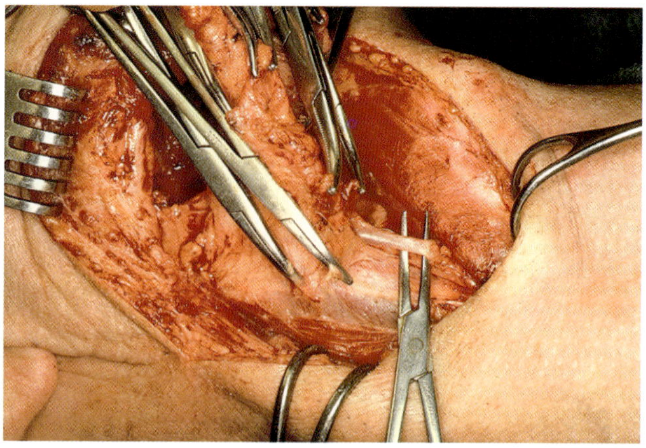

Figure 9.32 The pharyngeal veins are divided and ligated.

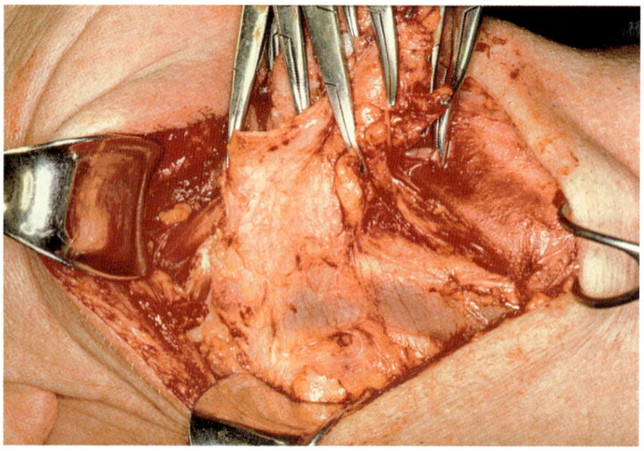

Figure 9.33 Lateral retraction of the sternocleidomastoid muscle exposes the jugulodigastric lymph nodes.

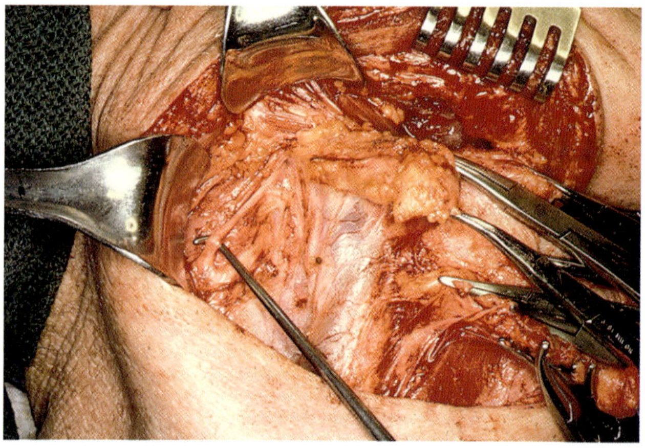

Figure 9.34 The lymph nodes at the apex of the posterior triangle are dissected out, carefully preserving the spinal accessory nerve.

9.34). Once the accessory nerve is identified, the lymph nodes posterolateral to it are dissected and passed beneath the nerve anteriorly to remain in continuity with the rest of the specimen. The upper end of the jugular vein is now nearly fully cleared of deep jugular, jugulodigastric, and upper accessory chain lymph nodes.

Dissection of the apex of the posterior triangle clearly shows the upper end of the internal jugular vein and the occipital artery.

The highest root of the cervical plexus is exposed with further dissection of the eleventh nerve and removal of lymph nodes in the jugulodigastric region. The posterior boundary of the supraomohyoid neck dissection in this area is rather arbitrary, since no specific anatomical landmarks exist to define the extent of posterior triangle lymph node dissection, so clinical judgment must be exercised to decide on the extent of their removal.

Dissection of the accessory chain lymph nodes posterior to the internal jugular vein at the apex of the posterior triangle is now complete (Fig. 9.35). The entire jugular vein is exposed with the posterior belly of the digastric muscle retracted cephalad. The common facial vein is now divided as it enters the internal jugular vein and is ligated (Fig. 9.36). Dissection continues anteriorly, carefully identifying and preserving the hypoglossal nerve as well as the descendens hypoglossi, the nerve supply to the strap muscles.

The descendens hypoglossi is shown in Fig. 9.37 as it comes off the hypoglossal nerve and runs anteroinferiorly. Dissection also continues along the medial aspect of the carotid sheath, exposing the carotid bulb. The surgical specimen mobilized so far consists of the contents of the submandibular triangle, lymph nodes from the jugulodigastric region and the apex of the posterior triangle of the neck, as well as the upper deep jugular lymph nodes. The specimen is reflected anteriorly.

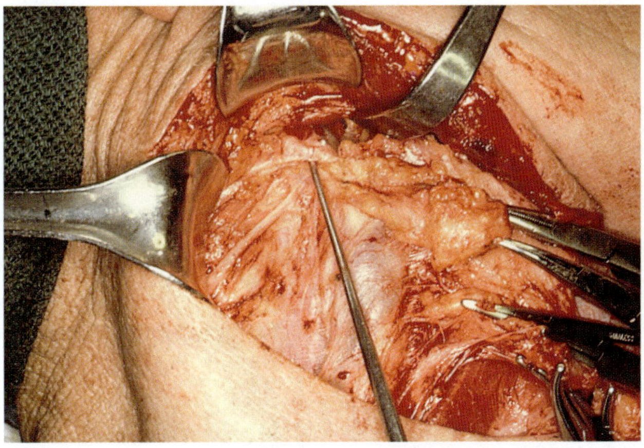

Figure 9.35 The occipital artery is seen crossing the internal jugular vein near its upper end.

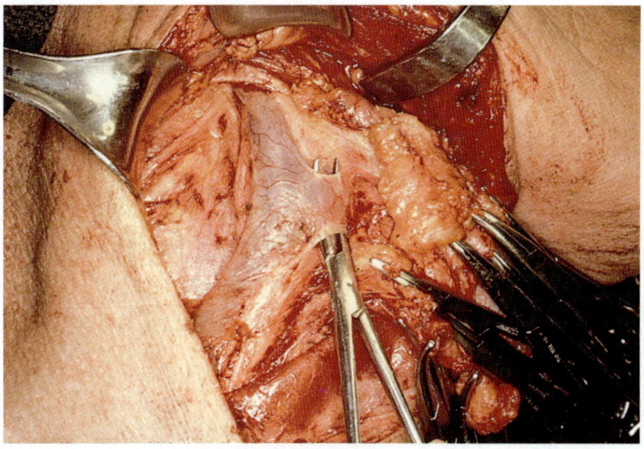

Figure 9.36 The common facial vein is divided and ligated.

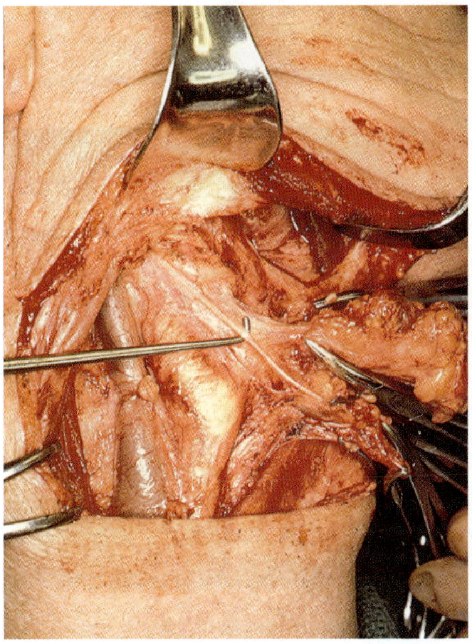

Figure 9.37 The descendens hypoglossi coming off the hypoglossal nerve is preserved.

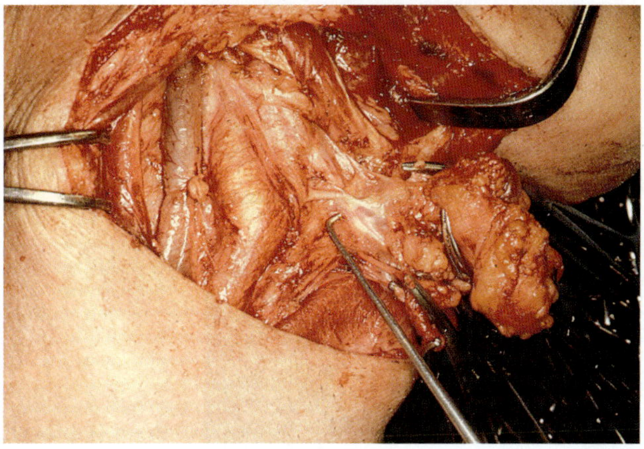

Figure 9.38 The specimen is reflected anteriorly showing the carotid bifurcation.

Dissection is now continued caudad towards the apex of the supraomohyoid triangle, at the junction where the superior belly of the omohyoid muscle meets the sternomastoid muscle (Fig. 9.38). A loop retractor is placed to expose the lower part of the carotid sheath from where midjugular lymph nodes are dissected out and reflected cephalad. Dissection continues further medially, exposing the origin of the superior thyroid artery which is preserved, but the superior thyroid vein will have to be sacrificed since this was previously divided from the internal jugular vein. The final attachments of the specimen in the region of the thyrohyoid membrane and the insertion of the strap muscles over the hyoid bone are divided by electrocautery.

The surgical field following removal of the specimen shows complete clearance of the supraomohyoid triangle (Fig. 9.39). The anatomical structures demonstrated here are the anterior and posterior bellies of the digastric and myelohyoid muscles. The lingual and hypoglossal nerves as well as the marginal branch of the facial nerve are also seen in the submandibular triangle. The superior belly of the omohyoid, sternohyoid, and the stylohyoid muscles, as well as the bifurcation of the carotid artery, are also in clear view. Note that the lymph nodes from levels II and III along the internal jugular vein are all dissected off with the specimen. The posterior and inferior views of the surgical field demonstrate the accessory nerve as well as branches of the cervical plexus, and the lower end of the supraomohyoid triangle where the sternomastoid and the omohyoid muscles cross each other (Fig. 9.40).

The wound is now irrigated with Bacitracin solution. A single suction drain is inserted through a separate stab incision and is placed parallel to the anterior border of the sternomastoid muscle up to the submandibular triangle (Fig. 9.41). The drain is secured in place with a silk suture to the skin at the

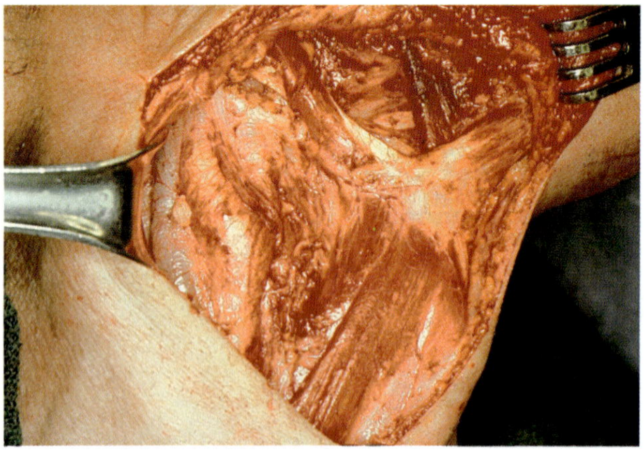

Figure 9.39 The surgical field following removal of the specimen.

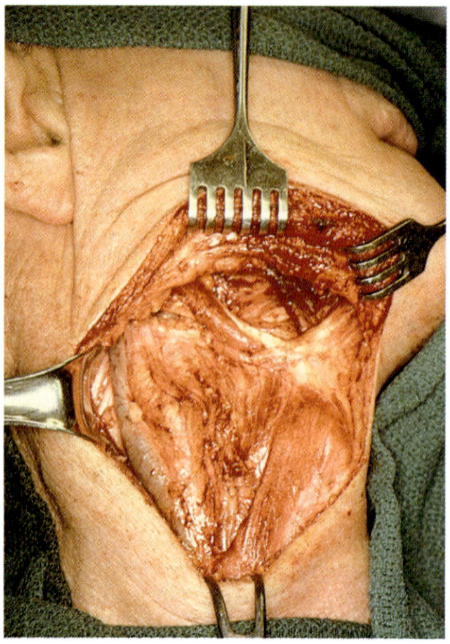

Figure 9.40 Posterior part of the surgical field shows the spinal accessory nerve and the roots of the cervical plexus.

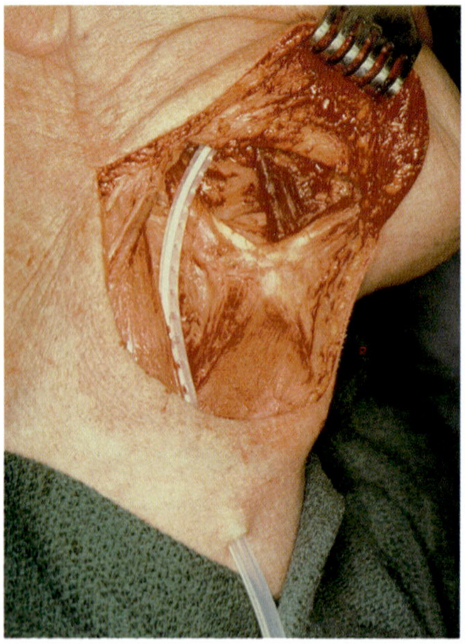

Figure 9.41 A single suction drain is placed parallel to the anterior border of the sterno-cleidomastoid muscle.

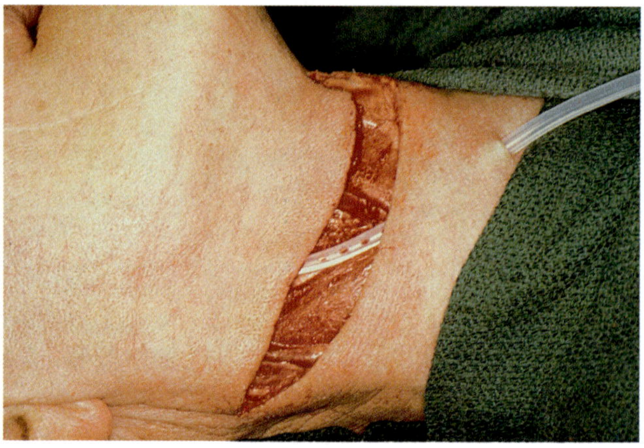

Figure 9.42 The skin incision is closed in two layers.

site of entry, and the incision closed in two layers using 3/0 chromic catgut interrupted sutures for platysma and 5/0 nylon interrupted sutures for skin (Fig. 9.42). Blood loss during this operative procedure should be minimal. The postoperative appearance of the patient demonstrates that there is essentially no esthetic or functional deformity following this operation (Fig. 9.43).

Jugular neck dissection

This operation is usually performed in conjunction with resection of the primary tumor of the oropharynx, larynx, or hypopharynx.[27,46,61,95] Jugular node dissection may be performed on the ipsilateral side for lesions which are unilateral in its mucosal extent, or it may be performed bilaterally for those lesions which cross the midline to involve both sides of the laryngopharyngeal mucosa. The operative procedure is usually performed through the same incision employed for resection of the primary tumor, which is usually a transverse incision along an upper neck skin crease in the region of the thyrohyoid membrane, extending from the posterior border of the sternocleidomastoid muscle on one side of the neck to that on the other side of the neck.

Following skin incision, the platysma is divided throughout the entire length of the incision and upper and lower skin flaps are elevated in the usual fashion, exposing the anterior border of the sternocleidomastoid muscle in its entirety from the region of the posterior belly of the digastric muscle cephalad to the insertion of the sternal head caudad. There is no particular virtue in performing jugular node dissection in continuity with resection of the primary tumor, since technically it may be somewhat awkward to perform. In as much as all internal jugular chains of lymph nodes at levels II, III, and IV are excised in a monobloc fashion, the oncologic purpose of this operation is served. The

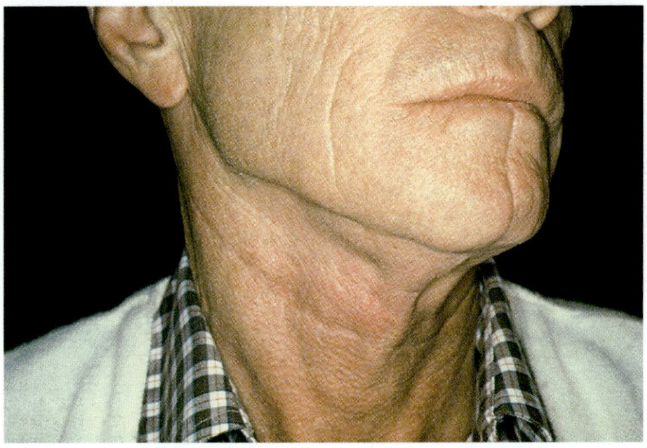

Figure 9.43 Postoperative appearance of the patient after supraomohyoid neck dissection.

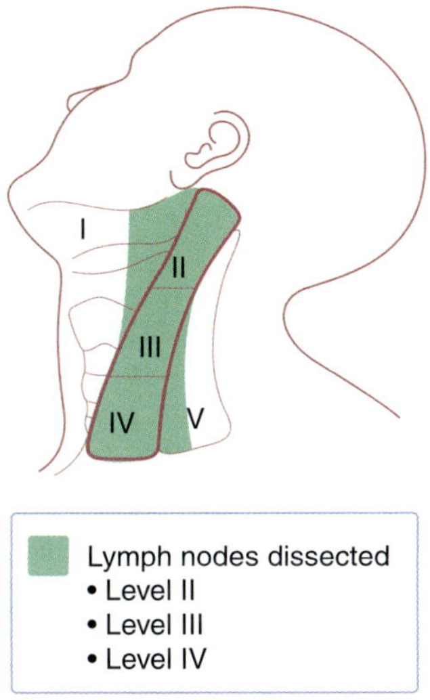

Figure 9.44 Jugular neck dissection. Lymph nodes dissected: levels II, III and IV.

extent of the nodal tissue to be cleared is shown in Fig. 9.44. The internal jugular group of lymph nodes which lie anteriorly, laterally and posterior to the internal jugular vein are excised in a monobloc fashion. This, by necessity, will require clearance of lymph nodes at least up to the posterior border of the sternocleidomastoid muscle from the internal jugular chain.

The operative procedure begins with incision of the fascia along the anterior border of the sternocleidomastoid muscle, which is grasped with hemostats to permit retraction of the sternomastoid muscle posteriorly. This dissection continues on the undersurface of the sternocleidomastoid muscle all the way up to its posterior border. During the course of this part of the operation, the blood supply to the sternocleidomastoid muscle from branches of the occipital artery and superior thyroid artery will be encountered. These vessels are carefully divided and ligated. Once this is accomplished, the entire sternocleidomastoid muscle can be retracted with Richardson retractors posteriorly, totally exposing the internal jugular lymph nodes from the jugulo-digastric region cephalad to the supraclavicular region caudad.

Dissection begins at the upper end, clearing the lymph nodes which are posterior to the accessory nerve as it exits from the jugular foramen. These lymph nodes are covered by the upper end of the sternocleidomastoid muscle and lie over the splenius capitus and levator scapulae muscles in the floor of the posterior triangle of the neck. Meticulous dissection of these lymph nodes allows delivery from beneath the accessory nerve anteriorly to remain in continuity with the jugulo-digastric group of lymph nodes. Similarly dissection of lymph nodes overlying the sensory roots of the cervical plexus is undertaken, exposing the sensory roots, and the dissection is carefully continued up to the lateral border of the internal jugular vein to keep these lymph nodes in continuity with the deep jugular lymph nodes. Clearance of the accessory chain of lymph nodes and exposure of all the cervical roots are essential to provide satisfactory clearance of contiguous lymph nodes in the posterior triangle.

At this juncture, dissection continues anterolateral to the internal jugular vein, clearing all the lymph nodes and freeing up the internal jugular vein in its entirety from the jugular foramen cephalad and to the supraclavicular region caudad. In so doing, the tendon of the omohyoid muscle is divided. No attempt is made to continue the dissection of lymph nodes in the submandibular triangle, leaving the submandibular salivary gland intact. Several pharyngeal branches of the internal jugular vein and the common facial vein, however, will have to be divided and ligated to facilitate dissection of the upper jugular lymph nodes. By meticulous alternate blunt and sharp dissection, the hypoglossal nerve, the desendens hypoglossi, and the branches of the superior thyroid artery are identified and carefully preserved, delivering the specimen.

The specimen shown in Fig. 9.45 demonstrates monobloc excision of the bilateral internal jugular group of lymph nodes from levels II, III and IV. To facilitate accurate description of the excised lymph nodes, it is important to apply numerical tags to the lymph nodes depicting levels II, III, and IV. This would facilitate proper analysis of the surgical specimen to render an accurate histopathologic report. If bilateral jugular node

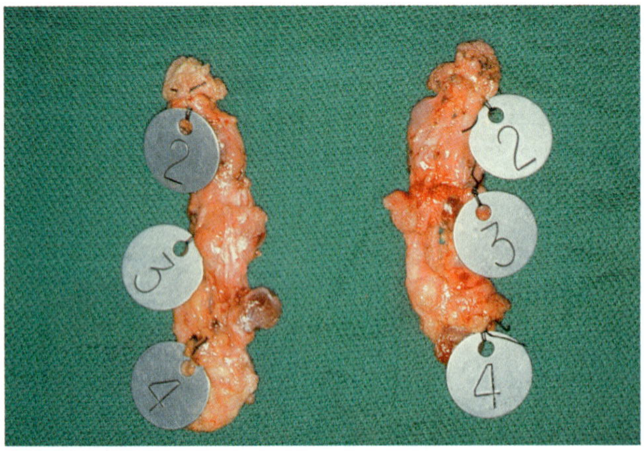

Figure 9.45 Specimen of bilateral jugular lymph node dissections, clearing levels II, III and IV.

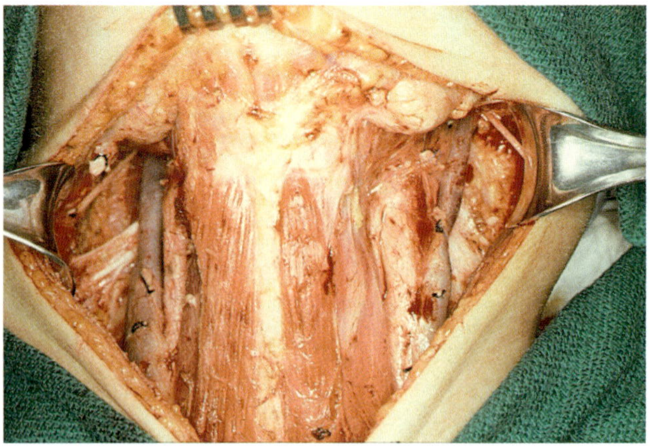

Figure 9.46 Surgical field following bilateral jugular neck dissections.

dissection is undertaken, then the surgical specimen should also indicate whether it is from the left or the right hand side.

The surgical field following bilateral jugular neck dissections performed in this patient with carcinoma of the posterior pharyngeal wall is shown in Fig. 9.46. Note complete clearance of internal jugular lymph nodes, exposing the internal jugular vein in its entirety. Roots of the cervical plexus in the posterior triangle are exposed. Submandibular salivary glands are seen cephalad. Suction drains are placed appropriately and the incision is closed in layers in the usual manner. The functional and esthetic impact of this surgical procedure is essentially none. However, the histologic information derived from analysis of the surgical specimen allows accurate pathologic staging of the primary tumor to select patients who would require adjuvant postoperative radiation therapy.

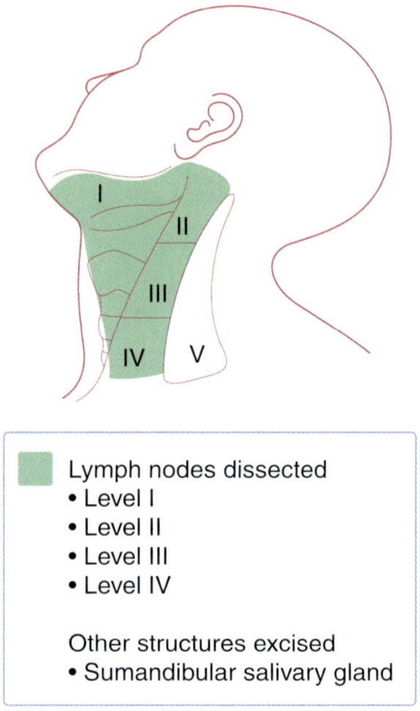

Figure 9.47 Selective anterior triangle neck dissection. Lymph nodes dissected: levels I, II, III and IV. Other structures excised: submandibular salivary gland.

Anterior triangle neck dissection

This extended selective neck dissection may ultimately prove to be the ideal elective operation for patients at risk of nodal metastases from primary cancers of the oral cavity and oropharynx (Fig. 9.47). This operation would also address the risk of skip metastases to level IV in some patients with primary tumors of the oral tongue.[64] In fact, this operation may even prove to be equally satisfactory as a therapeutic neck dissection in patients with limited neck disease (N1). Clearly the role of anterior triangle neck dissection as a therapeutic procedure for patients with N1 disease needs to be studied by a prospective randomized trial, comparing it with modified radical neck dissection type I. On observational statistical grounds, it should prove to be satisfactory since the incidence of posterior triangle lymph node metastasis from primary tumors of the oral cavity is exceedingly low.[65]

The incision for this operation is usually transverse, along a midcervical skin crease. This incision is somewhat lower than that for supraomohyoid neck dissection to provide access to level IV lymph nodes. The remaining steps of the operation are well described above under supraomohyoid and jugular neck dissections. If the operation is performed in a therapeutic setting for oral primaries, or in an elective setting for laryngo-pharyngeal primaries,

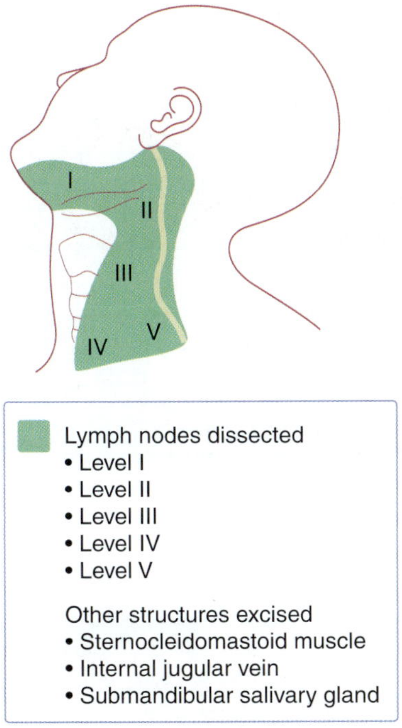

Figure 9.48 Modified radical neck dissection, type I. Lymph nodes dissected: levels I, II, III, IV and V. Other structures excised: sternocleidomastoid muscle; internal jugular vein; submandibular salivary gland. Preserved: spinal accessory nerve.

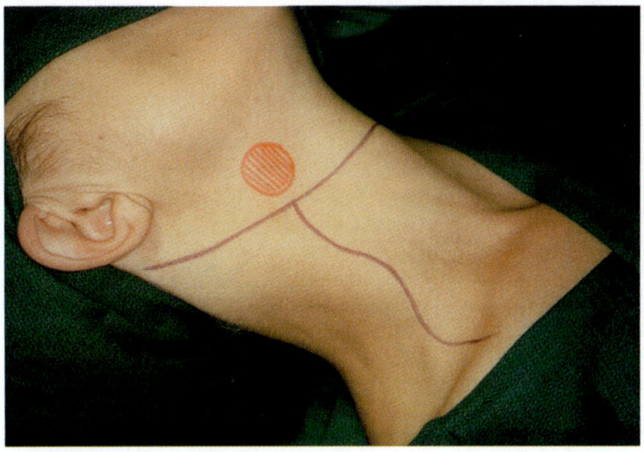

Figure 9.49 Skin incision for modified radical neck dissection type I, in a patient with cancer of the tongue.

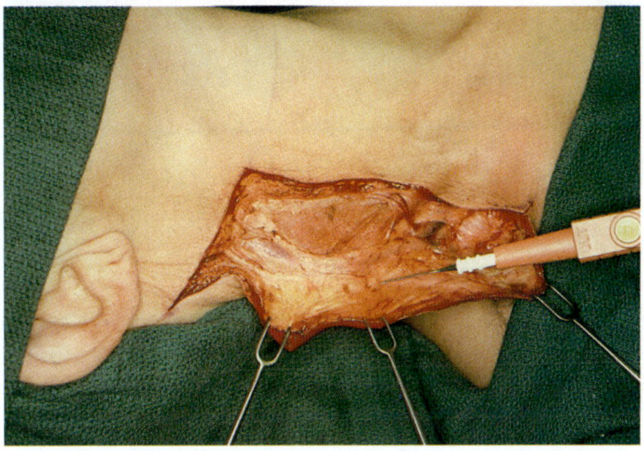

Figure 9.50 The operation begins with elevation of the posterior skin flap.

then particular attention should be paid to adequate clearance of jugular lymph nodes lateral to the internal jugular vein, overlying the roots of the cervical plexus.[92]

Modified radical neck dissection type I (MRND-I)

This operative procedure comprehensively clears cervical lymph nodes at all five levels in the neck, but selectively preserves only *one* anatomic structure, which is the spinal accessory nerve (Fig. 9.48). The patient shown here had a primary carcinoma of the tongue treated previously and she now presents with a clinically apparent metastatic lymph node at level II. The location of the lymph node is shown in relation to the outline of the lower border of the mandible (Fig. 9.49). In patients with such a limited extent of metastatic disease, or in others with palpable metastatic nodes located in the anterior triangle of the neck, sparing the spinal accessory nerve is considered feasible as long as gross metastatic disease does not involve the accessory nerve. The skin incision is at least two fingerbreadths below the angle of the mandible, with a curvaceous, vertical limb posterior to the carotid artery.

The posterior skin flap is elevated first, keeping it just on the undersurface of the platysma (Fig. 9.50). Meticulous attention should be paid as elevation of the lateral aspect of the skin flap approaches the anterior border of the trapezius muscle in the lower part of the neck, since the accessory nerve enters the muscle in this region. The flap is elevated well over the anterior border of the trapezius muscle to expose at least 1 cm of its anterolateral surface. On occasion, elevation of the superior part of the skin flap may have to be withheld if the accessory nerve is found to enter the trapezius muscle high in the neck rather than in its usual lower location. At this point, the accessory nerve is identified as it enters the trapezius muscle, using a hemostat and spreading technique to prevent injury to the nerve (Fig. 9.51).

Once identified, the nerve is traced cephalad by careful and meticulous sharp dissection. It becomes

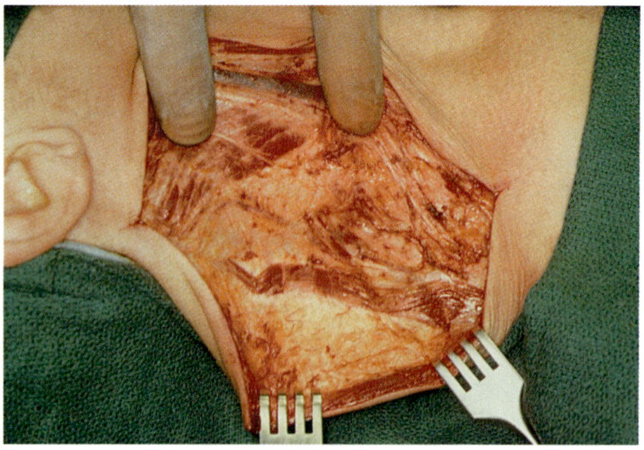

Figure 9.51 The posterior skin flap is elevated until the anterior border of the trapezius muscle.

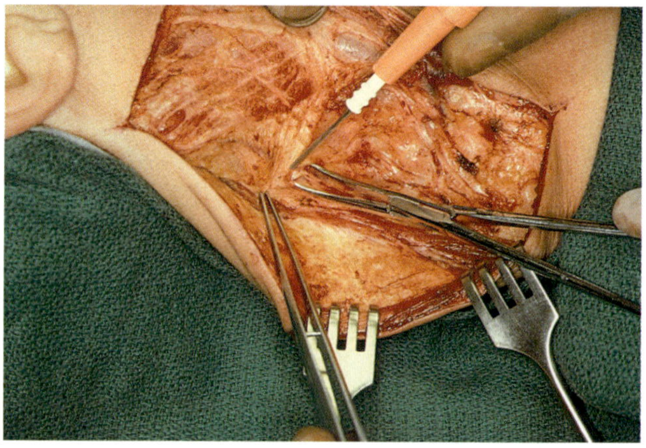

Figure 9.52 The spinal accessory nerve is meticulously dissected through the soft tissues of the posterior triangle.

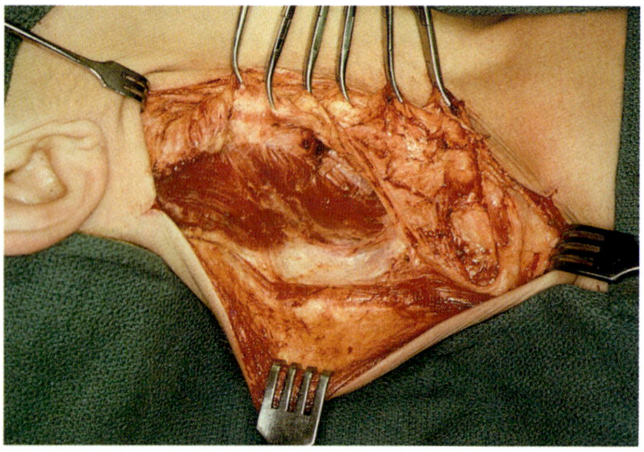

Figure 9.53 The nodal tissue overlying the splenius capitis and levator scapulae muscles is dissected.

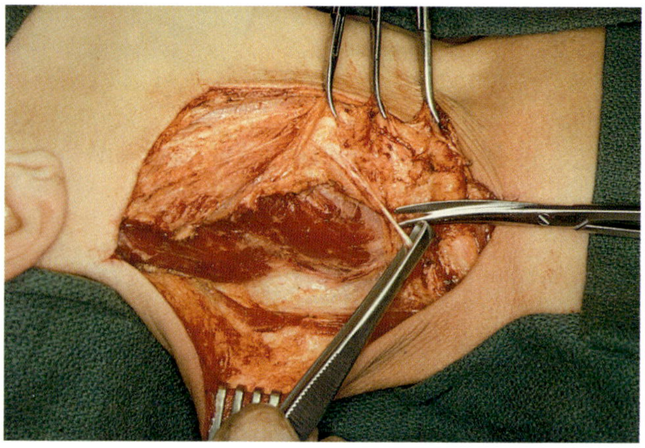

Figure 9.54 The spinal accessory nerve is freed from the nodal tissue in the posterior triangle of the neck.

necessary to split the contents of the posterior triangle of the neck to dissect the nerve out of the posterior triangle (Fig. 9.52). Dissection of the accessory nerve through the posterior triangle continues until the nerve emerges from the posterior border of the sternomastoid muscle (Fig. 9.53). At this point the muscle is divided in order to trace the nerve further cephalad. The posterior half of the upper part of the sternomastoid muscle is divided, with care taken to keep the nerve in view at all times during its division.

The anterior portion of the divided sternomastoid muscle is retracted anteriorly, while the posterior part is retracted posteriorly (Fig. 9.54). As dissection of the accessory nerve through the sternomastoid muscle and deep to it proceeds cephalad, the sternomastoid branch of the accessory nerve comes into view. This branch is sacrificed, which facilitates further dissection of the nerve up to the jugular foramen.

Dissection of the nerve continues further cephalad near the upper end of the jugular vein in a plane deep to the posterior belly of the digastric muscle (Fig. 9.55). The entire nerve is now exposed from its exit at the skull base up to its entry in the trapezius muscle. Dissection of the nerve, however, requires splitting the specimen in the posterior triangle and the upper half of the sternomastoid muscle in the upper part of the neck. Therefore, if gross metastatic nodes are found adherent to the nerve along its course, it should not be preserved.

The nerve is completely free at this point. Using a nerve hook, it is lifted up and the dissected contents of the posterior triangle of the neck are pushed from behind the nerve and pulled out anteriorly (Fig. 9.56). The specimen from the dissected posterior triangle is pushed from behind the nerve into the anterior aspect of the surgical field to remain in continuity with the rest of the specimen. The nerve is allowed to rest on the

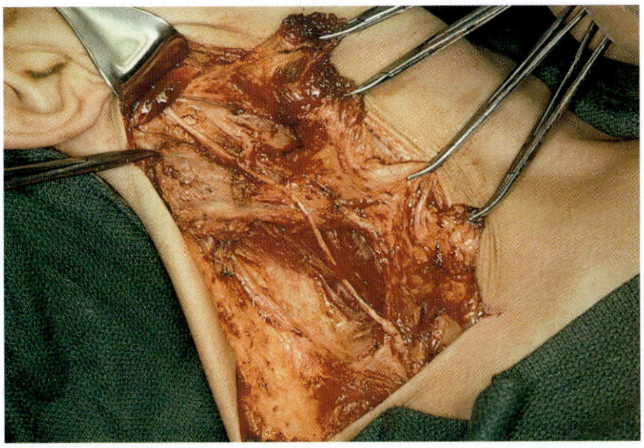

Figure 9.55 The spinal accessory nerve is dissected and freed up throughout its course in the neck.

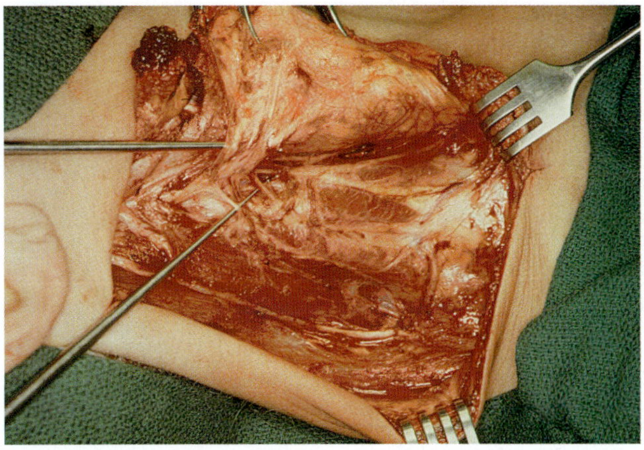

Figure 9.56 Dissected nodal tissue from the posterior triangle is passed under the nerve anteriorly.

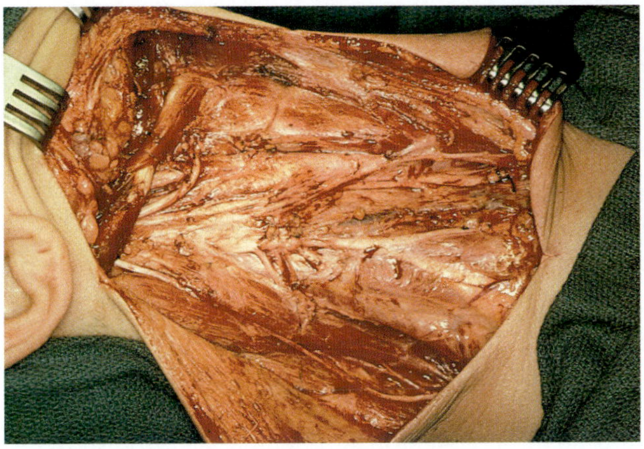

Figure 9.57 Surgical field showing comprehensive clearance of all five levels of lymph nodes with preservation of the spinal accessory nerve.

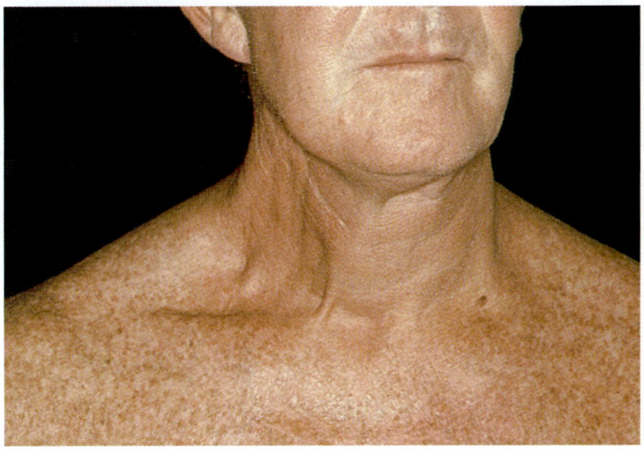

Figure 9.58 Postoperative appearance following modified radical neck dissection Type I. Note absence of shoulder droop.

exposed, clean musculature of the floor of the posterior triangle of the neck.

The rest of the neck dissection continues as described in classical radical neck dissection. All other steps of the operative procedure are exactly the same, removing all other structures as described for a radical neck dissection. The surgical field at the conclusion of the operation is similar to a classical radical dissection, except for the accessory nerve which is preserved in its entirety as seen in the lower part of the surgical field (Fig. 9.57). Suction drains are placed in the wound after irrigation and the incisions are closed in the usual way.

The postoperative appearance of the patient approximately 6 months following MRND-I is shown in Fig. 9.58. Note the absence of dropped shoulder. The contour of the trapezius muscle is preserved, demonstrating that the nerve supply to the muscle is maintained intact, preserving the shoulder function. The patient is able to raise his shoulders all the way up. The only esthetic debility is due to loss of the sternomastoid muscle and soft tissues.

Modified radical neck dissection type II (MRND-II)

This operative procedure is similar to modified radical neck dissection type III, preserving the sternocleidomastoid muscle and the spinal accessory nerve but selectively sacrificing the internal jugular vein (Fig. 9.59). The indications for this operation are massive metastatic disease from differentiated carcinoma of the thyroid gland grossly involving the internal jugular vein, or metastatic squamous cell carcinoma selectively invading the internal jugular vein in the mid-cervical or lower cervical region. All the steps of the operative procedure are otherwise essentially similar to those described for MRND-III.

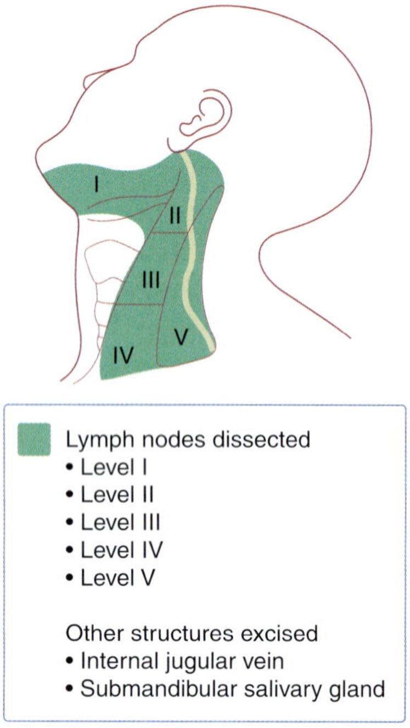

Figure 9.59 Modified radical neck dissection, type II. Lymph nodes dissected: levels I, II, III, IV and V. Other structures excised: internal jugular vein; submandibular salivary gland. Preserved: sternocleidomastoid muscle; spinal accessory nerve.

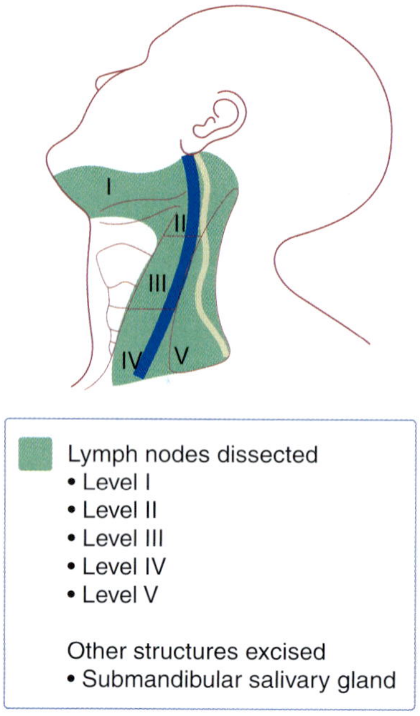

Figure 9.60 Modified radical neck dissection, type III. Lymph nodes dissected: levels I, II, III, IV and V. Other structures excised: submandibular salivary gland. Preserved: sternocleidomastoid muscle; internal jugular vein; spinal accessory nerve.

Modified radical neck dissection type III (MRND-III)

This operation comprehensively clears lymph nodes from all five levels in the lateral neck, preserving the sternocleidomastoid muscle, spinal accessory nerve, and the internal jugular vein (Fig. 9.60), and it is usually indicated in patients with metastatic lymph nodes from well-differentiated carcinomas of the thyroid gland. It is not a satisfactory operation for metastatic squamous cell carcinoma or metastatic adenocarcinoma of salivary gland origin.

The surgical field of a patient who has undergone total thyroidectomy and a comprehensive modified neck dissection type III (MRND-III) for metastatic papillary carcinoma of the thyroid is shown in Fig. 9.61. The technical details of the steps of the operation are similar to that described for other neck dissections. On the anterior view of the surgical field, clearance of the central compartment of the neck following a radical, total thyroidectomy is clearly seen. Complete dissection of the tracheo-esophageal groove lymph nodes on both sides is accomplished, preserving the right lower parathyroid gland with its vascular pedicle. Both carotid sheaths are opened and the deep jugular nodes in the central compartment of the neck on the right hand side are also cleared. The sternomastoid muscle on the left side is retracted laterally, showing clearance of the cervical lymph nodes in the central compartment.

The lateral view of the surgical field from the patient's left hand side, with the sternomastoid muscle retracted posteriorly, shows complete clearance of the tracheoesophageal groove lymph nodes. The recurrent laryngeal nerve is preserved. Lymph nodes in the central compartment and jugular chain are excised en bloc with the primary lesion. The laterally retracted sternomastoid muscle exposes the contents of the carotid sheath, demonstrating total clearance of lymph nodes from the anterior triangle of the neck (Fig. 9.62).

The lateral view of the surgical field with the sternomastoid muscle now retracted anteriorly demonstrates the carotid sheath with its contents clearly dissected (Fig. 9.63). All the lymph nodes lateral to the carotid sheath and from the posterior triangle of the neck are completely removed. Note that the vagus, phrenic and accessory nerves in the lower part of the surgical field overlying the trapezius muscle are carefully preserved.

Since this operation has to be performed with the sternomastoid muscle intact, it is often difficult to

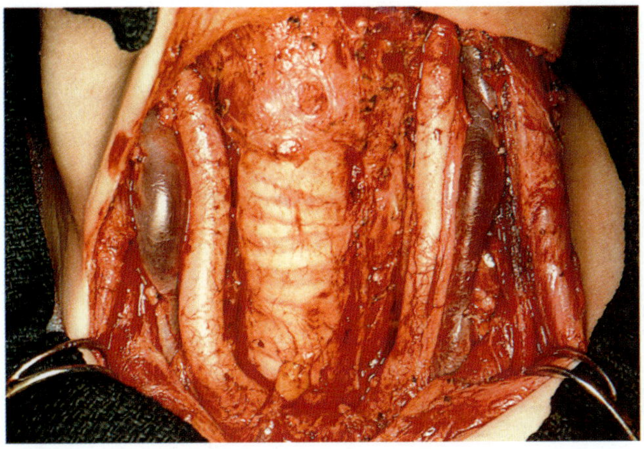

Figure 9.61 Anterior view of the surgical field after total thyroidectomy and MRND-III.

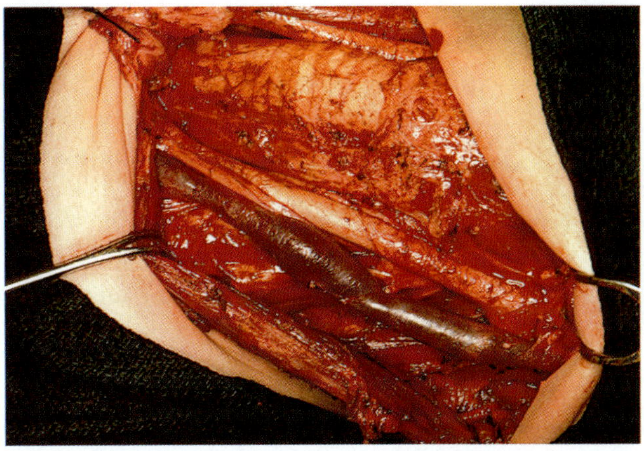

Figure 9.62 Lateral view of the surgical field after total thyroidectomy and MRND-III, showing clearance of the anterior triangle of the neck.

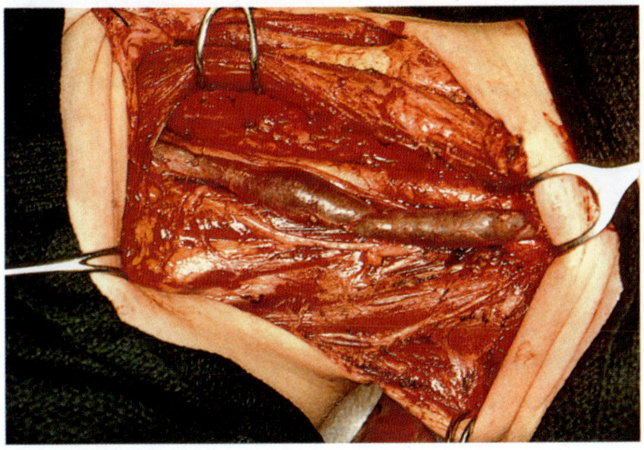

Figure 9.63 Lateral view of the surgical field after total thyroidectomy and MRND-III, showing clearance of the posterior triangle of the neck.

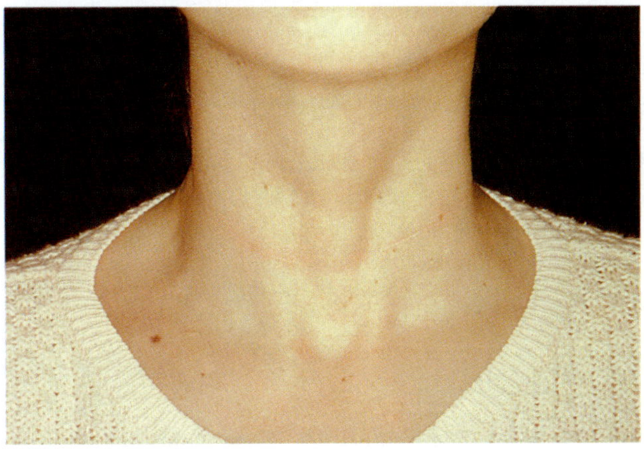

Figure 9.64 Postoperative appearance of the patient after total thyroidectomy and bilateral MRND-III.

keep the surgical specimen in continuity as a monobloc resection. The contents of the anterior triangle of the neck and the primary tumor may be resected en bloc, while lymph nodes from the posterior triangle may be removed as a separate specimen. Wound closure with suction drains is similar to previous surgical procedures on the neck.

The postoperative appearance of the patient approximately 6 months after bilateral modified radical neck dissections type III (MRND-III), with total thyroidectomy for papillary carcinoma of the thyroid with bilateral neck node metastasis, is shown in Fig. 9.64. Note that the surgical procedure in this patient was performed through a single transverse incision in the lower part of the neck at the level of the cricoid cartilage, extending from the trapezius muscle on one side to that on the opposite side.

Classical radical neck dissection (RND)

The classic radical neck dissection has been the gold standard for surgical treatment of clinically apparent, metastatic cervical lymph nodes. It comprehensively clears lymph nodes from levels I, II, III, IV and V, but also requires sacrifice of the sternocleidomastoid muscle, spinal accessory nerve, internal jugular vein, and the submandibular salivary gland (Fig. 9.65). However, due to significant postoperative esthetic deformity and functional disability, the operation is currently recommended only when appropriate indications are present, as discussed before. A variety of incisions have been described for completing a radical neck dissection. However, a single, trifurcate T-shaped incision is preferred (Fig. 9.66). The transverse limb of the T begins at the mastoid process and follows an upper neck skin crease, remaining at least two fingerbreadths below

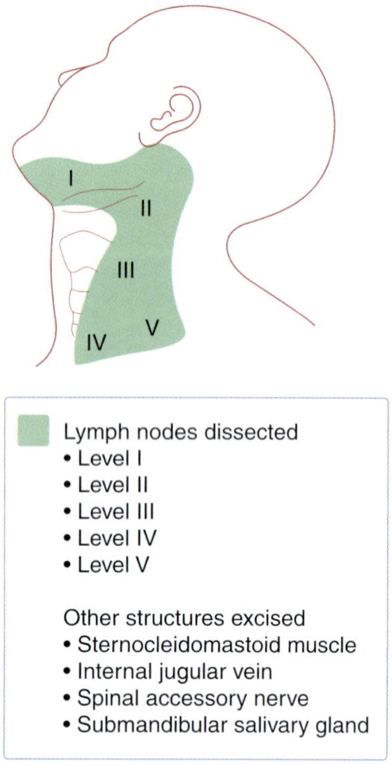

Figure 9.65 Radical neck dissection. Lymph nodes dissected: levels I, II, III, IV, and V. Other structures excised: sternocleidomastoid muscle; internal jugular vein; spinal accessory nerve; submandibular salivary gland.

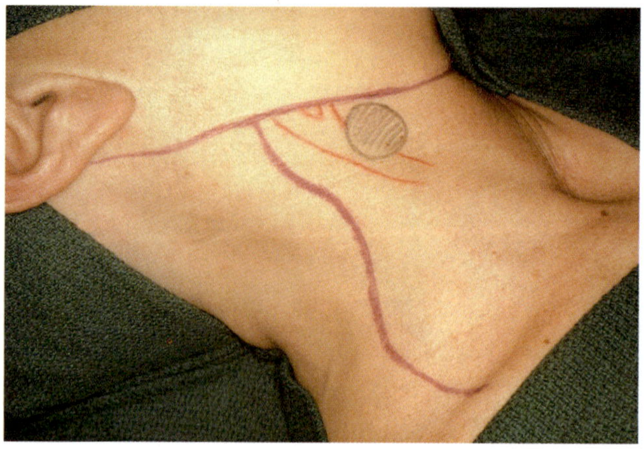

Figure 9.66 A single trifurcate incision is preferred.

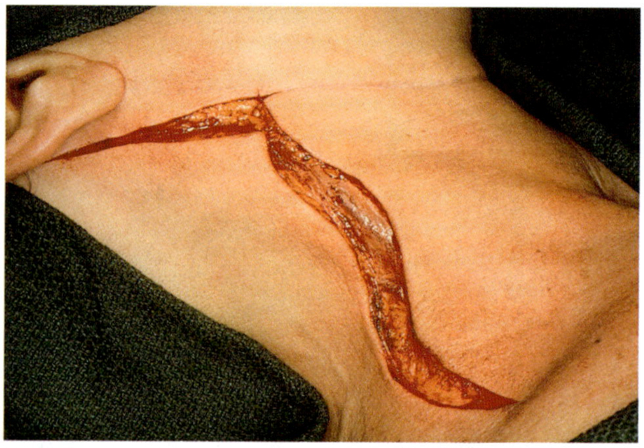

Figure 9.67 The operation is begun with elevation of only the posterior flap and dissection of the posterior triangle of the neck first.

the angle of the mandible. The incision extends across the midline up to the anterior border of the opposite sternomastoid muscle. At about the midpoint of the transverse incision near the posterior border of the sternomastoid muscle, the vertical limb of the T incision is begun. This vertical limb is curvaceous and ends at the midclavicular point. The incision provides adequate exposure for completion of a radical neck dissection; it is suitable both for bilateral radical neck dissections with a similar incision on the opposite side of the neck and for a pectoralis major myocutaneous flap, since the vertical limb can be safely extended down on the anterior chest wall for elevation of the myocutaneous flap. Since the blood supply to the three skin flaps resulting from this incision is not disturbed, marginal necrosis at the trifurcation of the skin incision is rarely seen. The trifurcation of the incision is shown marked out on the skin here in relation to the carotid artery. The trifurcation point should be kept posterior to the carotid artery when feasible. This incision provides the necessary exposure by elevation of the posterior, anterior, and superior skin flaps.

The dissection begins with elevation of the posterior skin flap. The incision begins with the posterior half of the transverse incision at the mastoid process and continues with the vertical incision beyond the trifurcation point (Fig. 9.67). The anterior and superior skin flaps are not elevated at this time. The skin incision is made with a scalpel, but the rest of the dissection is carried out with an electrocautery. The skin incision is deepened through the platysma, but if grossly enlarged lymph nodes are present, and there is suspicion of extension of disease beyond the capsule of the lymph nodes, then the flap is elevated superficial to the platysma muscle, which is sacrificed. Electrocautery aids rapid elevation of the posterior skin flap. Several skin hooks are employed to retract the posterior skin flap, while countertraction is provided by the second assistant over the soft tissues in the neck. The plane of dissection is along the undersurface of the platysma muscle. The posterior skin flap is elevated until the anterior border of the trapezius muscle is identified, and exposed all the way from the mastoid process down to the clavicle. It is important to remember that platysma is not present all the way up to the trapezius muscle and therefore meticulous attention should be paid to remain in the proper subcutaneous plane beyond the platysma to maintain uniform thickness of the skin flap.

Rake retractors are now employed to retract the posterior skin flap (Fig. 9.68). Soft tissues anterior to the trapezius muscle are now grasped with several hemostats, which are used to provide traction on the surgical specimen. Dissection proceeds along the floor of the posterior triangle of the neck, exposing each successive muscle with anterior elevation of the specimen. The superior attachment of the sternomastoid muscle is detached from the mastoid process and retracted anteriorly. The plane of dissection continues just anterior to the anterior border of each successive muscle in the posterior triangle of the neck. The splenius capitis and levator scapulae muscles are then exposed. Several small veins have to be divided and ligated as this dissection proceeds anteriorly. In the lower part of the neck, the transverse cervical artery and its accompanying vein are identified, divided between clamps and ligated. Likewise, the posterior belly of the omohyoid muscle is divided in the floor of the posterior triangle of the neck and its anterior stump is retracted medially. Dissection continues medially, exposing the posterior scalene muscle. The lower end of the external jugular vein is divided between clamps near the clavicle and its stump is ligated.

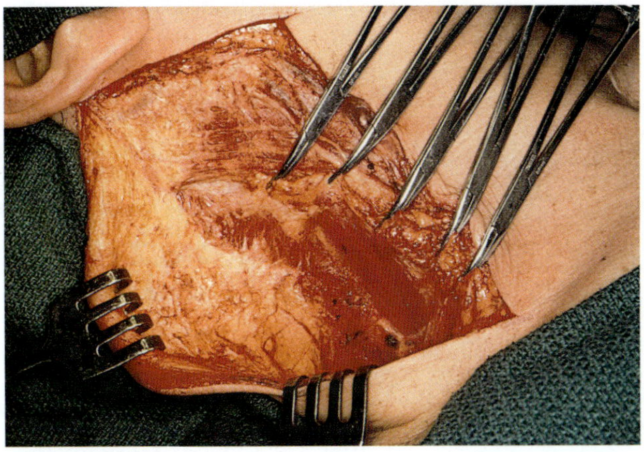

Figure 9.68 Nodal tissue anterior to the trapezius muscle from the posterior triangle is dissected and retracted anteriorly.

As the scalene muscles are exposed, roots of the cervical plexus come into view (Fig. 9.69). However, these are left intact until the phrenic nerve is identified lying on the anterior aspect of the scalenus anticus muscle. Similarly, motor branches of the cervical plexus providing nerve supply to the posterior compartment muscles should be carefully preserved. The cutaneous branches of the cervical plexus are transected, leaving short stumps to prevent injury to the phrenic nerve. The cutaneous branches of the cervical roots carry with them small blood vessels and therefore these stumps should be ligated. In the lower part of the posterior triangle of the neck, the brachial plexus comes into view. Dissection over this is easy because there is a plane of loose areolar tissue between the cervical lymph nodes and the supraclavicular fat pad contained within the deep cervical fascia. Dissection of the posterior triangle of the neck is now complete. The specimen mobilized so far is now reflected posteriorly (Fig. 9.70). A dry gauze pad is placed on the musculature of the posterior triangle of the neck over which the surgical specimen is allowed to rest.

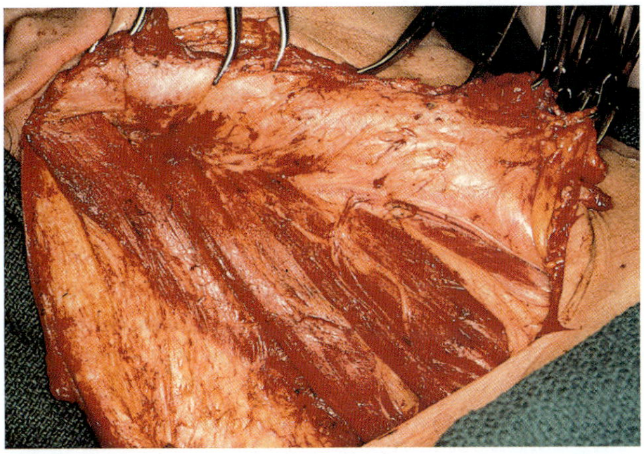

Figure 9.69 Dissection of posterior triangle is complete with exposure of the cervical roots and brachial plexus.

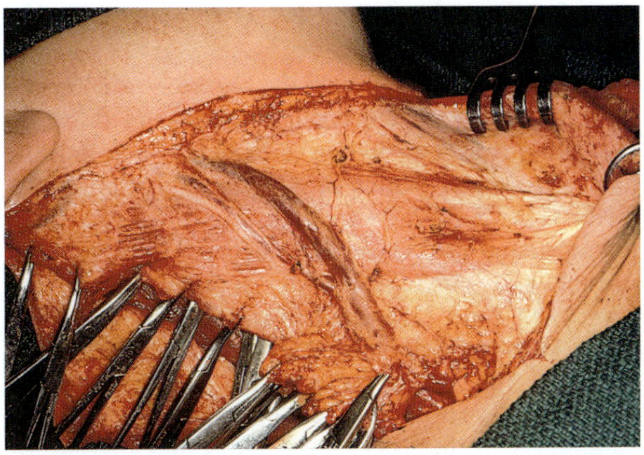

Figure 9.70 The anterior skin flap is elevated to the midline to expose the lower end of the sternocleidomastoid muscle.

Attention is now focused on the anterior skin flap. The transverse skin incision is completed by extending it from the trifurcation point up to the medial end,

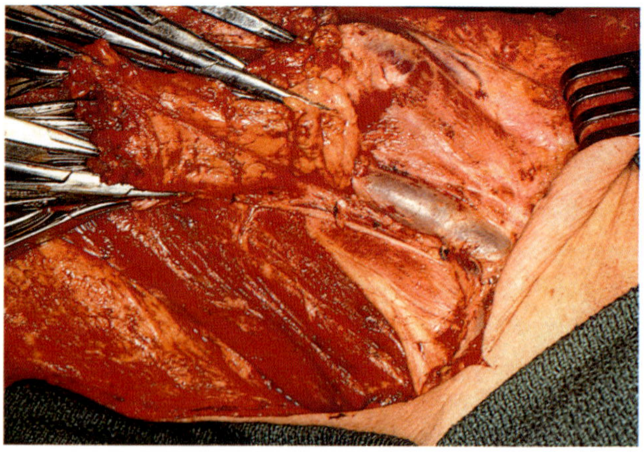

Figure 9.71 The sternocleidomastoid muscle is detached from its lower attachment and retracted cephalad exposing the carotid sheath.

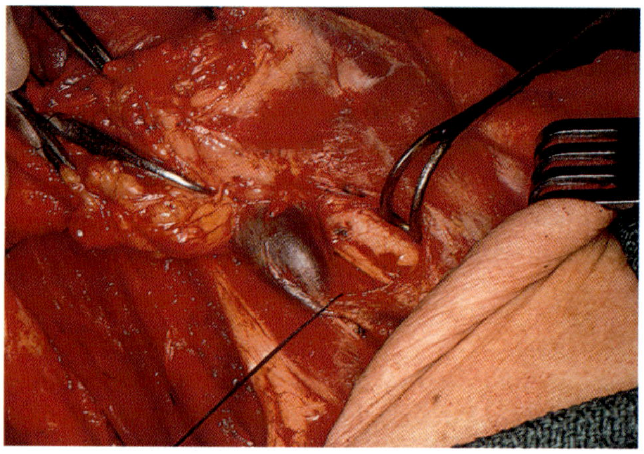

Figure 9.72 The internal jugular vein is divided and ligated after identification of the vagus nerve in the carotid sheath.

deepening through the platysma. The anterior skin flap is retracted medially by the use of skin hooks and rake retractors. The use of electrocautery permits rapid elevation of this skin flap through the loose plane of areolar tissue lying deep to the platysma muscle. Several cutaneous vessels are encountered during elevation and these are electrocoagulated. The skin flap is elevated up to the medial border of the omohyoid muscle superiorly and up to the medial border of the sternomastoid muscle at its attachment to the manubrium sterni inferiorly. A large loop retractor is now used to expose the sternal end of the sternomastoid muscle which facilitates complete elevation of the anterior skin flap. Using electrocautery with the cutting current, the tendon of the sternomastoid muscle is divided from the sternal end, and the rest of the muscular attachment on the manubrium and the clavicle is divided using coagulating current. There is a plane of loose areolar tissue containing fat between the carotid sheath and the posterior aspect of the sternomastoid muscle, so the latter can be safely divided by electrocautery.

Several small vessels enter the anterior skin flap as it is elevated near the clavicle. These are branches from the first perforating branch of the internal mammary artery, which provide blood supply to the lower skin flap. These are carefully preserved. Once the sternomastoid muscle is detached from both its sternal and clavicular ends, it is grasped with hemostats and retracted cephalad. The fascia between the carotid sheath and the strap muscles is incised with a scalpel. A small loop retractor is used to retract the strap muscles medially to expose the common carotid artery and the vagus nerve. By alternate blunt and sharp dissection, the areolar tissue of the carotid sheath is divided circumferentially around the internal jugular vein (Fig. 9.71). At this juncture, the proximal ends of the transverse cervical artery and vein are identified, divided and ligated. Lymphatic vessels present in the vicinity of the jugular vein are carefully identified, divided and ligated. On the left hand side of the neck, the thoracic duct requires special attention. It should be meticulously identified, carefully dissected, divided and ligated in order to prevent chyle leak and fistula. Lymph nodes contained in loose areolar tissue behind the internal jugular vein are dissected and pulled out at this time to remain in continuity with the rest of the specimen. During this dissection, the phrenic nerve should be carefully protected and kept out of harm's way.

The small loop retractor placed on the strap muscles is now pulled to expose the common carotid artery and the vagus nerve (Fig. 9.72). The internal jugular vein should not be ligated until after both the carotid artery and nerve are identified and retracted medially. The vein is doubly ligated, divided in between and its proximal stump is suture ligated.

The middle thyroid vein usually seen at this point entering the medial aspect of the internal jugular vein is divided and ligated. Dissection now proceeds along the lateral border of the carotid sheath remaining posterior to the vein but anterolateral to the vagus nerve. This is a relatively avascular plane and one can safely divide the carotid sheath along this plane all the way up to the base of the skull. As dissection proceeds cephalad, minor vessels in the carotid sheath may cause bleeding, which is easily controlled with electrocoagulation (Fig. 9.73).

Dissection of the lateral aspect of the carotid sheath in the upper part of the neck brings the hypoglossal

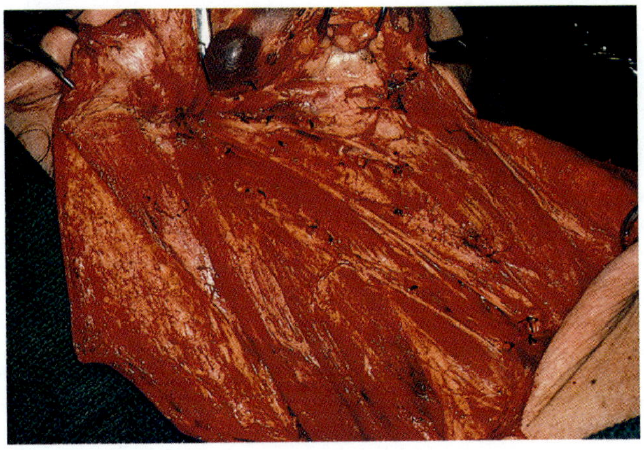

Figure 9.73 Dissection proceeds along the carotid sheath cephalad, protecting the vagus nerve until the hypoglossal nerve is identified.

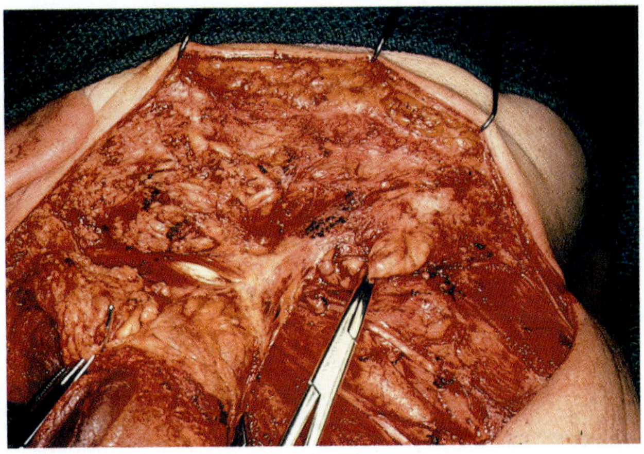

Figure 9.74 The upper skin flap is elevated and dissection of the submandibular triangle completed, carefully preserving the mandibular branch of the facial nerve.

nerve into view. On the medial aspect of the carotid sheath, the dissection is carried cephalad along the medial border of the superior belly of the omohyoid muscle up to the hyoid bone, from which it is detached. Small blood vessels running along the descendens hypoglossi are divided and ligated. The superior thyroid artery is preserved but the superior thyroid vein will have to be divided and ligated. A dry gauze pad is now placed on the surgical field and the entire specimen is allowed to rest over the gauze pad.

The superior skin flap is now elevated in the usual fashion and is retained close to the platysma. The mandibular branch of the facial nerve is located in the fascia over the submandibular salivary gland, approximately two fingerbreadths below and two fingerbreadths anterior to the angle of the mandible. The nerve is carefully identified, dissected off the fascia, and retracted cephalad with the skin flap. The facial vessels are divided and ligated (Fig. 9.74). The contents of the submandibular triangle are dissected off by dividing the secretomotor fibers to the submandibular salivary gland and Wharton's duct but preserving the lingual and hypoglossal nerves. The submandiblar gland and level I lymph nodes are thus reflected caudad to remain in continuity with the rest of the specimen. Several pharyngeal veins along the digastric tendon and the posterior belly of the digastric muscle are divided and ligated. At this juncture the hypoglossal nerve should be carefully dissected, protected and preserved. Finally, the tail of the parotid gland is separated or transected along the superior border of the posterior belly of the digastric muscle. During division of the tail of the parotid gland, the posterior facial vein and several arterial branches of the occipital artery have to be divided and ligated.

The posterior belly of the digastric muscle is now retracted cephalad with a deep, right-angled retractor, bringing into view the occipital artery which runs across the internal jugular vein anteriorly at right angles to it. If the occipital artery is high behind the digastric muscle it may be left alone, but if it is quite low it will have to be divided and ligated. The adipose tissue and lymph nodes lateral to the internal jugular vein under the sternomastoid muscle are dissected out. This is easily accomplished once the tendon of the sternomastoid muscle is detached from the mastoid process.

The accessory nerve is divided near the jugular foramen and its proximal stump is ligated as there is a small vessel running with the nerve. Finally, the upper end of the internal jugular vein is skeletonized and the vein is doubly ligated and divided. The surgical specimen is now delivered.

The surgical field following radical neck dissection shows clearance of all five levels of lymph nodes as previously described, along with loss of the sternomastoid muscle, internal jugular vein, spinal accessory nerve and the submandibular salivary gland (Fig. 9.75). The wound is now irrigated with Bacitracin solution. Meticulous hemostasis must be ensured prior to closure of the wound. Two suction drains are now inserted through separate stab incisions (Fig. 9.76). One drain overlies the anterior border of the trapezius muscle in the posterior triangle, and is retained there through a loop of chromic catgut suture between the skin flap and the trapezius muscle; another is maintained over the strap muscles, anteriorly, and is retained by a loop of catgut suture. The rest of the skin wound is closed in two layers using 3/0 chromic catgut interrupted sutures for platysma and 5/0 nylon sutures for skin

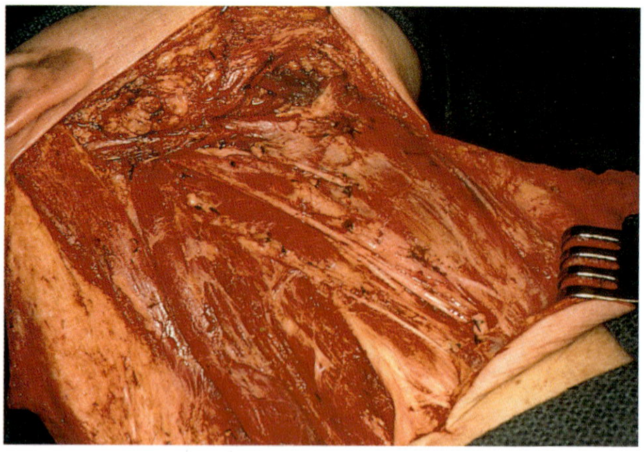

Figure 9.75 The surgical field following removal of the specimen.

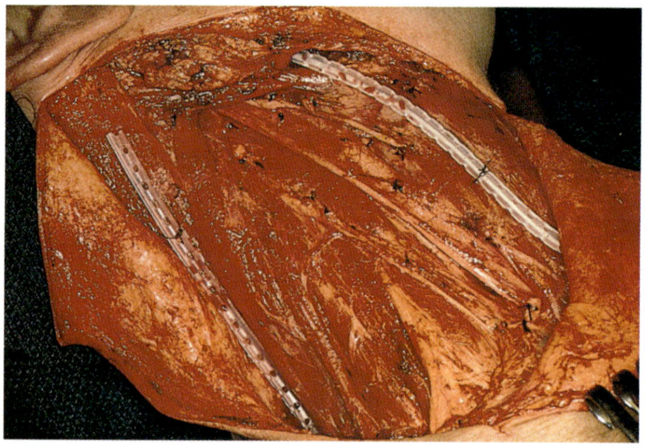

Figure 9.76 Two suction drains are inserted and appropriately positioned.

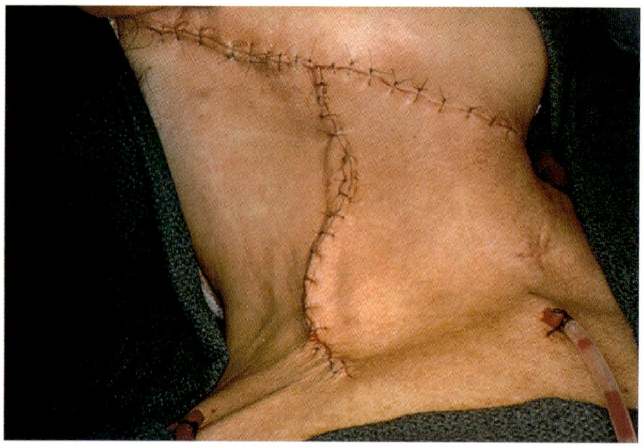

Figure 9.77 The incision is closed in two layers with interrupted sutures.

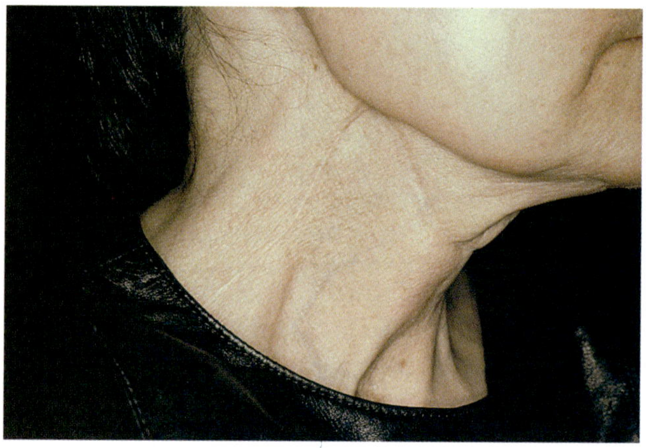

Figure 9.78 Postoperative appearance of the patient, six months following classical radical neck dissection.

(Fig. 9.77). It is vital for the suction drains to be on continuous suction while the wound is being closed.

As soon as the last skin sutures are applied, the wound should be made airtight, allowing the skin flaps to remain completely down and snug to the deeper tissues by suction through the drains. If suction in this manner is not maintained, minor venous oozing will allow the flaps to become lifted, causing collection of hematoma and clotting of blood in drainage tubes which will, in turn, initiate new venous oozing, leading to a larger hematoma. The suction drains are retained until the volume of serous drainage is minimal.

The postoperative appearance of the patient approximately 6 months after surgery shows a well-healed scar with esthetic deformity due to loss of sternomastoid muscle (Fig. 9.78). The functional disability is due to inability to abduct the shoulder beyond 90° cephalad. This is due to loss of function of the trapezius muscle. In addition to this, the imbalance of shoulder musculature due to the paralyzed trapezius muscle causes drooping of the shoulder (Fig. 9.79). When bilateral radical neck dissections are performed with sacrifice of the internal jugular vein on both sides for tumor of the oral cavity or oropharynx, chronic lymphedema of the face and swelling result. Although venous drainage is initially compromised, within a few weeks collateral venous drainage through the pharyngeal veins is restored as long as the anatomy of the central compartment is not disturbed. However, chronic lymphedema of the face with thickening of the subdermal plane and cutaneous telangiectasia remains (Fig. 9.80). On the other hand, when simultaneous bilateral radical neck dissections are performed in conjunction with laryngectomy, acute venous obstruction to intracranial and extracranial venous drainage occurs. This leads to the development of massive venous and lymphatic edema of the face in the postoperative period (Fig. 9.81).

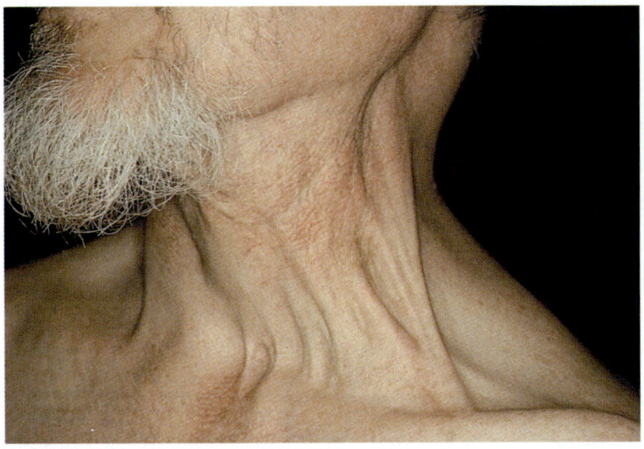

Figure 9.79 Drooping shoulder and fibrotic scar following radical neck dissection.

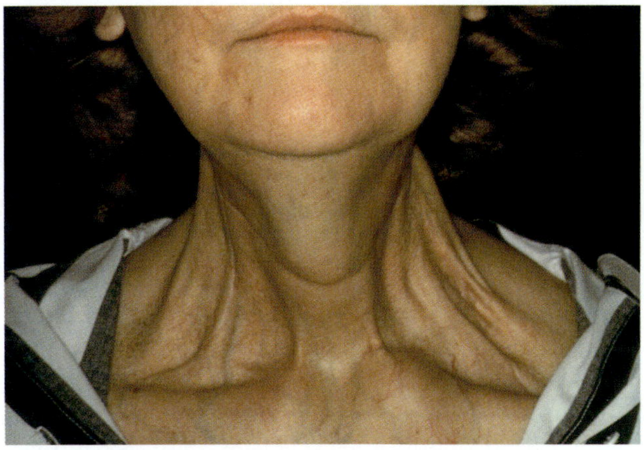

Figure 9.80 Chronic lymphedema and venous telangiectasia following bilateral radical neck dissections for oral cancer.

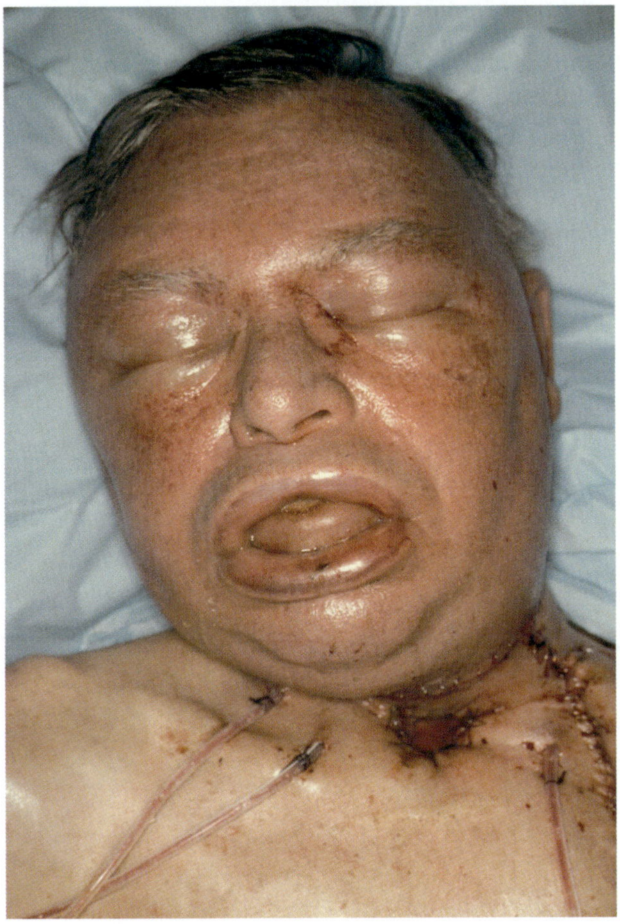

Figure 9.81 Massive edema due to venous obstruction immediately following total laryngectomy and bilateral radical neck dissections.

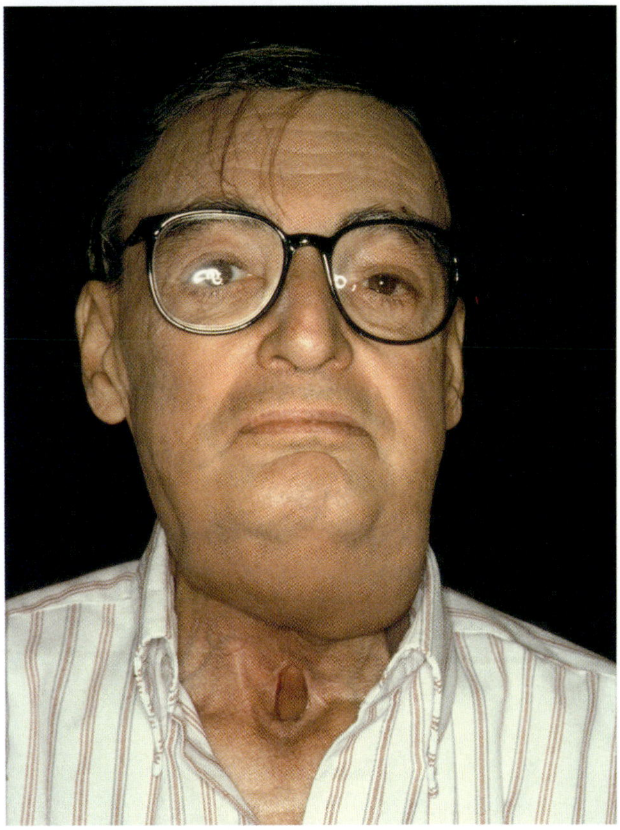

Figure 9.82 The same patient shown in Fig. 9.81, one year following surgery.

Although, with the passage of time, collateral venous drainage is established through Batson's prevertebral venous plexus, the extent of venous and lymphatic edema leaves significant facial swelling for a long time (Fig. 9.82). In addition to this, the operative mortality of such a massive resection is significant and therefore, when feasible, bilateral radical neck dissections in conjunction with pharyngolaryngectomy as a single stage procedure should be avoided. Patients undergoing classic radical neck dissection require an intensive program of postoperative physiotherapy for rehabilitation of shoulder function and to avoid a painful and stiff shoulder joint.

Results of treatment

As indicated earlier, the single most important factor in the prognosis of squamous cell carcinoma of the head and neck is the presence or absence of cervical lymph node metastasis.[2–21] Cure rates for patients with cervical lymph node metastasis are nearly one-half of those achieved in patients who present with tumors localized at the primary site. The extent of nodal metastasis in the neck clearly has an impact on prognosis. Patients with N_1 disease in the neck have a better prognosis compared to those with N_2, and N_3 disease (Fig. 9.83). In addition to this, the presence of capsular rupture and extranodal spread also have an adverse impact on prognosis.[12,14,55,57,58] Thus, regional failure in the dissected neck depends on the extent of nodal disease. Patients undergoing neck dissection for N_0 neck have the lowest risk of local recurrence compared to those with N_1, N_2 and N_3 disease. Patients with multiple level involvement develop recurrence in the dissected neck twice as often as those with single level involvement. Adjuvant postoperative radiation therapy, however, significantly improves regional control in the dissected neck.[81–86] This improvement in regional control is seen in patients with limited neck disease (N_1) as well as in patients with extensive nodal disease (N_2B) (Fig. 9.84).

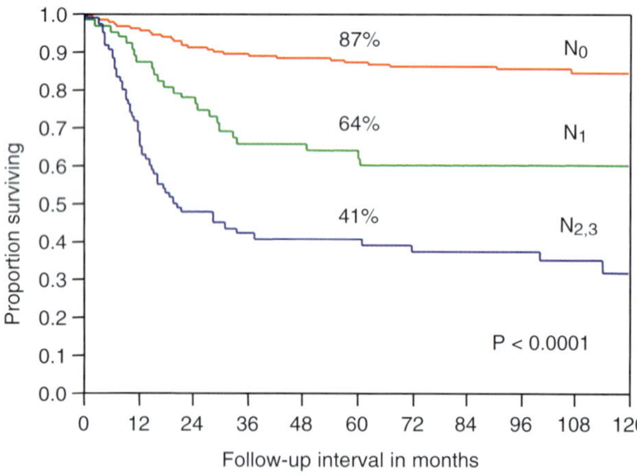

Figure 9.83 5-year disease-specific survival in patients with oral cancer according to N stage (MSKCC 1986–95)

Significant functional and esthetic morbidity following classic radical neck dissection led to modification of the operation to reduce morbidity without compromising regional control rates or survival.[19,43,46,87–93] Modified radical neck dissection type I (MRND-I) achieves that goal without an adverse impact on prognosis. Five-year survival rates, regional failure rates in the dissected neck, and the location of recurrence are comparable in patients with palpable metastatic disease undergoing classic radical neck dissection and modified radical neck dissection with preservation of the spinal accessory nerve (MRND-I) (Fig. 9.85). Regional recurrence rates in the dissected neck following classical radical neck dissection and

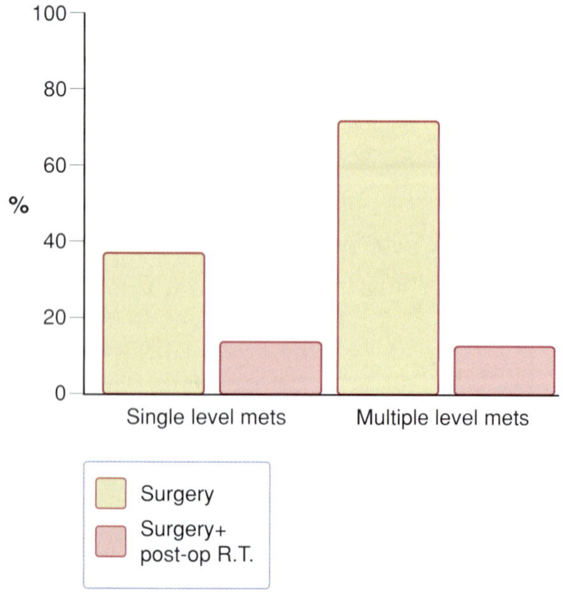

Figure 9.84 Regional failure in the neck after neck dissection with and without postoperative radiotherapy.

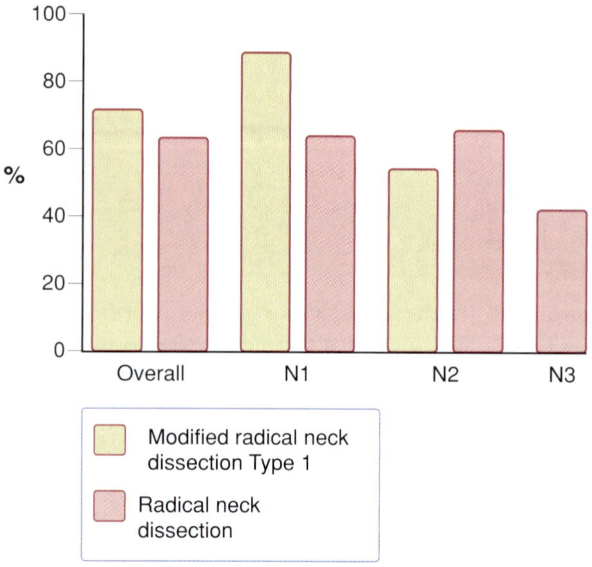

Figure 9.85 Overall 5-year survival after therapeutic neck dissection.

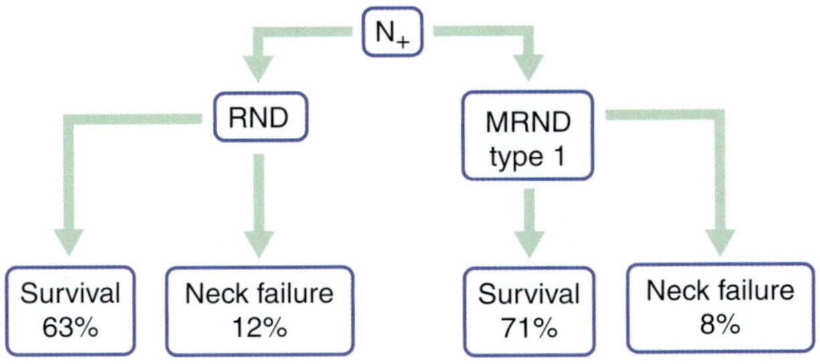

Figure 9.86 Survival and regional failure after RND and MRND type I in patients with palpable neck metastases.

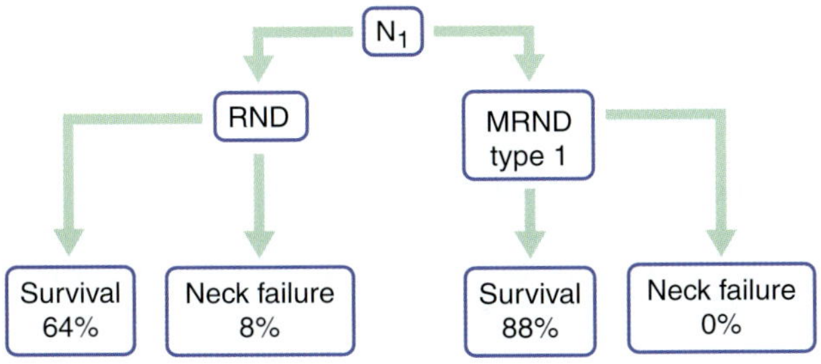

Figure 9.87 Survival and regional failure after RND and MRND type I with N_1 disease.

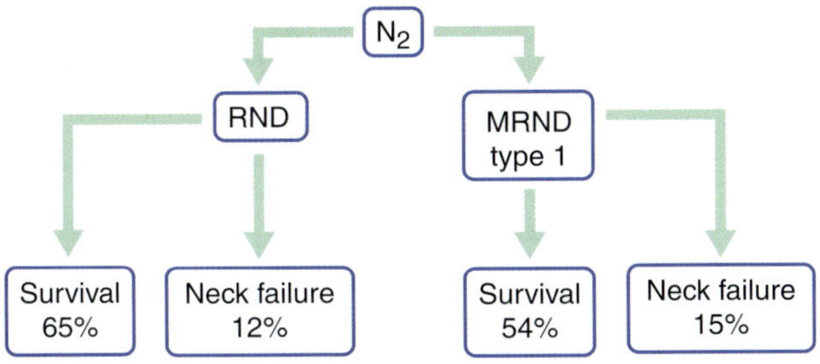

Figure 9.88 Survival and regional failure after RND and MRND type I with N_2 disease.

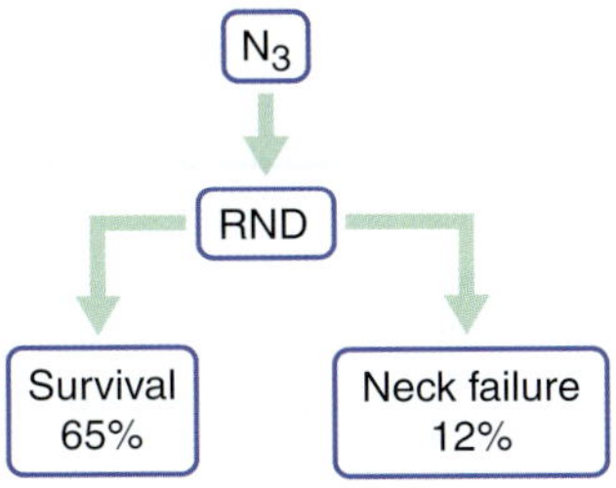

Figure 9.89 Survival and regional failure after RND with N_3 disease.

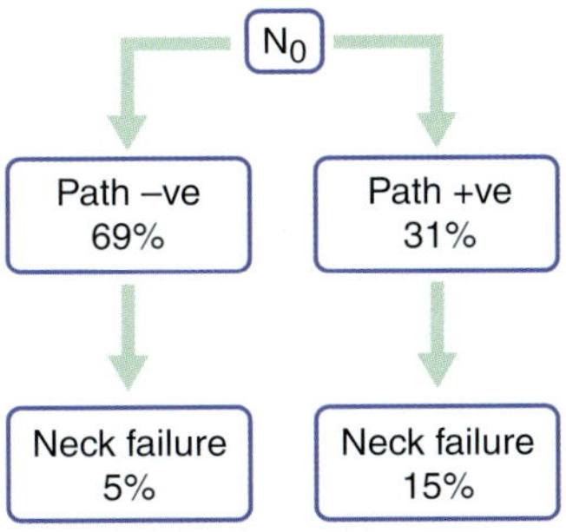

Figure 9.90 Regional failure after supraomohyoid neck dissection.

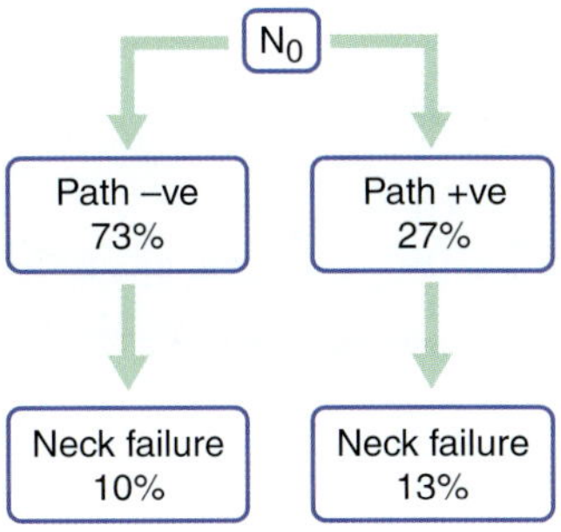

Figure 9.91 Regional failure after jugular neck dissection.

MRND-I are comparable (Fig. 9.86). Similarly, regional failure rates in patients undergoing classic radical neck dissection and modified radical neck dissection type I for N_1 and N_2 disease are also comparable (Figs 9.87, 9.88). The presence of extranodal spread by metastatic disease does not seem to influence regional recurrence rates following classic radical neck dissection or MRND-I as long as the accessory nerve is not directly involved by cancer. At present, it is felt inadvisable to perform modified radical neck dissection type I for N_3 disease. However, regional recurrence rates for patients undergoing classic radical neck dissection for N_3 disease are shown in Fig. 9.89.

Selective neck dissections in patients with N_0 neck provide accurate pathologic staging of the regional lymph nodes at risk of micrometastasis and offers regional control rates comparable to those obtained with more radical operative procedures. However, in order to achieve comparable regional control rates, postoperative radiation therapy should be employed when indicated. Regional control rates following supraomohyoid neck dissection for cancers of the oral cavity and jugular node dissection for cancers of oropharynx are shown in Figs 9.90 and 9.91.

The current philosophy in the management of cervical lymph nodes in squamous carcinomas of the head and neck region is to perform a comprehensive modified radical neck dissection type I, preserving the spinal accessory nerve in patients with grossly enlarged lymph nodes as long as the nerve is not involved by metastatic disease. A selective neck dissection is recommended in patients who have at least a 10 to 15% risk of having micrometastasis in the N_0 neck on the basis of the characteristics of the primary tumor. Postoperative radiation therapy is recommended in all patients with multiple metastatic lymph nodes, extranodal spread of tumor, or where other ominous histopathologic features are present.

The distribution of various types of neck dissections performed by the Head and Neck Service at

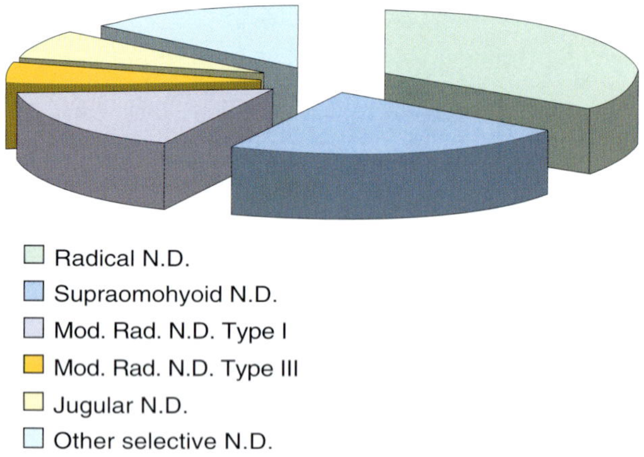

Figure 9.92 Distribution of types of neck dissection (MSKCC 1984–2000: 4864 patients).

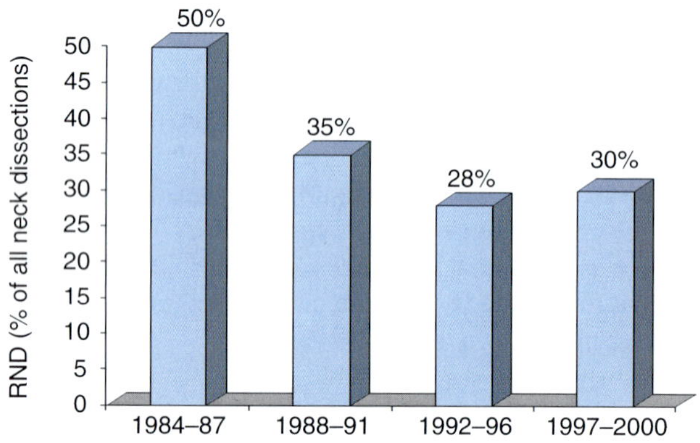

Figure 9.93 Declining incidence of radical neck dissection by time period (MSKCC 1984–2000).

Memorial Sloan–Kettering Cancer Center (MSKCC) from 1984 to 2000 is shown in Fig. 9.92. Over the same period, the number of patients undergoing a classic radical neck dissection declined and an increasing number of patients underwent modifications in neck dissection for management of cervical lymph node metastasis (Fig. 9.93).

References

1. Martin H, Del Valle BD, Ehrlich H et al. Neck dissection. Cancer 1951; 4: 441–449
2. Shah J. Management of cervical lymph nodes in patients with squamous cell carcinoma of the head and neck. In: Ariyan S (ed.). Cancer of the head and neck. St Louis: CV Mosby, 1986
3. Shah J. Cervical lymph node metastasis, its diagnostic, therapeutic, and prognostic implications. Oncology 1990; 4: 61–69
4. Shah J. Cervical lymph nodes. In: Head and neck surgery, 2nd edn. London: Mosby-Wolfe, 1996: 355–392
5. Shah J, Medina J, Shaha A. Cervical lymph node metastasis. Curr Probl Surg 1993; 30: 273–344
6. Bloom ND, Spiro RH. Carcinoma of the cheek mucosa. A retrospective analysis. Am J Surg 1980; 140: 556–559
7. Grandi C, Alloisio M, Moglia D et al. Prognostic significance of lymphatic spread in head and neck carcinomas: therapeutic implications. Head Neck Surg 1985; 8: 67–73
8. Heller KS, Shah JP. Carcinoma of the lip. Am J Surg 1979; 138: 600–603
9. Johnson CD, Hill I, Vela J. Squamous cell carcinoma of the floor of the mouth with invasion of the mandible. J Gt Houst Dent Soc 1994; 66: 13–14
10. Maddox WA, Sherlock EC, Evans WB. Cancer of the tongue: review of thirteen-year experience—1955–1968. Am Surg 1971; 37: 624–650
11. Schleuning AJd, Summers GW. Carcinoma of the tongue: review of 220 cases. Laryngoscope 1972; 82: 1446–1454
12. Shah JP, Cendon RA, Farr HW, Strong EW. Carcinoma of the oral cavity. Factors affecting treatment failure at the primary site and neck. Am J Surg 1976; 132: 504–507
13. Shaha AR, Spiro RH, Shah JP, Strong EW. Squamous carcinoma of the floor of the mouth. Am J Surg 1984; 148: 455–459
14. Silver CE, Moisa II. Elective treatment of the neck in cancer of the oral tongue. Semin Surg Oncol 1991; 7: 14–19
15. Snow GB, Annyas AA, van Slooten EA, Bartelink H, Hart AA. Prognostic factors of neck node metastasis. Clin Otolaryngol 1982; 7: 185–192
16. Soo KC, Spiro RH, King W, Harvey W, Strong EW. Squamous carcinoma of the gums. Am J Surg 1988; 156: 281–285
17. Spiro RH. Squamous cancer of the tongue. CA Cancer J Clin 1985; 35: 252–256
18. Zitsch RPd. Carcinoma of the lip. Otolaryngol Clin North Am 1993; 26: 265–277
19. Houck JR, Medina JE. Management of cervical lymph nodes in squamous carcinomas of the head and neck. Semin Surg Oncol 1995; 11: 228–239
20. Richard JM, Sancho-Garnier H, Micheau C, Saravane D, Cachin Y. Prognostic factors in cervical lymph node metastasis in upper respiratory and digestive tract carcinomas: study of 1,713 cases during a 15-year period. Laryngoscope 1987; 97: 97–101
21. Leemans CR, Tiwari R, Nauta JJ, van der Waal I, Snow GB. Regional lymph node involvement and its significance in the development of distant metastases in head and neck carcinoma. Cancer 1993; 71: 452–456
22. Ho CM, Lam KH, Wei WI, Lau WF. Treatment of neck nodes in oral cancer. Surg Oncol 1992; 1: 73–78
23. Leemans CR, Tiwari R, Nauta JJ, van der Waal I, Snow GB. Recurrence at the primary site in head and neck cancer and the significance of neck lymph node metastases as a prognostic factor. Cancer 1994; 73: 187–190
24. Shah JP, Strong E, Spiro RH, Vikram B. Surgical grand rounds. Neck dissection: current status and future possibilities. Clin Bull 1981; 11: 25–33

25. Snow GB, Patel P, Leemans CR, Tiwari R. Management of cervical lymph nodes in patients with head and neck cancer. Eur Arch Otorhinolaryngol 1992; 249: 187–194
26. Snow GB, van den Brekel MW, Leemans CR, Patel P. Surgical management of cervical lymph nodes in patients with oral and oropharyngeal cancer. Recent Results Cancer Res 1994; 134: 43–55
27. Spiro RH, Alfonso AE, Farr HW, Strong EW. Cervical node metastasis from epidermoid carcinoma of the oral cavity and oropharynx. A critical assessment of current staging. Am J Surg 1974; 128: 562–567
28. Spiro RH. The management of neck nodes in head and neck cancer: a surgeon's view. Bull N Y Acad Med 1985; 61: 629–637
29. Vikram B, Strong EW, Shah JP, Spiro R. Failure in the neck following multimodality treatment for advanced head and neck cancer. Head Neck Surg 1984; 6: 724–729
30. Lore JM, Jr. Early diagnosis and treatment of head and neck cancer [editorial]. CA Cancer J Clin 1995; 45: 325–327
31. Whitehurst JO, Droulias CA. Surgical treatment of squamous cell carcinoma of the oral tongue: factors influencing survival. Arch Otolaryngol 1977; 103: 212–215
32. From the Centers for Disease Control. Current trends: deaths from oral cavity and pharyngeal cancer—United States, 1987. JAMA 1990; 264: 678
33. Sankaranarayanan R. Oral cancer in India: an epidemiologic and clinical review. Oral Surg Oral Med Oral Pathol 1990; 69: 325–330
34. Hindle I, Downer MC, Speight PM. The epidemiology of oral cancer. Br J Oral Maxillofac Surg 1996; 34: 471–476
35. Hoffman HT, Karnell LH, Funk GF, Robinson RA, Menck HR. The National Cancer Data Base report on cancer of the head and neck. Arch Otolaryngol Head Neck Surg 1998; 124: 951–962
36. Boyle P, Macfarlane GJ, Zheng T, Maisonneuve P, Evstifeeva T, Scully C. Recent advances in epidemiology of head and neck cancer. Curr Opin Oncol 1992; 4: 471–477
37. Baden E. Prevention of cancer of the oral cavity and pharynx. CA Cancer J Clin 1987; 37: 49–62
38. Mashberg A, Samit A. Early diagnosis of asymptomatic oral and oropharyngeal squamous cancers. CA Cancer J Clin 1995; 45: 328–351
39. Mashberg A, Samit AM. Early detection, diagnosis, and management of oral and oropharyngeal cancer [see comments]. CA Cancer J Clin 1989; 39: 67–88
40. Plesko I, Obsitnikova A, Vlasak V. Increasing occurrence of oropharyngeal cancers among males in Slovakia. Neoplasma 1997; 44: 77–83
41. Swango PA. Cancers of the oral cavity and pharynx in the United States: an epidemiologic overview. J Public Health Dent 1996; 56: 309–318
42. Shah J, Andersen P. Evolving role of modifications in neck dissections for oral squamous cell carcinoma. Br J Oral Maxillofac Surg 1995; 33: 3–8
43. Shah JP, Andersen PE. The impact of patterns of nodal metastasis on modifications of neck dissection. Ann Surg Oncol 1994; 1: 521–532
44 Shah J. Indications, rationale, and techniques in neck dissection. In: Najarian J, Delaney J (eds). Progress in cancer surgery. St Louis: Mosby Year Book; 1991: 262–273
45. Shah JP, Candela FC, Poddar AK. The patterns of cervical lymph node metastases from squamous carcinoma of the oral cavity. Cancer 1990; 66: 109–113
46. Shah JP. Patterns of cervical lymph node metastasis from squamous carcinomas of the upper aerodigestive tract. Am J Surg 1990; 160: 405–409
47. Robbins KT. Classification of neck dissection: current concepts and future considerations [in process citation]. Otolaryngol Clin North Am 1998; 31: 639–655
48. Robbins KT, Medina JE, Wolfe GT, Levine PA, Sessions RB, Pruet CW. Standardizing neck dissection terminology. Official report of the Academy's Committee for Head and Neck Surgery and Oncology [see comments]. Arch Otolaryngol Head Neck Surg 1991; 117: 601–605
49. Medina JE. A rational classification of neck dissections. Otolaryngol Head Neck Surg 1989; 100: 169–176
50. Medina JE, Byers RM. Supraomohyoid neck dissection: rationale, indications, and surgical technique. Head Neck 1989; 11: 111–122
51. Lindberg R. Distribution of cervical node metastasis from squamous cell carcinoma of the upper respiratory and digestive tracts. Cancer 1972; 29: 1446–1449
52. Ballantyne A. Significance of retropharyngeal nodes in cancer of the head and neck. Am J Surg 1964; 108: 500–503
53. Kalnins IK, Leonard AG, Sako K, Razack MS, Shedd DP. Correlation between prognosis and degree of lymph node involvement in carcinoma of the oral cavity. Am J Surg 1977; 134: 450–454
54. Tytor M, Olofsson J. Prognostic factors in oral cavity carcinomas. Acta Otolaryngol Suppl 1992; 492: 75–78
55. Johnson JT, Myers EN, Bedetti CD, Barnes EL, Schramm VL Jr, Thearle PB. Cervical lymph node metastases. Incidence and implications of extracapsular carcinoma. Arch Otolaryngol 1985; 111: 534–537
56. Andersen PE, Cambronero E, Shaha AR, Shah JP. The extent of neck disease after regional failure during observation of the N0 neck. Am J Surg 1996; 172: 689–691
57. Alvi A, Johnson JT. Extracapsular spread in the clinically negative neck (N0): implications and outcome. Otolaryngol Head Neck Surg 1996; 114: 65–70
58. Zelefsky MJ, Harrison LB, Fass DE et al. Postoperative radiotherapy for oral cavity cancers: impact of anatomic subsite on treatment outcome. Head Neck 1990; 12: 470–475
59. Carter RL, Barr LC, O'Brien CJ, Soo KC, Shaw HJ. Transcapsular spread of metastatic squamous cell carcinoma from cervical lymph nodes. Am J Surg 1985; 150: 495–499
60. Byers RM, El-Naggar AK, Lee YY et al. Can we detect or predict the presence of occult nodal metastases in patients with squamous carcinoma of the oral tongue? Head Neck 1998; 20: 138–144

61. Candela FC, Kothari K, Shah JP. Patterns of cervical node metastases from squamous carcinoma of the oropharynx and hypopharynx. Head Neck 1990; 12: 197–203
62. Cummings C, Goepfert H, Myers E. Squamous cell carcinoma of the base of the tongue. Head Neck Surg 1986; 9: 56–59
63. Leemans CR, Engelbrecht WJ, Tiwari R et al. Carcinoma of the soft palate and anterior tonsillar pillar. Laryngoscope 1994; 104: 1477–1481
64. Byers RM, Weber RS, Andrews T, McGill D, Kare R, Wolf P. Frequency and therapeutic implications of 'skip metastases' in the neck from squamous carcinoma of the oral tongue [see comments]. Head Neck 1997; 19: 14–19
65. Davidson BJ, Kulkarny V, Delacure MD, Shah JP. Posterior triangle metastases of squamous cell carcinoma of the upper aerodigestive tract. Am J Surg 1993; 166: 395–398
66. van den Brekel MW, Castelijns JA, Stel HV et al. Occult metastatic neck disease: detection with US and US-guided fine- needle aspiration. Radiology 1991; 180: 457–461
67. Shaha A, Webber C, Marti J. Fine-needle aspiration in the diagnosis of cervical lymphadenopathy. Am J Surg 1986; 152: 420–423
68. van den Brekel MW, Stel HV, Castelijns JA et al. Cervical lymph node metastasis: assessment of radiologic criteria. Radiology 1990; 177: 379–384
69. van den Brekel MW, Castelijns JA, Stel HV et al. Detection and characterization of metastatic cervical adenopathy by MR imaging: comparison of different MR techniques. J Comput Assist Tomogr 1990; 14: 581–589
70. van den Brekel MW, Stel HV, Castelijns JA, Croll GJ, Snow GB. Lymph node staging in patients with clinically negative neck examinations by ultrasound and ultrasound-guided aspiration cytology. Am J Surg 1991; 162: 362–366
71. van den Brekel MW, Castelijns JA, Croll GA et al. Magnetic resonance imaging vs palpation of cervical lymph node metastasis. Arch Otolaryngol Head Neck Surg 1991; 117: 663–673
72. van den Brekel MW, Snow GB. Assessment of lymph node metastases in the neck. Eur J Cancer B Oral Oncol 1994; 2: 88–92
73. Shah J, Kraus D. Radical neck dissection and its modifications. In: Donohue J, Heerden JV, Monson J (eds) Atlas of surgical oncology. Cambridge, Massachussetts: Blackwell Science, 1994
74. Martin H. The case for prophylactic neck dissection. CA Cancer J Clin 1951; 4: 92–97
75. Hughes CJ, Gallo O, Spiro RH, Shah JP. Management of occult neck metastases in oral cavity squamous carcinoma. Am J Surg 1993; 166: 380–383
76. Ho CM, Lam KH, Wei WI, Lau SK, Lam LK. Occult lymph node metastasis in small oral tongue cancers. Head Neck 1992; 14: 359–363
77. Kurita H, Kurashina K, Minemura T, Kotani A. Pitfalls in the treatment of delayed lymph-node metastases after control of small tongue carcinomas. Int J Oral Maxillofac Surg 1995; 24: 356–360
78. van den Brekel MW, van der Waal I, Meijer CJ, Freeman JL, Castelijns JA, Snow GB. The incidence of micro-metastases in neck dissection specimens obtained from elective neck dissections. Laryngoscope 1996; 106: 987–991
79. McGuirt WF Jr, Johnson JT, Myers EN, Rothfield R, Wagner R. Floor of mouth carcinoma. The management of the clinically negative neck. Arch Otolaryngol Head Neck Surg 1995; 121: 278–282
80. Yuen AP, Wei WI, Wong YM, Tang KC. Elective neck dissection versus observation in the treatment of early oral tongue carcinoma. Head Neck 1997; 19: 583–588
81. Vandenbrouck C, Sancho-Garnier H, Chassagne D, Saravane D, Cachin Y, Micheau C. Elective versus therapeutic radical neck dissection in epidermoid carcinoma of the oral cavity: results of a randomized clinical trial. Cancer 1980; 46: 386–390
82. Vikram B. Adjuvant therapy in head and neck cancer. CA Cancer J Clin 1998; 48: 199–209
83. Bartelink H, Breur K, Hart G, Annyas B, van Slooten E, Snow G. The value of postoperative radiotherapy as an adjuvant to radical neck dissection. Cancer 1983; 52: 1008–1013
84. Peters LJ, Goepfert H, Ang KK et al. Evaluation of the dose for postoperative radiation therapy of head and neck cancer: first report of a prospective randomized trial. Int J Radiat Oncol Biol Phys 1993; 26: 3–11
85. Strong EW, Henschke UK, Nickson JJ, Frazell EL, Tollefsen HR, Hilaris BS. Preoperative x-ray therapy as an adjunct to radical neck dissection. Cancer 1966; 19: 1509–1516
86. Strong EW. Preoperative radiation and radical neck dissection. Surg Clin North Am 1969; 49: 271–276
87. Kraus DH, Rosenberg DB, Davidson BJ et al. Supraspinal accessory lymph node metastases in supraomohyoid neck dissection. Am J Surg 1996; 172: 646–649
88. Remmler D, Byers R, Scheetz J et al. A prospective study of shoulder disability resulting from radical and modified neck dissections. Head Neck Surg 1986; 8: 280–286
89. Sobol S, Jensen C, Sawyer Wd, Costiloe P, Thong N. Objective comparison of physical dysfunction after neck dissection. Am J Surg 1985; 150: 503–509
90. Leipzig B, Suen JY, English JL, Barnes J, Hooper M. Functional evaluation of the spinal accessory nerve after neck dissection. Am J Surg 1983; 146: 526–530
91. DeSanto LW, Beahrs OH. Modified and complete neck dissection in the treatment of squamous cell carcinoma of the head and neck. Surg Gynecol Obstet 1988; 167: 259–269
92. Spiro RH, Gallo O, Shah JP. Selective jugular node dissection in patients with squamous carcinoma of the larynx or pharynx. Am J Surg 1993; 166: 399–402
93. Lingeman RE, Helmus C, Stephens R, Ulm J. Neck dissection: radical or conservative. Ann Otol Rhinol Laryngol 1977; 86: 737–744
94. Byers RM. Modified neck dissection. A study of 967 cases from 1970 to 1980. Am J Surg 1985; 150: 414–421
95. Byers RM, Wolf PF, Ballantyne AJ. Rationale for elective modified neck dissection. Head Neck Surg 1988; 10: 160–167

96. Spiro JD, Spiro RH, Shah JP, Sessions RB, Strong EW. Critical assessment of supraomohyoid neck dissection. Am J Surg 1988; 156: 286–289
97. Spiro RH, Strong EW, Shah JP. Classification of neck dissection: variations on a new theme. Am J Surg 1994; 168: 415–418
98. Spiro RH, Morgan GJ, Strong EW, Shah JP. Supraomohyoid neck dissection. Am J Surg 1996; 172: 650–653
99. Suen JY, Goepfert H. Standardization of neck dissection nomenclature. Head Neck Surg 1987; 10: 75–77

10 Surgical approaches to the oral cavity

John F Carew, Bhuvanesh Singh and Jatin P Shah

A variety of surgical approaches are available for resection of primary oral cavity tumors, including per oral, mandibulotomy, lower cheek flap, visor flap, and upper cheek flap approaches, as shown in Fig. 10.1. The selection of a particular approach depends on several factors, including the tumor size and site, depth of infiltration, and proximity to mandible or maxilla.[1–21] Access for oncological resection should not be compromised by efforts to minimize the extent of the procedure.

Excision of small primary lesions in the oral cavity can be accomplished under local anesthesia. However, resection of most oral cavity tumors requires general endotracheal anesthesia and adequate muscle relaxation. Nasotracheal intubation is preferable in this setting, since it facilitates surgical access and instrumentation of the oral cavity during surgery. Per oral intubation and endotracheal tube fixation with tape can distort facial skin lines, resulting in misplaced incisions. Accordingly, surgical incisions are marked out prior to endotracheal intubation. In patients with bulky, potentially obstructive oropharyngeal tumors, a preliminary tracheostomy is performed under local anesthesia, prior to the induction of general anesthesia.

Ideally, the patient is placed on the operating table in the supine position with the upper half of the body elevated at 30° (Fig. 10.2). The head and neck region is draped according to whether the planned operative approach is solely intra-oral or will require external incision either on the face or the neck. A transparent plastic drape is used to isolate the anesthetic tubing, with care taken to ensure that the patient's eyes, nose and endotracheal tube are clearly visible to both the surgeon and the anesthesiologist (Fig. 10.3).

Per oral surgical approach

Surgical treatment for many tumors of the oral cavity can be performed safely via an open mouth approach, provided the tumor is small and easily accessible (Fig. 10.4). Thus, small primary tumors of the oral tongue, floor of mouth, gum, cheek mucosa and hard or soft palate are suitable for per oral excision. However, in patients with oral apertures inadequate to provide access to the tumor, alternative approaches are required to allow for satisfactory resection.

Partial glossectomy

All T1 and most T2 lesions of the oral tongue, that is the anterior two-thirds of the tongue, are suitable for a partial glossectomy through the open mouth. Tumors involving the lateral aspect of the oral tongue are amenable to a wedge excision oriented in a transverse fashion. Longitudinally oriented excision of a large tumor results in an elongated narrow tongue which often impairs speech and interferes with mastication. In contrast, transversely oriented wedge resections foreshorten the tongue, resulting in functionally and cosmetically superior results.

The procedure is best performed by electrocautery. First, the cutting current is used to incise the mucosa of the tongue, both on its superior and inferior aspects. Following the mucosal incision, coagulating current is used for resection of the underlying musculature of the tongue. Minor bleeding points in the musculature of the tongue are electrocoagulated while major branches of the

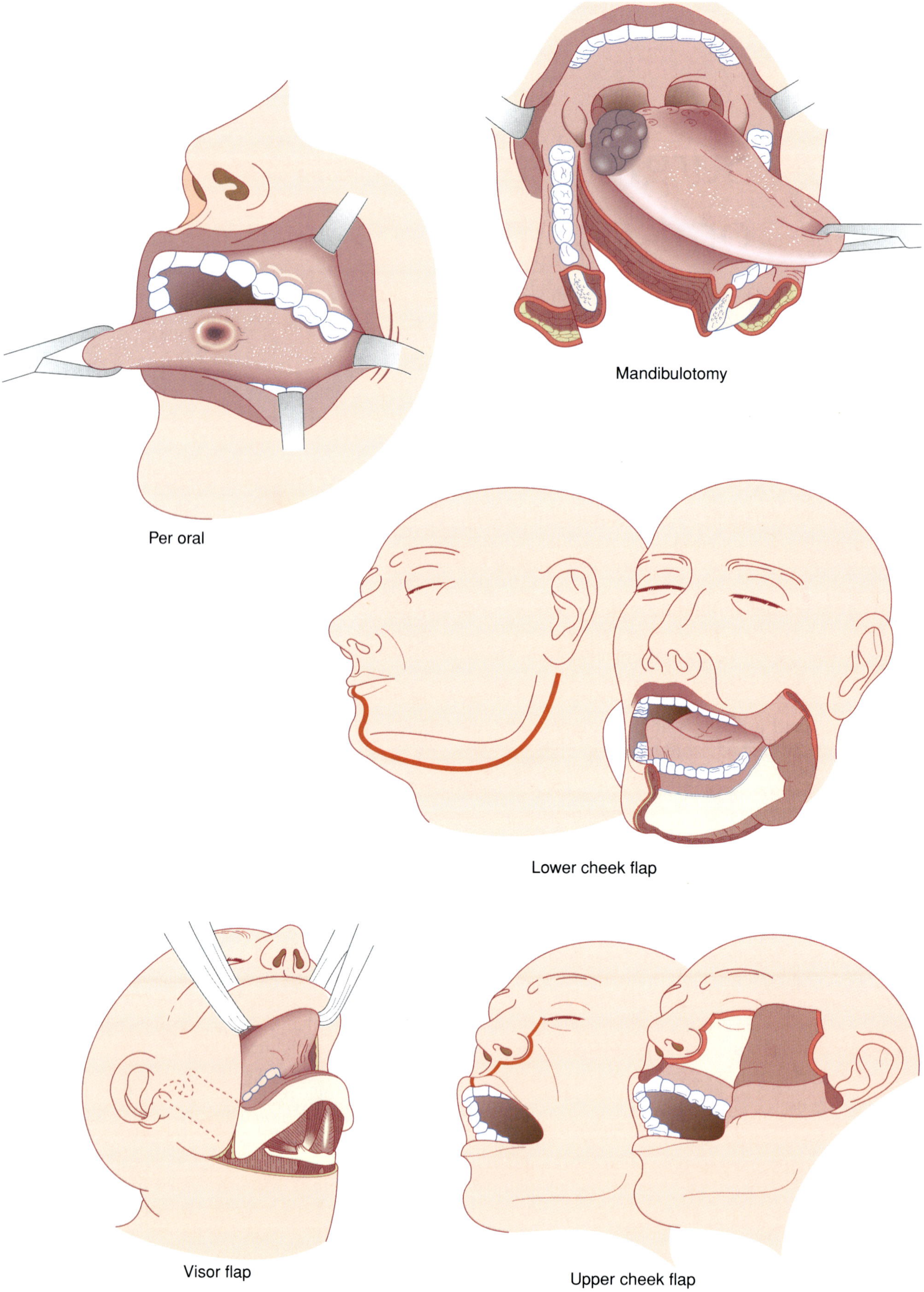

Figure 10.1 Surgical approaches to the oral cavity.

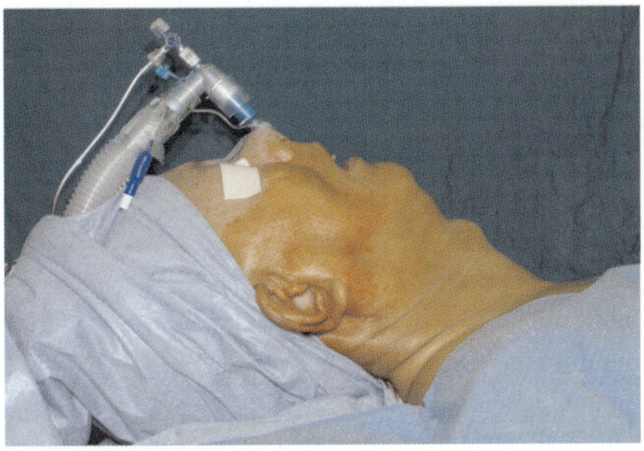

Figure 10.2 Position of the patient on the operating table.

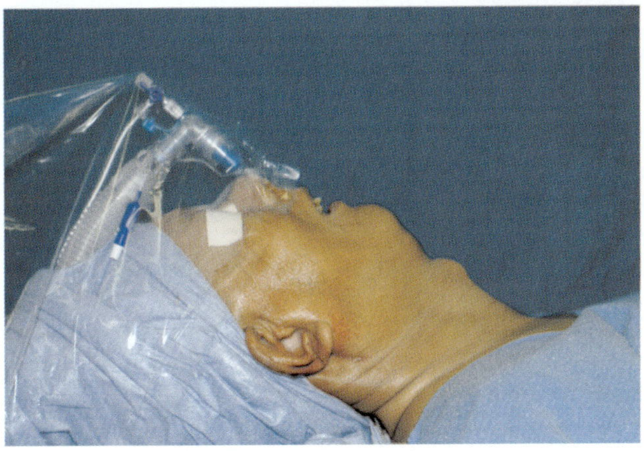

Figure 10.3 A transparent plastic drape provides a view of the anesthetic tubing and eyes.

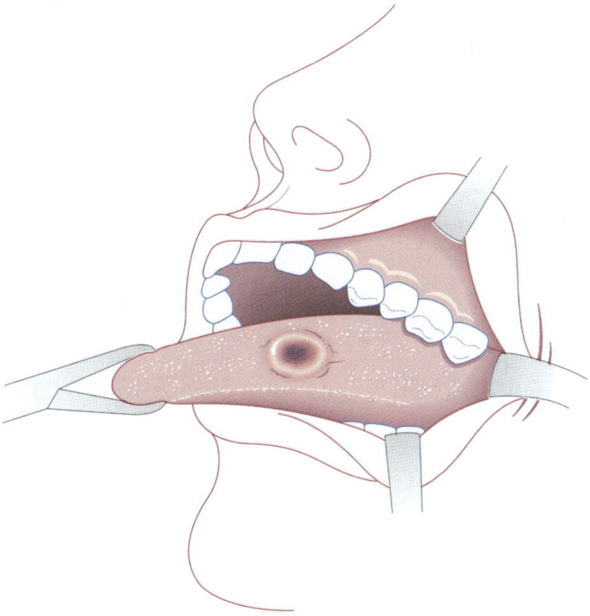

Figure 10.4 Per oral approach.

lingual artery are ligated with chromic catgut. The excision should include a generous margin of the mucosa adjacent to the tumor and a full complement of the thickness of the musculature of the tongue surrounding the palpable tumor. Frozen sections are taken from the mucosal margins, as well as from the depth of the surgical defect, to ensure adequate excision of the primary tumor. Repair of the surgical defect follows confirmation of negative margins by frozen section and attainment of complete hemostasis. A two-layered closure is performed using interrupted 000 chromic catgut sutures to approximate the musculature and the superior and inferior mucosal aspects of the tongue. A skin hook is used to retract the apex of the wedge-shaped surgical defect for transverse orientation of the closure. Blood loss during the procedure is negligible. The patient can take clear liquids by mouth within 24 to 48 hours and is allowed a puréed diet on the third postoperative day. Most patients will be able to tolerate a soft diet by the end of the week. Initially there is some degree of speech impairment which improves as healing progresses and mobility of the tongue improves.

The lesion shown in Fig. 10.5 is an ulcerated, endophytic 2.5 cm carcinoma involving the right lateral border of the anterior and middle one-third of the tongue. The tumor does not extend across the midline nor does it involve the adjacent floor of the mouth. Mobility of the tongue is not restricted. The steps of the operation are shown schematically in Fig. 10.6.

The procedure is performed under general anesthesia with nasotracheal intubation. The oral cavity is isolated and cleaned with Betadine solution (Purdue Frederick, Connecticut, USA). A wedge-shaped incision is illustrated in Fig. 10.7. The surgical specimen demonstrates full-thickness, three-dimensional

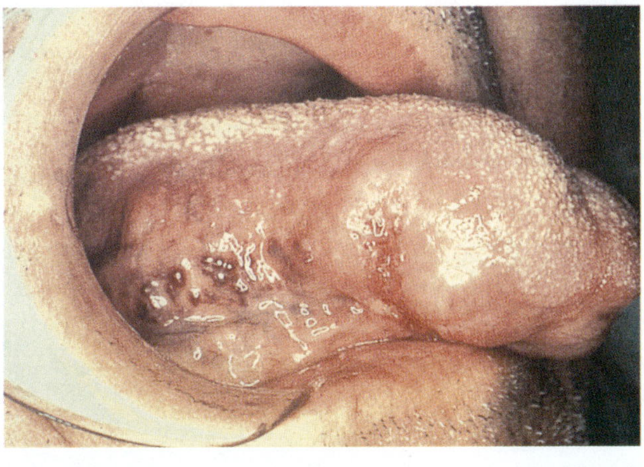

Figure 10.5 Squamous carcinoma of the lateral border of oral tongue.

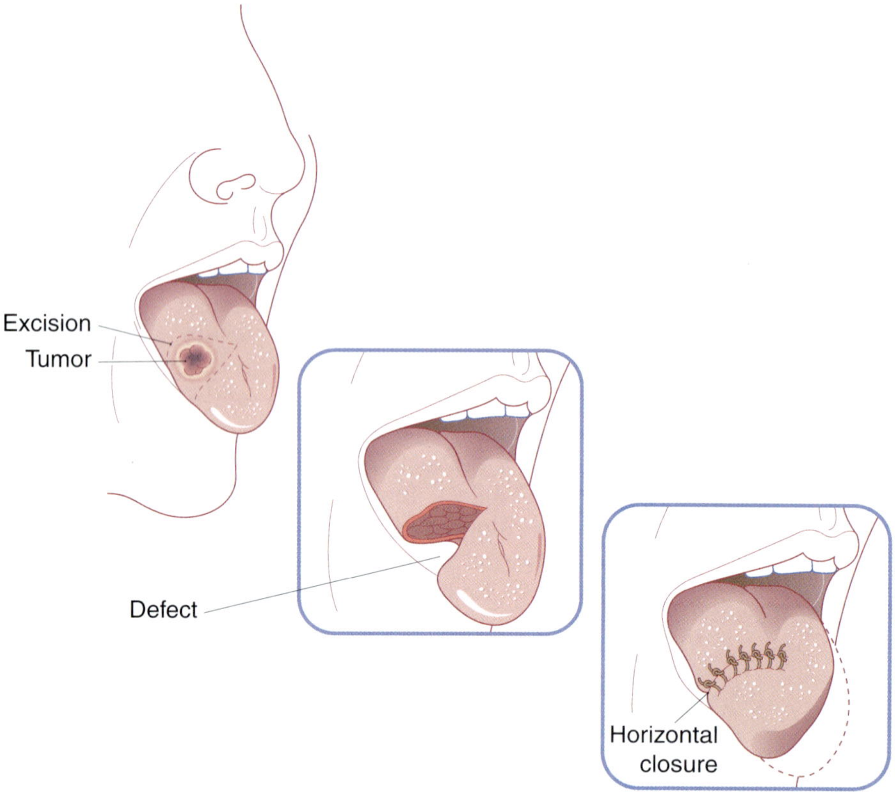

Figure 10.6 Transversely oriented wedge resection of tongue tumor.

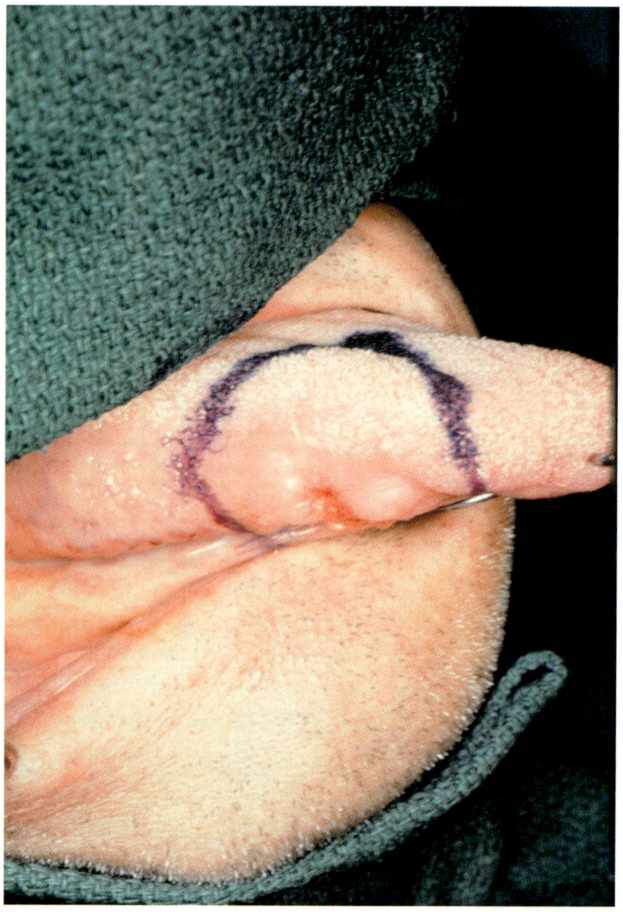

Figure 10.7 Surgical excision is outlined.

resection of the tumor of the oral tongue with adequate mucosal and soft tissue margins (Fig. 10.8). The surgical defect demonstrates satisfactory excision of the primary tumor (Fig. 10.9). A two-layered closure is performed with interrupted catgut sutures. The postoperative appearance of the tongue approximately 3 months after partial glossectomy is shown in Fig. 10.10. Note the transverse scar at the suture line, giving a normal configuration of the oral tongue. The patient now has practically no speech impairment and is able to tolerate all types of food by mouth.

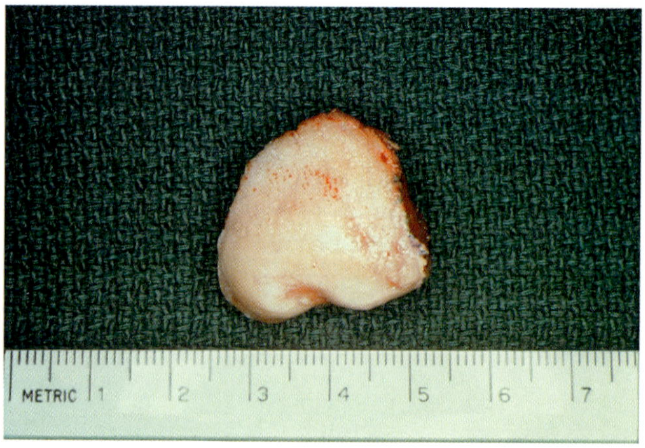

Figure 10.8 Wedge shaped surgical specimen.

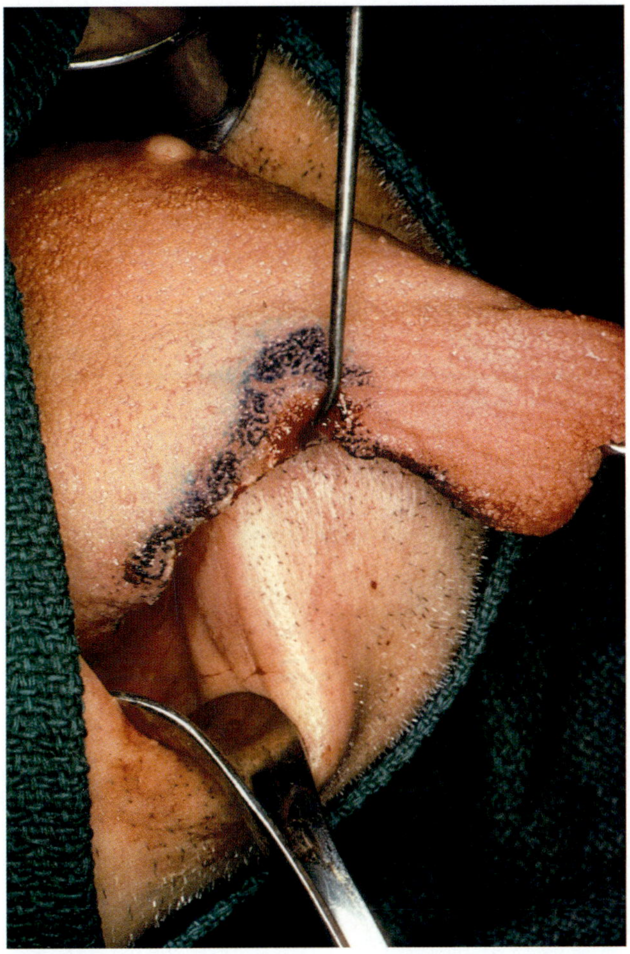

Figure 10.9 Wedge shaped surgical defect.

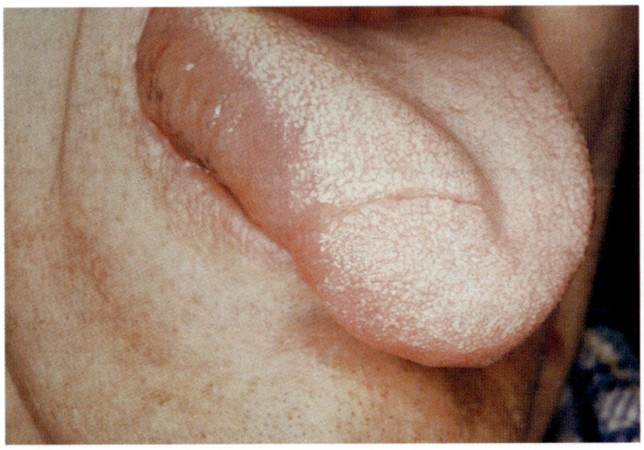

Figure 10.10 Postoperative appearance of the tongue at 3 months.

Excision of floor of mouth and skin graft

Peroral excision can be performed for superficial lesions of the floor of the mouth, cheek mucosa or soft palate, leaving the surgical defect open to granulate and heal by secondary intention. However,

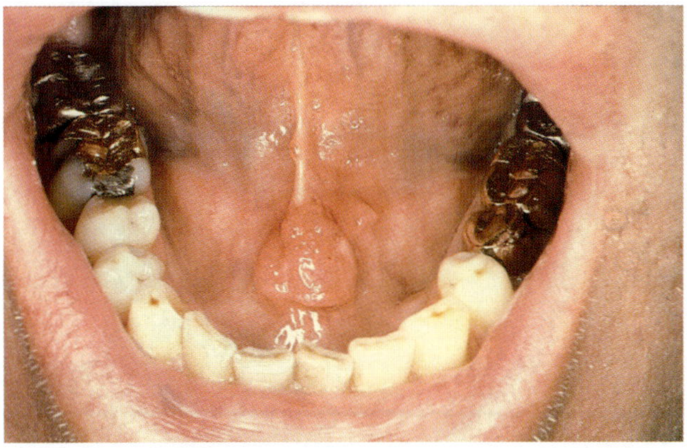

Figure 10.11 Squamous carcinoma of the anterior floor of the mouth.

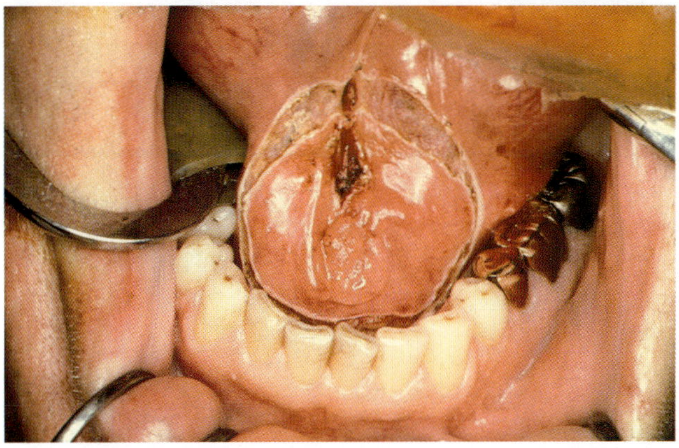

Figure 10.12 A circumferential mucosal incision is placed.

when such an excision is in critical areas where mobility is essential, or when the depth of excision extends to the underlying musculature, then healing by secondary intention leads to fibrosis and contracture, causing impairment of function. In these cases, it is desirable to cover such surgical defects with a full-thickness skin graft.

The patient shown in Fig. 10.11 has squamous carcinoma of the anterior floor of the mouth invading the openings of the Wharton's ducts on both sides. A generous margin around the tumor is obtained by the incision outlined with electrocautery (Fig. 10.12). Excision of the lesion, including the underlying sublingual glands, is performed in a three-dimensional fashion (Fig. 10.13). Note that the Wharton's ducts are isolated bilaterally. The ducts are transected and tagged with a suture and the specimen is delivered. The surgical defect shows the underlying genioglossus muscle (Fig. 10.14).

The full-thickness skin graft is harvested from one of several areas, including the supraclavicular area of the neck. The skin graft is appropriately trimmed and sutured to the mucosal edges of the surgical defect using 000 chromic catgut interrupted sutures

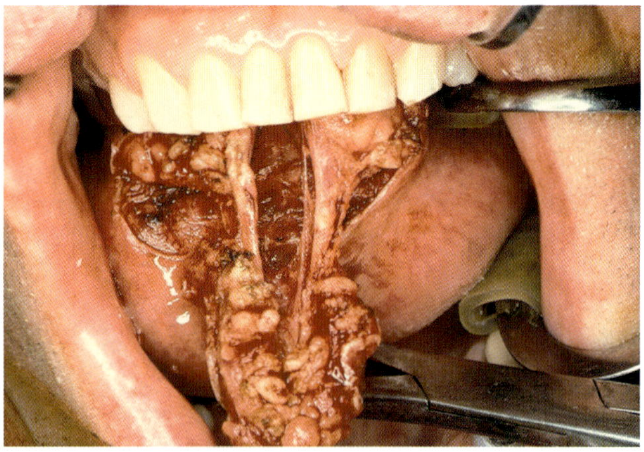

Figure 10.13 Wharton's ducts are dissected.

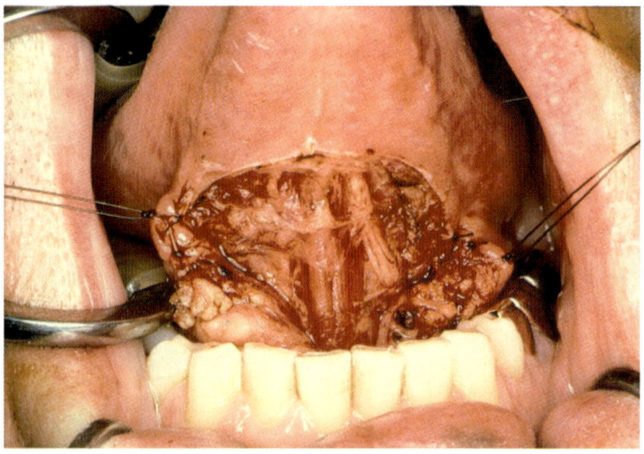

Figure 10.14 Wharton's ducts are resected and transposed.

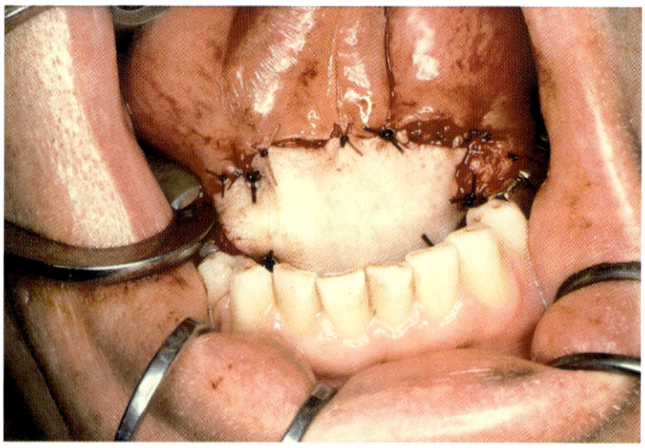

Figure 10.15 A skin graft is applied to the defect.

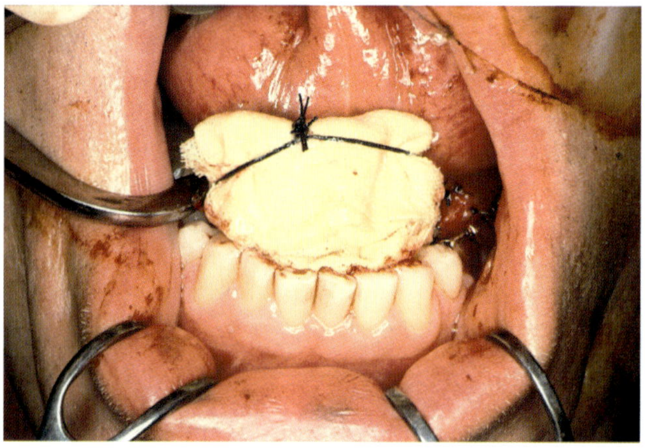

Figure 10.16 Bolus dressing holds the skin graft in position.

(Fig. 10.15). Several stab incisions are made in the skin graft after it is sutured in place, to permit drainage of blood and/or serum that may accumulate beneath the graft. A xeroform gauze bolster is made to fit the area of the skin graft and is anchored in position with 00 silk tie-over sutures (Fig. 10.16). The patient is not allowed to take anything by mouth until the bolster dressing is removed at approximately one week. Optimal oral hygiene is maintained with oral irrigation until the graft has satisfactorily healed. The patient can then take clear liquids and purėed foods by mouth. The postoperative appearance of the skin graft at approximately 8 weeks following surgery shows complete healing with normal mobility of the tongue, with no deficit in mastication or clarity of speech (Fig. 10.17).

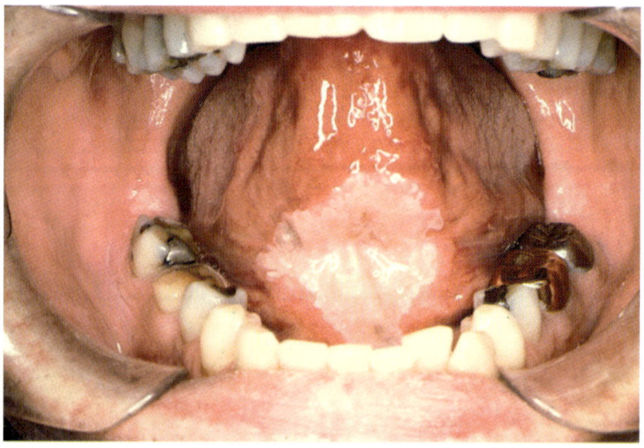

Figure 10.17 Healed skin graft at eight weeks following surgery.

Per oral partial maxillectomy

Consideration for per oral tumor excision can also be extended to small tumors of dentoalveolar or mucosal origin of the upper alveolus via a per oral partial maxillectomy. However, it is important to remember that adequate radiographic assessment of the extent of bony involvement by the tumor is mandatory prior to embarking on this surgical procedure.

For anterior maxillary lesions, the first stage in the surgical procedure is to outline a circular incision in the mucosa around the visible tumor by electrocautery. The mucosal incision is then deepened through the soft tissue up to the underlying bone. The bone cuts are made using a high-speed power saw, and the specimen is fractured by the use of osteotomes. Every effort is made to achieve a monobloc removal and to avoid fragmentation of the specimen. The interior of the maxillary antrum is inspected for any pathology after completion of the tumor excision. If the mucosa of the antrum appears edematous then it is curetted out as far as possible. If the mucosa appears normal and there is no other pathology within the maxillary antrum, then it is best left undisturbed.

Resection of posterior alveolar and maxillary tubercle lesions can also be accomplished in a similar manner. However, the pterygoid muscles will be exposed in the surgical defect, requiring skin grafting to avoid fibrosis and resultant trismus. A split-thickness skin graft is harvested from a suitable donor site and sutured to the edges of the mucosal defect with absorbable sutures. The graft is held in position with xeroform gauze packing and a dental obturator. If grafting is not required, then the maxillary antrum is packed with xeroform gauze and a temporary dental obturator is wired to the remaining teeth. The packing is left in position for approximately one week, but the patient can take liquids and puréed food by mouth from the first postoperative day. While the packing is in place, optimal oral hygiene is maintained by frequent oral irrigations and sprays in the oral cavity with half strength hydrogen peroxide solution. The surgical dental obturator and the packing are removed after one week, and an interim dental obturator with a soft liner is fabricated, which is used until soft tissue healing is complete.

The patient shown in Fig. 10.18 has a squamous carcinoma arising on the labial surface of the upper gum. The tumor is adherent to the underlying alveolar process of the maxilla. A CT scan shows minimal bone destruction (Fig. 10.19). The surgical specimen shows the canine and premolar teeth with a generous margin of mucosa, soft tissue and bone around the resected tumor (Fig. 10.20). The postoperative view of the oral cavity approximately 3 months after the surgical procedure shows a well-healed surgical defect leading to the maxillary antrum (Fig. 10.21). The permanent

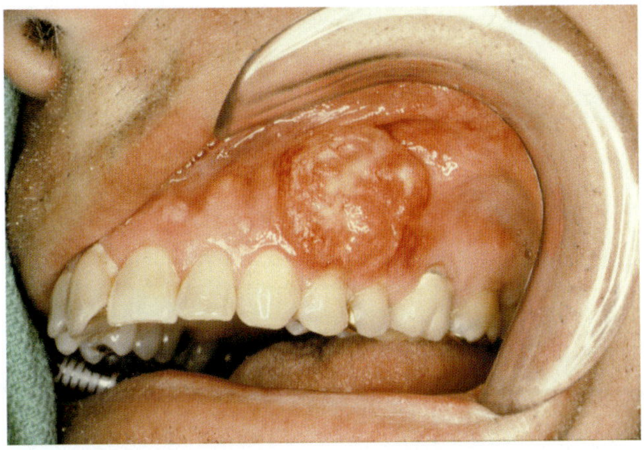

Figure 10.18 Squamous carcinoma of left upper gum.

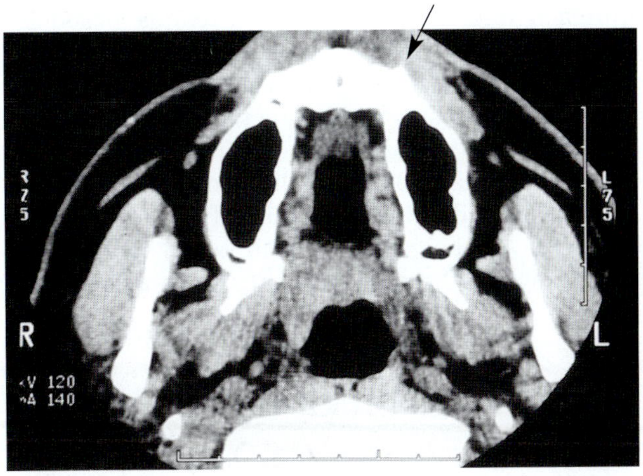

Figure 10.19 A CT scan showing minimal bone erosion.

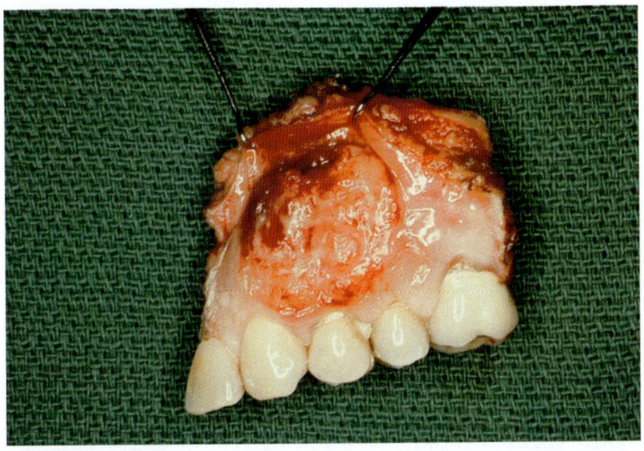

Figure 10.20 Surgical specimen showing adequate margins in all three dimensions.

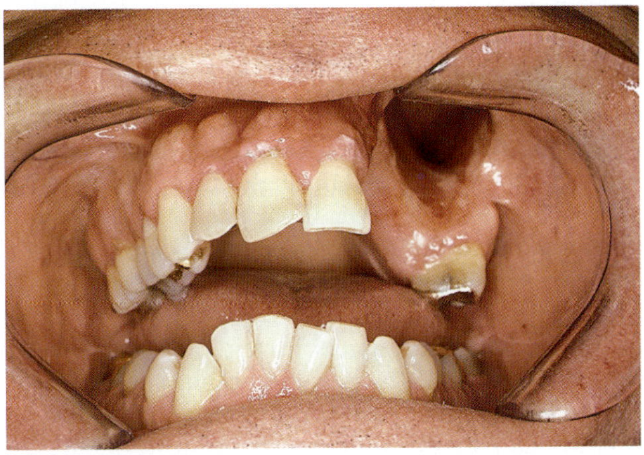

Figure 10.21 Healed surgical defect three months following surgery.

dental obturator is now made which provides a plug to obliterate the opening of the maxillary antrum in the oral cavity and replaces the missing teeth (Fig. 10.22). The patient is able to tolerate a regular diet by mouth and has no functional impairment with mastication or speech (Fig. 10.23).

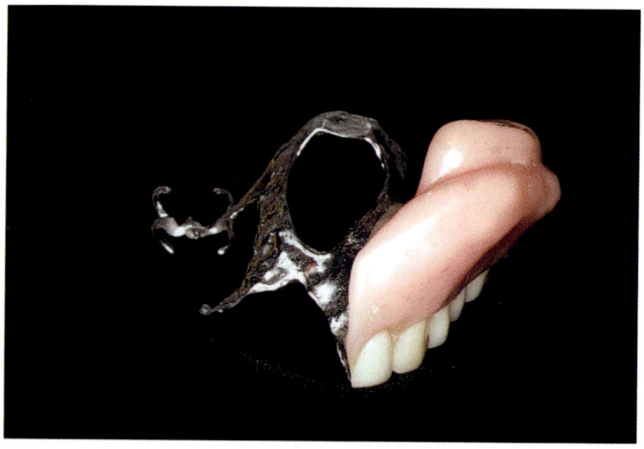

Figure 10.22 The dental obturator.

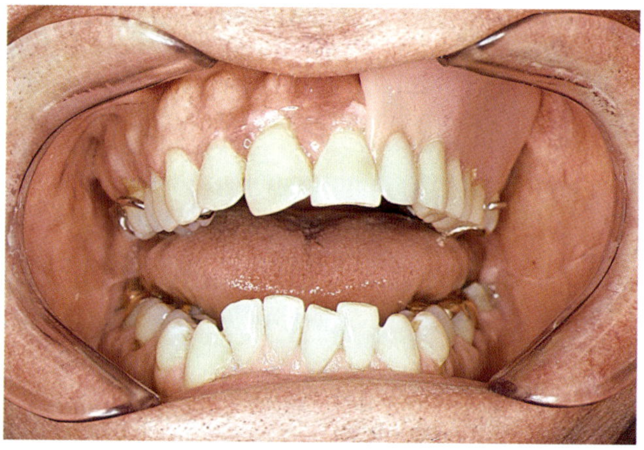

Figure 10.23 The dental obturator in place in the oral cavity.

Management of the mandible

Careful assessment of the mandible for invasion by tumor is essential for appropriate surgical treatment planning. The mandible is considered at risk when the primary tumor overlies, is adherent to, or lies in proximity to it. Careful examination under anesthesia by bimanual palpation is the most important aspect of mandibular assessment. Radiographic evaluation should be used to supplement findings of clinical evaluation.[22–29]

In addition to the risk for tumor involvement, management of the mandible also needs to be considered in large primary tumors of the oral cavity or oropharynx that are not accessible through the open mouth or even through a lower cheek flap approach due to anatomical restrictions posed by the mandible. In the past, uninvolved mandible in such cases was routinely resected to gain access to the primary tumor to perform a composite resection ('commando' operation). However, sacrifice of uninvolved mandible to gain access to the oral cavity for facilitating resection of large intra-oral tumors is no longer acceptable, since mandibulotomy provides the necessary exposure for resection.

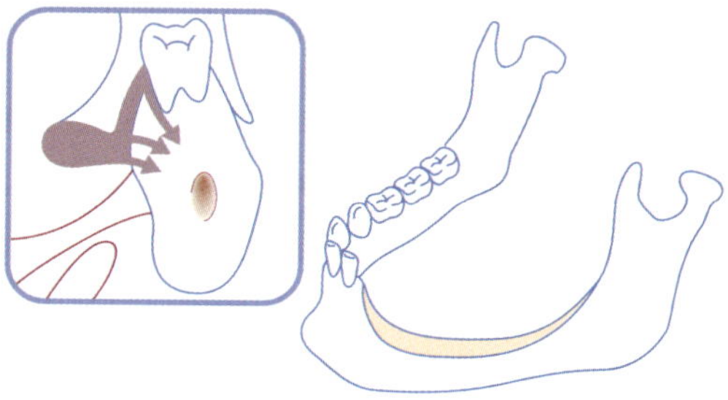

Figure 10.24

Tumor invasion of the mandible

In order to assess the need for and the extent of mandible resection required to encompass the primary tumor, it is essential to understand the process of invasion of the mandible by tumor.[22,28,30–35] Primary carcinomas of the oral cavity extend along the surface mucosa and the submucosal soft tissues to approach the attached lingual, buccal, and labial gingiva. From this point, tumors do not extend directly through intact periosteum and cortical bone towards the cancellous part of the mandible since the periosteum acts as a significant protective barrier.[30,31,35] Instead, the tumor advances from the attached gingiva towards the alveolus. In patients with teeth, tumors invade the mandible by extending through the dental sockets and advance into the cancellous part of the bone (Fig. 10.24). In edentulous patients, tumors extend up to the alveolar process than infiltrate the dental pores in the alveolar process to extend to the cancellous part of

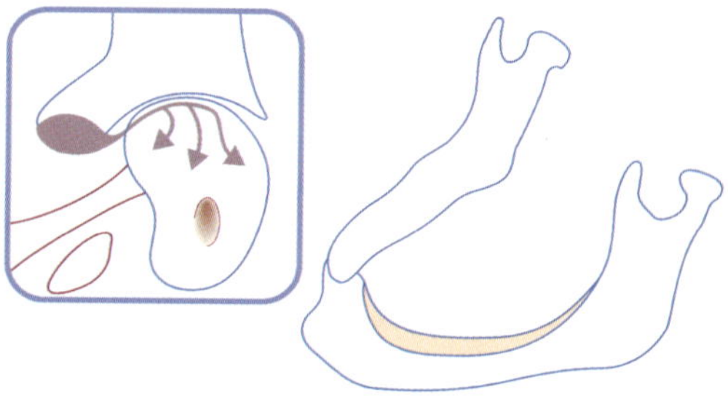

Figure 10.25 Mandible invasion by oral cancer. Marginal mandibulectomy is feasible for minimal erosion of the alveolar process.

the mandible (Fig. 10.25). In patients who have been previously irradiated, the periosteal barrier is weak and direct invasion through the lingual plate of the mandible may take place.[30,31]

In non-irradiated, dentate patients with early invasion of the mandible, marginal mandibulectomy is feasible since the cortical part of the mandible inferior to the roots of the teeth remains uninvolved and can be spared safely[36–38] (Fig. 10.26). In edentulous patients, however, the feasibility of marginal mandibulectomy depends on the vertical height of the body of the mandible. With aging, the alveolar process recedes and the mandibular canal comes closer and closer to the surface of the alveolar process. As shown in Fig. 10.27, the resorption of the alveolar process eventually leads to a 'pipestem' mandible. It is almost impossible to perform a satisfactory marginal mandibulectomy in such patients since the probability of iatrogenic fracture or post-surgical spontaneous fracture of the remaining portion of the mandible is very high (Fig. 10.28). In select patients who have received previous radiotherapy, marginal mandibulectomy may be feasible, but it should be performed with extreme caution.

When the tumor extends to involve the cancellous part of the mandible, a segmental mandibulectomy must be performed (Fig. 10.29). Generally, segmental

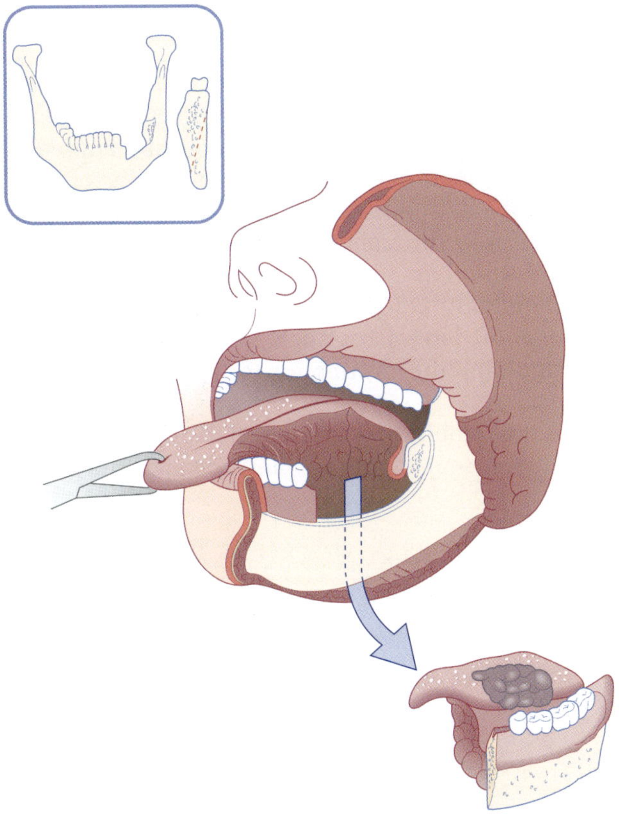

Figure 10.26 Marginal mandibulectomy.

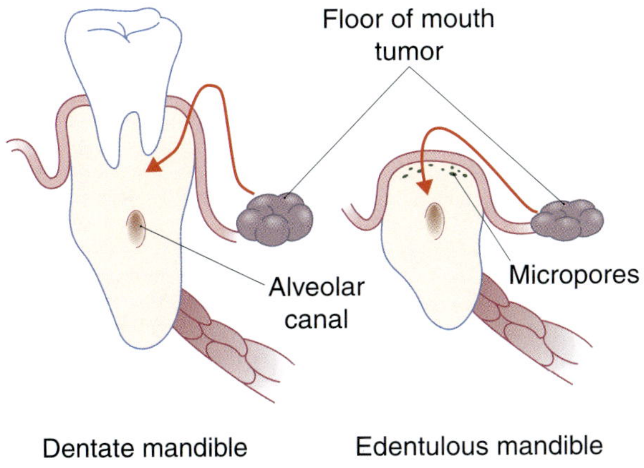

Figure 10.27 Feasibility of marginal mandibulectomy in dentate and edentulous mandible.

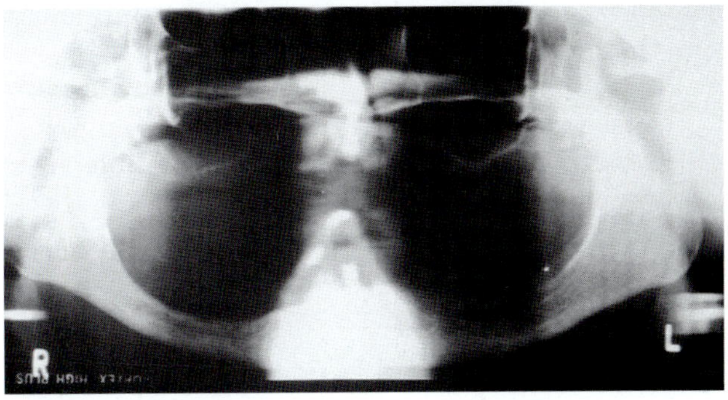

Figure 10.28 Pipe stem mandible.

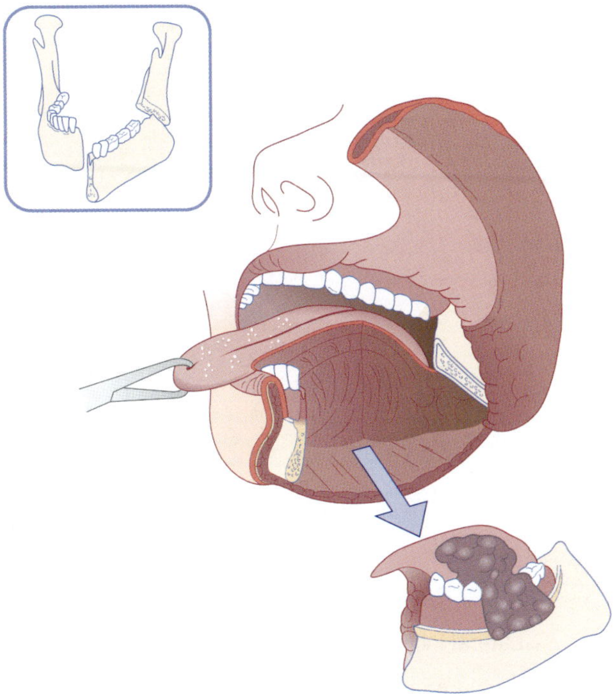

Figure 10.29 Segmental mandibulectomy.

mandibulectomy is also recommended in previously irradiated patients whose oral cancer is in close proximity to the mandible.[5,39,40] Consideration of segmental resection should also extend to cases having significant soft tissue involvement adjacent to the mandible, in association with a 'massive primary tumor'.

As mentioned earlier, segmental mandibulectomy should never be considered simply to gain access to primary cancers of the oral cavity or oropharynx not in the vicinity of the mandible.[12,13,41] In addition, since there are no lymphatic channels passing through the mandible, there is no need for an in continuity 'composite resection'.[12,13,42] Accordingly, the concept of the commando operation, with sacrifice of the normal uninvolved mandible to gain access to the primary tumors of the oral cavity or to accomplish an 'in continuity composite resection' cannot be justified.

The current indications for segmental mandibulectomy include:

1. Gross invasion by oral cancer;
2. Proximity of oral cancer to the mandible in a previously irradiated patient;
3. Primary bone tumor of the mandible;
4. Metastatic tumor to the mandible;
5. Invasion of the inferior alveolar nerve or canal by tumor; and
6. Massive soft tissue disease adjacent to the mandible.[2]

Elucidation of the process of tumor invasion of the mandible has enabled the development of mandible sparing approaches. These include mandibulotomy for gaining access to large tumors of the oral cavity or posteriorly located tumors in the oropharynx and marginal mandibulectomy, for minimal invasion of the alveolar process.

Mandibulotomy

Mandibulotomy or mandibular osteotomy is an excellent mandible sparing surgical approach designed to gain access to the oral cavity or oropharynx for resection of primary tumors otherwise not accessible through the open mouth or by the lower cheek flap approach[12,13,41] (Fig. 10.30). The mandibulotomy can be performed in one of three locations: (a) lateral (through the body or angle of the mandible), (b) midline, or (c) paramedian.

Lateral mandibulotomy has several disadvantages.[43] First, the muscular pull on the two segments of the

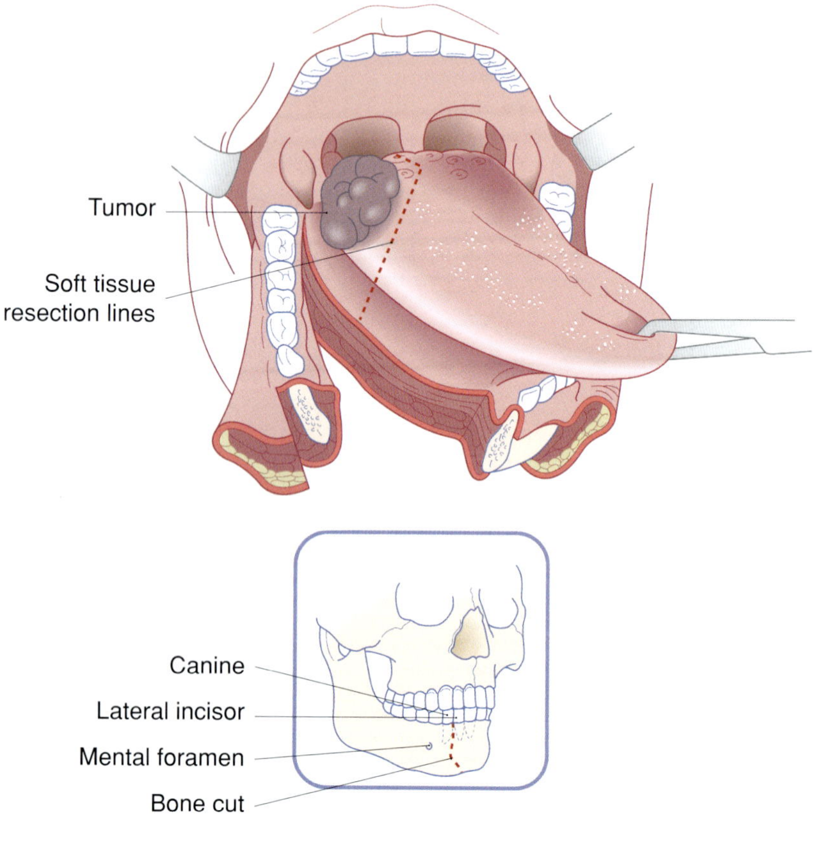

Figure 10.30 Paramedian mandibulotomy.

mandible is unequal, putting the mandibulotomy site under significant stress. This results in delayed healing and may necessitate intermaxillary fixation. Second, the presence of intermaxillary fixation restricts access to the suture line in the oral cavity for cleaning, leading to poor oral hygiene and an increased risk for sepsis and wound breakdown. Furthermore, lateral mandibulotomy poses several anatomic disadvantages. Denervation of the teeth distal to the mandibulotomy site and the skin of the chin is a direct consequence of the procedure, due to transection of the inferior alveolar nerve. Disruption of the endosteal blood supply is also a consequence of this approach, resulting in devascularization of the distal teeth, and the distal segment of the mandible. In addition, in patients needing postoperative radiation therapy, the mandibulotomy site is directly within the lateral portal of the radiation field, leading to delayed healing and complications at the mandibulotomy site.[44,45] For these reasons and the limited exposure afforded by the lateral mandibulotomy, this approach is not recommended.

By placing the site of mandibulotomy in the anterior midline, all of the disadvantages of lateral mandibulotomy are avoided.[39–41] However, in order to avoid exposure of the roots of both central incisor teeth and put them at the risk of extrusion, standard midline mandibulotomy requires extraction of one central incisor tooth. This alters the esthetic appearance of the lower dentition. In addition, since midline mandibulotomy requires division of muscles arising from the genial tubercle, that is the geniohyoid and genioglossus muscles, delayed recovery of the function of mastication and swallowing may occur. Therefore, a median mandibulotomy is also not recommended for access to oral tumors.

Mandibulotomy performed in a paramedian position avoids the disadvantages of lateral mandibulotomy as well as midline mandibulotomy.[45] The preferred site for paramedian mandibulotomy is between the lateral incisor and canine teeth. Since the roots of these two adjacent teeth diverge, bone cuts are performed without risking tooth loss.[2,39–41] Paramedian positioning of the mandibulotomy offers significant advantages, including wide exposure and preservation of the hyomandibular complex by avoiding division of the geniohyoid and genioglossus muscles. The mylohyoid is the only muscle that requires division, which results in minimal swallowing difficulties. Paramedian mandibulotomy does not cause denervation or devascularization of the skin of the chin or the teeth and mandible. Fixation at the mandibulotomy site is easy and the mandibulotomy site does not fall within the lateral portal of radiation therapy. Thus paramedian mandibulotomy is the optimal surgical approach for access to posteriorly located larger lesions of the oral cavity and tumors of the oropharynx.

Several non-tumor factors also impact on the selection of the mandibulotomy site which need to be assessed in the preoperative setting. Mandibulotomy through an area of septic teeth should be avoided. If another pathology is present at the proposed site of mandibulotomy, radiographic studies assist in the selection of an alternate site for mandibulotomy. Accordingly, in any patient requiring mandibulotomy, radiographic assessment of the mandible must be performed prior to surgery. A panoramic view of the mandible is usually satisfactory. If, however, facilities for a panoramic view are not available, then at least conventional lateral radiographs should be obtained prior to surgery.

Marginal mandibulectomy

The current indications for marginal mandibulectomy are: (a) for obtaining satisfactory three-dimensional margins around the primary tumor, (b) when the primary tumor approximates the mandible, and (c) for minimal erosion of the alveolar process of the mandible.[36–38,46–48] Marginal mandibulectomy is contraindicated when there is gross invasion into the cancellous part of the mandible or when there is massive soft tissue disease. This procedure is also contraindicated in patients with previously irradiated edentulous mandibles or with significant atrophy of the alveolar process resulting in 'pipestem mandible'.

Marginal mandibulectomy can be performed to resect the alveolar process, the lingual plate, or a combination of the alveolar process and lingual plate of the mandible for tumors of the anterior oral cavity. Marginal mandibulectomy can also be performed for lesions adjacent to the retromolar trigone whereupon the anterior aspect of the ascending ramus of the mandible including the coronoid process and the adjacent alveolar process of the body of the mandible are resected. Reverse marginal mandibulectomy is indicated in patients who have tumors of the cheek mucosa or soft tissue disease such as fixation or prevascular facial lymph nodes to the lower cortex of the mandible.

When performing a marginal mandibulectomy, right angled cuts should be avoided, since the angles create points of excessive stress leading to the risk of spontaneous fracture. The marginal mandibulectomy should be performed in a smooth curve to evenly distribute the stress at the site of resection (Fig. 10.31). Following marginal mandibulectomy, the exposed bone may be covered by primary closure of the mucosa of the tongue or floor of the mouth to the mucosa of the cheek. However, primary closure eliminates the lingual or the buccal

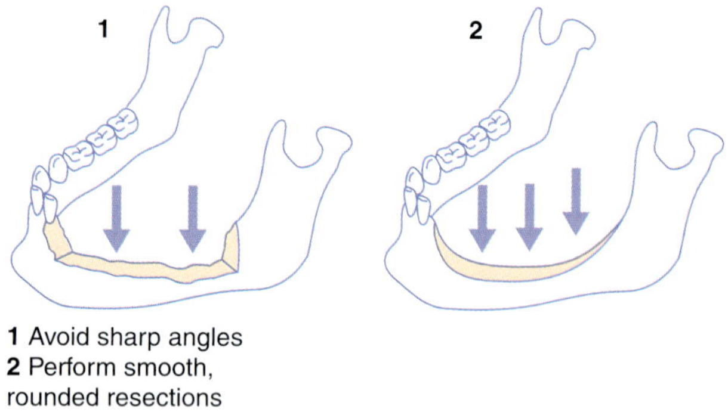

Figure 10.31 Technique of marginal mandibulectomy. It is essential to avoid sharp edges and to perform a smooth, rounded resection.

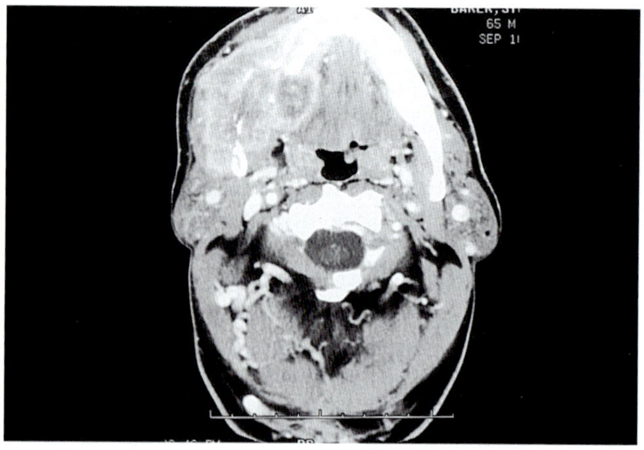

Figure 10.32 Gross destruction of the mandible by tumor.

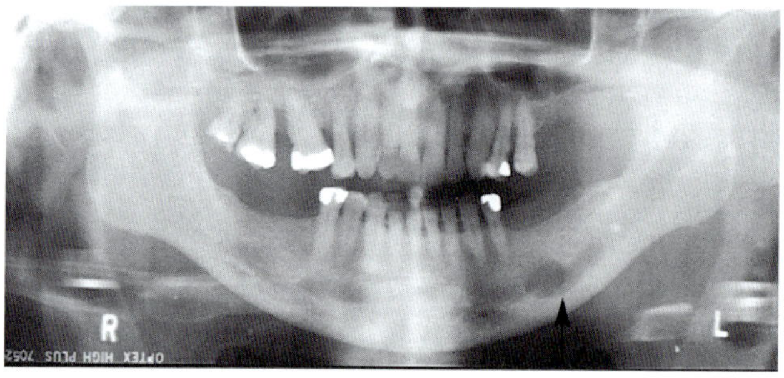

Figure 10.33 Invasion of inferior alveolar canal by tumor.

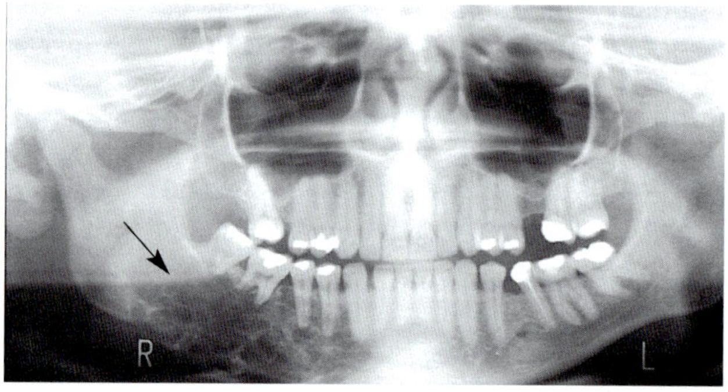

Figure 10.34 Panoramic X-ray showing gross invasion of mandible.

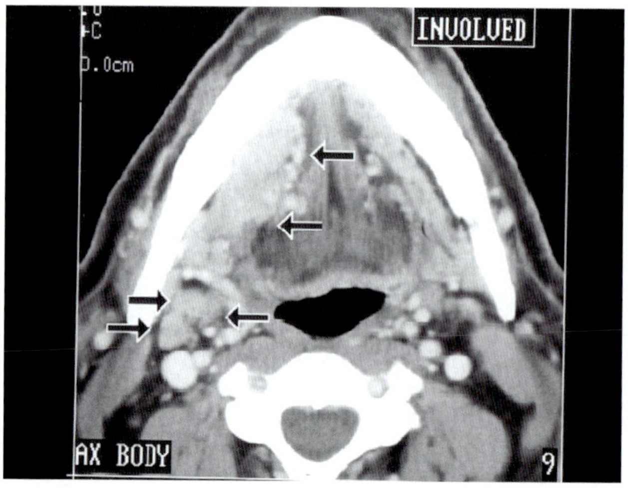

Figure 10.35 Extensive soft tissue disease adjacent to mandible.

sulcus and therefore fabrication and retention of a removable denture becomes exceedingly difficult. Alternatively, a skin graft can be applied directly over the exposed cancellous part of the mandible, which retains the sulci and the ability to wear a removable partial denture, which can be clasped to the remaining teeth. In edentulous patients, the ability to wear a denture over a marginally resected mandible is limited. The use of osseointegrated implants with a fixed denture should be considered when a removable partial denture at the site of marginal mandibulectomy is not feasible or not acceptable to the patient. When there is significant soft tissue and mucosal loss in addition to marginal mandibulectomy, a radial forearm free flap provides ideal lining and reconstruction of the soft tissue defect.

Segmental mandibulectomy

Resection of a segment of the mandible is required when there is gross bone destruction, tumor invasion in the cancellous part of the bone, invasion of the inferior alveolar canal, or primary or metastatic lesions involving the mandible[2,4,39] (Figs 10.32–10.34). Massive soft tissue involvement around the mandible also occasionally requires segmental mandibulectomy (Fig. 10.35). In a segmental mandibulectomy, the location of the segment of the mandible to be resected plays an important part in reconstruction and/or rehabilitation of the residual mandible. If any portion of the body of the mandible is resected and the remaining two stumps of the mandible are to be retained for secondary reconstruction, then fixation of the two segments of the mandible with a reconstruction plate (A–O plate) is required. Alternatively, primary reconstruction of the missing segment of the mandible can be undertaken with an appropriate microvascular free flap. If segmental mandibulectomy is performed on the posterior aspect of the body of the mandible up to the angle or the lower part of the ascending ramus, then the residual portion of the ascending ramus is not functional and is indeed a hindrance to adequate closure of the mouth. The unequal pull on the short stump of the ascending ramus of the mandible from the unopposed pterygoid muscles causes medial and cephalad deviation of the mandible towards the soft palate. With passage of time, this shift of the residual stump of the mandible causes pain and produces significant impairment in oral function. Therefore, if segmental mandibulectomy is performed on the posterior part of the body of the mandible beyond the angle into the ascending ramus, and if reconstruction is not planned, then the residual ascending ramus should be resected. On the other hand, if any immediate reconstruction of the mandible is planned, then every portion of the uninvolved mandible should be preserved to facilitate accurate reconstruction of the missing segment of mandible.

It is imperative that immediate reconstruction of the mandible is undertaken when segmental resection of the anterior arch of the mandible is performed. Reconstruction plates are not a satisfactory solution to replacement of the anterior arch of the mandible, as they are esthetically and functionally unacceptable and are invariably exposed in a majority of patients, requiring their subsequent removal. Therefore, whenever a resection of a segment of the anterior arch of the mandible is performed, immediate bone reconstruction is necessary and should be factored in surgical treatment planning.

Paramedian mandibulotomy for resection of cancer of the oral tongue

This procedure is best suited for resection of tumors of the base of the tongue. The patient shown here has squamous carcinoma of the posterior third of the tongue (Fig. 10.36). The patient is placed under general anesthesia with nasotracheal intubation on the operating table and adequate relaxation is obtained. An incision is planned, splitting the lower lip in the midline with extension of the incision up to the hyoid bone, at which point the incision extends lateral on the side of neck dissection along an upper neck skin crease (Fig. 10.37). Extension of the incision to the lateral aspect of the upper neck provides adequate exposure for an appropriate neck dissection as required.

Initially only the transverse part of the neck incision is made and in this patient a supraomohyoid neck dissection is completed (Fig. 10.38). The skin incision is then extended in the midline, dividing the chin and the lower lip through its full thickness up to the reflection of the mucosa at the

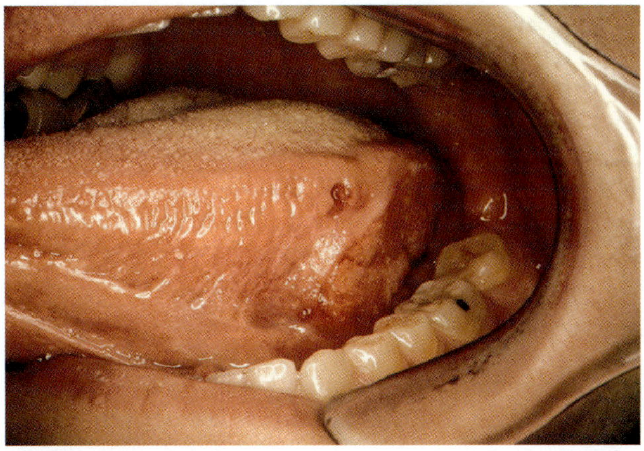

Figure 10.36 Squamous carcinoma of the posterior third of the tongue.

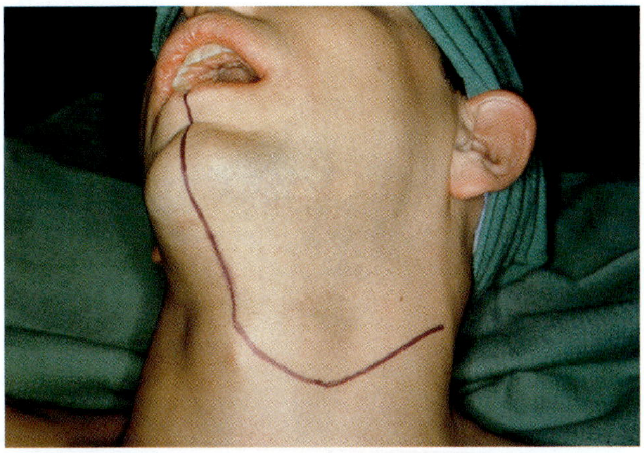

Figure 10.37 Lower lip-splitting incision with lateral extension.

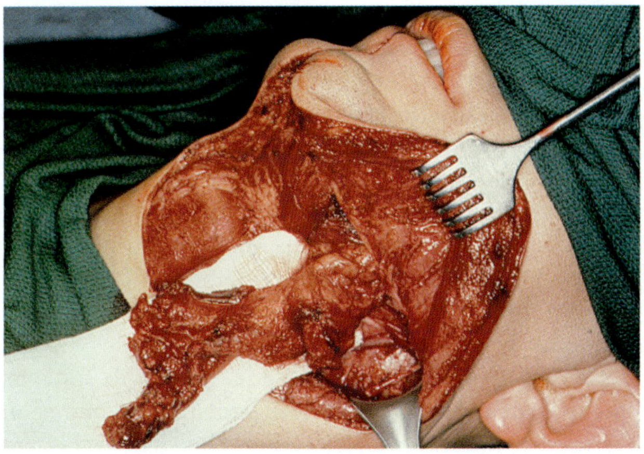

Figure 10.38 Supraomohyoid neck dissection is completed.

gingivolabial sulcus. Approximately 5 mm of labial mucosa at the gingivolabial sulcus is left attached to the gum to facilitate closure. At that point, an incision is made in the labial mucosa on the left hand side of the midline for a distance of approximately 2 cm and a short cheek flap is elevated (Fig. 10.39). All the soft tissue attachments of the chin are elevated from the anterior aspect of the mandible to a distance of approximately 3 cm from the midline on the left hand side, exposing the mandibulotomy site. Elevation of the cheek flap, however, should not extend up to the mental foramen, otherwise the mental nerve is exposed to injury, resulting in loss of sensation of the skin of the chin. Elevation of the left sided short cheek flap exposes the outer cortex and the inferior border of the mandible at the mandibulotomy site.

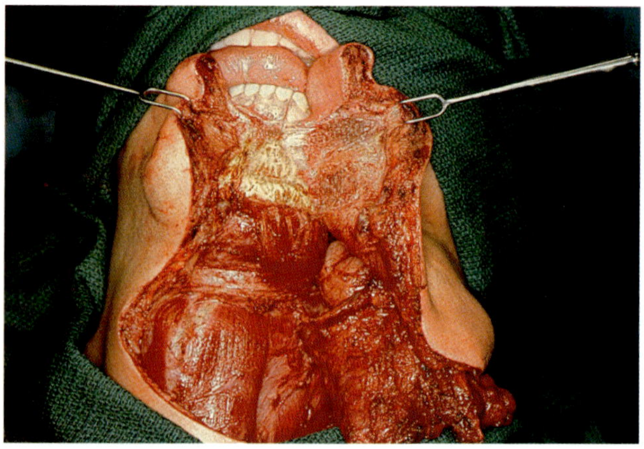

Figure 10.39 A short cheek flap is elevated to expose the mandible.

There are a variety of different ways in which an osteotomy may be performed to accomplish mandibulotomy. The mandible may be divided with a straight line vertical cut. This is not desirable since immobilization of the mandible is difficult due to the possibility of sliding motion at the site of the mandibulotomy, causing delayed union or malunion. Alternatively, the mandible may be divided in a step-ladder fashion to avoid upward and downward displacement. However, antero-posterior displacement would still be a problem with that approach. In addition, the transverse cut of a stepladder osteotomy may amputate or injure the roots of teeth at that site and devitalize them. The preferred approach therefore is a mandibulotomy performed in a zig-zag fashion, dividing the alveolar process between the lateral incisor and canine tooth in a vertical plane for a distance of approximately 10 mm, at which point the mandibulotomy incision in the bone is angled medially. The angulation in the osteotomy is below the level of the roots of adjacent teeth. The angled cut provides a more stable osteotomy for fixation. We prefer to use a high-speed power saw with an ultra-thin blade to make the mandibular cuts. However, prior to division of the bone, appropriate drill holes are placed for fixation of the mandibulotomy site using titanium miniplates. Two-plane fixation is necessary. A four-hole miniplate is placed on the outer cortex of mandible over the mandibulotomy site below the level of the roots of adjacent teeth. With the use of benders, the plate is appropriately bent and shaped to fit snugly over the mandibular surface. Four drill holes are now made through the plate holes in the mandible (Fig. 10.40). Another similar plate is shaped to fit over the lower border of the mandible and four drill holes are made in a vertical plane through the holes in the plate, but avoiding entry into adjacent tooth sockets. These plates are saved for use later in the operation for repair of the osteotomy site. The drill holes are placed before the osteotomy is performed to allow accurate reapproximation of the two ends of the mandible during closure, preserving the occlusal surfaces of the upper and lower dentition in perfect alignment. Accurate placement of both miniplates is vitally important to avoid injury to the roots of adjacent teeth. The mandible is divided exactly as planned using a high-speed power saw. Over-riding of the bone cuts at the angulation should be avoided to prevent iatrogenic fracture at the mandibulotomy site.

Once the mandible is divided, its two segments are retracted laterally with sharp retractors (Fig. 10.41). Brisk hemorrhage from each stump of the mandible is to be expected; however, this can be easily controlled with electrocautery or bone wax. Electrocautery is now used to divide the soft tissue and muscular attachments on the two sides of the mandible. As the two sides of the mandible are retracted, a mucosal incision is made in the floor of the mouth, leaving a cuff of approximately 1 cm of mucosa at the gingiva. This is essential to facilitate closure of the floor of the mouth (Fig. 10.42).

The mucosal incision in the floor of the mouth extends from the mandibulotomy site all the way up to the anterior pillar of the soft palate. If the incision has to be extended further posteriorly, it will require division of the lingual nerve which crosses the surgical field between the mandible and the lateral aspect of the tongue. The tongue is retracted medially in the oral cavity as the mandibular segment is retracted laterally, providing the necessary exposure.

The soft tissue attachments on the medial aspect of the mandible are divided and the two halves of the mandible are retracted (Fig. 10.43). The sublingual salivary gland is swept medially to remain attached to the tongue. Note that the mucosal incision in the floor of the mouth should retain a cuff of mucosa

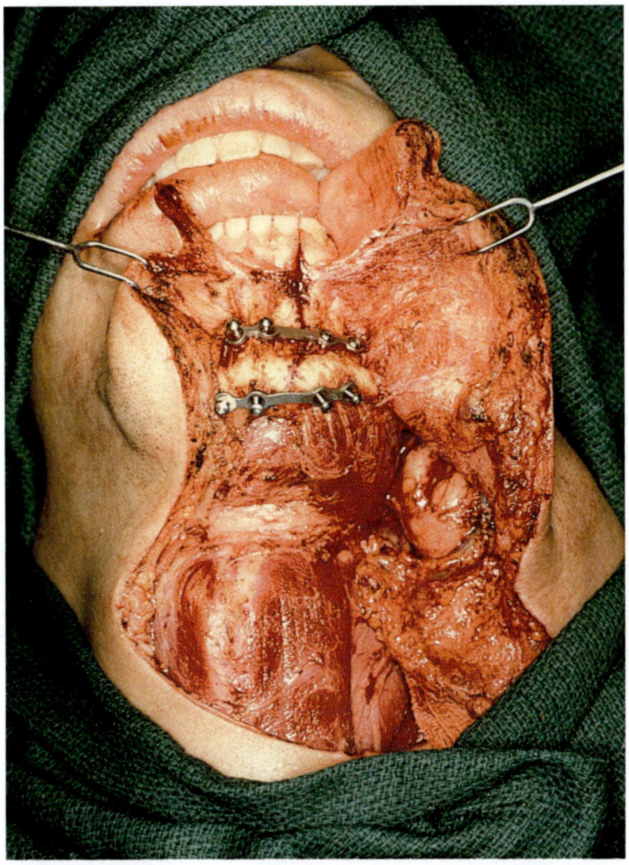

Figure 10.40 Drill holes for fixation are made prior to bone division.

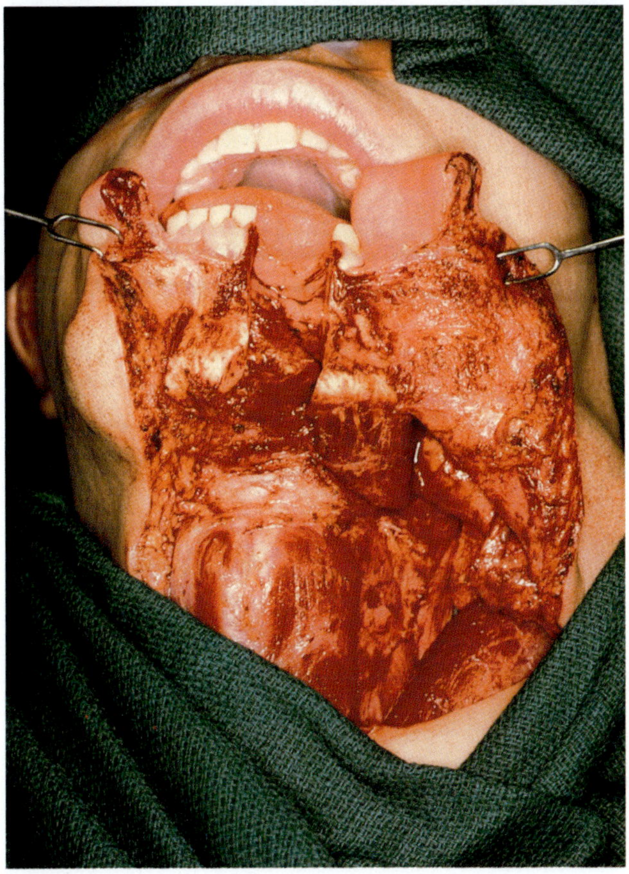

Figure 10.41 An angled osteotomy is performed.

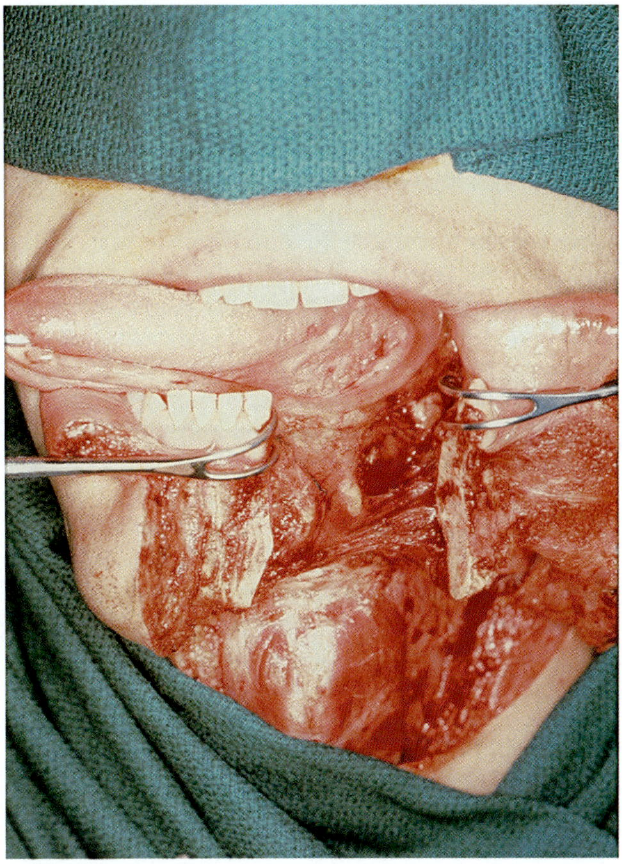

Figure 10.42 Incision in the mucosa of the floor of the mouth extends up to the soft palate.

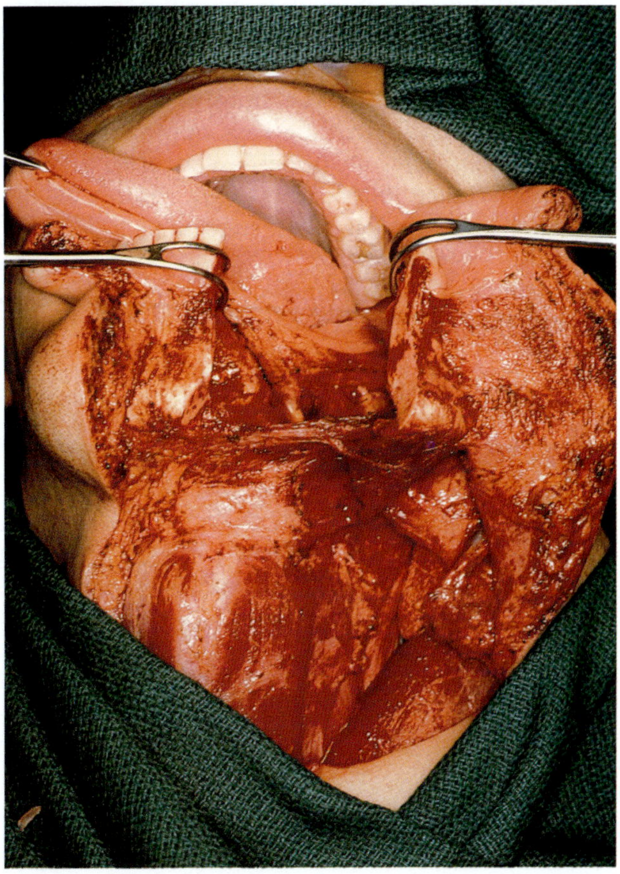

Figure 10.43 The mylohyoid muscle is exposed.

along the gingiva to facilitate closure. The mylohyoid muscle attached to the mandible is now exposed. It will have to be divided to permit mandibular 'swing' and further exposure. It is divided in its center by electrocautery, leaving its lateral half attached to the mandible. Complete division of the mylohyoid muscle permits sufficient swing of the mandible to provide exposure of the tumor in the surgical field (Fig. 10.44). The palpable extent of the tumor is examined and the proposed site of resection is marked out. A full thickness, through and through three-dimensional resection of the tumor is now performed using electrocautery with coagulating current. Note that the wedge-shaped resection is oriented transversely to permit reapproximation of the surgical defect by primary closure (Fig. 10.45). Brisk hemorrhage from the lingual artery and/or its branches is to be expected during resection of the tongue; however, this is easily controlled with appropriate measures.

Upon completion of the surgical resection, frozen sections are obtained from the lateral mucosal margins and the deep soft tissue margin of the surgical defect to ensure adequacy of resection (Fig. 10.46). A nasogastric feeding tube is inserted prior to beginning the closure. It is important to introduce the feeding tube at this point because if there is difficulty in the insertion of the tube after the wound is closed, then any digital manipulation may disrupt the suture line. A skin hook is placed at the apex of the wedge-shaped surgical defect on the dorsum of the tongue and traction is applied towards the right hand side. This allows the front of the tongue to draw posteriorly, providing easy approximation of the raw areas. Closure is performed in two layers using interrupted 00 chromic catgut sutures for the muscular layer as well as the mucosa.

Following repair of the tongue, the retracted left half of the mandible is brought back in its normal position. Closure of the mucosa of the lateral aspect of the tongue to the mucosa of the floor of the mouth on the gingiva is completed with interrupted chromic catgut sutures. As the closure proceeds anteriorly, the mandible draws closer and closer to the mandibulotomy site until complete mucosal closure of the floor of the mouth is accomplished. At this point, the mandibulotomy is repaired with fixation using the previously shaped miniplates (Fig. 10.47).

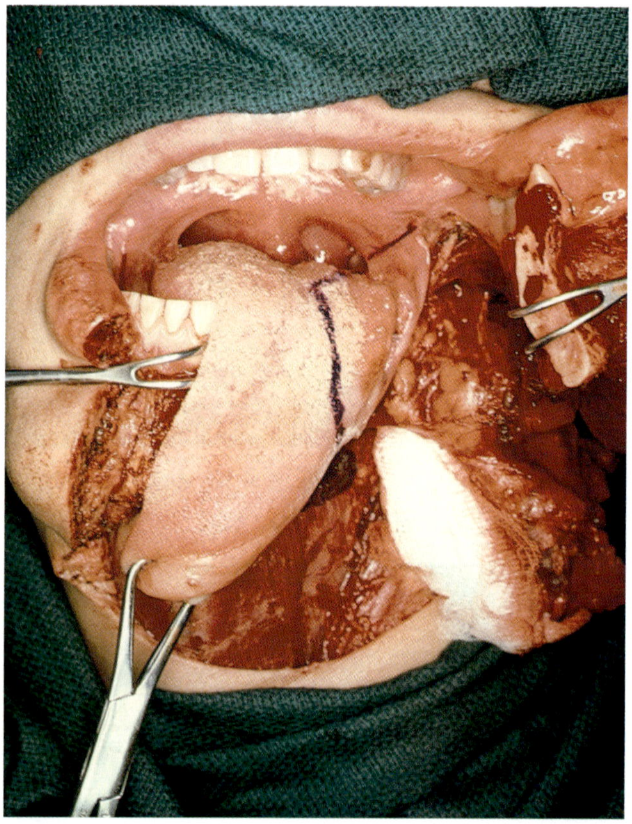

Figure 10.45 A transversely-oriented wedge resection is outlined.

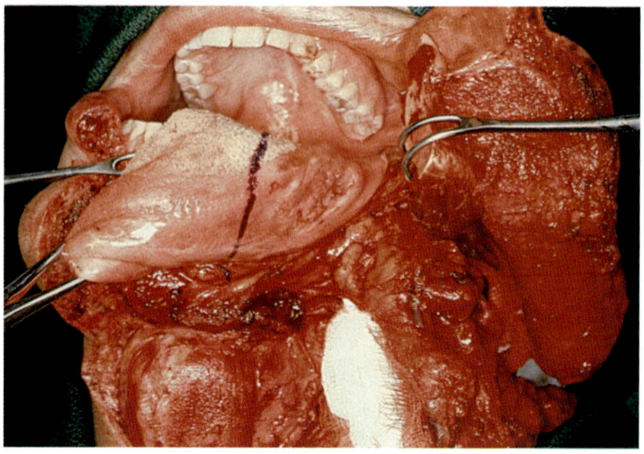

Figure 10.44 The tumor is exposed.

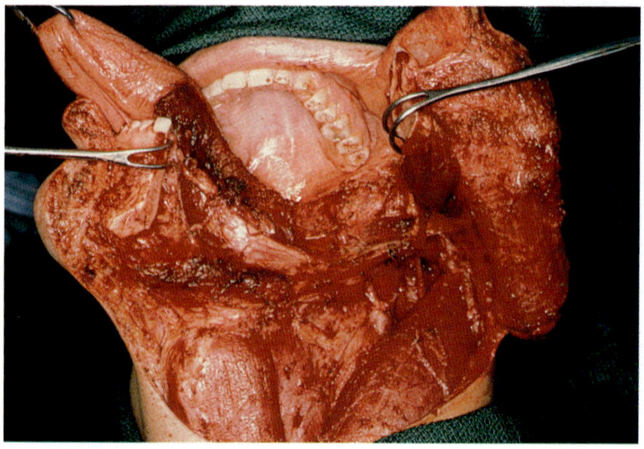

Figure 10.46 The surgical defect following resection.

A depth gauge is used to select the length of the screws for the miniplates. We prefer to use screws long enough to enter the lingual cortex of the mandible for the lateral plate. On the other hand, the miniplate on the lower border of the mandible is fixed with relatively short screws to avoid injury to the roots of the adjacent teeth. Every attempt is made to secure perfect alignment of the two ends of the mandible to restore normal occlusion. The screws are tightened snug but not too tight, otherwise the heads of the titanium screws will break.

If titanium miniplates and screws are not available, fixation of the mandible can be accomplished equally well using No. 24 gauge stainless steel wire.[49] In that case, four drill holes are made prior to mandibulotomy (Fig. 10.48). Two horizontal wires and one oblique wire are used to stabilize the mandible. The wires are twist-tied and the stumps are bent and buried to avoid exposure through soft tissues (Fig. 10.49). In the experience of the author, miniplate fixation and wire fixation following mandibulotomy work equally well. The rigidity of immobilization and postoperative complications are comparable with these two techniques.[49]

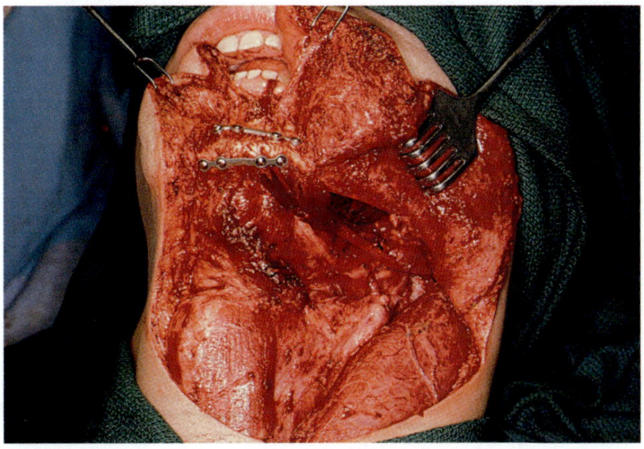

Figure 10.47 The mandibulotomy is reconstructed with miniplates.

Mucosal closure now begins by reapproximating the cut edge of the labial mucosa to the cuff of the mucosa at the gingivolabial sulcus on the alveolar process. This closure is accomplished using 000 chromic catgut interrupted sutures. Chromic catgut sutures are used for both the muscular layer and the mucosal layer of the lip, while nylon sutures are used for the skin and vermilion border. For perfect closure of the midline lip splitting incision, a fine nylon suture is first placed accurately, aligning the vermilion border. This suture is held as a retractor and closure of the labial mucosa progresses backwards from the vermilion border up to the gingivolabial sulcus. Interrupted sutures are placed to approximate the muscular layer in a similar fashion. Finally, accurate reapproximation of the skin of the lip and chin is essential to obtain an esthetically acceptable scar. The stumps of the divided mylohyoid muscle are reapproximated using interrupted chromic catgut sutures. Although this reapproximation is seldom accurate, it does permit reduction of the dead space in the submandibular region. In addition, the muscle provides support to the mucosal suture line in the floor of the mouth. A suction drain is placed in the wound and brought out through a separate stab incision. The neck incision is closed in two layers. The surgical specimen shows in-continuity resection of the primary tumor with the lymph nodes of levels I, II, and III from the supraomohyoid triangle and the intervening sublingual and submandibular salivary glands (Fig. 10.50).

In the postoperative period, the patient is maintained on nasogastric tube feeding for approximately one week, followed by a trial with puréed food to assess whether swallowing is successful. If, indeed, the patient is able to tolerate puréed food,

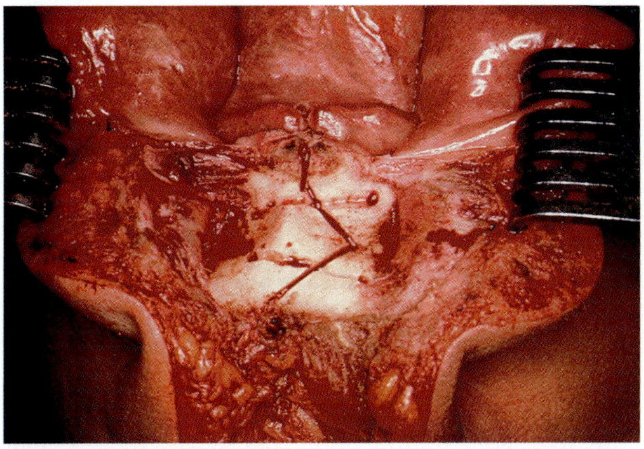

Figure 10.48 Mandibulotomy site and curfs for wire fixation.

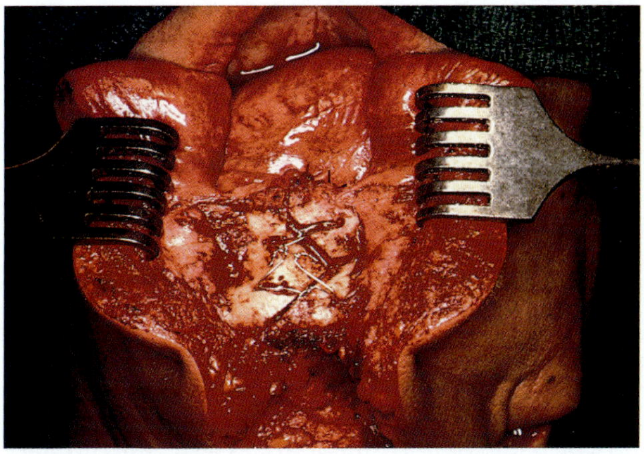

Figure 10.49 Mandibulotomy repair with wire fixation.

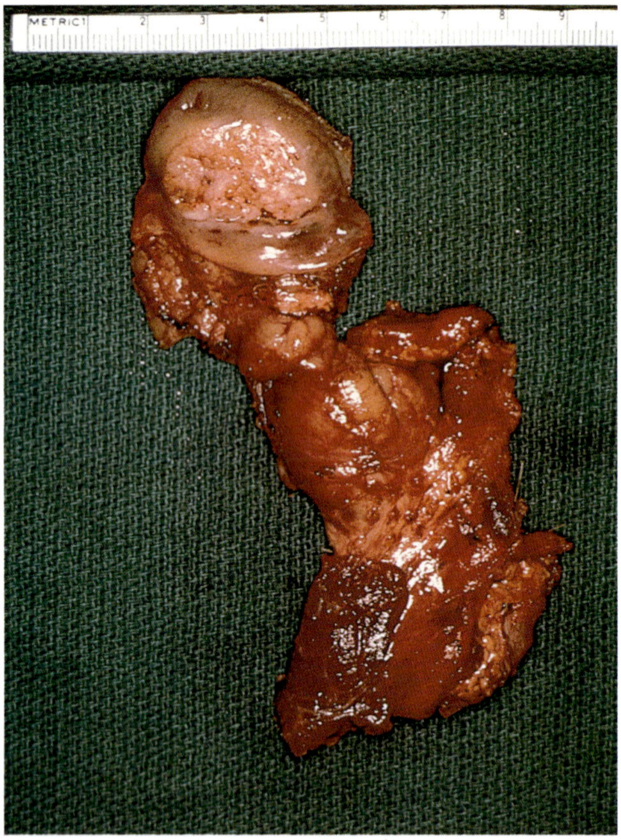

Figure 10.50 Surgical specimen showing primary tumor removed in continuity with regional lymph nodes.

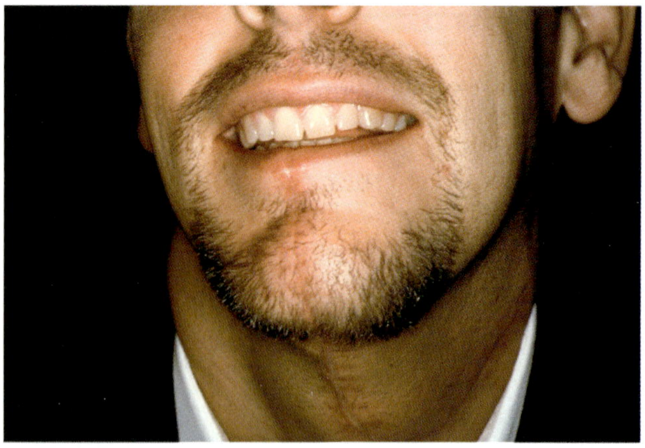

Figure 10.51 Postoperative view showing healed incision.

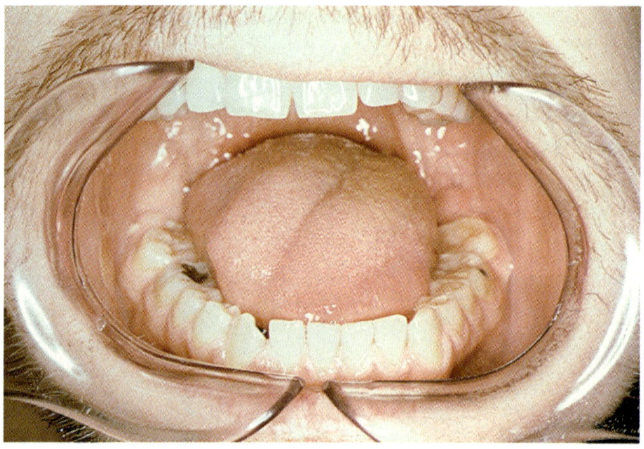

Figure 10.52 Postoperative intra-oral view.

then he is gradually advanced to a soft diet over the next few days.

A postoperative view of the patient 3 months after surgery shows a well-healed midline scar and esthetically acceptable external appearance (Fig. 10.51). The intra-oral view shows excellent shape and mobility of the tongue (Fig. 10.52).

Mandibulotomy approach for hemiglossectomy in continuity with radical neck dissection

Locally advanced primary tumors of the oral tongue can be resected in continuity with the regional lymph nodes in a monobloc fashion without the intervening mandible. For this to be accomplished, the primary tumor must not be adherent to or involve the mandible. The extirpation is achieved by first completing a comprehensive neck dissection, followed by a paramedian mandibulotomy to facilitate resection. Then the mandible is swung laterally on the side of the tumor to expose the primary tumor of the oral tongue. The hemiglossectomy is carried out with electrocautery. The primary tumor remains attached to the specimen of the right neck dissection, through the soft tissues and musculature of the floor of the mouth and the right submandibular and sublingual salivary glands as well as adjacent lymph nodes. A monobloc in-continuity resection can thus be performed without resecting the intervening mandible if it is not involved by the tumor. The resulting surgical defect usually requires reconstruction by bringing in soft tissue from elsewhere into the region, in the form of either a pedicled flap or microvascular free tissue transfer. Following restoration of the surgical defect, closure of the mucosal suture line is completed. The mandibulotomy site is repaired with miniplates and screws and the neck incision is closed in the usual fashion.

The patient shown in Fig. 10.53 has a T3 carcinoma of the lateral border of the oral tongue with clinically palpable lymph node metastases in the right hand side of the neck. The tumor does not involve

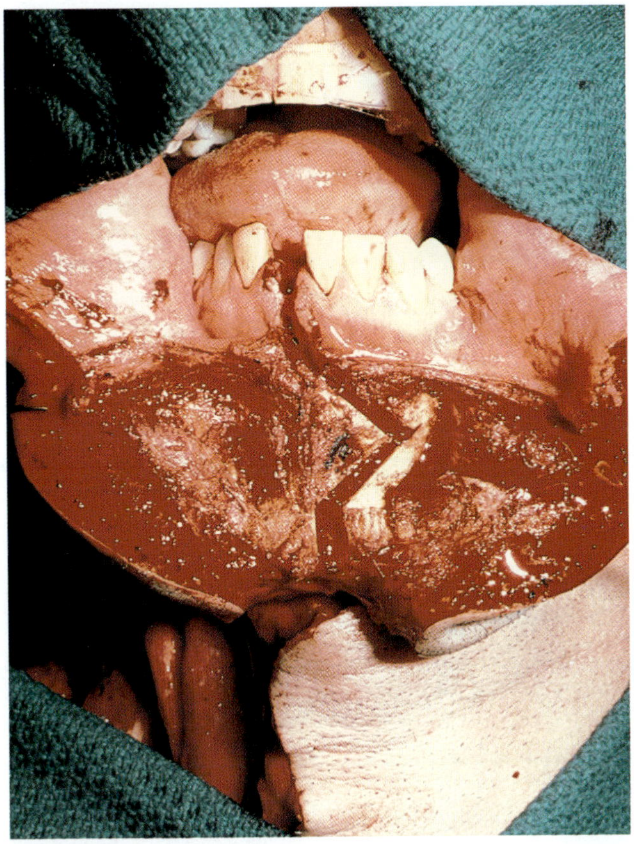

Figure 10.53 Paramedian mandibulotomy.

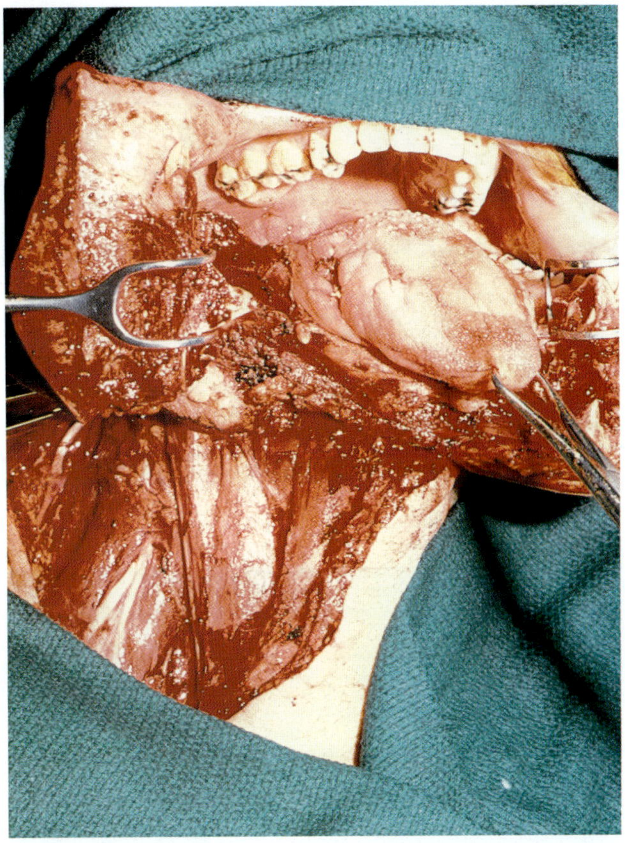

Figure 10.54 The primary tumor involves the right half of the tongue.

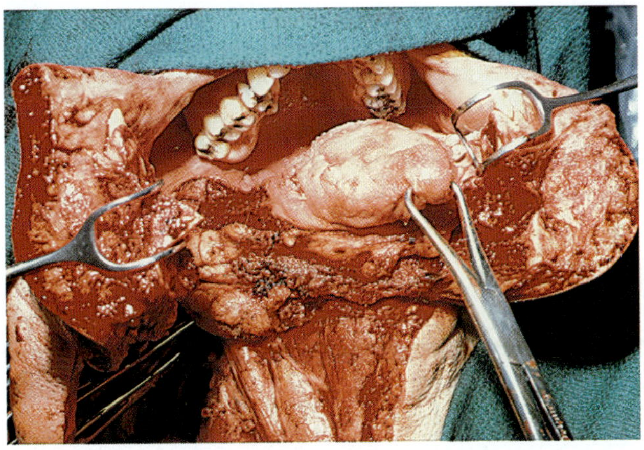

Figure 10.55 A right hemiglossectomy is performed.

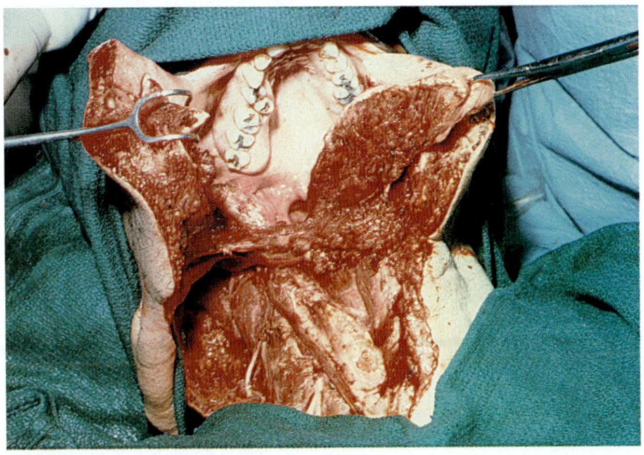

Figure 10.56 The surgical defect after tumor resection.

the floor of the mouth or the gingiva and, therefore, the mandible can be safely spared. A comprehensive right neck dissection sparing the accessory nerve is completed and a paramedian mandibulotomy is performed. The mandible is swung laterally exposing the primary tongue tumor (Fig. 10.54). Due to the extent of the tumor the patient requires a hemiglossectomy, extending from the tip up to and including a portion of the posterior third of the tongue on the right hand side (Fig. 10.55).

The surgical defect at the site of resection of the primary tumor shows the cut surface of the left half of the tongue from a lateral view (Fig. 10.56). The anterior view shows excision of the right half of the tongue (Fig. 10.57). The surgical specimen shows the primary tumor of the tongue resected in continuity with a right modified radical neck dissection, including the intervening soft tissues of the floor of the mouth and the submandibular triangle (Fig. 10.58).

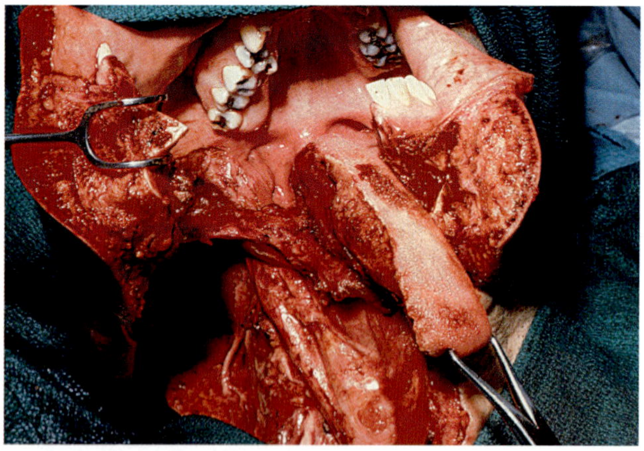

Figure 10.57 Right hemiglossectomy defect showing the remaining tongue.

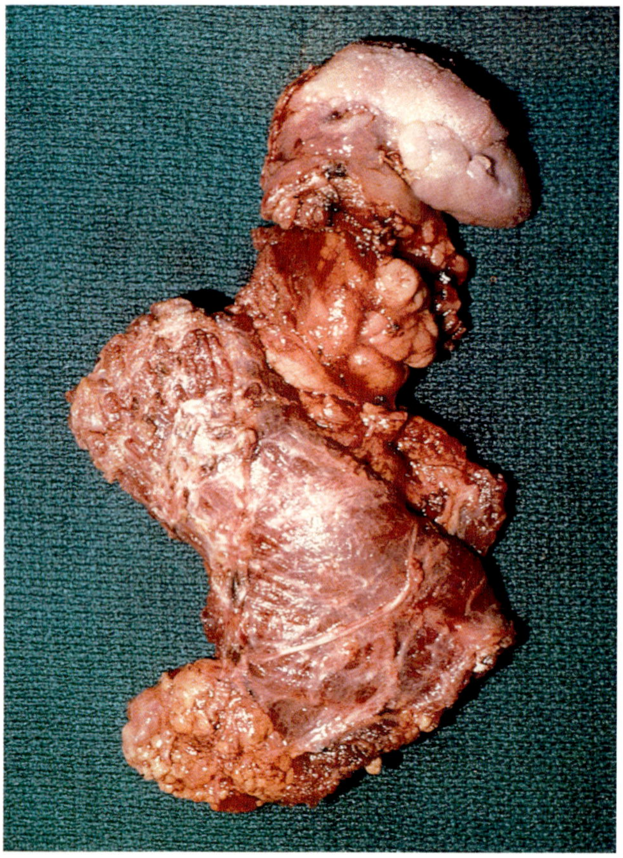

Figure 10.58 The surgical specimen of right hemiglossectomy and radical neck dissection done in continuity in a monobloc fashion.

The postoperative appearance of the oral cavity of the same patient shows perfect alignment of the two segments of the mandible and satisfactory reconstruction of the tongue, maintaining acceptable mobility for speech, mastication and swallowing (Fig. 10.59). The external appearance of the patient is shown in Fig. 10.60. Note that the external contour of the face is essentially unchanged.

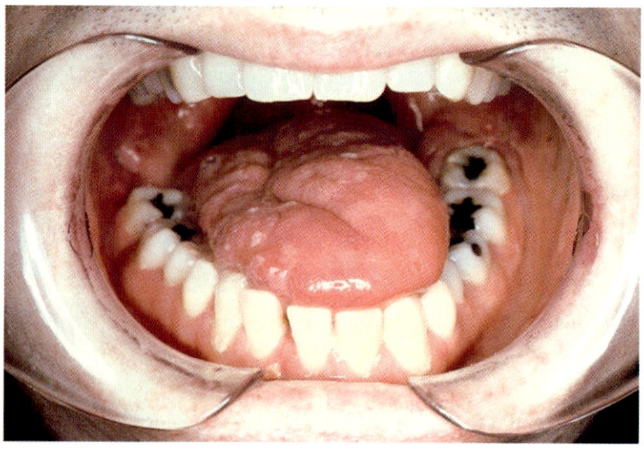

Figure 10.59 Postoperative intra-oral view showing the reconstructed tongue.

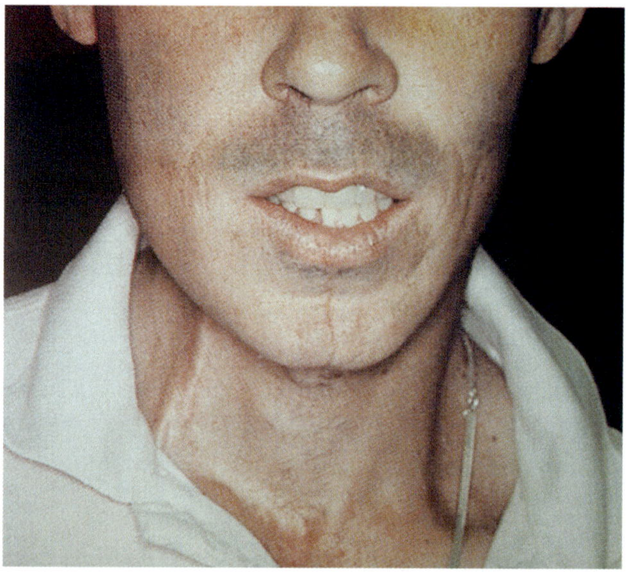

Figure 10.60 Postoperative picture of the patient showing well-healed incisions.

Mandible resection in the management of intra-oral cancer

Surgical resection of the mandible becomes necessary when a primary malignant tumor of the oral cavity extends to the gingiva over the alveolar process, or directly infiltrates into the mandible. If there is direct extension of the tumor from the alveolar process to the cancellous part of the mandible, or if contiguous tumor infiltration to the lingual or lateral cortex of the mandible is present, then a segmental mandibulectomy becomes necessary (Fig. 10.61). However, if a primary tumor of the oral cavity approximates the alveolar process or the lingual plate of the mandible, then resection of a part of the mandible, preserving its arch, is adequate

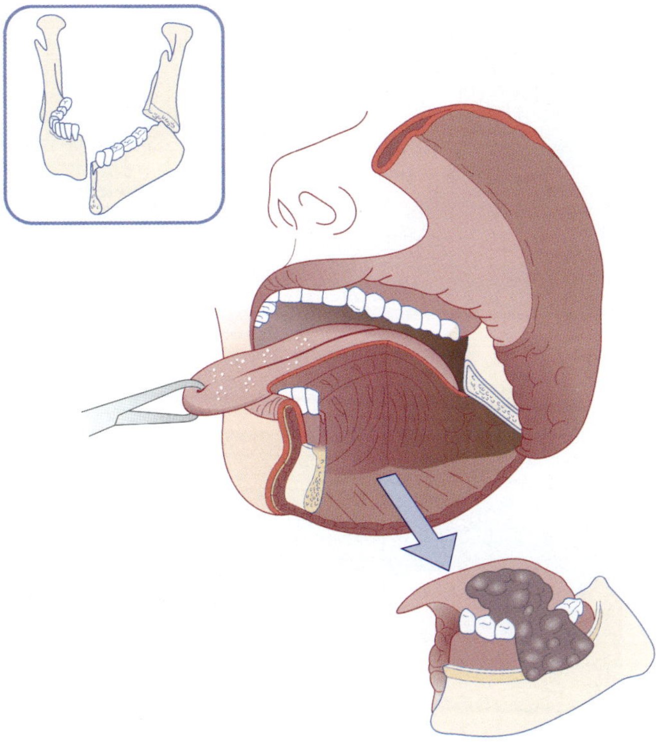

Figure 10.61 Segmental mandibulectomy.

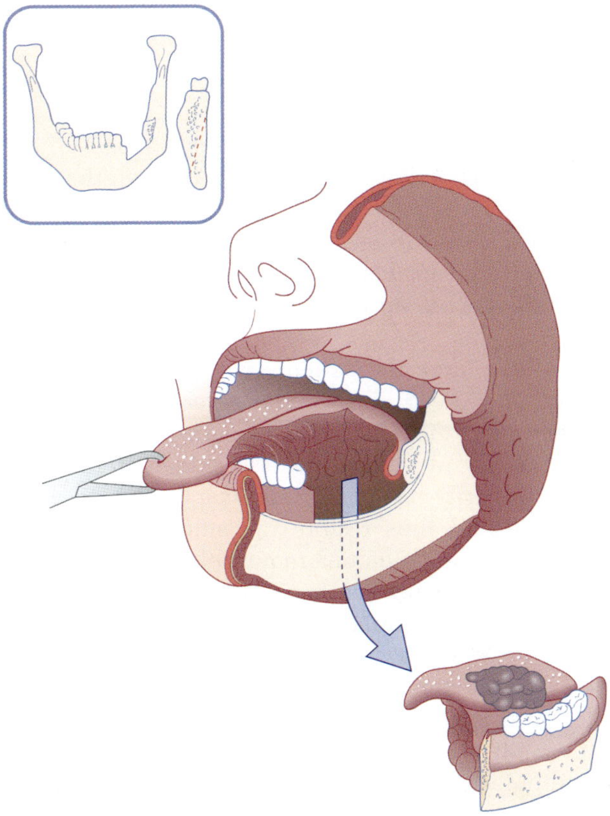

Figure 10.62 Marginal mandibulectomy.

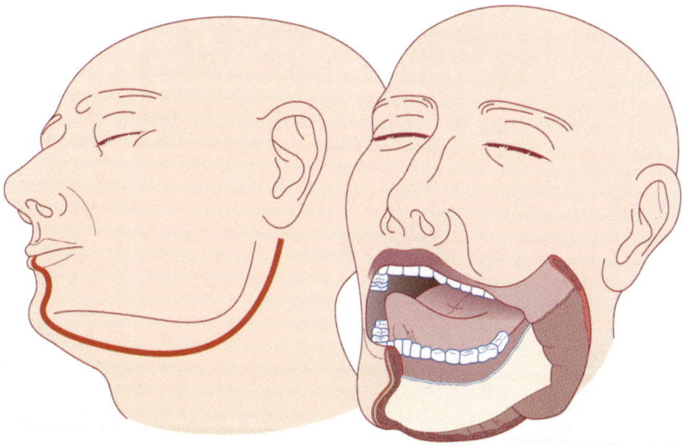

Figure 10.63 Lower cheek flap approach.

to obtain satisfactory margins around the primary tumor. In this clinical setting, segmental mandibulectomy is not indicated, but a marginal mandibulectomy proves to be satisfactory (Fig. 10.62).

A marginal mandibulectomy may include resection of the lingual plate or the alveolar process, or both, but still retains the continuity of the arch of the mandible by preserving its lower border and/or the lateral cortex. The routes of spread of intra-oral tumors in proximity to the mandible are such that marginal resection is feasible in either dentate or edentulous mandible.[30,31] This procedure produces minimal, if any, esthetic and functional deformity. Marginal mandibulotomy can be performed on any part of the mandible, that is the symphysis, body, or retromolar trigone.

Marginal mandibulectomy provides an oncologically sound three-dimensional resection of tumors of the oral cavity that approach, approximate, or superficially involve the mandible. The operative procedure leaves minimal esthetic and functional deformity, avoids the need for mandible reconstruction, and offers local control of cancer in properly selected patients, comparable to that achieved by segmental mandibulectomy.[39]

Marginal mandibulectomy can be performed safely through the open mouth for small lesions, particularly in the anterior aspect of the oral cavity. For larger lesions, a wider exposure is necessary for access to the primary tumor and its satisfactory resection. Either a low cheek flap approach or a visor flap approach may be employed. In most instances, the lower cheek flap approach is desirable since it provides satisfactory exposure and permits resection of the primary tumor and ipsilateral cervical lymph nodes (Fig. 10.63). The details of a variety of marginal mandibulectomy procedures are presented here.

Per oral marginal mandibulectomy

Small primary tumors of the anterior aspect of the lower gum are suitable for excision through the open mouth including the alveolar process, regardless of the presence or absence of teeth. This operation is also indicated for lesions of the floor of the mouth or cheek mucosa approaching the lower alveolus.

In the long term, the patient shown in the example below may need a secondary vestibuloplasty to create sulci to facilitate wearing a denture. Alternatively, a split thickness skin graft may be used primarily to cover the marginally resected mandible and thus restore the sulci. A vestibuloplasty and fabrication of a removable denture are not required if the patient is a suitable candidate for osseointegrated implants and a permanent fixed denture. Osseointegrated implants can be inserted either at the time of marginal mandibulectomy or later on if adequate vertical height of the remaining body of the mandible following marginal mandibulectomy is available. If the osseointegrated implants are inserted primarily, satisfactory coverage over the mandible should be secured to avoid exposure and loss of the implants.

The patient shown in Fig. 10.64 has a 1 cm, ulcerated, superficial carcinoma involving the alveolus of the edentulous mandible adjacent to her central incisor tooth. A panoramic radiograph of the mandible did not show any evidence of bone destruction beneath this lesion. This tumor is therefore suitable for a marginal mandibulectomy. The surgical specimen of marginal mandibulectomy accomplished through the open mouth is shown in Fig. 10.65. Note that satisfactory mucosal and soft tissue margins are secured as seen on the surface view of the specimen. On the side view, the height of the surgical specimen is shown with ample deep

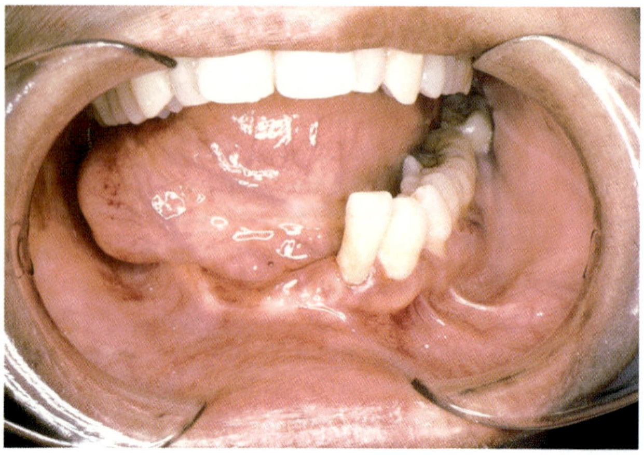

Figure 10.64 Superficial squamous carcinoma of lower gum.

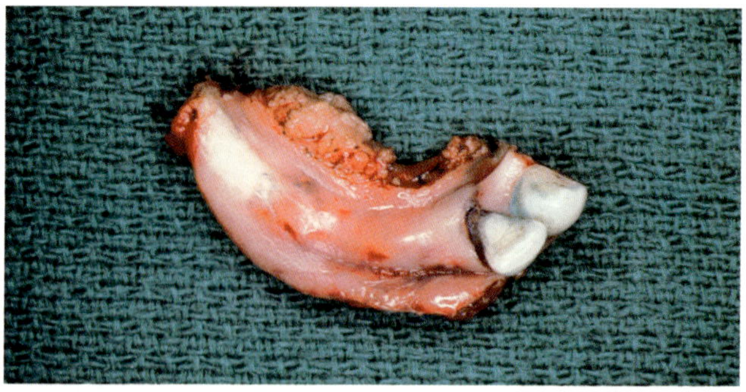

Figure 10.65 Specimen showing adequate mucosal margins.

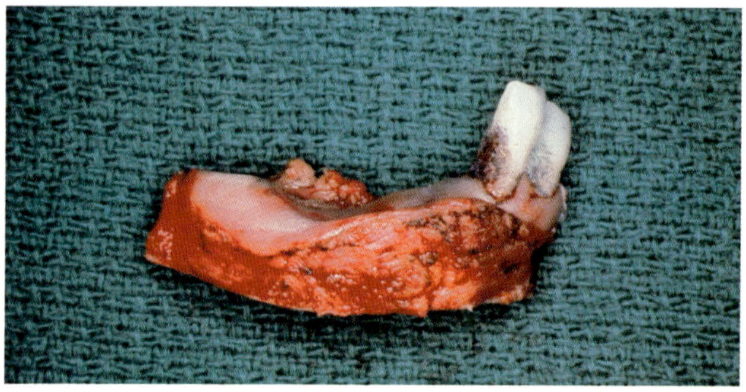

Figure 10.66 Specimen showing satisfactory deep margin.

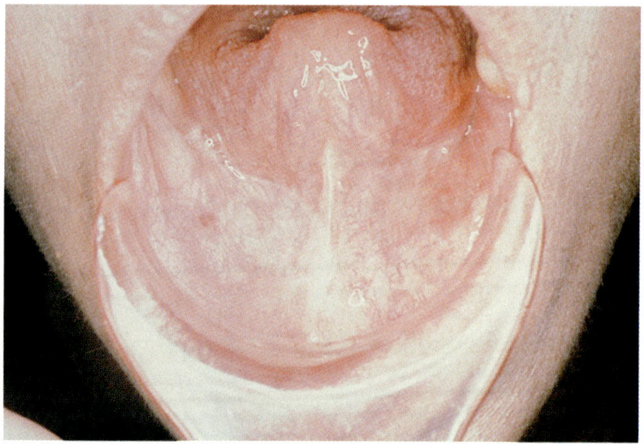

Figure 10.67 Postoperative intra-oral view.

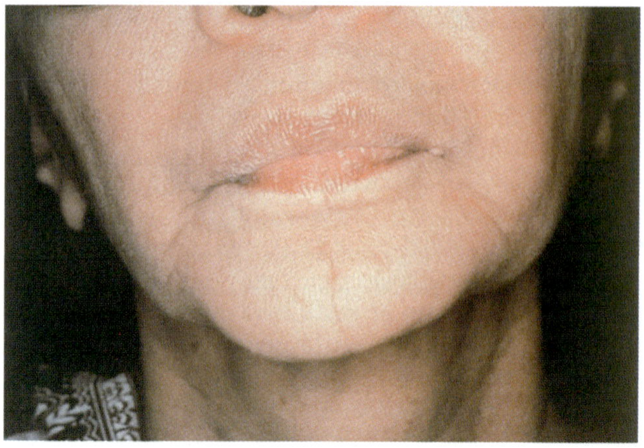

Figure 10.68 Postoperative external appearance.

bone margins for this superficial ulcerated carcinoma (Fig. 10.66). The surgical defect is repaired by primary closure of the mucosa of the floor of the mouth to the mucosa of the lower lip. Although the sulci at the site of the resected mandible in the floor of the mouth and the gingivolabial region are eliminated, the functional impairment in the immediate postoperative period is minimal. The postoperative appearance of the mouth at approximately one year shows a well-healed suture line (Fig. 10.67). Note the absence of gingivolabial sulcus, as well as flattening of the mucosa of the floor of the mouth. The external appearance of the patient, however, remains unchanged (Fig. 10.68).

Marginal mandibulectomy and repair with skin graft

The intra-oral photograph of a patient with carcinoma of the lower alveolus adjacent to her remaining teeth is shown in Fig. 10.69. The primary lesion is exophytic and relatively superficial, involving the alveolar process and attached gingiva of the adjacent teeth. A panoramic radiograph of the mandible fails to show any evidence of bone destruction (Fig. 10.70), and reveals the lesion and the extent of marginal mandibulectomy. Marginal mandibulectomy in this patient was performed using a lower cheek flap approach, splitting the lip in the midline to gain exposure of the lesion. A high-speed sagittal power saw is used to accomplish a marginal mandibulectomy in a smooth curved fashion to evenly distribute the stress at the site of bone resection. The surgical specimen shows a satisfactory three-dimensional resection of the primary tumor (Fig. 10.71). The surgical defect demonstrates a smooth, curved, marginal resection of the mandible with sufficient cortical bone remaining to provide stability to the mandible and to preserve the continuity of the arch of the mandible (Fig. 10.72). The surgical defect in this patient was repaired using a split-thickness skin graft. The skin graft usually heals satisfactorily and provides excellent coverage of the exposed bone (Fig. 10.73). Since the patient has remaining teeth in the lower dentition, a removable denture was fabricated which can be

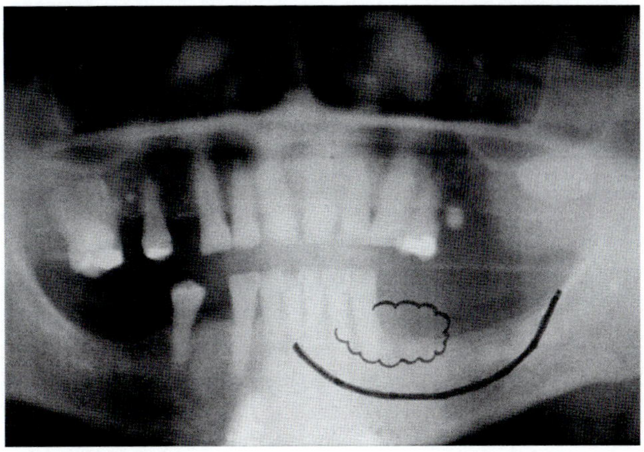

Figure 10.70 Panoramic x-ray of the mandible showing the location of the tumor and proposed marginal mandibulectomy.

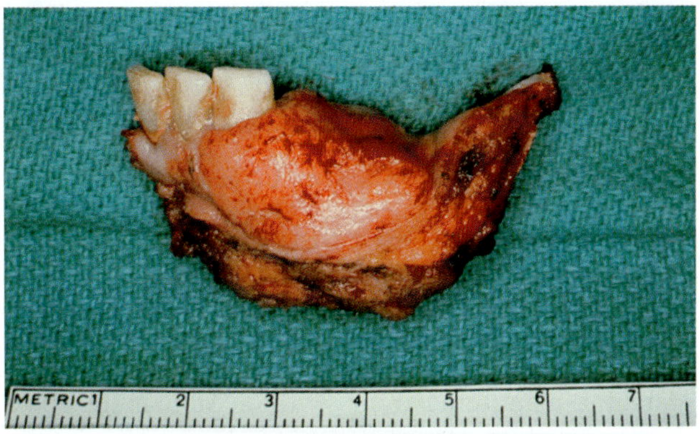

Figure 10.71 Surgical specimen of marginal mandibulectomy.

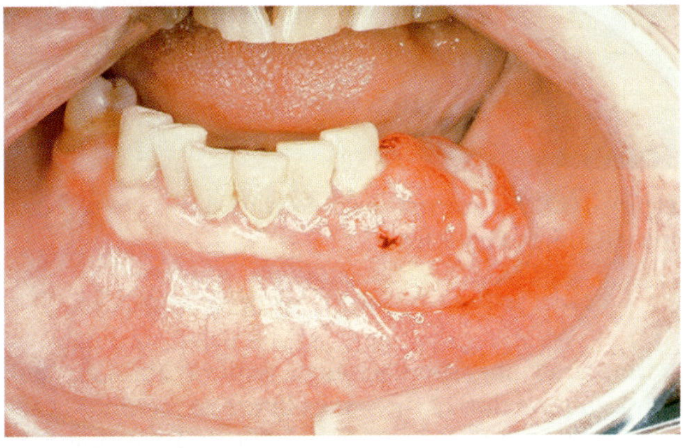

Figure 10.69 Squamous carcinoma of the lower alveolus.

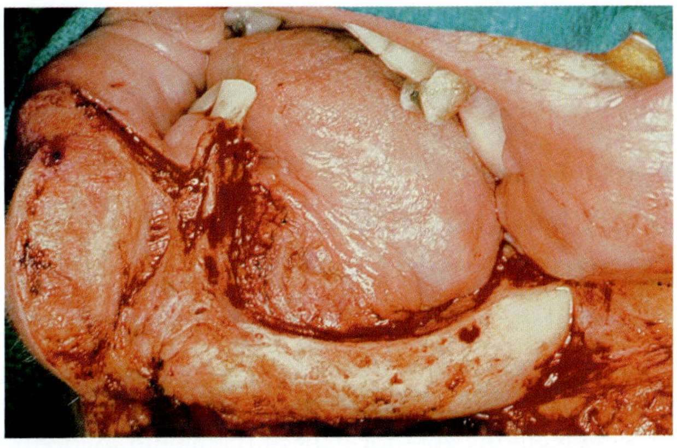

Figure 10.72 Surgical defect following marginal mandibulectomy.

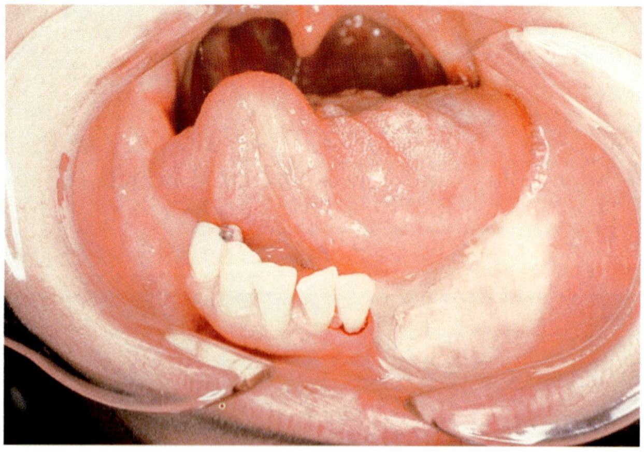

Figure 10.73 Healed skin graft over the marginally resected mandible.

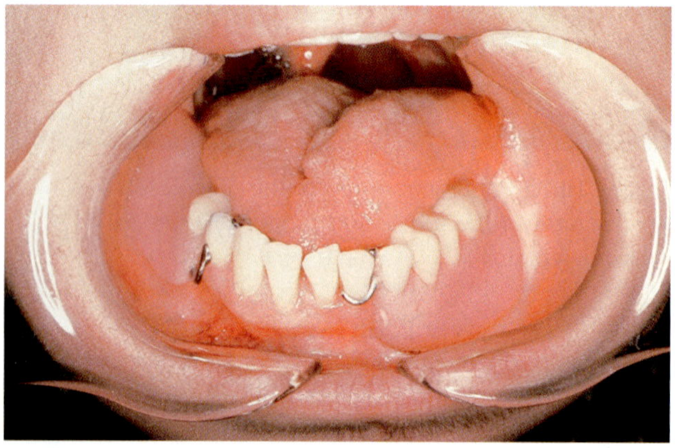

Figure 10.74 Partial denture at the site of marginal mandibulectomy.

clasped to the teeth to restore lower dentition (Fig. 10.74). Another patient, shown in Fig. 10.75, has osseointegrated implants placed at the site of marginal mandibulectomy with a permanent fixed denture in place. Her panoramic radiograph shown in Fig. 10.76, demonstrates satisfactory position of the implants in the mandible where marginal mandibulectomy was performed. The permanent dental implants restoring lower dentition are shown in Fig. 10.77. Thus, when feasible, osseointegrated implants should be considered for complete dental rehabilitation following marginal mandibulectomy.

Marginal mandibulectomy in continuity with radical neck dissection (pull-through operation)

The patient shown in Fig. 10.78 has squamous cell carcinoma of the anterior floor of the mouth involving the lingual gingiva. This procedure will accomplish resection of the floor of the mouth in conjunction with

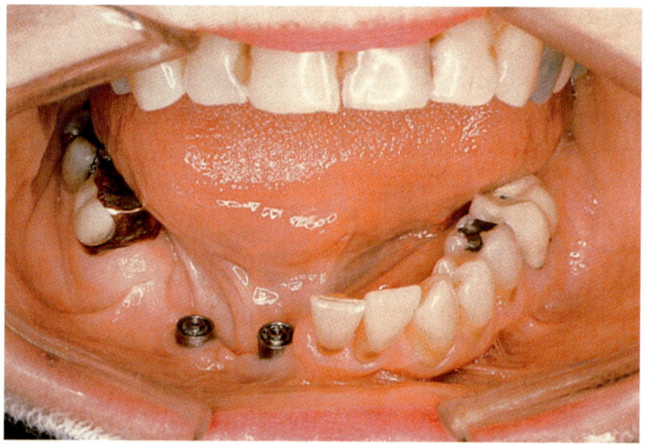

Figure 10.75 Osseointegrated implants at the site of marginal mandibulectomy.

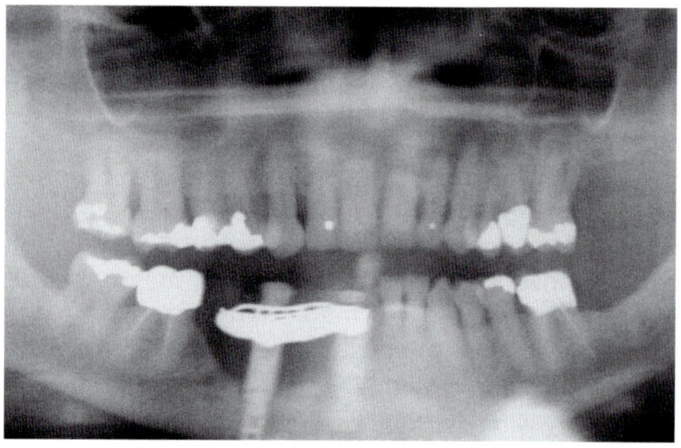

Figure 10.76 Panoramic x-ray showing the osseointegrated implants.

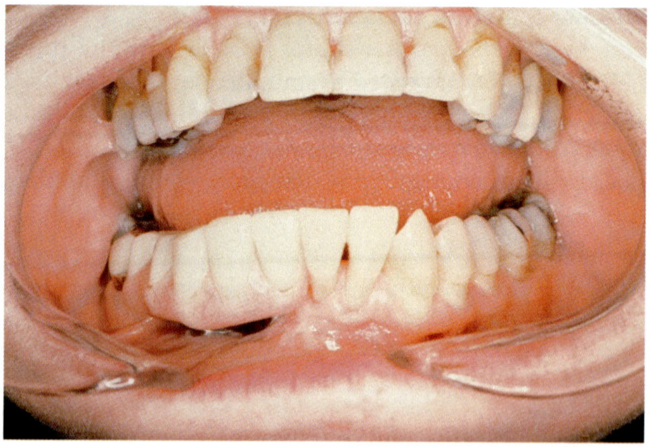

Figure 10.77 Permanent fixed denture at the site of marginal mandibulectomy.

a marginal mandibulectomy, with a through and through resection of the musculature of the floor of the mouth in continuity with a right neck dissection. The specimen of the primary tumor will be delivered in the neck in a pull-through fashion.

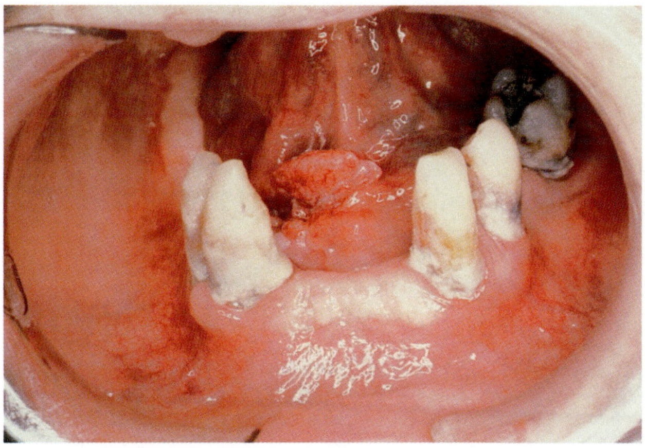

Figure 10.78 Squamous carcinoma of the anterior floor of the mouth.

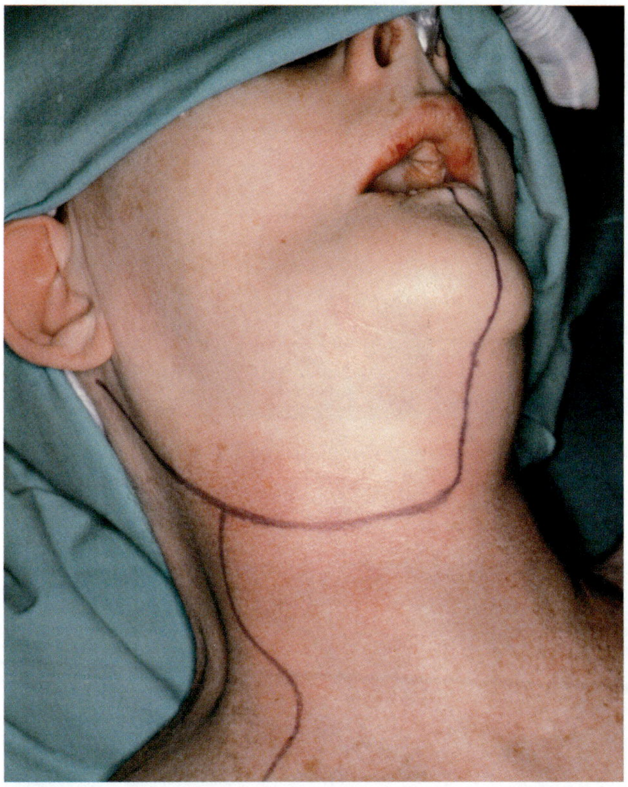

Figure 10.79 Planned incisions for resection of the primary tumor in continuity with a modified radical neck dissection.

The patient is placed on the operating table under general anesthesia with a nasotracheal tube. The incision begins at the tip of the mastoid process, curving anteriorly along an upper skin crease of the neck up to the midline where it curves cephalad, dividing the chin and the lower lip in the midline. A curvaceous vertical limb extends from about the midpoint of the transverse incision up to the clavicle to facilitate a modified or radical neck dissection, as indicated (Fig. 10.79).

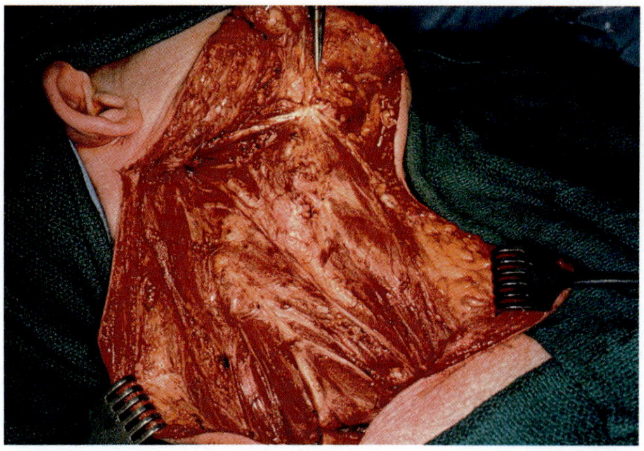

Figure 10.80 Dissection of lymph nodes from levels II–V is completed.

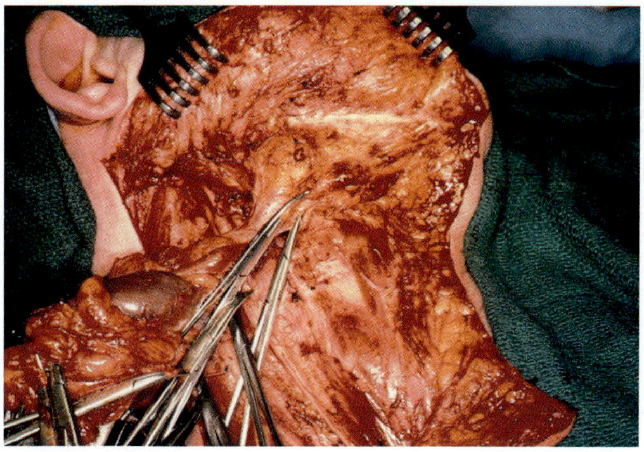

Figure 10.81 Dissection of level I lymph nodes in progress.

The neck dissection is completed in the usual fashion except for level 1, through which it remains attached to the primary tumor (Fig. 10.80). The specimen of the dissected neck is flipped towards the chin. All attachments of the specimen inferior and deep to the digastric tendon are divided at this point. The neck dissection specimen is now flipped back in the posterior part of the neck and dissection of level 1 is performed (Fig. 10.81). The upper neck flap is elevated and the mandibular branch of the facial nerve is carefully identified and preserved. Soft tissues overlying the body of the mandible are now incised by electrocautery, exposing the periosteum of the body of the mandible from the symphysis up to the insertion of the masseter muscle near the angle of the mandible. The rest of the skin incision, dividing the lower lip and the soft tissues of the chin, is now completed. An incision is made in the mucosa of the gingivobuccal sulcus from the midline up to the retromolar trigone (Fig. 10.82). Thus the lower cheek flap is elevated and the lateral cortex of the body of the mandible is exposed (Fig. 10.83).

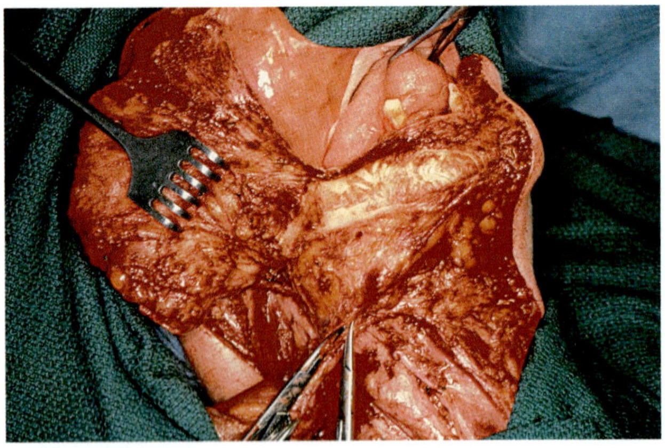

Figure 10.82 The lower cheek flap is elevated.

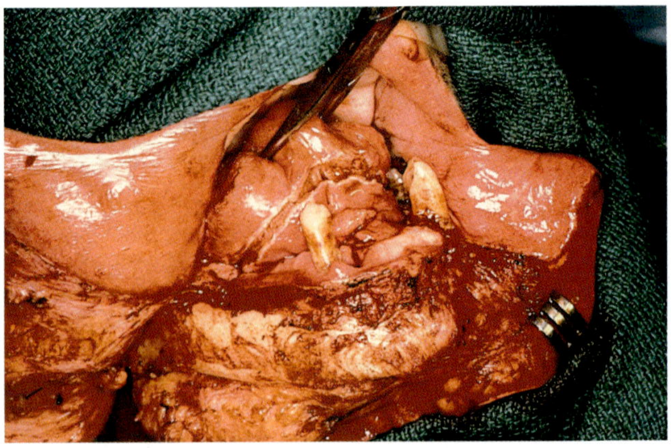

Figure 10.84 The mucosal incision around the tumor is deepened through the muscles of the tongue and floor of mouth.

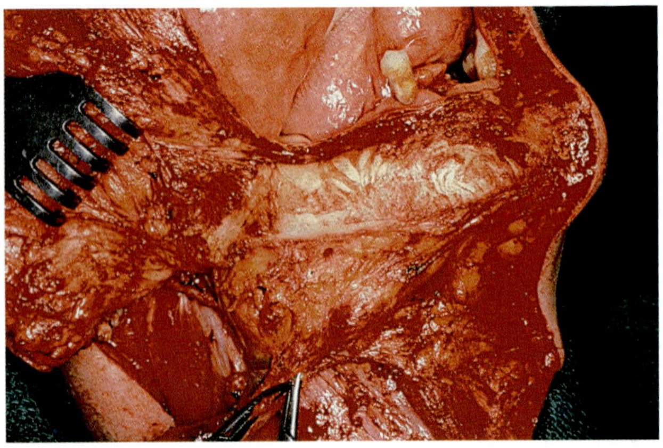

Figure 10.83 The lateral cortex of the mandible is exposed.

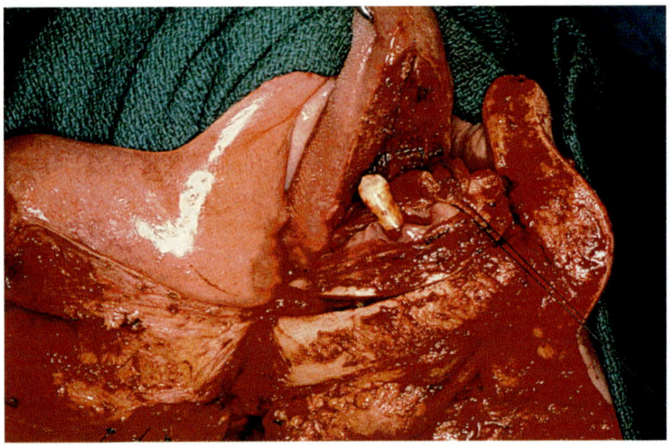

Figure 10.85 A marginal mandibulectomy is performed in an oblique plane.

The musculature of the undersurface of the tongue and the mucosa of the floor of the mouth are completely divided (Fig. 10.84). A power sagittal saw is now used to divide the mandible so that the specimen includes the alveolar process and as much of the lingual cortex of the mandible as possible. This is performed by cutting the mandible obliquely (Fig. 10.85). Such an oblique cut permits resection of the musculature of the floor of the mouth, which remains attached to the excised portion of the mandible in a monobloc fashion. The mandible is thus divided in an oblique sagittal plane, permitting resection of the alveolar process and a significant part of the lingual plate.

With the use of a skin hook, the portion of the mandible to be resected with the primary tumor is now retracted cephalad, demonstrating the muscular attachments at the genial tubercle (Fig. 10.86). The entire thickness of the musculature of the floor of the mouth is thus resected with the marginal mandibulectomy. Remaining soft tissue attachments between the resected part of the mandible and the patient are now detached using electrocautery. The specimen containing the primary tumor, resected portion of the mandible, and the musculature of the floor of the mouth, is now ready to be delivered through the mandibular arch to the right side of the neck. After its delivery in the neck, the specimen of the primary tumor still remains attached through

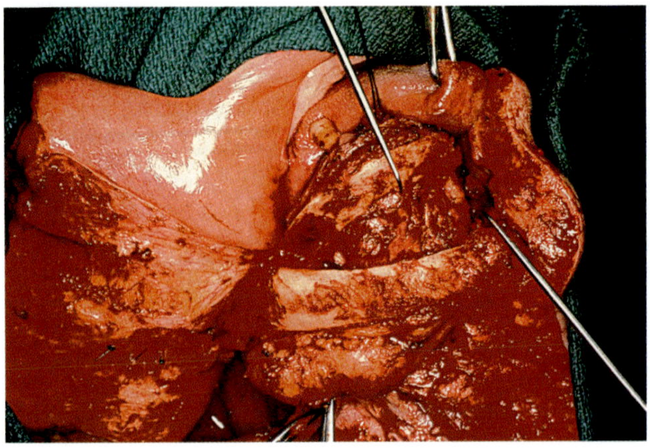

Figure 10.86 The muscles attached to the genial tubercle are excised in a monobloc fashion.

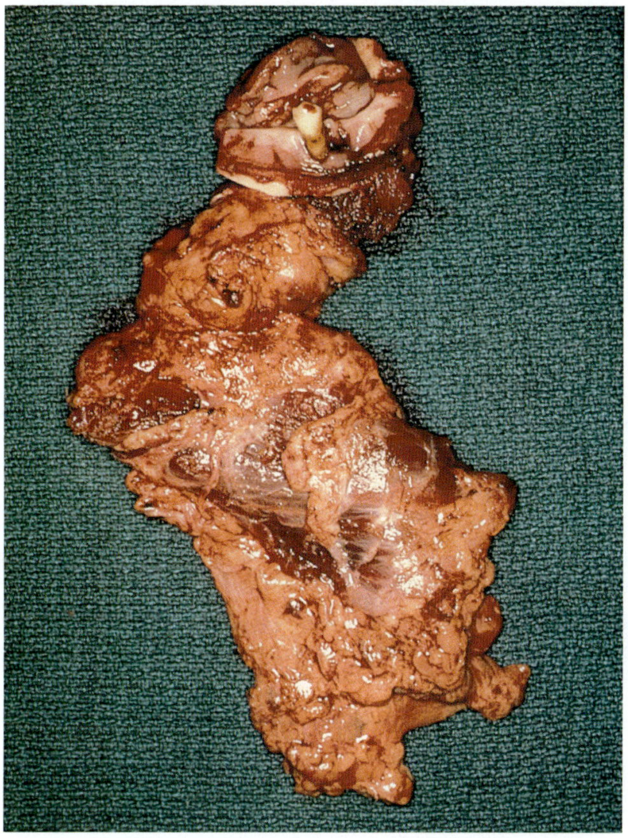

Figure 10.87 Specimen of the primary tumor removed with regional lymph nodes in continuity.

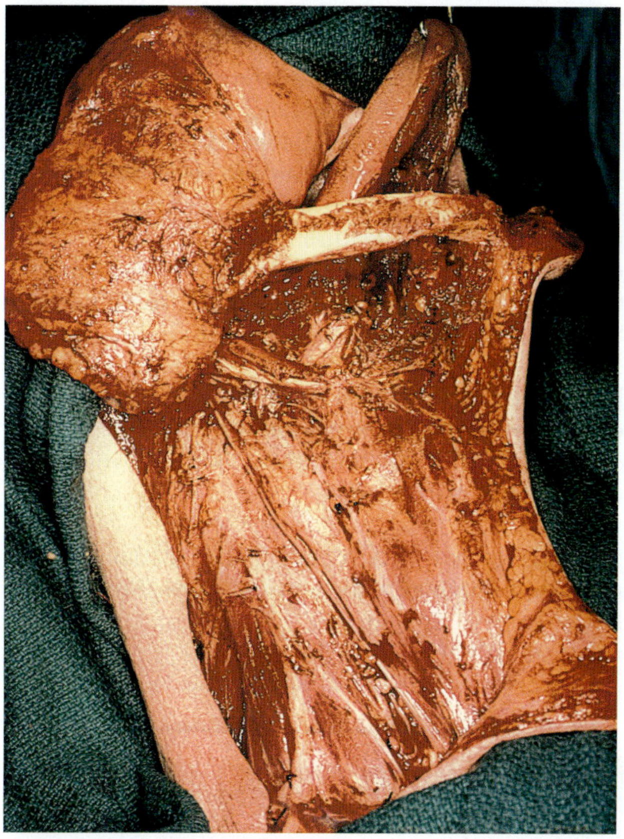

Figure 10.88 The surgical field showing a through-and-through defect at the primary site.

remaining fibers of the hyoglossus and geniohyoid muscles. Once these are divided, the primary tumor, resected in continuity with the contents of the dissected right side of the neck, is removed (Fig. 10.87).

The resulting surgical defect is seen in Fig. 10.88. A through and through defect of the floor of the mouth creates a communication between the oral cavity and the dissected neck on the right hand side.

A close-up view of the surgical defect at the primary site shows that the musculature of the undersurface of the anterior one-third of the tongue is excised in conjunction with the floor of the mouth to ensure a true three-dimensional resection (Fig. 10.89). However, the continuity of the arch of the mandible is preserved. Repair of the surgical defect thus created can be easily accomplished by primary closure, approximating the mucosa of the right cheek to the mucosa of the right lateral border of the tongue over the marginally resected mandible. As the closure continues anteriorly, the mucosa of the tip of the tongue is sutured to the mucosa of the lower lip up to the midline. Primary closure performed in this fashion, however, causes significant tethering of the tongue with severe impact on the clarity of speech, mastication, and swallowing

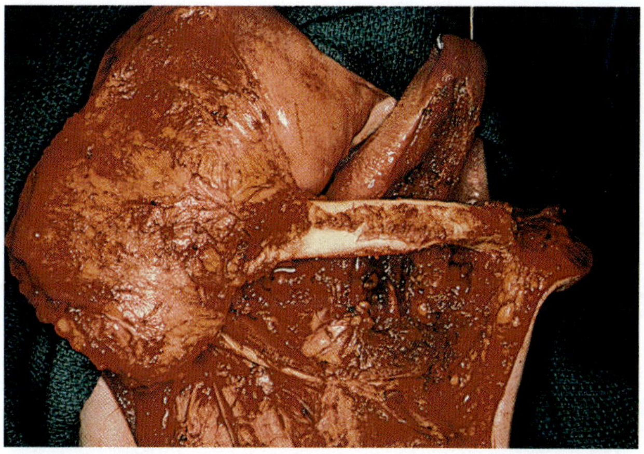

Figure 10.89 Close-up view of the surgical defect showing a three-dimensional resection of the primary tumor.

due to impaired mobility of the tongue. On the other hand, a surgical defect such as this is ideally suited for primary reconstruction using a radial forearm free flap. Alternatively, a skin graft can be employed to provide mucosal coverage in the anterior floor of the mouth. It must be noted, however, that if a skin graft is used, the healing process will be prolonged since satisfactory primary healing of the skin graft in this location for a defect of this magnitude seldom takes place. Therefore, when feasible, a radial forearm free flap should be used since it ensures primary healing and also provides just sufficient soft tissue to fill the through and through defect. If adequate vertical height of the marginally resected mandible is available, then this patient would be an ideal candidate for secondary placement of osseointegrated dental implants and a permanent fixed denture. Clearly such dental rehabilitation is functionally superior. If, however, this patient requires postoperative radiotherapy, then extreme caution should be exercised in placing osseointegrated implants in a marginally resected irradiated mandible. The risk for implant failure and osteoradionecrosis is significant. At this time, experience with osseointegrated implants in irradiated mandibles is limited.

This patient had a skin graft placed at the surgical site. This provided excellent coverage (Fig. 10.90). Postoperative appearance of the patient shows minimal esthetic deficit (Fig. 10.91).

Marginal mandibulectomy in an edentulous patient

When marginal mandibulectomy is performed in an edentulous patient, extreme caution must be exercised with regard to viability of the remaining mandible,[30,32] otherwise a pathological fracture is possible at that site. If such is feared to be the case, then the remaining mandible should be supported using a metallic plate as a buttress to prevent iatrogenic fracture.

Carcinoma of the retromolar trigone and the adjacent lower gingiva on the left hand side with invasion of the underlying cortical bone in an edentulous patient is shown in Fig. 10.92. Panoramic radiograph of the mandible shows cortical erosion at the retromolar trigone, requiring at least a marginal mandibulectomy (Fig. 10.93). A supraomohyoid neck dissection as a staging procedure is done and

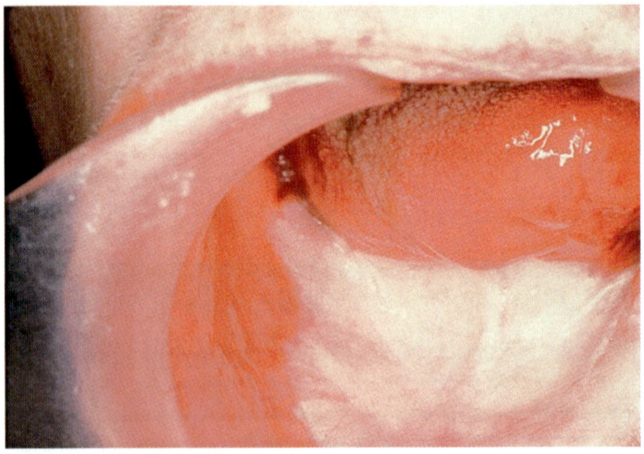

Figure 10.90 Healed skin graft at the site of resection.

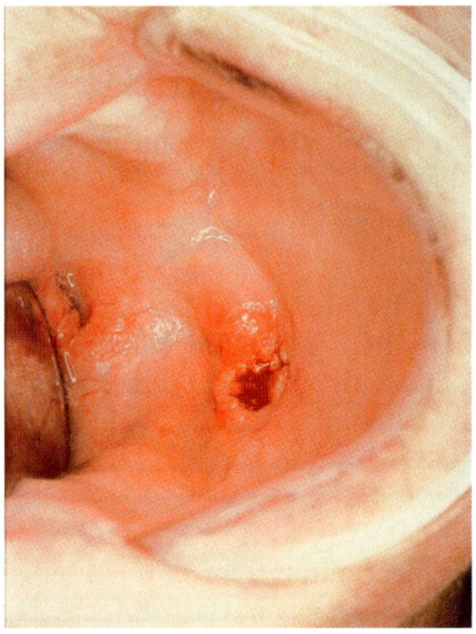

Figure 10.92 Carcinoma of retromolar gingiva.

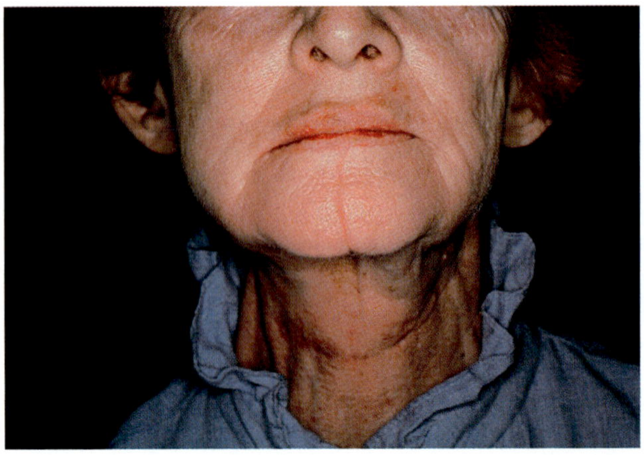

Figure 10.91 Postoperative appearance of the patient at one year.

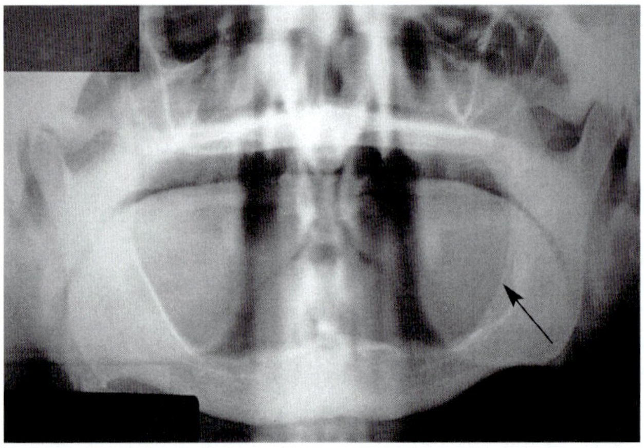

Figure 10.93 Panoramic x-ray showing minimal cortical erosion at left retromolar region.

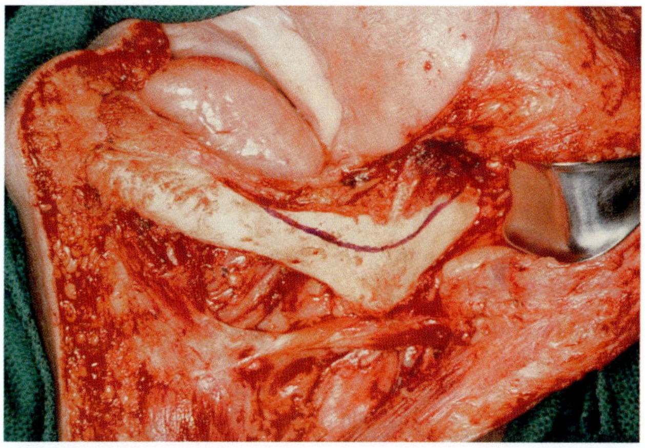

Figure 10.94 The proposed marginal mandibulectomy is outlined.

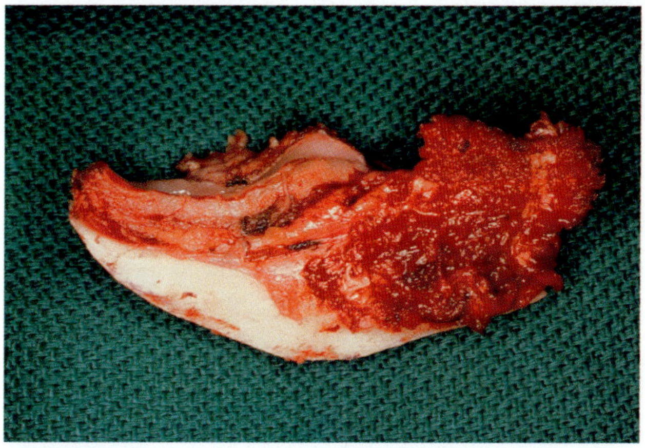

Figure 10.95 Specimen showing adequate deep margin.

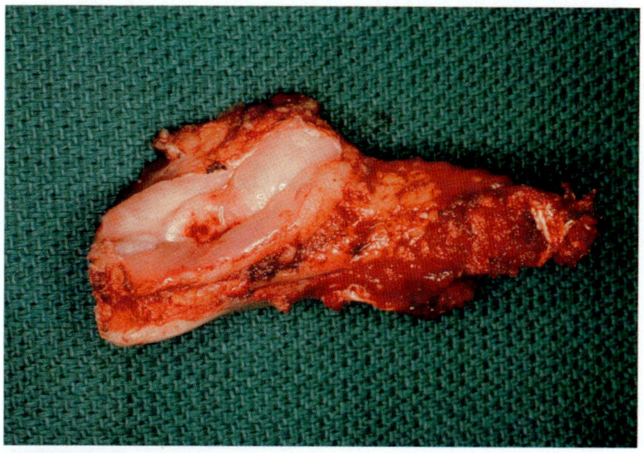

Figure 10.96 Specimen showing adequate mucosal margins.

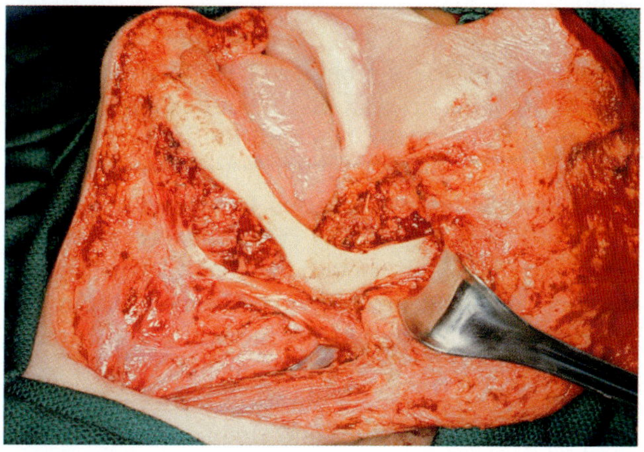

Figure 10.97 Surgical defect showing remaining edentulous mandible.

the lower cheek flap is elevated in the usual fashion so it remains lateral to the outer cortex of the mandible from the symphysis at the anterior midline up to the mandibular notch posteriorly. The extent of bone resection to be undertaken at the site of the primary tumor is marked on the ascending ramus and the posterior aspect of the body of the mandible (Fig. 10.94). Appropriate three-dimensional resection is then undertaken using a high-speed power saw with an ultra-thin blade. The surgical specimen viewed from the lateral aspect is shown in Fig. 10.95. Note a three-dimensional resection has been accomplished with a satisfactory deep margin to excise the superior cortex of the mandible in a monobloc fashion. The surface view of the surgical specimen shows adequate mucosal margins around the primary tumor (Fig. 10.96). The marginally resected mandible is smoothed out. Note that the remaining mandible is very thin, has a very limited height, and is at a risk for spontaneous fracture (Fig. 10.97). A long miniplate is therefore used to support the remaining mandible to prevent pathological fracture. The miniplate is appropriately shaped to fit

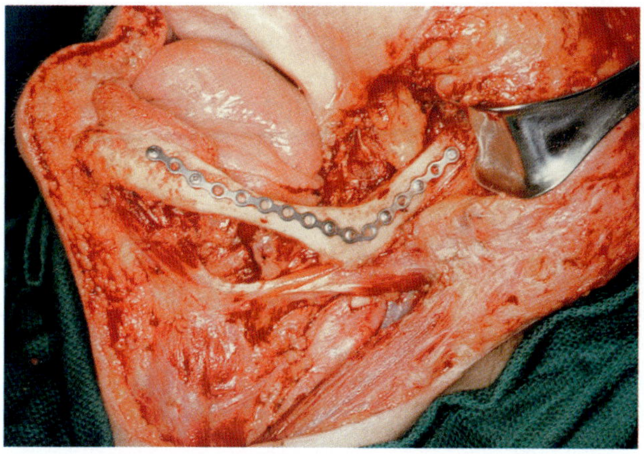

Figure 10.98 A long miniplate support is applied to the remaining mandible to prevent fracture.

the lateral cortex of the mandible extending from the ascending ramus up to the anterior aspect of the body of the mandible (Fig. 10.98). Several screws are used to hold the miniplate in position.

Marginal mandibulectomy with resection of the lower gum and reconstruction with an A–O plate and radial forearm free flap

When a large area of mucosa of the lower gum is involved by primary tumor, then clearly a secondary effort at reconstruction to provide surface lining in the oral cavity is essential. However, if the underlying bone is not involved, then a marginal mandibulectomy is technically feasible.

A primary verrucous carcinoma of the lower gum, extending from the region of the first molar tooth to the retromolar trigone, is shown in Fig. 10.99. Panoramic radiography of the mandible shows cortical erosion of the retromolar trigone region. The extent of bone resection is indicated on this radiograph (Fig. 10.100). A midline lower lip-splitting incision extended to the lateral aspect of the upper part of the neck is used to facilitate a supraomohyoid neck dissection (Fig. 10.101). A supraomohyoid neck dissection is completed and a marginal mandibulectomy is performed through a lower cheek flap approach. A monobloc resection is accomplished (Fig. 10.102). The medial surface view of the surgical specimen shows a large area of the mucosa of the lower gum and floor of the mouth as well as the cheek excised in a monobloc fashion, with the underlying mandible in continuity with the contents of the supraomohyoid neck dissection (Fig. 10.103). The surgical field shows the bony defect in the body and the ascending ramus of the mandible (Fig. 10.104). The remaining mandible is at a significant risk of spontaneous fracture unless it is supported by a metallic buttress. An A–O plate is used to support the residual mandible (Fig. 10.105).

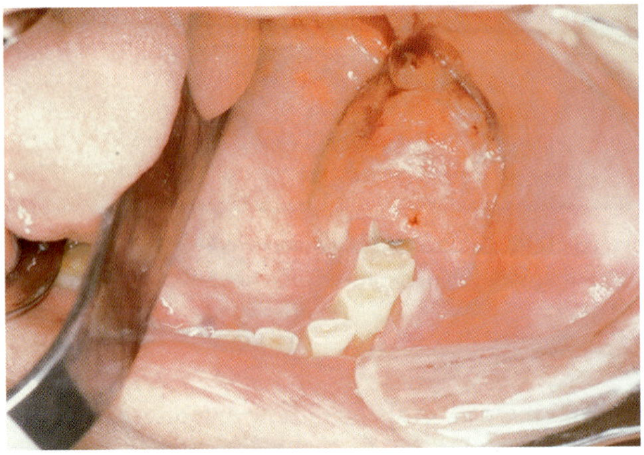

Figure 10.99 Verrucous carcinoma of the lower gum extending up to retromolar trigone.

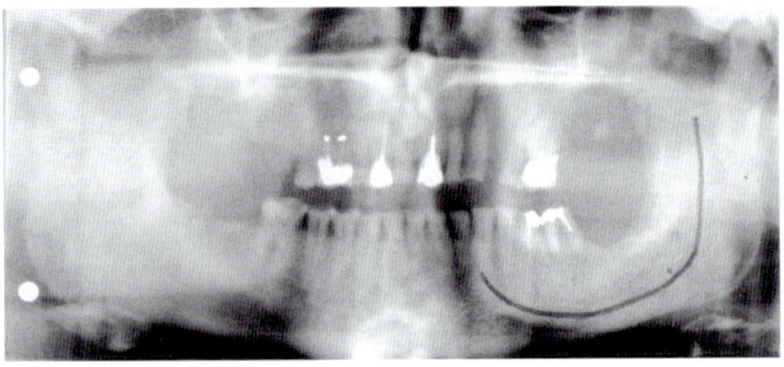

Figure 10.100 Proposed marginal mandibulectomy outlined on a panoramic x-ray.

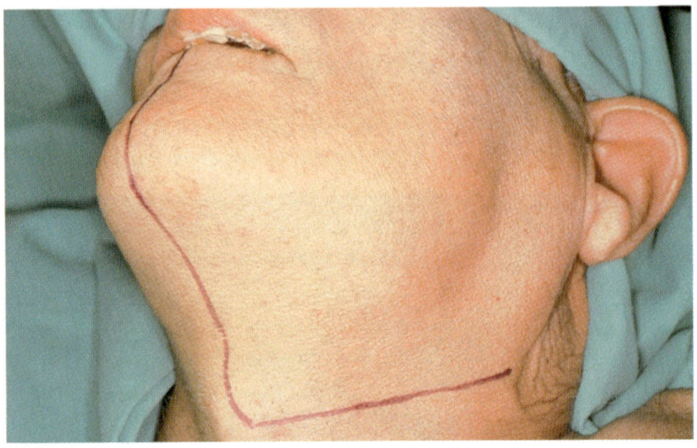

Figure 10.101 The skin incision is outlined for marginal mandibulectomy and modified neck dissection.

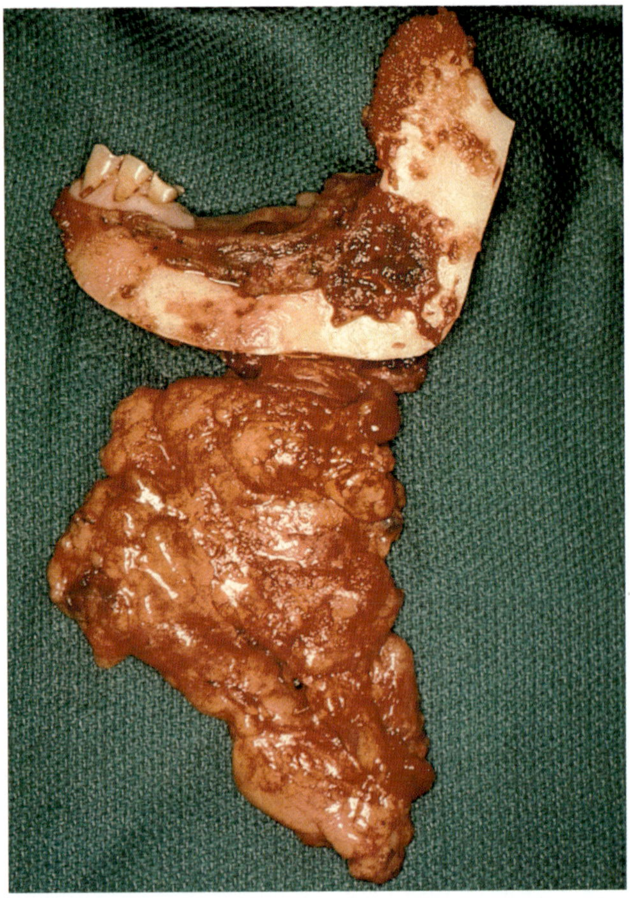

Figure 10.102 Specimen of an aggressive marginal mandibulectomy and supraomohyoid neck dissection.

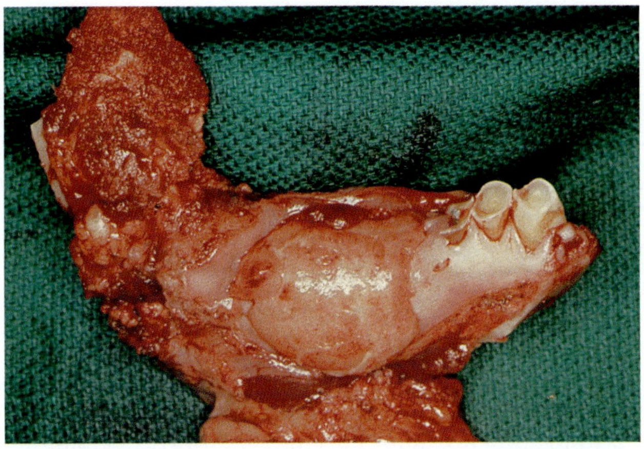

Figure 10.103 Specimen showing excision of a large mucosal surface.

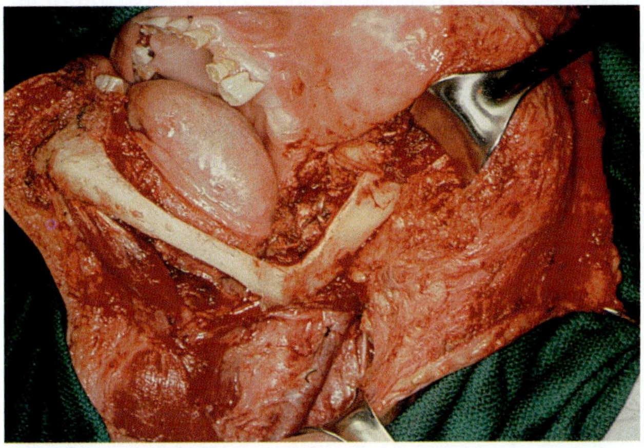

Figure 10.104 Surgical field showing residual mandible.

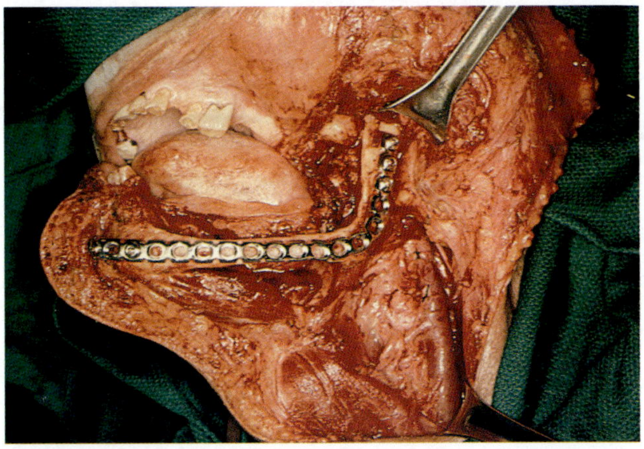

Figure 10.105 An AO plate is used to support the remaining mandible.

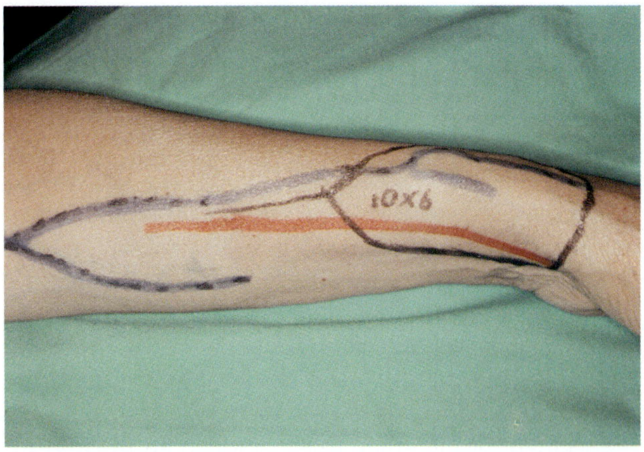

Figure 10.106 A radial forearm flap is used to reconstruct the mucosal defect.

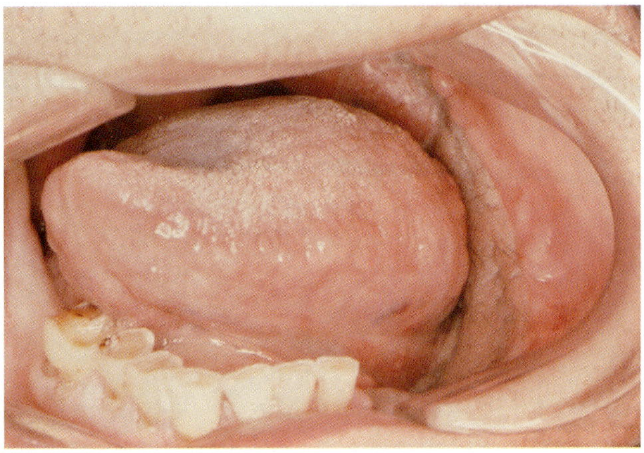

Figure 10.107 Postoperative intra-oral view showing the radial forearm flap.

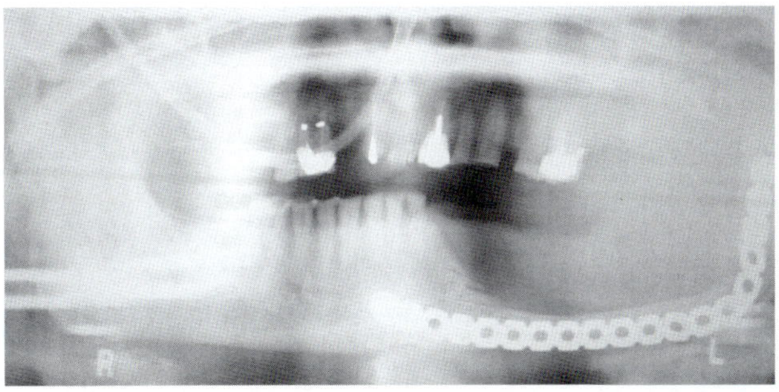

Figure 10.108 Postoperative panoramic x-ray showing the AO plate.

A fascio-cutaneous radial forearm free flap is elevated from the patient's left arm (Fig. 10.106). The free flap is used to resurface the lining of the oral cavity over the remaining portion of the mandible supported by the A–O plate. A postoperative intra-oral view of the patient shows primary healing of the radial forearm free flap providing excellent coverage of the lining in the oral cavity (Fig. 10.107).

A postoperative panoramic view of the mandible shows adequate placement of the A–O plate (Fig. 10.108).

Composite resection with segmental mandibulectomy (commando operation)

A composite resection with segmental mandibulectomy (commando operation) is indicated for primary tumors of the oral cavity which extend to involve the mandible (Fig. 10.109). On occasion, a composite resection may be indicated for patients with primary tumors having extensive soft tissue disease around the mandible that necessitates the sacrifice of an intervening segment of mandible to accomplish an in-continuity monobloc resection of the primary tumor in conjunction with neck dissection. Thus, a commando operation or a composite resection entails excision of the intra-oral primary tumor along with a segment of the mandible performed in conjunction with ipsilateral neck dissection as a monobloc surgical resection.

The patient shown in Fig. 10.110 has primary carcinoma of the lower gum with extension to the retromolar trigone and adjacent gingivo-buccal sulcus. He had received previous radiotherapy with a curative intent but the tumor persisted and hence the surgical procedure of composite resection was indicated. He has clinically palpable cervical lymph node metastasis. The incision for the operation is a standard trifurcate incision for neck dissection beginning at the tip of the mastoid process and curving anteriorly, remaining approximately two fingerbreaths below the body of the mandible up to the midline of the neck at the level of the hyoid bone (Fig. 10.111). At that point, the incision turns cephalad, dividing the skin and soft tissues of the chin and the lower lip in the midline. A vertical curvaceous component of the incision begins at the region of the posterior border of the sternocleidomastoid muscle on the transverse incision and it extends down to the clavicle at the midclavicular point. Due to the

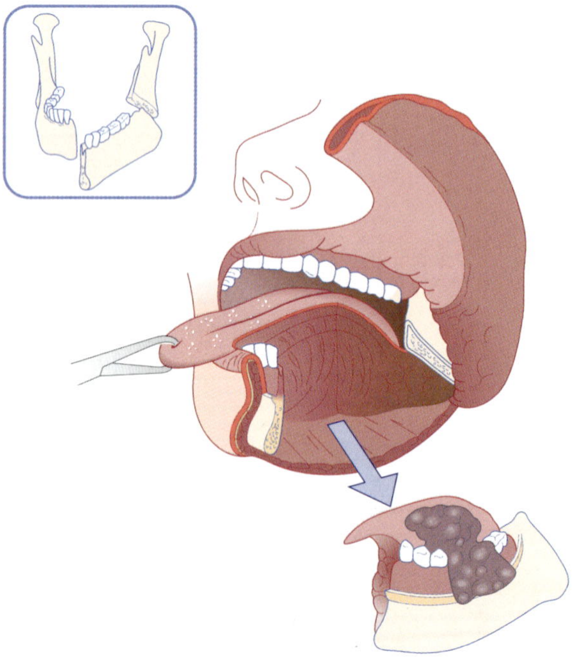

Figure 10.109 Segmental mandibulectomy.

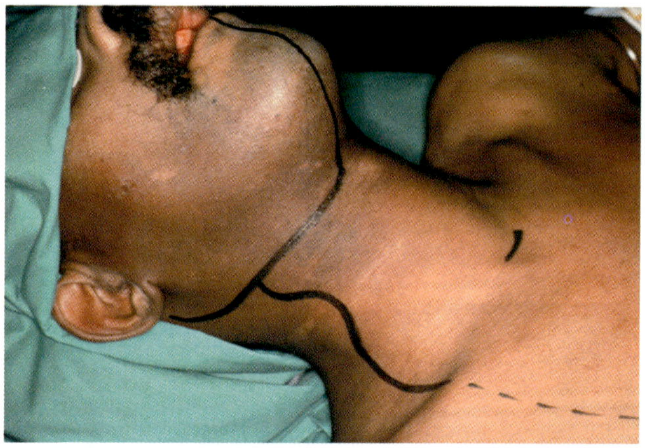

Figure 10.111 Skin incision outlined for composite resection of lower gum with neck dissection.

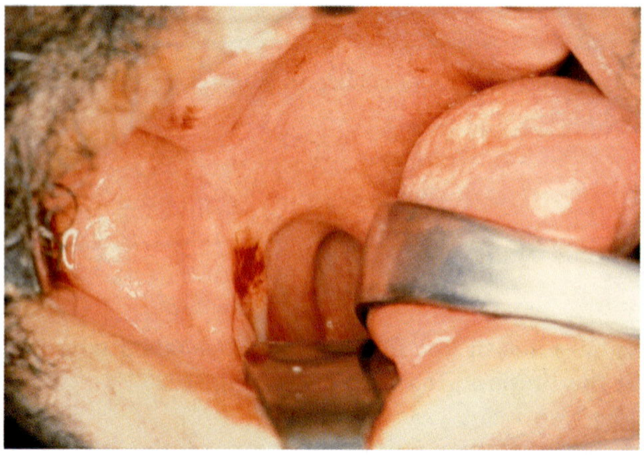

Figure 10.110 Previously irradiated squamous carcinoma of the lower gum.

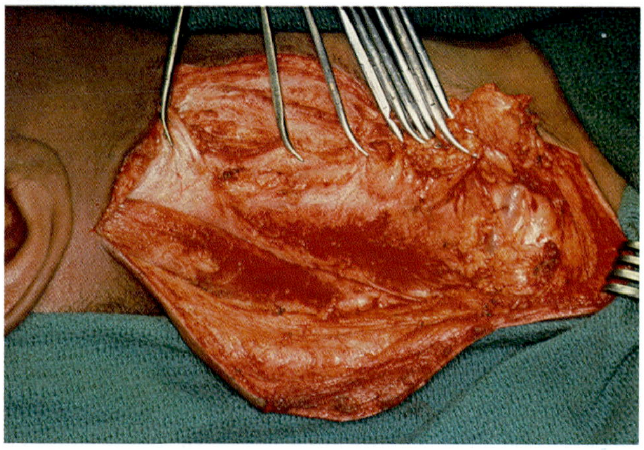

Figure 10.112 Neck dissection begins in the posterior triangle.

presence of clinically palpable cervical lymph nodes, this patient requires a comprehensive neck dissection. The sequential steps of various types of neck dissections are described in the chapter on the management of the neck. Dissection of the posterior triangle and lower neck is completed in the usual fashion, preserving the accessory nerve if it is not directly involved by metastatic disease (Fig. 10.112). The phrenic nerve is preserved and the cutaneous roots of the cervical plexus are divided (Fig. 10.113). The lower anterior skin flap is now elevated and the insertion of the sternomastoid muscle is detached from the sternum and the clavicle (Fig. 10.114). After ligation of the internal jugular vein at the lower end, dissection proceeds cephalad along the carotid sheath towards level 1 (Fig. 10.115). No attempt is made to dissect the contents of the submandibular triangle, which remain attached through the floor of the mouth and the soft tissues medial to the mandible to the primary site (Fig. 10.116).

At this point, the neck incision is extended cephalad in the midline, dividing the skin of the chin and the lower lip through its full thickness (Fig. 10.117). The upper skin flap of the neck dissection is now elevated, remaining deep to the platysma which is retained on the flap. Meticulous attention should be paid to identification and careful preservation of the marginal branch of the facial nerve to maintain the

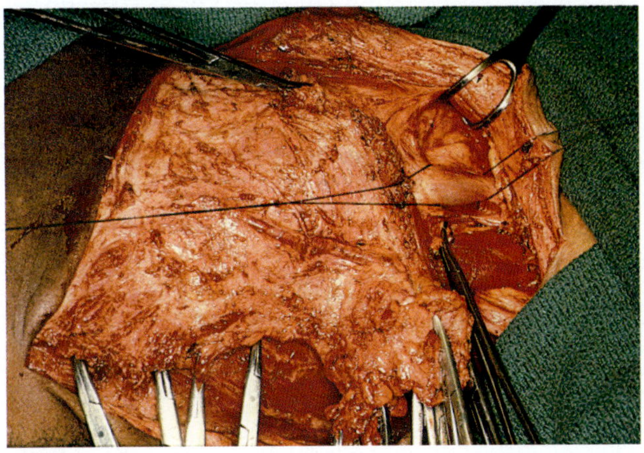

Figure 10.115 The internal jugular vein is doubly ligated and divided.

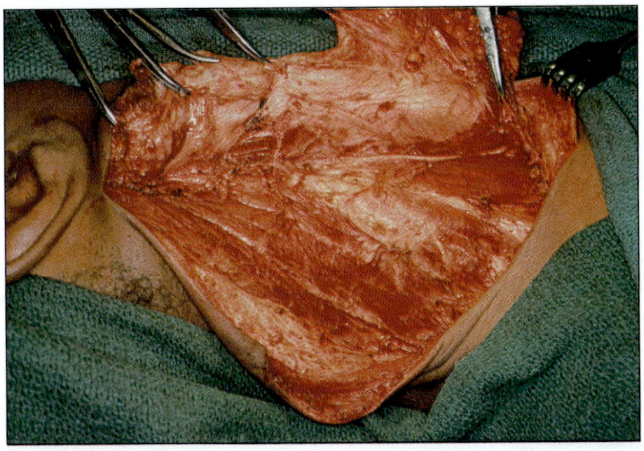

Figure 10.113 The accessory and phrenic nerves are preserved, but the cutaneous cervical roots are divided.

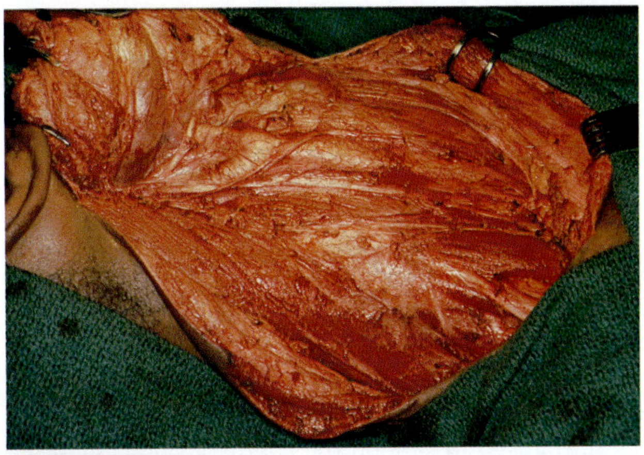

Figure 10.116 Dissection proceeds along the carotid sheath up to the hypoglossal nerve.

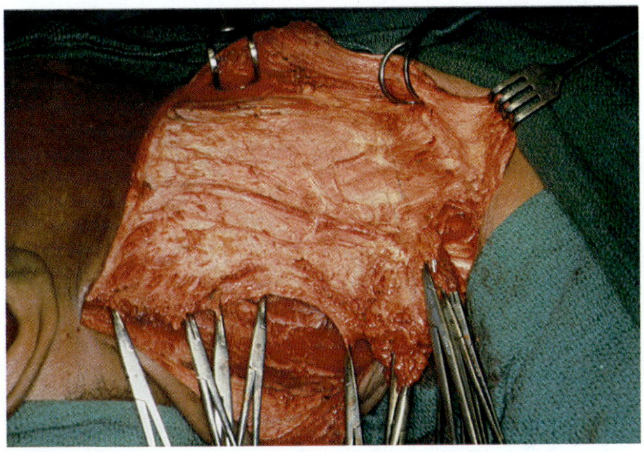

Figure 10.114 The anterior skin flap is elevated to expose the lower end of the sternomastoid muscle.

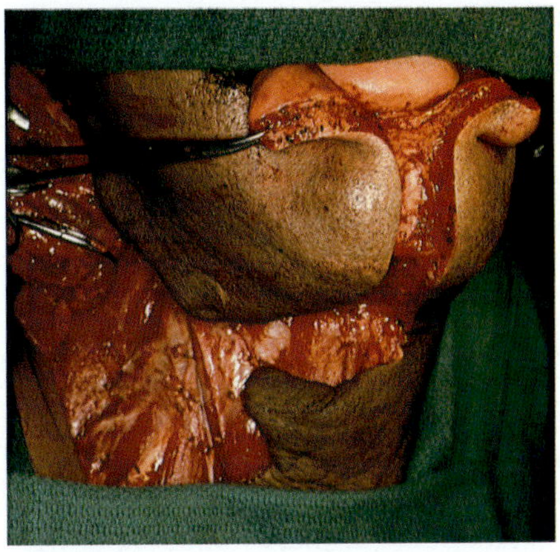

Figure 10.117 The lower lip is split in the midline and the outer cortex of the mandible is exposed.

function of the lower lip and competency of the oral cavity. The upper skin flap is elevated up to the lower border of the mandible, extending from the angle of the mandible all the way up to the midline of the chin. Division of the upper lip in the midline through its full thickness is now completed up to the anterior cortex of the mandible at the symphysis.

A mucosal incision is placed in the gingivobuccal sulcus, leaving adequate mucosal and soft tissue margins around the primary tumor (Fig. 10.118). In this patient the cheek flap is elevated, leaving all soft tissues including prevascular facial nodes attached to the mandible. The lateral surface of the masseter is exposed and the masseter is detached from the ascending ramus of the mandible up to the mandibular notch. This maneuver provides exposure of the entire lateral cortex of the mandible from the mandibular notch up to the midline at the symphysis menti. An appropriate site on the mandible for division is marked (Fig. 10.119).

The muscular attachments of the temporalis muscle over the coronoid process of the mandible are detached. A sagittal power saw is now used to divide the mandible through the ascending ramus. Brisk hemorrhage ensues from the two cut ends of the mandible following division of the condyloid process. Bone wax is used to control bleeding from the cut ends of the bone. Extreme caution should be exercised to prevent the power saw from cutting through the soft tissues medial to the mandible, otherwise excessive hemorrhage will result from laceration of the pterygoid muscles and the rich network of terminal branches of the internal maxillary artery. In order to avoid laceration of the soft tissues medial to the mandible, it is desirable to introduce a small malleable retractor medial to the condyloid process of the mandible before dividing the bone. Alternatively, a Mixter clamp may be introduced to support the condyloid process of the mandible and prevent the blade of the sagittal saw from lacerating the soft tissues situated medially. Attention is now focused on dividing the mandible distally at an appropriate place depending upon the site, size, and surface extent of the tumor as well as the extent of the soft tissue disease contiguous to the mandible. A straight cut through the body of the mandible is performed at the appropriate site. Bone wax is used again to control hemorrhage from the cut ends of the mandible. The mandible, having been divided at two places, permits its lateral retraction and exposure of the intra-oral tumor.

Using electrocautery, a mucosal incision is placed around the primary tumor with a generous cuff of normal mucosa to secure satisfactory margins. A three-dimensional resection of the primary tumor along with the adjacent floor of the mouth, underlying soft tissues and musculature of the tongue is performed with the use of electrocautery, remaining in continuity with the mandible and the contents of the dissected neck. Hemostasis is secured as the procedure proceeds by ligation or electrocoagulation of the bleeding points as they are encountered. The extent of mucosa and soft tissue resection clearly depends on the extent and invasive nature of the primary tumor and the involvement of the underlying musculature, soft tissues, and neurovascular bundles.

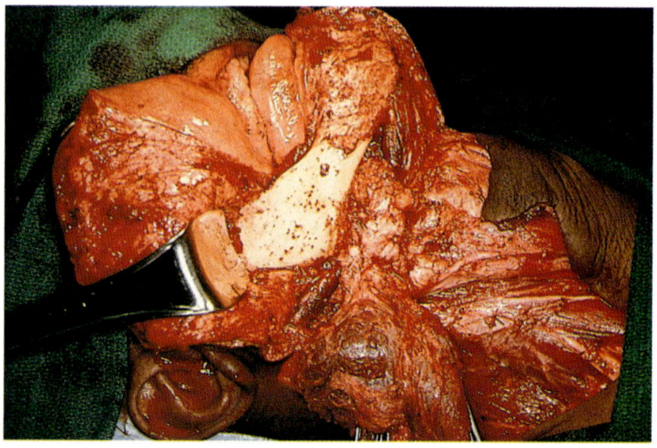

Figure 10.118 The lower cheek flap is elevated.

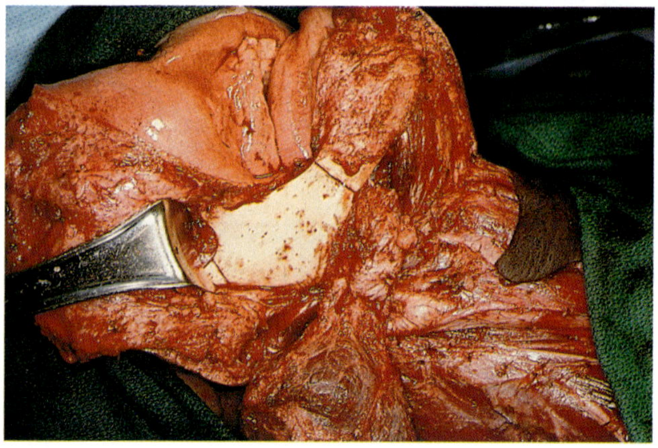

Figure 10.119 Mucosal incisions are placed around the tumor, and the extent of bone resection is outlined.

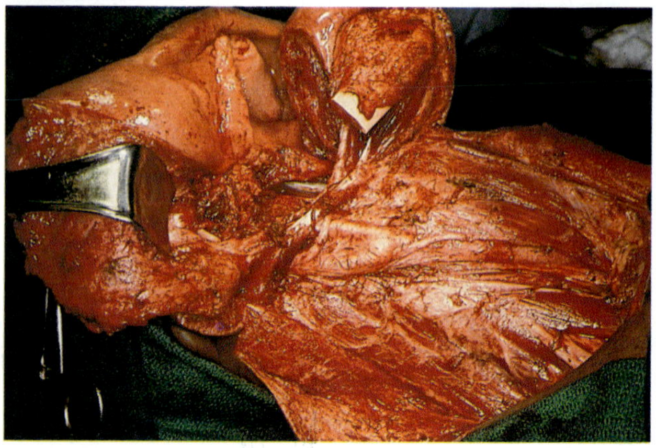

Figure 10.120 The surgical defect following composite resection.

After removal of the specimen, the surgical field shows a satisfactory monobloc resection of the primary tumor in conjunction with the contents of the dissected neck and the intervening soft tissues and lymphatics (Fig. 10.120). Frozen sections are obtained from appropriate areas according to the extent of the primary tumor and the judgment of the surgeon regarding the proximity of the tumor to the surgical margins, as seen in a close-up view (Fig. 10.121).

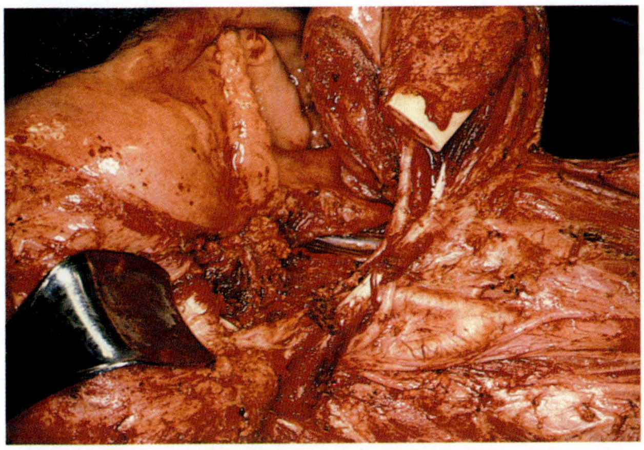

Figure 10.121 Close-up view of the surgical defect at the primary site.

The surgical specimen on its lateral aspect shows the masseter muscle and soft tissues overlying the angle of the mandible and the contents of the dissected neck with the sternomastoid muscle (Fig. 10.122). On its medial aspect, the primary tumor of the lower gum is seen, removed in continuity with neck dissection showing the internal jugular vein on the medial aspect of the specimen (Fig. 10.123).

If immediate reconstruction of the mandible and the mucosal lining is planned with a composite microvascular free flap, then the appropriate reconstructive procedure begins at this point. On the other hand, if no specific effort at reconstruction of the surgical defect is planned, then primary closure of the surgical defect should be performed.

A tracheostomy is done at the conclusion of the operation to facilitate clearance of pulmonary secretions postoperatively and for provision of a satisfactory airway to facilitate smooth postoperative recovery. Blood loss during this operative procedure is minimal. Blood transfusion is seldom necessary. If there is no tension on the suture line of the mucosa in the oral cavity, then primary healing should be expected within 1 to 2 weeks. At that point, the patient is started on puréed foods by mouth and gradually advanced to soft diet.

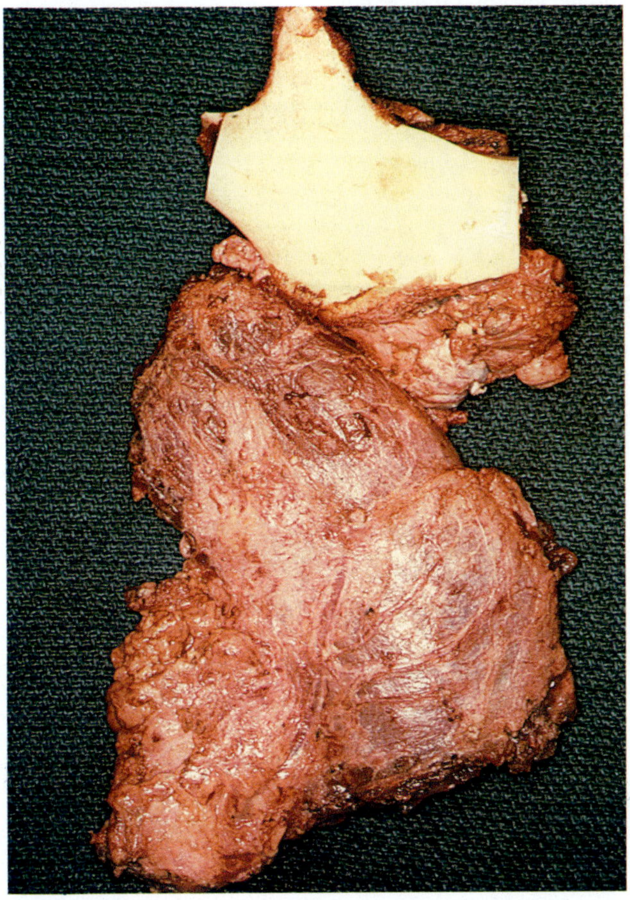

Figure 10.122 Lateral view of the surgical specimen.

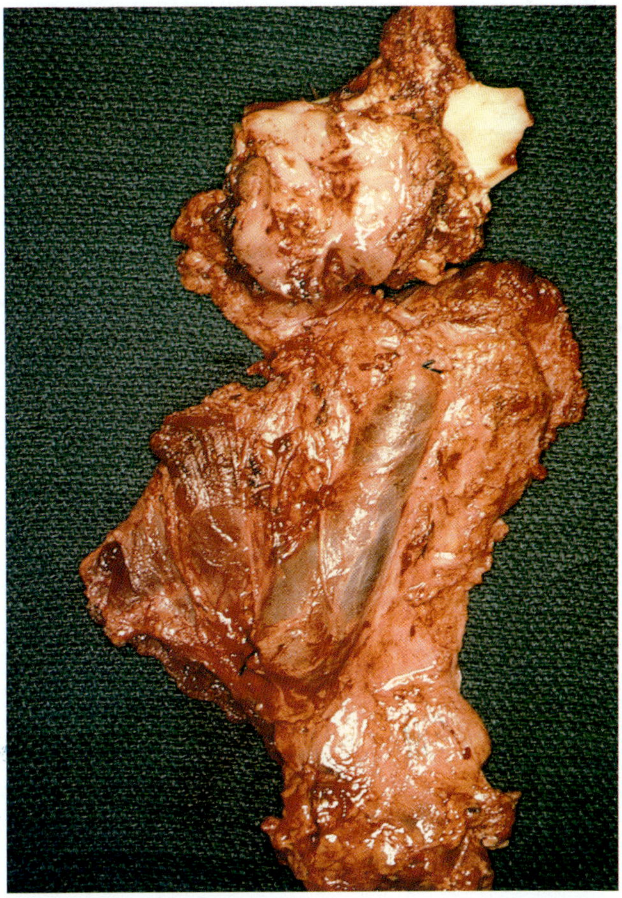

Figure 10.123 Medial view of the surgical specimen.

Visor flap approach for resection of tumors of the oral cavity

The advantage of a visor flap approach to the oral cavity is that it avoids splitting the lower lip and chin in the midline. The oral cavity is exposed via a single transverse skin incision extending from the mastoid process on one side to that on the other, along an upper neck skin crease. The visor flap requires a mucosal incision in the gingivobuccal and gingivolabial sulci, with division of all the soft tissues lateral to the mandible. This permits elevation and retraction of the visor flap to expose the oral cavity (Fig. 10.124). Although the exposure provided by the visor flap approach is satisfactory for tumors of the anterior oral cavity, it is clearly inadequate if a primary tumor of the oral cavity extends posteriorly to involve the middle third of the tongue or the region of the retromolar gingiva on either side. Another disadvantage of the visor flap is that it requires transection of both mental nerves, leading to anesthesia of the skin of the chin and lower lip. This may produce drooling in elderly patients.

A locally advanced primary carcinoma of the anterior floor of the mouth in a patient with direct extension to the edentulous mandible is shown in Fig. 10.125. The operative procedure planned here consists of a right radial neck dissection and a left supraomohyoid neck dissection together with (segmental mandibulectomy) resection of the anterior arch of the mandible with the floor of the mouth and undersurface of the tongue.

The dissected contents of the right hand side of the neck remain attached through level I to the undersurface of the mandible in the submental region. The supraomohyoid triangle on the left side of the neck is also dissected, with the specimen remaining attached to the primary tumor through the left submandibular triangle (Fig. 10.126). A close-up

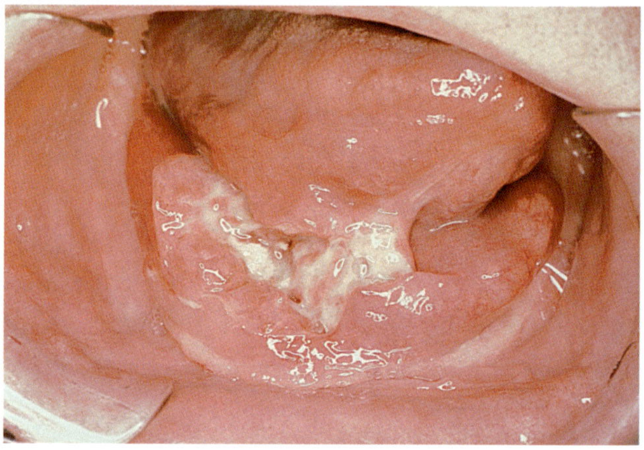

Figure 10.125 Squamous carcinoma of the floor of the mouth invading the mandible.

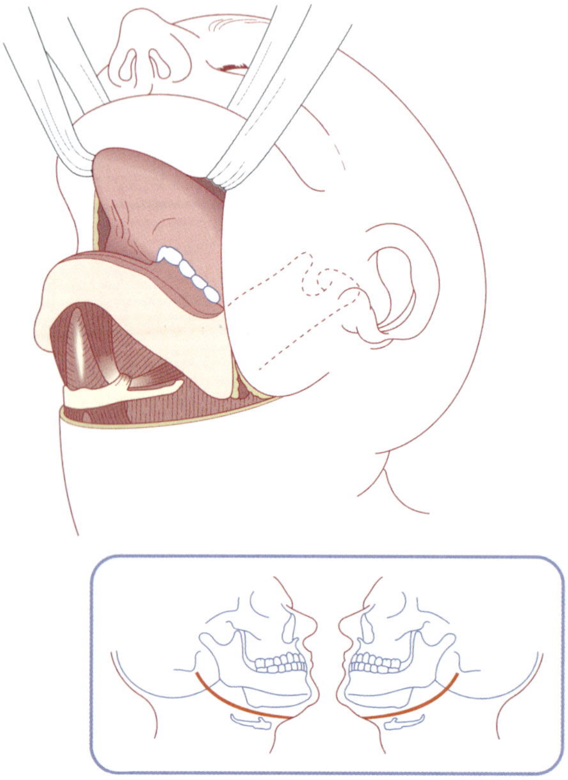

Figure 10.124 Visor flap approach.

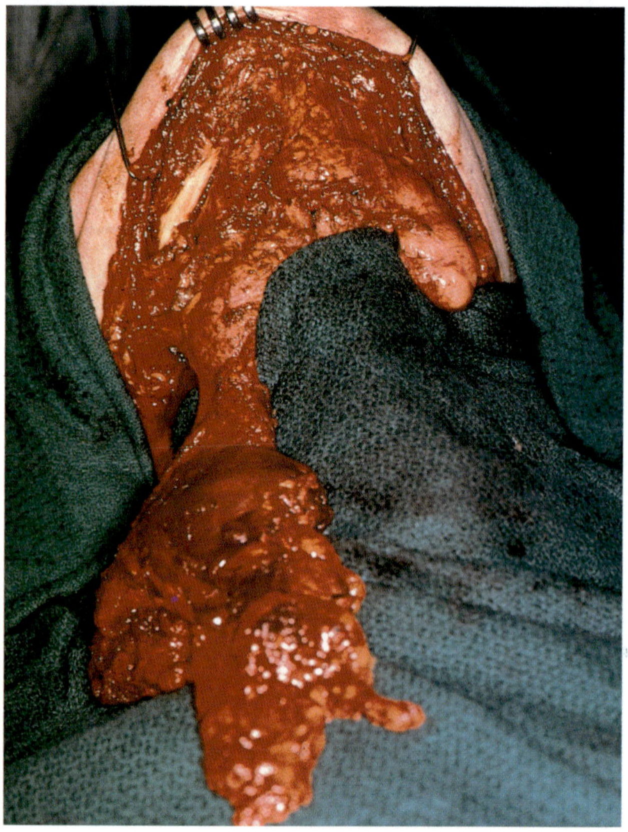

Figure 10.126 Bilateral neck dissections are completed.

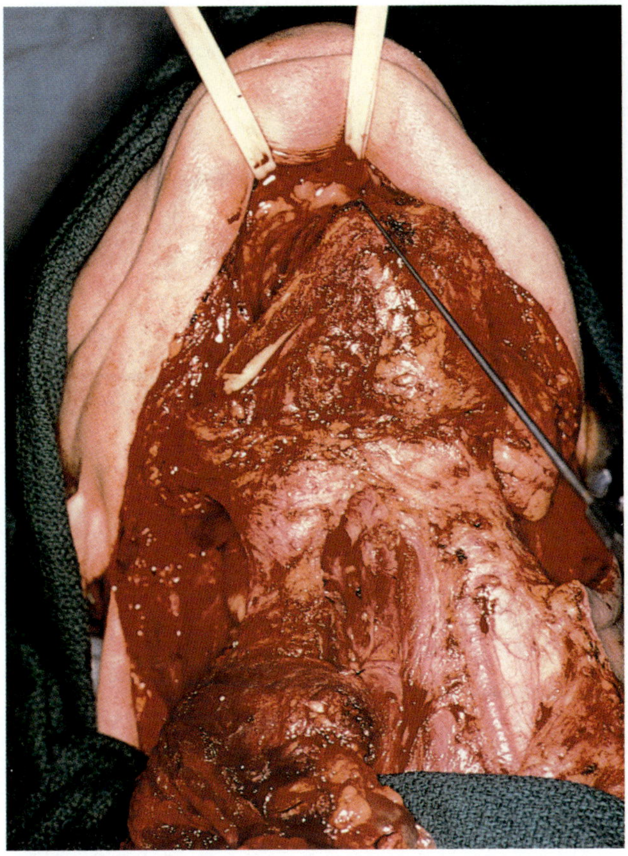

Figure 10.127 The dissected lymph nodes remain in continuity with the primary tumour at the submental region.

view of the exposed submental region is seen in Fig. 10.127. The visor flap is developed completely by connecting the mucosal incision in the gingivobuccal sulcus, beginning at the retromolar trigone on the right side and extending up to the left retromolar trigone. In the neck the visor flap is elevated up to the undersurface of the mandible from the angle of the mandible on one side up to the angle of the mandible on the other side. At this point, sharp retractors are used to retract the lower lip and the visor flap, facilitating division of the soft tissue attachments on the outer cortex of the mandible, to permit separation of the visor flap from the mandible. Two Penrose drains are now used to retract the visor flap towards the upper lip and expose the mandible and the oral cavity (Fig. 10.128).

The mandible is retracted caudad showing the primary tumor of the floor of the mouth. Note the limitations in gaining adequate exposure of the retromolar trigone with the visor flap. Mucosal incisions are now made on the undersurface of the tongue and in the floor of the mouth posterior to the tumor, securing adequate margins. The musculature of the undersurface of the tongue is divided with electrocautery up to the region of the angle of the mandible on both sides. At this point, a power sagittal saw is used to divide the mandible just anterior to the angle on the right hand side and just lateral to the mental foramen on the left hand side. Following division of the mandible, the remaining muscular attachments of the hyoglossus and the genioglossus muscles are divided. The specimen consists of the primary tumor of the floor of the mouth with the anterior arch of the mandible, and contents of the right radical neck dissection and left supraomohyoid neck dissection (Fig. 10.129). A close-up view of the specimen shows satisfactory mucosal and soft tissue margins around the primary tumor and a three-dimensional resection

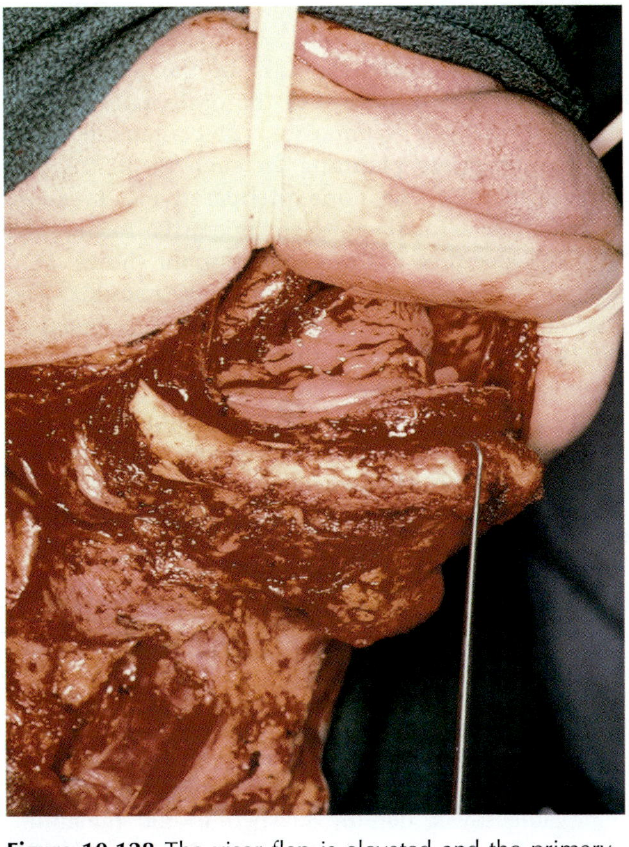

Figure 10.128 The visor flap is elevated and the primary tumor is exposed.

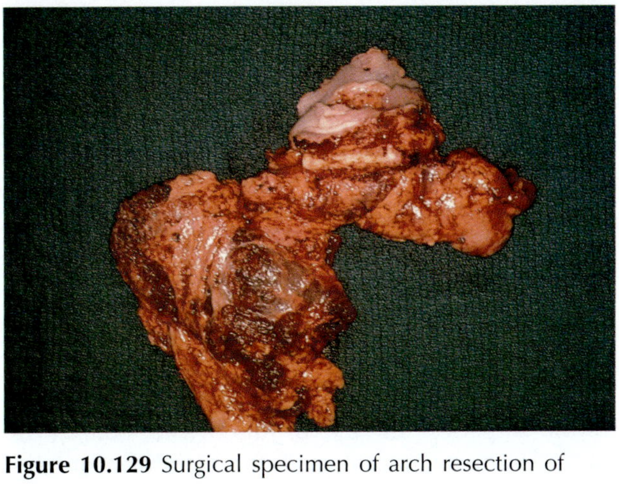

Figure 10.129 Surgical specimen of arch resection of mandible with bilateral neck dissections.

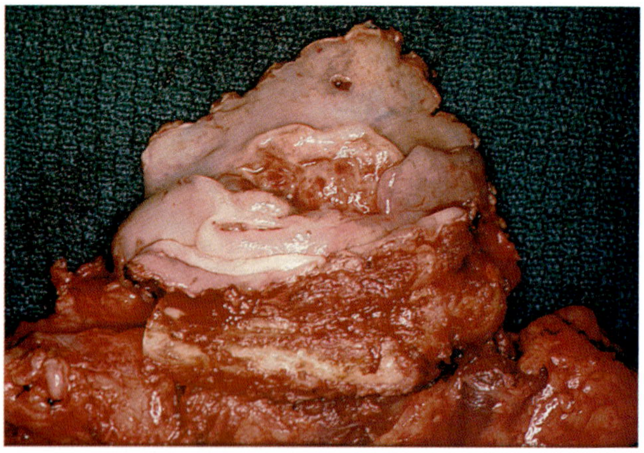

Figure 10.130 Close-up view of the specimen showing adequate three-dimensional resection.

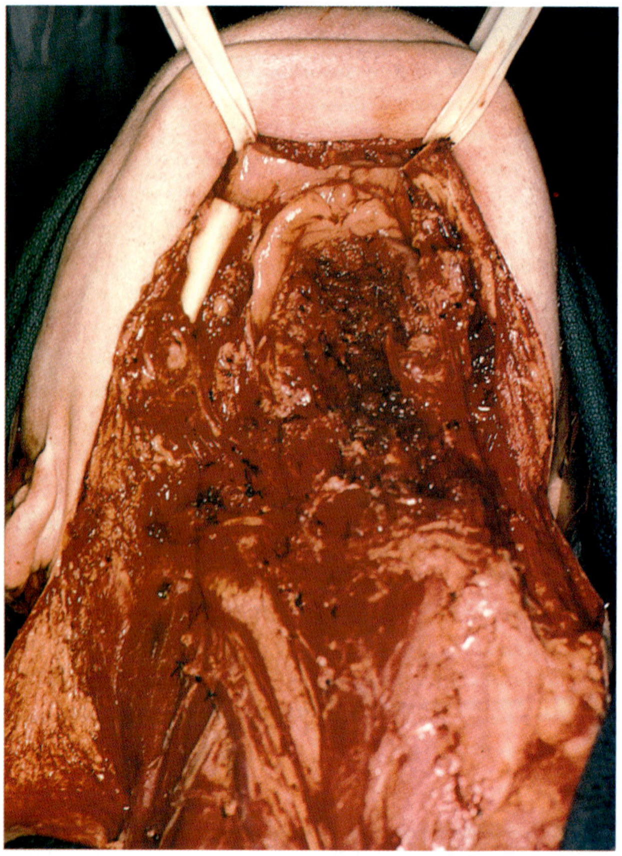

Figure 10.131 Surgical defect showing stumps of the mandible and tongue musculature.

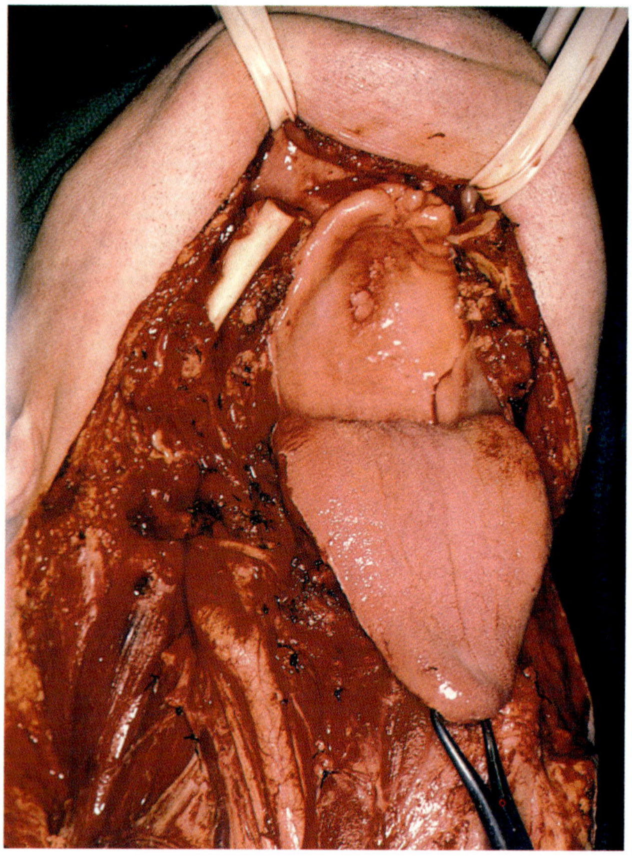

Figure 10.132 Surgical defect showing stumps of the mandible and tongue retracted down.

of the depth of the tumor in continuity with the mandible (Fig. 10.130).

The surgical defect shows the stumps of the mandible and the raw surface of the transected musculature of the tongue in its anterior and middle thirds, as well as the stumps of the muscles attached to the superior surface of the hyoid bone (Fig. 10.131). The two stumps of the mandible and the hard palate are seen with the tongue retracted anteriorly and inferiorly (Fig. 10.132). A surgical defect of this magnitude, with the loss of the arch of the mandible and soft tissues in the oral cavity, is best repaired with a composite osteocutaneous free flap. Appropriate planning for such reconstruction should therefore be done preoperatively in every instance for a satisfactory postoperative result. The surgical specimen of the resected tumor shows satisfactory mucosal, soft tissue and bony margins. The surgical defect thus created requires replacement of the bone and soft tissues in the floor of the mouth as well as the mucosal lining in the oral cavity. A composite free flap of a segment of fibula, with its attached muscles and overlying skin, is ideal for reconstruction of this defect.

Dental rehabilitation following mandible reconstruction

Complete anatomic and functional rehabilitation of the oral cavity following cancer ablation and reconstruction of the mandible requires either a satisfactory removable lower denture clasped to the remaining teeth or the use of osseointegrated implants to facilitate a permanent fixed denture.[50–53] The choice of dental rehabilitation is based on several factors, including the status of the oral cavity after tumor resection, available resources, and patient preferences.

If osseointegrated dental implants are to be used, we prefer that they be placed secondarily after satisfactory healing of the bone has occurred, rather than primarily at the time of free flap reconstruction of the mandible. A minimum of 12 months is allowed to elapse before osseointegrated implants are considered. A panoramic radiograph of the reconstructed mandible should show satisfactory bony union between the graft and the mandible and satisfactory bony healing of the graft at the sites of multiple osteotomies. Ideally, the placement of the implants should be performed by an appropriately trained oral surgeon. The first step is to assess the site for positioning of the implants. If metallic titanium plates and screws used for reconstruction of the mandible are impeding implant placement, then they are removed to clear that area to receive the implants.

The location and number of implants to be placed are best assessed by the oral surgeon, who will assume the responsibility of placement of the implants and their subsequent exposure, and the eventual fabrication and placement of the permanent fixed denture. Satisfactorily integrated implants are exposed between 4 to 6 months following placement. For details on the technical aspects of placement of osseointegrated implants, their subsequent exposure, and fabrication and fixation of a permanent fixed denture, the reader is referred to appropriate textbooks of oral surgery and dental implantology.

The patient shown in Fig. 10.133 had a central salivary carcinoma of the lower gum on the left hand side. His preoperative CT scan shows expansion of

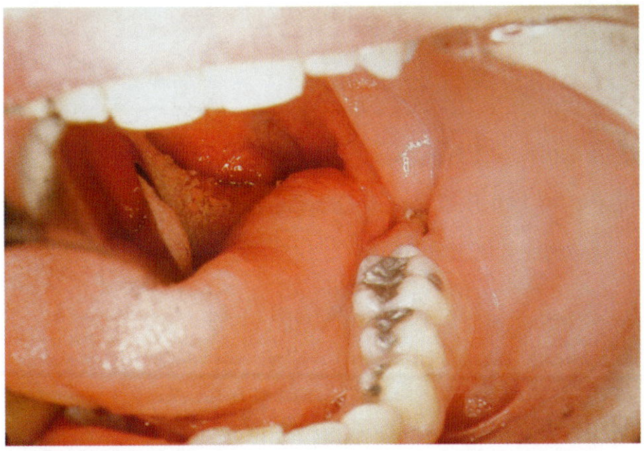

Figure 10.133 Intra-oral view of the left lower gum lesion.

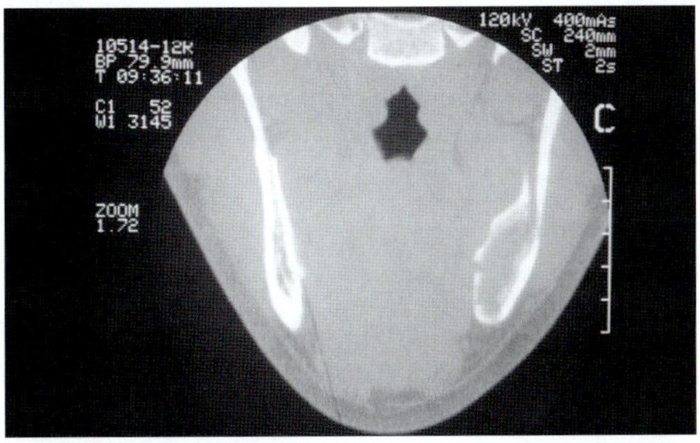

Figure 10.134 Coronal view of CT scan of the mandible showing an expansive lesion.

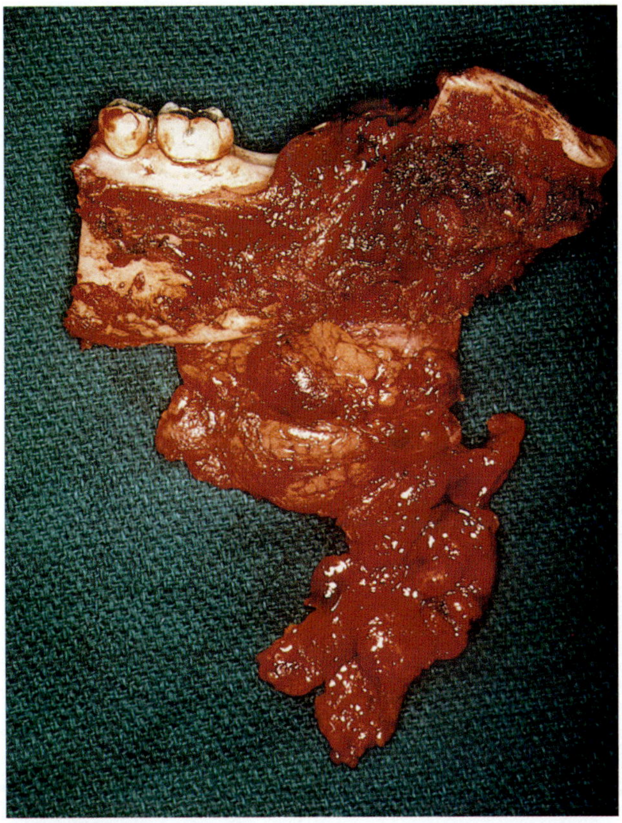

Figure 10.135 Surgical specimen of segmental mandibulectomy and supraomohyoid neck dissection.

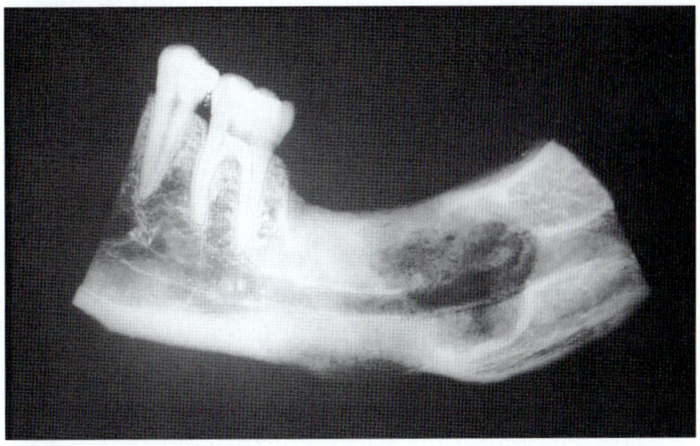

Figure 10.136 Plain radiograph of the specimen showing the lytic lesion.

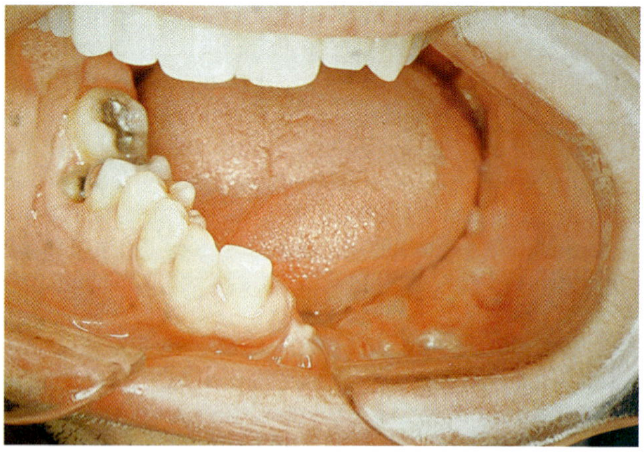

Figure 10.137 Postoperative intra-oral view showing primary healing.

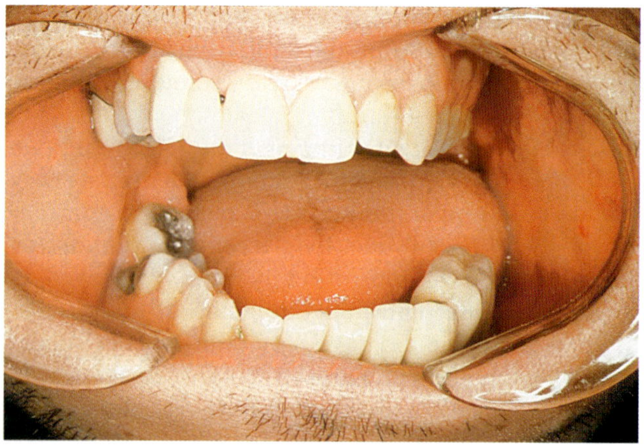

Figure 10.139 Intra-oral view showing permanent fixed denture.

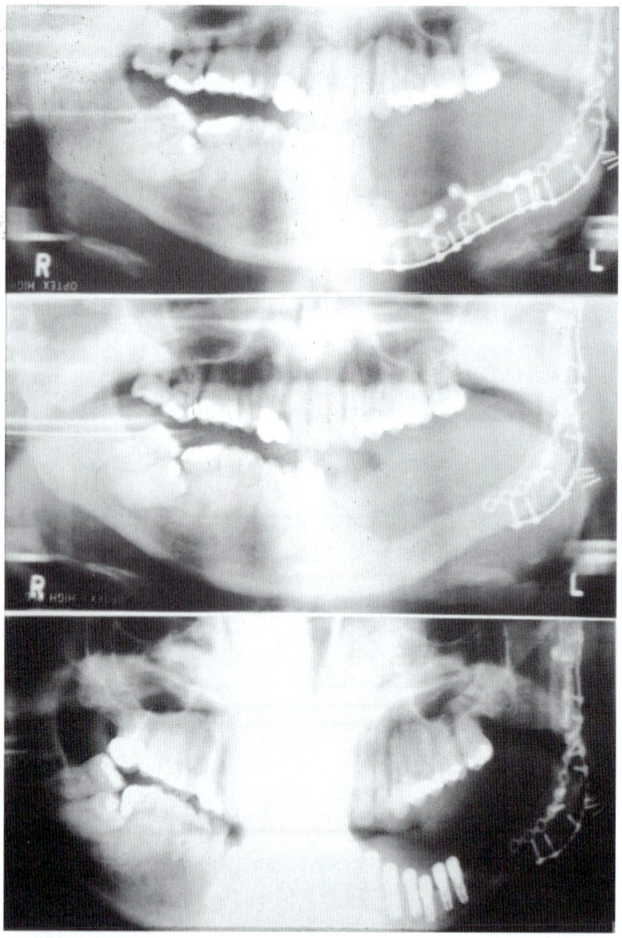

Figure 10.138 Serial postoperative panoramic x-rays of the mandible.

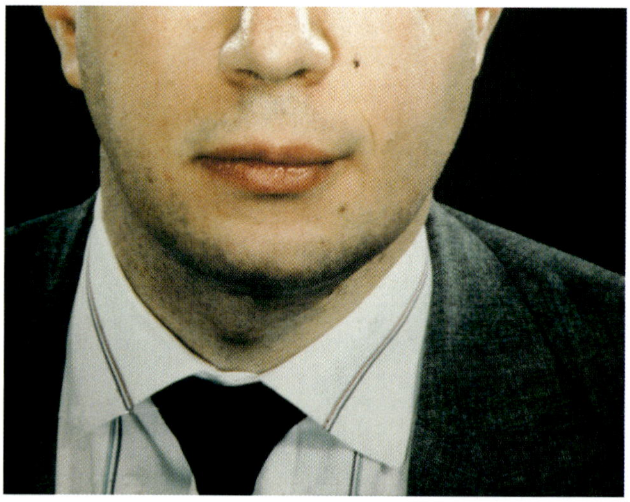

Figure 10.140 Postoperative appearance of the patient.

the involved mandible by tumor (Fig. 10.134). He underwent segmental mandibulectomy. The specimen is shown in Fig. 10.135. A radiograph of the specimen shows the extent of bone invasion (Fig. 10.136). The mandible was reconstructed with a free flap of fibula. The postoperative intra-oral picture shows satisfactory mucosal healing (Fig. 10.137).

Osseointegrated implants were placed after satisfactory healing. Serial panoramic views of the mandible show the immediate postoperative appearance of the reconstructed mandible after removal of plates and screws and after insertion of implants (Fig. 10.138). The finished permanent fixed denture is shown in Fig. 10.139. At this time, the patient is considered fully rehabilitated following ablative cancer surgery and reconstruction to restore form and function. His external appearance is seen in Fig. 10.140.

Resection of maxilla for primary tumors of oral cavity

Maxillary resection is included in the surgical treatment planning for primary epithelial tumors of the oral cavity arising on the hard palate, upper gum, upper gingivo-buccal sulcus and anterior aspect of the soft palate. If the primary tumor involves the underlying hard palate or the upper gum, then resection of the maxilla is mandatory. Maxillary resection should be considered even when a tumor is only adherent to or in direct contiguity with the maxilla. Maxillary resections range from simple alveolectomy (A), to palatal fenestration (B), and partial maxillectomy (C)[54] (Fig. 10.141). The extent of maxillary resection is dictated by the location and extent of the tumor. Radiographic evaluation can be used to supplement the assessment of bone invasion, but it must be remembered that early invasion is often not demonstrated on radiographic studies. Satisfactory evaluation of the hard palate requires CT scans in the coronal plane, with soft tissue and bone windows.

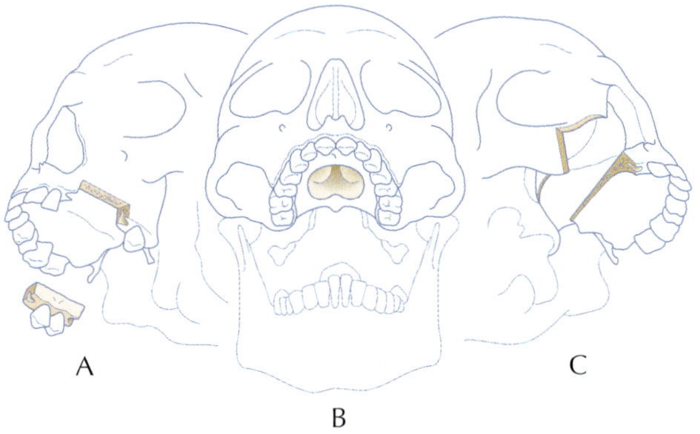

Figure 10.141 Maxilla resection. (A) alveolectomy; (B) palatal fenestration; (C) partial maxillectomy.

Assessment of the status of dentition in the vicinity of the primary tumor is vitally important and is performed in the preoperative setting. If any dental care is necessary, it is completed either preoperatively or intraoperatively, with appropriate assistance from a dental surgeon. Impressions of the upper alveolus and hard palate are obtained preoperatively if any part of the upper gum or hard palate is to be resected with resultant communication between the oral cavity and the nasal cavity or the maxillary antrum. The impressions are used to make dental cast models, which facilitate fabrication of an immediate surgical obturator to be used intraoperatively for restoration of the palatal defect.

The final dental prosthesis with teeth is fabricated approximately 3 months after surgery. This dental prosthesis effectively plugs the surgical defect and also incorporates the remaining denture. When inserted in the oral cavity, the prosthesis provides satisfactory restoration of speech and mastication. It is important to re-emphasize that in any type of surgery for primary tumors of the oral cavity where removal of the alveolar process or hard palate is indicated, continuous communication between the surgeon and the prosthodontist is essential for the satisfactory outcome of functional and esthetic rehabilitation.

Small lesions which are easily accessible through the open mouth can be resected in conjunction with a limited partial maxillectomy via the per oral approach. However, when access is difficult or the primary tumor is large, then the upper cheek flap approach is indicated. This requires a Weber–Ferguson incision with either a Lynch or a Diffenbach extension, depending on the location of the primary tumor and the exposure necessary. In most instances, if only the hard palate or the upper gum is to be resected, then neither the Lynch nor the Diffenbach extension is necessary.

A modification of the Weber–Ferguson incision is very important for esthetic reasons. The philtrum of the upper lip is divided exactly in the midline from the vermilion border up to the columella, where the incision turns laterally along the nasal vestibule and then follows the ala of the nostril and the lateral aspect of the nose. Esthetic improvement in the cosmetic appearance of the healed Weber–Ferguson incision can be obtained if modifications in the incisions are made respecting the nasal subunits (Fig. 10.142). The incision begins exactly in the midline dividing the philtrum. At the lower end of the columella, it turns lateral and into the floor of the nasal cavity. The incision then exits the nasal cavity, leaving a 60° notch in the floor of the nasal cavity where the triangular portion of the skin of the upper lip is inserted during closure. The incision then follows the crease of the nasal ala all the way up to its superomedial end on the lateral aspect of the nose. A sharp 90° turn of the incision then

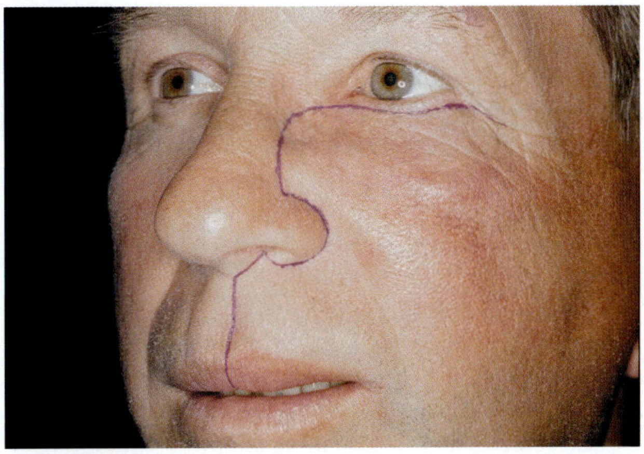
Figure 10.142 Modified Weber–Ferguson incision.

extends as a straight line on the lateral aspect of the nose overlying the nasal bone up to a point about 6–8 mm medial to the medial canthus. At this point, it may be extended up to the inferomedial end of the eyebrow (Lynch extension) or extended laterally just below the eyelashes up to the lateral canthus (subciliary extension). All the angles and corners of the incision are accurately aligned at the time of the closure to achieve a superior cosmetic result.

The patient shown here presented initially with a longstanding history of multifocal areas of hyperkeratoses and in situ carcinomas in the oral cavity. As seen in her intra-oral photograph, she had undergone excision of a superficial squamous cell carcinoma of the mucosa of the right cheek with skin graft coverage several years ago (Fig. 10.143). At this time, however, she developed a new primary carcinoma involving the right upper gingivo-buccal sulcus with extension of tumor almost up to the margin of the previously employed skin graft. The lesion involves the region of the maxillary tubercle of the upper alveolus on the right side. The tumor measures 2.5 × 1.5 cm in its surface dimension and appears to be deeply infiltrating the soft tissues. She also has a diffuse area of keratosis involving the junction of the hard and soft palate, which clinically appears to be benign. A conventional coronal tomogram of the hard palate through the region of the tumor shows erosion of the alveolar process on the right side with thinning out of the palatal bone (Fig. 10.144). Although there is no gross bone destruction, there is an indication of early invasion of the bone by tumor on this radiograph.

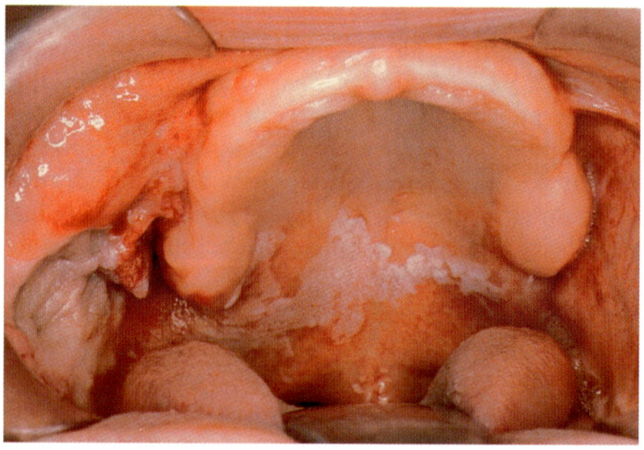

Figure 10.143 Intra-oral view of squamous carcinoma of the right upper gingivo-buccal sulcus.

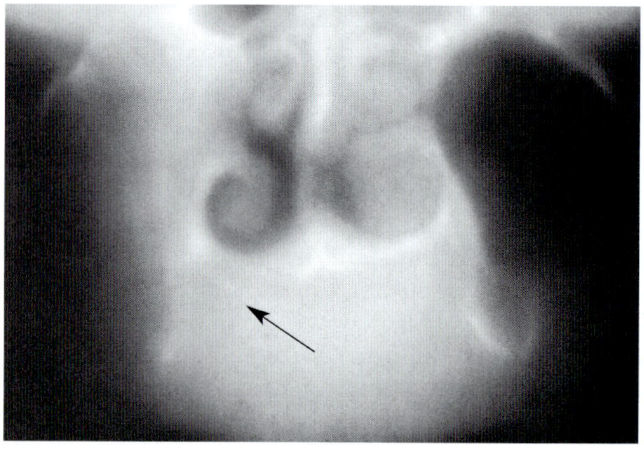

Figure 10.144 Coronal view of a conventional tomogram of the hard palate.

The surgical procedure necessary for resection of this tumor is a partial maxillectomy excising the alveolar process and hard palate on the right hand side, in conjunction with soft tissues of the cheek and the adjacent mucosa as well as the lower half of the right maxilla. General anesthesia is administered with the airway secured via an endotracheal tube introduced through the oral cavity. After satisfactory relaxation is obtained, the head and neck area is isolated as usual. The endotracheal tube is positioned at the left oral commissure and is secured in place with appropriate taping. A ceramic corneal shield is introduced into the right conjunctival sac to protect the cornea. A standard Weber–Ferguson incision is marked, as shown in Fig. 10.145, prior to induction of anesthesia and endotracheal intubation.

The skin incision is made with a scalpel, but afterwards electrocautery is used to divide the rest of the thickness of the upper cheek flap. The orbicularis oris and the musculature around the ala of the right nostril are divided with electrocautery up to the anterior surface of the maxilla (Fig. 10.146). Bleeding is usually controlled with electrocoagulation; however, major branches of the facial artery require ligation.

Following completion of the skin incision, a mucosal incision is made in the upper gingivo-labial and gingivo-buccal sulcus, leaving an appropriate cuff of mucosa attached to the hard palate as a margin around the periphery of the tumor (Fig. 10.147). A cuff of mucosa is left attached to any part of the gum which is to be retained for reapproximation of the cheek to the gum. On the other hand, if the gum is to be sacrificed, then the incision in the labial and buccal mucosa is placed with a satisfactory margin around the tumor (Fig. 10.148). Soft tissues of the cheek are then elevated, remaining directly over the anterior aspect of the bony wall of the maxillary antrum. As the cheek flap is elevated laterally and superiorly, the infra-orbital nerve exiting from the intra-orbital foramen comes into view. Care should be taken to preserve this nerve if possible, since its sacrifice will result in permanent anesthesia of the skin of the cheek.

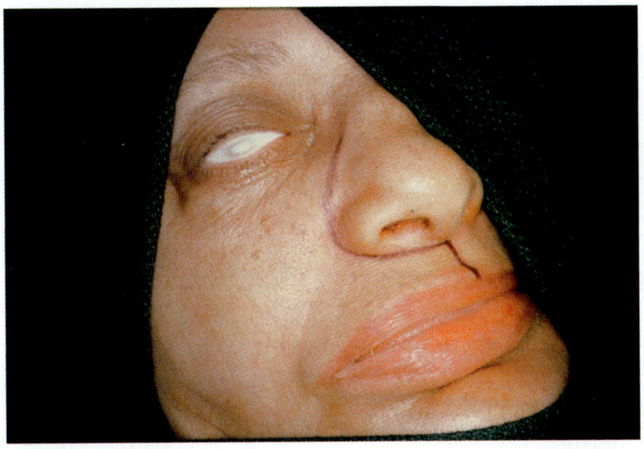

Figure 10.145 The standard Weber–Ferguson incision.

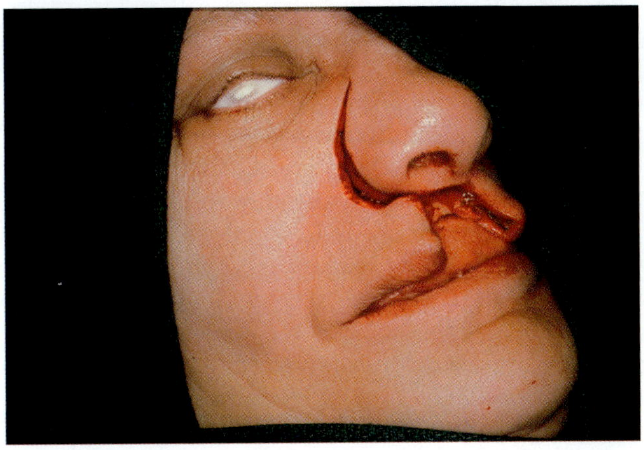

Figure 10.146 The upper lip is divided in the midline.

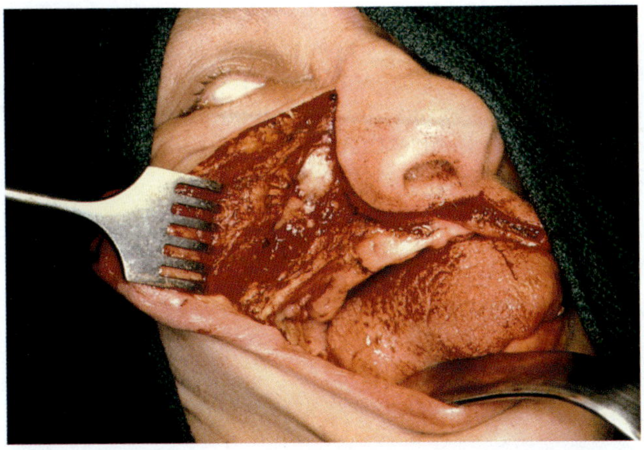

Figure 10.147 The right upper cheek flap is elevated.

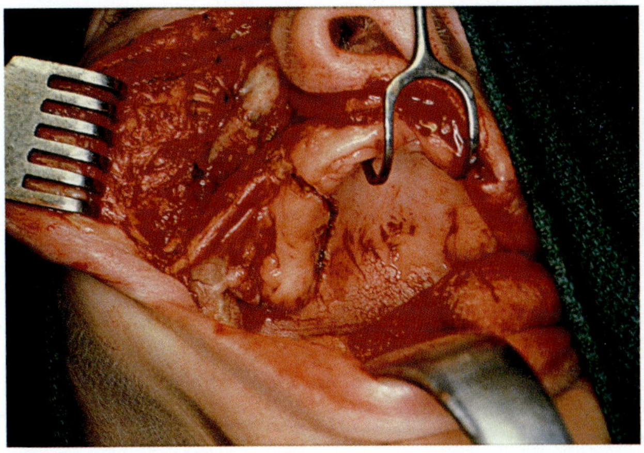

Figure 10.148 Mucosal incisions are marked out.

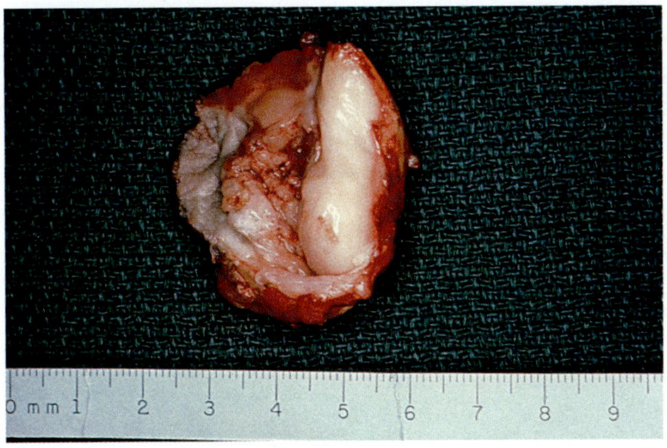

Figure 10.149 Surgical specimen showing adequate margins around the tumor.

Using electrocautery, an incision is now made in the mucosa of the upper gum and the hard palate to encompass the primary tumor circumferentially. The incision is deepened through the mucoperiosteum up to the underlying bone of the alveolar process and the hard palate. A power saw is then used to divide the alveolar process as well as the hard palate through the line of mucosal incision. Similarly, the anterior wall of the maxilla is divided with the saw. After all the bone cuts are made with the power saw, a small curved osteotome is used to fracture the remaining bony attachments to remove the specimen. Final soft tissue attachments of the specimen are divided using a Mayo scissors.

The surgical specimen shows complete removal of the primary tumor with a generous cuff of normal mucosa on all its margins and the alveolar process as its medial margin (Fig. 10.149). The surgical defect following removal of the specimen shows absence of the lower half of the maxilla and the posterior part of the alveolar process, creating a direct communication between the oral cavity and the maxillary antrum (Fig. 10.150). The surgical field is irrigated with Bacitracin solution. If the mucosa of the maxillary antrum is edematous, then it is curetted out to prevent any pseudopolyp formation. On the other hand, if this mucosa appears to be normal, it is best left alone. If the antral mucosa is retained, then a skin graft is not necessary.

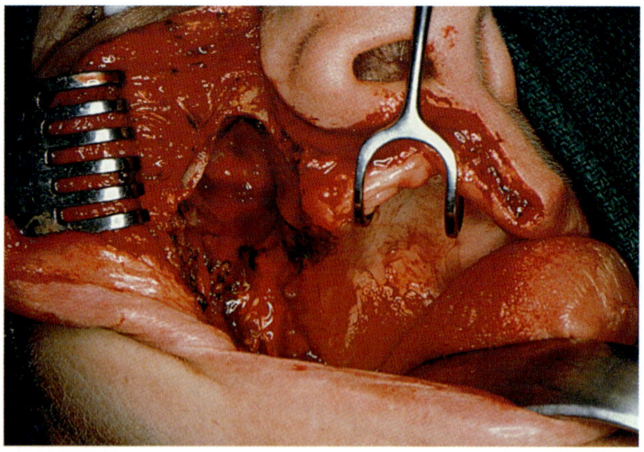

Figure 10.150 The surgical defect following removal of the tumor.

Sharp spicules of bone are smoothed out using a power drill with a fine burr. A split-thickness skin graft harvested from a suitable donor site is used in this patient for lining the denuded bone in the maxillary antrum and the soft tissues of the pterygoid fossa. The skin graft will facilitate speedy healing of the defect and provide a smooth lining over the raw areas.

The skin graft is sutured to the mucosal edges of the defect and draped over the maxillary antrum, where it is retained in position with a snug packing of xeroform gauze. The packing is placed tight enough to stretch the graft out entirely over the raw surfaces of the surgical defect.

A previously fabricated dental obturator is now wired to the alveolar process (Fig. 10.151). Since this patient is edentulous, multiple drill holes are made in the remaining alveolar process, through which wires are threaded to anchor the obturator. On the other hand, if teeth are present, then the obturator is wired to the remaining teeth to keep it in position. The obturator satisfactorily covers the surgical defect, holds the packing in position, and permits the patient to start oral alimentation postoperatively.

The incision is then closed in two layers. Chromic catgut interrupted sutures are used for approximation of the soft tissues and muscles. The mucosa of the cheek is reapproximated to the cuff of the mucosa left over the remaining alveolus with interrupted sutures. Meticulous attention must be paid in accurate reapproximation of the vermilion border of the upper lip, the philtrum, and the skin edges around the ala of the nose.

The skin incision is closed with 5/0 nylon interrupted sutures (Fig. 10.152). Dressings are not necessary but Bacitracin ointment is applied over the suture line. In the postoperative period the patient receives extra humidity with a vaporizer and mask, to prevent dryness of the oral cavity. Clear liquids are permitted by mouth the day following surgery and the patient proceeds to a puréed diet over the next 24 hours. The patient is instructed to use frequent oral irrigations to keep the maxillectomy defect clean. Irrigations of the oral cavity and the surgical site are necessary, particularly after every meal. Occasional minor bleeding episodes may occur from granulation tissue in the intermediate postoperative period while the skin graft is healing. However, once satisfactory healing is achieved, the defect remains clean. A postoperative photograph of the oral cavity, 3 months following surgery, shows a well-healed skin graft (Fig. 10.153). A permanent dental obturator is eventually fabricated (Fig. 10.154). The postoperative intra-oral view (Fig. 10.155) and external view of the patient (Fig. 10.156) show an excellent esthetic result.

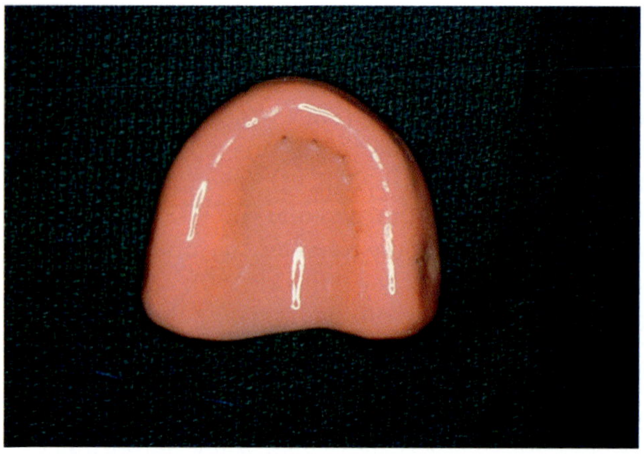

Figure 10.151 Immediate surgical dental obturator.

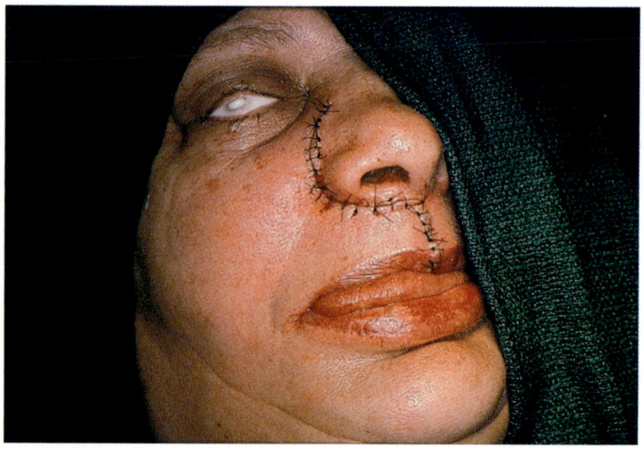

Figure 10.152 The incision is closed in two layers.

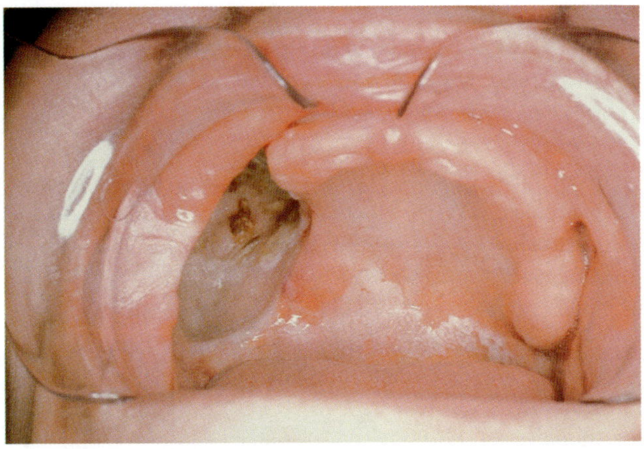

Figure 10.153 Postoperative intra-oral view showing a healed skin graft.

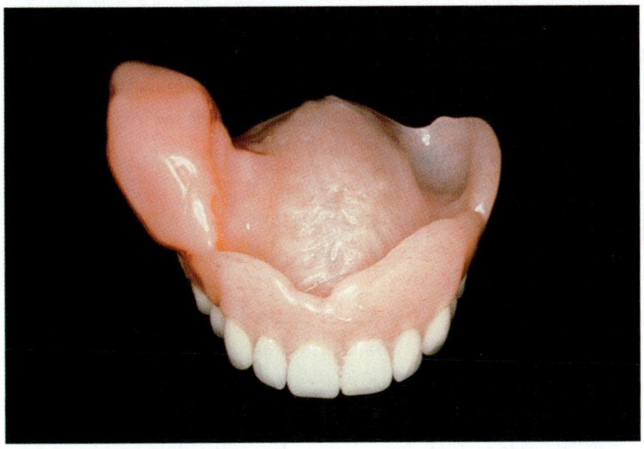

Figure 10.154 Permanent dental obturator.

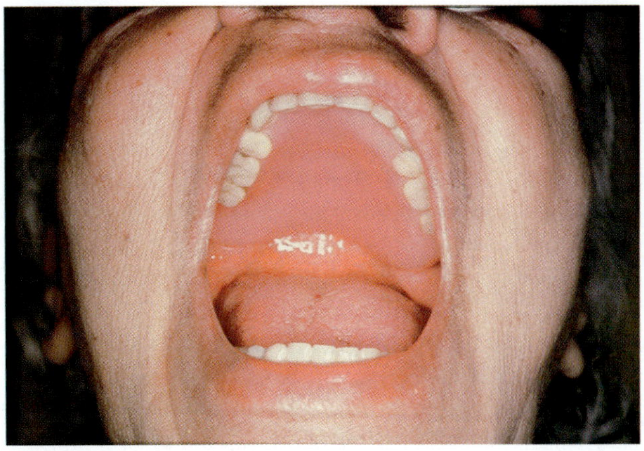

Figure 10.155 Dental obturator covering the maxillectomy defect.

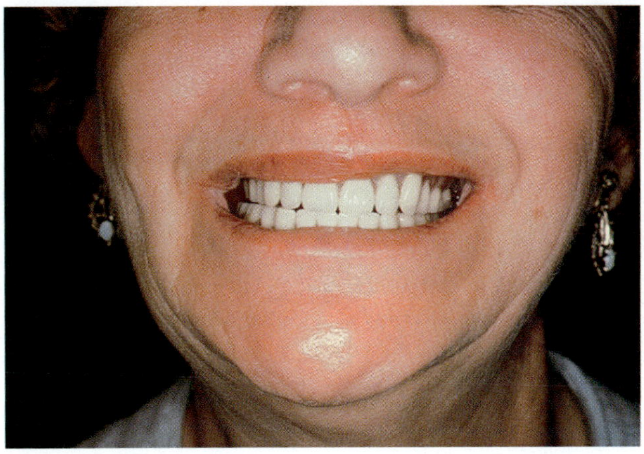

Figure 10.156 Postoperative appearance of the patient, with dental obturator.

References

1. Shah JP, Candela FC, Poddar AK. The patterns of cervical lymph node metastases from squamous carcinoma of the oral cavity. Cancer 1990; 66: 109–113
2. Shah JP. Surgical treatment of tumors of the oral cavity. In: Thawley S, Panje W (eds). Comprehensive management of head and neck tumors. Philadelphia: WB Saunders, 1986
3. Shah JP, Cendon RA, Farr HW, Strong EW. Carcinoma of the oral cavity: factors affecting treatment failure at the primary site and neck. Am J Surg 1976; 132: 504–507
4. Shaha AR, Spiro RH, Shah JP, Strong EW. Squamous carcinoma of the floor of the mouth. Am J Surg 1984; 148: 455–459
5. Shaha AR. Preoperative evaluation of the mandible in carcinoma of the floor of mouth. Head Neck 1991; 13: 398–402
6. Shaha AR. Preoperative evaluation of the mandible in patients with carcinoma of the floor of mouth. Head Neck 1991; 13: 398–402
7. Spiro RH, Strong EW. Epidermoid carcinoma of the mobile tongue. Treatment by partial glossectomy alone. Am J Surg 1971; 122: 707–710
8. Spiro RH, Strong EW. Epidermoid carcinoma of the oral cavity and oropharynx. Elective vs therapeutic radical neck dissection as treatment. Arch Surg 1973; 107: 382–384
9. Spiro RH, Strong EW. Discontinuous partial glossectomy and radical neck dissection in selected patients with epidermoid carcinoma of the mobile tongue. Am J Surg 1973; 126: 544–546
10. Spiro RH, Alfonso AE, Farr HW, Strong EW. Cervical node metastasis from epidermoid carcinoma of the oral cavity and oropharynx. A critical assessment of current staging. Am J Surg 1974; 128: 562–567
11. Spiro RH, Strong EW. Surgical treatment of cancer of the tongue. Surg Clin North Am 1974; 54: 759–765
12. Spiro RH, Gerold FP, Strong EW. Mandibular 'swing' approach for oral and oropharyngeal tumors. Head Neck Surg 1981; 3: 371–378

13. Spiro RH, Gerold FP, Shah JP, Sessions RB, Strong EW. Mandibulotomy approach to oropharyngeal tumors. Am J Surg 1985; 150: 466–469
14. Spiro RH. Squamous cancer of the tongue. CA Cancer J Clin 1985; 35: 252–256
15. Spiro RH, Huvos AG, Wong GY et al. Predictive value of tumor thickness in squamous carcinoma confined to the tongue and floor of the mouth. Am J Surg 1986; 152: 345–350
16. Leemans CR, Tiwari R, Nanta JJ, Snow GB. Discontinuous vs in-continuity neck dissection in carcinoma of the oral cavity. Arch Otolaryngol Head Neck Surg 1991; 117: 1003–1006
17. Leemans CR, Tiwari R, Nanta JJ, van der Waal I, Snow GB. Regional lymph node involvement and its significance in the development of distant metastases in head and neck carcinoma. Cancer 1993; 71: 452–456
18. Leemans CR, Engelbrecht WJ, Tiwari R et al. Carcinoma of the soft palate and anterior tonsillar pillar. Laryngoscope 1994; 104: 1477–1481
19. Leemans CR, Tiwari R, Nanta JJ, van der Waal I, Snow GB. Recurrence at the primary site in head and neck cancer and the significance of neck lymph node metastases as a prognostic factor. Cancer 1994; 73: 187–190
20. Guillamondegui OM, Oliver B, Hayden R. Cancer of the anterior floor of the mouth. Selective choice of treatment and analysis of failures. Am J Surg 1980; 140: 560–562
21. Byers RM, White D, Yue A. Squamous carcinoma of the oral cavity: choice of therapy. Curr Probl Cancer 1981; 6: 1–27
22. Brown JS, Browne RM. Factors influencing the patterns of invasion of the mandible by oral squamous cell carcinoma. Int J Oral Maxillofac Surg 1995; 24: 417–426
23. Campbell RS, Baker E, Chippindale AJ et al. MRI T staging of squamous cell carcinoma of the oral cavity: radiological–pathological correlation. Clin Radiol 1995; 50: 533–540
24. Chan KW, Merrick MV, Mitchell R. Bone SPECT to assess mandibular invasion by intraoral squamous-cell carcinomas. J Nucl Med 1996; 37: 42–45
25. Close LG, Merkel M, Burns DK, Schaefer SD. Computed tomography in the assessment of mandibular invasion by intraoral carcinoma. Ann Otol Rhinol Laryngol 1986; 95: 383–388
26. Curran AJ, Toner M, Quinn A, Wilson G, Timon C. Mandibular invasion diagnosed by SPECT. Clin Otolaryngol 1996; 21: 542–545
27. Muller H, Slootweg PJ. Mandibular invasion by oral squamous cell carcinoma. Clinical aspects. J Craniomaxillofac Surg 1990; 18: 80–84
28. Smyth DA, O'Dwyer TP, Keane CD, Stack J. Predicting mandibular invasion in mouth cancer [see comments]. Clin Otolaryngol 1996; 21: 265–268
29. Ator GA, Abemayor E, Lufkin RB, Hanafee WN, Ward PH. Evaluation of mandibular tumor invasion with magnetic resonance imaging. Arch Otolaryngol Head Neck Surg 1990; 116: 454–459
30. McGregor AD, MacDonald DG. Patterns of spread of squamous cell carcinoma to the ramus of the mandible. Head Neck 1993; 15: 440–444
31. McGregor AD, MacDonald DG. Routes of entry of squamous cell carcinoma to the mandible. Head Neck Surg 1988; 10: 294–301
32. Haribhakti VV. The dentate adult human mandible: an anatomic basis for surgical decision making. Plast Reconstr Surg 1996; 97: 536–541; discussion 542–543
33. Jones AS, England J, Hamilton J et al. Mandibular invasion in patients with oral and oropharyngeal squamous carcinoma. Clin Otolaryngol 1997; 22: 239–245
34. Slootweg PJ, Muller H. Mandibular invasion by oral squamous cell carcinoma. J Craniomaxillofac Surg 1989; 17: 69–74
35. Marchetta FC, Sako K, Murphy JB. The periosteum of the mandible and intraoral carcinoma. Am J Surg 1971; 122: 711–713
36. Shaha AR. Marginal mandibulectomy for carcinoma of the floor of the mouth. J Surg Oncol 1992; 49: 116–119
37. Barttelbort SW, Ariyan S. Mandible preservation with oral cavity carcinoma: rim mandibulectomy versus sagittal mandibulectomy. Am J Surg 1993; 166: 411–415
38. Barttelbort SW, Bahn SL, Ariyan SA. Rim mandibulectomy for cancer of the oral cavity. Am J Surg 1987; 154: 423–428
39. Dubner S, Heller KS. Local control of squamous cell carcinoma following marginal and segmental mandibulectomy. Head Neck 1993; 15: 29–32
40. Dubner S, Spiro RH. Median mandibulotomy: a critical assessment. Head Neck 1991; 13: 389–393
41. Shaha AR. Mandibulotomy and mandibulectomy in difficult tumors of the base of the tongue and oropharynx. Semin Surg Oncol 1991; 7: 25–30
42. Spiro RH, Spiro JD, Strong EW. Surgical approach to squamous carcinoma confined to the tongue and the floor of the mouth. Head Neck Surg 1986; 9: 27–31
43. Marunick M, Mahmassani O, Siddoway J, Klein B. Prospective analysis of masticatory function following lateral mandibulotomy. J Surg Oncol 1991; 47: 92–97
44. Altman K, Bailey BM. Non-union of mandibulotomy sites following irradiation for squamous cell carcinoma of the oral cavity. Br J Oral Maxillofac Surg 1996; 34: 62–65
45. Sullivan PK, Fabian R, Driscoll D. Mandibular osteotomies for tumor extirpation: the advantages of rigid fixation. Laryngoscope 1992; 102: 73–80
46. Beecroft WA, Sako K, Razack MS, Shedd DP. Mandible preservation in the treatment of cancer of the floor of the mouth. J Surg Oncol 1982; 19: 171–175
47. Fleming WB. Marginal resection of the mandible in treatment of cancer of the floor of the mouth. Aust N Z J Surg 1987; 57: 521–525
48. Randall CJ, Eyre J, Davies D, Walsh-Waring GP. Marginal mandibulectomy for malignant disease: indications, rationale, and results. J Laryngol Otol 1987; 101: 676–684
49. Shah JP, Kumaraswamy SV, Kulkarni V. Comparative evaluation of fixation methods after mandibulotomy for oropharyngeal tumors. Am J Surg 1993; 166: 431–434

50. Zlotolow IM, Huryn JM, Piro JD, Lenchewski E, Hidalgo DA. Osseointegrated implants and functional prosthetic rehabilitation in microvascular fibula free flap reconstructed mandibles. Am J Surg 1992; 164: 677–681
51. Mounsey RA, Boyd JB. Mandibular reconstruction with osseointegrated implants into the free vascularized radius [see comments]. Plast Reconstr Surg 1994; 94: 457–464
52. Butow KW, Duvenage JG. Implanto-orthognathic reconstructive surgery. A preliminary report. J Craniomaxillofac Surg 1993; 21: 326–334; discussion 335
53. Urken ML, Moscoso JF, Lawson W, Biller HF. A systematic approach to functional reconstruction of the oral cavity following partial and total glossectomy. Arch Otolaryngol Head Neck Surg 1994; 120: 589–601
54. Spiro RH, Strong EW, Shah JP. Maxillectomy and its classification. Head Neck 1997; 19: 309–314
55. Franceschi D, Gupta R, Spiro RH, Shah JP. Improved survival in the treatment of squamous carcinoma of the oral tongue. Am J Surg 1993; 166: 360–365
56. Tytor M, Olofsson J. Prognostic factors in oral cavity carcinomas. Acta Otolaryngol Suppl 1992; 492: 75–78
57. Snyderman CH, Wagner RL. Superiority of the T and N integer score (TANIS) staging system for squamous cell carcinoma of the oral cavity. Otolaryngol Head Neck Surg 1995; 112: 691–694
58. Kalnins IK, Leonard AG, Sako K, Razack MS, Shedd DP. Correlation between prognosis and degree of lymph node involvement in carcinoma of the oral cavity. Am J Surg 1977; 134: 450–454

11 Reconstructive surgery

John F Carew, Bhuvanesh Singh and Jatin P Shah

The esthetic and functional impact of major cancer ablative surgery in the head and neck region can be devastating for the patient. In order to restore form and function and totally rehabilitate the patient, the efforts necessary require reconstruction of anatomic defects created by ablative surgery to restore esthetic appearance and physiological function. In addition to these means of rehabilitation, psychosocial and vocational counseling help through support groups and emotional counseling are necessary for complete recovery. However, in reconstructive surgery two basic issues need to be addressed and they are esthetic and functional restoration. Examples of reconstructive efforts to restore esthetics include restoration of contour and appearance. Examples of functional restoration include speech, mastication, deglutition, and also restoration of oral competence for major surgery of the oral cavity and oropharynx.

The extent of tissue loss from cancer ablative surgery relates to the loss of soft tissue and bone (Fig. 11.1). The soft tissue loss may be due to loss of cutaneous or mucosal lining or the bulk of underlying soft tissues. Ideally, all bone losses should be replaced with bone reconstruction. However, the need for bone reconstruction depends on the site and the extent of bone resection, whether it is in the mandible or maxilla. In addition, planning of reconstructive surgery requires assessment of tissue loss which may be from mobile parts of the anatomy of the head and neck region or from immobile tissues. Special consideration is necessary for reconstruction of resected nerves, blood vessels, cartilage, and other structures critical to esthetics and function.

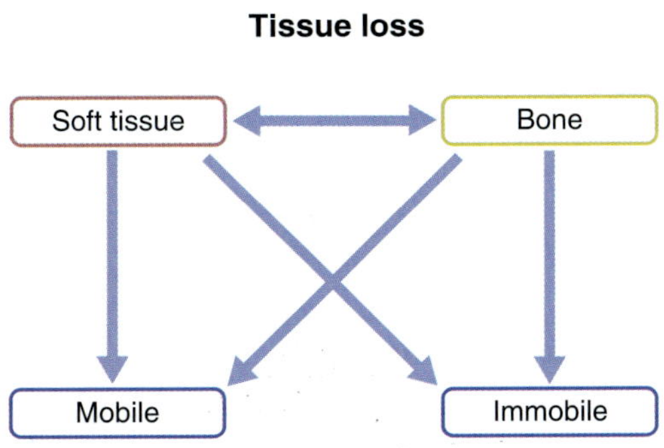

Figure 11.1 Tissue loss.

The surgical defect created by resection of a tumor in the head and neck region can usually be repaired by primary closure if the loss of tissue is modest. The defect may be due to loss of mucosa, skin, soft tissue, or bone, or loss of any combination of these tissues depending on the site, size, and extent of surgical resection. However, if primary closure is not feasible, then viable tissue should be brought over to repair the surgical defect. This may be done by mobilization of local tissues or transfer of adjacent tissues from the head and neck region, or by bringing in tissues from distant sites as free grafts or vascularized free tissue transfer. Examples of non-vascularized free grafts are skin, bone, cartilage, etc. Split- or full-thickness skin grafts are the most popular means of resurfacing large superficial surface defects of mucosa or skin in the head and neck region. Skin grafts in general are acceptable in relatively immobile parts of the face or oral cavity, for example the temple, middle third of the nose, and forehead on the face, and the hard palate, cheek, and floor of mouth in the oral cavity. On mobile parts of the oral cavity such as the tongue, however, free skin grafts are not preferred. The grafted area feels leathery and is non-sensate and, therefore, is exposed to the risk of repeated trauma during mastication. In such instances, surgical defect may be left open to granulate and spontaneously epithelialize. On the other hand, if there is substantial loss of the underlying muscle, then a flap is required.

Thus, the tissue flaps available for reconstruction of defects in the head and neck region may be local, regional or distant. The viability of a cutaneous flap depends on its blood supply, which may be axial or random.[1] In general, an axial flap is more reliable due to adequate perfusion from its identifiable vascular pedicle. The width to length ratio of an axial skin flap may be as great as 1:5 or more, depending on the particular flap chosen and its blood supply. In contrast, random flaps are less reliable due to the absence of an identifiable vessel supplying blood to the flap. A random flap is generally less reliable when the width to length ratio exceeds 1:2. Thus the applicability of random flaps is somewhat limited.

The identification of the myocutaneous circulation has resulted in the availability of a number of myocutaneous flaps which are reliable and have a wide range of application in the reconstruction of various defects, not only in the head and neck region but elsewhere in the body.[2–11] All myocutaneous flaps are considered axial since there is an identifiable vascular pedicle perfusing the flap, providing the blood supply to the underlying muscle and, through perpendicular perforators, to the overlying skin. The availability of the operating microscope and the development of vascular surgery in the earlier part of the twentieth century led to the development of microsutures and instrumentation for microsurgery which opened up the new field of microvascular free tissue transfer. Microvascular free flaps are also axial, since there is an identifiable vascular pedicle perfusing the flap. The reliability of the myocutaneous flaps and microvascular free flaps is therefore comparable to axial regional cutaneous flaps.

Planning of reconstructive surgery for a surgical defect should take place prior to the surgical resection. This is necessary since it will directly influence the surgical approach for resection of the tumor including the planning of the incisions and the availability of appropriate tissue to reconstruct the anticipated defect. Ideally, the head and neck surgeon should have sufficient training and familiarity with the application and techniques of local, regional and myocutaneous flaps in reconstructive surgery of the head and neck. Microvascular surgery requires special expertise by additional training and is best performed by a separate reconstructive surgical team. A well-trained head and neck surgeon with expertise in microvascular surgery is capable of doing the ablative cancer surgery as well as reconstructive surgery with free tissue transfer. However, it becomes a *tour de force* and an exhausting experience for a single surgical team to undertake major resection and microvascular reconstruction. If, however, the reconstructive surgery is to be undertaken by a second surgical team, then the reconstructive surgeon should evaluate the patient preoperatively and discuss the surgical treatment plan with the ablative head and neck surgeon.

Special considerations

Several special considerations arise for reconstructive surgery in various regions of the head and neck. These are considered individually.

Skin and soft tissues of the face

Loss of the superficial surface lining of the skin of the face or neck can be easily replaced with either a split- or a full-thickness skin graft. However, when major tissue loss entails resection of underlying soft tissues in addition to the overlying skin, then more elaborate reconstructive effort is required. The choices available for reconstruction of major three-dimensional defects of skin and soft tissues of the face and neck are regional cutaneous flaps, including forehead, cervical and delto-pectoral flaps.[12,13] Regional myocutaneous flaps such as the pectoralis major and vertical trapezius flap can also be used under select circumstances.[2–4,7,8,14] Examples of microvascular free flaps applicable in these situations include the radial forearm free flap,[15–17] latissimus dorsi free flap,[5] scapula free flap,[18,19] rectus abdominis,[20–23] and groin free flap.[24–27]

Oral cavity

The goals of reconstructive surgery of the oral cavity are related to functional restoration and esthetic appearance. The factors to be considered in functional reconstruction are oral competency, mobility of the tongue, clarity of speech, mastication, bolus transport, avoidance of nasal regurgitation and aspiration, and, when feasible, restoration of tactile sensations. Esthetic considerations include restoration of bony framework, soft tissue contour, chin protrusion, mobility of the lower jaw, and restoration of oral competence and skin sensations. Major ablative surgery for tumors of the oral cavity may result in loss of mucosa, submucosal soft tissues, underlying musculature, and the overlying skin or underlying bony framework. Superficial small defects of mucosa and underlying soft tissues in the oral cavity can be repaired by primary closure or a split thickness skin graft. More elaborate reconstruction using regional cutaneous or myocutaneous flaps or microvascular free flaps, particularly the radial forearm free flap, may be required to line a large area in the oral cavity. Resection of the upper alveolus seldom requires any major reconstructive effort since a dental prosthesis is usually satisfactory. However, if total obliteration of the communication between the oral cavity and nasal cavity or maxillary antrum is desired, then a microvascular free flap remains the only viable option to achieve that goal. Resection of the lower alveolus with marginal mandibulectomy usually does not require any special reconstructive effort to restore bone loss. Bone augmentation with hydroxyapatite and/or vestibuloplasty with skin graft may be necessary to restore sulci to facilitate fabrication and use of removable dentures. On the other hand, segmental mandibulectomy of any part of the mandible requires appropriate planning to reconstruct the resected bone with a short segment of non-vascularized free bone graft, a metallic plate, or a microvascular composite free flap of bone and soft tissues, with or without skin.

Reconstruction with flaps

Local flaps

Local flaps may be employed in the closure of small surgical defects which cannot be repaired primarily. A local flap may be mucosal or cutaneous depending on the location and need for repair of a particular situation. Examples of mucosal flaps are the tongue flap and pharyngeal wall flap. Both of these are myomucosal flaps. A palatal flap, on the other hand, is a mucoperiosteal flap.

The tongue flap has been used in the past for repair of a surgical defect of the oropharynx. The flap is usually based posteriorly and is frequently employed to repair defects in the tonsillar region and lateral pharyngeal wall. Since the blood supply to the flap is random, its dimensions are limited. This flap, however, produces functional disturbance in swallowing due to distortion in the anatomic configuration of the base of the tongue and its mobility, and therefore is not recommended for routine application in lateral pharyngeal defects.

The pharyngeal wall flap may be used for repair of surgical defects in the oropharynx or hypopharynx. A myomucosal flap from the posterior pharyngeal wall is usually rotated laterally to repair a defect of the lateral pharyngeal wall. The applicability of this flap is also limited because of its random blood supply, limited size, and limited arc of rotation. On the other hand, a palatal mucoperiosteal flap has a good blood supply from the palatine artery. This flap is quite reliable for the repair of small through-and-through palatal defects or for repair of a post-surgical oronasal fistula.

A number of local cutaneous flaps are available for repair of surgical defects on the skin of the face and neck. Examples of local flaps of the skin are the nasolabial flap, glabellar flap, rhomboid flap, bilobed flap, and cervical flap. The nasolabial flap is an axial flap based on the nasolabial branch of the facial artery. It may be based inferiorly or superiorly and is generally used to repair skin defects on the nose and upper lip. It may also be used to repair small intra-oral defects, but requires two stages to accomplish the goal. The rhomboid flap was described by Limberg, a mathematician, and is a random flap that is designed by including the planned resection in the shape of a rhomboid.[28] It rotates a local skin flap to fill the rhomboid defect. The bilobed flap is also a random flap and is often utilized for closure of superficial cheek defects. The cervical flap is also a random flap and is thus designed with a width to length ratio not exceeding 1:3 and uses tissue rotated up from the neck. It may be used to close superficial defects on the chin.

Regional cutaneous flaps

Regional cutaneous flaps are skin flaps which are available in the head and neck region for transfer from one area to another to cover a surgical defect which cannot be repaired by primary closure or by advancement of local tissues or local flaps. The most frequently used regional cutaneous flaps are the forehead flap, the anterior cervical flap, the posterior cervical flap, and the deltopectoral flap. The blood supply is axial to the forehead flap and is random to the cervical flap.[1,13] The blood supply to the deltopectoral flap is axial in its proximal part and random in its distal part.[12]

Forehead flap

The forehead flap uses a popular and extremely reliable axial cutaneous flap which is readily available for the repair of large surgical defects of the oral cavity and oropharynx. The blood supply to this cutaneous flap is axial and therefore it can be raised with a width to length ratio of up to 1:5. The forehead flap can be used for reconstruction of skin and soft tissue defects of the face, and mucosal defects of the oral cavity and pharynx. It may also be employed for reconstruction of through-and-through defects of the cheek and for reconstruction of the nose. Although the forehead flap is very reliable, it has several disadvantages. The major drawbacks of this flap are that it requires two stages for reconstruction of surgical defects and it leaves a significant esthetic deformity at the donor site on the forehead. This flap should only be employed in situations where other regional, distant or free flaps are either unavailable or inadvisable.

The patient shown in Fig. 11.2 has a locally advanced carcinoma involving the mucosa of the entire cheek. The infiltrating nature of the tumor has led to the involvement of soft tissues and the muscles of mastication, leading to trismus. The tumor extends up to the dermis of the overlying skin, requiring a through-and-through resection of the cheek along with the commissure of the mouth on the right hand side (Fig. 11.3). The patient also has palpable cervical lymph node metastases in the upper part of the neck, requiring a right neck dissection.

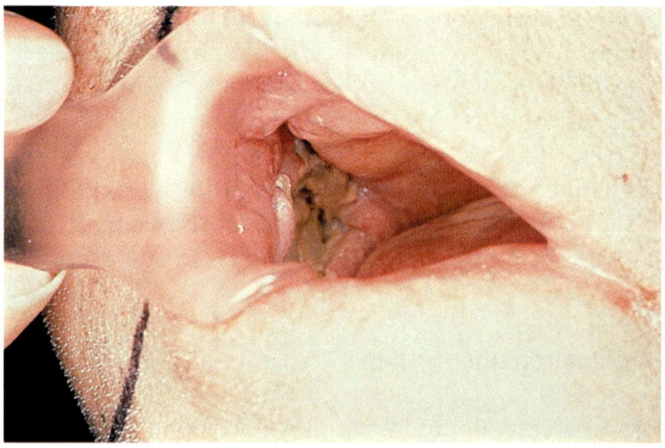

Figure 11.2 Locally advanced squamous carcinoma of cheek mucosa.

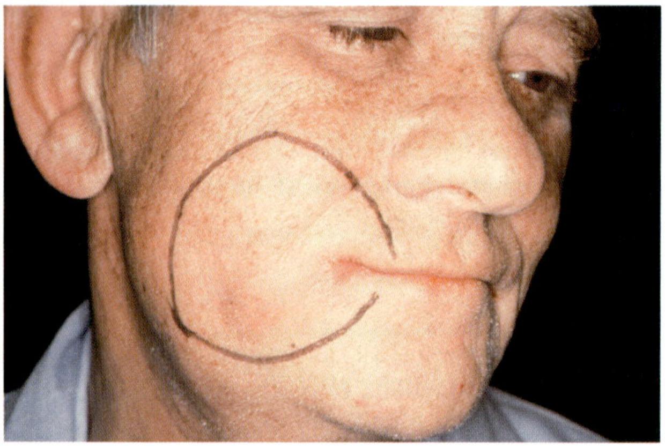

Figure 11.3 Extensive soft tissue invasion requiring a through-and-through resection.

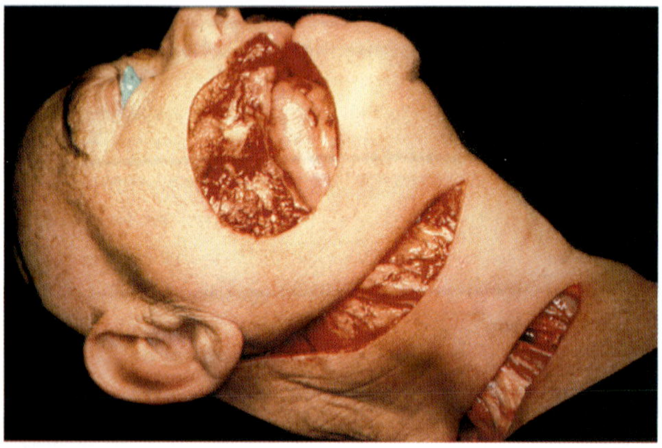

Figure 11.4 Surgical field following neck dissection and resection of the primary tumor.

The neck dissection has been completed through a MacFee incision. The recurrent tumor of the cheek is resected with a generous margin of skin, mucosa and soft tissues, in conjunction with segmental mandibulectomy and upper alveolectomy (Fig. 11.4). A close-up view of the surgical defect shows a through-and-through resection of the cheek with the exposed stumps of the pterygoid muscles

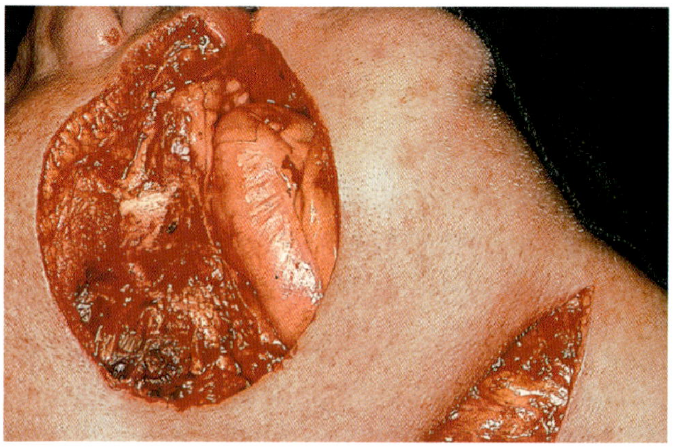

Figure 11.5 Through-and-through surgical defect at the primary site.

following segmental mandibulectomy (Fig. 11.5). The lateral border of the tongue is seen in the center of the surgical defect. The mucosal defect in the oral cavity extends from the floor of the mouth to the hard palate and from the labial mucosa anteriorly up to the anterior pillar of the soft palate posteriorly. A through-and-through defect is created by resection of this tumor.

The external aspect of the specimen shows the excised skin of the cheek, including a portion of the upper and lower lip, with monobloc excision of all the soft tissues and musculature of the cheek including the ascending ramus of the mandible and the specimen of neck dissection on the right-hand side (Fig. 11.6). A medial view of the specimen shows the ulcerated lesion with excised musculature attached to the resected mandible (Fig. 11.7).

The schematic plan of reconstruction of this full-thickness defect of the cheek is shown in Fig. 11.8. In the diagram, the outline of the forehead flap is shown with the tumor of the cheek requiring full-thickness resection. The forehead flap is elevated, extending from the left temporal region up to the right temporal region, carefully preserving the anterior branch of the superficial temporal artery and its accompanying vein, which form the vascular pedicle for the flap (Fig. 11.8A). The incisions for the flap follow the upper border of the eyebrows at the lower end and the hairline at the upper end. The distal incision is placed just lateral to the eyebrow in the temporal region. The flap is elevated superficial to the pericranium.

For transposition of the flap, a tunnel is created through the soft tissues of the zygomatic region by blunt and sharp dissection deep to the base of the flap and the upper border of the cheek defect (Fig. 11.8B). The plane of dissection should be lateral to the zygomatic arch. Extreme caution must be exercised, however, in developing this plane, which

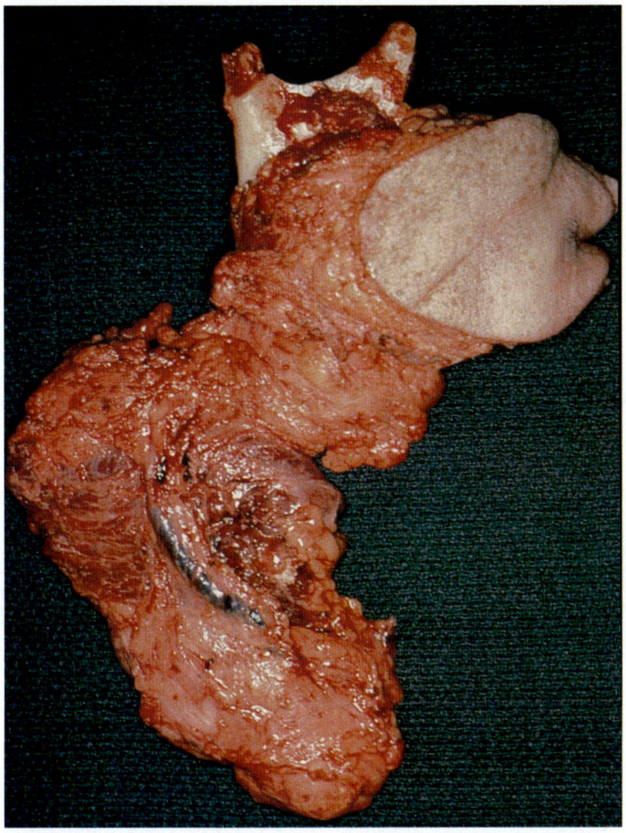

Figure 11.6 Surgical specimen of composite resection of cheek and mandible with neck dissection.

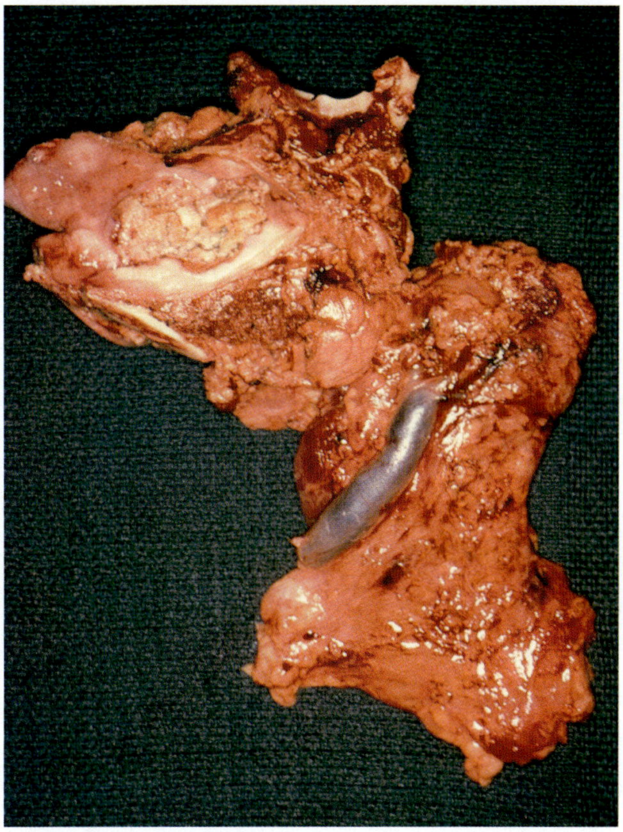

Figure 11.7 Intraoral view of the surgical specimen, showing the primary tumor.

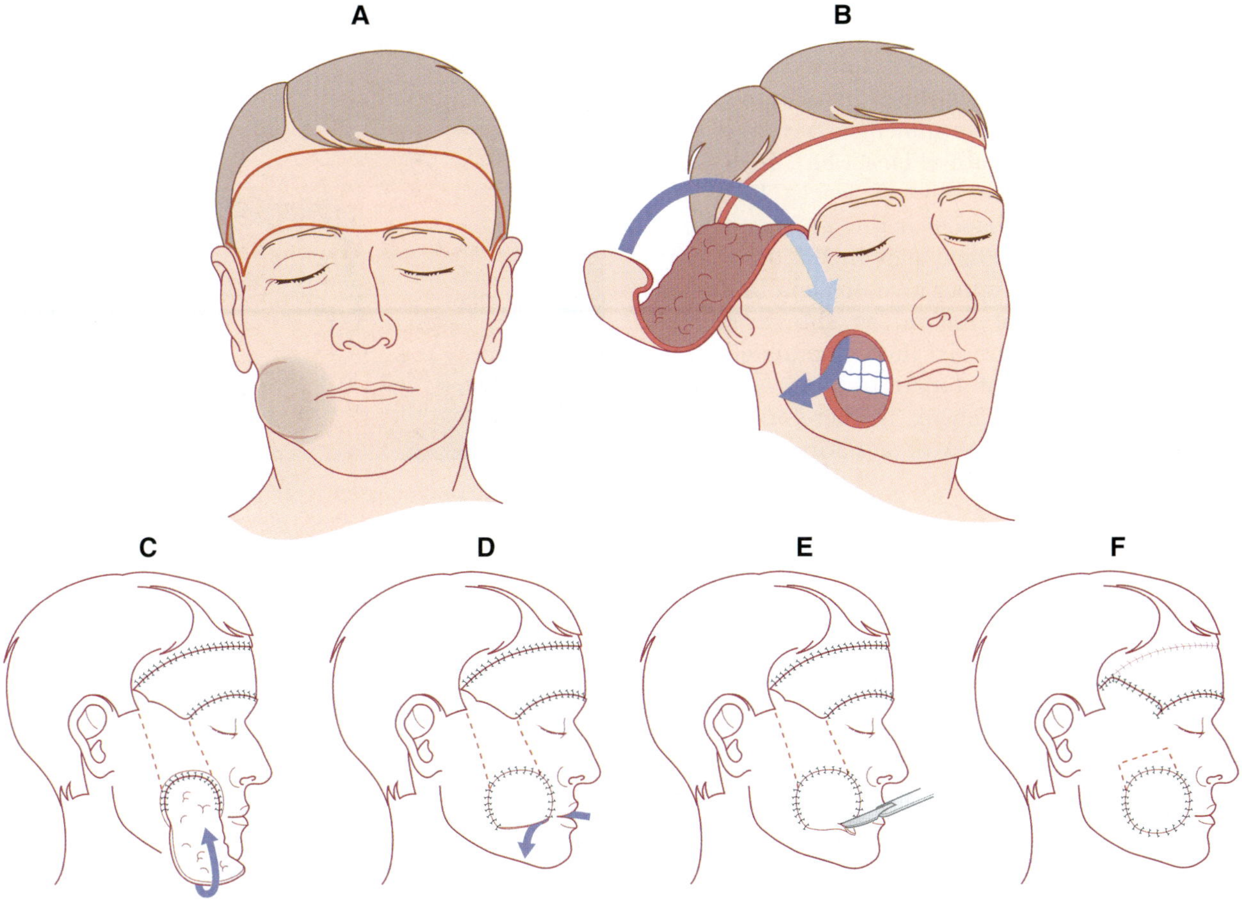

Figure 11.8 Folded forehead flap technique of cheek reconstruction.

should be superficial to the peripheral branches of the facial nerve. Every attempt must be made to remain in a subcutaneous plane, otherwise there is a risk of injury to the zygomatic branch of the facial nerve.

The flap is now folded 180° and delivered in the oral cavity, as shown in Fig. 11.8C. The skin aspect of the flap thus presents in the oral cavity, providing an inner lining to replace the excised cheek mucosa. The flap is then brought outside the cheek defect and turned 180° once again over itself in its distal part. The distal end of the flap is sutured to the margins of the skin defect as shown in Fig. 11.8D, leaving an orocutaneous fistula at the lower portion of the surgical defect. The mucosal margins of the defect in the oral cavity are sutured with the skin margins of the middle third of the flap in the oral cavity. This closure is not circumferential, since there will be a communication at the upper end with the temporal region where the flap was folded and turned in. So at the completion of this stage of the operation, the patient will have two orocutaneous fistulae, one in the lower part of the cheek and the other at the temporal region communicating with the oral cavity at the superior aspect of the right cheek.

In the second stage of the operation undertaken a few weeks later, the orocutaneous fistula of the cheek is closed by dividing the flap at the lower border of the cheek defect, and approximating the skin edges externally and the skin margin of the middle third of the flap to the edges of the mucosa of the floor of the mouth (Fig. 11.8E). In a third stage of the procedure, several weeks later, the proximal part of the flap near the zygomatic arch is transected. The proximal part in the oral cavity is transected near the upper alveolus and delivered back in the temporal region, as shown in Fig. 11.8F. Mucosal closure is then completed. The reconstructive effort of repair of a through-and-through defect of the cheek is therefore accomplished in three stages, over a period of 4 to 6 weeks.

The patient presented here, however, had a through-and-through defect of the cheek as well as excision of the oral commissure with resection of the lateral aspect of the upper and lower lip. In Fig. 11.9, the patient is shown following completion of the first stage of the operation with primary healing between the skin edges of the forehead flap and the cheek. Since the oral commissure is resected, the second fold of the flap is at the level of the oral commissure. This patient does not therefore have an orocutaneous fistula in the cheek, but has instead an incompetent oral commissure, as shown in Fig. 11.10.

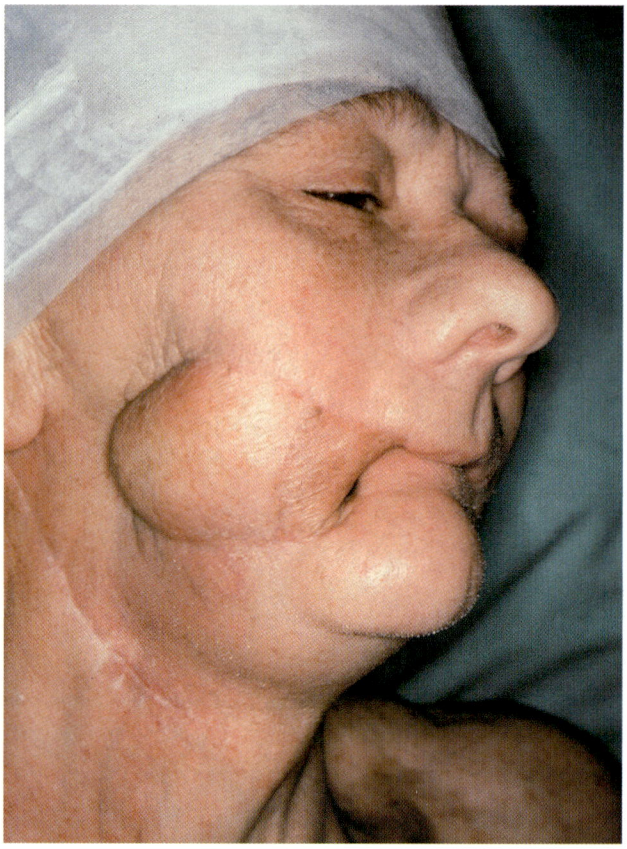

Figure 11.9 Postoperative view following completion of first stage of reconstruction.

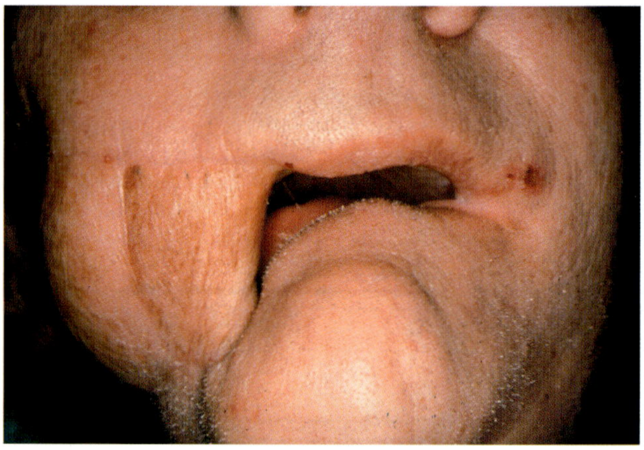

Figure 11.10 Incompetent oral commissure on the right-hand side.

Following the second stage of the operative procedure with division of the proximal part of the forehead flap in the oral cavity and the return of the excess flap to the forehead, this patient will need revision of the oral commissure to restore competency of the mouth.

Cervical flap

The cervical flap is a regional flap with a random pattern circulation.[13] It may be based superiorly or

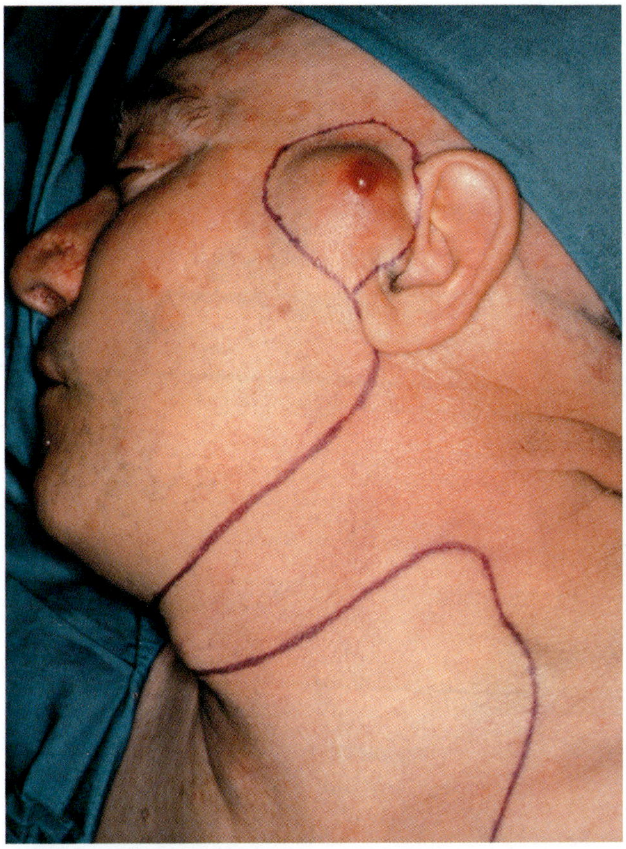

Figure 11.11 Outline of the cervical flap for repair of preauricular skin defect.

posteriorly and may thus be oriented in a vertical or a transverse plane. When the skin of the anterior aspect of the neck is used, it is called the anterior cervical flap, while if the skin of the posterior aspect of the neck is used it is called the posterior cervical flap or Mutter flap.[29] The cervical flap may be used to cover defects of the skin of the face and neck or it may be used intra-orally to repair mucosal defects of modest dimensions.

The superiorly- or posteriorly-based anterior cervical flap is an excellent regional flap, although it has several limitations. Since the blood supply to the flap is random, the width to length ratio should not exceed 1:3. The donor site deformity is minimal. If, however, the flap is wider than 4 to 5 cm, then primary closure of the donor site may not be possible.

The patient shown in Fig. 11.11 has a metastatic carcinoma in the left parotid region fungating through the skin, with palpable cervical lymph nodes from a primary squamous cell carcinoma of the skin of the left temple. The primary tumor was excised previously and at this time there is no evidence of recurrence at that site.

A radical neck dissection in conjunction with subtotal parotidectomy and excision of the skin of the

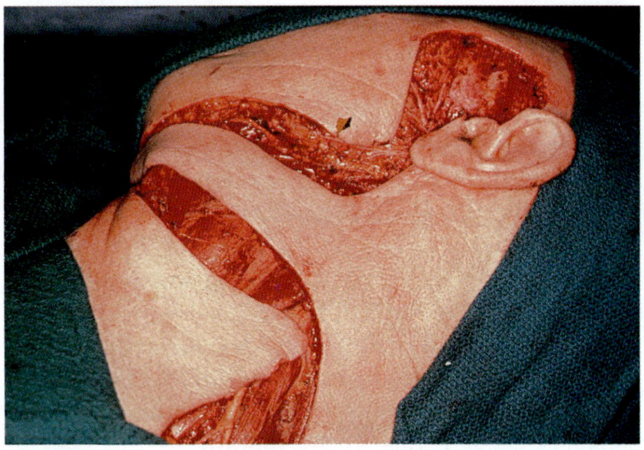

Figure 11.12 Surgical field following radical parotidectomy and neck dissection.

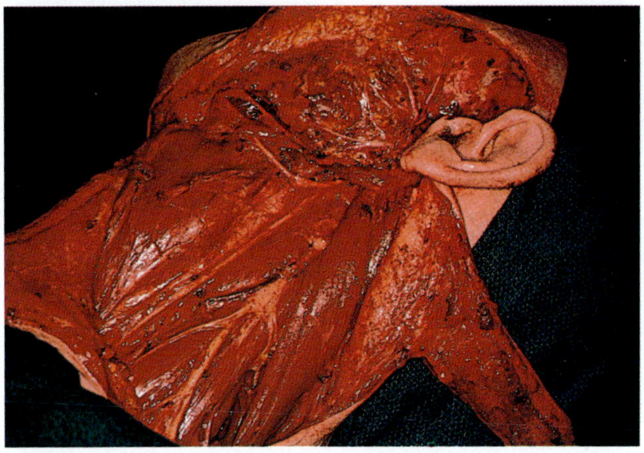

Figure 11.13 The elevated cervical flap.

pre-auricular region to remove all the metastatic disease in a monobloc fashion is planned. The incisions are shown in Fig. 11.11, encompassing the area of skin to be excised in conjunction with the outline of the cervical flap and remaining incision for completion of radical neck dissection.

The remainder of the operative procedure is completed with a standard radical neck dissection in conjunction with a subtotal parotidectomy, carefully dissecting and preserving the facial nerve but excising all the intraparotid and periparotid lymph nodes. The specimen shows the skin of the pre-auricular region excised in continuity with subtotal parotidectomy and en bloc removal of the contents of the dissected neck (Fig. 11.12).

The cervical flap is elevated first, followed by the rest of the skin flaps. In Fig. 11.13 the elevated cervical flap is shown, its blood supply deriving from the posterior aspect of the skin of the neck. Although this is a random flap, its width to length ratio is almost 1:3. However, the distal part of the flap will be trimmed off and discarded if necessary when the surgical defect is repaired. A close-up view of the parotid region shows the dissected facial nerve with each of its branches carefully preserved (Fig. 11.14).

The cervical flap is reflected out in Fig. 11.13 to show the dissected neck. Excessive mobilization of the posterior skin flap is avoided in order to preserve the blood supply to the cervical flap.

The cervical flap is now rotated cephalad (Fig. 11.15). The tip of the flap is brought up to the upper margin of the skin defect in the pre-auricular region. The flap is appropriately trimmed to fit the surgical defect. The donor site defect in the upper part of the neck is closed primarily by mobilizing the skin of the cheek and the skin of the lower part of the neck.

Completed closure is shown in Fig. 11.16. A satisfactory closure of the skin defect in the pre-auricular region is thus accomplished by the posteriorly based transverse cervical flap. Note the presence of a skin fold at the point of rotation of the cervical flap, producing a 'dog ear'. However, in time, this fold of skin usually flattens out and in most cases does not require revision. The surgical specimen is shown in Fig. 11.17.

A close-up view of the well-healed cervical flap is shown approximately 3 months following completion of postoperative radiation therapy (Fig. 11.18). Note that the flap not only provides excellent coverage but also has a very satisfactory color match, giving an acceptable esthetic appearance. The donor site has no deficit and heals just like a routine neck dissection.

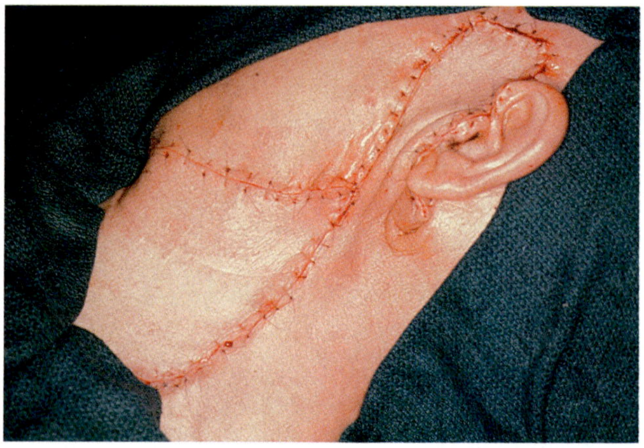

Figure 11.16 Closure of the surgical defect is completed.

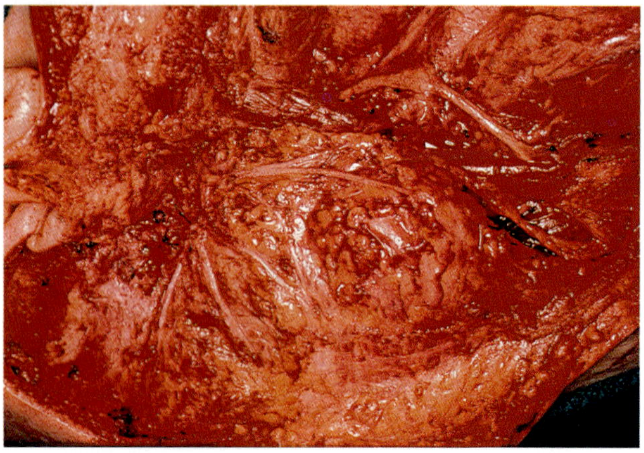

Figure 11.14 Close-up view of the surgical field showing facial nerve dissection.

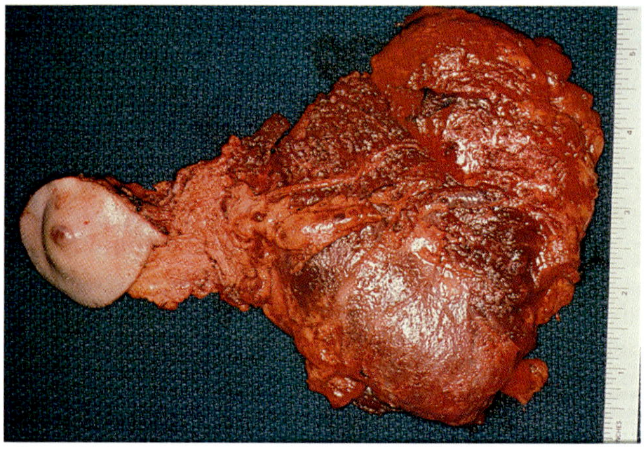

Figure 11.17 The specimen of preauricular skin, excision, parotidectomy and neck dissection.

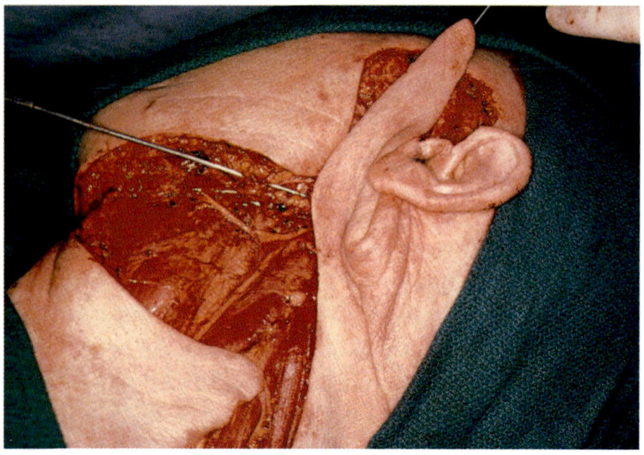

Figure 11.15 The cervical flap is rotated cephalad.

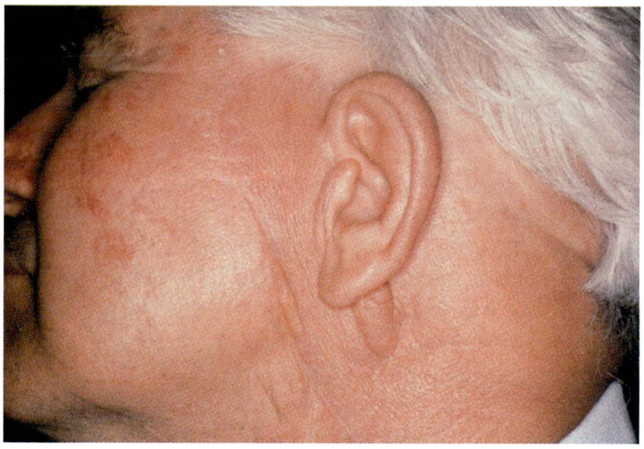

Figure 11.18 Postoperative view, three months later.

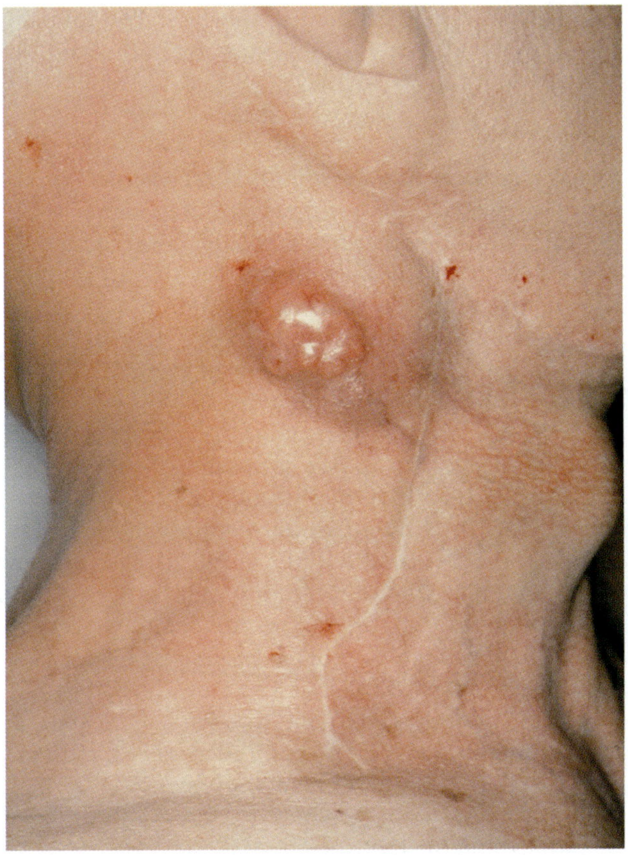

Figure 11.19 Recurrent metastatic carcinoma in a dissected neck.

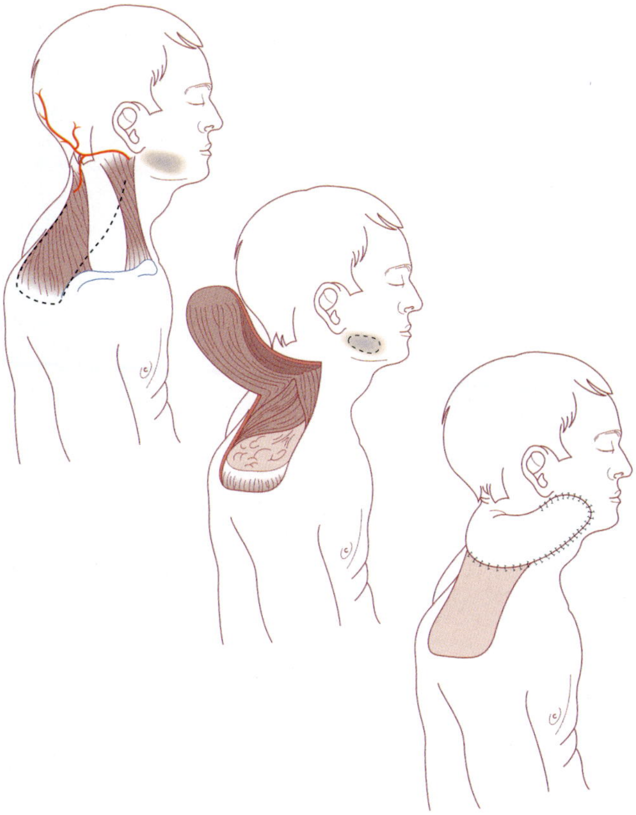

Figure 11.20 The posterior cervical flap (Mutter flap).

Posterior cervical flap (Mutter flap)

A superiorly based posterior cervical flap derives its blood supply from the occipital artery and the posterior auricular artery.[29] Although these are identifiable vessels, the blood supply to the distal part of the flap is random. The posterior cervical (Mutter) flap is a readily available regional flap for coverage of skin defects in the lateral aspect of the neck and the retromandibular area. However, it must be borne in mind that the flap has a random pattern circulation in its distal part and therefore its length is somewhat limited. It also requires a split-thickness skin graft for coverage of the donor site and therefore produces some degree of esthetic deformity.

The patient shown in Fig. 11.19 has recurrent metastatic carcinoma in the posterior aspect of the right side of the neck, which has been previously dissected and irradiated for metastatic disease. The recurrent cancer involves the skin of the neck and adjacent soft tissues, although it is mobile over the deeper soft tissues. Excision of this recurrent tumor will require sacrifice of a generous portion of the adjacent skin and the underlying soft tissues.

In Fig. 11.20 a schematic diagram of the posterior cervical flap and its anterior rotation is shown. The base of the flap should be kept wide enough to include the blood supply derived from the posterior auricular as well as the occipital arteries. However, the width to length ratio of this flap should not exceed 1:3. The donor site in the suprascapular region will require a split-thickness skin graft for coverage.

The patient is shown on the operating table in Fig. 11.21, with the area of skin excision and the proposed flap outlined. Note that the base of the flap extends from the mastoid process to the occiput. A wide three-dimensional excision of the recurrent tumor is performed with a generous margin of normal skin around the visible tumor and a portion of the underlying muscles from the floor of the posterior triangle of the neck as its deep margin. The carotid vessels are exposed in the surgical defect. The flap is elevated and rotated anteriorly to cover the surgical defect, protecting the carotid vessels. The donor site in the suprascapular region is covered with a split-thickness skin graft.

In Fig. 11.22 the patient is shown approximately 2 weeks following surgery. The late appearance of the well-healed flap approximately 3 months following surgery is shown in Fig. 11.23. This cervical flap has

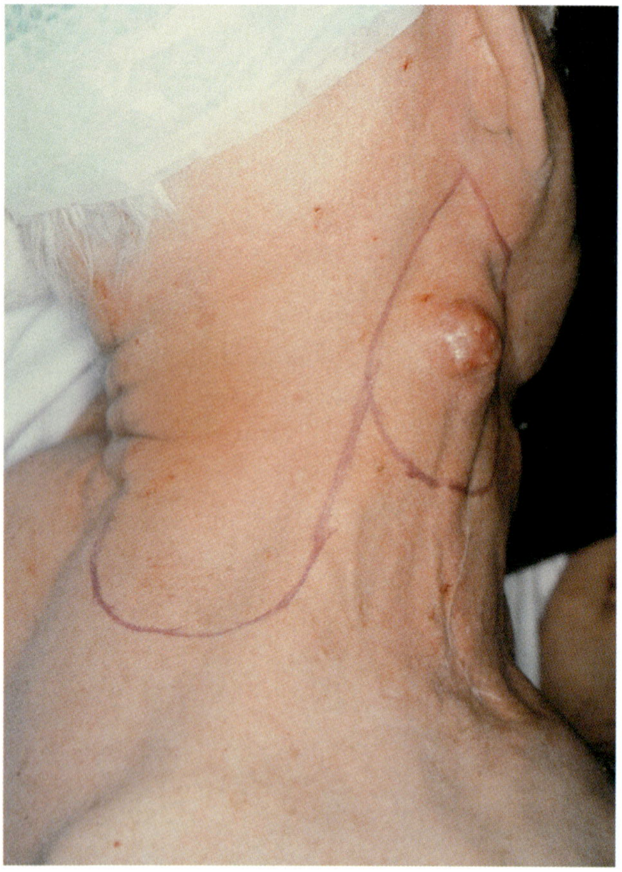

Figure 11.21 Outline of the cervical flap and skin resection.

thus provided an excellent coverage of the surgical defect with adequate soft tissues over the carotid vessels.

Anterior cervical flap for intra-oral reconstruction

A superiorly based anterior cervical flap can be used for intra-oral reconstruction of mucosal and soft tissue defects of the floor of the mouth and tongue. The blood supply to the flap is random and therefore its dimensions are limited. This flap is therefore applicable only in the repair of relatively small defects of the anterior oral cavity.

Although the cervical flap is acceptable for reconstruction of the floor of the mouth, it has several drawbacks. It is limited in its width, length and arc of rotation. The blood supply to the flap is random and therefore its viability is not ensured. The flap requires two-staged operations to complete reconstruction. Thus it is not a preferred choice for intra-oral reconstruction. The availability and applicability of this flap should, however, be kept in mind since it may be used under select circumstances. The optimal choice for reconstruction of similar defects in the oral cavity is the microvascular radial forearm free flap.

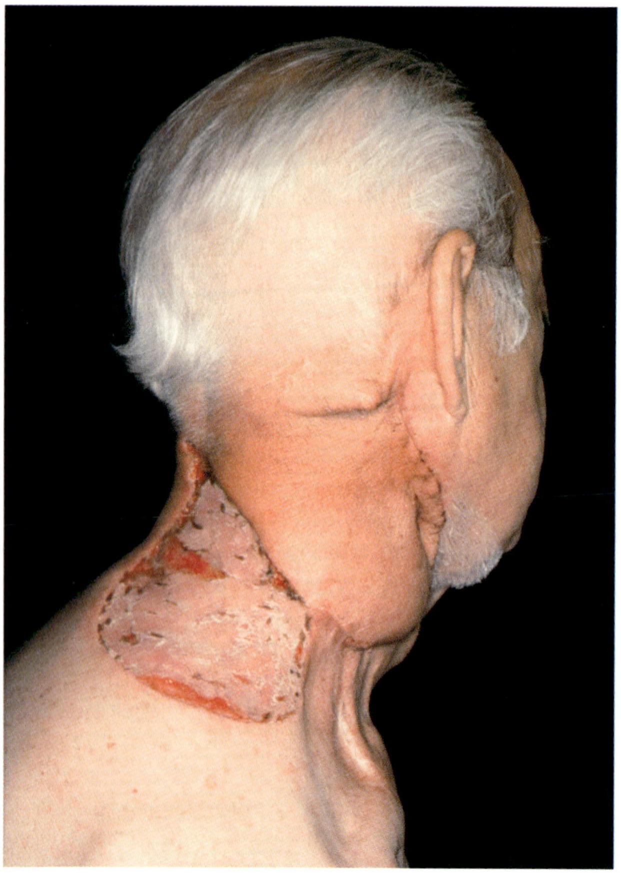

Figure 11.22 Postoperative view at three weeks.

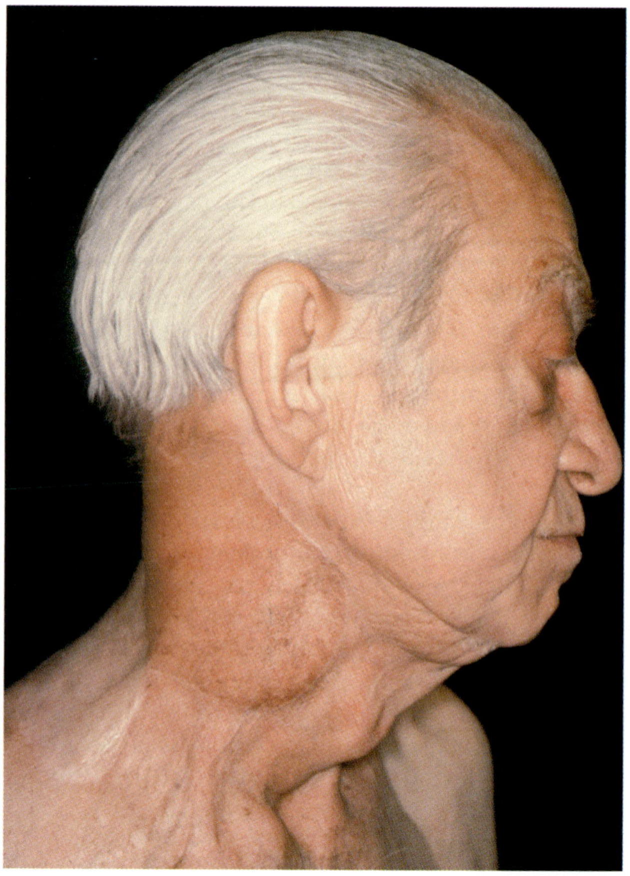

Figure 11.23 Postoperative view at six months.

Medially based deltopectoral flap

The medially based deltopectoral flap was considered in the past to be the work horse for reconstruction of oropharyngeal and pharyngo-esophageal defects.[9,12] The flap derives its primary blood supply from the perforating branches of the internal mammary artery through the second, third and fourth intercostal spaces. The proximal part of the flap therefore has an axial blood supply. However, the blood supply to the distal one-third of the deltopectoral flap is of a random pattern through the subdermal plexus. The skin overlying the deltoid region derives its blood supply from the anterior perforating branch of the acromiothoracic artery. This artery, however, is divided when the deltopectoral flap is elevated and therefore the distal third of the flap derives its blood supply through random pattern blood vessels of the subcutaneous plexus.

The deltopectoral flap can be used for surface coverage of large skin defects of the neck or parotid region. It may also be used for reconstruction of surface defects of the oral cavity or oropharynx. However, it has the disadvantage of requiring two staged procedures and there is a significant donor site deformity.

The deltopectoral flap is useful for pharyngeal reconstruction. Currently, however, it is not considered the optimal method for reconstruction of defects of the hypopharynx and cervical esophagus due to its several disadvantages. The operative procedure requires at least two stages. The incidence of suture line breakdown and fistulae is high and therefore in many instances more than two operations are required for complete restoration of the gullet. A donor site defect requires coverage with a split-thickness skin graft. There is significant delay from the time of resection of the primary tumor until restoration of the patient's ability to swallow by mouth. Stricture formation at the anastomosis between the neopharynx and the cervical esophagus is frequent, requiring either surgical repair, repeated dilatations or maintenance of the patient on a semisolid or liquid diet. For these reasons, the deltopectoral flap is currently not employed routinely in reconstruction of the hypopharynx or cervical esophagus. But it should still remain in the armamentarium of the head and neck surgeon for use under select circumstances. The current choices for pharyngo-esophageal reconstruction are a free segment of jejunum with microvascular anastomosis or gastric pull-up.

Myocutaneous flaps

The description of the myocutaneous circulation in the mid 1970s led to the development of several myocutaneous flaps which have been very popular for reconstruction of various defects in the head and neck region.[2,3] The pectoralis major, the anterior trapezius, the posterior or vertical trapezius and the latissimus dorsi are the most frequently used myocutaneous flaps for reconstruction in the head and neck region.[2–5,7,8,14] Every head and neck surgeon should be familiar with the pectoralis major myocutaneous flap, the most versatile amongst all myocutaneous flaps.

Pectoralis major myocutaneous flap

The pectoralis major myocutaneous flap is readily available for reconstruction of a variety of defects in the head and neck region.[2–4] The advantages of this flap are:

1. The surgical defect following resection can be repaired in one stage.
2. The flap provides a generous portion of skin and soft tissues.
3. The blood supply to the flap is consistent and therefore the flap is highly reliable.
4. Its arc of rotation is adequate for most oropharyngeal and facial defects.
5. The donor site can be closed primarily in most instances.
6. It may be used to provide both an inner and outer lining (two skin islands on the same muscle paddle).
7. The muscular component of the flap protects the carotid artery in the neck.
8. Technically, the flap is easy to elevate and hence requires very little specialized training on the part of the surgeon to accomplish the reconstructive effort.

The disadvantages of the pectoralis major myocutaneous flap are:

1. It can be too bulky, particularly when used in the oral cavity.
2. Its arc of rotation is limited for upper facial and oromaxillary defects.
3. There is distortion of symmetry at the donor site (not appealing in the female).
4. Shoulder function is impaired due to loss of pectoralis major muscle.
5. Distal skin on the flap is not reliable.

Figure 11.24 depicts the anatomic features of the pectoralis major myocutaneous flap. The area shown in blue is an area of skin which derives its blood supply through the pectoralis major myocutaneous circulation, so a skin flap of any dimension can be elevated from this area. Extension of the blue area towards the sternum may be considered under select circumstances if additional skin is necessary. The blood supply of the pectoralis major myocutaneous flap is derived from the descending branch of the

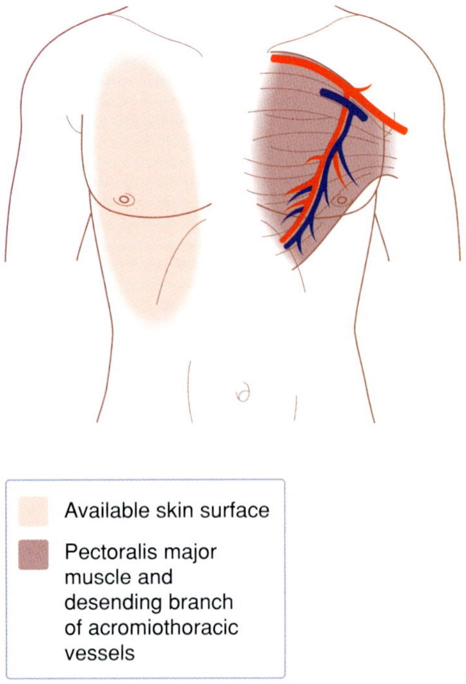

Figure 11.24 Anatomy of pectoralis major myocutaneous flap.

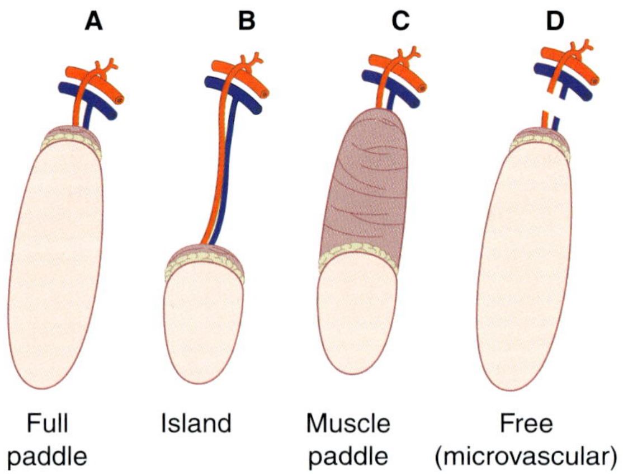

Figure 11.25 Types of flap.

acromiothoracic artery, as shown on the left side. This artery runs directly on the undersurface of the pectoralis major muscle. The acromiothoracic artery originates from the subclavian artery at about the midclavicular point and runs directly caudad towards the nipple. So a line joining the midclavicular point to the nipple is recommended for the surface marking of the vessel. One or two veins usually accompany this artery.

The pectoralis major myocutaneous flap may be elevated in a variety of ways, as shown in Fig. 11.25. It can be elevated in the manner of a full paddle as shown in Fig. 11.25A, with the dimensions of the skin matching the dimensions of the underlying pectoralis major muscle. It may be elevated like an island flap, as shown in Fig. 11.25B, or it may be elevated with a larger muscle paddle and a small island of skin, as shown in Fig. 11.25C. Finally, the pectoralis major myocutaneous flap may be elevated and the vascular pedicle divided for transfer of the whole unit with free microvascular anastomosis at the recipient site (Fig. 11.25D). In addition, the flap may be elevated with two islands of skin to provide an inner and outer lining. It may also be used as a muscle flap to protect the carotid artery or to provide bulk. A pectoralis osteomyocutaneous flap with the fourth or fifth rib can be elevated for mandible reconstruction, but it is not recommended since the blood supply to the ribs is tenuous and the rib is not a satisfactory bone for mandible reconstruction.

Each of the four variants of the pectoralis major myocutaneous flap described above is shown in

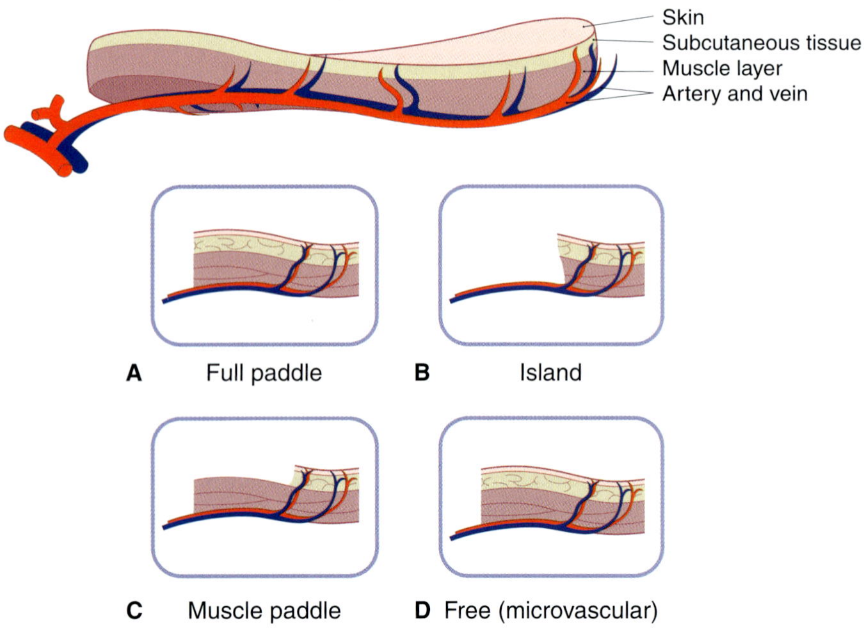

Figure 11.26 Anatomical details of flaps.

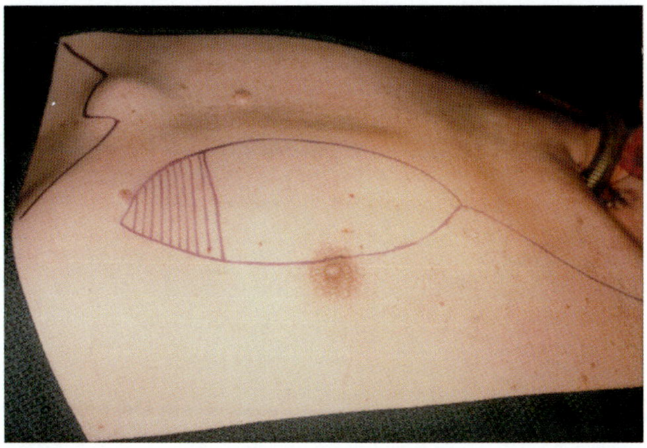

Figure 11.27 The outline of the pectoralis major myocutaneous flap is marked.

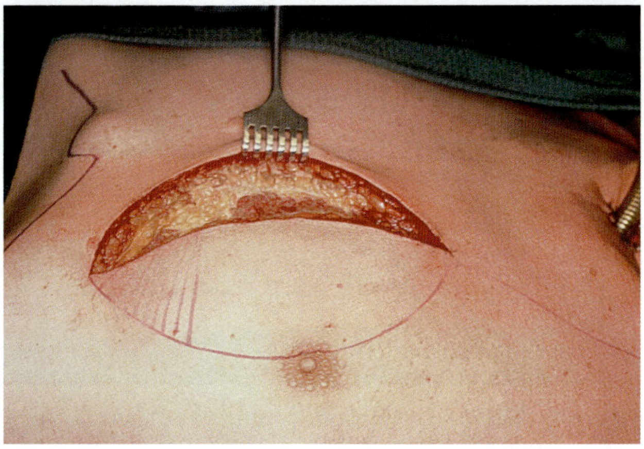

Figure 11.28 Elevation of the flap begins with the medial incision first.

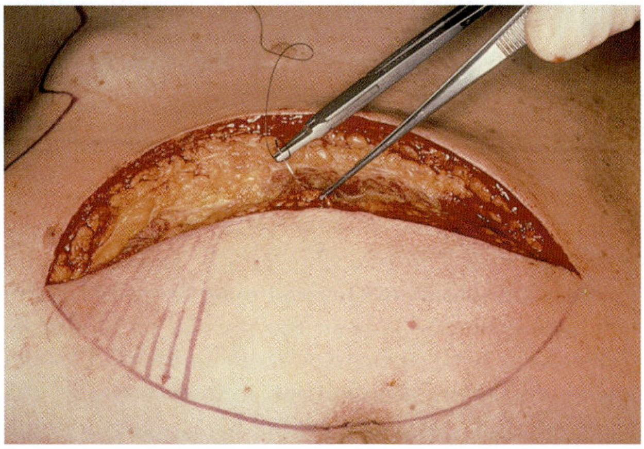

Figure 11.29 The pectoralis muscle is tacked to the subcutaneous soft tissues with sutures.

cross-section in Fig. 11.26, depicting the location of the feeding vessels and the perforating branches providing the blood supply to the overlying skin.

The technical details of the elevation of the flap are discussed here. In Fig. 11.27 the anterior chest wall of a patient who has undergone a laryngectomy and partial pharyngectomy for an advanced carcinoma of the larynx is shown. The pectoralis major myocutaneous flap will be used for repair of the partial pharyngeal defect. The outline of the flap is drawn on the skin. The shaded area on the distal part of the flap will be discarded so that the flap matches the shape of the defect. The length and width of the skin island of the myocutaneous flap as well as the length of its pedicle are determined by the site, size and shape of the surgical defect. The pivot for the flap is the midclavicular point. A tape or string is used to measure the distance from this point up to the most distal portion of the surgical defect. This is the distance from the midclavicular point up to the distal tip of the flap, which is marked out.

The approximate width and length of the flap are then estimated to match the defect and the proposed flap is drawn out on the skin of the anterior chest wall. The flap should never be elevated prior to resection of the tumor and assessment of the surgical defect. The exact dimensions and configuration of the defect are confirmed to match the outline of the flap. Any adjustments in the length and width of the skin island of the myocutaneous flap or the length of its pedicle are rechecked at this point before its elevation begins.

Elevation of the flap begins on its medial aspect first. The skin incision starts from the tip of the flap up to its proximal end on the medial aspect. The incision is deepened through the subcutaneous tissues and fat up to the underlying pectoralis major muscle. No attempt is made to retract the skin and subcutaneous tissues overlying the muscle in the area of the flap since it may produce undue traction on and avulsion of the perforating vessels. However, the margin of the skin overlying the sternum may be retracted to gain exposure if necessary (Fig. 11.28).

Using electrocautery, the underlying pectoralis major muscle is divided up to the intercostal spaces and the anterior surface of the underlying ribs throughout the length of the skin incision. At this point, several interrupted chromic catgut sutures are placed between the transected edge of the pectoralis major muscle and the subcutaneous tissue of its overlying skin (Fig. 11.29). Approximately eight to ten such sutures are placed on the medial edge of the pectoralis major myocutaneous flap. These sutures maintain the entire myocutaneous unit as one block of tissue, avoiding any undue tension, traction or laceration of the perforating vessels to the skin.

If the distal outline of the flap extends over the costal margin, then the pectoralis major muscle will not be present underneath the skin on the distal

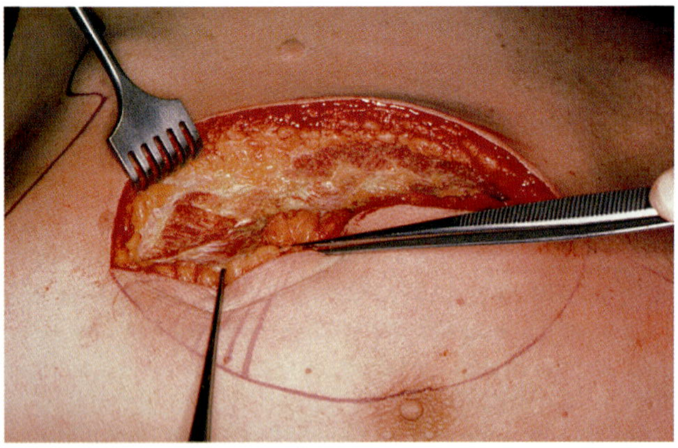

Figure 11.30 The anterior rectus sheath is incised and elevated as the deep layer of the flap.

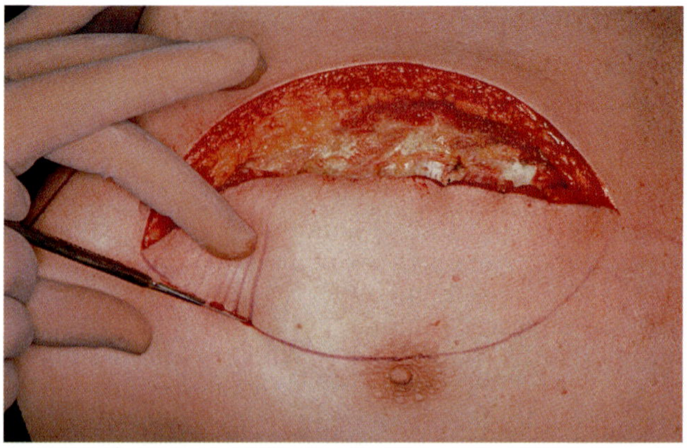

Figure 11.32 The lateral skin incision begins at the distal end of the flap.

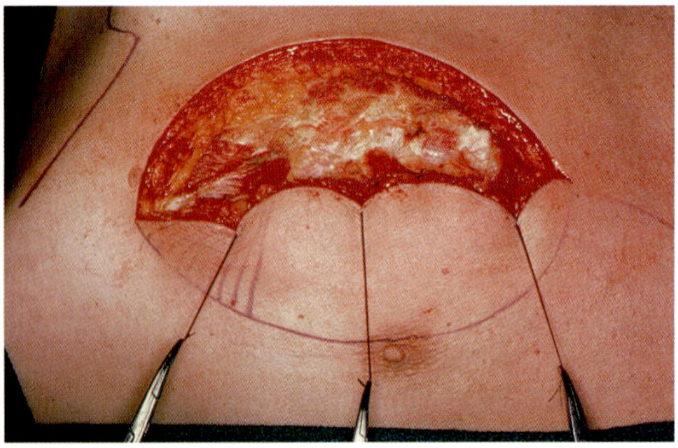

Figure 11.31 Elevation of the medial edge of the flap is completed.

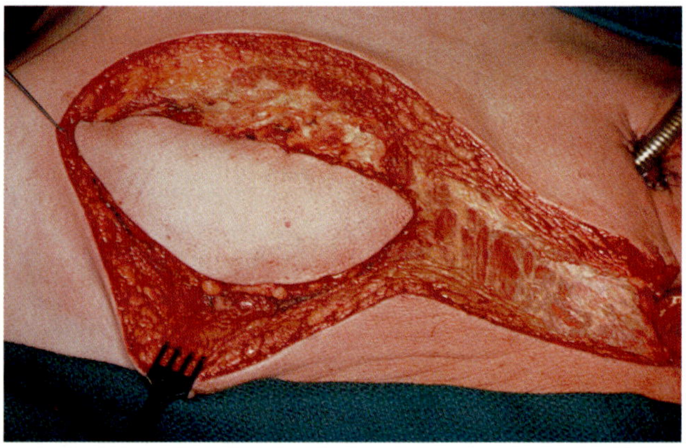

Figure 11.33 The lateral skin incision is extended up to the midclavicular point.

part. In that area, therefore, the myocutaneous flap should be elevated deep to the anterior rectus sheath, preserving the subdermal plexus and anastomotic vessels between the acromiothoracic artery and the superior gastric artery. The subcutaneous vascular plexus is thus preserved, providing the blood supply to the skin of the distal part of the flap. The anterior rectus sheath is thus incised along the skin incision of the distal part of the flap.

Elevation of the flap with the anterior rectus sheath is shown in Fig. 11.30. Interrupted chromic catgut sutures are also placed between the cut edge of the rectus sheath and the subcutaneous tissues in the distal part of the flap (Fig. 11.31). A skin incision is now taken along the outline of the lateral border of the myocutaneous flap (Fig. 11.32). The skin incision is deepened up to the pectoralis major muscle which is, however, not divided at this point. The incision around the island of skin is, however, circumferentially completed. Several catgut sutures similar to those on the medial aspect are put between the subcutaneous tissue and the anterior surface of the pectoralis major muscle to maintain the myocutaneous unit without any disruption. Division of the lateral aspect of the pectoralis major muscle along the incision for the skin island should be undertaken only after identification of the acromiothoracic vessels and their course on the posterior surface of the pectoralis major muscle.

From the proximal end of the skin island, a skin incision is taken up to the midclavicular point. This incision is deepened through the subcutaneous tissues to expose the anterior surface of the pectoralis major muscle (Fig. 11.33). The lateral and medial skin edges are elevated over the pectoralis to expose a generous area of the muscle paddle to be transferred with the myocutaneous flap. On the lateral side of the skin incision in the lower part, the anterior chest wall contains the breast tissue, which is elevated over the pectoralis major muscle (Fig. 11.34). This part of the skin of the anterior chest wall is elevated until the lower border of the pectoralis major muscle is identified.

Adequate mobilization of the skin flaps and soft tissues anterior to the pectoralis major muscle is now completed (Fig. 11.35). The fingers of one hand are now inserted deep to the pectoralis major muscle in a plane between the pectoralis major and pectoralis minor muscles, as shown in Fig. 11.36.

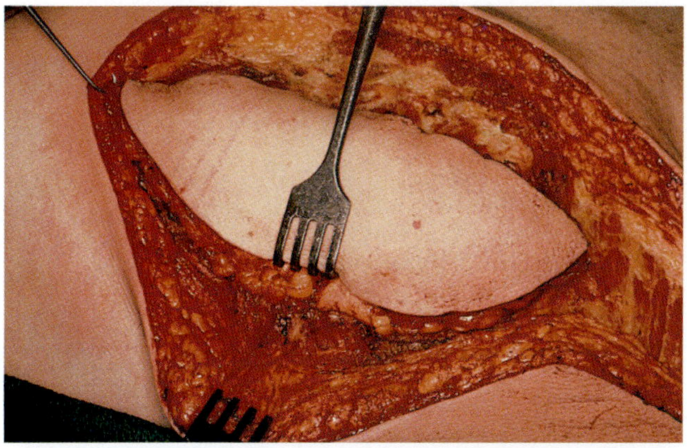

Figure 11.34 The lateral skin flap is elevated until the lower border of pectoralis muscle is exposed.

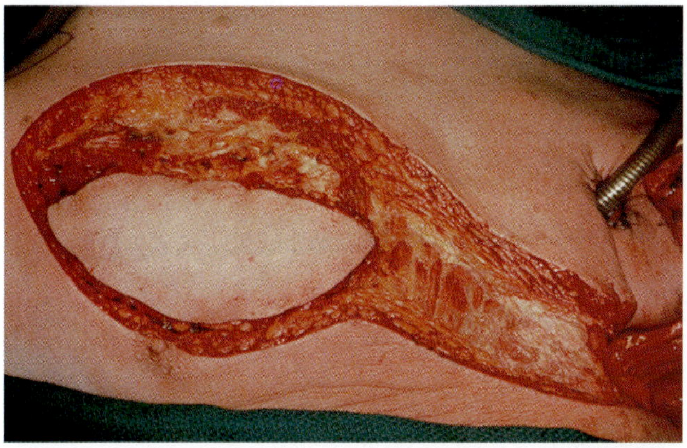

Figure 11.35 Elevation of the skin island is completed.

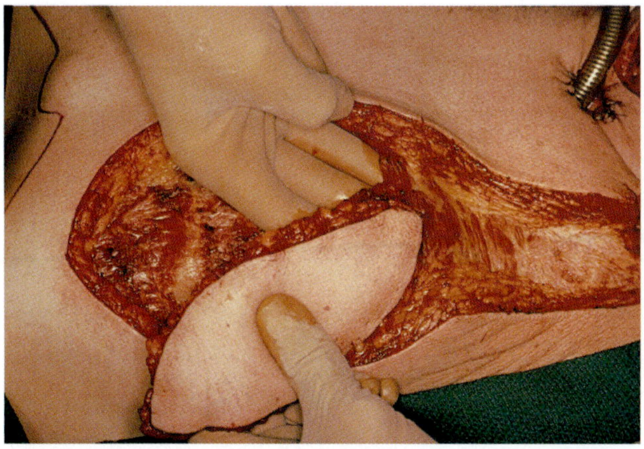

Figure 11.36 The pectoralis major is separated from the pectoralis minor by blunt digital dissection.

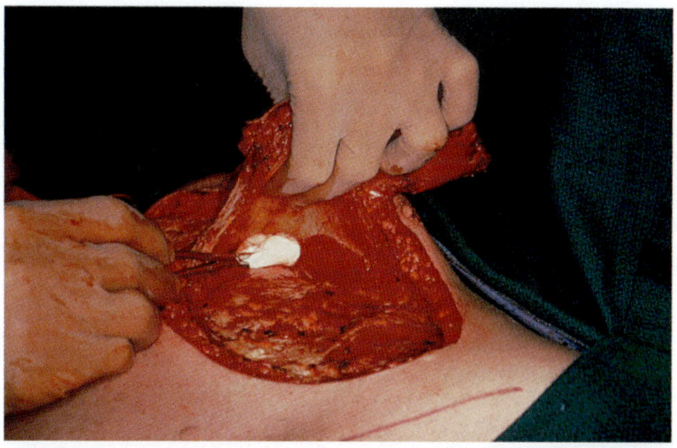

Figure 11.37 The acromiothoracic vessels are identified on the undersurface of the pectoralis major muscle.

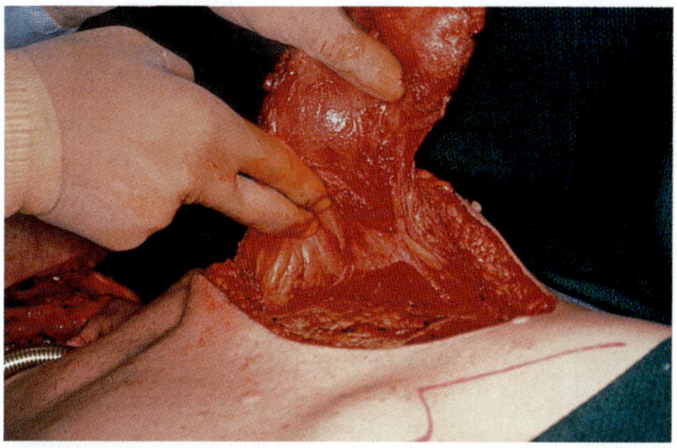

Figure 11.38 Close-up view of the undersurface of pectoralis major muscle.

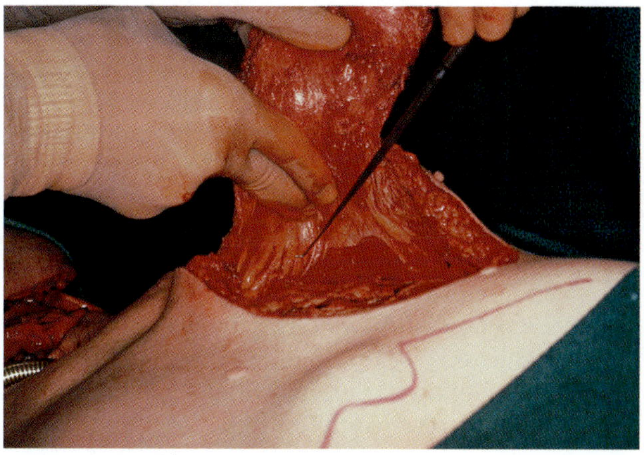

Figure 11.39 The descending branches of the acromiothoracic vessels.

Since this plane contains only loose areolar tissue, the pectoralis major is easily separated from the pectoralis minor muscle by blunt digital dissection.

The pectoral nerve which traverses from the pectoralis minor to the pectoralis major muscle in this plane is divided. The undersurface of the pectoralis major muscle is mobilized up to the clavicle, freeing up its entire posterior surface. The isolated portion of the myocutaneous flap is now lifted to expose the undersurface of the pectoralis major muscle. This enables identification of the acromiothoracic vessels at about the midclavicular point, viewed from the right-hand side of the patient (Fig. 11.37). A close-up view of that area is shown in Fig. 11.38, and the vascular pedicle is pointed out in Fig. 11.39.

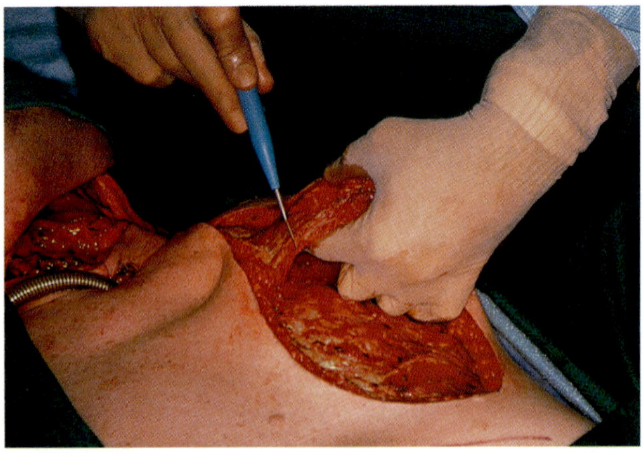

Figure 11.40 The vessels are protected and the medial aspect of the pectoralis major is divided up to the clavicle.

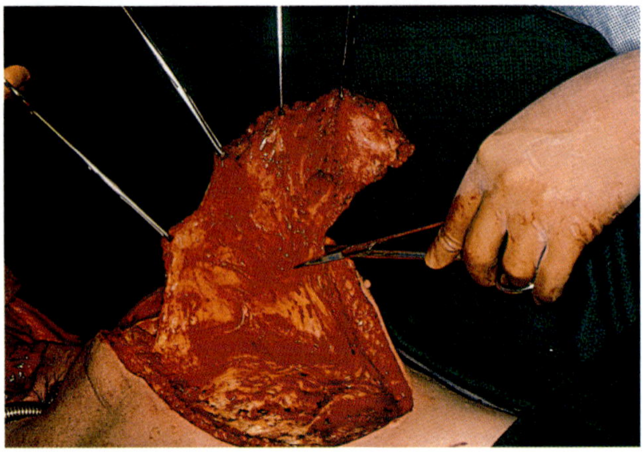

Figure 11.41 The lateral aspect of the pectoralis major is divided.

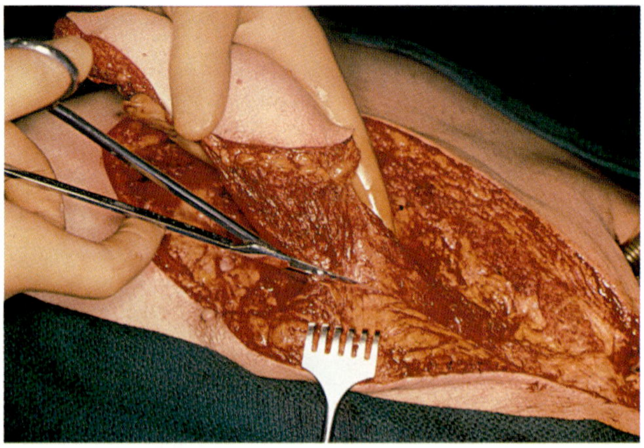

Figure 11.42 The vascular pedicle is protected during division of the pectoralis major muscle.

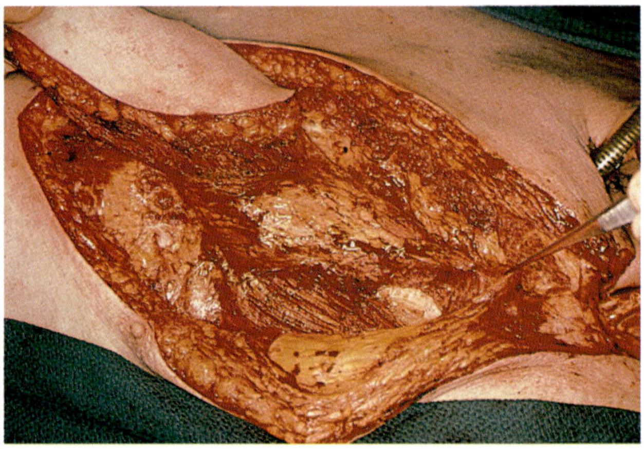

Figure 11.43 Laterally the muscle is also divided up to the clavicle.

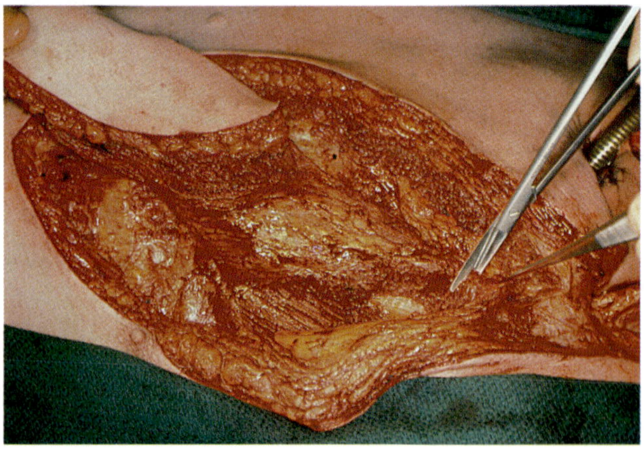

Figure 11.44 The clavicular attachment of the muscle is detached.

Once the location and course of the vessels are noted, the pectoralis major muscle is divided medial to the vessels with electrocautery up to the clavicle (Fig. 11.40). During this phase of the operation, several bleeders from the perforating branches of the internal mammary artery will be encountered, which are divided and ligated. Division of the medial aspect of the pectoralis major muscle permits further elevation and lateral rotation of the myocutaneous flap, exposing the undersurface of the muscle.

Now, under direct vision, keeping the vascular pedicle under view at all times, the pectoralis major muscle is divided, lateral to the vascular pedicle, using serrated scissors (Fig. 11.41). This could be done by electrocautery, but the use of scissors facilitates division of this thick bulk of muscle expeditiously. While dividing the pectoralis major muscle, the muscle paddle of the flap is reflected back and forth to retain an appropriate width of the muscle paddle and preserve its vascular pedicle without injury (Fig. 11.42). Division of the pectoralis major muscle lateral to the vascular pedicle is also performed all the way up to the clavicle (Fig. 11.43). The clavicular head of the pectoralis major muscle is detached from the clavicle to free up the flap completely on its vascular pedicle (Fig. 11.44).

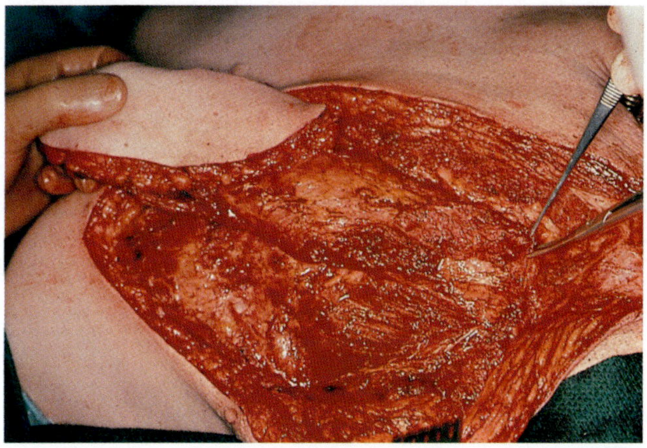

Figure 11.45 A plane is developed between the vascular pedicle and the undersurface of the muscle.

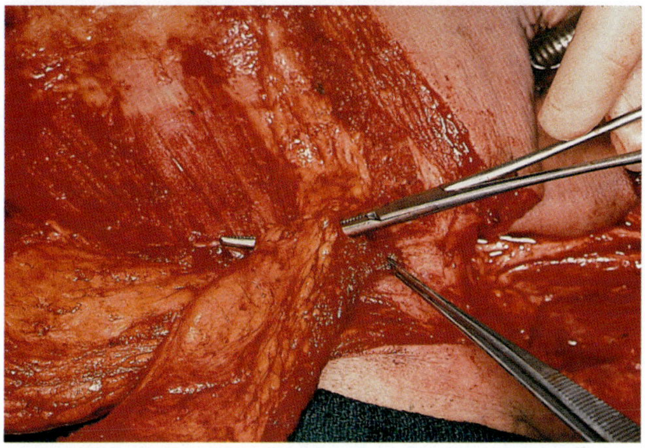

Figure 11.46 A Kelly clamp is used to separate the muscle from the vessels.

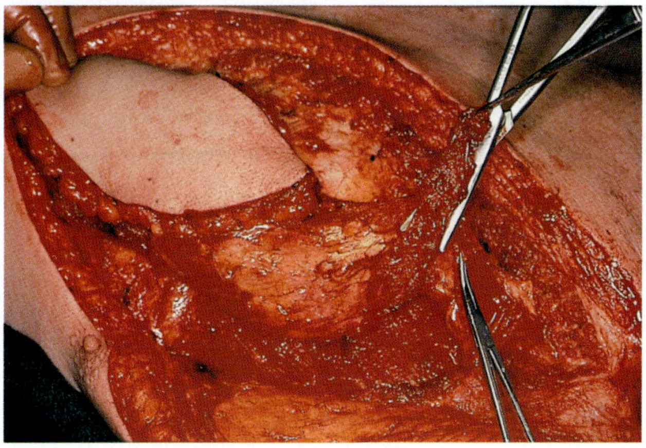

Figure 11.47 The overlying segment of muscle is excised.

At this point, the pectoralis major myocutaneous flap is ready for its rotation by 180° and its transfer to the neck for repair of the pharyngeal defect. However, if the myocutaneous flap is rotated as is, it will leave a thick muscular paddle crossing the clavicle, with an unsightly soft tissue bulge over the clavicle. A segment of the pectoralis major muscle overlying the vascular pedicle near the clavicle is therefore excised. The proximal part of the pedicle of the flap would then consist of only the blood vessels, making it an island myocutaneous flap. If, however, excision of this segment of the muscle is likely to traumatize the vascular pedicle, then it is best left alone and neither dissected nor isolated.

In order to create an island flap, the pedicle should be intact, non-traumatized and should have a good bounding pulse. First, the clavipectoral fascia is divided from the lower border of the clavicle (Fig. 11.45), freeing the clavicular attachments of the pectoralis major muscle. At this point, the flap is reflected cephalad to expose its undersurface and the vascular pedicle. A meticulous dissection is now undertaken in a plane between the vascular pedicle and the undersurface of the muscle paddle. There is usually a layer of fat and loose areolar tissue around the vessels, and a plane of dissection thus exists between the vascular pedicle and the muscle.

A Kelly clamp is inserted between the undersurface of the muscle and the vascular pedicle, which is elevated by the clamp (Fig. 11.46). The clamp is left between the vascular pedicle and the muscle and the pulsations of the vessels are confirmed by palpation. The flap is now returned to the anterior chest wall. The Kelly clamp is left in place and the overlying pectoralis major muscle is excised, preferably with serrated scissors (Fig. 11.47). Brisk hemorrhage from anterior branches of the vascular pedicle to this part of the muscle may be encountered. These branches are very carefully clamped and ligated without injuring or kinking the main vascular pedicle.

The island myocutaneous flap is now completely mobilized. The vascular pedicle is isolated to a length of approximately 2 inches from the undersurface of the clavicle up to the muscle paddle. The pedicle, the muscle paddle and the myocutaneous component of the whole flap fully mobilized are shown in Fig. 11.48. This flap is now ready for rotation at 180° on its axial plane to bring the skin surface of the flap for repair of the pharyngeal defect.

The mucosal defect following pharyngolaryngectomy is shown in Fig. 11.49. Note the absence of the anterior pharyngeal wall, which will be replaced by the rotated flap (Fig. 11.50). The proximal part of the skin island of the flap will thus be at the lower end of the pharyngeal defect and the distal part of the skin island approximates the upper end of the pharyngeal defect. Excess skin from the distal aspect of the skin island is trimmed

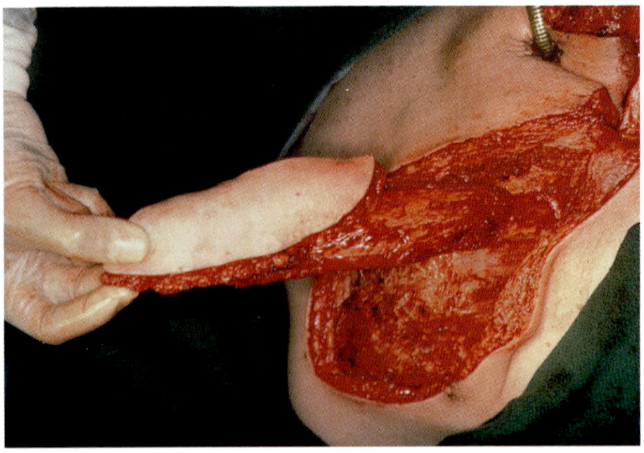

Figure 11.48 The island myocutaneous flap is now ready for rotation.

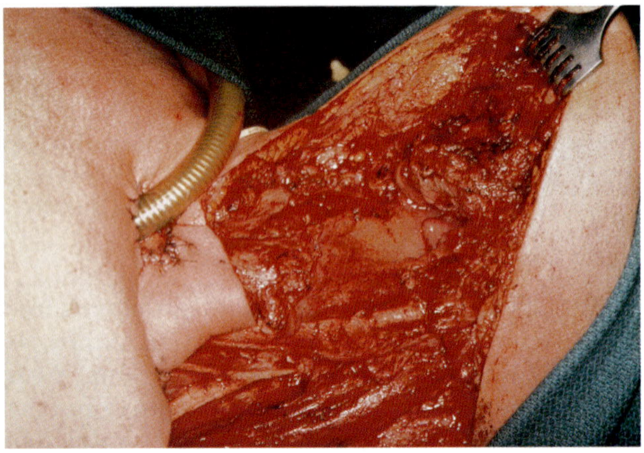

Figure 11.49 Anterior mucosal defect of the pharynx.

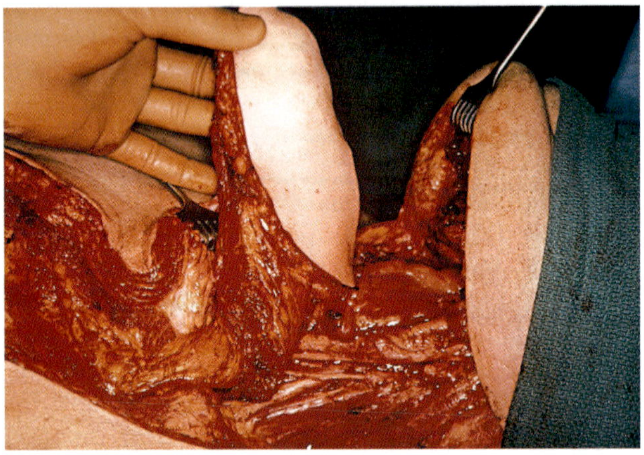

Figure 11.50 The flap is rotated to have the skin surface available for pharyngeal repair.

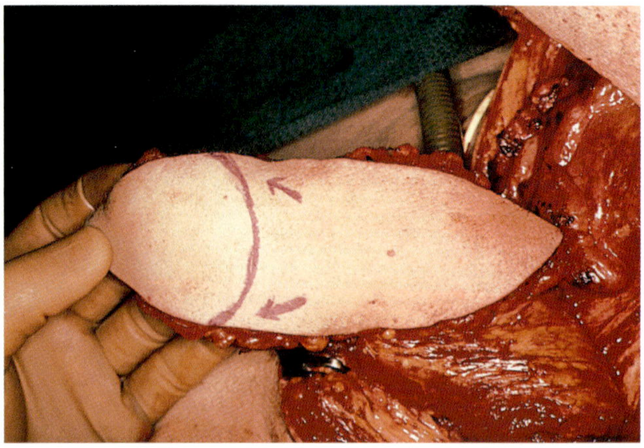

Figure 11.51 Excess skin from the distal part of the flap should be excised.

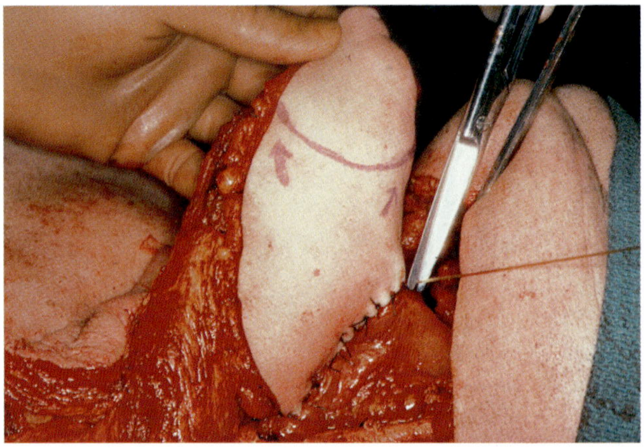

Figure 11.52 Closure of the pharyngeal defect begins at the lower end.

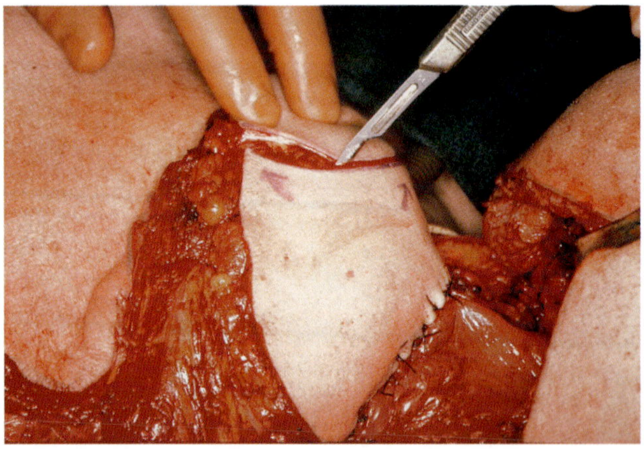

Figure 11.53 The excess distal skin is excised but the underlying muscle is preserved.

off as necessary. The distal part of the myocutaneous flap which needs trimming off is shown in Fig. 11.51. The anastomotic suture line begins at the lower end of the pharyngeal defect with interrupted 2/0 chromic catgut inverting sutures (Fig. 11.52).

After one lateral suture line is completed, a skin incision is placed on the previously outlined distal part of the flap which is to be excised (Fig. 11.53). Following the skin incision, the full thickness of the skin and subcutaneous tissue of that part of the flap is excised since it is redundant tissue (Fig. 11.54).

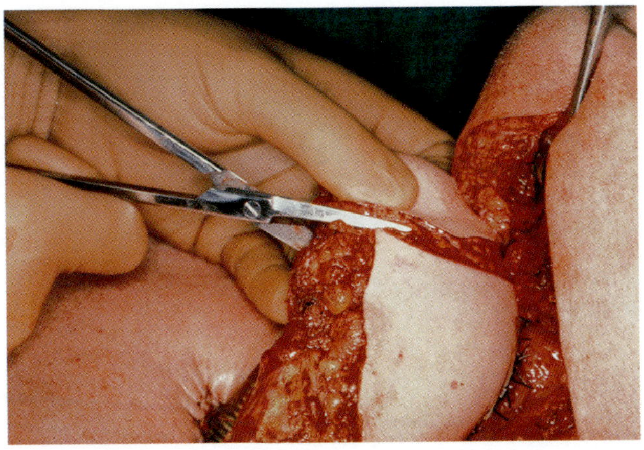

Figure 11.54 Excess skin and subcutaneous fat are excised from the distal part of the flap.

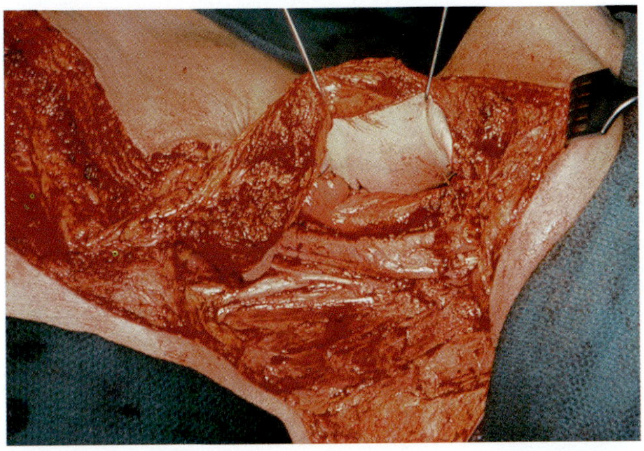

Figure 11.55 The remaining closure of the pharynx is completed with interrupted sutures.

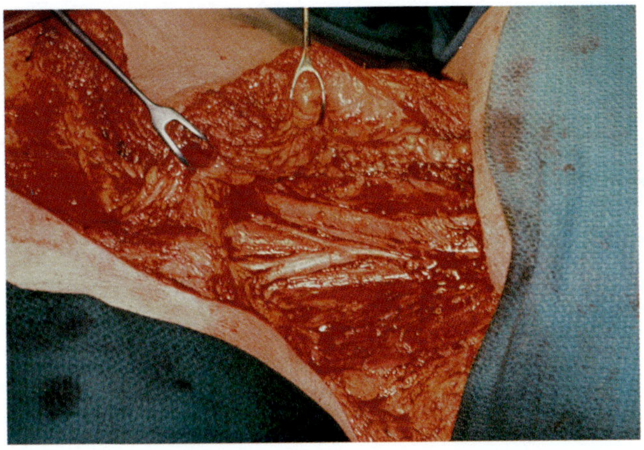

Figure 11.56 Pharyngeal closure is completed.

Closure of the pharynx is completed circumferentially with interrupted 2/0 chromic catgut inverting sutures (Fig. 11.55).

A nasogastric feeding tube is inserted prior to complete closure of the suture line. Completed

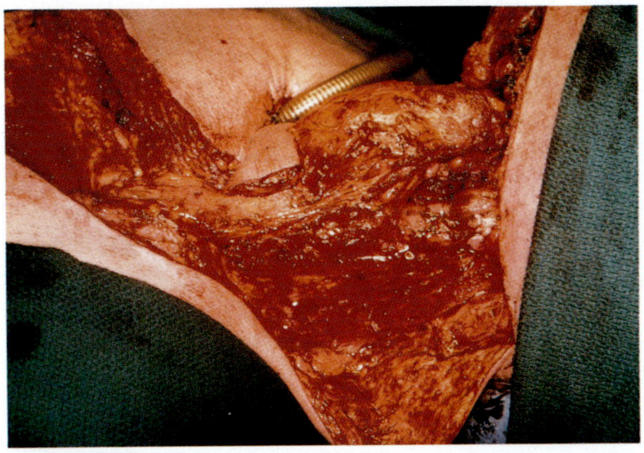

Figure 11.57 The muscle paddle is placed over the carotid artery to protect it.

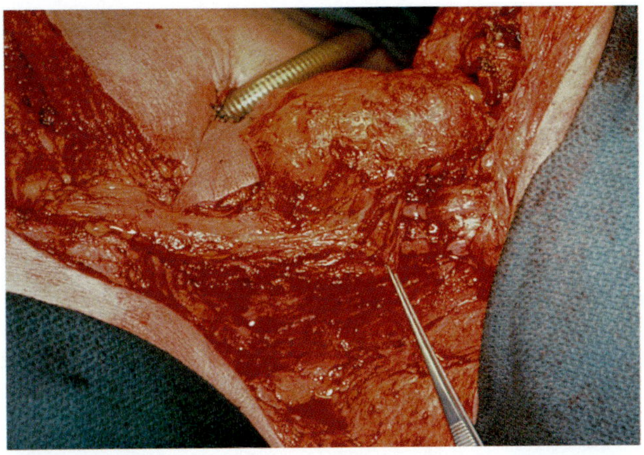

Figure 11.58 The lateral edge of the muscle paddle is tacked to the prevertebral fascia.

pharyngeal closure is shown in Fig. 11.56. Here, the muscle paddle is retracted with loop retractors to show the course of the common carotid artery.

The muscle paddle is splayed out to cover and protect the common carotid artery (Fig. 11.57). The lateral edge of the muscle paddle is stabilized with a few interrupted catgut sutures to the prevertebral fascia lateral to the carotid artery (Fig. 11.58). This is done without undue tension over the vascular pedicle.

The pectoralis major myocutaneous flap has thus provided complete restoration of the mucosal lining of the pharyngeal defect and its muscle paddle has provided protection to the carotid artery. The neck wounds are now closed in the usual fashion. Suction drains are placed in the neck and also on the anterior chest wall. The skin defect of the anterior chest wall is primarily closed in two layers.

Pectoralis major myocutaneous flap with two islands of skin

The pectoralis major myocutaneous flap provides a generous area of skin, as seen above, for transfer to

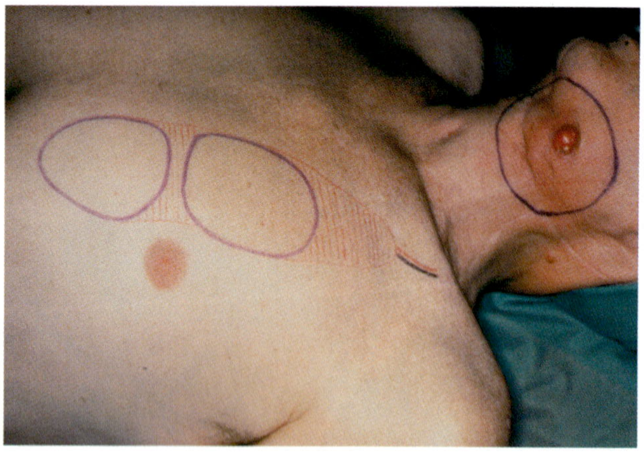

Figure 11.59 Two islands of skin outlined on the pectoralis myocutaneous flap.

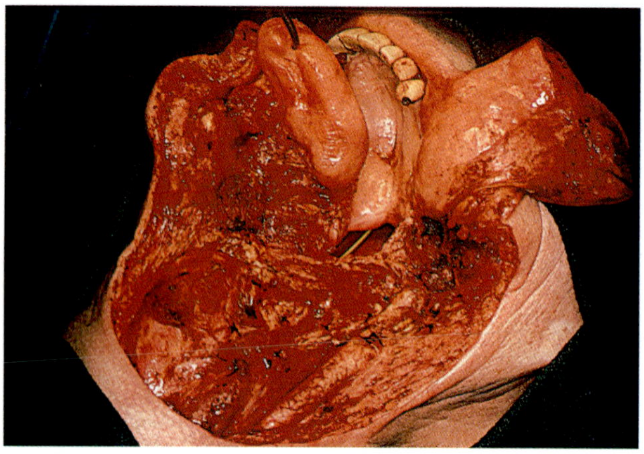

Figure 11.60 Surgical defect following through-and-through resection of recurrent cancer.

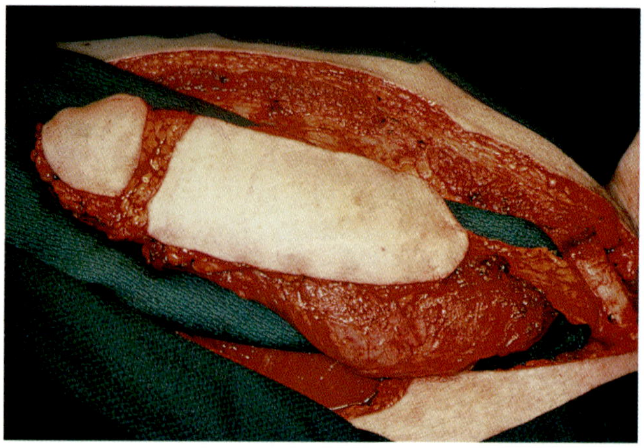

Figure 11.61 The pectoralis major myocutaneous flap is elevated with two islands of skin.

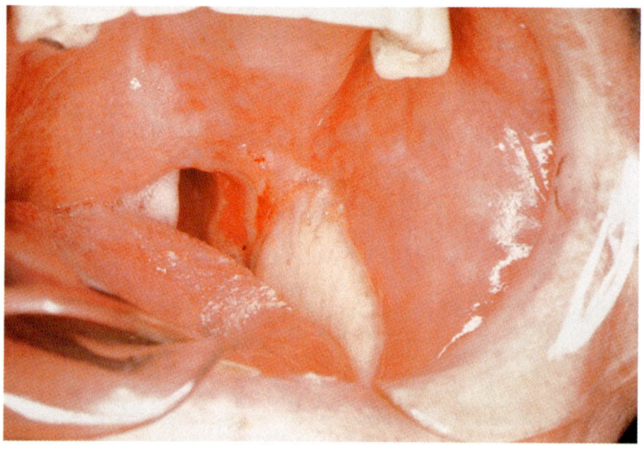

Figure 11.62 Postoperative intraoral view showing healed distal island of skin of the flap.

the head and neck region. So in situations where both internal (mucosal) lining and external (skin) coverage are required, two skin islands may be created on the same paddle of muscle for total one stage reconstruction of a through-and-through defect.

The patient shown in (Fig. 11.59) has recurrent carcinoma involving the floor of the mouth and the retromolar trigone area. He had previously undergone excision of the floor of the mouth and a left radical neck dissection followed by postoperative radiation therapy. The recurrent tumor is fungating through the skin of the neck. The area of skin and soft tissue for resection is outlined in the upper part of the neck. The pectoralis major myocutaneous flap is also outlined on the anterior chest wall on the left-hand side with two islands of skin. The distal skin island will be used for mucosal lining in the oral cavity and the proximal island for coverage of the skin defect of the neck.

A through-and-through resection in conjunction with segmental mandibulectomy, excision of the floor of the mouth and resection of a portion of the base of the tongue and anterior pillar of the soft palate is carried out (Fig. 11.60). Soft tissue resection in the upper part of the neck required sacrifice of the external carotid artery and the hypoglossal nerve as well as full-thickness resection of the musculature of the floor of the mouth. The exposed carotid artery can be seen in the surgical field.

The pectoralis major myocutaneous island flap is isolated with two islands of skin (Fig. 11.61). Note the vascular pedicle of the flap with a paddle of pectoralis muscle underlying the proximal island of the skin. The flap is reflected cephalad and rotated approximately 180° to bring the distal island in the oral cavity for mucosal closure. The proximal larger island of skin is appropriately trimmed for closure of the skin defect. A postoperative view of the oral cavity approximately 6 weeks following surgery shows a well-healed distal island of skin (Fig. 11.62). The proximal island of skin replaces the skin defect very satisfactorily with a well-healed skin incision (Fig. 11.63). The muscle paddle adequately protects the carotid artery.

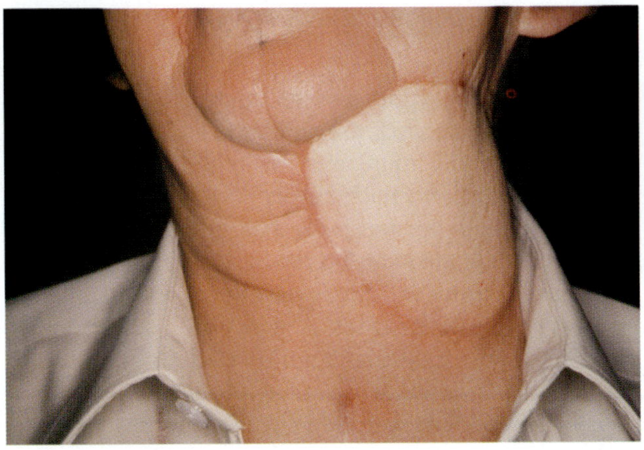

Figure 11.63 Postoperative external appearance, showing healed proximal island of skin of the flap.

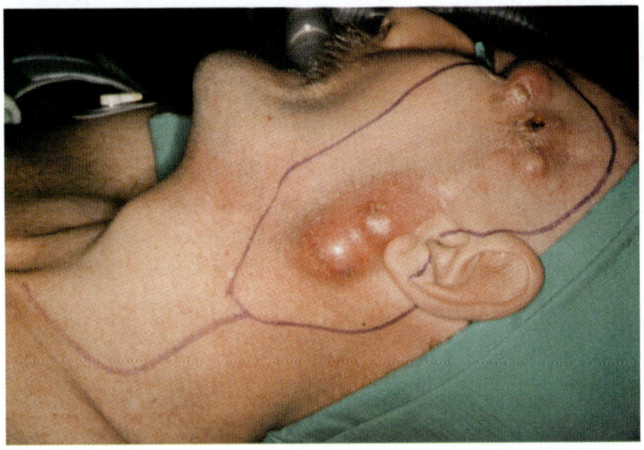

Figure 11.64 The extent of resection is outlined on the face.

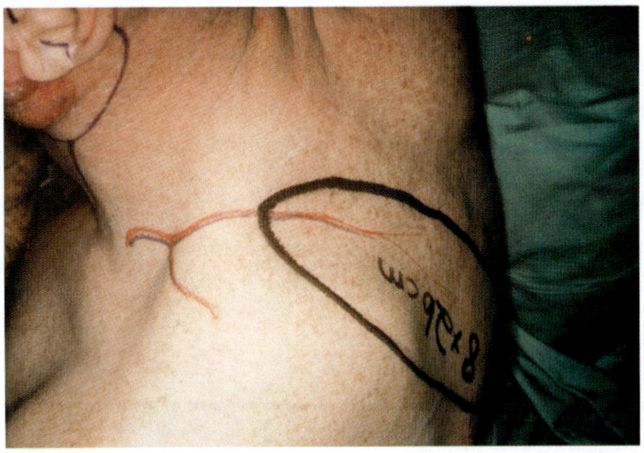

Figure 11.65 The flap is outlined. Note the course of the vascular pedicle.

A pectoralis major myocutaneous flap can thus be employed in situations where mucosal lining as well as skin coverage is necessary for through-and-through defects of the upper aerodigestive tract. When two islands of skin are planned for transfer on a paddle of the pectoralis major muscle, it is advisable not to divide the skin to create the two islands until after the flap is rotated up to the surgical defect. At that point, appropriate placement of the distal island to replace the mucosal defect is done first. Only then is the skin of the flap incised to make two islands of appropriate size. Division of the subcutaneous tissue up to the muscle is unnecessary since it may jeopardize blood vessels in the subcutaneous tissues going to the distal skin island.

Trapezius myocutaneous flap

The vascular anatomy of the circulation of the trapezius myocutaneous flap is similar to that described in the pectoralis major myocutaneous flap. However, the vascular pedicle is from the transverse cervical artery and its accompanying veins. While the feeding artery is constant and reliable, its venous drainage is not constant and sometimes inadequate. Two types of trapezius myocutaneous flaps are available.[7,14] The lateral trapezius myocutaneous flap overlying the acromioclavicular region has very limited application. The shortcoming of this flap is that the skin island is limited in its surface extent and the arc of rotation is very short. Therefore, application of the lateral trapezius myocutaneous flap in head and neck reconstruction is limited to small defects in the oral cavity or pharynx. The posterior or vertical trapezius myocutaneous flap, however, is more versatile. This flap is dependent on the descending branch of the transverse cervical artery deep to the trapezius muscle. One disadvantage is that the patient has to be positioned laterally to elevate the flap. This flap provides a generous amount of soft tissue and a large portion of skin island for repair of major surgical defects, particularly on the lateral aspect of the face, parotid region, mastoid region, and the temporoparietal region of the scalp. This flap is ideally suited for repair of surgical defects following radical parotidectomy, with or without temporal bone resection.

The patient shown in Fig. 11.64 had recurrent carcinoma of the parotid gland with clinically palpable cervical lymph node metastases and metastatic deposits involving the overlying skin in the retromandibular region and the upper part of the neck. The surgical resection required left radical neck dissection in conjunction with excision of a generous portion of skin of the neck and parotid region with radical total parotidectomy and segmental mandibulectomy with amputation of the external ear and partial temporal bone resection. In Fig. 11.65 the flap of appropriate dimensions is outlined. The technical steps of elevation of the trapezius myocutaneous flap are similar to those described in the section on the pectoralis major myocutaneous flap.

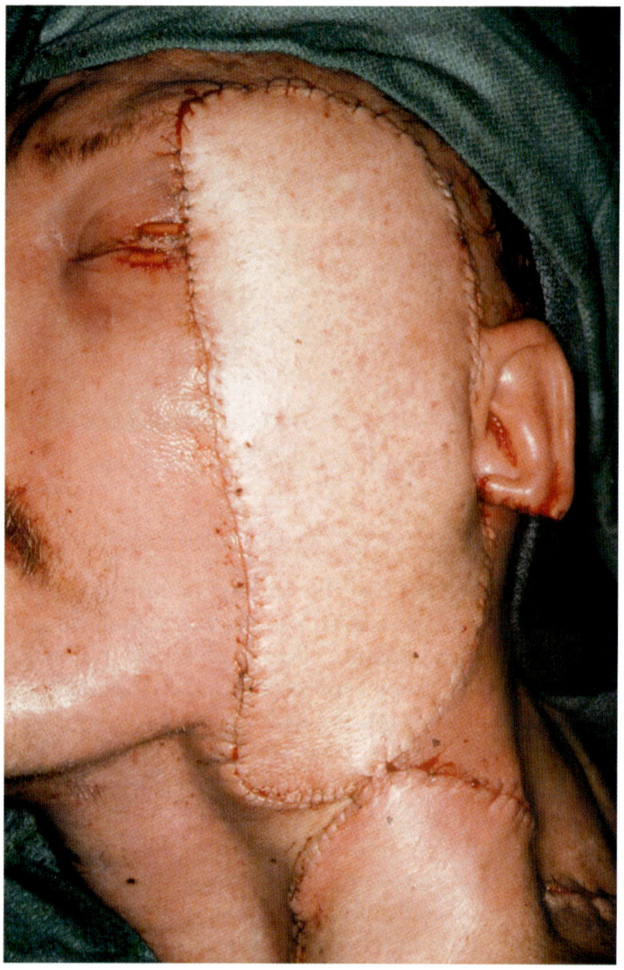

Figure 11.66 Complete closure of the skin and replacement of soft tissue is provided by the flap.

The vascular pedicle is usually identified in the region of the nape of the neck, where meticulous attention should be paid to delicate handling of the flap to avoid injury to the vascular pedicle and particularly the draining veins. To cover the surgical defect, the flap requires axial rotation of its pedicle by 90° to permit satisfactory placement of the flap. In Fig. 11.66 closure of the surgical defect is shown providing excellent one-stage repair of this massive soft tissue and skin defect of the lateral aspect of the face, mastoid region and temporoparietal scalp. The donor site defect is usually closed primarily.

Latissimus dorsi flap

A latissimus dorsi myocutaneous flap is also available for coverage of large soft tissue and skin defects in the head and neck region.[5] However, elevation of this flap requires repositioning of the patient and will often unduly increase the length of the operative procedure. Therefore, if other means of repair of the surgical defect are available, a latissimus dorsi myocutaneous flap is usually not preferred.

Microvascular free tissue transfer

The increasing application of microvascular surgery for free tissue transfer over the last 20 years has produced new dimensions in reconstructive techniques in head and neck surgery.[11,17,20,21,23,26,27,30–39] All types of defects created by resection of tumors in the head and neck area can be repaired by microvascular free tissue transfer. Although the applicability of microvascular techniques is universal, some degree of discretion, judgement and wisdom should be employed before microvascular free tissue transfer is chosen for reconstruction.

The success of microvascular free tissue transfer depends upon the technical perfection of the microsurgeon. It is essential that the microvascular surgeon has frequent and varied involvement in the field of microsurgery. It is extremely hazardous for a head and neck surgeon not formally trained in the field of microvascular surgery to embark upon microvascular free tissue transfer. If the head and neck surgeon is inadequately trained in microsurgery, or has not maintained his technical competence in the field, then it is advisable that a well-trained and competent microvascular surgeon be called upon to assume the responsibility of the microsurgical reconstructive aspects of a head and neck operative procedure.

Details of the techniques of microsurgery and the various fundamental aspects of microvascular training are beyond the scope of this book but the indications for microvascular free tissue transfer are discussed. A brief summary of the various types of microvascular free flaps available at the discretion of the head and neck surgeon is presented. Several examples of simple and composite free tissue transfer are shown.

The type of tissue necessary for the reconstruction of a particular defect depends on the type of tissue loss following resection of a tumor. Thus, major resection of a tumor in the head and neck region may result in loss of skin, soft tissues, mucosa, bone, cartilage, or any combination of these tissues. The microvascular free flap essential for reconstruction of a particular defect may therefore consist either of skin alone with its underlying fascia; skin and soft tissues such as muscles; skin, soft tissue and bone; soft tissue alone; soft tissue and bone; bone alone; or bone and skin. Various different combinations of tissues are available in several microvascular free flaps. The most commonly employed microvascular free flaps in the head and neck region are the radial forearm, rectus abdominis, fibula, jejunum, scapula, lattismus dorsi and iliac crest with or without skin of the groin.[11,17,20,21,23,26,27,30–39]

In the selection, design and fabrication of a microvascular free flap, the clinician needs to remember that merely plugging the hole, replacing bone for bone loss or providing skin coverage for a large skin defect is not sufficient. Adequate preoperative assessment is essential for understanding the nature of the anticipated surgical defect and an appropriate plan for the reconstructive effort should be developed before proceeding with the operation. Therefore, detailed communication between the ablative surgeon and the reconstructive surgeon is vitally important for the successful outcome of reconstructive surgery.

It is also important to remember that, whenever feasible, mucosa should be replaced with mucosa, bone with bone, and skin with skin. If, however, this is not feasible, then certain compromises may have to be made to achieve the most desired result. It is therefore essential that the microsurgeon has a proper understanding of the functional and esthetic impact of the planned resection, facilitating the choice of the most appropriate flap for the given situation. After the flap is harvested, it should be adequately tailored to fit the surgical defect. It should be shaped, contoured and appropriately set in the surgical defect to achieve the most desirable functional and esthetic result.

Indications for microvascular free tissue transfer

In clinical situations where local or regional tissues are unavailable or inadequate and the application of loco-regional tissues would result in significant functional or esthetic loss, then reconstructive surgery with microvascular free tissue transfer should be considered. Clearly, the potential for loco-regional control of cancer should be reasonably good to justify the effort required for microsurgical tissue transfer. Such a prolonged operative undertaking is rarely indicated in palliative situations.

Several patient factors also influence the choice of free tissue transfer for reconstruction. It is essential to have an adequate preoperative evaluation of the patient to assess the risk of a prolonged operative procedure which may take several hours. Therefore very elderly patients, particularly with poor cardiopulmonary status and significant comorbidities, are poor candidates for microvascular surgery. Patients with atherosclerotic disease of small vessels in peripheral arteries (especially for the fibula free flap) are suboptimal candidates for microvascular surgery. All other patients, if suitable to withstand a long operative procedure, are considered for microvascular free tissue transfer if appropriate indications exist for reconstruction of a major surgical defect in the head and neck area. Several examples are now shown to demonstrate the application of a variety of microvascular free flaps in the head and neck region.

Radial forearm free flap reconstruction of skin and soft tissues of the face

The patient shown in Fig. 11.67 had recurrent sweat gland carcinoma of the skin of the lateral aspect of her face and the preauricular region. She had previously undergone multiple surgical procedures with local rotation flaps. Thus, local and regional skin flaps are not available or suitable for repair of the surgical defect. Surgical resection in this patient required sacrifice of a generous portion of the skin and underlying soft tissues as well as a portion of the zygomatic arch where the tumor was adherent to the bone. The specimen is shown in Fig. 11.68. A subtotal parotidectomy with sacrifice of the upper division of the facial nerve was necessary to encompass a monobloc resection with negative margins. A facial nerve graft was not possible since a portion of the orbicularis oculi muscle had to be resected to

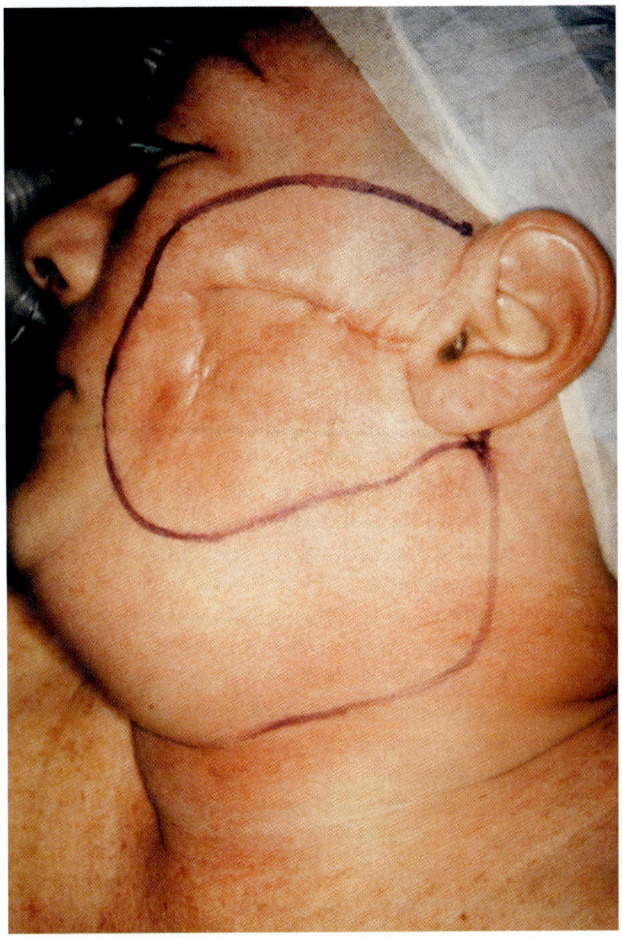

Figure 11.67 Outline of the skin incision for resection of tumor and neck dissection.

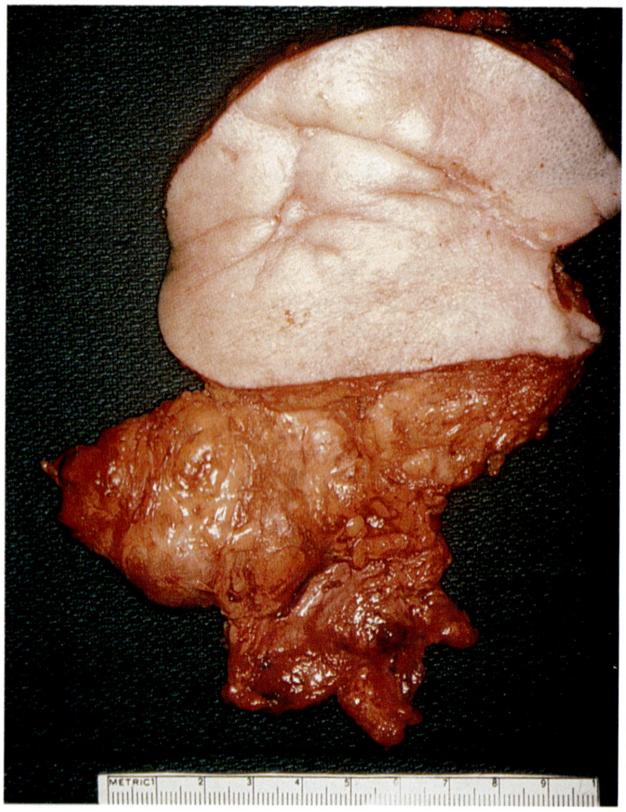

Figure 11.68 Surgical specimen of skin, parotid gland and neck dissection.

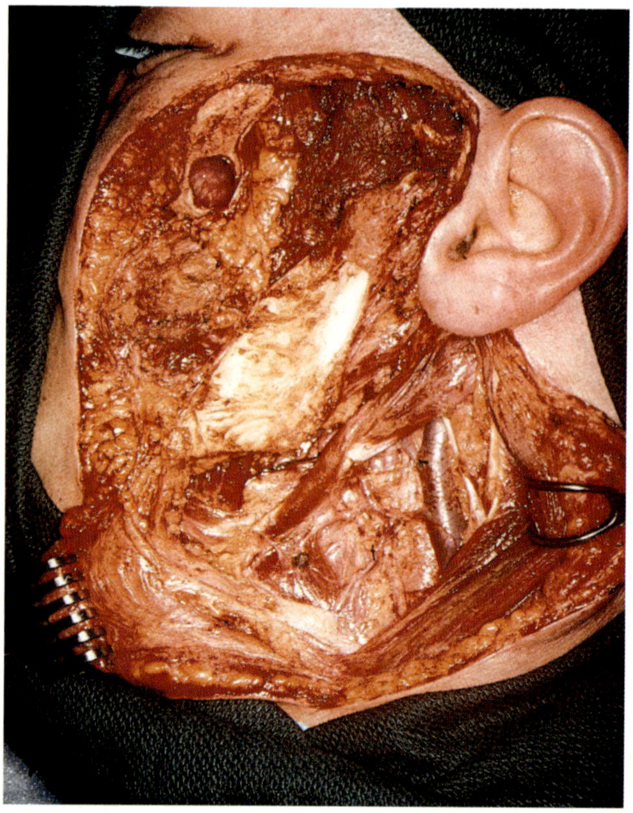

Figure 11.69 Surgical defect following resection of skin, parotid gland and masseter muscle.

encompass the recurrent tumor. A supraomohyoid neck dissection was performed in conjunction with resection of the recurrent tumor. The surgical defect is shown in Fig. 11.69.

A radial forearm free flap is outlined with its vascular pedicle which will be anastomosed to the facial artery and one of the tributaries of the internal jugular vein (Figs 11.70, 11.71). The donor site on the forearm requires a split-thickness skin graft for coverage of the defect. The postoperative appearance of the patient at three months is shown in Fig. 11.72. A very satisfactory repair of the surgical defect of skin and underlying soft tissues of the face is accomplished using a radial forearm free flap.

Another patient with dermatofibrosarcoma protuberans of the preauricular skin involving the parotid gland is shown in Fig. 11.73. This patient had previously undergone an attempt at surgical excision of this tumor by a superficial parotidectomy. However, residual tumor mandated a wider three-dimensional resection. A near total parotidectomy with excision of a generous portion of the overlying skin was performed. The facial nerve was dissected and carefully preserved. The surgical defect following resection of the specimen is shown in Fig. 11.74. A radial forearm flap is now used to repair the soft tissue and skin defect in the preauricular region.

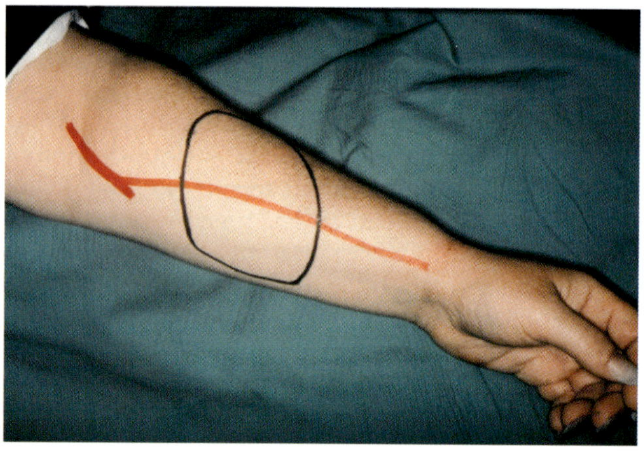

Figure 11.70 Outline of radial forearm free flap.

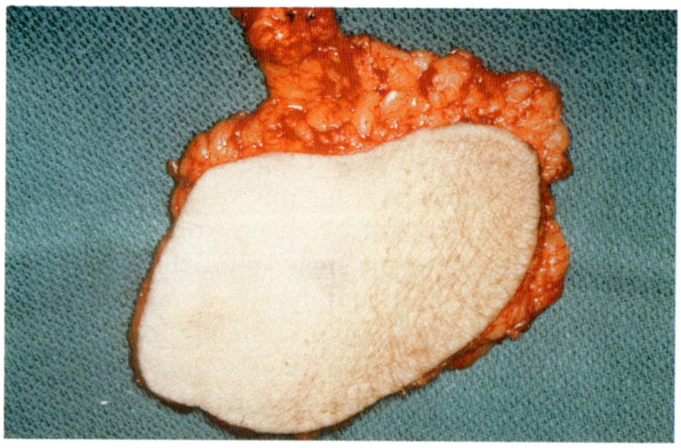

Figure 11.71 The isolated free flap with its vascular pedicle.

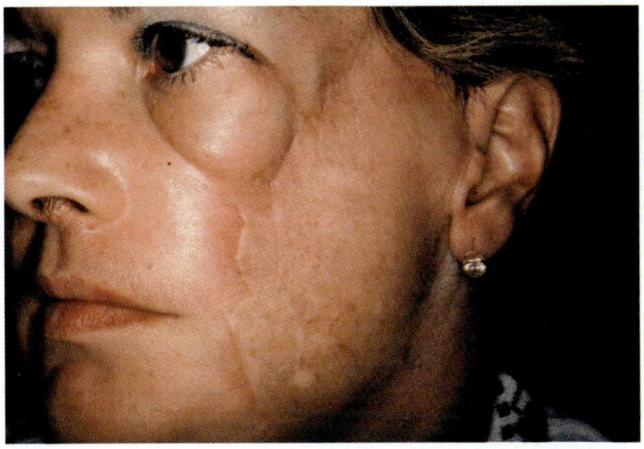

Figure 11.72 Postoperative appearance of the patient at three months.

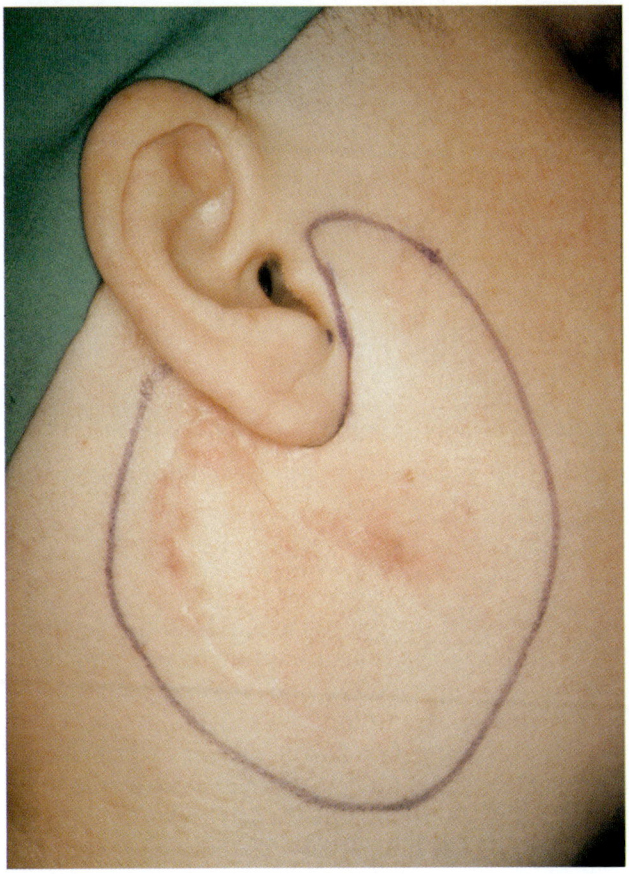

Figure 11.73 Dermatofibrosarcoma protuberans of parotid region.

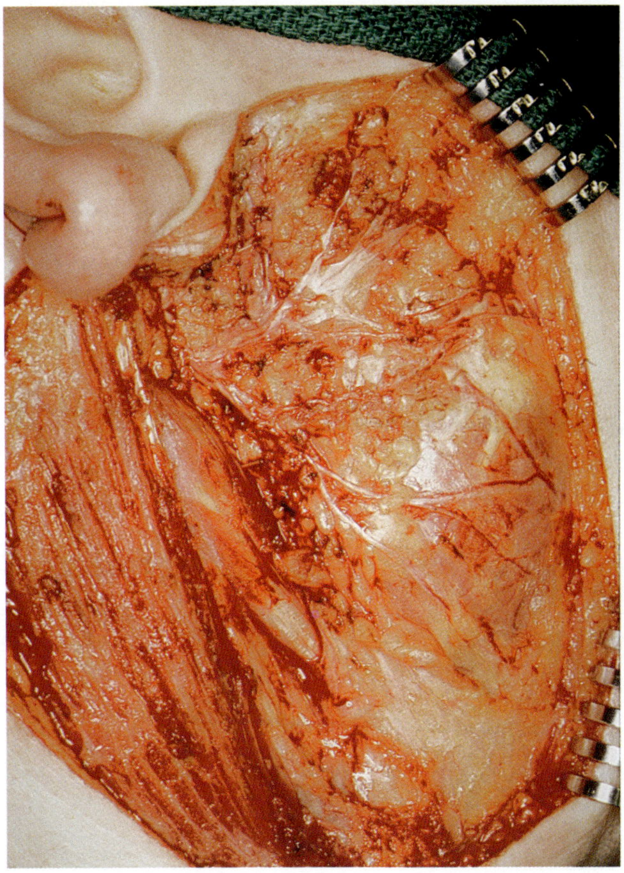

Figure 11.74 Surgical defect, showing preservation of the facial nerve.

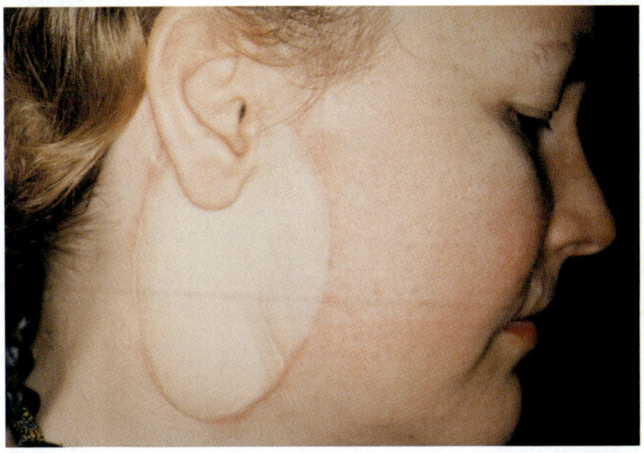

Figure 11.75 Postoperative appearance of the patient.

The postoperative appearance of the patient shows a very satisfactory coverage of the surgical defect (Fig. 11.75). The flap provides excellent esthetic restoration of this defect.

The radial forearm flap is currently considered to be the ideal free flap for reconstruction of mucosal and soft tissue defects in the oral cavity. The flap is highly reliable and is quite versatile for various applications of reconstructive techniques in the oral cavity. In Fig. 11.76, a radial forearm free flap is shown elevated with its vascular pedical isolated. The shape and dimensions of the flap can be highly variable and are generally suitable for any size surgical defect in the oral cavity. The patient whose oral cavity is shown in Fig. 11.77 demonstrates a radial forearm free flap used for reconstruction of the anterior half of the oral tongue. This patient required amputation of the anterior 50% of the oral tongue for squamous carcinoma. The radial forearm free

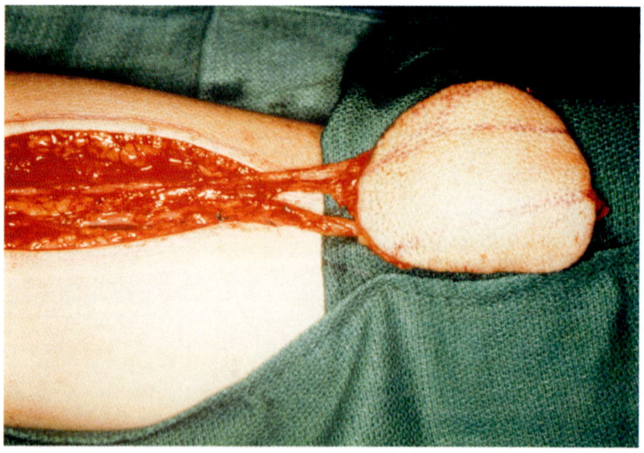

Figure 11.76 Radial forearm flap with its long vascular pedicle.

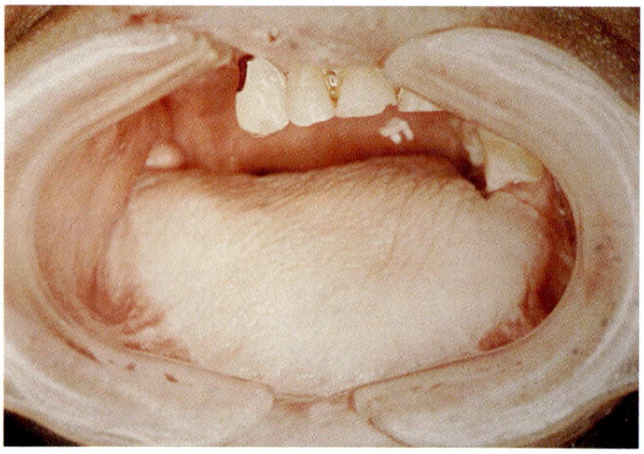

Figure 11.77 Radial forearm flap reconstruction of anterior half of oral tongue.

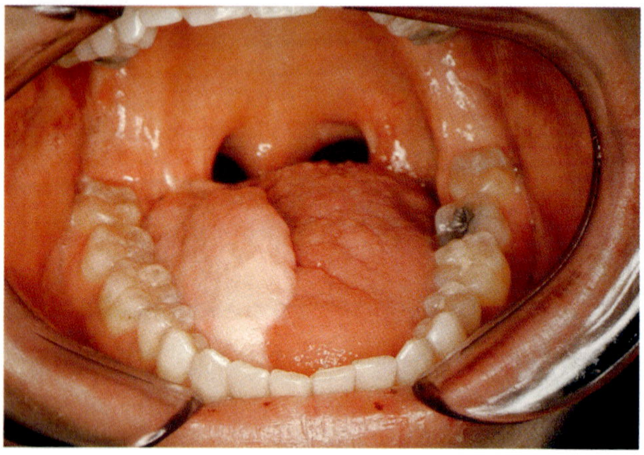

Figure 11.78 Radial forearm flap reconstruction of hemiglossectomy defect.

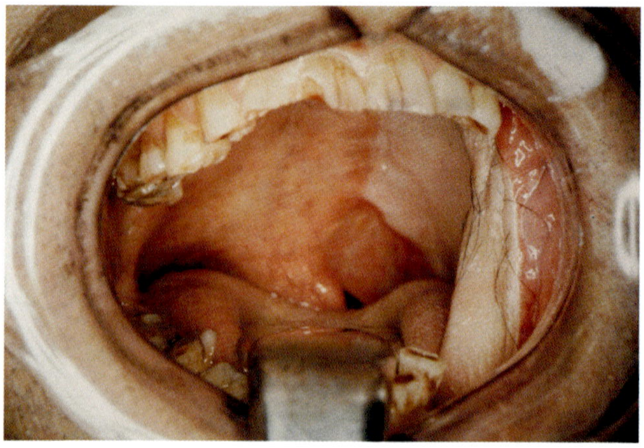

Figure 11.79 Reconstructed left cheek defect, with radial forearm flap.

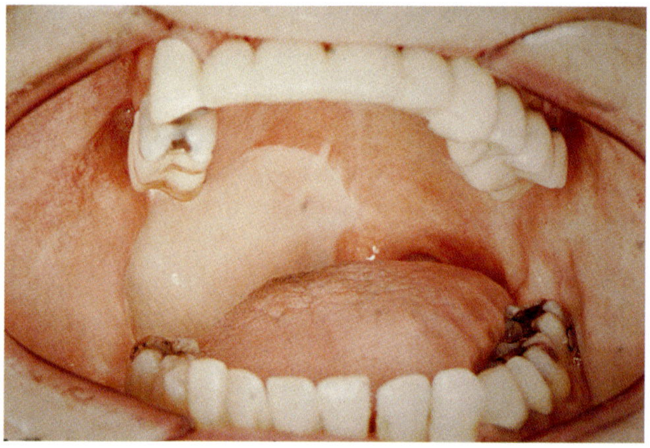

Figure 11.80 Radial forearm flap reconstruction after soft palate and tonsil resection.

flap has very satisfactorily replaced the resected tongue and provided lining, and has been effective in retaining the mobility of the remaining tongue. Another patient shown in Fig. 11.78 underwent right hemiglossectomy for squamous carcinoma. The radial forearm free flap has been used to reconstruct the right half of the oral tongue, which has retained the mobility of the remaining tongue and provided excellent lining coverage and volume replacement for the resected portion of the tongue. In Fig. 11.79 the radial forearm free flap is shown to reconstruct a surgical defect of the left cheek following resection of squamous carcinoma of the left cheek mucosa in conjunction with upper alveolectomy and marginal mandibulectomy. The flap has provided excellent surface coverage and maintains its supple soft consistency, thus permitting excellent mobility of the temporomandibular joint and assisting in prevention of trismus. The radial forearm free flap is also an excellent choice for repair of surgical defects of the oropharynx. In Fig. 11.80 a patient who underwent resection for carcinoma of the tonsil requiring excision of the tonsillar fossa, soft palate, lateral pharyngeal wall, and retromolar trigone is shown. The radial forearm free flap has provided excellent coverage of the mucosal defect and the soft tissue defect to restore anatomic continuity and maintain functional integrity of the velopharyngeal complex.

Reconstruction of the mandible

In order to achieve satisfactory restoration of form and function, reconstruction of the mandible requires several important considerations: functional, anatomic, and esthetic. The functional considerations are restoration of oral competence, mastication, speech, bolus transport and deglutition. Anatomic considerations are restoration of inter-incisor opening, restoration of inter-arch distance and inter-arch alignment, as well as adequate soft tissue replacement. Clearly, an excessive bulk of tissue must be avoided so that the airway is not compromised. The esthetic considerations include restoration of facial symmetry, lower facial height, projection of the chin, and avoidance of facial incisions.

The current options for mandible reconstruction are the use of non-vascularized bone, pedicled composite osteomyocutaneous flaps, metallic plates with local flaps, metallic plates with free flaps, and osteomyocutaneous microvascular free flaps. Defects of the posterior aspect of the body of the mandible near its angle or of the ascending ramus may be left alone without consideration of any major reconstructive effort in elderly or high-risk patients. The esthetic impact of this surgical defect is minimal, as shown in Fig. 11.81. On the other hand, resection of the anterior aspect of the body of the mandible, and particularly the anterior arch of the mandible, produces significant functional and esthetic loss which mandates an appropriate reconstructive effort to restore form and function (Fig. 11.82). A very small (up to 3 cm) segmental defect in the mandible without previous exposure to radiotherapy can be repaired with a non-vascularized bone graft, usually harvested from the iliac crest. Regional composite osteomyocutaneous flaps can be used for reconstruction of the mandible although the esthetic and functional result of such a reconstructive procedure is far from satisfactory. The use of metallic plates is indicated in elderly patients who are not suitable for microvascular free flaps or in patients whose prognosis is poor due to massive tumor. It is important to re-emphasize that if a metallic plate is used for reconstruction of the mandible, then adequate soft tissue support and skin coverage for mucosal lining should be provided to avoid exposure and extrusion of the metallic plate. Although the operative procedure is expeditious, the esthetic and functional result is not optimal.

Microvascular free flap mandible reconstruction clearly provides significant advantages in that it is highly successful, there is an unlimited volume of tissue available, and the harvested tissue can be fabricated to have an ideal configuration for restoration of the surgical defect.[11,15,18,30–34,37–40] The only disadvantage is that the operative procedure is quite long and requires the resources and commitment of a dedicated microvascular surgical and nursing team and operating room time. The currently available free flap options for mandible reconstruction are radius, scapula, ilium, and fibula.[11,15,18,30–34,37–40] Ideally, free flap mandible reconstruction should be done primarily at the time of surgical resection of the tumor since the reconstruction is very precise and the process of resection and reconstruction is

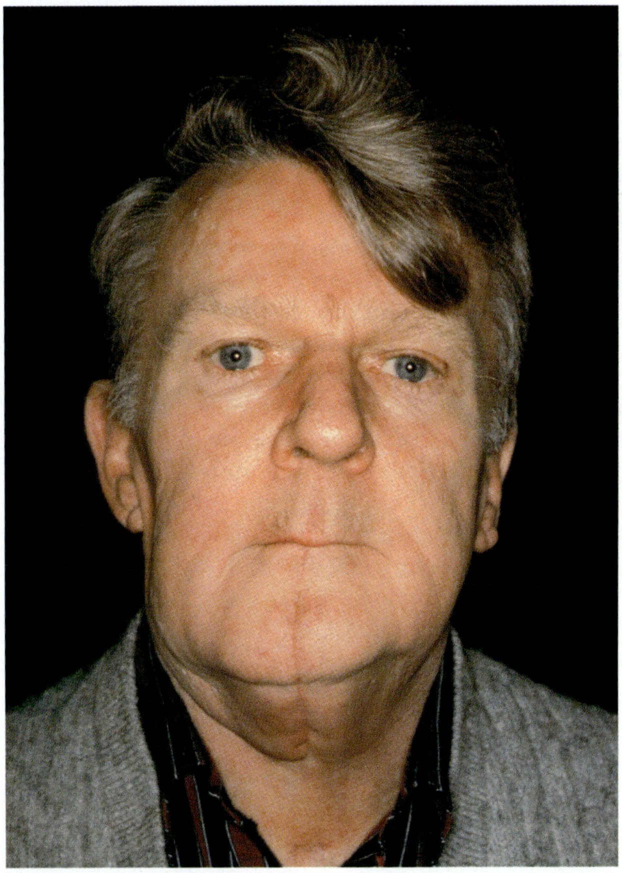

Figure 11.81 Facial appearance following resection of the ascending ramus of the mandible on the right-hand side.

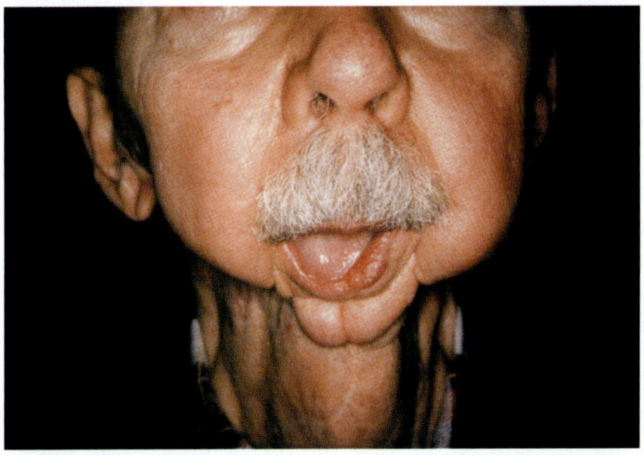

Figure 11.82 Facial appearance following resection of the anterior arch of mandible.

accomplished in a single operation and the patient does not have to live for a period of time with a deformity. The characteristics, advantages, disadvantages, and indications of various free flaps for mandible reconstruction are presented.

Radial forearm osteocutaneous free flap

The radial forearm osteocutaneous free flap offers excellent soft tissue characteristics.[15,37] The thickness of the skin is ideal, the abundant surface area of the skin is pliable and there is an excellent blood supply for the intra-oral lining. However, the length of bone available is limited and only one half of the circumference of the cortex of the bone can be harvested as a graft. The blood supply to this segment of bone is non-segmental and is therefore somewhat precarious. There is a potential for significant morbidity from this flap if there is a fracture at the donor site. The skin grafted appearance of the forearm is an esthetic disadvantage. The tendons in the forearm often become exposed and prolonged immobilization to prevent fracture may result in a stiff hand and wrist. Clearly, the advantage is that of an ideal skin flap with an ideal vascular pedicle, but with the disadvantage of an undesirable stock of bone. With these limitations, the indications for the radius free flap are surgical defects where there is a large mucosal area to be covered with only a short segment of lateral mandibular defect in the body or ascending ramus of the mandible.

An example of a radial forearm osteocutaneous free flap is shown in a patient who presented with recurrent carcinoma of the lower lip with metastatic lymph nodes fungating through the skin, adhering to the lateral cortex and undersurface of the body of the mandible (Fig. 11.83). The operative procedure required a left neck dissection in conjunction with a segmental mandibulectomy and excision of a generous portion of the overlying skin in a monobloc fashion. The surgical defect is shown in Fig. 11.84. A radial forearm osteocutaneous flap is outlined as shown in Fig. 11.85. The postoperative appearance of the patient following reconstruction of the defect with the radial forearm osteocutaneous free flap is shown in (Fig. 11.86). A quite satisfactory postoperative result is obtained with the radius free flap.

Scapula free flap

The scapula free flap is an ideal flap where one can obtain abundant soft tissue with separate skin and bone on the same vascular pedicle.[18,20] The blood vessels are reliable and there is minimal donor site morbidity. The bone characteristics of this flap are

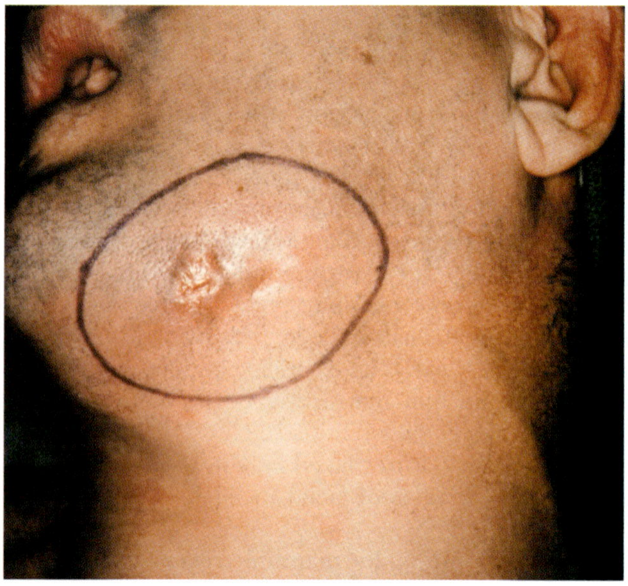

Figure 11.83 Metastatic carcinoma at level I, involving skin and mandible.

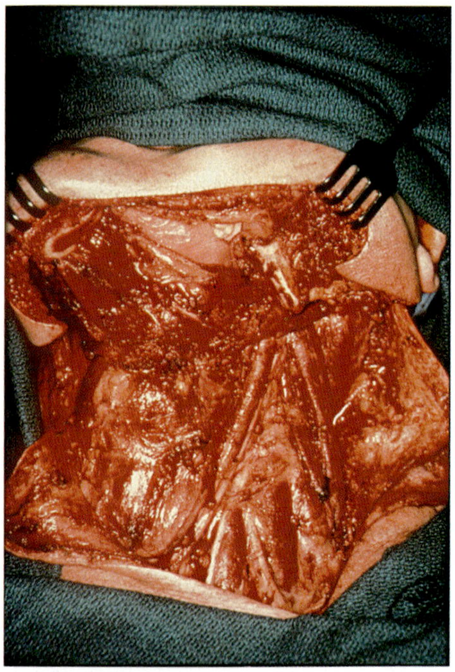

Figure 11.84 Surgical defect following monobloc resection of skin and mandible with neck dissection.

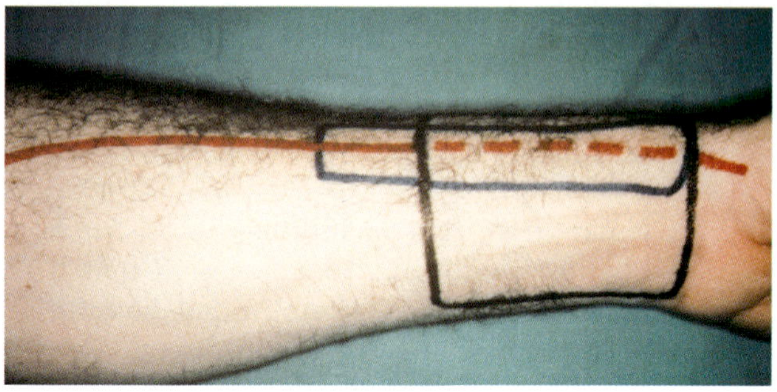

Figure 11.85 Outline of proposed radial forearm osteocutaneous flap.

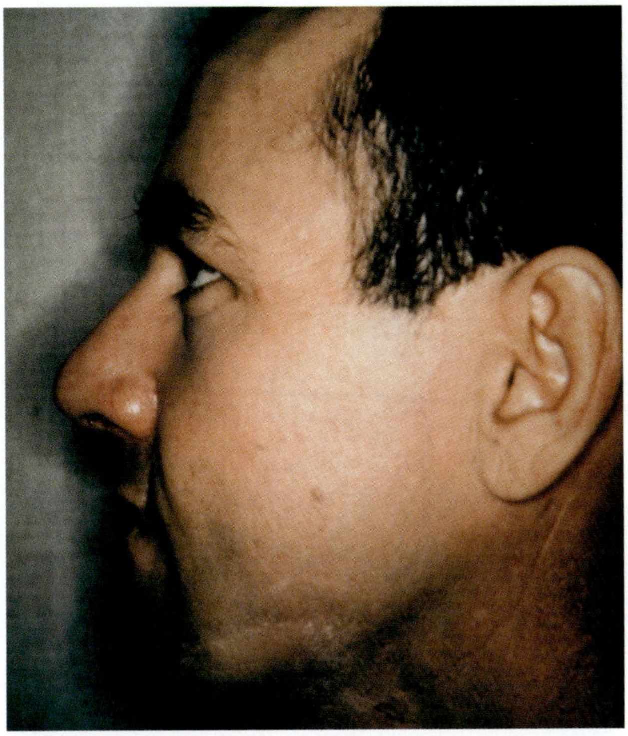

Figure 11.86 Postoperative appearance following composite radial forearm free flap reconstruction.

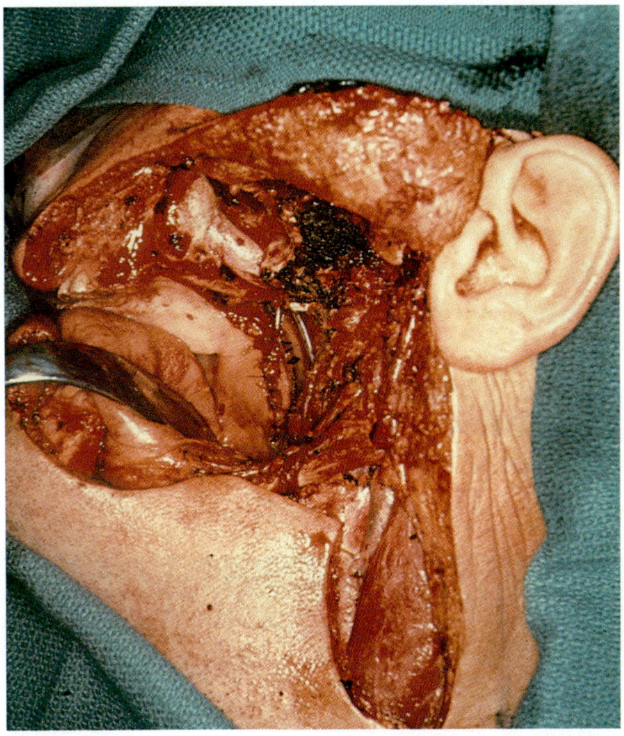

Figure 11.88 The surgical defect following composite resection of cheek with segmental mandibulectomy.

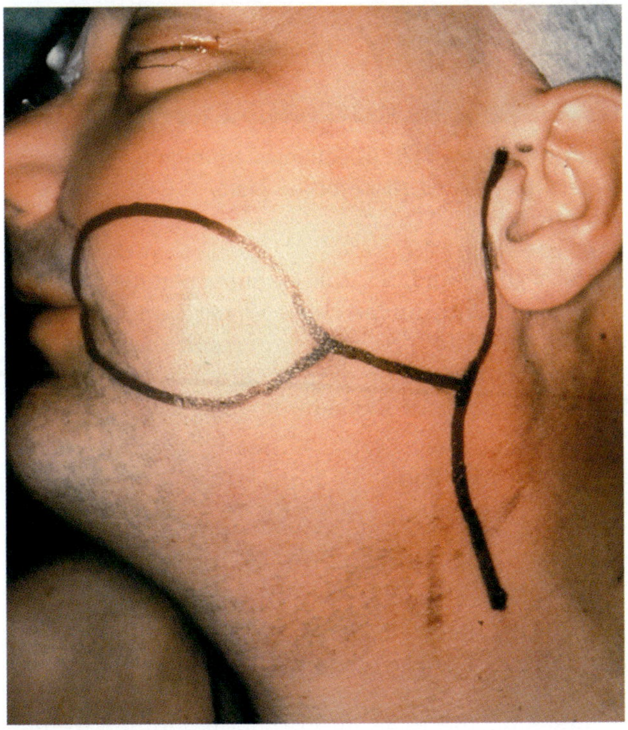

Figure 11.87 Outline of incisions for resection of sarcoma of left cheek.

not ideal as the thickness is barely adequate for osseointegrated implants and the maximum length that can be harvested is also limited (10–12 cm). The blood supply to this segment of bone is not segmental and therefore the use of multiple osteotomies to fabricate the appropriate shape of the mandible is hazardous. The soft tissue characteristics are ideal, with an unlimited size for the skin island. However, the skin is thick for intra-oral reconstruction and the color match is poor for replacement of the external facial skin. The disadvantages of this flap are the need for lateral positioning of the patient, which necessitates sequential resection and reconstruction. There is considerable amount of postoperative pain and shoulder stiffness and there is often prolonged serous drainage from the donor site. The indications for this flap are surgical defects where massive soft tissue replacement is not the priority.

An example of this is shown in a patient who had sarcoma of the left cheek with invasion of the underlying mandible. The surgical resection required segmental mandibulectomy with a three-dimensional through-and-through resection of the left cheek including the overlying skin (Fig. 11.87). The surgical defect is shown in Fig. 11.88. Reconstruction of this surgical defect requires replacement of the resected segment of the mandible, as well as a significant bulk of soft tissue to repair the defect of the cheek with lining for the buccal mucosa and the overlying skin of the cheek. The scapula free flap is outlined on the patient, who is in his right lateral position. The markings indicate the dimensions of the skin island as well as the underlying soft tissues and the segment of the bone which would be resected for reconstruction (Fig. 11.89). The prefabricated scapula free flap showing the reconstituted

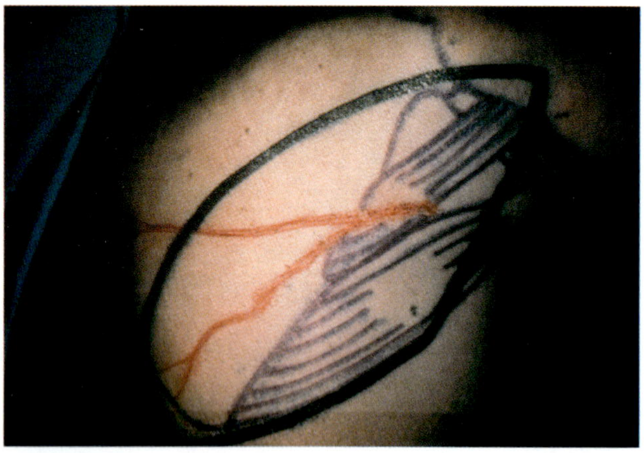

Figure 11.89 Outline of the proposed composite scapula free flap.

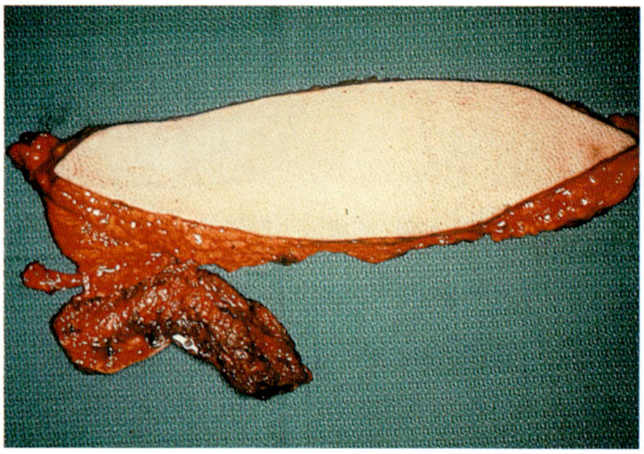

Figure 11.90 The prefabricated composite scapula free flap.

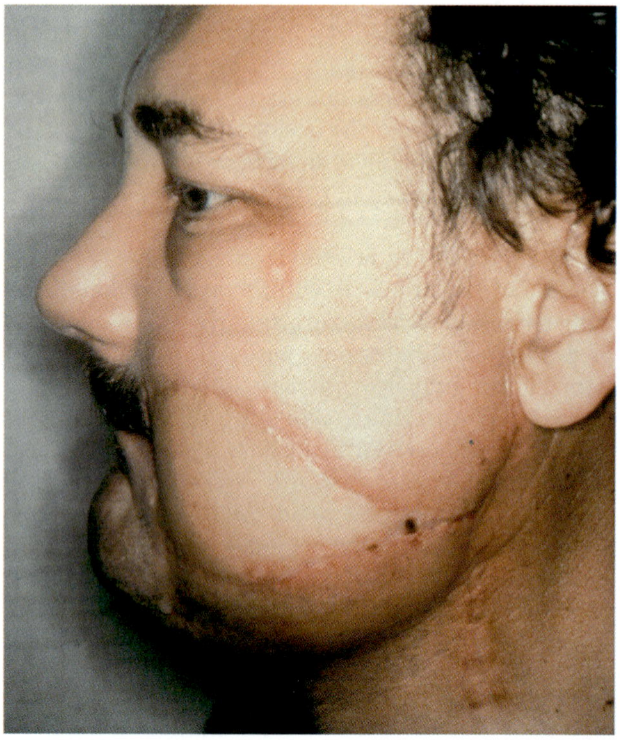

Figure 11.91 Postoperative appearance of the patient following reconstruction of the cheek and mandible.

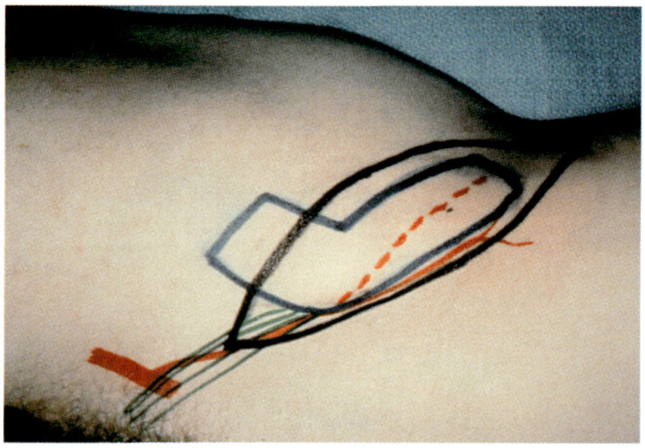

Figure 11.92 Outline of composite iliac free flap for reconstruction of the angle of the mandible.

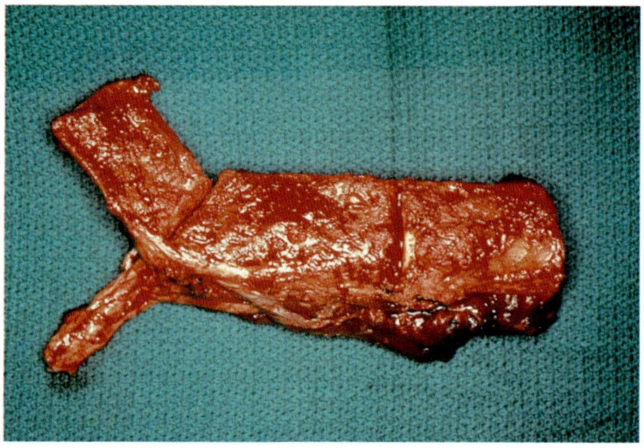

Figure 11.93 Multiple osteotomies are required to achieve the desired shape of the graft.

angle of the mandible, the vascular pedicle, and the skin island with underlying soft tissues is shown in Fig. 11.90. The postoperative result demonstrates satisfactory restoration of the contour of the chin and adequate lining for the skin defect (Fig. 11.91).

Iliac crest free flap

A composite flap of ilium with the overlying skin is of limited value in mandible reconstruction. Although the amount of the bone available is unlimited, the shape is of fixed characteristics and therefore unfavorable (Fig. 11.92). The blood supply to the bone is nonsegmental and the overlying skin is bulky, non-mobile, and often unreliable. In addition to this, there is significant morbidity at the donor site due to a difficult closure with associated pain leading to delayed mobilization. Some patients will develop a hernia at the donor site. Therefore, although abundant bone is available in the iliac free flap, its indications in mandible reconstruction are limited. In spite of these limitations, some reconstructive surgeons prefer the iliac crest free flap for mandible reconstruction, particularly for the lateral defect (Fig. 11.93).[31,34,41]

Fibula free flap

The fibula free flap is ideal for mandible reconstruction since the bone stock is appropriate and abundant, with just sufficient muscular attachment providing soft tissue, although the overlying skin in some patients (10%) could be unreliable.[19,32,33] The bone length is unlimited (up to 25 cm). The fibula has circumferential cortical bone and segmental blood supply making multiple osteotomies safe. Due to these anatomic characteristics, fabrication of the shape, angulation and curvature of the mandible can be achieved for all types of mandibular defects. In addition to this, the donor site is at a distant location and therefore extirpative surgery and harvest of the flap can be performed simultaneously, reducing the length of the operation.

Fibula free flap reconstruction of the hemimandible

Primary tumors of the mandible requiring resection of a segment of the bone with minimal or no soft tissue loss require specifically a microvascular free bone flap. Minimal or no soft tissue is required in this clinical setting.

The patient shown in Fig. 11.94 has an ossifying fibroma of the mandible requiring a right hemimandibulectomy. The tumor had been managed conservatively and observed over a period of time. However, demonstrable progression of the lesion and increasing pain required surgical treatment. A preoperative panoramic radiograph of the mandible shows diffuse patchy bone destruction involving the right hemimandible (Fig. 11.95).

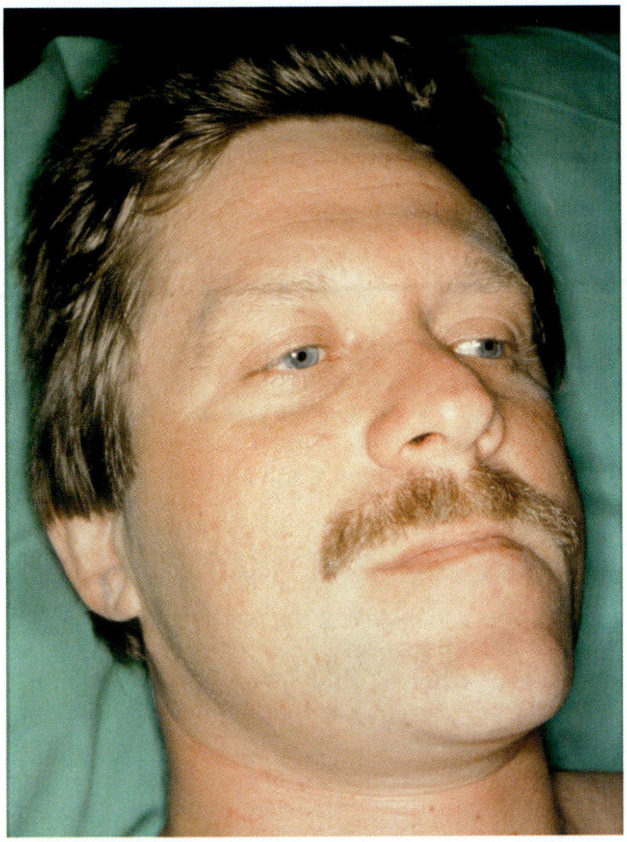

Figure 11.94 Patient with ossifying fibroma of the mandible on the right-hand side.

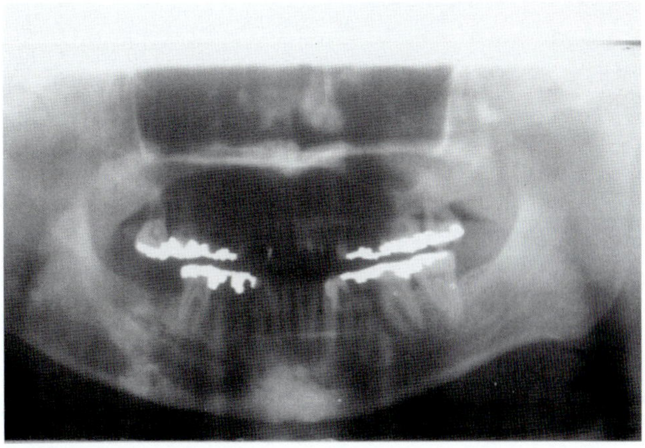

Figure 11.95 Panoramic x-ray of the mandible showing diffuse bone destruction on the right-hand side.

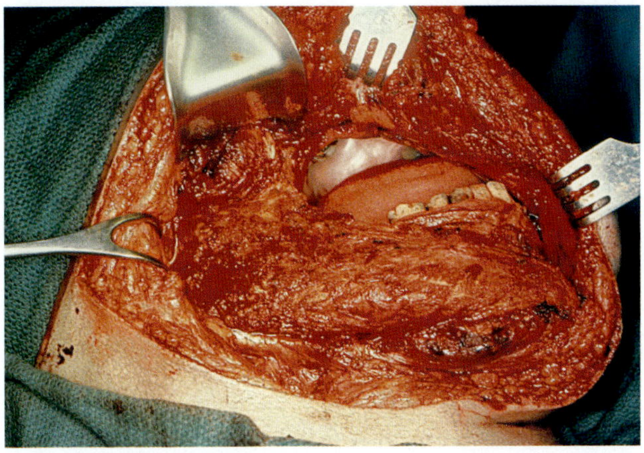

Figure 11.96 The right hemimandible is exposed through a visor flap approach.

For resection of the right hemimandible, a transverse incision is employed through an upper neck skin crease. The incision begins at the mastoid process and ends under the chin. The right lower cheek flap is elevated in the manner of a visor flap through an incision in the gingivolabial and gingivobuccal sulcus, providing adequate exposure of the right hemimandible (Fig. 11.96).

The mandible is divided just to the right of the midline anteriorly and is disarticulated from the temporomandibular joint. Thus, a true right hemimandibulectomy is performed for this patient. The optimal reconstruction for the resected hemimandible is performed using a microvascular free

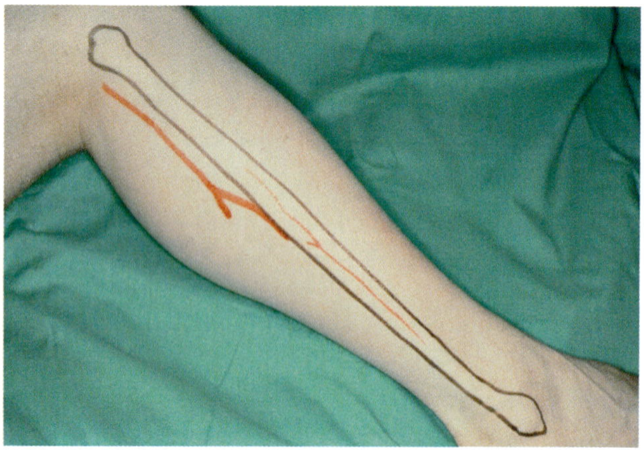

Figure 11.97 Outline of the fibula and the vascular pedicle of the flap.

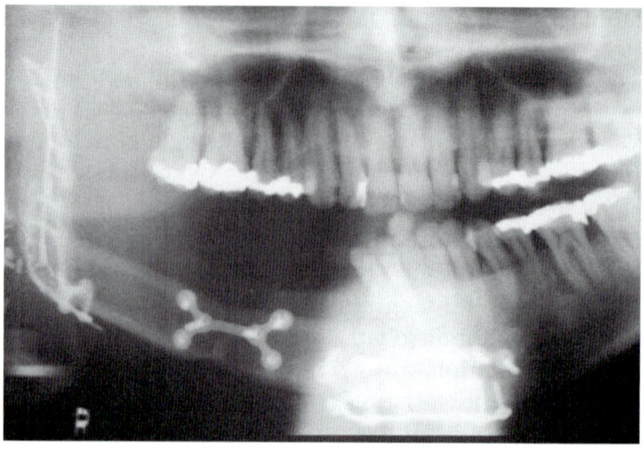

Figure 11.99 Postoperative panoramic x-ray showing reconstructed mandible.

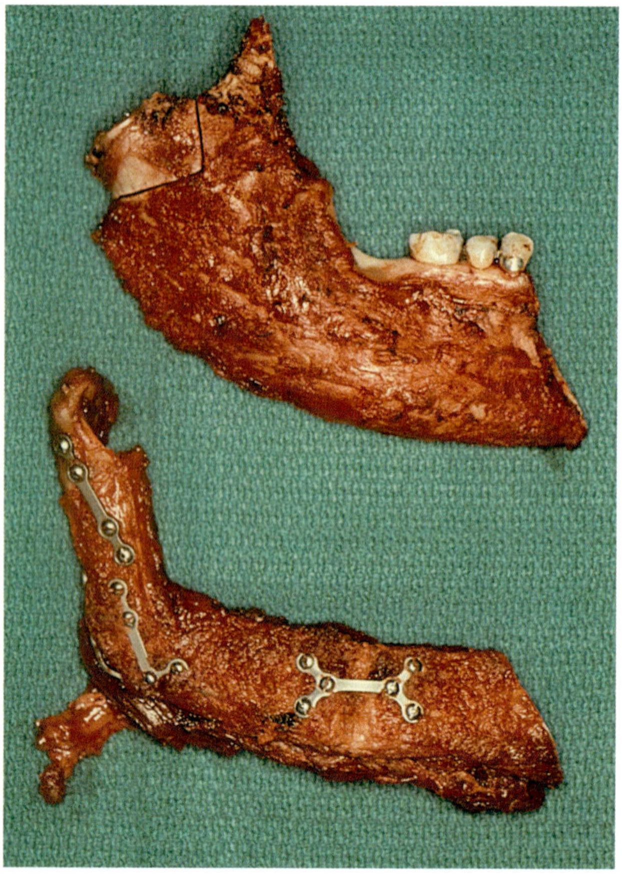

Figure 11.98 Surgical specimen of hemimandibulectomy and matching fabrication of fibula free flap.

flap of fibula (Fig. 11.97). The blood supply to the fibula is derived from the peroneal artery. A segment of the fibula with its attached musculature and the feeding vessel is isolated. The fibula is now contoured and shaped to match the resected mandible ex vivo.

Multiple osteotomies are performed in the fibula and are appropriately positioned to match the shape of the resected mandible (Fig. 11.98). Ultimate precision is exercised during these osteotomies to ensure the blood supply to the bone which is not disturbed. The shape and contour of the osteotomized fibula are maintained with the use of several miniplates and screws. The condyle of the resected mandible which is uninvolved by the disease process is amputated from the specimen and attached to the graft to form a new temporomandibular joint. The condyle is fixed to the fibula with a miniplate. Microvascular anastomoses are then completed. The temporomandibular joint is reconstituted and the graft is anchored to the stump of the mandible with miniplates. The patient is kept in intermaxillary fixation for only 2 weeks.

A postoperative panoramic view of the mandible shows the graft well aligned (Fig. 11.99). The postoperative appearance of the patient approximately three months following surgery shows a well-healed incision with a very gratifying esthetic result (Fig. 11.100). This patient's ability to open his mouth and chew food is now normal. Note that excessive soft tissue bulk is avoided in this type of reconstructive procedure since there was minimal soft tissue loss following resection of the tumor. The esthetic reconstruction of the hemimandible is at this point complete. Functional reconstruction requires osseo-integrated implants for fixed dentures in the future.

Fibula free flap reconstruction following composite resection for carcinoma of the lower gum

The patient shown in Fig. 11.101 has a locally advanced carcinoma of the lower gum involving the region of the molar teeth. A composite resection with hemimandibulectomy is performed to resect the primary tumor with adjacent soft tissues in continuity with right neck dissection. The surgical specimen is shown in Fig. 11.102. The microvascular composite free flap is fabricated with appropriate osteotomies of the fibula to create the shape of

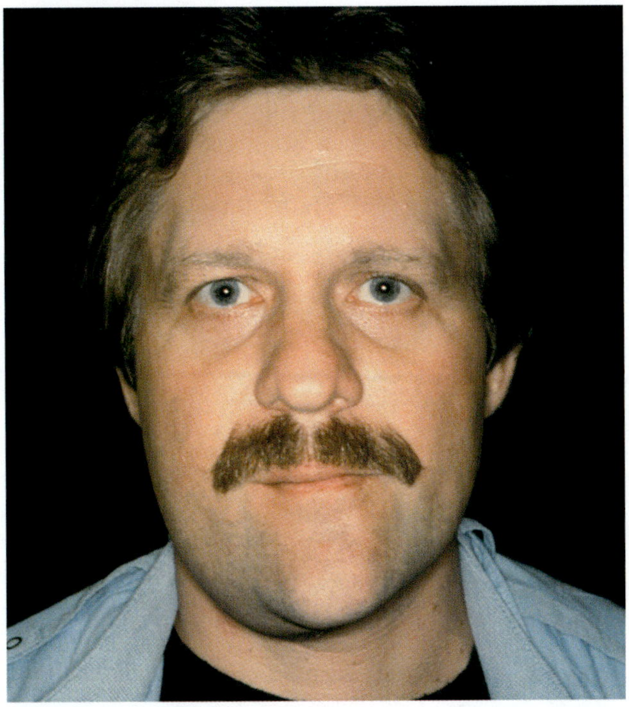

Figure 11.100 Postoperative appearance three months following mandible reconstruction.

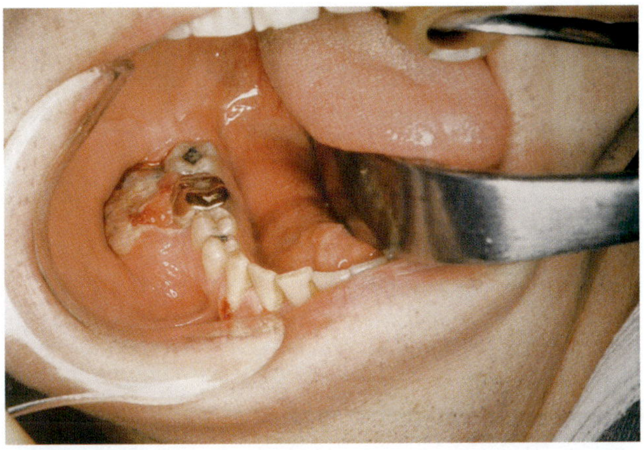

Figure 11.101 Intraoral view showing squamous carcinoma of the lower gum.

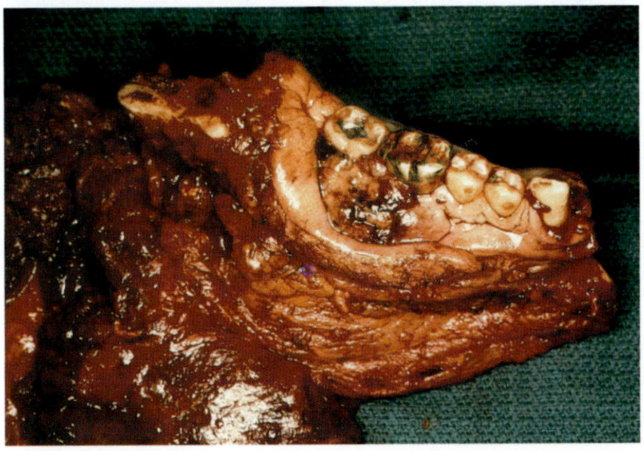

Figure 11.102 Surgical specimen of segmental mandibulectomy with neck dissection.

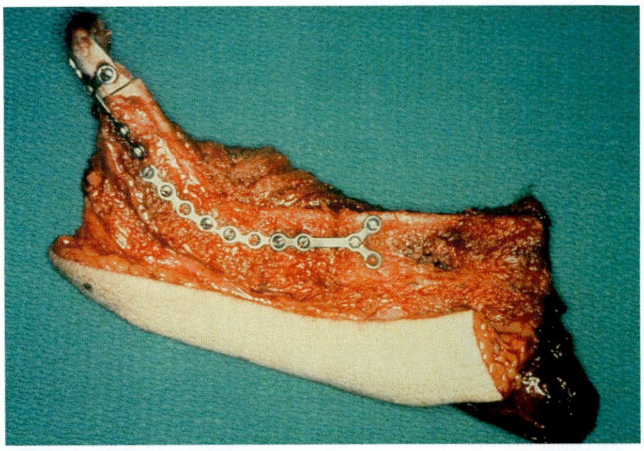

Figure 11.103 Contoured composite fibula free flap, ready for reconstruction.

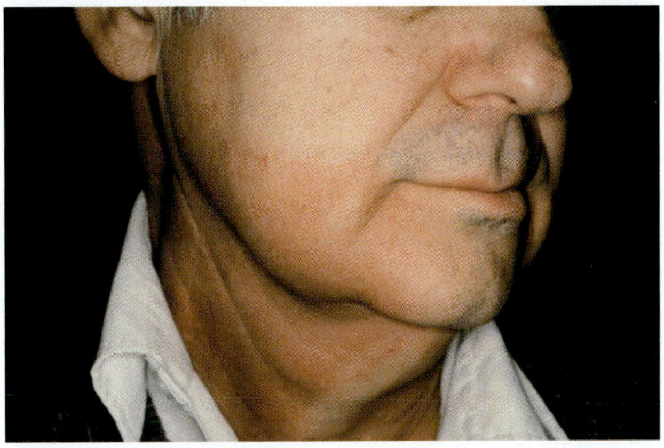

Figure 11.104 Postoperative appearance of the patient following mandible reconstruction.

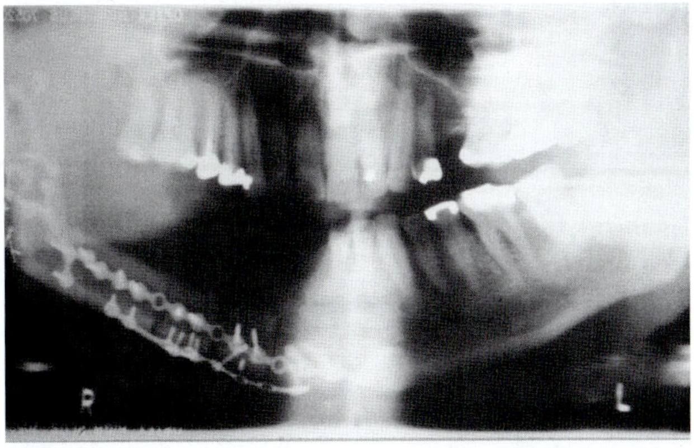

Figure 11.105 Postoperative panoramic x-ray of mandible, showing the fibula free flap.

the mandible with attached soft tissues and overlying skin to provide lining in the oral cavity (Fig. 11.103). The postoperative appearance of the patient shows restoration of the contour and the continuity of the mandible (Fig. 11.104). A panoramic radiograph of the mandible shows the fibula free flap inset and attached to the remaining mandible with miniplates and screws (Fig. 11.105).

Reconstruction of hemimandibulectomy and hemiglossectomy defect following composite resection for locally advanced carcinoma of the oral tongue

The patient whose surgical defect is shown in Fig. 11.106 had locally advanced carcinoma of the oral tongue with extension to the floor of the mouth and fixation to the lingual plate of the mandible requiring a hemiglossectomy in conjunction with hemimandibulectomy and right neck dissection. A prefabricated fibula free flap composite graft is shown in Fig. 11.107. Multiple osteotomies are performed in the fibula to create the shape

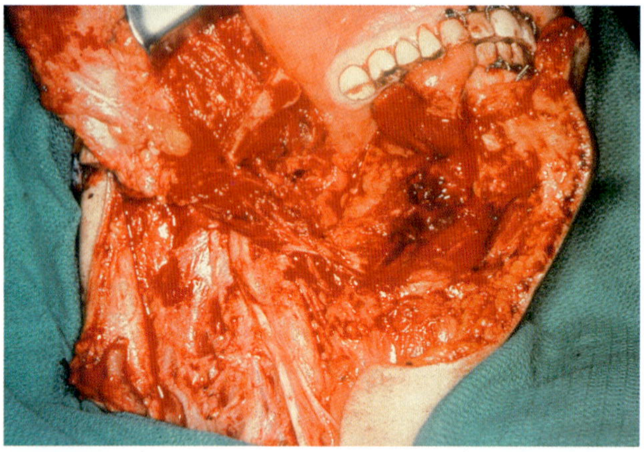

Figure 11.106 Surgical defect of hemiglossectomy, hemimandibulectomy and neck dissection.

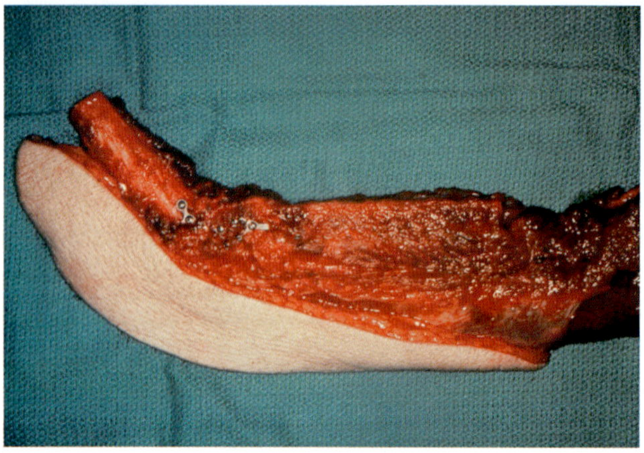

Figure 11.107 Composite fibula free flap prepared for reconstruction.

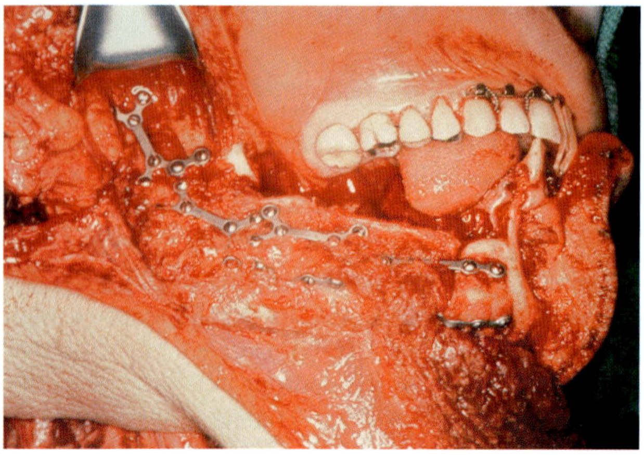

Figure 11.108 The hemimandibulectomy defect is reconstructed.

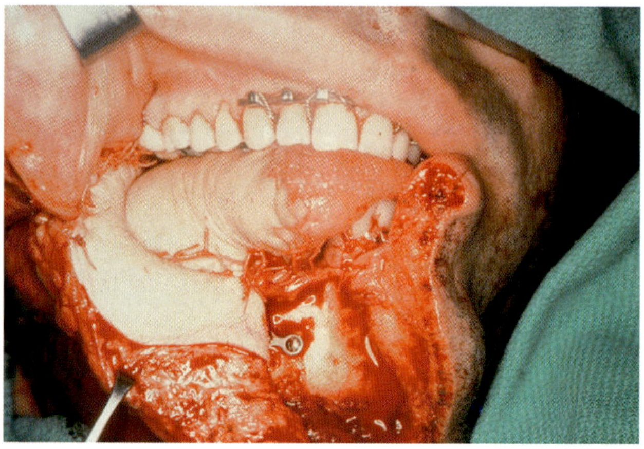

Figure 11.109 The hemiglossectomy reconstruction in progress.

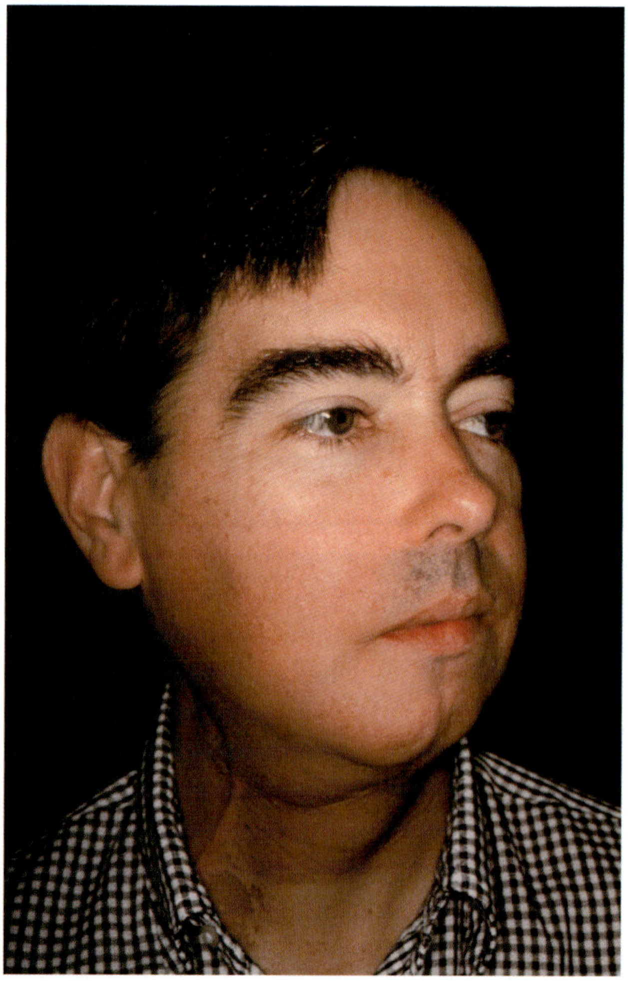

Figure 11.110 Postoperative appearance of the patient at three months.

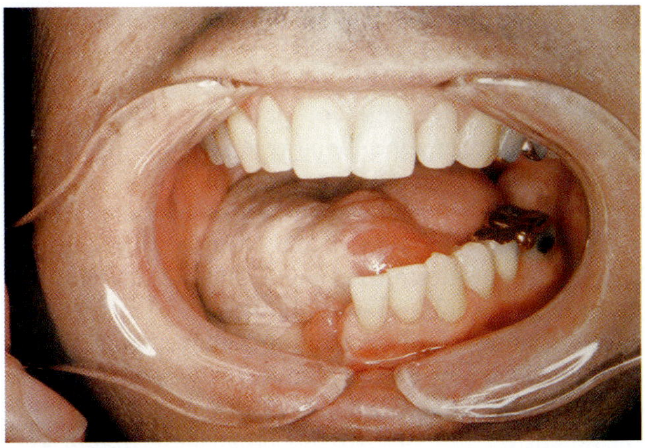

Figure 11.111 Postoperative intraoral view showing reconstructed tongue on the right-hand side.

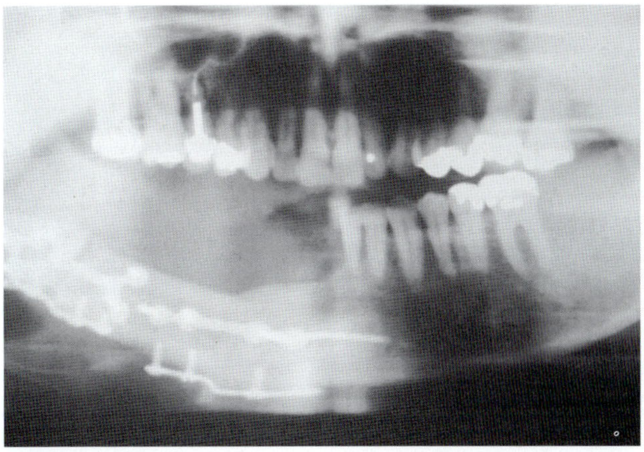

Figure 11.112 Postoperative panoramic x-ray showing reconstructed mandible.

of the mandible. The mandible reconstruction is completed first by fixation of the graft to the remaining mandible (Fig. 11.108). The soft tissues and overlying skin remain attached to the bone and will provide lining for the lower gum, floor of the mouth, and for reconstruction of the resected half of the tongue on the right hand side (Fig. 11.109). The postoperative view of the patient shows restoration of the contour and continuity of the mandible (Fig. 11.110). The intra-oral view shows the reconstructed half of the oral tongue on the right-hand side with restored mobility and shape of the oral tongue (Fig. 11.111). A postoperative panoramic radiograph shows accurate alignment of the reconstructed mandible (Fig. 11.112).

Reconstruction of the anterior arch of the mandible

A preoperative photograph of a 17-year-old male with chondrosarcoma of the anterior arch of the mandible is shown in Fig. 11.113. This patient's CT scans in the coronal and axial planes show an intra-osseous lesion with a honeycomb-like appearance, which is typical for a chondrosarcoma (Fig. 11.114). Biopsy of this lesion confirmed it to be a low grade chondrosarcoma. Resection of the anterior arch of the mandible is performed, extending from the level of the first molar tooth on the right-hand side to the level of the second premolar tooth on the left-hand side. The surgical specimen shows a complete monobloc resection of the anterior arch of the mandible (Fig. 11.115). The bone defect is repaired using a fibula free flap with multiple osteotomies. The postoperative appearance of the patient shows perfect restoration of the contour and shape of the face and projection of the chin (Fig. 11.116). Comparison of the preoperative and postoperative panorex of the mandible shows exact restoration of the anterior arch of the mandible (Fig. 11.117).

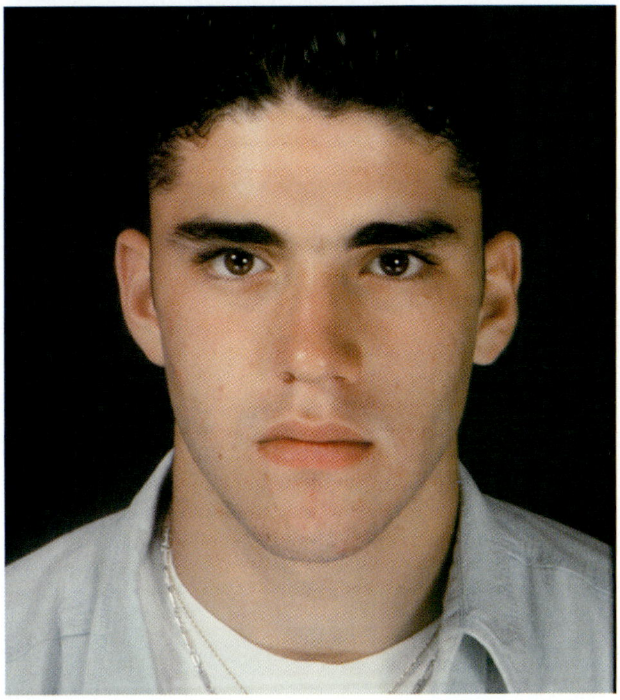

Figure 11.113 Patient with chondrosarcoma of the anterior arch of mandible.

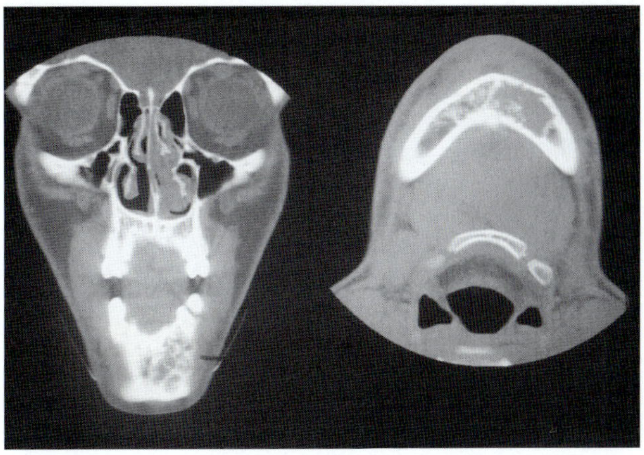

Figure 11.114 Coronal and axial views of the CT scan of the mandible showing chondrosarcoma.

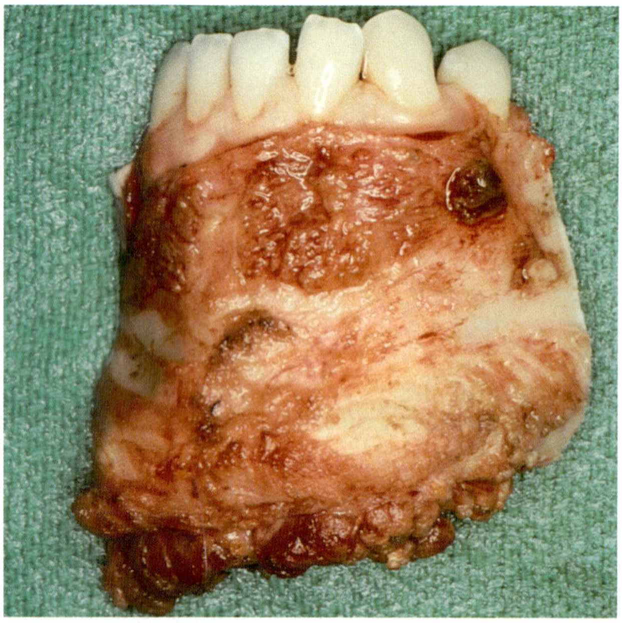

Figure 11.115 Specimen of the anterior arch of the mandible.

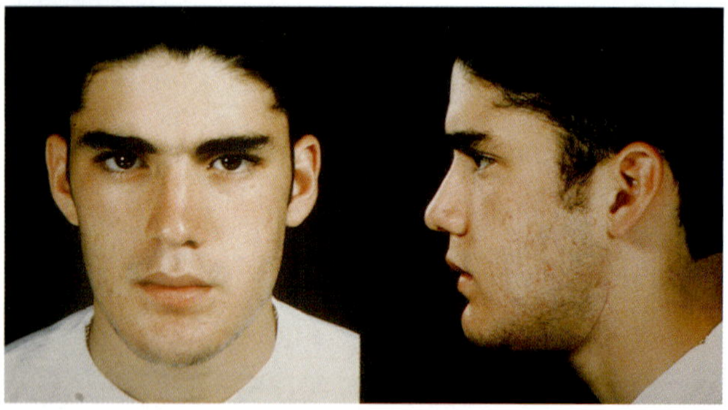

Figure 11.116 Frontal and lateral views of the face following reconstruction of the anterior arch.

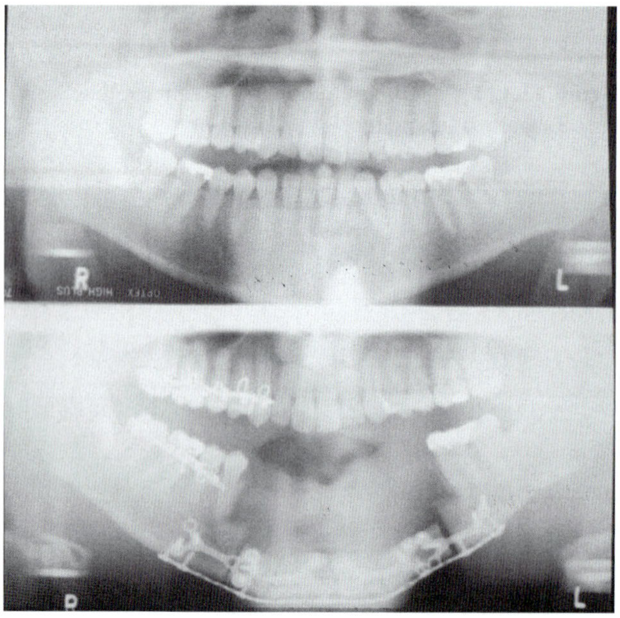

Figure 11.117 Pre- and postoperative panoramic x-rays, showing accurate alignment of the fibula free flap.

Osseointegrated implants in the reconstructed mandible

The obvious advantages of proceeding with osseointegrated implants for dental restoration in the reconstructed mandible are improvement in the esthetic appearance of the patient, restoration of the clarity of speech, and restoration of oral competence and the function of mastication. However, the requirement for successful osseointegration of the implants is the availability of adequate soft tissue coverage (i.e. soft and pliable) over the bone. Implants in irradiated bone should be considered with extreme caution. The vertical height of the bone should be at least 10 mm and the width of the bone approximately 5 to 6 mm. Clearly the best candidates are those who are free of disease and who have accurate reconstruction of the resected mandible. Patients with defects of the anterior arch of the mandible and those in whom no skin island is required for lining in the oral cavity are ideal candidates. A reconstructed mandible with fibula is ideal due to adequate dimensions of the bone. The time of osseointegration in the fibula is approximately the same as in edentulous normal mandible, and therefore the success rate is very high. However, before proceeding with implementation of osseointegrated implants, satisfactory bone healing must be demonstrated. This usually takes 9 to 12 months following fibula free flap mandible reconstruction. In addition to this, the miniplates and screws in the region of the site of implants must be removed before the implants are placed. Thus, it may take up to 2 years before osseointegrated implants are completed with placement of the teeth to achieve total mandible reconstruction and rehabilitation.

Some reconstructive surgeons prefer placement of dental implants in the fibula primarily at the time of mandible reconstruction. This clearly saves time and offers the patient early dental rehabilitation. However, we feel that accurate alignment of the implants at the time of mandible reconstruction is difficult and usually unsatisfactory, leading to poor esthetic dental rehabilitation. In addition to this, metallic implants in the graft may produce bone complications secondary to postoperative radiotherapy, which most of these patients need. For these reasons, we favor secondary dental rehabilitation with osseointegrated implants after all treatment is finished, adequate healing of the bone graft is achieved, and a sufficient disease-free interval has elapsed.

The patient whose left lower gum is shown in Fig. 11.118 underwent resection of the body of the mandible for a central salivary carcinoma of the lower gum. A preoperative CT scan shows the lesion in the left-hand side of the mandible (Fig. 11.119). The surgical specimen is shown in Fig. 11.120. Fibula free flap reconstruction was accomplished

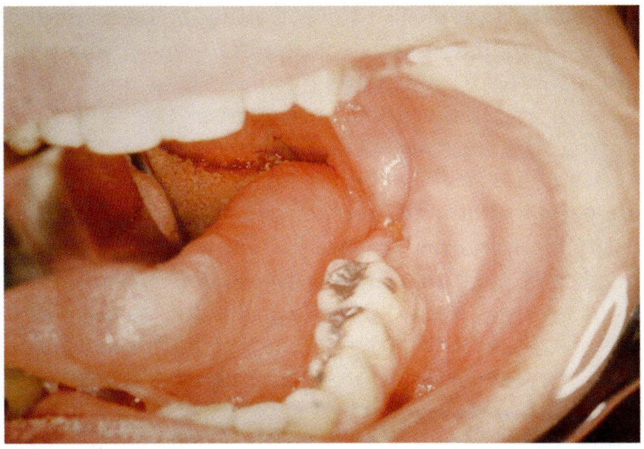

Figure 11.118 Intra-oral view of the left lower gum.

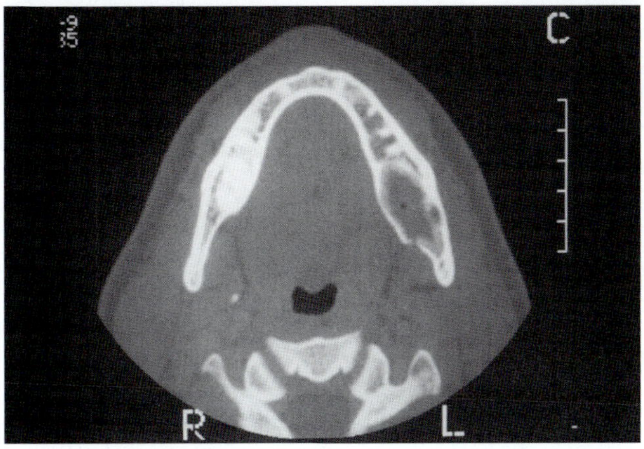

Figure 11.119 Axial view of the CT scan showing the bone destructive lesion.

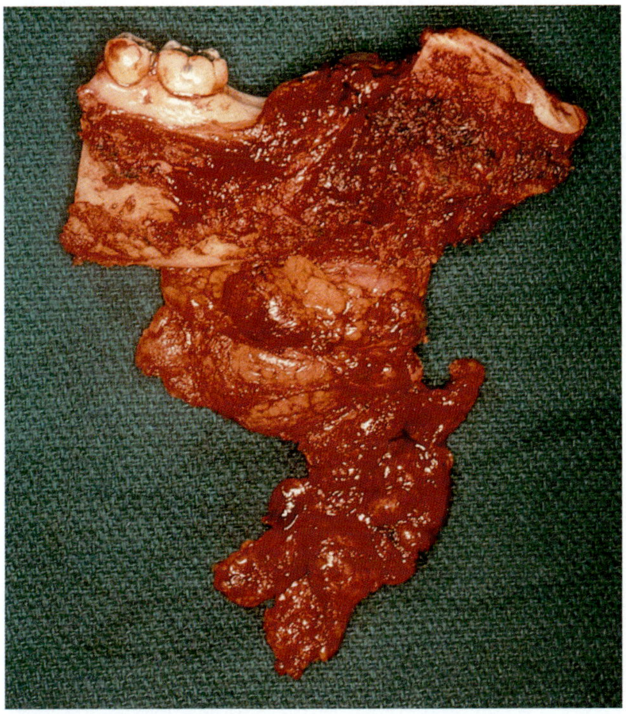

Figure 11.120 Surgical specimen of segmental mandibulectomy and supraomohyoid neck dissection.

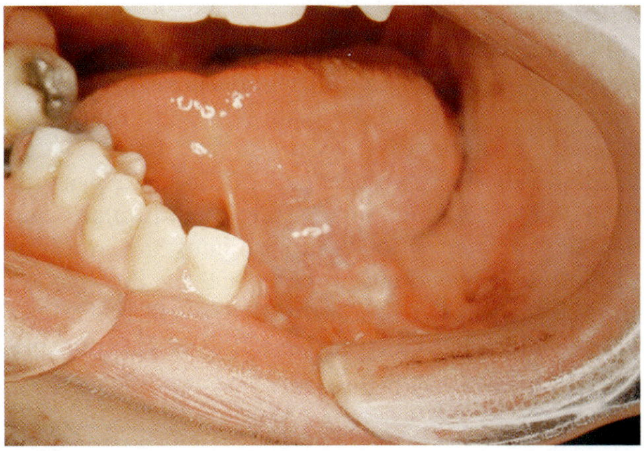

Figure 11.121 Postoperative intra-oral view showing primary healing of mucosa.

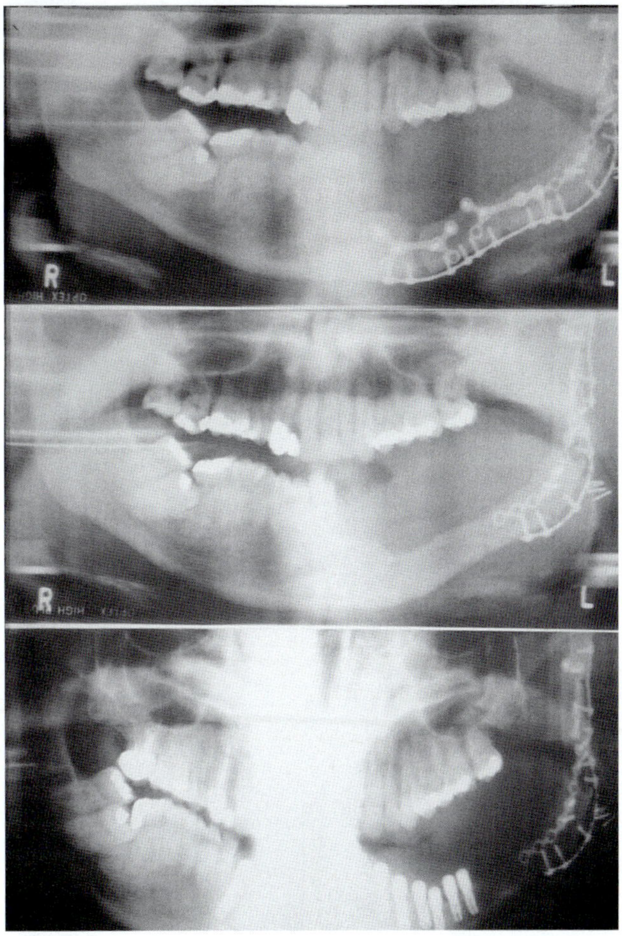

A

B

C

Figure 11.122 Postoperative panoramic x-rays: (A) immediately after reconstruction; (B) after removal of screws and plates; (C) with osseointegrated implants.

with accurate alignment of the reconstructed bone. A postoperative intra-oral photograph shows satisfactory mucosal healing (Fig. 11.121). The panoramic radiographs shown in Fig. 11.122 demonstrate immediate restoration of the continuity of the mandible with the fibula free flap. The intermediate radiograph shows satisfactory bone healing and removal of the plates and screws prior to osseointegrated implants and the third panoramic radiograph shows implants placed in the anterior aspect of the reconstructed body of the mandible on the left-hand side. A postoperative view of the patient after implants shows the placement of the teeth over the implants achieving total oral, mandibular, and dental reconstruction and rehabilitation (Fig. 11.123). The external appearance of the patient shows the restored contour of the face (Fig. 11.124). This is the ideal that can be achieved in appropriate candidates requiring resection and reconstruction of the mandible with a fibula free flap.

An increasing proportion of patients have undergone immediate reconstruction of the mandible with microvascular free flaps at the Head and Neck Service at Memorial Sloan-Kettering Cancer Center during the period 1985–2000[20] (Figs 11.125 and 11.126). A variety of other microvascular free flaps are used for immediate reconstruction of other surgical defects following cancer ablative surgery in the head and neck region. Microvascular surgery is an exciting new field and its application in the head and neck area is limitless. What we have seen in the past 15 years is just the beginning of a whole new era in a promising field of surgery.

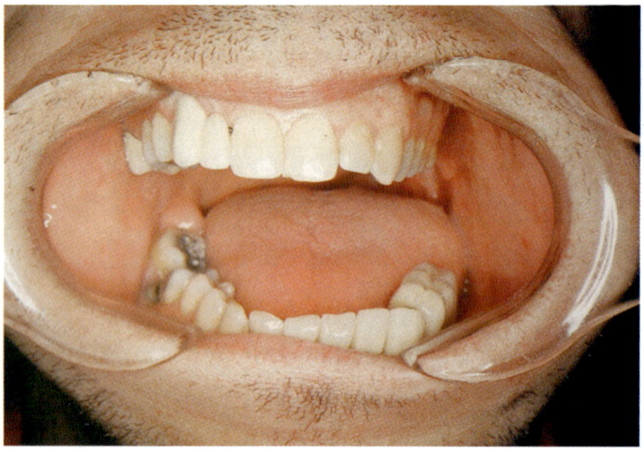

Figure 11.123 Intra-oral view after placement of dental implants.

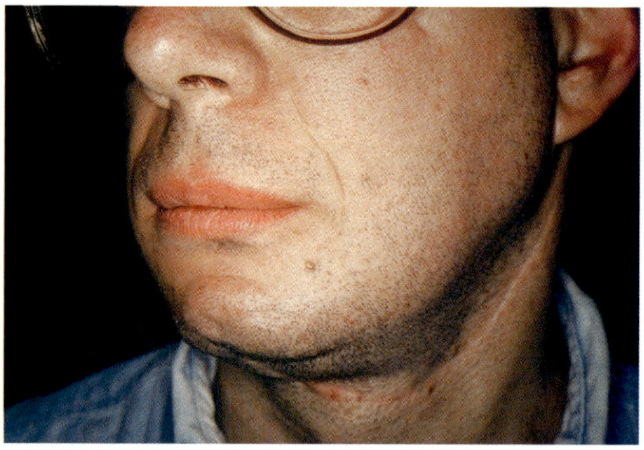

Figure 11.124 Restored facial contour, two years following surgery.

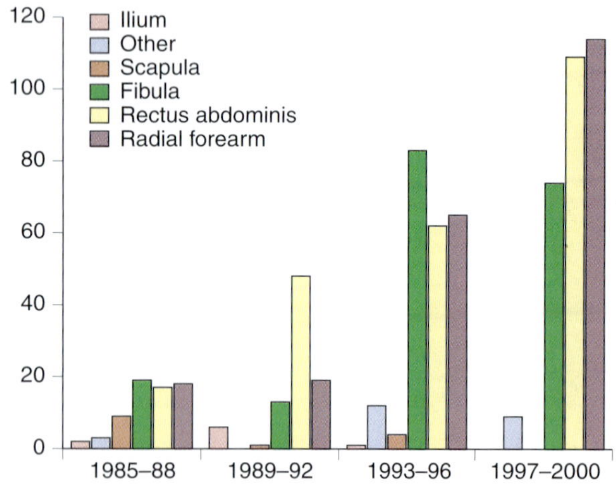

Data points

	1985–88	1989–92	1993–96	1997–2000
Ilium	2	6	1	0
Other	3	0	12	9
Scapula	9	1	4	0
Fibula	19	13	83	74
Rectus abdominis	17	48	62	109
Radial forearm	18	19	65	114

Figure 11.125 Types of free flaps used for oral cavity reconstruction at Memorial Sloan–Kettering Cancer Center.

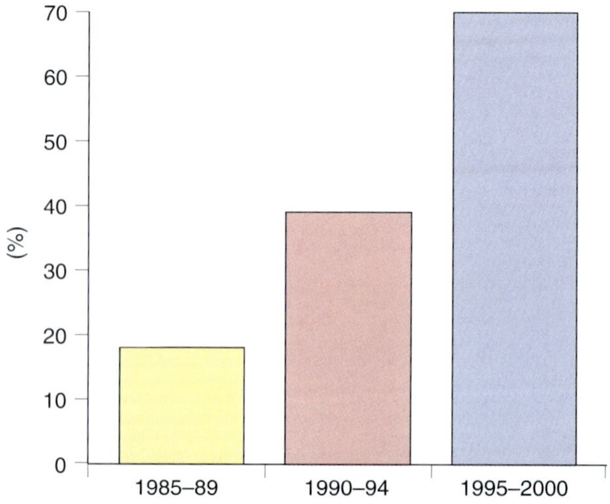

Data points	1985–89	1990–94	1995–2000
Free flaps	18%	39%	70%

Figure 11.126 Percentage of mandibular defects reconstructed with free flaps at Memorial Sloan–Kettering Cancer Center during three time periods.

References

1. McGregor IA, Morgan G. Axial and random pattern flaps. Br J Plast Surg 1973; 26: 202–213
2. Ariyan S. Further experiences with the pectoralis major myocutaneous flap for the immediate repair of defects from excisions of head and neck cancers. Plast Reconstr Surg 1979; 64: 605–612
3. Baek SM, Biller HF, Krespi YP, Lawson W. The pectoralis major myocutaneous island flap for reconstruction of the head and neck. Head Neck Surg 1979; 1: 293–300
4. Baek SM, Lawson W, Biller HF. An analysis of 133 pectoralis major myocutaneous flaps. Plast Reconstr Surg 1982; 69: 460–469
5. Barton FE Jr, Spicer TE, Byrd HS. Head and neck reconstruction with the latissimus dorsi myocutaneous flap: anatomic observations and report of 60 cases. Plast Reconstr Surg 1983; 71: 199–204
6. Conley J, Gullane PJ. The sternocleidomastoid muscle flap. Head Neck Surg 1980; 2: 308–311
7. Demergasso F, Piazza MV. Trapezius myocutaneous flap in reconstructive surgery for head and neck cancer: an original technique. Am J Surg 1979; 138: 533–536
8. Gregor RT, Davidge-Pitts KJ. Trapezius osteomyocutaneous flap for mandibular reconstruction. Arch Otolaryngol 1985; 111: 198–203
9. Shah JP, Shemen L, Spiro RH, Strong EW. Selecting variants in pharyngeal reconstruction. Ann Otol Rhinol Laryngol 1984; 93(4 Pt 1): 318–321
10. Shah JP, Haribhakti V, Loree TR, Sutaria P. Complications of the pectoralis major myocutaneous flap in head and neck reconstruction. Am J Surg 1990; 160: 352–355
11. Urken ML, Vickery C, Weinberg H, Buchbinder D, Lawson W, Biller HF. The internal oblique-iliac crest osseomyocutaneous free flap in oromandibular reconstruction. Report of 20 cases. Arch Otolaryngol Head Neck Surg 1989; 115: 339–349
12. Bakamijan VY, Long M, Rigg B. Experience with the medially based deltopectoral flap in reconstructuve surgery of the head and neck. Br J Plast Surg 1971; 24: 174–183
13. Farr HW, Jean-Gilles B, Die A. Cervical island skin flap repair of oral and pharyngeal defects in the composite operation for cancer. Am J Surg 1969; 118: 759–763
14. Netterville JL, Wood DE. The lower trapezius flap. Vascular anatomy and surgical technique. Arch Otolaryngol Head Neck Surg 1991; 117: 73–76
15. Boyd JB, Rosen I, Rotstein L, et al. The iliac crest and the radial forearm flap in vascularized oromandibular reconstruction. Am J Surg 1990; 159: 301–308
16. Soutar DS, Scheker LR, Tanner NS, McGregor IA. The radial forearm flap: a versatile method for intra-oral reconstruction. Br J Plast Surg 1983; 36: 1–8
17. Urken ML, Weinberg H, Vickery C, Biller HF. The neurofasciocutaneous radial forearm flap in head and neck reconstruction: a preliminary report. Laryngoscope 1990; 100(2 Pt 1): 161–173
18. Swartz WM, Banis JC, Newton ED, Ramasastry SS, Jones NF, Acland R. The osteocutaneous scapular flap for mandibular and maxillary reconstruction. Plast Reconstr Surg 1986; 77: 530–545
19. Taylor GI. The current status of free vascularized bone grafts. Clin Plast Surg 1983; 10: 185–209
20. Disa JJ, Hu QY, Hidalgo DA. Retrospective review of 400 consecutive free flap reconstructions for oncologic surgical defects. Ann Surg Oncol 1997; 4: 663–669
21. Kroll SS, Baldwin BJ. Head and neck reconstruction with the rectus abdominis free flap. Clin Plast Surg 1994; 21: 97–105
22. Cordeiro PG, Santamaria E. The extended, pedicled rectus abdominis free tissue transfer for head and neck reconstruction. Ann Plast Surg 1997; 39: 53–59
23. Wanamaker JR, Burkey BB. Overview of the rectus abdominis myocutaneous flap in head and neck reconstruction. Facial Plast Surg 1996; 12: 45–50
24. Koshima I, Yamamoto H, Hosoda M, Moriguchi T, Orita Y, Nagayama H. Free combined composite flaps using the lateral circumflex femoral system for repair of massive defects of the head and neck regions: an introduction to the chimeric flap principle. Plast Reconstr Surg 1993; 92: 411–420
25. Karcher H, Hellbom B, Radner H. The osteomusculocutaneous musculoperitoneal groin flap in head and neck reconstruction. J Reconstr Microsurg 1989; 5: 31–35
26. Harrison TJ, Quillen CG. Free osteocutaneous groin flap in the reconstruction of large mandibular defects. A case study. Arch Otolaryngol 1983; 109: 485–488
27. Serafin D, Rios AV, Georgiade N. Fourteen free groin flap transfers. Plast Reconstr Surg 1976; 57: 707–715
28. Lister GD, Gibson T. Closure of rhomboid skin defects: the flaps of Limberg and Dufourmentel. Br J Plast Surg 1972; 25: 300–314
29. Mutter T. Cases of deformity from burns relieved by operation. Am J Med Sci 1842; 4: 66
30. Daniel RK. Mandibular reconstruction with free tissue transfers. Ann Plast Surg 1978; 1: 346–371
31. David DJ, Tan E, Katsaros J, Sheen R. Mandibular reconstruction with vascularized iliac crest: a 10-year experience. Plast Reconstr Surg 1988; 82: 792–803
32. Hidalgo DA. Fibula free flap: a new method of mandible reconstruction. Plast Reconstr Surg 1989; 84: 71–79
33. Hidalgo DA. Aesthetic improvements in free-flap mandible reconstruction. Plast Reconstr Surg 1991; 88: 574–585; discussion 586–587
34. Jewer DD, Boyd JB, Manktelow RT et al. Orofacial and mandibular reconstruction with the iliac crest free flap: a review of 60 cases and a new method of classification [see comments]. Plast Reconstr Surg 1989; 84: 391–403; discussion 404–405
35. Katsaros J, Schusterman M, Beppu M, Banis JC Jr, Acland RD. The lateral upper arm flap: anatomy and clinical applications. Ann Plast Surg 1984; 12: 489–500
36. MacLeod AM, Robinson DW. Reconstruction of defects involving the mandible and floor of mouth by free

osteo-cutaneous flaps derived from the foot. Br J Plast Surg 1982; 35: 239–246
37. Soutar DS, Widdowson WP. Immediate reconstruction of the mandible using a vascularized segment of radius. Head Neck Surg 1986; 8: 232–246
38. Urken ML, Buchbinder D, Weinberg H et al. Functional evaluation following microvascular oromandibular reconstruction of the oral cancer patient: a comparative study of reconstructed and nonreconstructed patients [see comments]. Laryngoscope 1991; 101: 935–950
39. Urken ML. Composite free flaps in oromandibular reconstruction. Review of the literature. Arch Otolaryngol Head Neck Surg 1991; 117: 724–732
40. Riediger D. Restoration of masticatory function by microsurgically revascularized iliac crest bone grafts using enosseous implants. Plast Reconstr Surg 1988; 81: 861–877
41. Taylor GI. Reconstruction of the mandible with free composite iliac bone grafts. Ann Plast Surg 1982; 9: 361–376

12 Radiotherapy and chemotherapy

John Glaholm

Radiotherapy

Biological effects: basic principles

The origin of the therapeutic use of ionizing radiation dates from the end of the nineteenth century, following the discovery of radium by Marie and Pierre Curie. It became apparent that rapidly dividing tissues, including malignant tumours, could be selectively destroyed by this process. Radiotherapy initially developed from diagnostic radiology using low energy X-ray equipment for external beam delivery and from radium as a means of administering interstitial or intracavitary therapeutic irradiation. Ionization of atoms in living tissue by therapeutic doses of such electromagnetic radiation is thought primarily to cause nuclear DNA damage which, if irreparable, may result in cell death. The mechanism of action is therefore relatively unselective between tumour and normal tissue, with a narrow therapeutic index (Fig. 12.1). Radiotherapy techniques have consequently been developed to enhance the therapeutic ratio by physical methods using multiple beams directed at the tumour volume in order to minimize the radiation dose to surrounding normal tissues (Fig. 12.2) and by delivering the total dose of radiation in multiple fractions over a period of several weeks. Conventional radiotherapy fractionation schedules vary considerably, particularly throughout the UK, and have primarily been determined by treatment equipment resource limitations rather than by science.[1]

A number of radiobiological factors are considered important in the response of normal tissues and tumours to radiotherapy and are implicated in the effects of fractionated irradiation.[2] *Repair* is the phenomenon of cellular recovery which takes place over several hours following exposure to ionizing radiation and is a significant factor in normal tissue tolerance when the interval between fractionated doses of irradiation is reduced below the 'conventional' 24-hour period. *Repopulation* of surviving normal and tumour cell clonogens occurs during the multiple weeks of conventional radiotherapy fractionation. This may result in reduced tumour control when treatment schedules are protracted as a result of accelerated tumour clonogen repopulation,[3] or when gaps are inadvertently or deliberately introduced in a course of radiotherapy. Clinical or radiological tumour volume doubling time is not an accurate surrogate for measuring tumour clonogen proliferation because a tumour is also composed of normal stromal cells and non-dividing, resting, tumour cells. To account for this and for the cell loss factor, which can be high in squamous cancers, the parameter of *potential doubling time* has been developed to represent tumour clonogen replication more

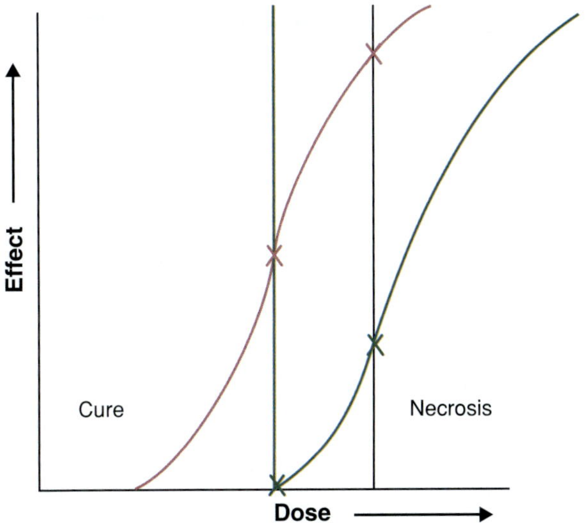

Figure 12.1 Radiation dose response curves: theoretical sigmoid tumour dose response and risk of late tissue necrosis.

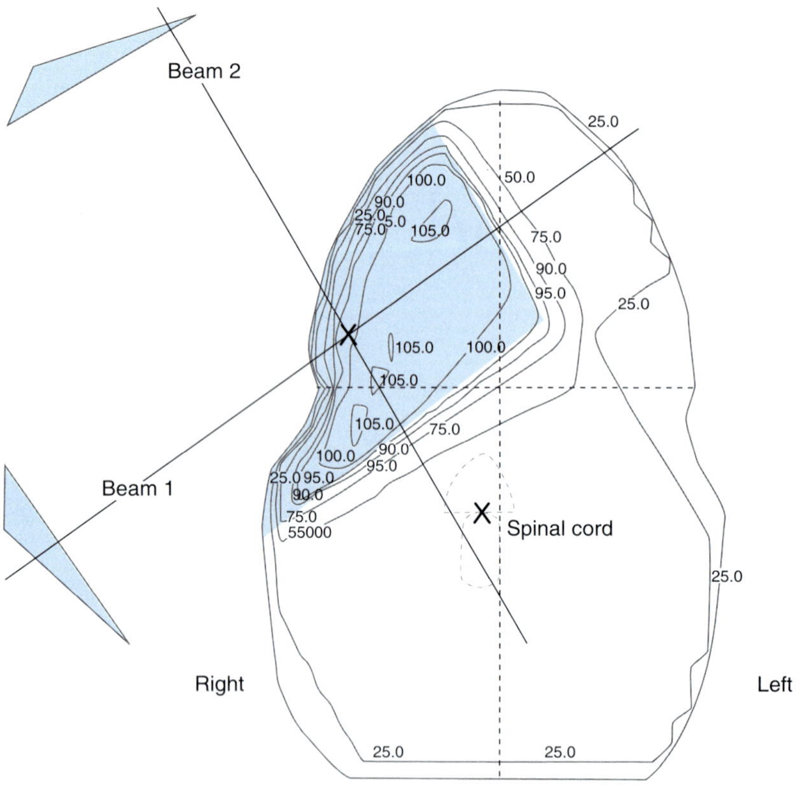

Figure 12.2 Floor of mouth radiation isodose distribution; anterior and posterior oblique wedged fields.

clearly and it may become useful in predicting control by radiotherapy.[2]

The damaging effects of ionizing radiation are highly dependent upon the presence of oxygen such that well-oxygenated clonogenic cells are up to three-fold more sensitive than anoxic cells.[4] Tumour specimens examined by Thomlinson and Gray in 1955 demonstrated lung cancer tumour cells growing concentrically around blood vessels. Cells at least 200 microns distant from a vessel were frequently necrotic and hence non-viable, with intermediate layers of viable although presumably hypoxic and by inference radioresistant cells.[5] Such chronic hypoxia is therefore a result of restricted oxygen diffusion within the tumour. More recently evidence has suggested that transient or acute hypoxia may result from transitory closure of intra-tumoural blood vessels.[6] In contrast, normal tissues, as a rule, are well oxygenated. Therefore the process of *reoxygenation* of tumours during fractionated radiotherapy may be an important factor in tumour control. These radiobiological factors have now been investigated in head and neck cancer clinical trials and will be discussed later in this chapter. Other phenomena which may be clinically important are the *recruitment* of resting cells into the cycling pool and *redistribution* of cycling cells into radiosensitive phases of the cell cycle.

The biological effects of ionizing radiation on normal tissues depend upon their cellular kinetics and repair capacity, the quality (energy) and type of radiation, for example, low linear energy transfer (LET) gamma ray, X-ray and megavoltage electron irradiation, where there is relatively sparse energy deposition in tissues, or high LET irradiation such as with fast neutrons,[7] the overall dose and time of a course of irradiation, the dose per fraction and the interval between each fraction.

Normal tissue reactions can be broadly divided into early and late. Early reactions typically occur within 3 to 9 weeks and result from mitotic arrest of rapidly dividing cells, mucosa, skin, taste buds, facial hair. The clinical course is usually transient and repopulation of the normal tissue will typically be achieved within 4 to 6 weeks after the completion of a course of radiotherapy unless permanent damage has resulted from excessive radiation dosage resulting in consequential damage. The sensitivity of this process to fraction size and type of irradiation is relatively low, but is enhanced by shortening the overall radiotherapy fractionation schedule. Late reactions typically occur beyond 12 weeks and can progress or become apparent over several years. Damage may result from vascular injury with subsequent healing by fibrosis in peripheral tissues and by gliosis in the central nervous system. The effect is irreversible. Late reactions are relatively more sensitive than early reactions to larger radiation doses per fraction and to high LET irradiation. Salivary gland cells deserve special mention as they are highly sensitive to ionizing radiation and undergo programmed, 'apoptotic', cell death at relatively low doses, unlike most normal and tumour cells which die upon attempted cell division, 'mitotic', cell death. Dissociation between early, reversible, and late, irreversible, tissue reactions may therefore result when changes are made in dose, time, fractionation and LET of irradiation.

Mathematical models have been used to describe the relationship between total isoeffective dose and the dose per fraction in clinical radiotherapy. The linear quadratic (LQ) model, in which the effect is represented by both a linear and a quadratic function of dose, provides a method of dose equivalence calculation for early and late reactions.[8] Nevertheless, such models are at best approximate mathematical fits for biological phenomena and must be interpreted with caution when applied to the clinical setting.

With new developments in radiation dose fractionation, the investigation of radiosensitizers and the addition of adjuvant chemotherapy, it has become increasingly important to be able to score late tissue effects accurately and in the past few years several independent systems have been devised. However, a consensus conference in San Francisco has now recommended a uniform scoring system for Late Effects on Normal Tissues, LENT. The system accounts for late effects on vital organs with clearly defined endpoints in terms of somatic and genetic effects and second malignant tumours. The scoring system defines four major categories, Subjective, Objective, Management and Analytic, hence the acronym SOMA.[9,10] As will be discussed later, several strategies have now been investigated in an attempt to enhance the therapeutic ratio by increasing tumour control, possibly at the cost of intensified early tissue reaction but without enhanced late tissue damage.

External beam radiotherapy

Modern megavoltage external beam radiotherapy linear accelerators (Fig. 12.3) which produce X-ray energies of 4 to 6 million volts are ideal for head and neck irradiation and have largely superseded cobalt-60 units. Megavoltage photon beams have several physical and biological advantages compared to earlier kilovoltage X-rays. Beam definition and direction are precise, there is sparing of surface tissues incident to the beam and the depth of penetration is high. The radiation dose absorbed by bone is low, similar to soft tissue, which is associated with a much reduced risk of osteoradionecrosis. Head and neck irradiation is usually undertaken using a custom made transparent plastic localization shell (Fig. 12.4), which allows the patient to be positioned to an accuracy of within 2–3 mm. Multiple beams can therefore be directed, repeatedly and reproducibly, at the tumour during a course of fractionated radiotherapy. Computerized planning allows rapid summation of each radiation beam which can be arranged in order to ensure a uniform dose distribution within the tumour, while

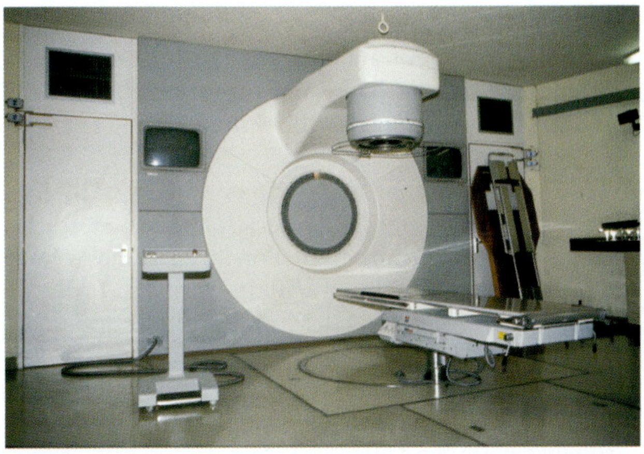

Figure 12.3 Multiple energy medical linear accelerator.

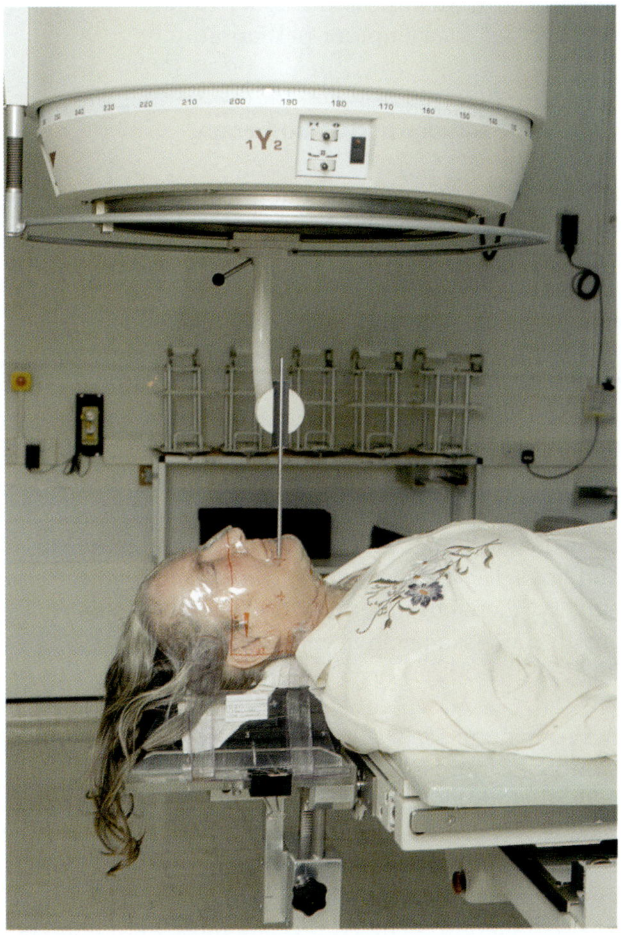

Figure 12.4 Patient positioned in the beam localization shell.

minimizing radiation exposure of surrounding critical structures, such as the spinal cord and lens of the eye.

High-energy medical linear accelerators can also be used to produce megavoltage electron beams whose radiobiological properties in tumours and normal tissues are analogous to megavoltage X-rays. Electrons are charged particles and therefore their penetration into tissue is limited, with a rapid fall-off in dose at depths which depend upon the chosen electron energy. This modality is particularly useful for treating tumours overlying dose-limiting critical normal structures such as the spinal cord.

Overall dose, number of fractions and overall time must all be taken into consideration when defining a radical dose of irradiation. For laryngopharyngeal cancer, dose fractionation schedules of the order of 50 Gray in 16 fractions, 55 Gray in 20 fractions and 66 Gray in 33 fractions, given over time periods of 3 to 6.5 weeks respectively, have been found to be equivalent with reference to tumour control, survival, acute and late toxicity.[11] External beam radiotherapy has proven successful for the treatment of many types and sites of head and neck malignancy, being used radically for smaller tumours, often in conjunction with surgery in more advanced disease and for symptom palliation.

Combined surgery and radiotherapy

In order to eradicate a tumour it is a logical assumption that all tumour clonogenic cells must be eliminated. The relatively low therapeutic index for radiotherapy is such that even doses near to maximum normal tissue tolerance are unable to achieve 100% control of small (< 1 cm) tumours, for example T1 glottic squamous cell carcinoma. Therefore, as the volume of the primary tumour and/or nodal metastases increases and hence the tumour clonogenic population, the probability of achieving control with radiotherapy decreases, an effect which has been clinically demonstrated in the treatment of oropharyngeal[12] and laryngeal carcinomas.[13,14] The frequency of salvage surgery therefore increases and is associated with significant postoperative morbidity of up to 40% in head and neck cancer.[15,16]

Surgery alone for stage III and IV disease has been compared retrospectively with surgery and postoperative radiotherapy by Vikram et al. at Memorial Sloane Kettering Cancer Center. Primary site recurrence occurred in 39% of patients with negative histological resection margins and in 73% with positive margins. The recurrence rates were reduced by elective postoperative radiotherapy to 2% and 10.5%, respectively. Furthermore, recurrence rates were higher when radiotherapy was delayed more than 6 weeks after surgery suggesting that significant tumour repopulation occurs during such a time interval.[17]

A planned combined surgical and radiotherapeutic approach in patients with larger tumour volumes, either at the primary site or in the neck, is therefore appropriate. Elective postoperative radiotherapy, rather than preoperative radiotherapy, has become standard practice following the results of the RTOG 73-03 phase III trial. In this series, 277 patients with head and neck squamous cancer were randomized to preoperative irradiation of 50 Gray in 25 fractions versus postoperative irradiation of 60 Gray in 30 fractions, the lower preoperative radiation dose being chosen because a previous study had shown excessive surgical morbidity following the use of 60 Gray preoperatively in 30 fractions. The 2-year recurrence rates were 31% for preoperative compared to only 18% for postoperative irradiation, with very low associated morbidity.[18] Therefore a postoperative dose of 60 Gray in 30 fractions, or a biological equivalent such as 50 Gray in 20 fractions, has become the standard for postoperative irradiation in the head and neck.

The Scottish/Yorkshire phase III trial, which randomized patients with operable, locally advanced oral cancer between radical radiotherapy with surgery reserved for salvage versus elective surgery and postoperative radiotherapy, was significant. Stopping rules had been introduced into the trial design and were applied by the Data Monitoring Committee at an early stage because of excess mortality and cancer deaths in the radical radiotherapy arm.[19] To this author's knowledge, it is the first reported trial of its kind and the result, although perhaps disappointing, nevertheless much strengthens the case for a planned combined modality approach in patients with larger tumour volumes either at the primary site or in the neck.

Treatment interruption during external beam radiotherapy

Clinical evidence is now accumulating concerning the risk of reduced tumour control rates as a consequence of tumour repopulation resulting from gaps during a course of radiotherapy. Such interruptions may be unplanned, as a result of radiation mucositis or problems intercurrent with a patient's health, or due to machine breakdown. Planned interruptions include machine service and public holidays and have also been deliberately included in split-course radiation treatment schedules in both a prospective randomized trial[20] and a retrospective trial[21] for laryngeal cancer, which resulted in significantly lower local control rates compared to conventional continuous treatment. A review of 971 patients treated for supraglottic carcinoma using 6–7 week daily fractionation schedules reported significant reduction in local control rate in patients with gaps in treatment, the most profound effects being associated with early gaps before day 19 or later gaps beyond 29 days.[22] A similar outcome has been reported for 162 patients treated for T3 carcinoma of the oropharynx and larynx with hyperfractionated and moderately accelerated radiotherapy in which a mid course gap of more than 14 days adversely affected local control.[23] Control rates using shorter daily fractionation schedules over 4 weeks may also be adversely affected by gaps. Duncan et al., in a series of 383 laryngeal cancer patients, have shown a two-fold increase in local relapse rates and a four-fold increase in laryngeal cancer deaths when treatment exceeded 30 days as a result of treatment interruption.[24] Decreased local control rates for laryngeal cancer may be similar whether caused by protracted fractionation or by treatment interruption and the effect may be greater for larger, more advanced tumours.[25] Another series using a similar 4-week daily radiation fractionation schedule for laryngeal cancer confirmed the adverse effect of the treatment gap, but also suggested that the number of gaps during a treatment course may be an independent prognostic variable (van Daesdonk et al. personal communication). The magnitude of the effect has been estimated by a review of the existing data for a number of disease sites including head and neck and suggests a 1.6% decrease in local control probability per day of treatment prolongation, although the value may be as high as 5% for individual patients. The report suggests methods of compensating for gaps in treatment.[26]

Interstitial irradiation (brachytherapy)

Therapeutic irradiation can also be delivered by direct insertion or implantation of radioactive sources into a tumour and for many years has been used successfully as a single modality for treating small volume oral cavity tumours, T1 and T2, up to approximately 3 cm in diameter. Various gamma ray emitting isotopes have been employed for this purpose, beginning with radium-226 at the beginning of the twentieth century and subsequently caesium-137 needles, which require less shielding. However, these rigid application systems require manual positioning and insertion of live sources with unavoidable operator exposure to ionizing radiation and consequently it is difficult to achieve ideal implant geometry. In recent years the iridium-192 wire has been introduced.[27] This is a platinum-coated material which can be cut and shaped as required. The emitted gamma ray energy of 412 kV is relatively low so that only 2 cm of lead shielding provides satisfactory protection. The operator inserts non-radioactive titanium guides (Figs 12.5, 12.6) or hollow plastic tubes into the tumour-bearing tissue under general or local anaesthesia. The geometry is then checked using image intensifier equipment (Fig. 12.7) and modified if necessary before the

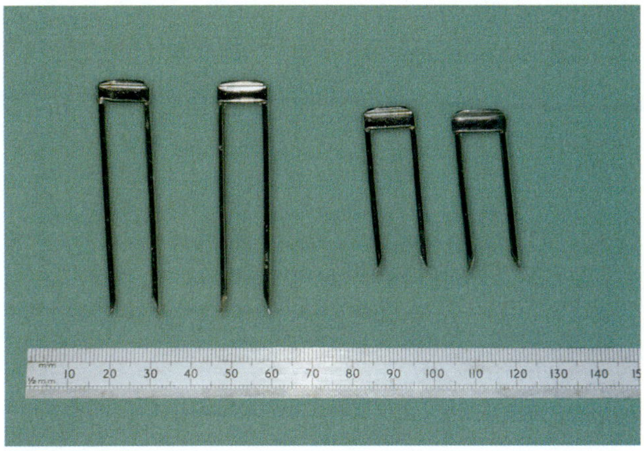

Figure 12.5 Titanium guides (hairpin type).

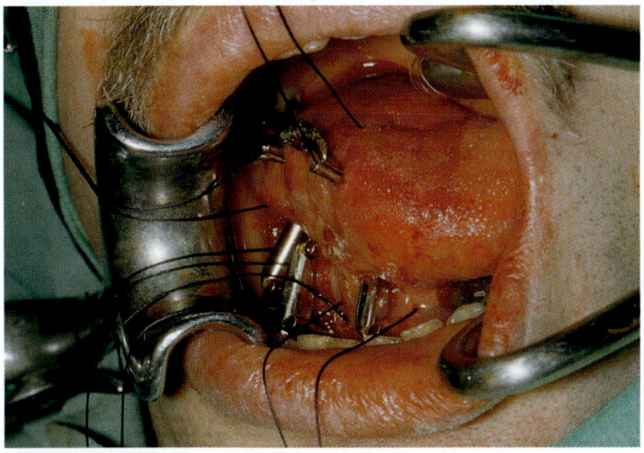

Figure 12.6 Titanium guides inserted into a floor of mouth tumour.

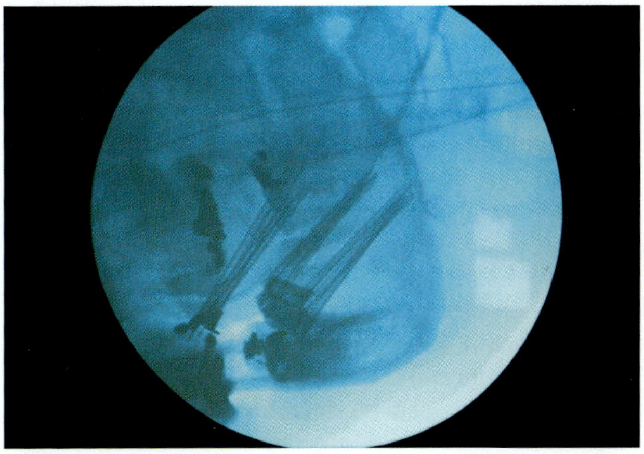

Figure 12.7 Image intensifier verification of titanium guide insertion.

iridium wire is afterloaded (Fig. 12.8), the titanium guides are removed, the wire is sutured into place and the hollow tube system directly afterloaded for the duration of the implant. Radiographs are taken (Fig. 12.9), from which co-ordinates of the implanted wires can be used for computer calculations of the three-dimensional dosimetry.

Staff radiation exposure is therefore reduced but not eliminated by this manually afterloaded technique and patients require nursing care for the duration of the implant, which is usually between 6 and 7 days for a radical dose of 60 Gray. The low dose rate of these techniques, delivering between 0.4 and 0.5 Gray per hour, has proven to be safe and very effective with high rates of local control equivalent to surgery.[28] This form of radiotherapy delivers radical irradiation by continuous low dose rate (LDR) and may be considered biologically equivalent to giving a very large number of extremely small fractions over a short, approximately one week, period. The high therapeutic ratio and hence efficacy of this technique may therefore be anticipated from radiobiological principles because late tissue damage and the adverse effects of tumour repopulation should be minimized. Reported rates of mandibular necrosis are low, although an incidence as high as 10% was reported in patients undergoing brachytherapy for floor of mouth and oral tongue tumours, which was significantly correlated with dose rate and volume irradiated.[29]

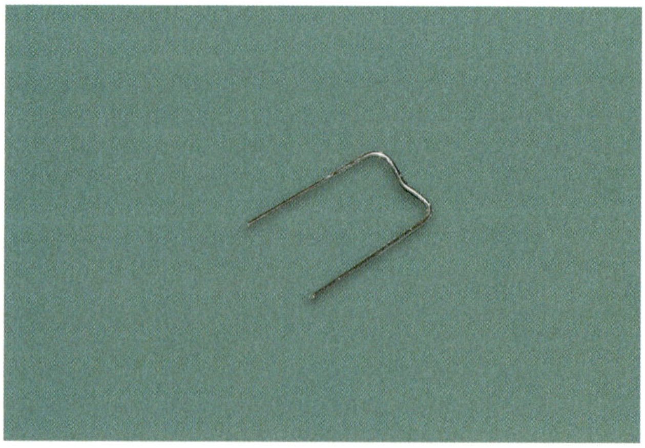

Figure 12.8 Iridium wire (hairpin type).

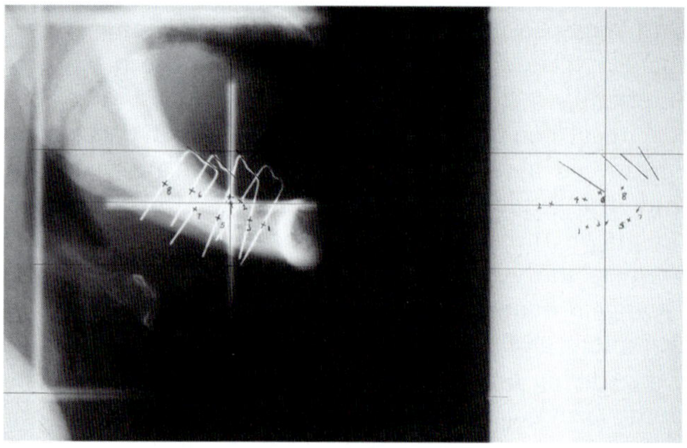

Figure 12.9 Simulator verification film of lateral view of inserted iridium wire.

In order to avoid operator exposure to ionizing radiation completely, remote afterloading methods have been developed using sophisticated computerized equipment (Fig. 12.10). Radioactive sources are transferred by remote control through flexible connecting conduits coupled to hollow guides or tube systems inserted into the patient's tumour. As it is necessary to maintain direct connection with the patient for the duration of radiation exposure, continuous low dose rate systems equivalent to the manual methods previously described have mostly proven impractical for the treatment of head and neck cancers. High dose rate (HDR) systems have therefore been developed which deliver > 0.1 Gray per minute, similar to external beam irradiation, with treatment times lasting a few minutes to deliver doses of the order of 2 Gray per treatment. The radiobiology is therefore more closely analogous to external beam radiotherapy with similar risks of late tissue damage and therefore treatment must be appropriately fractionated. An interval of several hours between each radiation exposure is required to allow for normal tissue DNA repair, during which time the patient can be detached from the restraint of the source connecting conduit. This method has been most commonly used for delivering relatively small boost doses to the tumour following external beam radiotherapy rather than the entire radical treatment dose. However, a phase III trial from Osaka University has reported results on 29 patients with T1, T2, N0 oral tongue cancer randomized between conventional LDR Brachytherapy (15 patients), delivering 70 Gray continuously over 4 to 8 days, and HDR brachytherapy (14 patients), giving

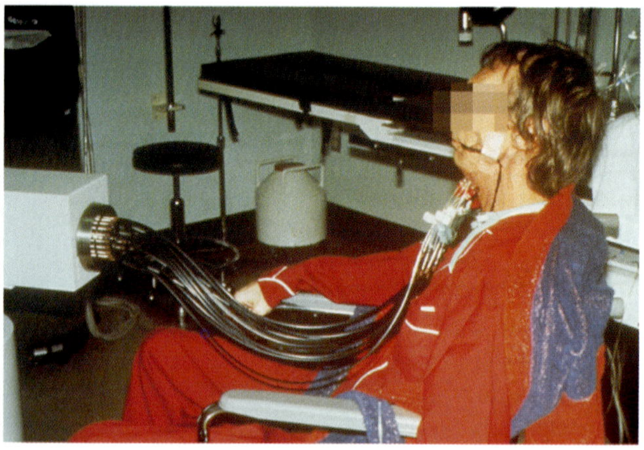

Figure 12.10 'Selectron' high dose rate remote afterloading unit (courtesy of Nucletron).

60 Gray in 10 fractions over 6 days, with a minimum of 6 hours between each treatment. The 2-year local control rates were not significantly different: 86% LDR group and 100% HDR group. Neck relapse rates of 26% and 21%, respectively, were also similar in both groups.[30] Of note, significant late tissue damage was not reported, however the treatment volumes were relatively small and caution must be exercised before the HDR technique is applied to larger irradiation volumes.

Combined external beam and interstitial brachytherapy

Early stage oral cancer can be treated with interstitial brachytherapy alone or combined with external beam radiotherapy. However, data exist which support the importance of delivering all or a majority of the dose by the interstitial method, although it must be conceded that to date there are no published randomized trials. Pernot et al. reported a series of 147 patients with T2 N0 squamous carcinoma of the oral tongue; 70 patients treated with interstitial irradiation alone achieved a 5-year local control rate of 89.8% compared to 50.6% for 77 patients treated with combined external beam and interstitial irradiation. The advantage was also reflected by higher rates of locoregional control and disease specific survival.[31] Other studies have also shown a correlation between local control rates and the proportion of irradiation given by interstitial implant.[32,33] The combined approach should perhaps only be selected for treating larger T2 tumours or where the depth of infiltration, or degree of histological de-differentiation, is considered to be associated with a significant risk of subclinical, microscopic, nodal disease. In such cases, external beam irradiation is used to treat both the primary tumour and the neck electively, to a dose of 50 Gray in 25 fractions or the biological equivalent, with interstitial irradiation delivering an additional 30 Gray over 3 to 4 days as a boost to the primary tumour. The author uses interstitial irradiation followed immediately by external beam radiotherapy in order to deliver the highest proportion of the overall dose within the first few days of the treatment programme with the anticipated effect of minimizing tumour repopulation.

Radiotherapy for verrucous carcinoma

Traditionally, radiotherapy was considered to be contraindicated for the treatment of verrucous carcinoma because of early reports of inferior control rates compared to that achieved by surgery and a risk of anaplastic transformation which was attributed to the effects of ionizing irradiation. However, more recent data clearly refute this conclusion. A series of 53 patients with verrucous oral cancer has been reported by Jyothirmayi et al., in which 42 patients underwent primary radiotherapy and 11 primary surgery. Complete response rates were achieved in 76% of irradiated patients with actuarial 5-year disease-free and overall survival of 66% and 86%, respectively, compared to corresponding survival parameters for a series of well-differentiated squamous carcinomas of 43% and 56%. Survival results for patients treated with primary surgery were similar and none of the 16 patients who recurred after radiotherapy had anaplastic transformation.[34] The weight of evidence is now strongly in support of radiotherapy for verrucous cancers of the oral cavity and for other sites in the head and neck.[35,36]

Treatment by site and stage

Lip and oral cancer

Carcinoma of the lip

The lower lip is most commonly affected by squamous carcinoma as a result of excessive sun exposure and historically was associated with prolonged thermal damage caused by clay pipe smoking. Patients most frequently present with early stage disease and in a reported series of 299 patients from Bordeaux, the incidence of nodal metastases was only 5.6% for T1 and T2 tumours, rising to 17.6% for T3 tumours.[37]

T1 tumours can be readily excised with primary closure, which provides excellent cosmesis and avoids a fractionated course of radiotherapy with resultant mucositis. Larger, T2, tumours usually require surgical flap repair following excision and are treated equally effectively with external beam radiotherapy using directly applied electron or orthovoltage (250–300 kV) photon fields. Gingival shielding is used to reduce mucositis and to minimize the risk of bone and dental damage. A radical dose of irradiation, that is 50 Gray in 15 fractions or the biological equivalent, will achieve high local control rates of up to 95% (Figs. 12.11, 12.12).[38,39] Because of the low incidence of subclinical nodal disease it is unnecessary to treat the neck electively.

The choice between radiotherapy and surgery must be carefully considered in younger patients because the late development of tissue atrophy and telangiectasia may detract from the longer term cosmetic result. T3 tumours may also be treated with radical radiotherapy, although local control rates decrease with increasing tumour size. Prophylactic neck irradiation is recommended in consideration of the

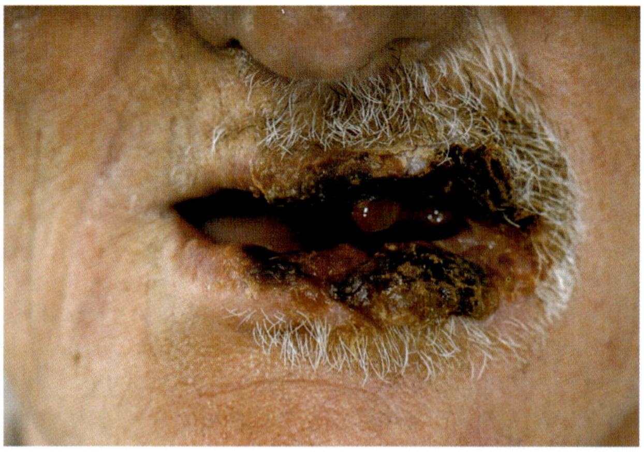

Figure 12.11 Extensive squamous carcinoma involving upper and lower lips.

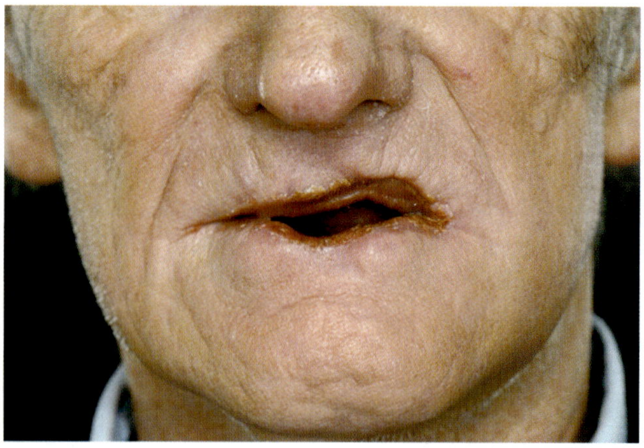

Figure 12.12 Complete response following radical external beam radiotherapy.

higher incidence of nodal metastases. Patients with deeply infiltrating T4 tumours or macroscopic nodal metastases who are considered suitable for radical treatment should be managed with combined surgery and postoperative radiotherapy.

Carcinoma of the floor of the mouth

The floor of the mouth is a complex site owing to the proximity of the mandible and the potential for deep infiltration. Tumour thickness may be a more important prognostic factor than T stage and disease-related death is rare when tumours are 2 mm or less,[40] similarly lymph node involvement is uncommon in tumours less than 1.5 mm in thickness.[41] Careful assessment, preferably during examination under anaesthesia, and imaging using CT and MRI are important for selecting the appropriate treatment.

Early T1 tumours at least 5 mm clear of the mandible can be treated effectively by interstitial

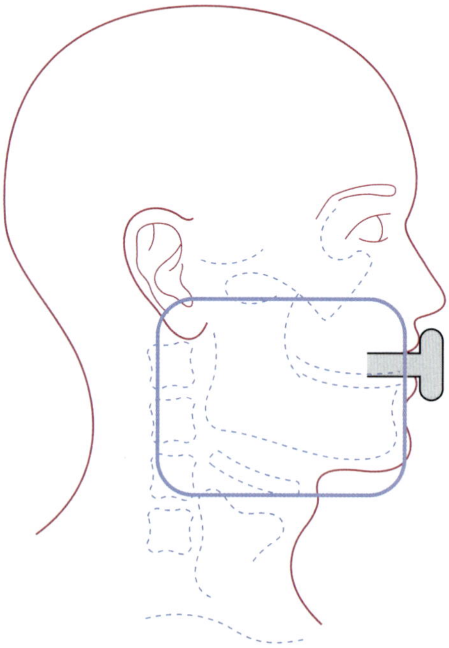

Figure 12.13 Floor of mouth external beam irradiation for lateralized tumour: lateral perspective. Note use of mouth insert.

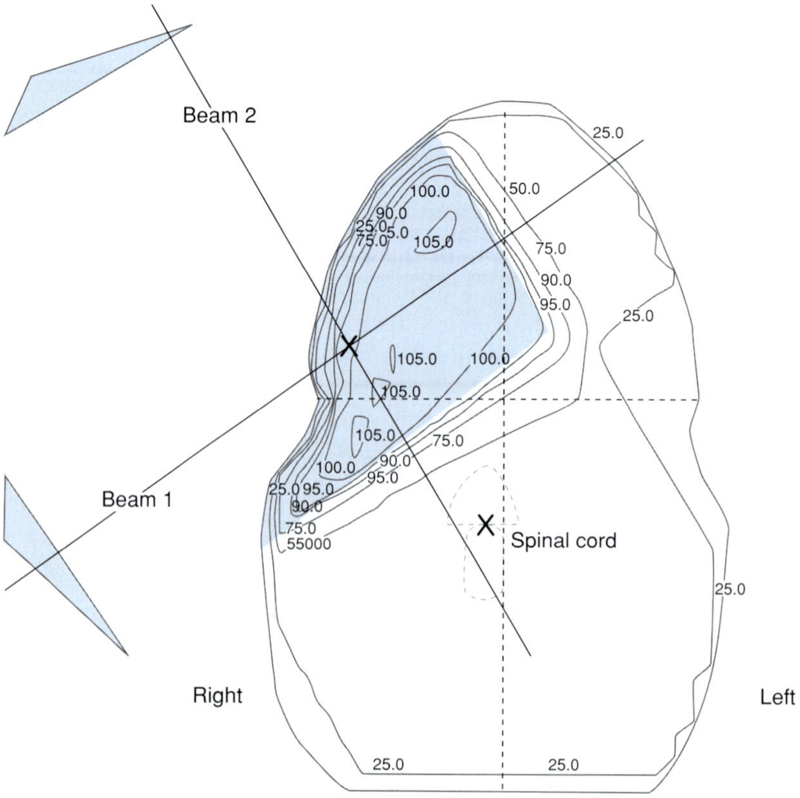

Figure 12.14 Floor of mouth radiation isodose distribution for lateralized tumour; anterior and posterior oblique fields.

implant alone with high rates of local control of approximately 90%. Significant late morbidity is rare because of the small volume of tissue irradiated and the relatively low dose exposure to the mandible compared to external beam radiotherapy. However, if the implant lies close to the duct of the submandibular salivary gland scarring can occasionally result in outflow obstruction which requires surgical intervention. Larger T2 tumours or tumours > 2 mm thickness which are at least 1 cm clear of the midline are probably most appropriately treated with a combination of implant and external beam radiotherapy to include the ipsilateral lymph node drainage which achieves local control rates of 80–85%.[42] The beam arrangement uses anterior and posterior oblique fields in order to avoid significant irradiation to the contralateral parotid salivary gland and hence minimize the risk of significant xerostomia (Figs 12.13, 12.14). Lesions closer to or crossing the midline will require prophylactic bilateral neck irradiation and tumours too close to the mandible for implantation should be treated with external beam irradiation alone.

T3 tumours and T4 tumours, when considered operable, are most appropriately treated with surgery and postoperative radiotherapy,[43] bone infiltration in particular being a contraindication for radical radiotherapy alone as tumour control rates are very low.

Carcinoma of the oral tongue

The oral part of the tongue comprises the anterior two-thirds and lies anterior to the cirumvallate papillae, each side having lateralized lymphatic drainage. As for the floor of the mouth, careful assessment and imaging are essential because tumours may be more deeply infiltrating than anticipated from routine clinical examination.

T1 and small T2 tumours up to 3.5 cm diameter which are at least 1 cm clear of the midline can be effectively treated with interstitial implant irradiation; 5-year local control rates are equivalent to surgery: T1 85–95% and T2 80–85%. Tumours on the tip of the tongue are difficult to implant because of the position and mobility and are best treated by surgical excision. T3 tumours are usually treated by combined implant and external beam radiotherapy including the ipsilateral lymph node drainage (Figs 12.15–12.18). Corresponding control rates of between 35% and 50% are reported.[42]

Following interstitial brachytherapy, soft tissue ulcers can occur at the irradiated site in up to 30% of patients, however most heal within 18 months and the late functional and cosmetic results are excellent.[44,45] When surgery is considered for T3 or operable T4 tumours, postoperative irradiation may improve control rates and should include the operative bed and the lymphatic drainage.[46]

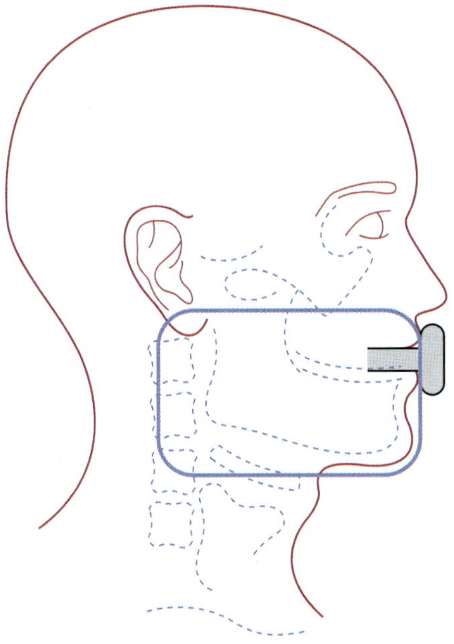

Figure 12.15 External beam irradiation of anterior two-thirds of tongue for anterolateral tumour: lateral perspective. Note use of mouth insert.

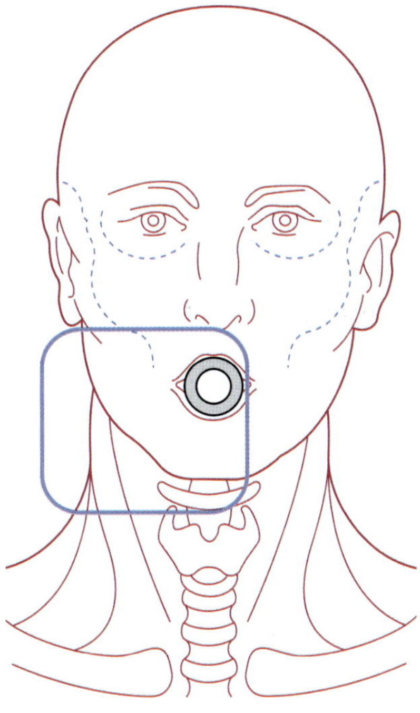

Figure 12.16 External beam irradiation of anterior two-thirds of tongue for anterolateral tumour: anterior perspective. Note use of mouth insert.

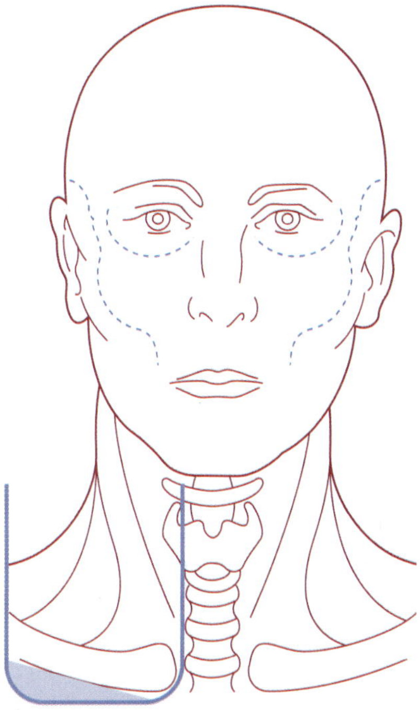

Figure 12.17 Anterior radiation field for ipsilateral lower neck irradiation.

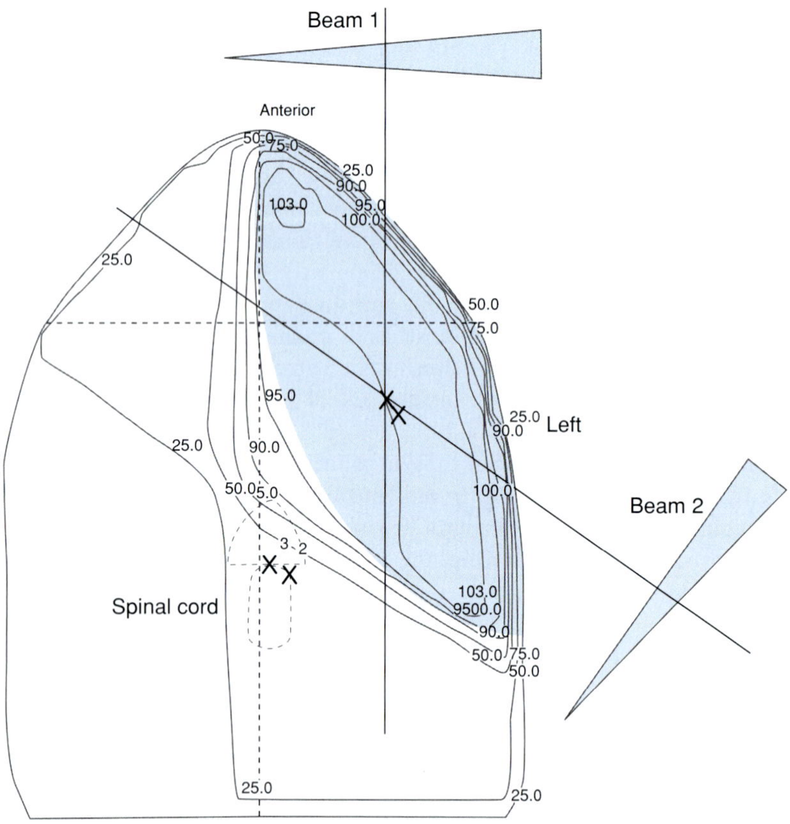

Figure 12.18 Anterior two-thirds of tongue: isodose distribution for anterolateral tumour.

Carcinoma of the buccal mucosa

Squamous carcinoma of the buccal mucosa is associated with betel nut chewing and the use of various forms of oral tobacco as well as with smoking and alcohol consumption, which have a synergistic interaction. The disease therefore has a high incidence in the Indian subcontinent. Lesions at this site commonly present early and lymph node metastasis is uncommon in small tumours. Posterior lesions must be carefully assessed for extension into the retromolar and pterygoid fossae.

External beam radiotherapy is most commonly used for T1 and T2 tumours using ipsilateral anterior and posterior oblique fields to encompass the primary lesion with a 2 cm margin; it is unnecessary to irradiate lymph nodes prophylactically. T1 and T2 tumours at least 1 cm clear of bone can also be treated effectively with an interstitial implant with high rates of local control using modern iridium wire techniques.[47]

Larger T3 and operable T4 tumours are more appropriately treated with surgery and postoperative radiotherapy[48] and a randomized trial from India has reported 68% disease-free survival using the combined approach compared to 38% for the group treated with surgery alone.[49]

Carcinoma of the lower alveolar mucosa

Because of the close proximity of this site to the underlying mandible, bone invasion occurs relatively early in the natural history, usually as a result of spread down the periodontal membrane. Imaging, with OPG, CT and MRI, is particularly important.

T1 and T2 tumours are most frequently treated with external beam irradiation using anterior and posterior oblique fields with a greater than 70% probability of local control. Interstitial irradiation using the afterloaded flexible tubing system described previously is an effective alternative.[42] Tumours not extending beyond the inferior alveolar canal or with only superficial bone invasion may be effectively treated with marginal mandibular resection.[50]

However, the more common advanced tumours with more extensive bone invasion require surgery and postoperative radiotherapy to include prophylactic lymph node irradiation. Overall results of treatment have historically been relatively poor with control rates of approximately 25%,[51] although one series has reported 3-year disease-free survival of 68% for T4, N1 tumours using hemimandibulectomy, supra-omohyoid dissection and postoperative radiotherapy.[52]

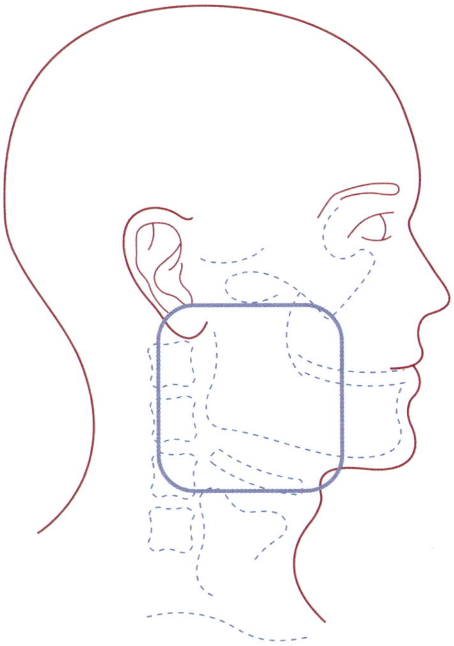

Figure 12.19 Oropharyngeal irradiation: lateral opposing fields.

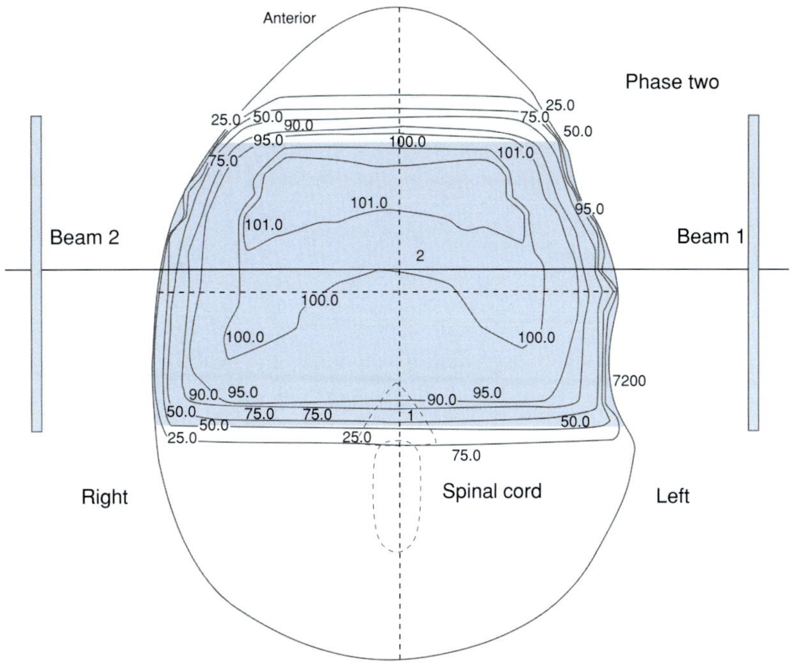

Figure 12.20 Oropharyngeal irradiation: opposing radiation field isodose distribution radiation.

Carcinoma of the retromolar trigone and anterior faucial pillar

Tumours at this site spread early along the mandibular ramus and can track superiorly into the pterygoid fossa. Careful clinical and imaging assessments are necessary as for the other areas. T1 amd T2 tumours can be effectively treated with external beam radiotherapy using anterior oblique and posterior oblique fields. It is important to include the anterior border of the mandibular ramus and the pterygoid fossa superiorly to the skull base with elective irradiation to the ipsilateral lymph node drainage.

More advanced tumours, particularly where there is bone involvement, require surgery and postoperative radiotherapy. An overall 2-year local control rate of the order of 75% can be achieved.[51]

Oropharyngeal carcinoma

Oropharyngeal structures other than the tonsilar fossae have bilateral lymphatic drainage and carcinomas are associated with a higher incidence of lymph node metastases which may therefore be bilateral even when the primary tumour is relatively small. The treatment techniques depend upon the site and stage of disease and prognosis is generally worse than for oral cavity carcinomas. Careful assessment and imaging with CT and MRI are important in the oropharynx because of the risks of nodal metastases, of spread into the parapharyngeal space in the case of tonsilar tumours and the potential for extension of tongue base tumours into the pre-epiglottic space.

Radiotherapy techniques are similar whichever site is being treated, with the exception of small lateralized tonsilar carcinomas, and bilateral radiation fields are used to treat the whole oropharynx including prophylactic nodal irradiation. Xerostomia is therefore a common long-term side effect of treatment because of inevitable bilateral parotid irradiation (Figs 12.19, 12.20). Overall 5-year local control as high as 73% has been reported for oropharyngeal cancers treated with radical radiotherapy.[53]

Carcinoma of the tonsil

Small tonsilar fossa tumours, T1 and T2, N0, which have not invaded the tongue base and are clear of the midline of the soft palate are effectively treated with radical radiotherapy. Anterior and posterior oblique fields are used to minimize exposure of the contralateral parotid salivary gland and therefore reduce the risk of xerostomia (Figs 12.21, 12.22). The ipsilateral upper deep cervical (tonsilar) nodes and submandibular nodes are irradiated electively. Cosmetic and functional results can be excellent (Figs 12.23, 12.24). Massachusetts General Hospital has reported 5-year actuarial local control and disease-free survival rates of 91% and 77% for T1 and T2 tumours, respectively, in a large series of patients[54] and 2-year local control rates of 81% have also been reported in a series of 53 similar stage patients with tonsilar carcinomas treated at the University of Virginia.[55]

T3 tumours can also be effectively treated with radical radiotherapy with 5-year actuarial local

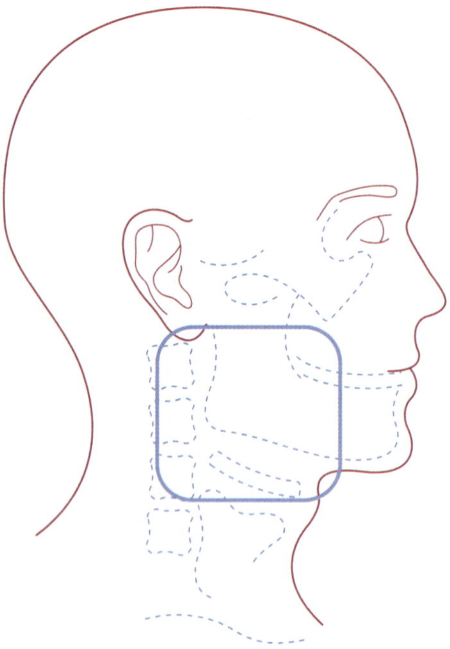

Figure 12.21 T1, T2, N0 tonsilar carcinoma external beam irradiation: lateral perspective.

control and disease free survival rates of 80% and 68%, respectively, using a twice daily hyperfractionated radiotherapy schedule,[54] although similarly high control rates have also been reported with more conventional radiation fractionation.[56] Where the primary tumour has invaded the tongue base or crossed the palatal midline, bilateral elective lymph node irradiation is essential. A radical dose of irradiation, that is 66 Gray in 33 fractions, 55 Gray in 20 fractions or the biological equivalent, is essential for adequate tumour control, particularly in larger tumours as highlighted by the poor results for radiotherapy reported by O'Brien et al. from Royal Prince Albert Hospital, Australia, where suboptimal dose fractionation schedules had historically been used.[57]

Large T4 tumours considered operable are probably best treated by combined surgery, often using free tissue transfer techniques, followed by postoperative radiotherapy. In a series of 120 patients with advanced disease in which 70 were treated with primary surgery followed by irradiation and 50 were treated with radical radiotherapy and salvage surgery, the 3-year survival rates were 58% and 38%, respectively.[58] Where ipsilateral lymph node involvement has occurred there is a significant risk of contralateral subclinical nodal disease because of lymphatic shunting and bilateral lymph node irradiation is important irrespective of the size of the primary tumour.

Carcinoma of the tongue base

The tongue base differs from the anterior oral tongue in having bilateral lymphatic drainage and tumours are more frequently advanced at presentation by a

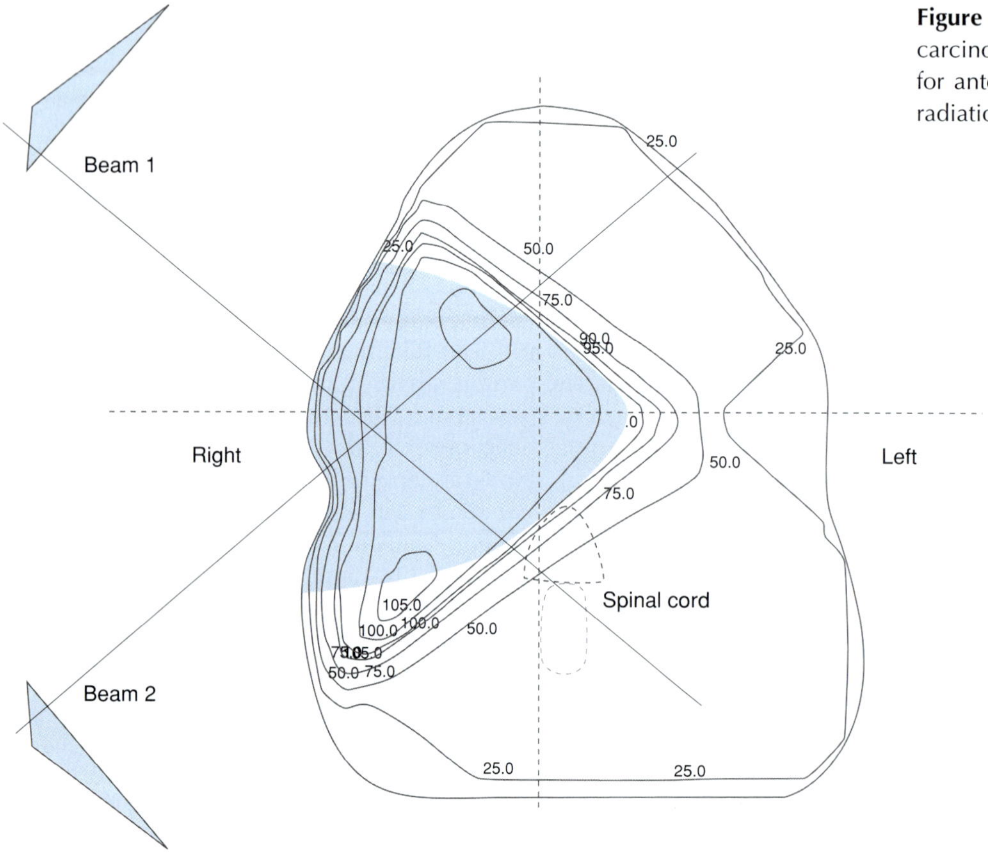

Figure 12.22 T1, T2, N0 tonsilar carcinoma: isodose distribution for anterior and posterior oblique radiation field arrangement.

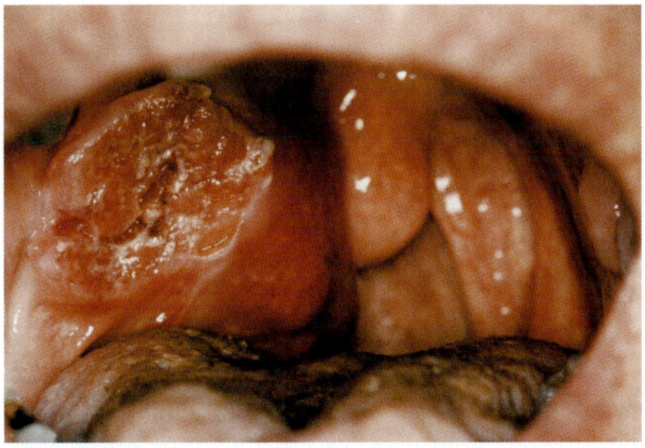

Figure 12.23 T2, N0 squamous carcinoma of tonsil at presentation.

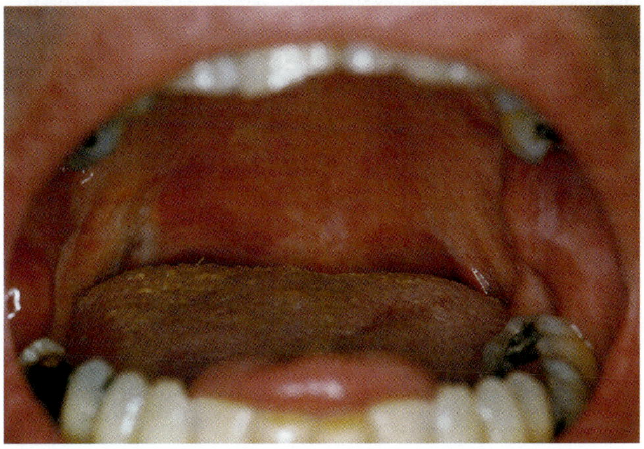

Figure 12.24 T2, N0 squamous carcinoma of tonsil 3 months after completion of radical radiotherapy.

factor of 2. The difference in prognosis appears to be related to stage and hence tumour volume at presentation rather than to an inherently more aggressive behaviour and treatment responses for the two parts of the tongue are probably similar stage for stage.[59] Radical tongue base surgery can be particularly mutilating, with significant dysfunctional sequelae especially when laryngectomy is also required. Radical radiotherapy to the primary site with bilateral prophylactic nodal irradiation is an effective treatment for early stage T1 and T2 tumours and can be used successfully for T3 disease. A published series from the University of Florida has reported 5-year local control rates of 90% for T1, 92% for T2 and 73% for T3 tumours, however the control rate for T4 tumours was only 35%.[60] Interstitial brachytherapy using the hollow tube system afterloaded with iridium[42] or by permanent implantation of radioactive iodine 125 seeds can also be effective in achieving high rates of control.[61]

Early stage exophytic tumours are more responsive and more effectively controlled with radiotherapy than are deeply invasive tumours,[62] presumably this is a reflection of disease volume. Weber et al. reported 2-year primary site control rates of 84% and 58%, respectively. A higher 2-year control rate was noted for deeply invasive disease using surgery and postoperative radiotherapy (79%) than with radiotherapy alone (55%).[63] For larger infiltrating T3 tumours and for T4 tumours, a combined approach of surgery and postoperative radiotherapy may therefore be more appropriate.

Carcinoma of the soft palate and posterior pharyngeal wall

The soft palate and posterior pharyngeal wall are the least common sites for carcinoma of the oropharynx. The soft palate is a muscular mobile structure which acts as a valve to close off the posterior nasal space. Surgical removal can result in problems with nasal regurgitation and nasal speech. Medini et al. reported a 3-year disease-free survival following radical radiotherapy for T1 and T2 tumours of more than 95%, falling to 65% for T3 tumours with a poor survival rate for those with advanced T4 disease.[64]

Posterior pharyngeal wall carcinoma more frequently presents as advanced disease with a longer clinical history and overall control and survival rates with radiotherapy are correspondingly lower when compared to tumours of the soft palate.[65] One of the largest published series of 74 patients treated with radiotherapy alone has reported disease-specific survival rates of 85–100% for early stage I and II disease and 40–60% for more advanced stage II and IV disease, with overall survival rates which are approximately 20% lower. Twice daily hyperfractionated radiotherapy was used in a subgroup of patients which the authors suggest may have produced superior control compared to conventional fractionation, however the study was not randomized.[66]

For advanced disease, combined surgery and postoperative radiotherapy may offer advantages because salvage surgery following high dose irradiation has been associated with high rates of complications and recurrence at this site.[67]

Management of the neck

The frequency and pattern of neck node disease depends upon the primary site, T stage and histological tumour grade. The incidence of subclinical nodal metastasis is less than 10% for cancers of the lip and rises to between 20 and 35% for cancers of the floor of the mouth and oral tongue, the lower figure corresponding to the incidence of subclinical neck disease following neck dissection and the higher to neck relapse in patients managed by surveillance.[68,69] T stage is correlated with incidence of nodal metastasis, and in a series of 346 patients with oral cavity tumours the frequency of subclinical disease at neck dissection was found to be 20% for T1 and 33% for T2 tumours.[70]

For cancers of the oropharynx, particularly the tongue base and posterior pharyngeal wall, the incidence of subclinical nodal disease rises further to 30–45%.[71] High grade primary tumours metastasize to nodes more frequently than low grade tumours, with a higher risk of lower neck node involvement.[72] Oral cancers, particularly of the tongue and floor of mouth, are also associated with an unexpectedly high incidence of skip metastases as a result of the direct lymphatic pathway to lower neck nodes. Byers et al. have reported a 15.8% incidence of metastasis to levels III and IV nodes in the absence of disease in levels I and II in a series of 277 patients with squamous carcinoma of the oral tongue, which has clear therapeutic implications.[73]

The N0 neck

Three therapeutic options may be considered for management of the clinically and radiologically negative neck. Active surveillance is most clearly appropriate for tumours of the lip, small T1 tumours of the oral tongue and thin (< 2 mm) tumours of the floor of mouth, which are all associated with a low incidence of nodal metastasis. For other primary sites a higher risk of nodal relapse of up to 45% must be expected, of which 60% of patients will be successfully salvaged. Early studies have suggested a higher incidence of distant metastases in patients with neck failure, which has been cited as a rationale for elective neck treatment,[74–76] however none of these were prospective randomized trials and it is possible that the observation is simply an epiphenomenon since patients with locoregional relapse may have an inherently higher rate of distant metastatic disease. Nevertheless, a significant benefit of surveillance is that it avoids treatment-related morbidity in the majority of cases and may be safe providing a patient's compliance with follow-up can be assured. Elective neck dissection is an alternative, which is undoubtedly effective in achieving high rates of disease control in the neck, although only two randomized trials have addressed this issue, neither of which were large enough to provide clearly significant results.[77,78] However, morbidity can be significant following either radical or modified radical neck dissection, with disfigurement, persistent shoulder pain and stiffness.

Elective neck irradiation studies have shown clear dose, time and fractionation control rates for subclinical neck disease. The seminal work of Gilbert Fletcher demonstrated that approximately 95% of subclinical neck disease could be controlled by a dose of 45–50 Gray in 25 daily fractions.[79] More recent reports are confirmatory and have shown a threshold at 45 Gray in 25 fractions, or the biological equivalent, below which control rates decrease significantly.[80,81] The inference that such doses of irradiation should almost totally eliminate subclinical neck disease is perhaps at variance with clinical experience, the explanation being that the reported control rates excluded patients with recurrence at the primary site because local failure was considered to be a potential for nodal reseeding. The overall control rates are therefore lower than suggested. Only one prospective randomized trial has addressed the role of elective irradiation in 204 patients with oral cancer. The requirement for salvage neck dissection was 14% in the patients whose necks were irradiated to a dose of 40 Gray in 15 fractions compared to 25% in the observed control group, with no difference in overall survival. Unfortunately, the number of patients was too small to demonstrate a clear significant difference.[82]

The late morbidity from elective irradiation is less than for surgery and the majority of patients will have normal appearance and function, however in a small proportion (< 5%) of patients, unpredictable significant tissue fibrosis is observed. A logical management policy is therefore to offer elective nodal irradiation, including the whole neck in oral tongue and floor of mouth cancers, whenever there is a significant (> 15%) risk of subclinical nodal disease and when the primary tumour is to be treated with radiotherapy. The most common technique uses an anterior radiation field or, in larger patients, opposing anterior–posterior fields with shielding of the midline structures including the sensitive spinal cord (Figs 12.25, 12.26).

The involved neck

Involved nodes are frequently diagnosed by fine needle aspirate cytology. Excisional or incisional biopsy has been considered hazardous because of early reports suggesting higher rates of recurrence, distant metastases and wound necrosis.[83,84] Ellis et al., at the University of Florida, have reported a series of 508 patients with head and neck squamous carcinoma, 66 of whom underwent open neck node biopsy prior to definitive radiotherapy. Rates of neck control, distant metastasis and cause-specific survival did not differ significantly from 442 patients who had not undergone nodal biopsy.[85] A further report from the same centre has demonstrated 95% 5- and 10-year control rates in the neck following single node excision followed by high

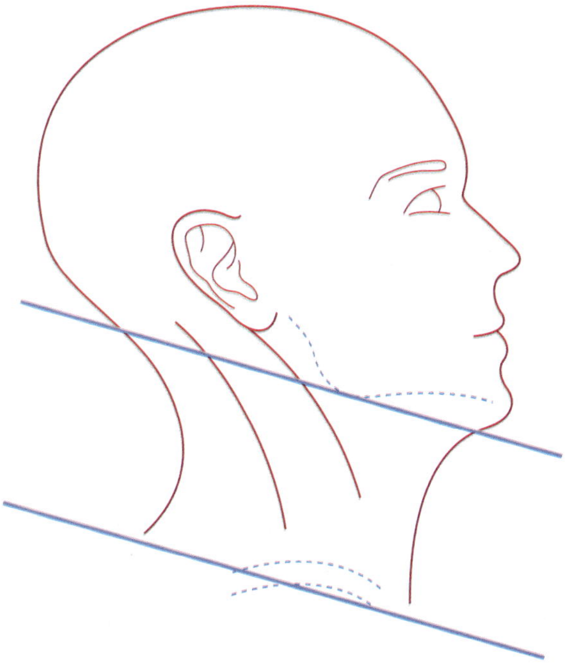

Figure 12.25 Lateral perspective of anterior neck irradiation fields.

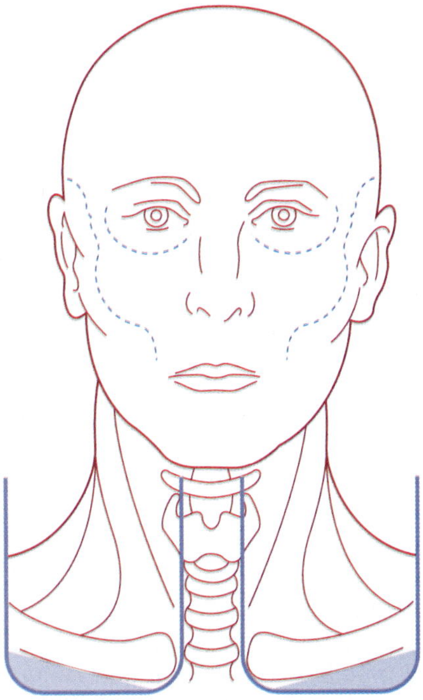

Figure 12.26 Anterior perspective of bilateral neck irradiation fields showing shielding to the spinal cord and to the lung apices.

dose postoperative radiotherapy in a series of 44 patients, with no apparent increase in the risk of distant metastasis,[86] which emphasizes the importance of radiotherapy following such diagnostic procedures.

Macroscopic nodal disease can be treated with radical radiotherapy using the same doses as for the primary tumour. High control rates are achieved for small volume disease and involved nodes of up to 1 cm can be eradicated effectively in patients whose primary tumours are treated with radiotherapy.[87] However, control rates diminish as nodal size increases, with reported 10-year disease-free survival rates of 60% for lymph nodes of 3 cm or less, 36% for 4–6 cm lymph nodes and 20% for lymph nodes greater than 6 cm in patients with squamous cell carcinoma of the head and neck.[88] Although observation of the neck has been advocated after complete nodal response, reserving surgery for neck salvage,[89] recurrence following neck irradiation tends to be diffuse rather than developing as discrete nodes, probably because radiotherapy disrupts lymph node capsules and normal tissue planes, consequently salvage rates are lower than for the non-irradiated neck.

The most frequent approach in patients with operable nodal disease is therefore neck dissection. Postoperative irradiation is indicated when more than two nodes are involved or if there is evidence of capsular invasion, which has been shown to reduce the rate of neck recurrence.[90,91] A radiation dose of 60 Gray in 30 daily fractions,[92] or a biologically equivalent dose such as 50 Gray in 20 daily fractions, is required to achieve high rates of control. The doses required are larger than those required for elective irradiation, which may be the result of relative tissue hypoxia and hence radioresistance in the neck following major surgery.

Fixed and inoperable nodal disease

Nodal fixity does not necessarily imply inoperability, unless the disease is attached to the skull base or to the deep tissues of the posterior triangle. Such patients typically present with large volume disease and have a poor prognosis. Radical surgery alone in an attempt to resect fixed disease is usually unsuccessful.[93] Radiotherapy to a dose of 50 Gray in 25 fractions, or the biological equivalent, or induction chemotherapy may be used in fitter patients in an attempt to render the mass operable, although neither technique has been proven to increase survival. Innovative techniques using intraoperative irradiation[94] and combined radiotherapy and hyperthermia[95] have shown promise. However, for the majority of patients the only option is high-dose radiotherapy to the primary site and the nodal mass in an attempt to provide a period of effective palliation and delay the onset of pain and disease fungation.

Adverse effects of radiotherapy

Radiation mucositis

The timing and severity of radiation mucositis depends upon the treatment dose, time, fractionation, extent of irradiated mucosa and continued smoking and alcohol consumption. With conventional once daily radiation schedules the onset usually occurs towards the end of the second week of treatment, or a few days after an interstitial implant, rising to a peak towards the end or a few days after completion. Shorter fractionation regimens are usually associated with more severe reactions, although of shorter duration. Re-epithelialization may commence before the end of treatment and is usually complete by 6 weeks. Radiation mucositis frequently causes swallowing difficulties and patients should be advised to avoid excessively hot, cold or spicy food, smoking or drinking alcohol. Symptomatic measures include a topical anaesthetic agent such as mucaine, soluble aspirin in a mucilage suspension and sucralfate suspension which can be particularly effective,[96] either alone or in combination. Oral morphine suspension, having both local and systemic analgesic effects, is also frequently used to relieve the pain of mucositis. In severe cases nasogastric feeding may be necessary and it is important for the patient to be assessed by experienced dieticians. In patients where treatment volumes are large and significant reactions are anticipated it may be advisable to consider prophylactic percutaneous insertion of a feeding gastrostomy tube in order to maintain nutrition until the radiation reaction has settled.[97]

Xerostomia

Significant xerostomia occurs when major salivary glands are included in the irradiation volume and is therefore a more common complication of oropharyngeal than oral cancer irradiation. Salivary tissue is particularly sensitive and temporary xerostomia will occur if a dose of 20 Gray in 10 fractions is given, with a high risk of permanent damage when doses exceed 30 Gray in 15 fractions. Quality of life can be adversely affected by this complication and dietary changes may be necessary for patients unable to masticate and swallow dry foods satisfactorily. Artificial saliva preparations have been used for many years with variable success, although relief is short lived and frequent application is required. A small volume of dietary fat melted on the tongue can lubricate the oral mucosa and relieve the sensation of dryness, particularly at night. More recently oral, systemically absorbed, pilocarpine tablets have been used with a degree of success, as they can stimulate salivation effectively with objective and subjective improvement in a significant proportion of patients.[98] However, there is a clear dose response and systemic toxicity is common at higher doses, with up to 55% of patients experiencing excessive sweating, urinary frequency, lacrimation and rhinitis at therapeutic doses of 5 mg three times daily or higher.[99] Topical pilocarpine in pastille form may be effective in alleviating xerostomia with a lower incidence of systemic side effects and improved patient tolerance.[100] To date there are no proven effective measures for preventing radiation induced xerostomia and although there have been early reports of long term benefits from pilocarpine administered during and after radiotherapy,[101,102] the results require confirmation in larger randomized prospective trials.

Taste impairment

Taste impairment occurs soon after radiotherapy is commenced and has been shown to correlate with the volume of tongue within the radiation field, presumably a result of radiation effects upon taste buds, and does not appear to be related to major salivary gland irradiation. However, the majority of patients recover most or all taste sensation over a period of months following treatment completion.[103]

Dental care

Dental caries associated with radiation are typically marginal and develop rapidly (Fig. 12.27). The mechanism of damage is uncertain but probably involves direct damage to the pulp and enamel organ and changes in composition and pH reduction of saliva, resulting in excessive plaque formation. Furthermore, subtle changes in taste sensation coupled with increased salivary viscosity following salivary gland irradiation may result in patients changing to a low residue, high carbohydrate diet, which also increases the risk of carie formation. Trauma to irradiated bone by dental extraction or as a result of damage from periodontal disease, even

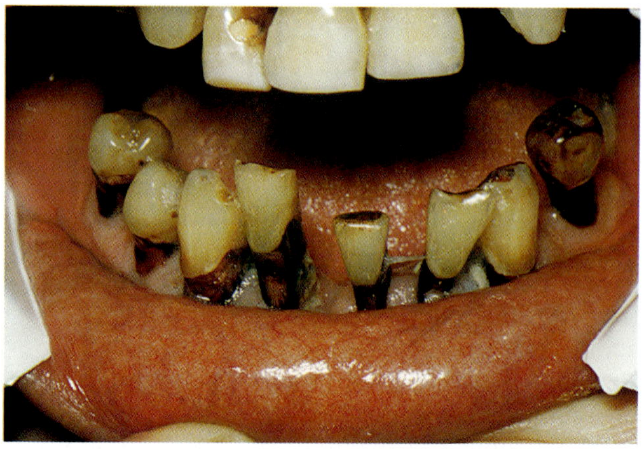

Figure 12.27 Dental caries following oropharyngeal irradiation. Note typical marginal involvement.

years after treatment, will stimulate osteoblast cell division and hence may promote mitotic cell death, leading to osteoradionecrosis. The risk to the mandible is greater than to the maxilla by a ratio of 24:1, which probably reflects the relatively poor vascular supply to the former and also depends upon the radiation dose and the volume of bone irradiated.[104] It is therefore important to undertake major restorative dentistry or dental extraction before commencing radiotherapy and to reduce the risk of subsequent carie formation.[105] Rigorous preventative measures are essential, and the dental hygienist has a particularly important role in after-care. Regular use of a fluoride dental paste or high fluoride content toothpaste is recommended,[106] together with meticulous oral hygiene and appropriate dietary advice.

Treatment of established osteoradionecrosis

Once established, osteoradionecrosis should initially be treated conservatively. Concurrent infection is thought to be a significant factor in pathogenesis and antibiotic therapy should be commenced. Tetracyclines are recommended as they are preferentially absorbed by bone and metronidazole may be added for the treatment of anaerobic organisms. A sequestrum which may form should be gently removed. Such measures have been reported to promote resolution in approximately 50% of patients,[107] however the additional use of hyperbaric oxygen therapy may further improve results by 15–20%,[108,109] although there are no reported prospective randomized trials. Patients must be carefully selected because as many as 36, twice daily, treatments may be required and in many countries treatment facilities are limited such that travelling distances may be considerable, necessitating residential care. The long-term prognosis for osteoradionecrosis following initially successful conservative treatment is reasonably good, with up to 60% of patients remaining free from recurrence of this complication.[110] More radical surgical removal is required for those patients with persistent radionecrosis who fail to respond to conservative measures, with reconstruction using corticocancellous bone particulate grafts or microvascular osseous tissue transfer, depending upon the clinical circumstances.[111]

Osteo-integrated implantation has become a standard technique for dental restoration and has been used successfully in previously irradiated patients. Esser and Wagner have reported an osteoradionecrosis incidence of only 3.4% in a series of 221 mandibular implants following postoperative radiotherapy, with a 5-year actuarial success rate of approximately 80% without the use of prophylactic hyperbaric oxygen therapy.[112] Meticulous care and avoidance of infection are important for the success of these procedures and it may be advisable to delay implantation for at least 5 months after radiotherapy.[113]

Developments in radiotherapy

Modification of tumour hypoxia

Cellular hypoxia is considered to be an important factor in the control of head and neck cancer. Two principle avenues of research have been pursued in radiotherapy in an endeavour to increase the therapeutic ratio and improve control rates and survival, using methods to increase tumour oxygenation either by hyperbaric oxygen or oxygen mimetic hypoxic cell sensitizers, or by modified radiation fractionation. Several large randomized trials have been undertaken and it is now possible to begin to draw conclusions from the results. The medical research trial of hyperbaric oxygen therapy for head and neck cancers, reported by Henk in 1977, randomized 49 patients to hyperbaric oxygen or conventional radiotherapy in air, with respective 2-year local control rates of 45% and 27% and 5-year survival rates of 38% and 27%. These results were statistically significant and included patients with oral and oropharyngeal cancers, although patients with very large tumours (> 5 cm) failed to benefit.[114] However, at least half of the patients considered for hyperbaric oxygen are medically unfit for the procedure, which is also complex, time consuming and costly, hence subsequent interest in the technique has been somewhat limited.

As an alternative, a group of bioreductive nitroimidazole drugs, which mimic oxygen but have greater tissue perfusion characteristics, has now been investigated in prospective randomized trials in head and neck cancer. The first drug designed specifically for this purpose, misonidazole, has been assessed in two large trials: the RTOG study with 306 patients,[115] and the Danish study with 626 patients.[116] Both failed to demonstrate overall benefit compared to their control groups, although subgroup analysis of the larger trial suggested benefit in 304 patients with oropharyngeal cancer. Similarly disappointing results were demonstrated by the EORTC randomized trial of three fractions per day with misonidazole.[117] A successor agent, etanidazole, has also been investigated in the RTOG ETA trial, which randomized 521 patients,[118] and in a multicentre European trial with 374 patients.[119] Once again, neither trial was able to demonstrate overall benefit, although in the RTOG study a subgroup of patients with early nodal disease appeared to show a positive result.[120]

Both of these nitroimidazole drugs were dose limited in humans because of problems with neurotoxicity, which may be a reason why the results of earlier animal studies have not been realized in the clinical setting. However, the Danish nimorazole trial, DHANCA 5, reported a significantly improved local control rate of 46% compared to 32% for drug placebo controls in 288 patients undergoing radical radiotherapy for supraglottic laryngeal and pharyngeal carcinoma, with an apparent additive effect of haemoglobin concentration. The rationale for selecting this drug was its reduced neurotoxicity and hence patient tolerance of higher doses, despite the fact that it has a lower sensitizing effect (sensitizer enhancement ratio) then misonidazole or etanidazole,[121] and these exciting results undoubtedly justify further investigation. More recently a new bioreductive agent, tirapazamine, has been developed, which undergoes selective electron reduction in hypoxic conditions, forming free radicals, which result in cell death. This agent has been shown to potentiate the cytotoxicity of ionizing radiation and of several chemotherapeutic drugs, in particular the platinum compounds and taxanes. Phase I studies have now been completed with results from phase II trials awaited.[122]

Another approach in an attempt to modify tissue hypoxia has used nicotinamide, which causes vasodilatation, with the objective of reducing transient or acute hypoxia, and the breathing of carbogen in order to overcome chronic hypoxia. These agents are well tolerated, although nicotinamide can cause impairment of renal function and should not be given concomitantly with nephrotoxic drugs. Preliminary results have been promising, although the approach requires confirmation by large randomized trials.

Anaemia has been closely correlated to reduced radiotherapy control rates and survival.[123] The effect appears to be independent of disease stage. A secondary analysis of the aforementioned RTOG 85-27 trial for advanced cancer indicated 5-year survival of 35.7% for patients with 'normal' haemoglobin levels compared to 21.7% for those with anaemia defined as < 14.5 g/dl for men and < 13 gm for women.[124] Similarly, reduction of approximately 30% in local control has been shown for patients with T1 and T2 glottic cancer, although the 'threshold' in this study was haemoglobin of 12 g/dl.[125] However, the mechanism of action of anaemia is uncertain and may not simply be related to tissue hypoxia as the same effect has been shown for surgically treated patients,[126] and may be an epiphenomenon related to patient performance status. Nonetheless, in the absence of a clear explanation for this phenomenon it would be wise to correct anaemia in patients undergoing radiotherapy for head and neck cancer.

Modified radiation fractionation

A more scientific approach to radiation fractionation, based upon known biological principles, is a relatively recent innovation. A number of radiobiological factors, which may influence the response of both normal tissue and tumours to ionizing radiation, have now been investigated by randomized clinical trials of modified radiation fractionation. The intention of these approaches has been to increase the narrow therapeutic ratio of tumour versus normal tissue damage.

Repopulation of normal and tumour cell clonogens occurs during the multiple weeks of conventional 5-day per week radiotherapy because cell damage from therapeutic ionizing radiation is a phenomenon of probability. During each treatment exposure only a proportion of tumour clonogenic cells will sustain lethal damage, and surviving cells continue to divide and multiply. Tumour eradication will only be successful once all have been eliminated, until which time tumor repopulation will continue. Furthermore, evidence has emerged that tumor repopulation during a period of fractionated radiotherapy may actually accelerate after the first four weeks of treatment.[127] Tumour control may therefore be compromised when fractionation schedules are protracted or when gaps are inadvertently or deliberately introduced into a course of radiotherapy. Loss of locoregional control may range from 1.6% to 6% for each day of delay.[128,129]

Normal tissue reactions to ionizing radiation can be broadly divided into early and late. Early reactions typically occur within the first few weeks of fractionated radiotherapy and are manifest by mucositis, taste loss, skin erythema and skin desquamation resulting from mitotic arrest of rapidly dividing cells. Healing usually occurs within a period of 4–6 weeks following treatment completion unless excessively high doses of radiation have been given over short time periods, following which consequential damage may occur as a result of excessive normal epithelial stem cell depletion. Late tissue reactions, which occur beyond three months following treatment and which may progress over many years, are manifest by tissue fibrosis or, in the extreme, radionecrosis. Late reactions are relatively more sensitive than early reactions to large radiation doses per fraction and to high LET radiation such as fast neutrons. Consequently, small doses per fraction of conventional megavoltage x-irradiation reduce the probability of late effects. Conventional fractionation delivers each dose with a minimum 24-hour interval. However, multiple fractions per day will, by definition, demand shorter interfraction intervals, in which case sufficient time must be allowed for tissue repair (a minimum of six hours is usually accepted, although tissue such as the CNS may require a longer period for repair).[130]

Accelerated radiotherapy fractionation is achieved by reducing the overall treatment time while maintaining the same or a similar number of treatment fractions as for conventional radiotherapy, with the objective of counteracting repopulation and thereby improving tumour control. The most extreme examples have used multiple fractions per day throughout treatment. Jackson et al reported excessive grade 4 acute mucosal toxicity with 66 Gy delivered in 3.5 weeks compared to the conventional arm of 6.5. As a consequence the trial was closed after entering only 82 patients. An anticipated improvement in local control at 3 years could not be demonstrated, perhaps because of the small number of patients.[131] Dose reduction in the accelerated arm reduces toxicity; however, a recently reported trial of 350 patients failed to demonstrate significant improvement in disease-free survival, disease-specific survival or locoregional control.[132]

Less extreme compression of overall treatment time has been achieved by delivering six fractions per week, either treating on a Saturday or a twice per day treatment on one day of the standard working week. Thereby the overall 6.5 week schedule is reduced by one to two weeks. Two large randomized trials have addressed this approach. The Danish DAHANCA 7/8 trials, which recruited over 500 patients, have together demonstrated a 15% improvement in local control for the accelerated arm compared to conventional 5 fraction per week radiotherapy, although to date overall survival is not significantly different.[133] However, Hliniak et al have very recently reported a trial of similar design randomizing 350 patients, which has failed to show a significant improvement in local control for the accelerated arm despite more severe early toxicity, albeit of short duration. The smaller number of patients might explain the negative result compared to DAHANCA.[134] Nevertheless, when the next logical step was taken to avoid all weekend breaks by using a seven-day per week treatment schedule, the result was an unacceptable 22% rate of consequential damage with positive tumour control endpoints. Three year local tumour control was improved from 37% to 82% and overall survival from 32% to 78% respectively for the control and accelerated arms of the study. The authors state that reducing the dose per treatment fraction from 2.0 to 1.8 Gy eliminated the phenomenon of consequential damage.[135] Perhaps one of the most important messages from this trial is the demonstration of the criticality of seemingly small changes in radiation dose fractionation.

Hyperfractionated radiotherapy employs a larger number of fractions compared to a conventional schedule given over the same period of time, and is also achieved by giving multiple fractions per day. For a given overall dose the reduced radiation dose per fraction results in a lesser risk of late tissue damage. The extrapolation of this approach therefore allows a higher overall dose to be given without incurring excessive late damage, with the objective of improving tumour control. An unqualified example of this approach is exemplified by the EORTC 22791 trial, which compared a hyperfractionated schedule of 80.5 Gy given in 70 fractions (twice per day) over seven weeks to a conventional dose of 70 Gy using 35–40 daily fractions in 356 patients with oropharyngeal cancer. Five year local control was increased from 40% to 59% with a trend towards increased survival but without incurring a higher risk of late tissue damage.[136] Such an early and imposing result has not led to widespread adoption of this approach because of the considerable demand upon resources and upon patients' psychological tolerance for undergoing 70 radiation treatment sessions. The results have been corroborated by an overview of several other trials showing improvement in long-term locoregional control and reduction in odds of death,[137] although the largest trial by Sanchiz et al analysed in this overview has been criticized for the low dose of 60 Gy used in the conventional arm.[138]

Accelerated hyperfractionation aims to achieve both objectives of minimizing the effects of tumour clonogen repopulation and of late tissue damage. Variations on this theme have now been evaluated in a number of large trials. The RTOG have recently published results of a four-arm trial investigating hyperfractionation, accelerated fractionation with concomitant boost (twice daily for last 12 treatment days) and acceleration with a two week rest during treatment compared to conventional fractionation. Both hyperfractionation (81.6 Gy in 68 fractions over seven weeks) and concomitant boost (72 Gy in 42 fractions over six weeks) have demonstrated improved local control compared to the control arm, although overall survival is similar in all arms. Acute effects were enhanced, although to date there has been no significant increase in late effects.[139] The EORTC trial 22851 randomized 512 patients with advanced head and neck cancer to an accelerated hyperfractionated schedule of 72 Gy in 45 fractions over five weeks, or to the conventional schedule of 70 Gy in 35 fractions over seven weeks. Locoregional control was improved by 13%. However, this was at the expense of a 14% risk of severe late tissue damage including two cases of radiation myelitis, another example of unacceptable damage resulting from relatively small changes in dose and fractionation.[140] Perhaps the most radical approach is exemplified by the CHART trial which to date is one of the largest head and neck radiotherapy fractionation trials. A total of 918 patients were randomized between conventional fractionation 66 Gy in 33 fractions over 6.5 weeks and a highly accelerated and hyperfractionated schedule of 54 Gy in 36 fractions over 12 days. Unfortunately there was no significant difference in control or survival parameters between the control and experimental of the trial. However, late effects appear to be less frequent for CHART, suggesting that the overall radiation dose reduction was perhaps greater than necessary.[141] A similar accelerated and hyperfractionated schedule has been applied in the postoperative setting. Seventy patients with locally advanced head and neck cancer were randomized to receive 46.2 Gy over 12 days; three fractions per day of 1.4 Gy with a six hour interfraction interval for six days per week or a conventional dose of 60 Gy for five days per week over six weeks. Improved three-year locoregional control rates of 88% versus 57% were achieved, although overall survival rates of 60% versus 46% were not statistically significant. Both early and late reactions were enhanced in the experimental arm, the latter considered to have resulted from a higher incidence of consequential damage. The study also indicated that optimal results were achieved if the interval between surgery and radiotherapy did not exceed six weeks and when the overall treatment time was within ten weeks.[142]

Combined chemotherapy/radiotherapy

The combination of chemotherapy and radiotherapy has been extensively investigated in head and neck cancer over the last three decades. The rationale was founded upon high response rates in patients with squamous head and neck cancer to a variety of chemotherapy agents including methotrexate, vinblastine, bleomycin, 5-fluorouracil, cisplatin, carboplatin and the taxoids, either alone or in combination.[143] The combination of cisplatin and 5-fluorouracil demonstrated complete response rates of up to 50% in previously untreated patients.[144] Such response rates equal those reported for other solid tumours, such as breast carcinoma, and there has therefore been considerable interest and enthusiasm for both adjuvant and palliative chemotherapy in head and neck cancer.

Neo-adjuvant or 'induction' chemotherapy schedules have most commonly been employed in an attempt to downstage disease prior to definitive local therapies and to reduce the incidence of distant metastases. Alternatively chemotherapy has been given, simultaneously with radiotherapy, subsequently as an adjuvant or in combination. The danger of bias from historical control or case matched control studies is no better exemplified than for head and neck cancer, with the majority of early published non-randomized trials strongly supporting the case for neoadjuvant chemotherapy. An important clinical objective has been to achieve 'organ preservation' by avoiding ablative surgery in advanced disease. The Veterans Affairs Study randomized patients between induction chemotherapy followed by radiotherapy versus surgery followed by postoperative radiotherapy. Those receiving chemotherapy underwent surgery and radiotherapy if a partial response was not achieved. Two-thirds of the patients treated in the conservation arm retained their larynx, although overall survival was the same.[145] The trial has been heavily criticized for the absence of a radiotherapy-alone arm. Consequently, Intergroup trial R91-11 was initiated, comparing induction chemotherapy and radiotherapy versus concurrent chemotherapy and radiotherapy versus radiotherapy alone. An interim report has failed to indicate an overall survival benefit from chemotherapy. However, laryngectomy-free survival is significantly longer with concomitant chemotherapy, compared to radiotherapy alone, although induction chemotherapy offers no advantage. Both chemotherapy arms appear to reduce the incidence of distant metastases. These results must be regarded as preliminary and further follow-up is necessary.[146] Similar criticism can be levelled at the EORTC trial reported by Lefebvre, which investigated pyriform sinus cancer using a similar strategy and resulted in a comparable conclusion, albeit with a lower (35%) rate of pharyngeal preservation.[147]

A large number of randomized trials designed to investigate these approaches have now been reported and have drawn conflicting conclusions, primarily because the majority are of small sample size. In such a circumstance we can be guided by meta-analysis. One of the first to be published was by Stell and Rawson in 1990, which analysed 23 randomized trials of adjuvant chemotherapy in squamous carcinoma of the head and neck, none of which were individually large enough to detect the anticipated survival improvement of the order of 5%. The average response rate in four induction studies was 47%, yet overall there was no significant reduction in cancer mortality with this approach. Only synchronous and/or maintenance trials appeared to confer benefit. Perhaps unexpectedly, cisplatinum-containing regimens offered no benefit and patients treated with the commonly used vinblastine, bleomycin and methotrexate combination fared worse. While the incidence of locoregional recurrence was reduced in the chemotherapy arms, the distant metastasis rate was unchanged. Toxicity was poorly reported in these trials; however the average mortality rate in nine series was an alarming 6.5%.[148]

Reasons for the failure of the neoadjuvant approach to increase survival are unclear and several hypotheses have been suggested. The concept that tumours treated with chemotherapy may become more aggressive despite apparent downstaging is supported by a study of tumour cell kinetics using flow cytometry in 97 patients with oropharyngeal cancer, which demonstrated significantly increased mean labelling indices and shorter potential doubling times following induction chemotherapy compared to pretreatment measurements, particularly in poorly responding tumours.[149] Alternatively, the possible benefits of neoadjuvant chemotherapy for responding patients may be offset by the adverse effect of delaying surgery or radiotherapy in non-responding patients. A potential survival advantage may also be eroded by excess mortality associated with the high incidence of intercurrent disease, mainly second tumours and vascular disease, in this group of patients, which may be further offset by toxic related deaths resulting from chemotherapy. It is therefore logical to conclude that the reasons for failure are multifactorial.

Over the last decade many more trials have reached maturity. The meta-analysis of 54 randomized trials published by Munro in 1995 reiterated Stell's findings, with neoadjuvant chemotherapy conferring a small survival rate difference of 3.7% with 95% confidence intervals of 0.9–6.5%. However, single-agent simultaneous chemotherapy increased survival by 12.1% with a corresponding confidence interval of 5–19%. Once more, cisplatinum-containing schedules failed to confer a survival advantage.[150] By 2000, results of almost 11 000 patients from 63 randomized trials had become available, and formed the basis for a large meta-analysis based upon individual patient data. Pignon et al reported a 4% survival benefit at five years for chemotherapy overall. Neoadjuvant and adjuvant chemotherapy failed to confer a significant survival advantage, whereas a gain of 8% was achieved using 'concurrent' combinations. However, the authors affirm that clear conclusions could not be drawn because of the heterogeneity of the results. Most of the effect appears to relate to improved local and regional disease control, with less conclusive evidence for a reduction in the incidence of distant metastases.[151] Following the disappointment with neoadjuvant chemotherapy, more recent trials have investigated the 'synchronous' approach. A recent systematic review of 18 such trials including 3192 patients has reported a relative risk reduction of 11% with this methodology. Of particular interest, platinum-based regimens, involving almost half of this patient complement, were found to be most effective.[152] Many more such trials are now reaching maturity and further analyses will undoubtedly follow.

A note of caution is warranted; acute toxicity is enhanced by most regimens of simultaneous chemoradiotherapy and will be self-limiting with appropriate patient support. However, if we are to improve the therapeutic ratio for locoregional disease control we must ensure that late effects are not enhanced pro rata. Very few of these trials have collected late effect data. Nineteen simultaneous trials reported in the Munro meta-analysis were examined by Henk who found that late effects were indeed enhanced, suggesting that chemotherapy may merely be dose modifying. This implies that the same objective might be achieved by using a higher dose of irradiation given the limited efficacy of systemic chemotherapy for reducing the risk of metastatic disease, and would also have the advantage of avoiding systemic toxicity.[153] As a conclusion, adjuvant chemotherapy for head and neck cancer should not be used routinely outside the context of appropriate clinical trials, and future trials must closely assess both acute and late toxicity, perhaps with the inclusion of radiation dose escalation as a randomization.

Combined modified radiation fractionation and simultaneous chemotherapy

The most recent generation of randomized clinical trials have been designed to investigate the potential for further improvement by combining modified fractionation with simultaneous chemotherapy. Enhanced acute and late toxicities are a major concern with such intensive treatment and have been carefully documented in most of these studies. Pure hyperfractionation with or without cisplatinum and 5-fluorouracil in a trial of 122 patients reported by Brizel has been shown to improve locoregional control from 44–70%, albeit with a high risk of confluent mucositis in both arms of the trial.[154] Jeremic, using a similar approach with 77 Gy given in 35 fractions over seven weeks with or without low dose daily cisplatinum, achieved an overall survival improvement from 49–68% without incurring increased early or late toxicity. Distant metastasis-free survival was also improved by the combined modalities.[155]

The most intensive approach of combining simultaneous chemotherapy with hyperfractionation and acceleration has also been investigated. Dobrovski compared conventional fractionation to a hyperfractionated and accelerated radiotherapy with mitomycin C. Locoregional control was increased without an increase in mucosal toxicity, although haematological toxicity was significantly greater in those receiving chemotherapy. The inclusion of two variables in the experimental arm, namely altered fractionation and chemotherapy, make it impossible to determine which of these agents was responsible for improving disease control, and such trial design should be avoided.[156] However, the most recently reported trial by Starr, comparing hyperfractionated acceleration and chemotherapy using 5-fluorouracil and carboplatin in 263 patients, has failed to show significant improvements in locoregional control despite the 'intensity' of the combined arm. Of significance, GCSF was added as a second randomization with the intention of reducing mucositis, and resulted in decreased tumour control, possibly a result of tumour colonogen stimulation by the growth factor.[157] Results to date are therefore somewhat conflicting, perhaps reflecting the heterogeneity of approach, and require longer-term follow-up before clear conclusions can be drawn.

Conformal radiotherapy and intensity modulated radiotherapy: 'back to basics'

The discussion so far has focused upon biological and biochemical methods for modifying and modulating radiotherapy delivered by conventional 'crudely' shaped radiation beams directed at the tumour target. Logic dictates that in order to achieve maximum radiation dose to tumour with minimum dose to surrounding normal tissue, the beams should 'conform' as closely as possible to the shape of the tumour, which are by no means simple cuboidal, cylindrical or even spheroidal structures. This is even more difficult when associated tumour masses coexist in close proximity, for example a primary tumour with locally involved nodes.

Such techniques may allow significantly increased dose delivery to tumour volume whilst considerably reducing dosage to closely surrounding normal tissue, in the hope of improving both tumour control and normal tissue tolerance. The possibility of delivering a high dose of radiotherapy to the nasopharynx or oropharynx with selective sparing of critical structures such as major salivary glands can now be realized by using the combined techniques of conformal radiotherapy and intensity-modulated radiotherapy. These techniques are in their relative infancy, and much radiobiological work must be undertaken in order to ensure that the results realize their potential. Nevertheless, preliminary results are most encouraging.[158,159] These techniques will undoubtedly be included in future fractionation and combined modality studies, with the ultimate aim of achieving even greater enhancement of the therapeutic ratio between tumour and normal tissue.

The role of palliative chemotherapy may be similarly contentious. The high rates of clinical response achieved with chemotherapy as single agents or in combination have led to their frequent use in patients with advanced and frequently previously treated disease. However, clinical outcome measures have been crude and many trials have focused upon complete and partial response rates as their primary study endpoints. One of the most active drug combinations, cisplatinum and 5-fluorouracil, has clearly shown superior response rates compared to single agent methotrexate in a randomized trial, but at the cost of significantly increased toxicity and with no improvement in overall survival.[160] A review of trials of palliative chemotherapy has not shown a clear overall survival advantage for more active drug combinations, if indeed any survival advantage for chemotherapy over supportive care alone, and warns of the potential folly of assuming that tumour response is a valid surrogate for symptom control.[161] A review of single agent palliative chemotherapy suggests that carboplatin may offer relatively high response rates with minimal toxicity, and therefore hopefully optimal symptom relief (Munro A, personal communication).

The tools for quality of life measurement, FACT G&HN, EORTC QLQC30+HN35 and University of Washington, which include both general questions and specific questions relating to head and neck cancer, are currently being evaluated. The palliative value of chemotherapy for such advanced disease must be judged by such quality of life measurement as the principle endpoint and not by response rates nor necessarily by survival rates. A future trial design will include randomization to best supportive care in addition to active chemotherapy agents, with careful measurement of patients' quality of life as the primary endpoint (Glaholm J, personal communication) once more emphasizing the importance of treating such patients within the context of a well-designed clinical trial.

References

1. Priestman TJ, Bullimore JA, Godden TP, Deutsch GP. The Royal College of Radiologists Fractionation Survey. Clin Oncol 1989; 1: 39–46
2. Steel GG. Basic clinical radiobiology. London: Edward Arnold, 1993: 35
3. Withers HR, Taylor JMG, Maciejewski B. The hazard of accelerated tumour clonogen repopulation during radiotherapy. Acta Oncol 1988; 27: 131–146
4. Denekamp J. Physiological hypoxia and its influence on radiotherapy. In: Steel GG, Adams GE, Horwich A (eds). The biological basis of radiotherapy, 2nd edn. New York: Elselvier Science, 1989
5. Thomlinson RH, Gray LH. The histological structure of some human lung cancers and the possible implications for radiotherapy. Br J Cancer 1955; 9: 539–549
6. Horsman MR, Overgaard J. Overcoming tumour radioresistance resulting from acute hypoxia. Eur J Cancer 1992; 28: 717–718

7. Steel GG. Basic clinical radiobiology. London: Edward Arnold, 1993: 227
8. Steel GG. Basic clinical radiobiology. London: Edward Arnold, 1993: 55–80
9. Anon. LENT SOMA tables. Radiother. Oncol 1995; 35: 17–60
10. Anon. LENT SOMA scales for all anatomic sites. Int J Radiat Oncol Biol Phys 1995; 31: 1049–1091
11. Wiernik G, Alcock CJ, Bates TD. First interim progress report on the second British Institute of Radiology fractionation study: short versus long overall treatment times for radiotherapy of carcinoma of the laryngopharynx. Br J Radiol 1989; 62: 450–456
12. Bentzen SM, Johansen LV, Overgaard J et al. Clinical radiobiology of squamous carcinoma of the oropharynx. Int J Radiat Oncol Biol Phys 1991; 20: 1197–1206
13. Pameijer FA, Mancuso AA, Mendenhall WM et al. Can pretreatment computed tomography predict local control in T3 squamous cell carcinoma of the glottic larynx treated with definitive radiotherapy? Int J Radiat Oncol Biol Phys 1997; 15, 37: 1011–1211
14. Mendenhall WM, Parsons JT, Mancuso AA et al. Radiotherapy for squamous cell carcinoma of the supraglottic larynx: an alternative strategy to surgery. Head Neck 1996; 18: 24–35
15. Davidson J, Keane T, Brown D et al. Surgical salvage after radiotherapy for advanced laryngopharyngeal carcinoma. Arch Otolaryngol Head Neck Surg 1997; 123: 420–424
16. Croll GA, Gerritsen GJ, Tiwari RM, Snow GB. Primary radiotherapy with surgery in reserve for advanced laryngeal carcinoma. Results and complications. Eur J Surg Oncol 1989; 15: 350–360
17. Vikram B, Strong EW, Shah JP, Shapiro R. Failure at the primary site following multi-modality treatment in advanced head and neck cancer. Head Neck Surg 1984; 6: 720–723
18. Tupchong L, Scott CB, Blitzer PH et al. Randomised study of preoperative versus postoperative radiotherapy for head and neck squamous carcinoma, final results of trial RTOG 73-03. Int J Radiat Biol Phys 1991; 20: 21–28
19. Robertson AJ, Soutar DS, Paul J et al. Early closure of a randomised trial: Surgery and postoperative radiotherapy versus radiotherapy in the management of intraoral tumours. Clin Oncol (R Coll Radiol) 1998; 10: 155–160
20. Hansen HS, Overgaard J, Overgaard M et al. Continuous versus split course radiotherapy of advanced supraglottic carcinoma. Experience from the Danish head and neck cancer study. Abstract A:0235, Second World Congress on Laryngeal Cancer, 20–24 February 1994, Sydney, Australia
21. Amdur RJ, Parsons JT, Mendenhall WM, Million RR, Cassisi NJ. Split-course versus continuous course irradiation in the postoperative setting for squamous cell carcinoma of the head and neck. Int J Radiat Oncol Biol Phys 1989; 17: 279–285
22. Skaladowski K, Law MG, Maciejewski B, Steel GG. Planned and unplanned gaps in radiotherapy: the importance of gap position and gap duration. Radiother Oncol 1994; 30: 109–120
23. Wang CC, Efird J, Nakfoor B, Martins P. Local control of T3 carcinomas after accelerated fractionation: a look at the gap. Int J Radiat Oncol Biol Phys 1996; 35: 439–441
24. Duncan W, MacDougal RH, Kerr GR, Downing D. Adverse effects of treatment gaps in the outcome of radiotherapy for laryngeal cancer. Radiother Oncol 1996; 41: 203–207
25. Robertson C, Robertson AG, Hendry JH et al. Similar decreases in local tumour control are calculated for treatment protraction and for interruptions in the radiotherapy of carcinoma of the larynx in four centres. Int J Radiat Oncol Biol Phys 1998; 40: 319–329
26. Hendry JH, Betzen SM, Dale RG et al. A modelled comparison of the effects of using different ways to compensate for missed treatment days in radiotherapy. Clin Oncol (R Coll Radiol) 1996; 8: 297–307
27. Pierquin B, Dutreix A, Paine CH, Chassagne D, Marinello G, Ash D. The Paris system of interstitial radiation therapy. Acta Radiol Oncol Radiat Phys Biol (Sweden) 1978, 17: 33–48
28. Ash D. Overview of interstitial therapy. Br J Radiol (Suppl) 1988; 22: 79–82
29. Lozza L, Cerrotta A, Gardani G et al. Analysis of risk factors for mandibular bone radionecrosis after exclusive low dose rate brachytherapy for oral cancer. Radiother Oncol 1997; 44: 143–147
30. Inoue T, InoueT, Teshima T et al. Phase III trial of high and low dose rate interstitial radiotherapy for early oral tongue cancer. Int J Radiat Oncol Biol Phys 1996; 36: 1201–1204
31. Pernot M, Malisard L, Aletti P, Hoffsetter S, Forcard JJ, Bey P. Iridium-192 brachytherapy in the management of 147 T2 N0 oral tongue carcinomas treated with irradiation alone: comparison of two treatment techniques. Radiother Oncol 1992; 23: 223–228
32. Wendt CD, Peters LJ, Delclos L et al. Primary radiotherapy in the treatment of stage I and II oral tongue cancers: importance of the proportion of therapy delivered with interstitial therapy. Int J Radiat Oncol Biol Phys 1990; 18: 1287–1292
33. Mendenhall WM, Parsons JT, Stringer SP et al. T2 oral tongue carcinoma treated with radiotherapy: analysis of local control and complications. Radiother Oncol 1989; 16: 275–281
34. Jyothirmayi R, Sankaranarayanan R, Varghese C et al. Radiotherapy in the treatment of verrucous carcinoma of the oral cavity. Oral Oncology 1977; 33: 124–128
35. Vidyasagar MS, Fernandes DJ, Kasturi DP. Radiotherapy and verrucous carcinoma of the oral cavity: a study of 107 cases. Acta Oncol 1992; 31: 43–47
36. O'Sullivan B, Warde P, Keane T et al. Outcome following radiotherapy in verrucous carcinoma of the larynx. Int J Radiat Oncol Biol Phys 1995; 32: 611–617
37. Cowen D, Essomba M, Richaud P. Treatment of

cervical lymph nodes in lip cancers. Bull Cancer Radiother 1990; 77: 111–117
38. Sykes AJ, Allan E, Irwin C. Squamous carcinoma of the lip: the role of electron treatment. Clin Oncol (R Coll Radiol) 1996; 8: 384–386
39. de Visscher JG, Grond AJ, Botke G et al. Results of radiotherapy for squamous cell carcinoma of the vermillion border of the lower lip. A retrospective analysis of 108 patients. Radiother Oncol 1996; 39: 9–14
40. Spiro RH, Huvos AG, Wong GY et al. Predictive value of tumour thickness in squamous carcinoma confined to the tongue and floor of mouth. Am J Surg 1986; 152: 345–350
41. Mohit-Tabatabai MA, Sobel HJ, Rush BF et al. Relation of thickness of floor of mouth stage I and II cancers to regional metastasis. Am J Surg 1986; 152: 351–353
42. Gerbaulet A, Haie-Meder C, Marsiglaia U. Role of brachytherapy in treatment of head and neck cancers: Institute Gustave-Roussy experience with 1140 patients. In: Mould RF, Betterman JJ, Martinez AA, Speiser BL (eds). Brachytherapy from radium to optimization. Nucletron Int, 1994: Chapter 12, 101–120
43. Hichs WL Jr, Loree TR, Garcia RI. Squamous cell carcinoma of the floor of mouth: a 20 year review, Head Neck 1997; 19: 400–405
44. Henk JM. Treatment of oral cancer by interstitial irradiation using iridium-192. Br J Oral Maxillofac Surg 1992; 30: 355–359
45. Podd TJ, Carton AT, Barrie R et al. Treatment of oral cancers using iridium-192 interstitial irradiation. Br J Oral Maxillofac Surg 1994; 31: 207–213
46. Franceschi D, Gupta R, Spiro RH et al. Improved survival in the treatment of squamous carcinoma of the oral tongue. Am J Surg 1993; 166: 360–365
47. Lapeyre M, Peiffert D, Malisard L et al. An original technique of brachytherapy in the treatment of epidermoid carcinomas of the buccal mucosa. Int J Radiat Oncol Biol Phys 1995; 33: 447–454
48. Liubaev VL, Brzhezovski VZh, Amparaliev NM. [The importance of the surgical treatment method in cancer of the oral mucosa with the primary tumour 4 cm in size and larger.] Stomatologiia (Mosk) 1992; 1: 56–58
49. Mishra RC, Singh DN, Mishra TK. Post-operative radiotherapy in carcinoma of the buccal mucosa, a prospective randomised trial. Eur J Surg Oncol 1996; 22: 502–504
50. Totsuka Y, Usui Y, Tei K et al. Results of surgical treatments for squamous carcinoma of the lower alveolus: segmental vs marginal resection. Head Neck 1991; 13: 114–120
51. Langdon JD, Harvey PW, Rapidis AD et al. Oral cancer: the behaviour and response to treatment of 194 cases. J Maxillofac Surg 1977; 5: 221–237
52. Kannan V, Anantha N, Kumaraswamy SV. A prospective study of radiation and surgery in stage IV carcinoma of the lower alveolus. Radiotherapy and Oncology '95, Meeting abstract, Association of Radiation Oncologists of India, 16th Annual Meeting and Roentgen Centenary Celebration, 2–4 February 1995, Kerala, India: 245
53. Fein DA, Lee WR, Amos WR. Oropharyngeal carcinoma treated with radiotherapy: a 30 year experience. Int J Radiat Oncol Biol Phys 1996; 34: 289–296
54. Wang CC, Montgomery W, Efind J. Local control of oropharyngeal carcinoma by irradiation alone. Laryngoscope 1995; 105: 1258
55. Moose BD, Kelly MD, Levine P, et al. Definitive radiotherapy for T1 and T2 squamous carcinoma of the tonsil. Head Neck 1995; 17: 334–338
56. Foote RL, Hilgenfeld RU, Kunselman SJ et al. Radiation therapy for carcinoma of the tonsil. Mayo Clinic Proc 1994; 69: 525–531
57. O'Brien CJ, Castle GK, Stevens GN. Limitations of radiotherapy in the definitive treatment of squamous carcinoma of the tonsilar fossa. Aust N Z Surg 1992; 62: 709–713
58. Gehanno P, Depondt J, Guedon C. Primary and salvage surgery for cancer of the tonsilar region: a retrospective study of 120 patients. Head Neck 1993; 15: 185–189
59. Nason RW, Anderson BJ, Gujrathi DS. A retrospective comparison of treatment outcome in the posterior and anterior tongue. Am J Surg 1996; 172: 665–670
60. Hinerman RW, Parsons JT, Mendenhall WM et al. External beam irradiation alone or combined with neck dissection for base of tongue carcinoma: an alternative to primary surgery. Laryngoscope 1994; 104: 1466–1470
61. Horowitz EM, Frazier AJ, Martinez AA. Excellent functional outcome in patients with squamous cell carcinoma of the base of the tongue treated with external radiation and interstitial iodine 125 boosts. Cancer 1996; 1: 78: 948–957
62. Inakami K, Satou T, Yoshino K. A clinical study of squamous carcinoma of the tongue base. Nippon Jibiinkoka Gakkai Kaiho 1996; 99: 1010–1015
63. Weber RS, Gidley P, Morrison WH et al. Treatment selection for carcinoma of the base of tongue. Am J Surg 1990; 160: 415–419
64. Medini E, Medini A, Gapany M. External beam radiation therapy for squamous carcinoma of the soft palate. Int J Radiat Oncol Biol Phys 1997; 38: 507–511
65. Mak-Kregar S, Keus RB, Balm AJ et al. Carcinoma of the soft palate and posterior oropharyngeal wall. Clin Otolaryngol 1994; 19: 22–27
66. Chang L, Stevens KR, Moss WT et al.. Squamous cell carcinoma of the pharyngeal walls treated with radiotherapy. Int J Radiat Oncol Biol Phys 1996; 35: 477–483
67. Rodriguez J, Point D, Brunin F et al. Surgery of the oropharynx after radiotherapy. Bull Cancer Radiother 1996; 83: 24–30
68. Turner SL, Slevin NJ, Gupta NK et al. Radical external beam radiotherapy for 333 squamous carcinomas of the oral cavity—evaluation of late morbidity and a watch policy for the clinically negative neck. Radiother Oncol 1996; 41: 21–29
69. McGuirt WF Jr, Johnson JT, Myers EN et al. Floor of mouth carcinoma. The management of the clinically

negative neck. Arch Otolaryngol Head Neck Surg 1995; 121: 278–282
70. Pernot M, Verhaeghe JL, Guillemin F et al. Evaluation of the importance of systemic neck dissection in carcinoma of the oral cavity treated by brachytherapy alone for the primary lesion (apropos of a series of patients). Bull Cancer Radiother 1995; 82: 311–317
71. Byers RM, Wolf PF, Ballantyre AJ. Rationale for elective modified neck dissection. Head Neck Surg 1988; 10: 160–167
72. Umeda M, Yokoo S, Take Y et al. Lymph node metastasis in squamous cell carcinoma of the oral cavity: correlation between histologic features and the prevalence of metastasis. Head Neck 1992; 14: 263–272
73. Byers RM, Weber RS, Andrews T et al. Frequency and therapeutic implications of skip metastasis in the neck from squamous carcinoma of the oral tongue. Head Neck 1997; 19: 14–19
74. Jesse RH, Ballantyne AJ, Larson D. Radical or modified neck dissection: a therapeutic dilemma. Am J Surg 1978; 136: 516–519
75. Northrop MF, Fletcher GH, Jesse RH et al. Evolution of neck disease in patients with primary squamous carcinoma of the oral tongue, floor of mouth, and palatine arch, and clinically positive nodes neither fixed nor bilateral. Cancer 1972; 29: 23–30
76. Votava C Jr, Fletcher GH, Jesse RH Jr et al. Management of cervical nodes, either fixed or bilateral, from squamous cell carcinoma of the oral cavity and faucial arch. Radiology 1972; 105: 417–420
77. Vandenbrouck C, Sancho-Garnier H, Chassagne D et al. Elective vs therapeutic radical neck dissection in epidermoid carcinoma of the oral cavity: results of a randomised clinical trial. Cancer 1980; 46: 386–390
78. Fakih AR, Rao RS, Borges AM et al. Elective versus therapeutic neck dissection in early carcinoma of the oral tongue. Am J Surg 1989; 158: 309–313
79. Fletcher GH. Irradiation of sub-clinical disease in the draining lymphatics. Int J Radiat Oncol Biol Phys 1984; 10: 939–942
80. Mendenhall WM, Parsons JT, Million RR. Elective lower neck irradiation: 5,000 cGray/25 fractions versus 4,050 cGray/15 fractions. Int J Radiat Oncol Biol Phys 1988; 15: 439–440
81. Mendenhall WM, Million RR. Elective neck irradiation for squamous cell carcinoma of the head and neck: analysis of time dose factors and causes of failure. Int J Radiat Oncol Biol Phys 1986; 12: 741–746
82. Gleave E.N. Management of metastatic cervical nodes. Proceedings of the Edinburgh Surgical Festival 1980: 4–5
83. Martin H, Romieu C. The diagnostic significance of 'a lump in the neck'. Postgrad Med 1952; 11: 491–500
84. McGuirt WF, McCabe BF. Significance of node biopsy before definitive treatment of cervical metastatic carcinoma. Laryngoscope 1978; 88: 594–597
85. Ellis ER, Mendenhall WM, Rao PV et al. Incisional or excisional biopsy before definitive radiotherapy alone or followed by neck dissection. Head Neck 1991; 13: 177–183
86. Mack Y, Parsons JT, Mendenhall WM. Squamous cell carcinoma of the head and neck: management after excisional biopsy. Int J Radiat Oncol Biol Phys 1993; 25: 619–622
87. Varghese C, Sankaranrayanan R, Nair B et al. Predictors of neck node control in radically irradiated squamous carcinoma of the oropharynx and laryngopharynx. Head Neck 1993; 15: 105–108
88. Gomez PJP, Rodriguez R, Rijo GJ et al. Control of neck nodes in squamous cell carcinoma of the head and neck by radiotherapy: prognostic factors. Otolaryngology 1992; 17: 163–169
89. Peters LJ, Weber RS, Morrison WH et al. Neck surgery in patients with primary oropharyngeal cancer treated by radiotherapy. Head Neck 1996; 18: 552–559
90. Huang DT, Johnson CR, Schmidt-Ullrich R et al. Postoperative radiotherapy in head and neck carcinoma with extracapsular lymph node extension and/or positive resection margins: a comparative study. Int J Radiat Oncol Biol Phys 1992; 23: 737–742
91. Leemans CR, Tiwari R, van der Waal I et al. The efficacy of comprehensive neck dissection with or without postoperative radiotherapy in nodal metastases of squamous cell carcinoma of the upper respiratory and digestive tracts. Laryngoscope 1990; 100: 1194–1198
92. Ampil F, Datta R, Shockley W. Adjuvant postoperative external beam radiotherapy in head and neck cancer. J Oral Maxillofac Surg 1988; 46: 569–573
93. Ho CM, Lam KH, Wie WI et al. Treatment of neck nodes in oral cancer. Surg Oncol 1992; 1: 73–78
94. Garret P, Rate W, Freeman S et al. Intraoperative radiation in head and neck tumours. Meeting abstract, Seventh Annual Brachytherapy Symposium: Focus on intraoperative radiation therapy and high dose rate brachytherapy, 17–19 September 1993, Columbus, Ohio
95. Valdagni R, Amichetti M. Report of long term follow-up in a randomized trial comparing radiation therapy plus hyperthermia to metastatic lymph nodes in stage IV head and neck patients. Int J Radiat Oncol Biol 1994; 28: 163–169
96. Sur RK, Kochhar R, Singh DP. Oral sucralfate in acute radiation oesophagitis. Acta Oncol 1994; 33: 62–63
97. Lees J. Nasogastric and percutaneous endoscopic gastrostomy in head and neck cancer patients receiving radiotherapy treatment at a regional oncology unit: a two year study. Eur J Cancer Care 1997; 6: 45–49
98. Rieke JW, Hafermann MD, Johnson JT et al. Oral pilocarpine for radiation-induced xerostomia: integrated efficacy and safety results from two prospective randomised trials. Int J Radiat Oncol Biol Phys 1995; 31: 661–669
99. Jacobs CD, van der Pas M. A multicentre maintenance study of oral pilocarpine tablets for radiation-induced xerostomia. Oncology (Huntingt) 1996; 10 (Suppl 3): 16–20
100. Hamlar DD, Schuller DE, Gahbauer RA. Determination of the efficacy of topical oral pilocarpine for postirradiation xerostomia in patients with head and neck cancer. Laryngoscope 1996; 106: 972–976

101. Zimmerman RP, Mark RJ, Tran LM. Concomitant pilocarpine during head and neck irradiation is associated with decreased posttreatment xerostomia. Int J Radiat Oncol Biol Phys 1997; 37: 571–575
102. LeVeque F, Fontanesi J, Devi S. Salivary gland sheltering using concurrent pilocarpine (PC) in irradiated head and neck cancer patients [Meeting abstract]. Proc Annu Meet Am Soc Clin Oncol 1996; 15: A1665
103. Fernando IN, Patel T, Billingham I et al. The effect of head and neck irradiation on taste dysfunction. Clin Oncol (Royal College Radiol) 1995; 7: 173–178
104. Perrier M, Moeller P. Osteoradionecrosis. A review of the literature. Schweiz Monatsschr Zahnmed 1994; 104: 271–277
105. Singh N, Scully C, Joyston-Bechal S. Oral complications of cancer therapies: prevention and managment. Clin Oncol (R Coll Radiol) 1996; 8: 15–24
106. Horiot JC, Wambersie A. Prevention of dental caries and of osteoradionecrosis in patients irradiated in oncology. Rev Belg Med Dent 1991; 46: 72–86
107. Wong JK, Wood RE, McClean M. Conservative management of osteoradionecrosis. Oral Surg Oral Med Oral Pathol Oral Radiol Endod 1997; 84: 16–21
108. van Merkesteyn JP, Bakker DJ, Borgmeijer-Hoelen AM. Hyperbaric oxygen treatment of osteoradionecrosis of the mandible. Experience in 29 patients. Oral Med Oral Pathol Oral Radiol Endod 1996; 81: 265–266
109. McKenzie MR, Wong FL, Epstein JB et al. Hyperbaric oxygen and postradiation necrosis of the mandible. Eur J Cancer B Oral Oncol 1993; 29B: 201–207
110. Epstein J, van der Meij E, McKenzie M et al. Postradiation osteonecrosis of the mandible: a long term follow-up study. Oral Med Oral Pathol Oral Radiol Endod 1997; 83: 657–662
111. Constantino PD, Friedman CD, Steinberg MJ. Irradiated bone and its management. Otolaryngol Clin North Am 1995; 28: 1021–1038
112. Esser E, Wagner W. Dental implants following radical oral surgery and adjuvant radiotherapy. Int J Oral Maxillofac Implants 1997; 12: 552–557
113. Brogniez V, Lejuste P, Pecheur A et al. Prosthetic dental rehabilitation on osseointegrated implants placed in irradiate mandibular bone. Apropos of 50 implants in 17 patients treated over a period of 5 years. Rev Stomatol Chir Maxillofac 1996; 97: 288–294
114. Henk JM, Smith CW. Radiotherapy and hyperbaric oxygen in head and neck cancer. Interim report of the second trial. Lancet 1977; ii: 104
115. Fazekas J, Pajak TF, Wasserman T et al. Failure of misonidazole-sensitized radiotherapy to impact upon stage III–IV squamous cancers of the head and neck. Int J Radiat Oncol Biol Phys 1987; 13: 1155–1160
116. Overgaard J, Hansen HS, Anderson AP. Misonidazole combined with split-course radiotherapy in the treatment of invasive carcinoma of larynx and pharynx: report from the DAHANCA 2 study. Int J Radiat Oncol boil Phys 1989; 16: 1065–1068
117. Van den Bogaert W, van der Schueren E, Horiot JC et al. The EORTC randomized trial of three fractions per day and misonidazole in advanced head and neck cancer: prognostic factors. Radiother Oncol 1995; 35: 100–106
118. Lee DJ, Cosmatos D, Marcial VA. Results of an RTOG phase III trial (RTOG 85-27) comparing radiotherapy plus etanidazole with radiotherapy alone for locally advanced head and neck carcinomas. Int J Radiat Oncol Biol Phys 1995; 32: 567–576
119. Eschwege F, Sancho-Garnier H, Chassagne D. Results of a European trial of etanidazole combined with radiotherapy in head and neck carcinomas. Int J Radiat Oncol Biol Phys 1997; 39: 275–281
120. Lee DJ, Mioni M, Guiliano J et al. Hypoxic sensitiser and cytoxin for head and neck cancer. Ann Acad Med Singapore 1996; 25: 397–404
121. Overgaard J, Sand Hansen H, Lindelov B et al. Nimorazole as a hypoxic radiosensitiser in the treatment of supraglottic larynx and pharynx carcinoma. First report from the Danish head and neck cancer study (DAHANCA) protocol 5–85. Radiotherapy Oncol 1991; 20 (Suppl 1): 143–149
122. Gandara DR, Lara PN, Goldberg Z et al. Tirapazamine: the prototype for a novel class of therapeutic agents targeting tumor hypoxia. Semin Oncol 2002; 29: 102–109
123. Kumar P. Impact of anemia in patients with head and neck cancer. Oncologist 2000; 5: 13–18
124. Lee WR, Berkeley B, Marcial V et al. Anemia is associated with decreased survival and increased locoregional failure in patients with locally advanced head and neck carcinoma: a secondary analysis of RTOG 85-27. Int J Radiat Oncol Biol Phys 1998; 45: 1069–1075
125. Maciejewski A, Rutowski T, Skladowski K et al. The effectiveness of radiotherapy and the prognostic value of Hb level for patients with early glottic cancer (T1N0, T2N0). Otolaryngol Pol 1998; 52: 23–28
126. Lutterbach J, Guttenberger R. Anemia is associated with decreased local control of surgically treated squamous carcinomas of the glottic larynx. Int J Radiat Oncol Biol Phys 2000; 48: 1345–1350
127. Withers HR, Taylor JM, Maciejewski B. The hazard of accelerated tumor clonogen repopulation during radiotherapy. Acta Oncol 1988; 27: 131–146
128. Skaladowski K, Law MG, Maciejewski B, Steel GG. Planned and unplanned gaps in radiotherapy: the importance of gap position and gap duration. Radiother Oncol 1994; 30: 109–120
129. Robertson C, Robertson AG, Hendry JH et al. Similar decreases in local control are calculated for treatment protraction and for interruptions in the radiotherapy of carcinoma of the larynx in four centers. Int J Radiat Oncol Biol Phys 1998; 40: 319–329
130. Dische S, Saunders MI. Continuous hyperfractionated radiotherapy (CHART): an interim report upon late morbidity. Radiother Oncol 1989; 16: 65–72
131. Jackson SM, Weir LM, Hay JH et al. A randomised trial of accelerated versus conventional radiotherapy in

head and neck cancer. Radiother Oncol 1997; 43: 39–46

132. Poulsen MG, Denham JW, Peters LJ et al. A randomised trial of accelerated and conventional radiotherapy for stage III and IV squamous carcinoma of the head and neck: a Trans-Tasman Radiation Oncology Group Study. Radiother Oncol 2001; 60: 113–122
133. Overgaard J, Alsner J, Erikson J et al. Importance of overall treatment time for the response to radiotherapy in patients with squamous cell carcinoma of the head and neck. Rays 2000; 25: 313–319
134. Hliniak A, Gwiazdowska B, Szutkowski Z et al. A multicentre randomized/controlled trial of a conventional versus modestly accelerated radiotherapy in laryngeal cancer: influence of a one week shortening in overall time. Radiother Oncol 2002; 62: 1–10
135. Skaladowski K, Maciejewski B, Golen B et al. Randomised clinical trial of 7–day continuous accelerated irradiation (CAIR) of head and neck cancer report on 3-year tumour control and normal tissue toxicity. Radiother Oncol 2000; 55: 101–110
136. Horiot JC, Le Fur R, N'Guyen T et al. Hyperfractionated versus conventional fractionation in oropharyngeal carcinoma: final analysis of a randomized trial of the EORTC co-operative group of radiotherapy. Radiother Oncol 1992; 25: 231–241
137. Stuschke M, Thames HD. Hyperfractionated radiotherapy of human tumours: overview of the randomised clinical trials. Int J Radiat Oncol Biol Phys 1997; 37: 259–267
138. Sanchiz F, Milla A, Torner J et al. Single fraction per day versus two fractions per day radiochemotherapy in the treatment of head and neck cancer. Int J Radiat Oncol Biol Phys 1990; 19: 1347–1350
139. Fu KK, Pajak TF, Trotti A et al. A radiation therapy oncology group (RTOG) phase III randomized study to compare hyperfraction and two variants of accelerated fractionation to standard fractionation radiotherapy for head and neck squamous cell carcinoma: first report of RTOG 0993. Int J Radiat Oncol Biol Phys 2000; 48: 7–16
140. Horiot JC, Bontemps P, van den Bogaert W. Accelerated fractionation (AF) compared to conventional fractionation (CF) improves locoregional control in the radiotherapy of advanced head and neck cancers: results of the EORTC 22851 randomised trial. Radiother Oncol 1997; 44: 111–121.
141. Dische, Saunders MI. Continuous, hyoperfractionated, accelerated radiotherapy (CHART): an interim report upon late morbidity. Radiother Oncol 1989; 16: 65–72
142. Awwad HK, Lotayef M, Shouman T et al Accelerated hyperfractionation (AHF) compared to conventional fractionation (CF) in the postoperative radiotherapy of advanced head and neck cancer: influence of proliferation. Br J Cancer 2002; 86: 517–523
143. Stupp R, Weichselbaum RR, Vokes EE. Combined modality therapy of head and neck cancer in Seminars in Oncology 1994; 21: 349–358
144. Kish JA, Ensley JF, Jacobs J et al. A randomised trial of cisplatin (CACP) + 5-fluorouracil (5-FU) infusion and CACP + 5-FU bolus for recurrent and advanced squamous cell carcinoma of the head and neck. Cancer 1985; 56: 2740–2744
145. Spaulding MB, Fischer SG, Wolf GT. Tumor response, toxicity and survival after neoadjuvant organ-preserving chemotherapy for advanced laryngeal cancer. The department of Veterans Affairs Cooperative Laryngeal Cancer Study Group. J Clin Oncol 1994; 12: 1592–1599
146. Wolf TG. Commentary. Phase III trial to preserve the larynx: induction chemotherapy and radiotherapy versus concurrent chemotherapy and radiotherapy versus radiotherapy — Intergroup Trial R01–11. Clin Oncol 2001; 19: 28S–31S
147. Lefebre JL, Chevalier D, Luboinski B. Larynx preservation in pyriform sinus cancer: preliminary results of a European Organisation for Research and Treatment of Cancer phase III trial. EORTC head and neck cancer cooperative group. J Natl Cancer Inst 1996; 88: 890–899
148. Stell PM, Rawson NS. Adjuvant chemotherapy in head and neck cancer. Br J Cancer 1990; 61: 779–787
149. Bouris J, Wilson G, Wibault P et al. Rapid tumour cell proliferation after induction chemotherapy in oropharyngeal cancer. Laryngoscope 1994; 104: 468–472
150. Munro AJ. An overview of randomised controlled trials of adjuvant chemotherapy in head and neck cancer. Br J Cancer 1995; 72: 83–91
151. Pignon JP, Bourhis J, Domenge C. Chemotherapy added to locoregional treatment for head and neck squamous cell carcinoma: three meta-analyses of updated individual data. MACH-NC Collaborative Group. Meta-analysis of chemotherapy on head and neck cancer. Lancet 2000; 355: 949–955
152. Browman GP, Hodson DI, Mackenzie RJ et al. Choosing a concomitant chemotherapy regimen for squamous cell head and neck cancer. A systematic review of the published literature with subgroup analysis. Head Neck 2001; 23: 579–589
153. Henk JM. Controlled trials of synchronous chemotherapy with radiotherapy in head and neck cancer: overview of radiation morbidity. Clin Oncol (R Coll Radiol) 1997; 9: 308–312
154. Brizel DM, Albers ME, Fischer SR et al. Hyperfractionated irradiation with or without concurrent chemotherapy for locally advanced head and neck cancer. N Engl J Med 1998; 18: 1798–1804
155. Jeremic B, Shimbamoto Y, Milicic B et al. Hyperfractionated radiation therapy with or without concurrent low-dose daily cisplatinum in locally advanced squamous cell carcinoma of the head and neck: a prospective randomized trial. J Clin Oncol 2000; 18: 1458–1464
156. Dobrovski W, Naude J. Continuous hyperfractionated accelerated radiotherapy with/without mitomycin C in head and neck cancers. Radiother Oncol 2000; 57: 119–124

157. Staar S, Rudat V, Stuetzer H et al. Intensified hyperfractionated accelerated radiotherapy limits the additional benefit of simultaneous chemotherapy — results of a multicentric randomized German trial in advanced head and neck cancer. Int J Radiat Oncol Biol Phys 2001; 50: 1161–1171
158. Tubiana M, Eschwege F. Conformal radiotherapy and intensity-modulated radiotherapy — clinical data. Acta Oncol 2000; 39: 555–567
159. van Dieren EB, Nowak PJ, Wijers OB et al. Beam intensity modulation using tissue compensators or dynamic multileaf collimation in three-dimensional conformal radiotherapy of primary cancers of the oropharynx and larynx, including the elective neck. Int J Radiat Oncol Biol Phys 2000; 45: 1299–1309
160. Forastiere AA, Metch B, Schuller DE et al. Randomised comparison of cisplatin plus fluorouracil and carboplatin plus fluorouracil versus methotrexate in advanced squamous cell carcinoma of the head and neck: a Southwest Oncology Group study. J Clin Oncol 1992; 10: 1245–1251
161. Browman GP, Cronin L. Standard chemotherapy in squamous cell head and neck cancer: what we have learned from randomised trials. Sem Oncol 1994; 21: 311–319

13 Complications of treatment and their management

Bhuvanesh Singh and Jatin P Shah

The typical history of tobacco and alcohol abuse inherent to the population of patients developing head and neck cancer, combined with the clean-contaminated nature of oral cancer surgery, results in a significantly elevated risk for developing complications.[1–4] In general, surgical complications in oral cancer patients can be classified into those related to the surgical wound or those involving systemic structures.

Systemic complications

Systemic complications are the most common type associated with oral cancer surgery, with the presence of baseline comorbid conditions being the most important predictor.[5,6] Age by itself is not an important factor, but older patients tend to be more sensitive to the effects of comorbid conditions, and tend to develop more severe complications.[4,7–9]

Systemic complications most commonly involve the pulmonary system, and arise in about 15% of cases.[6,10,11] The co-existence of advanced medical disease, such as chronic obstructive pulmonary disease, combined with active tobacco use is the most important predictor for the development of a pulmonary complication.[6,11] The risk can be reduced if the patient gives up tobacco use preoperatively, pulmonary optimization, intensive postoperative pulmonary toilet and early ambulation.[6,12]

Other systemic complications are much less common. Myocardial infarction occurs in fewer than 1% of patients undergoing head and neck surgery, and is mainly related to pre-existing cardiac disease.[5,13] Central nervous system complications, including cerebrovascular accidents (CVA), meningitis and cerebrospinal fluid leaks, are rare unless skull base surgery or carotid artery manipulation or resection is performed.[14–16] Resection of the carotid artery should be performed in highly selected patients, with respect to both patient and tumor parameters. Angiographic balloon occlusion studies may help to identify patients at higher risk for CVA.

Surgical complications

Several factors are associated with an increased risk for the development of surgical complications, the most important of which are the type and extent of surgery, baseline medical status, presence of prior irradiation to the surgical bed, and factors related to surgical technique.[17–19] Surgical complications may be classified temporally into four groups, including intraoperative, early postoperative, late postoperative, and delayed complications. Careful preoperative assessment and meticulous surgical technique, combined with careful operative planning, can prevent many of the observed complications associated with surgery for oral cancer.

Intraoperative anesthesia complications

Anesthesia-related complications are rare with the use of modern anesthetic drugs and advancements in monitoring techniques. However, when they occur they can be life threatening if not identified and treated promptly.[20–22] Intraoperative airway complications are of primary concern and are mainly due to shifting of the endotracheal tube. The use of clear plastic head and neck drapes to cordon off the endotracheal tube, allowing its direct visualization throughout, is desirable. If the tube is dislodged or disconnected during the procedure, it should be promptly repositioned or an emergency tracheostomy may be performed if necessary. Once in place, the endotracheal tube should be secured firmly with tape and tracheostomy tubes sutured to the skin to minimize the risk of dislodgement. When a tracheostomy tube has been placed in emergency or if the procedure is complicated, a post-procedure chest radiograph should be performed to rule out the presence of pneumothorax.[23,24]

Volume overload is the next most common intraoperative problem associated with anesthetic management, and can lead to increased risks of pulmonary and wound complications.[20–22] This risk can be minimized by limiting intravenous fluid to a volume sufficient to maintain an adequate urine output. Less common complications include intraoperative bradycardia and hypotension, which can result from manipulation of the carotid bifurcation during neck surgery. This can be counteracted by the injection of lidocaine into the adventitia in the region of the carotid bifurcation.

Intraoperative surgical complications

Most intraoperative complications are associated with flaws in surgical technique, resulting in inadvertent injury to nerves and blood vessels. The marginal mandibular nerve is at greatest risk for iatrogenic injury, which can result from direct physical trauma or from stretching associated with dissection and flap retraction. The accessory nerve is similarly at risk in supraomohyoid and modified neck dissections. Injury to the greater auricular nerve, cervical plexus branches, and lower cranial nerves may occur during neck dissection. The lingual nerve may be injured in posterior floor of mouth resections. Most commonly, injury to nerves results from devascularization associated with circumferential dissection and stretching or by direct physical trauma. Limiting the extent of circumferential dissection does not appear to reduce the risk. In fact, patient perception of shoulder dysfunction after supraomohyoid or modified radical neck dissection with accessory nerve preservation is similar in incidence and severity.

Vascular injury requiring repair or ligation of the vessels, including the internal jugular vein and common carotid artery, may also occur. However, inadvertent trauma can be minimized by meticulous attention to surgical technique and maintenance of a dry surgical field throughout the procedure. If significant bleeding is anticipated, preliminary ligation of the feeding vessel may be performed during the neck dissection, for example ligation of the lingual artery for tongue resections.

Inadequate planning also results in intraoperative complications. Skin or mucosal slough can be prevented by careful planning of incisions to avoid an acute angle, gentle handling of tissues, and planned placement of sutures to avoid devitalization. If significant wound slough occurs, it can be managed conservatively after debridement and packing. However, if the carotid artery is exposed, then regional or distant tissue transfer should be used to close the defect and reduce the risk of carotid blowout.

Similarly, overaggressive marginal mandibulectomy can result in iatrogenic fractures of the mandible. The risk of fracture can be minimized by planning resections to avoid sharp angles and maintaining the mandibular height of approximately 1 cm. In addition to this, the use of a sharp, well-controlled, high-speed saw allows for controlled and safe resections, avoiding fractures associated with the use of chisels to wedge and lever the specimen. If a fracture occurs, immediate repair should be performed using miniplates or wires.

Chyle fistulae can result from injury to the cervical portion of the thoracic duct. Typically the duct is located in the lower portion of the left neck, but can extend as far as 5 cm superior to the clavicle and occur in the right neck in a small number of cases (< 5%). If injury to the duct is identified in the operating room, attempts should be made to isolate the injury and suture ligation performed. It is important to remember that the cervical thoracic duct is not a single structure, but rather has many tributaries, making several independent injuries possible. If injury to the duct is identified in the postoperative period, the dietary content should be modified and the volume of drainage followed. If the chyle output is over 600 ml per day, re-exploration and ligature is indicated. In cases with lower output, observation and conservative management will usually be sufficient for treatment.

Immediate postoperative complications

The main complication in the immediate postoperative period is collection of blood or serum under the flap. This can result from non-functioning suction catheters or inadequate hemostasis. The placement of suction drains should not substitute for the attainment of hemostasis, as this will invariably result in the development of complications. The role of suction catheters is to evacuate fluid and keep the neck flaps in close apposition to the underlying tissue, thereby improving healing and decreasing the risk of infection. To minimize the risk of blockage, drains should be inserted during the final closure of the wound and immediately placed on high, continuous suction. The wound should be irrigated thoroughly to remove any clots and debris prior to drain placement. If a small collection develops after removal of the drains, needle aspiration is performed. However, large accumulations or reaccumulations require opening, cleaning, and packing of the wound.

Airway compromise in the immediate postoperative setting may be caused by many different factors. Laryngeal intubation trauma may cause edema or hematoma resulting in early postoperative stridor. Investigation should include fiberoptic exmination to assess vocal cord function and ascertain the extent of airway compromise. In severe cases, intubation or tracheostomy should be performed. In less ominous cases, treatment with humidified oxygen and intravenous steroids may be attempted in a monitored setting. Other, less common causes of airway compromise include tracheostomy tube plugging, pneumothorax, and aspiration.

Although uncommon, the use of microvascular free tissue transfer introduces new avenues for complication development.[25–27] A pale appearance of the graft, combined with reduced temperature, delayed capillary refill, and delayed or absent bleeding to pin prick in the early postoperative period represents acute arterial obstruction. This usually results from technical errors in performing the anastomosis. Management requires immediate return to the operating room for exploration of the anastomosis and appropriate intervention. Flap congestion, with dark bleeding on pin prick typically occurring a few days after surgery, represents problems with the venous anastomosis. Conservative management, with the possible use of medical leeches, may lead to resolution. However, in severe cases re-exploration may be indicated.

Nasal alar necrosis secondary to malpositioned nasogastric feeding tubes can result in significant cosmetic deformity. In addition, prolonged tube placement can also foster the development of ipsilateral sinusitis. Early nasogastric tube removal should be planned, and proper positioning maintained while it is in place.

Late postoperative complications

Wound infections and fistulae are the most important complication in the late postoperative period, occurring in over 25–50% of complex cases.[28,29] The rate of wound infection associated with oral cancer surgery can be effectively reduced by the administration of preoperative antibiotics.[30–37] The choice of antibiotic is not as important as the time course in which it is administered. Ideally, prophylactic antibiotics are started 1–2 hours prior to the skin incision.[34] Cephalosporins (Ancef) and metronidazole (Flagyl) are usually given for clean-contaminated cases in the preoperative holding area. A second course of antibiotics is given in the operating room for cases lasting greater than 8 hours. In uncomplicated cases, prophylactic antibiotics only need be continued for 24–48 hours postoperatively.[32] However, the duration of therapy may need to be extended in high-risk cases.

Once they develop, mild wound infections can be treated by antibiotic therapy alone. However, it must be kept in mind that signs of local infection at the wound site may represent a more serious underlying infection. If suppuration is suspected, the wound should be opened widely and cleaned and appropriate cultures instigated. Empiric broad-spectrum antibiotic therapy, directed against oral flora, should be administered, since most infections associated with oral cancer surgery are polymicrobial. The choice of antibiotic should be modified according to the culture results, when available. The presence of a fistula should be suspected with all cases of wound suppuration, especially when associated with salivary drainage. Other non-specific manifestations of fistulization include fever, pain, and leukocytosis. Fistula development is associated with technical problems in closure of the mucosa, advanced tumors, and wound healing problems resulting from poor nutrition, diabetes mellitus, or prior radiation exposure. The risk of fistulization can be reduced by minimizing technical errors, including performance of a tension-free closure, avoidance of devitalization of mucosal edges, and adequate apposition with inversion of the mucosal edges.[29,38] The use of free tissue transfer to close complex defects may further decrease the rate of fistulization. Preoperative nutritional optimization should also be considered in selected cases, as it improves wound healing.[18,19,39–41] The role of previous radiation therapy in the development of wound breakdown and salivary fistulae may be debated. However, there is a consensus that fistulae in irradiated patients heal at significantly slower rates and often require surgical intervention for closure.[42,43] Initial management of salivary fistulae consists of wide opening, debridement, cleaning, and packing of the wound, along with the correction of the aggravating factors, when identified. Carotid coverage is performed in cases where it is exposed in the wound. For unresolving or large fistulae, regional or distant tissue transfer should be considered.

Exposure of the mandible may develop consequent to wound dehiscence or fistulization. Management is based on the severity of the problem. If minimal exposure is present, without hardware exposure, it can be managed with local wound care. In cases of extensive exposure, hardware removal, wound debridement, and mandibular stabilization may be required through an open approach. Non-union can also result from infection and improper immobilization. If left untreated, non-union can be the nidus for more severe infections, including osteomyelitis. Treatment consists of open debridement and restabilization of the mandibular fragments.

Delayed complications

A host of problems can occur in the delayed setting. Dysphagia can result from neurological injuries to cranial nerves V, IX, X, XII or from direct anatomical insults, as in glossectomy or partial laryngeal and pharyngeal surgery. The addition of postoperative radiation therapy amplifies the magnitude of dysphagia. Little can be done to avert these surgical sequelae, but anticipation and aggressive management are warranted if problems develop. If significant anatomical resections are planned, consideration should be given to early placement of a gastrostomy tube to maintain adequate nutrition.

Dysphagia assessment should be performed in collaboration with a speech and swallowing therapist.[44–46] It must be kept in mind that swallowing is accomplished through a complex series of interrelated reflex mechanisms, which can be disrupted by sensory, qualitative, and anatomical changes.[46–48] A thorough examination analysing the impact and extent of anatomic deficits and cranial nerve dysfunctions is performed, supplemented by functional fiberoptic examination of swallowing where possible. Modified barium swallow is used to identify the location and severity of the swallowing deficit and facilitate its treatment.

Anatomic resections resulting in significant loss in oral and pharyngeal soft tissue volume can cause problems with bolus formation and progression beyond the oral phase of swallowing.[44–46] Tongue resection and denervation is a particularly difficult problem, resulting in significant deficits in both speech and swallowing rehabilitation. A palatal drop prosthesis can be used to compensate for soft tissue volume loss of tongue to improve swallowing.[49] Dental rehabilitation with dentures or osseointegrated implants also plays a significant role in improving deglutition. Conversely, neurological deficits are difficult to treat and require intensive swallowing therapy, with modifications in swallowing techniques to allow for partial restoration of swallowing function.

Trismus can be a significant dilemma in this population, causing problems with deglutition and oral hygiene, as well as limitations in oral and pharyngeal examinations.[50–54] Once trismus develops it is difficult to reverse, therefore preventative management is best. The use of skin grafts and flaps can limit fibrosis in cases with exposure of pterygoid muscles. This results in significant reduction of trismus development. Aggressive jaw exercises, beginning in the immediate postoperative period and continued for several months, are of significant benefit. Oral rehabilitation exercises should also be initiated in patients receiving radiation to the pterygoid region to prevent fibrosis of the muscles of mastication.

Shoulder weakness and deformity are predictable sequelae in all patients undergoing radical neck dissection, consequent to sacrifice of the accessory nerve.[55–63] The severity of shoulder dysfunction, however, is intensified with denervation of the nerve supply to the other supporting musculature, including the rhomboids and levator scapulae.[47] The nerve supply to the latter is at greatest risk as it is derived from the cervical plexus in the neck. Functional deficit results from both pain on movement of the scapulohumeral joint and an inability to fully abduct the arm due to loss of muscular action. Treatment involves a combination of intensive physical therapy and pain control.[55]

Xerostomia is a consequence of radiation therapy that can have several significant long-term sequelae, including tooth decay and perigingival caries. Regular and lifelong use of fluoride gel is necessary to reduce the risk of dental caries. Dental sepsis can lead to progression of infection into the mandible or maxilla, resulting in the development of osteoradionecrosis.[50] Although it can involve the maxilla, the highest risk of osteoradionecrosis is in the mandible.[50–53,64] The risk can be effectively reduced by the maintenance of optimal oral hygiene, combined with avoidance of dental manipulation and procedures. Ideally, dental care and procedures in irradiated mandibles should be provided by dentists and oral surgeons experienced in the management of these patients. The treatment of osteoradionecrosis is conservative, with significant attention given to oral hygiene, wound debridement, and removal of sequestrum. Rarely, mandibulectomy may be necessary in cases unresponsive to conservative management.[65] Although it appears promising, the benefit from the use of hyperbaric oxygen therapy, both for prevention and treatment, needs to be well established.[65]

Sensory loss following neck dissections can be particularly troublesome. This results from injury to the branches of the greater auricular nerve and the cervical plexus.[66] The resultant deficit extends from the ear to the chest. Gradual resolution of much of the deficit can be anticipated with time, but patients should initially avoid exposure to extremes of temperature in the region. Many other long-term complications can occur, including scar contractures, neuroma formation, Frey's syndrome, reflex sympathetic dystrophy, and dysgeusia, but are relatively rare.[67–69]

References

1. Singh B, Bhaya M, Stern J et al. Validation of the Charlson comorbidity index in patients with head and neck cancer: a multi-institutional study. Laryngoscope 1997; 107: 1469–1475
2. Singh B, Bhaya M, Stern J et al. Impact of comorbidity on outcome of young patients with head and neck squamous cell carcinoma. Head Neck 1998; 20: 1–7
3. Funk GF, Hoffman HT, Karnell LH et al. Cost-identification analysis in oral cavity cancer management. Otolaryngol Head Neck Surg 1998; 118: 211–220
4. Shaari CM, Buchbinder D, Costantino PD et al. Complications of microvascular head and neck surgery in the elderly. Arch Otolaryngol Head Neck Surg 1998; 124: 407–411
5. Papac RJ. Medical aspects of head and neck cancer. Cancer Invest 1985; 3: 435–444
6. McCulloch TM, Jensen NF, Girod DA, Tsue TT, Weymuller EA Jr. Risk factors for pulmonary complications in the postoperative head and neck surgery patient. Head Neck 1997; 19: 372–377
7. Singh B, Cordeiro PG, Santamaria E et al. Factors associated with complications in microvascular reconstruction of head and neck defects. Plast Reconstr Surg 1999; 103: 403–411
8. Hosking MP, Warner MA, Lobdell CM, Offord KP, Melton LJ 3rd. Outcomes of surgery in patients 90 years of age and older [see comments]. JAMA 1989; 261: 1909–1915
9. Hosking MP, Lobdell CM, Warner MA, Offord KP, Melton LJ 3rd. Anaesthesia for patients over 90 years of age. Outcomes after regional and general anaesthetic techniques for two common surgical procedures [see comments]. Anaesthesia 1989; 44: 142–147
10. Weber RS, Hankins P, Rosenbaum B, Raad I. Nonwound infections following head and neck oncologic surgery. Laryngoscope 1993; 103: 22–27
11. Rao MK, Reilley TE, Schuller DG, Young DC. Analysis of risk factors for postoperative pulmonary complications in head and neck surgery. Laryngoscope 1992; 102: 45–47
12. Warner MA, Offord KP, Warner ME et al. Role of preoperative cessation of smoking and other factors in postoperative pulmonary complications: a blinded prospective study of coronary artery bypass patients. Mayo Clin Proc 1989; 64: 609–616
13. Jacobs C. The internist in the management of head and neck cancer. Ann Intern Med 1990; 113: 771–778
14. Snyderman CH, D'Amico F. Outcome of carotid artery resection for neoplastic disease: a meta-analysis [see comments]. Am J Otolaryngol 1992; 13: 373–380
15. Bilsky MH, Kraus DH, Strong EW et al. Extended anterior craniofacial resection for intracranial extension of malignant tumors. Am J Surg 1997; 174: 565–568
16. Shah JP, Kraus DH, Bilsky MH et al. Craniofacial resection for malignant tumors involving the anterior skull base. Arch Otolaryngol Head Neck Surg 1997; 123: 1312–1317
17. Johnson JT, Bloomer WD. Effect of prior radiotherapy on postsurgical wound infection. Head Neck 1989; 11: 132–136
18. Copeland EM 3rd, Daly JM, Dudrick SJ. Nutritional concepts in the treatment of head and neck malignancies. Head Neck Surg 1979; 1: 350–365
19. Copeland EM 3rd, Daly JM, Ota DM, Dudrick SJ. Nutrition, cancer, and intravenous hyperalimentation. Cancer 1979; 43 (Suppl): 2108–2116
20. Cox RG. The anesthetic management of patients undergoing free flap reconstructive surgery following resection of head and neck neoplasms—a review of 64 patients [letter]. Ann R Coll Surg Engl 1989; 71: 143–144
21. Inglis MS, Robbie DS, Edwards JM, Breach NM. The anaesthetic management of patients undergoing free flap reconstructive surgery following resection of head and neck neoplasms—a review of 64 patients. Ann R Coll Surg Engl 1988; 70: 235–238
22. Manson PN, Saunders JR Jr. Anesthesia in head and neck surgery. Head and neck cancer surgery and maxillofacial trauma. Clin Plast Surg 1985; 12: 115–122
23. Beahrs OH. Complications of surgery of the head and neck. Surg Clin North Am 1977; 57: 823–829
24. Barlow DW, Weymuller EA Jr, Wood DE. Tracheotomy and the role of postoperative chest radiography in adult patients. Ann Otol Rhinol Laryngol 1994; 103: 665–668
25. Hidalgo DA, Disa JJ, Cordeiro PG, Hu QY. A review of 716 consecutive free flaps for oncologic surgical defects: refinement in donor-site selection and technique. Plast Reconstr Surg 1998; 102: 722–732; discussion 733–734
26. Khouri RK, Cooley BC, Kunselman AR et al. A prospective study of microvascular free-flap surgery and outcome. Plast Reconstr Surg 1998; 102: 711–721
27. al Qattan MM, Boyd JB. Complications in head and neck microsurgery. Microsurgery 1993; 14: 187–195
28. Cohen M, Marschall MA, Greager JD. Early, aggressive management of postoperative oropharyngocutaneous fistulas. Plast Reconstr Surg 1992; 89: 56–61; discussion 62–63
29. Friess CC, Fontaine DJ, Kornblut AD. Complications of therapy for oral malignant disease. Otolaryngol Clin North Am 1979; 12: 175–181
30. Johnson JT, Schuller DE, SIlver F et al. Antibiotic prophylaxis in high-risk head and neck surgery: one-day vs. five-day therapy. Otolaryngol Head Neck Surg 1986; 95: 554–557
31. Girod DA, McCulloch TM, Tsue TT, Weymuller EA Jr. Risk factors for complications in clean-contaminated head and neck surgical procedures. Head Neck 1995; 17: 7–13
32. Fee WE Jr, Glenn M, Handon C, Hopp ML. One day vs. two days of prophylactic antibiotics in patients undergoing major head and neck surgery. Laryngoscope 1984; 94: 612–614
33. Clayman GL, Raad II, Hankins PD, Weber RS.

Bacteriologic profile of surgical infection after antibiotic prophylaxis. Head Neck 1993; 15: 526–531
34. Classen DC, Evans RS, Pestotnik SL et al. The timing of prophylactic administration of antibiotics and the risk of surgical-wound infection [see comments]. N Engl J Med 1992; 326: 281–286
35. Brown BM, Johnson JT, Wagner RL. Etiologic factors in head and neck wound infections. Laryngoscope 1987; 97: 587–590
36. Blair EA, Johnson JT, Wagner RL, Carrau RL, Bizakis JG. Cost analysis of antibiotic prophylaxis in clean head and neck surgery. Arch Otolaryngol Head Neck Surg 1995; 121: 269–271
37. Becker GD. Identification and management of the patient at high risk for wound infection. Head Neck Surg 1986; 8: 205–210
38. Krause CJ, Smits RG, McCabe BF. Complications associated with combined therapy of oral and pharyngeal neoplasms. Ann Otol Rhinol Laryngol 1972; 81: 496–500
39. Dudrick SJ, Copeland EM 3rd, Daly JM et al. A clinical review of nutritional support of the patient. J Parenter Enteral Nutr 1979; 3: 444–451
40. Daly JM, Reynolds HM, Dudrick SJ, Copeland EM 3rd. Effects of nutritional repletion on host and tumor response to chemotherapy. Curr Surg 1979; 36: 138–143
41. Daly JM, Dudrick SJ, Copeland EMD. Evaluation of nutritional indices as prognostic indicators in the cancer patient. Cancer 1979; 43: 925–931
42. Shemen LJ, Spiro RH. Complications following laryngectomy. Head Neck Surg 1986; 8: 185–191
43. Weingrad DN, Spiro RH. Complications after laryngectomy. Am J Surg 1983; 146: 517–520
44. Poertner LC, Coleman RF. Swallowing therapy in adults. Otolaryngol Clin North Am 1998; 31: 561–579
45. Machin J, Shaw C. A multidisciplinary approach to head and neck cancer. Eur J Cancer Care (Engl) 1998; 7: 93–96
46. Kronenberger MB, Meyers AD. Dysphagia following head and neck cancer surgery. Dysphagia 1994; 9: 236–244
47. Bigliani LU, Compito CA, Duralde XA, Wolfe IN. Transfer of the levator scapulae, rhomboid major, and rhomboid minor for paralysis of the trapezius. J Bone Joint Surg Am 1996; 78: 1534–1540
48. Valdez IH, Fox PC. Interactions of the salivary and gastrointestinal systems. II. Effects of salivary gland dysfunction on the gastrointestinal tract. Dig Dis 1991; 9: 210–218
49. Johnson JT, Aramany MA, Myers EN. Palatal neoplasms: reconstruction considerations. Otolaryngol Clin North Am 1983; 16: 441–456
50. Whitmyer CC, Waskowski JC, Iffland HA. Radiotherapy and oral sequelae: preventive and management protocols [published erratum appears in J Dent Hyg 1997; 71: 96]. J Dent Hyg 1997; 71: 23–29
51. Jansma J, Vissink A, Spijkervet FK et al. Protocol for the prevention and treatment of oral sequelae resulting from head and neck radiation therapy. Cancer 1992; 70: 2171–2180
52. Dreizen S. Oral complications of cancer therapies. Description and incidence of oral complications. NCI Monogr 1990; 9: 11–15
53. Maxymiw WG, Wood RE. The role of dentistry in head and neck radiation therapy [see comments]. J Can Dent Assoc 1989; 55: 193–198
54. Cohen SG, Quinn PD. Facial trismus and myofascial pain associated with infections and malignant disease. Report of five cases. Oral Surg Oral Med Oral Pathol 1988; 65: 538–544
55. Saunders WH, Johnson EW. Rehabilitation of the shoulder after radical neck dissection. Ann Otol Rhinol Laryngol 1975; 84: 812–816
56. Sobol S, Jensen C, Sawyer W 2nd, Costiloe P, Thong N. Objective comparison of physical dysfunction after neck dissection. Am J Surg 1985; 150: 503–509
57. Ariyan S. Functional radical neck dissection. Plast Reconstr Surg 1980; 65: 768–776
58. Hill JH, Olson NR. The surgical anatomy of the spinal accessory nerve and the internal branch of the superior laryngeal nerve. Laryngoscope 1979; 89: 1935–1942
59. Wright TA. Accessory spinal nerve injury. Clin Orthop 1975; 108: 15–18
60. Nori S, Soo KC, Green RF, Strong EW, Miodownik S. Utilization of intraoperative electroneurography to understand the innervation of the trapezius muscle. Muscle Nerve 1997; 20: 279–285
61. Zibordi F, Baiocco F, Bascelli C, Bini A, Canepa A. Spinal accessory nerve function following neck dissection. Ann Otol Rhinol Laryngol 1988; 97: 83–86
62. Short SO, Kaplan JN, Laramore GE, Cummings CW. Shoulder pain and function after neck dissection with or without preservation of the spinal accessory nerve. Am J Surg 1984; 148: 478–482
63. Leipzig B, Suen JY, English JL, Barnes J, Hooper M. Functional evaluation of the spinal accessory nerve after neck dissection. Am J Surg 1983; 146: 526–530
64. Marx RE. Osteoradionecrosis: a new concept of its pathophysiology. J Oral Maxillofac Surg 1983; 41: 283–288
65. Shaha AR, Cordeiro PG, Hidalgo DA et al. Resection and immediate microvascular reconstruction in the management of osteoradionecrosis of the mandible. Head Neck 1997; 19: 406–411
66. Swift TR. Involvement of peripheral nerves in radical neck dissection. Am J Surg 1970; 119: 694–698
67. Kiroglu MM, Sarpel T, Ozberk P, Soylu L, Cetik F, Aydogan LB. Reflex sympathetic dystrophy following neck dissections. Am J Otolaryngol 1997; 18: 103–106
68. Teague A, Akhtar S, Phillips J. Frey's syndrome following submandibular gland excision: an unusual postoperative complication. ORL J Otorhinolaryngol Relat Spec 1998; 60: 346–348
69. Hays LL. The Frey syndrome: a review and double blind evaluation of the topical use of a new anticholinergic agent. Laryngoscope 1978; 88: 796–824

14 Palliative care for head and neck cancer

Robert Dunlop

Introduction

This book reviews the advances which have been made in the management of patients with head and neck cancer. The accuracy of staging and diagnosis has been improved by technological advances such as flexible endoscopy and CT/MRI scanning. Treatments have been improved with the development of new surgical techniques, radiotherapy treatments such as hyperfractionation, and chemotherapy regimens. Combined modality therapies are constantly being refined, along with improvements in supportive measures to reduce treatment morbidity. Research continues to suggest new alternatives. All of these developments have brought new life and new hope for this group of patients.

However, despite all of these advances, some patients with head and neck cancer will die of their disease. Lifestyle and other factors may lead to patients presenting with advanced, incurable disease. In some cases, the disease relapses and progresses despite treatment. Traditionally, these patients were told 'nothing more can be done', which left the patients and families on their own to manage the worst part of the illness. In response to this situation in the UK, Dame Cicely Saunders founded the modern hospice movement by opening St Christopher's Hospice in 1967. Since then, the new specialty of palliative care has, in many countries, emerged into the field of cancer medicine.[1]

This chapter is about palliative care, which is the care of patients who have progressive incurable disease and the care of their families. Even in the face of incurable disease, when cancer treatment options have been exhausted, patients can still find meaning and purpose in their lives. Relatives can also find support for their anguish, the strength to cope, and the capacity to recover after the patient dies.

What is palliative care?

Palliative care is defined by the World Health Organization as:

> The active total care of patients whose disease is not responsive to curative treatment. Control of pain, of other symptoms, and of psychological, social, and spiritual problems is paramount. The goal of palliative care is achievement of the best quality of life for patients and their families. Many aspects of palliative care are also applicable earlier in the course of the illness in conjunction with anticancer treatment.[2]

The term 'palliative' was first used shortly after the hospice movement began because of the connotations of the word hospice. In many countries, hospices had been founded by religious orders solely for the care of dying patients. This led to a narrow interpretation of hospice care, heavily loaded with popular fears and misconceptions. These misapprehensions posed a serious barrier to the spread of the modern hospice movement.

The early pioneers of the hospice movement chose the word 'palliative' because of its derivation from the Latin word for cloak.[3] This image characterized the process of relieving patients' symptoms without being able to treat the underlying disease process. However, oncologists also describe some anticancer treatments as 'palliative', meaning that surgery, radiotherapy, or chemotherapy is being used to reduce tumour load with no expectation of cure. Active treatment with palliative intent may lead to symptom control if the cancer responds. If the disease does not regress, the patient's symptoms will continue unabated, or be compounded by side-effects from treatment. Because of the potential for confusion in terminology (which has clouded the clinical interface between palliative care services and clinical oncology), the broader meaning of palliative care will pertain throughout this chapter unless the word 'palliative' immediately precedes an anticancer treatment, for example palliative radiotherapy.

Palliative care is characterized by the following:[4]

1. The patient and the family are the focus of care. Cancer should not be thought of as a biological entity which affects a patient. The family (which means any other person significant to the patient) will also be profoundly affected, even after the patient dies. Palliative care recognizes that family needs are just as important as patient needs. This does not mean that patient confidentiality must be compromised; relatives can be encouraged to share their worries without jeopardizing patient wishes.
2. Physical, psychological, social, and spiritual needs are all important. Cancer patients and their families experience a multitude of problems, not just physical symptoms. Whatever the problem—physical, psycho-social or spiritual—palliative care seeks to provide support. Head and neck cancer patients frequently develop local symptoms such as pain and difficulty swallowing. Distant effects include anorexia, weakness and nausea. Relatives caring for patients also develop physical symptoms, particularly fatigue. Many will develop a physical illness, particularly during the bereavement period. Psychological needs include a wide range of powerful emotions, including sadness, depression, anxiety, fear, guilt and anger. These needs are often exacerbated by a perceived lack of information. Social isolation is common, particularly with the disfigurement and speech difficulties associated with head and neck cancers, and their treatment. Families are often burdened by the financial consequences of the illness. Existential issues may be profound as patients and families struggle for some sense of meaning.
3. Multidisciplinary teamwork is needed to meet the variety of needs. With such a wide range of needs experienced by patients and families, palliative care requires the close collaboration of many different professional disciplines including doctors, nurses, social workers, physiotherapists, occupational therapists, clergy and pharmacists. With head and neck cancers, dieticians, speech therapists and camouflage specialists also have a role to play. In specialist palliative care services, multiskilling is encouraged across disciplines. For example, nurse specialists are able to assess pain, make limited diagnoses and advise on medication changes. Increasingly, specialist palliative care services are working more closely with medical oncologists, radiotherapists, and pain clinics. For effective team working, team members must keep focused on the needs of the patients and families.[5] Communication is also crucial.
4. Availability of support 24 hours per day, seven days a week. The effects of cancer are not confined to outpatient visits or hospital admissions. Day or night, terminally ill patients and their families can experience problems. Support must be constantly available, particularly in the community. Ideally, smooth continuity of care should be available between hospital, hospice and community.
5. Bereavement follow-up. Grief and bereavement have significant effects on the relatives. Not everyone needs support but specialist palliative care services identify those at risk of prolonged or abnormal grieving. Counselling is then provided.[6–8] This chapter will not deal with bereavement care but it is an important component of palliative care.

Specialist palliative care services

The number and range of palliative care services has grown rapidly since the opening of St Christopher's Hospice. Unfortunately, the traditional view of hospices as places for the care of the dying still holds sway with the general public and many health professionals. However, in the UK most cancer patients who die are supported at home by community-based palliative care teams working with primary health care services. Another major development is the presence of advisory hospital support teams.[9] These teams work in acute hospitals, providing advice to the doctors and nurses. More recently, academic departments have been created and palliative medicine has become a separate specialty, marking the coming of age of the modern hospice movement.

In the beginning, hospices were developed physically apart from hospitals. This facilitated development of the principals and practices of palliative care. Hospital support teams and academic units have enabled palliative care to merge back into mainstream medicine. Now, patients with cancer should be able to enjoy the advantages of active anticancer treatments along with expert symptom control and psychosocial support. Unfortunately, this is prevented in the USA by the current reimbursement structures, particularly the Medicare Hospice Benefit.

Head and neck cancers

There are a variety of cancers which affect the head and neck, including squamous cell carcinoma and variants, lymphomas, salivary gland tumours and other tumours such as melanoma, basal cell carcinoma, sarcomas, etc.[10] The anticancer options vary according to factors such as histology, site, stage and the general condition of the patient. These issues are dealt with elsewhere in this book. Palliative care practitioners need to be familiar with the variety of options.

It is important for palliative care physicians to know about the various patterns and sites of spread. Within the head and neck, cancers may involve the orbit, base of skull, sinuses, palate, naso- and oropharynx, cheeks, tongue, floor of mouth, mandible, cranial nerves, cervical oesophagus, upper airways and lymph nodes. Distant spread can occur, most commonly to lungs, liver and bones. Paraneoplastic effects are common with advanced disease, for example anorexia and weight loss. The palliative care needs of patients are determined by the local and distant sites of spread, in combination with the paraneoplastic effects. However, anticancer treatments and other illnesses such as postherpetic neuralgia can mimic the effects of cancer. The palliative care of any cancer patient starts with a careful assessment.

Palliative care assessment

Any new symptom or psychosocial need should be thoroughly evaluated. For patients with advanced cancer, a detailed history and clinical evaluation is just as important as it is for patients being staged at first presentation. There is no justification for medical nihilism in the face of progressive disease, just as patients should not be denied palliative care just because they are still receiving active treatment. Health professionals need to be more interested in patients with progressive disease, not less interested.

Patients often under-report their needs. Sometimes, this is because they accept that symptoms such as pain are inevitable. Frequently, patients also avoid telling doctors for fear of upsetting or bothering them. It is important to give patients and families enough time, especially if there are communication difficulties as a result of the cancer or the treatment. This is difficult in a busy clinic or family practice, which is why multidisciplinary teamwork is needed. A palliative care nurse specialist can spend more time during or after the clinic.

The psychosocial assessment also takes time, often on several occasions. Attributions need to be surfaced; these are the meanings which patients and families attribute to symptoms such as pain.[11] Other issues which need time to unravel include information needs, the importance of cultural and religious beliefs, past experiences of relatives or friends who have died of cancer and enquiry about the effects of the illness on the family.

For symptom control problems, diagnostic tests may be helpful but must be tailored to the patient's physical condition. A clinical diagnosis will be adequate for patients who are imminently dying. Unfortunately, symptom control treatments are often withheld until a diagnosis is made. For example, patients are left to suffer pain while awaiting test results, when an analgesic could be started even before the tests are commenced.

Symptom control for head and neck cancer

The symptoms experienced by patients with advanced cancer relate to the local effects of the disease at various sites and to the general paraneoplastic effects which occur remotely.[12] This section will review the palliative care treatments for the symptoms of head and neck cancer. Wherever possible, palliative care treatments should be combined with treatments against the cancer. As clinicians become more confident with palliative care options, they become less reliant on using anticancer treatments when these have clearly failed. Radiotherapy, chemotherapy, surgery and nonmalignant conditions can mimic the effects of advanced cancer.

There are several general principles of symptom control. Most cancer symptoms are chronic and unremitting, which requires chronic therapy given regularly. Once a symptom is relieved, the aim of chronic therapy is to prevent it recurring. Each patient should have treatment that is individually tailored, taking into account patient preferences, the lower tolerance of advanced cancer patients to side-effects, age and other factors affecting drug clearance and the presence of other symptoms. Head and neck cancer patients often have difficult swallowing, which requires the use of different preparations or routes of administration. Multiple drug therapies are often needed, emphasizing the need to choose once daily formulations and to use medications which can treat more than one symptom. Any treatment plan should be discussed with the patient and family, then written down. Regular follow-up is crucial and the family should be given contact telephone numbers for support in the community.

Local effects of head and neck cancer

Pain

Pain is often the presenting symptom of head and neck cancers. It usually becomes more prevalent and more severe when the disease progresses. Patients frequently have more than one pain; each pain should be appraised separately. Factors to be elicited include: site, intensity, qualitative descriptors, onset and temporal pattern, relieving and aggravating factors and association with sleep disturbance. Pain charts offer a systematic way of collecting and monitoring this information. If possible, pain sites should be examined carefully, checking for tenderness, inflammation and altered sensation or allodynia, when light touch induces pain. The signs of acute pain, such as pallor, sweating and tachycardia, are rarely present, which often leads clinicians to erroneously discount patients' complaints of severe or persistent pain.

Pain can be usefully categorized as somatic, visceral and neuropathic in origin. Somatic pain can be further subdivided into superficial and deep somatic pain. Visceral pain implies spread to visceral organs such as liver, which is relatively infrequent with head and neck cancers. Neuropathic pain usually arises from damage to peripheral and cranial nerves; regional sympathetically-mediated pain and central pain are very rare with head and neck cancers. The history and clinical features often distinguish the types of pain.

Pharmacotherapy for pain is based on the analgesic 'stepladder' developed by the World Health Organization.[2] This approach has been validated in multinational trials.[13–15] Simple analgesics, such as paracetamol combined with a non-steroidal anti-inflammatory drug (NSAID), are used first, then supplemented with a weak opioid, progressing to a strong opioid if pain is not relieved. Adjuvant treatments are considered for specific pain problems. The logical stepwise approach is illustrated in Fig. 14.1.

Superficial pain (Fig. 14.2)

Superficial pain has a sharp stinging quality which is well localized. Prostaglandins, bradykinins and a variety of other chemical mediators play an important role in generating the pain, which is transmitted by small-diameter myelinated nerve fibres. Superficial pain is often associated with ulceration or clinical signs of inflammation such as redness, swelling and heat at the site of the pain.

Head and neck cancers often ulcerate mucous membranes. Rarely, subcutaneous metastases will be exquisitely tender. Secondary bacterial infection can exacerbate pain. Radiotherapy and chemotherapy also cause painful mucositis. Ulceration may be so extensive and so painful that the patient is unable to eat or drink. Secondary fungal and bacterial infections will compound this problem. Mucositis may also occur with herpetic infection. Patients with advanced cancer are very prone to developing painful inflammation and ulceration over pressure areas.

Treatment

Painful malignant nodules should be treated with local excision if possible. Radiotherapy may also be helpful for single nodules and for confluent areas of

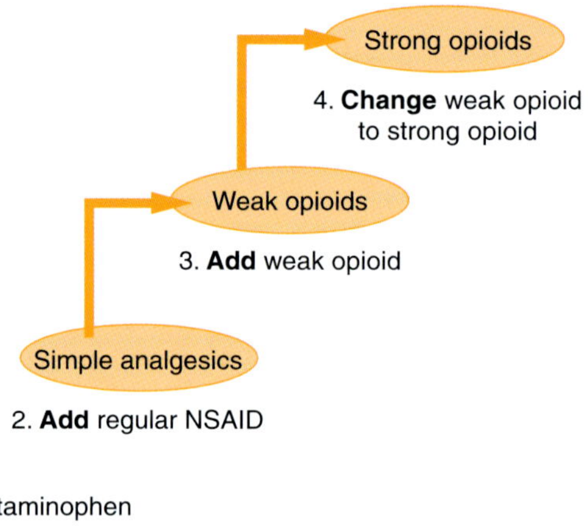

Figure 14.1 Analgesic 'stepladder'.

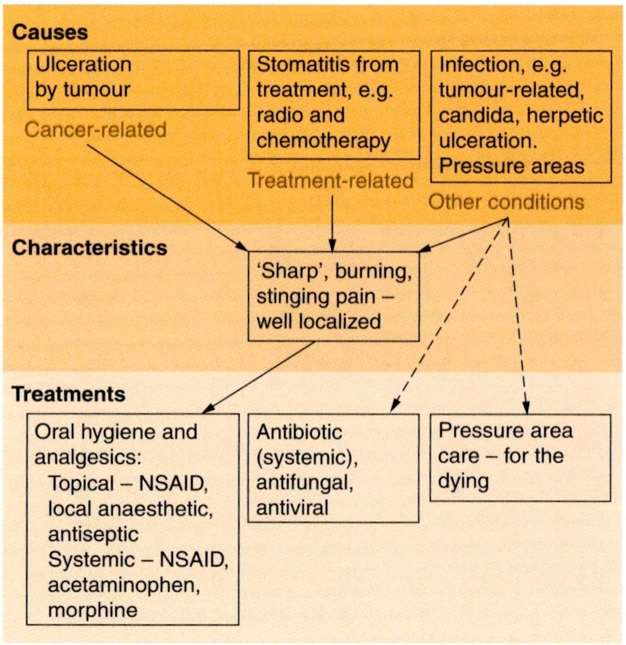

Figure 14.2 Superficial somatic pain.

local recurrence. However, these treatments are of limited use if there are multiple discrete nodules. Whenever infection is complicating tumour fungation and is contributing to pain, appropriate antibiotics should be given. Secondary infection is usually from anaerobes, hence the unpleasant odour that often occurs. Topical antibiotics such as metronidazole can be used, but oral antibiotics are preferable.

Superficial pain is usually treated with simple analgesics (Table 14.1). Malignant nodules or ulcers can sometimes be treated with a topical NSAID. The gel is gently applied and then covered with a non-absorbent dressing. Another useful topical analgesic is the eutectic mixture of local anaesthetics (EMLA) lignocaine and prilocaine. Unfortunately, some patients will develop a skin reaction. Thermoreversible gels offer an exciting new treatment for painful skin ulceration. These gels are liquid when cooled but solidify when warmed. Upon contact with a malignant ulcer, the gel conforms to the surface of the ulcer to produce a plastic-like coating. Local anaesthetics can be mixed with the gel to improve the analgesic effect. Morphine can be administered topically. Opioid receptors are associated with superficial inflammation, suggesting that morphine may act locally. The rubifacient creams such as capsaicin which rely on counter-irritation for pain relief should be avoided.

While the above measures can be used for painful pressure areas, prevention is the best form of management. The requirement for analgesics can be minimized with frequent turning of very weak patients and the use of pressure-relieving mattresses. If a painful ulcer does develop, topical NSAIDs can be very effective. Antibiotics may be necessary, but patients are often too ill to take oral medications. The cachexia process, which is the usual cause of the weakness, prevents ulcer healing; only rarely is this a feasible objective.

Prevention is also the best way of managing painful mucositis. Good mouth care with frequent antiseptic mouth washes and the regular prophylactic use of antifungal agents will minimize ulceration. Topical NSAID, steroid and local anaesthetic preparations may be used for established painful ulcers. Rarely, oral morphine may be necessary. Some patients benefit from a trial of acyclovir therapy for herpes infection.

Deep somatic pain (Fig. 14.3)

Deep somatic structures include muscle and bone. Pain arising in these organs is transmitted by larger, unmyelinated nerve fibres. It is usually described as dull and aching. The pain is relatively well localized but spreads across a wider area than superficial pain. In some instances, deep pain is referred. Tenderness may occur over the site of deep pain but signs of inflammation are rare, unless superficial spread of the cancer has also occurred. This frequently happens with head and neck cancers, which may arise superficially but quickly spread into the subjacent muscle and bone.

Table 14.1 Use of simple analgesics

- Acetaminophen (paracetamol):
  - 1000 mg regularly 6-hourly
  - available as tablets, capsules, elixir and suppositories
  - tablets are difficult to swallow; elixir has unpleasant taste
  - limited effectiveness, usually necessary to add other analgesics
- NSAIDs:
  - wide variety of preparations; choice depends on cost and convenience to patient
  - preferably once daily formulation
  - tablets should be small and coated so that they are easy to swallow
  - continue with suppositories or injections when patient is dying
  - caution in the elderly, renal or liver impairment, peptic ulcer
  - cytoprotective agents often coprescribed

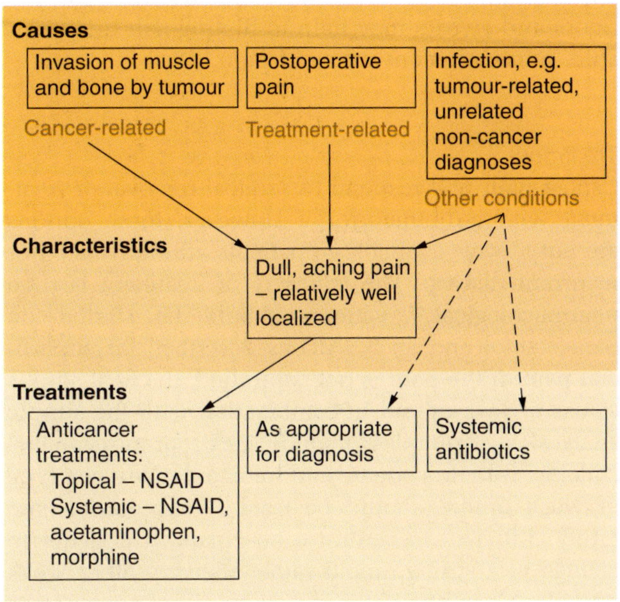

Figure 14.3 Deep somatic pain.

Causes
Deep somatic pain usually occurs as a result of local infiltration of soft tissue and muscles by head and neck cancers. Invasion of the jaw muscles will cause the tetanic pain of trismus. Lymph node metastases in the neck will also cause pain if they become large enough. Raised intracranial pressure can occur with metastatic brain tumours. The resultant headache is caused by tension on the falx and the meninges. Meningeal spread can also produce a headache associated with neck stiffness and cranial nerve signs. Rarely, a tumour invading the base of skull or cribriform plate will cause a CSF leak. This can cause headache which is exacerbated by sitting or standing, as well as bacterial meningitis.

Skeletal metastases may occur with head and neck cancers. The usual sites are vertebral bodies, followed by pelvis, femurs, ribs, skull and humerii. Bone destruction will eventually lead to fracture or collapse. Back or neck pain should prompt a review of spinal cord function to exclude evidence of cord compression. Radiographs of the painful site may reveal bone destruction (osteolysis). However, there may be no visible abnormality. Bone scintigraphy will highlight areas of bone reaction. MRI scans are most likely to detect metastases, including intramedullary spread.

Co-existing non-malignant conditions can cause deep somatic pain, such as arthritis. Patients recovering from major cancer surgery may experience deep somatic pain for several days despite successful removal of the cancer. Deep-seated soft tissue abscesses can produce constant pain as well as other features of advanced cancer such as anorexia, weakness and weight loss. Localized inflammatory changes may not be visible, making it very difficult to distinguish from tumour recurrence. Fevers, rigors and sweats may help to distinguish this treatable, non-malignant cause of pain.

Treatment
Cancer pain will respond to surgical removal or treatment with radiotherapy.[16,17] However, these options are not always available to patients with advanced or recurrent disease. The mainstay of treatment is then pharmacological.[18] Patients should be started on paracetamol and an NSAID as described for superficial pain. If the pain is not controlled, the next step is to use a weak opioid in combination with the simple analgesics. Examples include dextropropoxyphene, codeine, dihydrocodeine and tramadol. Only one type of weak opioid should be tried. Weak opioids are rarely sufficient to control cancer pain. It is better to change to a strong opioid rather than try other weak opioids. Morphine is the strong opioid of choice. It is usually given orally (Table 14.2).

Table 14.2 Using oral morphine

- Begin with elixir or immediate release tablets
- Starting dose is 10 mg 4 hourly if transferring from weak opioid—*a lower dose (2.5–5 mg) is needed for the elderly*
- Give regularly, not 'as required', for constant pain
- Wait for at least 24 hours before increasing the dose—*increase the dose by 30–50%*
- Titrate until pain is relieved, then transfer to slow-release preparations
- Use anti-emetics to prevent nausea (usually for 1st week of treatment)
- Prescribe aperients

Although most patients will only require oral medications, alternative routes may be needed. With head and neck cancers, patients may be unable to swallow tablets or liquids. Dying patients usually cannot swallow medications. Morphine can be given rectally, and by subcutaneous (not intramuscular) injection. The epidural and intrathecal route are rarely used, when appropriate doses of opioids cause unacceptable side-effects when given by other routes.[19] Failure of oral morphine to relieve pain is not an indication for epidural morphine.

Drowsiness may occur when patients first start morphine. They should be warned of the possibility but advised that the effect usually wears off after 2 or 3 days. If a patient is very worried by this, a smaller starting dose can be used (2.5 mg 4 hourly). When drowsiness persists, the dose of morphine should be lowered. If a balance cannot be struck between pain relief and drowsiness, an alternative opioid (Table 14.3) or some other analgesic strategy such as neural blockade should be tried. Patients who are dying become drowsy as part of the disease process. Their drowsiness should not be attributed to morphine. The family will need reassurance that the morphine is not responsible.

Table 14.3 Alternative opioids

- Methadone—*needs careful titration because of variable half-life*
- Hydromorphone—*available in slow-release preparations*
- Phenazocine
- Oxycodone
- Fentanyl—*given transdermally*

DO NOT use pethidine (meperidine) or pentazocine

Nausea and vomiting may occur in 50% of patients who start oral morphine. A regular anti-emetic should be started at the same time as the morphine: haloperidol 1.5 mg once or twice daily, metoclopramide 10 mg 6 hourly or cyclizine 50 mg 8 hourly. Morphine-induced nausea is usually temporary and the anti-emetics can often be reviewed and stopped after 3 to 4 days. Constipation is universal with opioids. A bowel softener (such as sodium docusate) and stimulant (such as senna) should always be prescribed with regular morphine.[18]

Whenever a strong opioid is prescribed, time should be spent with the patient and family eliciting their fears and reassuring them. They are usually worried about the traditional myths surrounding the use of morphine (Table 14.4). Careful explanations about how the morphine is to be used should be written down. Patients and families will need reassurance that extra doses of morphine can be given for breakthrough and incident pain without risk of overdosage.

Deep-seated infections associated with cancer can often be successfully managed with prolonged courses of oral antibiotics if surgical drainage is not feasible. Rotating courses of clindamycin and co-amoxiclav are easily tolerated and give the necessary anaerobic cover. A significant improvement in quality of life is possible, with some patients recovering from a 'terminal' decline.

Neural blockade (nerve blocks) has a limited role with head and neck cancers. Most blocks have a limited duration of effect, usually less than 2 months, and may exacerbate neuropathic pain (see below). There may be a role in selected cases, for example when patients cannot tolerate or do not want to take oral medications. The procedures are technically difficult and specialist advice should be sought from a pain clinic.[20]

Table 14.4 Myths about morphine

- Morphine causes 'addiction'—*patients may experience physical dependence but psychological dependence is very rare*
- Morphine causes respiratory depression, premature death—*not when given orally and titrated according to pain*
- Using morphine too soon will negate effectiveness later—*up to 50% of patients will be maintained on a stable dose; frequent dose escalation is uncommon*
- Morphine causes sedation—*not when titrated appropriately. Sedation is usually due to the effects of advanced cancer*

Visceral pain

Visceral pain usually has a dull aching quality. It may occur with mediastinal involvement. Occasionally, head and neck cancers spread to the liver, causing pain in the right upper quadrant of the abdomen. Pharmacological treatments are similar to those described for deep somatic pain.

Neuropathic pain (Fig. 14.4)

Neuropathic pain (nerve pain) is caused by damage to nerves, usually by direct invasion with cancer. Nerve pain is frequently not recognized. This means that appropriate treatments are often not used. The pain is described as burning, stabbing or shooting, like 'electric shocks'. It occurs in the distribution of cranial nerves, dermatomes or peripheral nerves, depending on where the damage occurs. Clinical examination will reveal signs of nerve damage, such as reduced or heightened sensation. Sometimes, gently stroking the skin will trigger pain (allodynia).

Causes

Nerve pain is commonly caused by cancer directly compressing and damaging nerves.[21] Head and neck cancers will often affect several nerves. Surgery can cause nerve damage. The history is often needed to distinguish a postsurgical cause from cancer recurrence. With the former, the pain starts soon after the operation; with the latter, the pain will start several months later. Investigations may be unreliable because of postoperative scarring and distortion. Too often, patients with recurrent disease have been repeatedly reassured despite worsening pain. A high index of suspicion is needed until the diagnosis is confirmed. This ensures that adequate analgesic

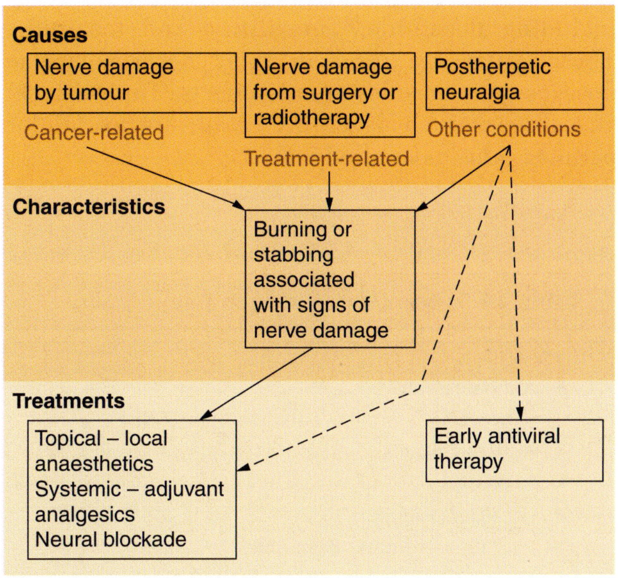

Figure 14.4 Neuropathic pain.

treatment is started in the interim. Nerve damage can result from the delayed effects of radiotherapy but this is very uncommon. The most common non-malignant cause of nerve pain is postherpetic neuralgia.

Treatment

Anticancer treatments can be less effective for nerve pain. If nerves have been infiltrated, the possibility of surgical resection is reduced. Radiotherapy and chemotherapy can relieve nerve pain, but their efficacy is reduced if fibrosis is associated with the malignant process. Usually, any beneficial effect on nerve pain is more short-lived than for other types of pain.

A wide range of drug therapies is available for nerve pain (Table 14.5). The most effective combination has to be individualized for each patient. The simple analgesics and the opioids should be started first. However, nerve pain is rarely contained by morphine. Other analgesics should be added to improve the quality and duration of analgesia. Antidepressants[22] must be started with a low dose, such as amitriptyline 10–25 mg at night. The dose is increased every 2 or 3 days until the pain is relieved or side-effects such as drowsiness and dry mouth occur. Several anticonvulsants are effective for nerve pain,[23] including carbamazepine, sodium valproate and clonazepam. The choice of anticonvulsant will depend on the preference of the doctor. The initial dose should be kept low and then built up gradually, as for amitriptyline, to minimize drowsiness. Steroids have been recommended on the basis that they reduce perineural oedema. They are also helpful for other symptoms of cancer, particularly nausea and anorexia. Recent interest has centred on the membrane-stabilizing antiarrhythmic drugs including flecainide,[24] mexilitine and tocainide. These drugs are used in their normal cardiac dosages and cause fewer side-effects. Topical local anaesthetics such as EMLA cream are useful for patients who have allodynia.

Table 14.5 Adjuvants for neuropathic pain

- Antidepressants:
  tricyclics are more effective than SSRIs
- Anticonvulsants
- Steroids
- Local anaesthetics:
  oral—mexilitine, flecainide
  topical—EMLA

Other symptoms

Haemorrhage

Minor bleeding is not uncommon from fungating head and neck cancers. Although direct invasion of blood vessels is the usual cause, other reasons for bleeding include thrombocytopenia associated with chemotherapy, infection and pulmonary embolism. This may present as external haemorrhage, epistaxis, blood-stained saliva or haemoptysis, depending on the site of the tumour. Occasionally, massive haemorrhage from the internal carotid artery is the cause of death. Fortunately, more radical surgery and radiotherapy appears to have reduced the incidence of this complication.

The best form of treatment is prevention. Appropriate anticancer management is important. If the disease cannot be controlled, then infection associated with malignant ulceration should be treated. When tumour erosion of the internal carotid is likely, some surgeons will ligate the artery. Minor bleeding may be reduced with topical adrenalin or thrombotic agents. Systemic antifibrinolytic agents should be avoided, as they can cause stroke and myocardial infarction in patients who are at risk for atherosclerotic vascular disease. Most instances of epistaxis will be fleeting and resolve spontaneously. Keeping the patient calm and advising bed rest are helpful general measures if epistaxis is more persistent.

When massive haemorrhage occurs, it is usually fatal within minutes. The patient quickly loses consciousness after the bleeding starts. An injection of morphine or benzodiazepine may relieve any distress, but it is often better to stay with the patient than go to get an injection. Some families can be taught to manage this complication at home if they have adequate support. If the patient dies unexpectedly, then bereavement follow-up will be needed.

Airway obstruction

Obstruction of the nasal passages is usually tolerated by patients. Mouth breathing may cause mouth dryness (see below). However, head and neck cancers can obstruct the oropharynx, larnyx and trachea. This causes severe anxiety and respiratory distress. Tracheostomy is the usual treatment. High-dose steroids can be used as a temporizing measure if any delay is expected. If airway obstruction occurs in patients who are dying from advanced disease, opioids and tranquilizers will be needed to relieve distress.

Dysphagia

Difficulty in swallowing is often associated with head and neck cancers. Advanced local disease can obstruct swallowing directly. Cranial nerve involvement may cause problems. The effects of aggressive surgery will also cause functional disturbances in deglutition. Mouth dryness will exacerbate any difficulties, as will the acute effects of radiotherapy, causing mucositis for example. Some patients manage with suitable modification of diet. However, alternative methods of nutritional support may be needed. Fine-bore nasogastric tubes are used less commonly now. Percutaneous gastrostomy is now easy to perform and is better tolerated by most patients. If a patient requires ongoing enteral feeding, then a reduction in intake should be considered when the patient reaches the terminal phase. Corticosteroids have been reported to improve swallowing in some patients with head and neck cancer.[25]

Dry mouth

Xerostomia is a very common symptom.[26] The usual cause is iatrogenic. Radiotherapy to the oral cavity diminishes salivary gland function. The saliva also becomes more viscous. Some medications cause dry mouth, including morphine and amitriptyline which are used for analgesia. Patients often drink more water but this provides minimal relief. Artificial saliva can be helpful, although it has to be used frequently to be effective. Pilocarpine can stimulate salivary flow, even after radiotherapy. However, the side-effects such as sweating are more likely to be troublesome for terminally ill patients. Chewing gum can improve dry mouth but is not always feasible after oral surgery or with advanced oral cancer.

Orocutaneous fistulae and drooling

When salivary function is normal, orocutaneous fistulae or difficulty in swallowing can cause troublesome drooling. With more than 1 litre of saliva being produced per day, patients can be severely embarrassed by drooling. In some cases, aspiration occurs which may lead to pneumonia. Anticholinergic drugs are often used to reduce salivary production. Antidepressants, transdermal scopolamine and oral glycopyrronium can be effective, provided systemic side-effects do not occur.[27] Radiotherapy may sometimes be helpful. The dose needed is lower than that used for anticancer treatment. The salivary branch of the facial nerve can be surgically transected using an approach through the middle ear. However, this option is only useful for patients with a longer prognosis who have failed other treatments.

Lymphoedema

Lymphatic drainage may be impaired by previous surgery, radiotherapy and disease recurrence. This causes swelling of the lip, tongue, submandibular region or neck. Sometimes the swelling may be severe enough to obstruct breathing and swallowing. Steroids and diuretics are often recommended but have little effect. Indeed, diuretics may make patients feel more unwell. Gentle massage at the outer edges of the lymphoedema may promote transfer of lymph into areas that are well drained, but this is also of limited value.

Breathlessness

Breathlessness is a very distressing symptom, both to patients and to carers.[28] There are many different causes (Table 14.6). Other factors such as fear, depression and anxiety can aggravate breathlessness. The distress associated with breathlessness can be extreme. Patients often describe fear of choking and suffocation. Anxiety may even cause dyspnoea.

Some treatments can improve the underlying cause of dyspnoea. Antibiotics should be used when chest infection contributes to breathlessness. Oral antibiotics should cover the possibility of anaerobic infection if the patient has been aspirating. Bronchodilators may be worth trying, given that many patients with head and neck cancer have been cigarette smokers. Symptomatic anaemia (haemoglobin less that 9.0 g/l) should be treated with transfusion, unless the patient is imminently dying. Steroids can have a non-specific effect to improve dyspnoea in addition to bronchodilator effects. Anticoagulants are rarely appropriate for symptomatic pulmonary emboli because of the risk of haemorrhage.

Low doses of opioids are often used orally to ease distress from breathlessness. Recent interest in nebulized morphine has not been supported by trials. Benzodiazepine, buspirone and synthetic cannabinoids have also been used to relieve the anxiety associated with dyspnoea. Nebulized bupivacaine is not helpful for dyspnoea but can

Table 14.6 Causes of breathlessness

- Cancer-related:
  - upper airways and tracheal compression; SVCO
  - lung mestastases
- Other causes:
  - anaemia
  - chest infection
  - chronic obstructive pulmonary disease
  - pulmonary embolism
  - severe cachexia

relieve distressing cough. Oxygen can reduce breathlessness in patients with advanced cancer. The effect is modest, and continuous oxygen causes dryness of the mouth and throat.

Systemic effects of head and neck cancers

Head and neck cancers can produce systemic symptoms, even in the absence of distant metastases. Advanced locoregional disease can produce anorexia, fatigue and drowsiness. Steroid therapy or high-dose progestagens can palliate these symptoms for a time. Both of these treatments increase appetite, which may be a problem if the patient has trouble swallowing.

Confusion, agitated delirium and restlessness are also associated with advanced disease.[29] Other causes such as hypercalcaemia have to be considered and treated appropriately. However, in dying patients it is necessary to use major tranquilizers such as haloperidol or midazolam to ensure that death is peaceful.

Summary

Patients with incurable head and neck cancer experience many problems. Physical symptoms are common, including pain, dysphagia, dry mouth, haemorrhage and general weakness. In addition, psychological, social and spiritual issues become more prominent with progressive disease. The families and other significant carers are also affected by cancer, even into the bereavement period. Although these problems often seem insurmountable, there is no longer any justification for patients and families to be told that 'nothing more can be done' when active treatments fail. This chapter describes how palliative care offers many strategies for controlling symptoms. Team work enables the broader needs of patients and families to be addressed.[30]

References

1. Greer DS, Mor V, Kastenbaum R (eds). The hospice experiment. Baltimore: Johns Hopkins Press, 1988
2. World Health Organization. Cancer pain relief and palliative care. Technical report series 804. Geneva: World Health Organization, 1990
3. Saunders C. The evolution of the hospices. In: Mann RD (ed.). The history of the management of pain: from early principles to present practice. Carnforth: Parthenon, 1988: 36–94
4. Saunders C. Hospice care. In: Ajemian I, Mount BM (eds). The R.V.H. manual on palliative/hospice care. New York: Arno Press, 1980: 21–26
5. Dunlop RJ. Cancer: palliative care. London: Springer-Verlag, 1998: 111–120
6. Parkes CM. Bereavement counselling: Does it work? Br Med J 1980; 281: 3–6
7. Parkes CM. Evaluation of a bereavement service. J Prevent Psych 1981; 1: 179–188
8. Doka KJ, Davidson JD. Living with grief: Who we are, how we grieve. Philadelphia: Brunner/Mazel, 1998
9. Dunlop RJ, Hockley JM. Hospital-based palliative care teams: The hospital/hospice interface. Oxford: Oxford University Press, 1998
10. Sidransky D, Schantz SP, Harrison LB et al. Cancer of the head and neck. In: DeVita VT, Hellman S, Rosenberg S (eds). Cancer: principles and practice of oncology, 5th edn. Philadelphia: Lippincott-Raven. 1997: 735–847
11. Billings JA. Outpatient management of advanced cancer. Philadelphia: Lippincott, 1985
12. Dunlop RJ, Campbell CW. Cytokines and advanced cancer. J Pain Symptom Manage 2000; 20: 214–232
13. Schug SA, Zech D, Dorr U. Cancer pain management according to WHO analgesic guidelines. J Pain Sympt Mgmt 1990; 5: 27–32
14. Takeda F. Results of field-testing in Japan of WHO draft interim guidelines on relief of cancer pain. Pain Clin 1986; 1: 83–89
15. Walker VA, Hoskin PJ, Hanks GWC et al. Evaluation of WHO analgesic guidelines for cancer pain in a hospital-based palliative care unit. J Pain Sympt Mgmt 1988; 3: 145–149
16. Price P, Hoskin PJ, Easton D et al. Prospective randomised trial of single and multifraction schedules in the treatment of painful bony metastases. Radiother Oncol 1986; 6: 247–255
17. Jacox AK, Carr DB, Payne R et al. Management of cancer pain. Clinical practice guidelines no. 9. AHCPR publications no. 94-0592. Rockville, Md: Agency for Health Care Policy and Research, 1994.
18. Foley KM. The treatment of cancer pain. N Engl J Med 1985; 313: 84–95
19. Sykes N, Baines M. Gastrointestinal symptoms in oncology. In: Dunlop RJ (ed.). Cancer: palliative care. London: Springer-Verlag, 1998: 49–63
20. Cousins MJ, Bridenbaugh PO. Neural blockade in clinical anaesthesia and management, 3rd edn. New York: Lippincott-Raven, 1998
21. Tasker RR. Deafferentation pain syndromes: introduction. New York: Raven Press, 1991
22. McQuay HJ, Tramer N, Nye DA et al. A systematic review of antidepressants in neuropathic pain. Pain 1996; 68: 217–227
23. McQuay HJ, Carroll D, Jadad AR et al. Anticonvulsant drugs for management of pain: a systematic review. Br Med J 1995; 311: 1047–1052

24. Dunlop RJ, Davies RJ, Hockley JM et al. Analgesic effects of oral flecainide. Lancet 1988; 1: 420–421
25. Sykes NP, Baines MJ, Carter RL. Clinical and pathological study of dysphagia conservatively managed in patients with advanced malignant disease. Lancet 1988; ii: 726–728
26. Davies AN. Xerostomia. Eur J Cancer Care 1997; 6: 209–214
27. Dunlop RJ. Transdermal hyoscine and drooling. Palliat Med 1990; 4: 328–329
28. Ahmedzai S. Palliation of respiratory symptoms. In: Doyle D, Hanks GWC, MacDonald N (eds). Oxford textbook of palliative medicine. Oxford: Oxford Unniversity Press, 1998: 583–616
29. Dunlop RJ. When palliative care fails to control suffering. J Palliat Care 1994; 2: 28–30
30. Farsides B, Dunlop RJ. Is there such a thing as a life not worth living? BMJ 2001; 322: 1481–1483

III Outcomes and Follow-up

15 Results of treatment

Snehal G Patel and Jatin P Shah

The majority of patients with tumors of the oral cavity are treated with surgery and/or radiation therapy. Patients with early stage tumors are usually treated with a single modality, most commonly surgery, while those with advanced stage disease are treated with a combination of surgery and adjuvant postoperative radiation therapy.

In order to provide contemporary data reflecting outcomes of therapy from a tertiary care cancer center, we have prospectively analyzed patients treated at Memorial Sloan–Kettering Cancer Center from 1986–95. These patients were treated by a multidisciplinary 'disease management team' with relatively uniform treatment philosophies. The initial evaluation data, operative details, pathology reports and longitudinal follow-up data are prospectively maintained on a computerized 'Disease Management System' database.

During the 10-year period between 1986–95, 595 previously untreated patients received surgery with or without postoperative radiotherapy for invasive squamous cell carcinoma (SCC) of the oral cavity. Clinical and pathology data were entered into a computer database (Microsoft Access 2000) and statistical analysis was carried out using a commercially available computer software package (JMP 4.0, SAS Institute Inc., Cary NC). The follow-up interval was calculated in months from the date of initial surgery to the date of last follow-up or death, and the disease-free interval was calculated from the date of initial surgery to the date of first recurrence. For disease-specific survival, patients who died of non-oral cancer related causes (64 patients, 11%) and those who were alive with disease at the last follow-up (8 patients, 1%) were censored. Patients who died with a secondary primary malignancy (SPM) of the head and neck area (10 patients, 2%) were considered as having died of the disease. Overall, disease-specific and relapse-free survival rates were calculated by the Kaplan–Meier method, and univariate comparisons were performed using the log-rank test. A p value of 0.05 or less was considered statistically significant and all significant factors were entered into multivariate analysis using the Cox proportional hazard model.

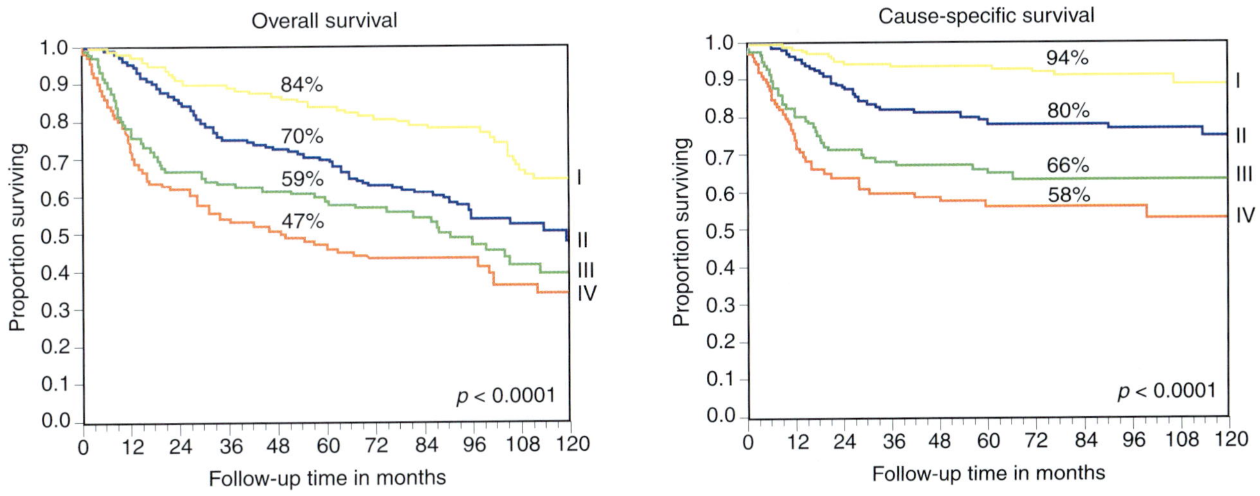

Figure 15.1 The clinical stage of the disease is a significant predictor of outcome in SCC of the oral cavity.

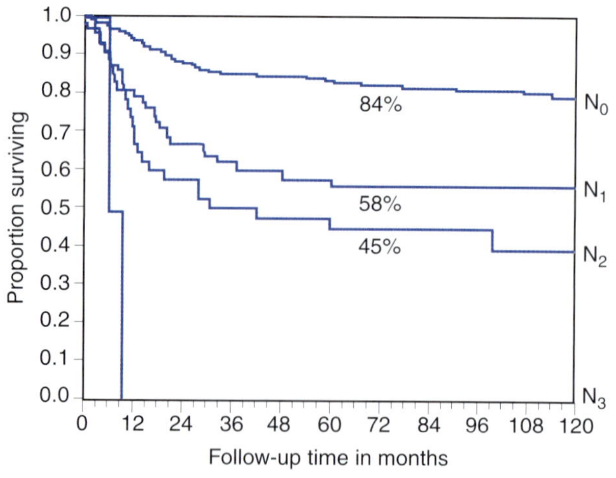

Figure 15.2 Impact of clinically palpable lymph node metastasis on disease-specific survival in squamous cell carcinoma of the oral cavity.

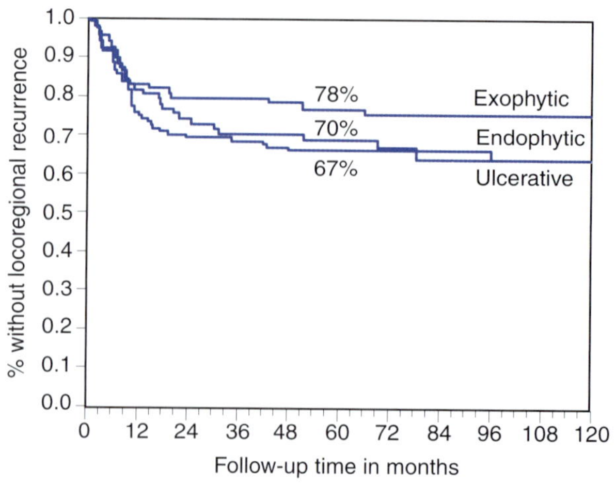

Figure 15.3 Endophytic, infiltrative tumors have poorer locoregional control rates compared to exophytic tumors.

For the purpose of this discussion, we have also included data from the National cancer DataBase (NCDB) of the Commission on Cancer of the American College of Surgeons. This database is supported by the American Cancer Society and the National Tumor Registrars Association. Over 1400 hospitals across the US voluntarily contribute data each year to this national database. Data analysis is performed at the American College of Surgeons.[1] This information offers national trends in therapeutic choices and outcomes data that reflect cross-sectional observations nationwide in the US.

Not surprisingly, the clinical stage of the tumor is an important factor predicting survival in patients with oral cavity cancer (Fig. 15.1). However, the presence of clinically positive lymph nodes is probably the single most important factor in determining outcome (Fig. 15.2).

Clinical predictors

Aside from regional lymph node metastasis, there are several other ominous clinical signs related to the primary tumor in patients presenting with oral cavity cancer, that imply locally advanced disease. The first is trismus, which suggests that the pterygoid, temporalis or masseter muscle have become involved. Another ominous sign is reduced tongue mobility, which suggests invasion of the deep musculature of the tongue or the hypoglossal nerve. Finally, patients with tumours displaying an ulcerative or infiltrative pattern of growth, rather than an exophytic pattern, have a poor prognosis (Fig. 15.3). When a tumour has grown to an extent where the skin is involved, the chance of cure is relatively low.

Locoregional control

Approximately a third of patients (29%) treated for oral cavity cancer fail treatment, and locoregional recurrence is the most common pattern of failure (Fig. 15.4). The rate of local control after treatment of tumors of the oral cavity can be related to several factors. The status of the surgical margins is probably the single most important factor determining local control (Fig. 15.5). It is interesting that in one report margins were classified as positive if they met one of the following four criteria:[2]

1. Close margin (tumor within 0.5 cm),
2. Premalignant change in the margin,
3. In situ carcinoma in the margin, and
4. Invasive microscopic cancer at the margin.

A significant aspect of margin assessment and reporting is that, after resection and processing, the average specimen has been shown to shrink by approximately 30%.[3] A lesion resected with a margin of 8 mm in vivo will thus be reported to have a margin of 5.3 mm on final pathology. The implication of this observation is that adequacy at surgical resection is more reliably assessed by examining margins from the surgical defect after resection of the specimen, rather than from the specimen alone. Nevertheless, the appearance of microscopic tumor cells at or near the margin of resection is of concern and warrants consideration of further wider resec-

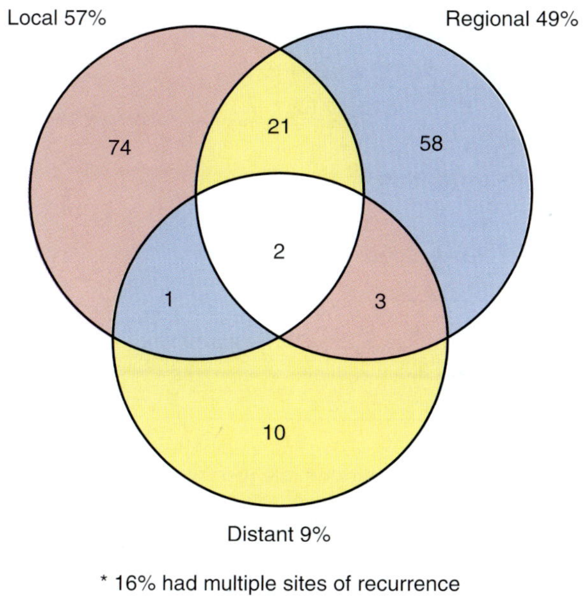

Figure 15.4 Patterns of failure in patients that failed treatment for cancer of the oral cavity. Treatment failure was noted in 171/595 patients (29%).

tion if feasible, and/or adjuvant treatment to improve local control.

In patients with close or positive surgical margins, adjuvant radiation therapy in doses of 60 Gy or more yields local control rates comparable to those in patients with negative margins.[4] When patients who received a dose of 60 Gy or more were analyzed as a subgroup, the control rate exceeded 90%.[3] An interesting caveat to this, however, is that the efficacy of postoperative radiation therapy was dependent on the site of the primary tumor; floor of mouth tumors had a better 5-year local control rate compared to oral tongue tumors (89% versus 62%). In spite of the general efficacy of postoperative radiation therapy, it is crucial for the surgeon to strive for adequate total resection of the tumor, especially for cancers of the oral tongue (as this data suggests).

Another histopathological sign that has been correlated with local control is the presence of perineural invasion. Patients with histologic evidence of perineural invasion have a lower control rate (77%) compared to others (91%).[5] When perineural invasion is seen in the specimen, consideration should be given to the use of adjuvant radiation therapy to enhance local control.

Various features of the primary lesion have also been utilized to predict the risk of occult cervical lymph node metastasis that in turn directly relates

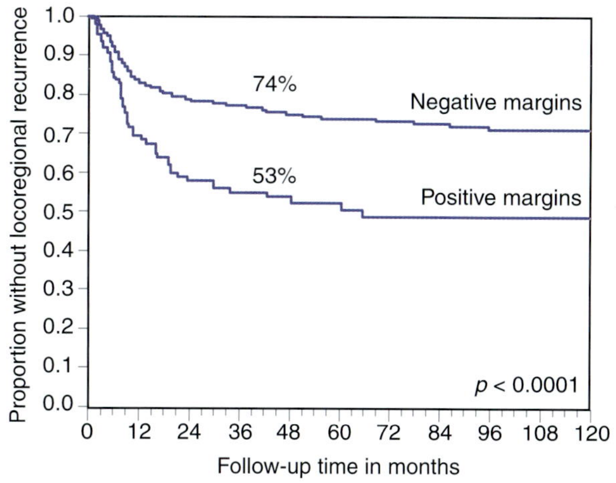

Figure 15.5 Local control rates drop significantly in patients with positive surgical margins.

to survival. The thickness of the primary tumor is one of the most predictive and reliable methods currently available to the clinician for estimating the risk of regional lymph node involvement,[6] Thus, patients with deeply infiltrative tumors will have a higher rate of lymph node metastasis and thus a lower rate of survival (Fig. 15.6). These findings have been duplicated by others.[7,8]

Survival and prognostic factors

Surgery and radiation therapy are the mainstays of treatment of oral cavity cancer, and 'equivalent' results have been reported using either modality for early stage tumors. It is, however, important to note that most early oral cancers can be easily surgically

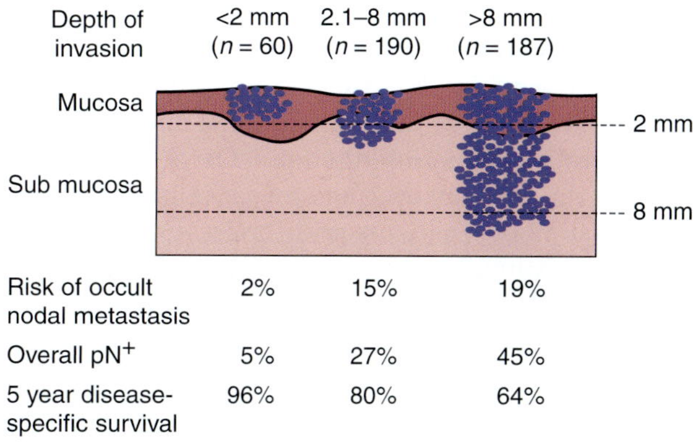

Figure 15.6 The depth of invasion of the primary tumor is a significant predictor of nodal metastasis and disease-specific survival.

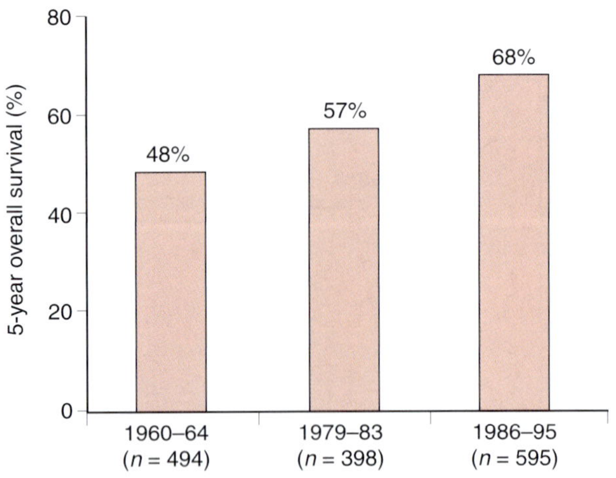

Figure 15.7 Improving outcomes in oral cavity cancer: results of treatment in three cohorts treated during different time periods at Memorial Sloan–Kettering Cancer Center (1960–95).

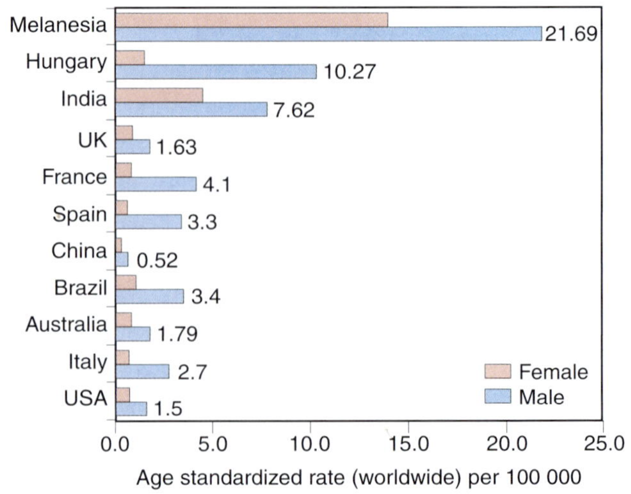

Figure 15.8 Estimated mortality rates for the year 2000 in patients treated for squamous carcinoma of the oral cavity (age-standardized (worldwide) death rates per 100 000 population). Data source: Ferlay J, Bray F, Pisani P, Parkin DM. GLOBOCAN 2000: Cancer incidence, mortality and prevalence worldwide, version 1.0. IARC CancerBase No. 5. Lyon: IARCPress, 2001. Limited version available from: URL:http://www.dep.iarc.fr/globocan/globocan.htm.

resected with minimal functional impact, whereas the morbidity associated with radiation therapy, e.g. xerostomia, loss of taste, life-long risk to dentition, can be considerable. For more advanced tumors, the two modalities are used in combination; our preference in tumors of the oral cavity is to employ radiation therapy in a postoperative adjuvant setting.

The overall 5-year survival in a recently analyzed cohort of patients at Memorial Sloan–Kettering Cancer Center was 68%. This represents a modest but appreciable improvement in our treatment results over the years (Fig. 15.7). Although a direct comparison of this nature is statistically irrelevant, it does provide some insight into trends. Factors that may have contributed to better results include: downstaging of the primary tumor due to earlier detection; enhanced ability to resect large tumors and reconstruct large and complex defects, particularly with the availability of microvascular free flaps; improved understanding of the patterns of regional lymphatic metastatic pathways; more aggressive regional therapy, including increasing use of elective selective neck dissections; and the use of postoperative radiation therapy. On a nationwide basis in the US, however, the 5-year relative survival in almost 59 000 patients with oral cancer analyzed by the National Cancer DataBase (NCDB) was reported to be 49.8% for squamous cell carcinoma.[1] This may be a better reflection of outcome of therapy, since it represents national data from all parts of the United States, and not institutional data from a leading tertiary care cancer center. Mortality rates from oral cancer also vary according to geographic location, and certain high-incidence regions such as Melanesia, Eastern Europe and India have considerably higher rates compared to the rest of the world (Fig. 15.8).

Patients with oral carcinoma are generally older and are more likely to suffer other comorbid conditions secondary to tobacco and alcohol abuse, that may contribute to outcome. This is reflected in the fact that the 5-year disease-specific survival (77%) is better than the corresponding overall survival (68%) (Fig. 15.9). The proportion of patients dying from

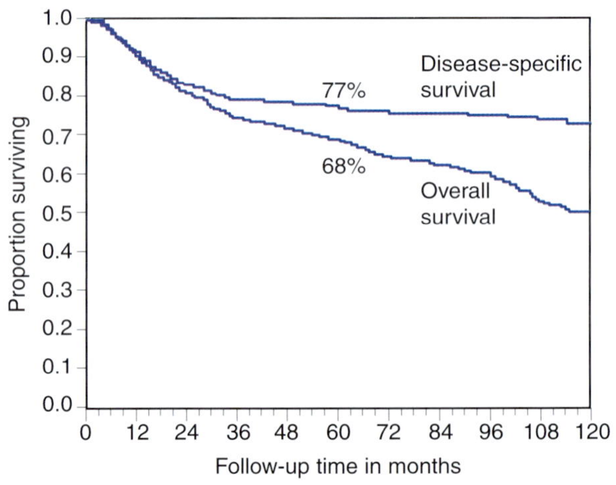

Figure 15.9 5-year overall and disease-specific survival in a recent cohort of patients with oral cavity cancer treated at Memorial Sloan–Kettering Cancer Center.

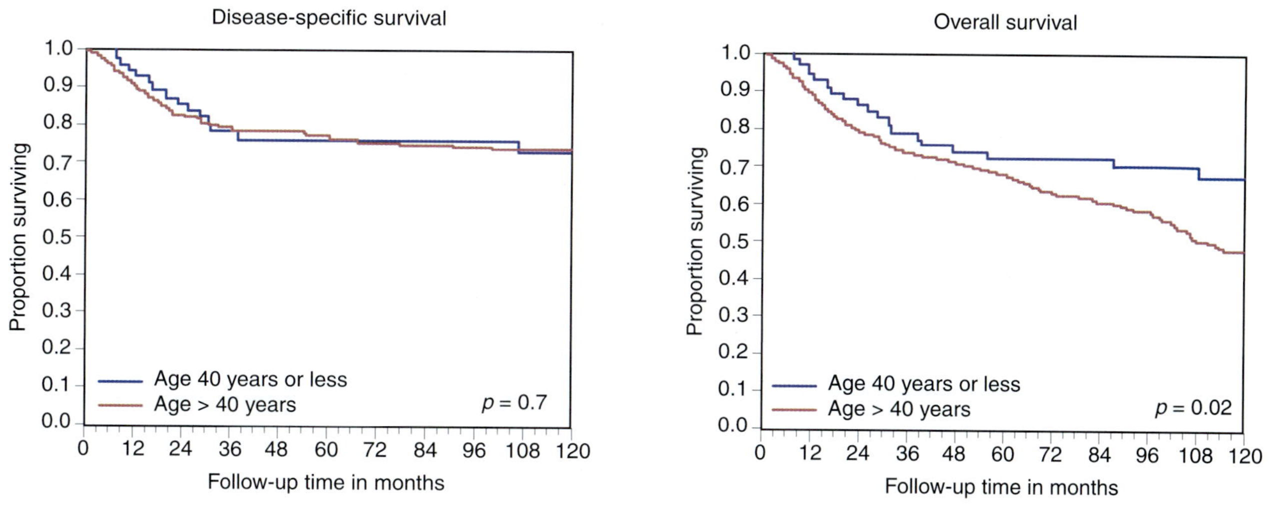

Figure 15.10 Overall survival is poorer in older patients while disease-specific survival is comparable to younger patients.

other causes has been reported to have increased from 14.1% at 5 years to approximately 50% at 10 years after treatment.[1] There are reports speculating that oral cavity tumors in younger patients are more aggressive than similar tumors in older patients. When patients are stratified for stage, however, the survival is not statistically different between the older and younger groups. In our experience, disease-specific survival was comparable while overall survival was poorer in older patients (Fig. 15.10). A similar finding was reported in the NCDB study.[1] These observations underscore the importance of comorbid conditions as determinants of outcome in patients with oral carcinoma.

There is some suspicion that tumors in some younger patients who do not have the usual risk factors behave differently from the tobacco and/or alcohol-associated tumors in the older age group.[9] These tumors may be related to the human papilloma virus (HPV) and are reported to have a better prognosis than tobacco/alcohol-induced carcinomas.[10] On the other hand, a subset of pathologically aggressive tumors that have a worse prognosis have been reported in patients younger than 35 years in age, especially females who do not have associated behavioral risk factors. It is unclear if these patients have biologically distinct tumors and/or if these differences are related to the host's immune status.[11,12]

A significantly worse outcome has been reported for African-Americans, compared to Caucasians, and for males compared to females after treatment for squamous carcinoma of the oral cavity.[1] Although the socioeconomic status of the host may contribute to ethnicity-related differences, the role of other factors such as aggressive tumor biology, host vulnerability, compliance with treatment and social support remain unclear. Hormonal, genetic, immunologic, and behavioral and compliance issues may be related to the better survival reported in women.[13]

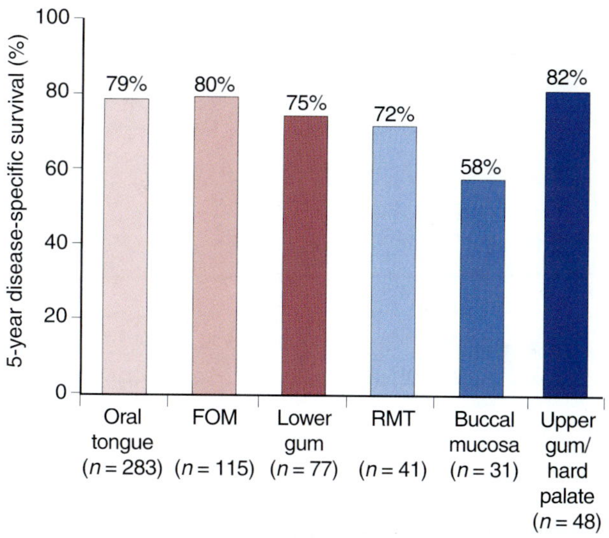

Figure 15.11 Disease-specific survival is related to the site of the primary tumor within the oral cavity.

The site of the tumor within the oral cavity can influence outcome (Fig. 15.11). For example, patients with tumors arising in the buccal mucosa and retromolar trigone have a poorer outcome compared with patients with tumors in other sites. This observation may be less related to the inherent biology of the tumor but rather to other factors such

Table 15.1 Overall 5-year survival (%) in patients with cancer of the floor of the mouth

Series	Total no. of patients	Stage I	Stage II	Stage III	Stage IV
Harrold, 1971[15]	634	69	49	25	7
Panje, 1980[16]	103	57	60	43	19
Nason, 1989[17]	198	69	64	46	26
Shaha, 1984[18]	320	88	80	66	32
Fu, 1976[19]	153	83	71	43	10
Pernot, 1996[20]	207	(T_1)	(T_2)	(T_3)	–
		71	42	35	
MSKCC, 2001[21]	61	82	56	49	55

Table 15.2 Overall 5-year survival (%) in patients with cancer of the tongue

Series	Total no. of patients	Stage I	Stage II	Stage III	Stage IV
Callery, 1984[22]	252	75	60	40	20
Decroix, 1981[23]	602	59	45	25	13
Wallner, 1986[24]	424	68	50	33	20
Ildstad, 1983[25]	122	48	48	18	26
O'Brien, 1986[26]	97	73	62	–	–
Pernot, 1996[20]	565	(T_1)	(T_2)	(T_3)	–
		70	42	29	
MSKCC, 2002[21]	283	84	73	59	27

as proximity of the tumor to bone (retromolar trigone or alveolus), or the density of lymphatics (tongue). Tables 15.1 and 15.2 list some results of treatment in patients treated for cancers of the floor of the mouth and oral tongue reported in the literature. Histologic variants of squamous cell carcinoma will also have vastly different clinical behavior and survival. Verrucous carcinoma of the oral cavity tends to have an indolent course and carries a relatively low potential for regional lymph node metastasis. The survival for patients with verrucous carcinoma is more favorable than for patients with invasive squamous cell carcinoma, and better survival rates have been reported using surgery compared to radiation therapy for oral verrucous tumors.[14]

The clinical and pathological stages of the tumor are obviously important determinants of outcome, but the presence of nodal metastasis is the single most powerful predictor of survival (Fig. 15.2). While the T stage measures the primary tumor in two dimensions, the depth of invasion represents the third dimension that relates to risk for lymph node metastasis (Fig. 15.6). Deeply infiltrative tumors have significantly higher locoregional recurrence rate and poorer outcome compared to more superficial tumors (Fig. 15.12).

Complete surgical excision of the tumor, achieving negative surgical margins, is crucial to locoregional control and disease-specific survival (Fig. 15.13). Various other parameters such as perineural and vascular invasion and the grade of the primary tumor have been reported to be significant prognostic factors. However, positive surgical margins and lymph node metastasis are the only independent predictors on multivariate analysis of locoregional control and disease-specific survival in patients with squamous carcinoma of the oral cavity. While the majority of oral cavity tumors are squamous cell carcinomas, a vast array of other tumor histologies

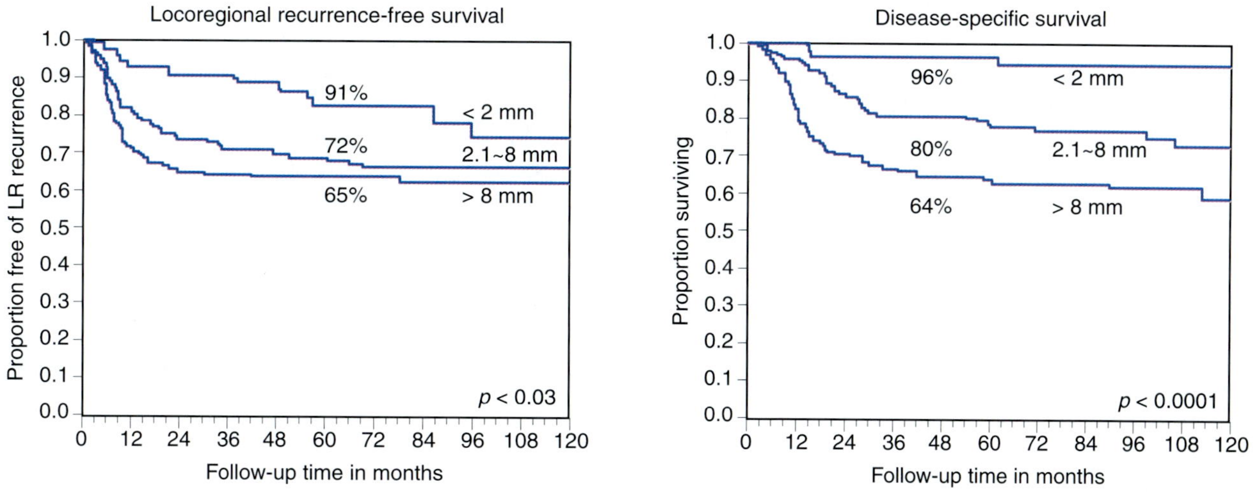

Figure 15.12 Deeply infiltrative tumors are more difficult to control locoregionally and have a poorer outcome compared to superficial tumors.

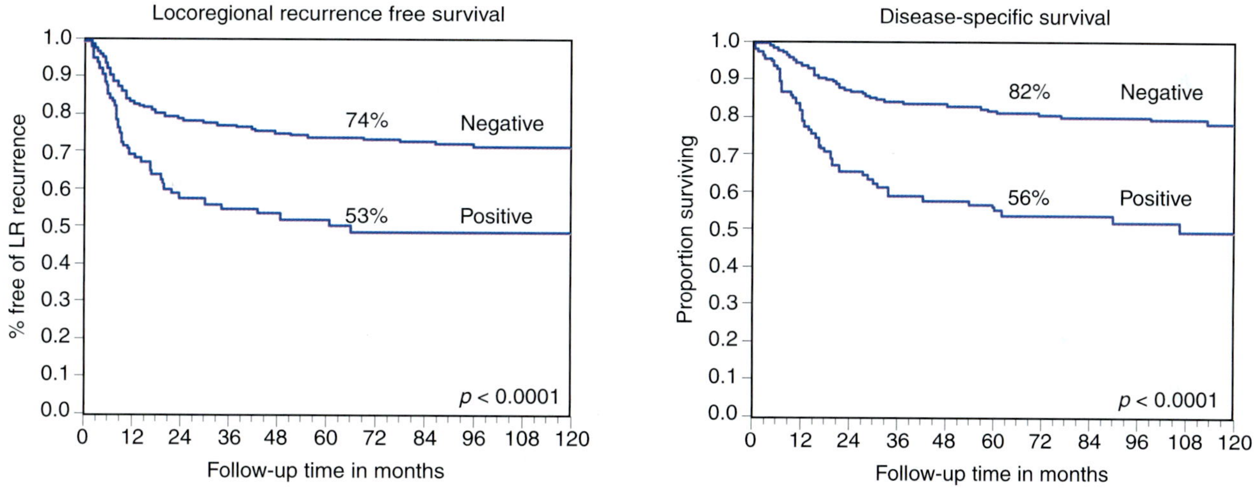

Figure 15.13 Positive surgical margins are significant predictors of locoregional failure and disease-specific survival.

may occur in this location. Minor salivary gland tumors, sarcomas, metastatic tumors, lymphomas, osseous tumors of the skeletal framework, and mucosal melanomas represent a few of the possibilities. Although the principles of surgical treatment for these tumors remain similar, the treatment and outcome in all of these are widely divergent and beyond the scope of this chapter.

References

1. Funk GF, Karnell LH, Robinson RA et al. Presentation, treatment, and outcome of oral cavity cancer: a National Cancer DataBase report. Head Neck 2002; 24: 165–180
2. Loree TR, Strong EW. Significance of positive margins in oral cavity squamous carcinoma. Am J Surg 1990; 160: 410–414
3. Carew JF et al. Unpublished data, 1999
4. Zelefsky MJ, Harrison LB, Fass DE et al. Postoperative radiation therapy for squamous cell carcinoma of the oral cavity and oropharynx: impact of therapy on patients with positive surgical margins. Int J Radiat Oncol Biol Phys 1993; 25: 17–21
5. Fagan JJ, Collins B, Barnes L et al.Perineural invasion in squamous cell carcinoma of the head and neck. Arch Otolaryngol Head Neck Surg 1998; 124: 637–640
6. Spiro RH, Huvos AG, Wong GY et al. Predictive value of tumor thickness in squamous carcinoma confined to the tongue and floor of the mouth. Am J Surg 1986; 152: 345–350.
7. Mohit-Tabatabai MA, Sobel HJ, Rush BF, Mashberg A. Relation of thickness of floor of mouth stage I and II

cancers to regional metastasis. Am J Surg 1986; 152: 351–353
8. Yuen AP, Lam KY, Wei W et al. A comparison of the prognostic significance of tumor diameter, length, width, thickness, area, volume, and clinicopathological features of oral tongue carcinoma. Am J Surg 2000; 180: 139–143
9. Koch WM, Lango M, Sewell D et al. Head and neck cancer in nonsmokers: a distinct clinical and molecular entity. Laryngoscope 1999; 109: 1544–1551
10. Gillison ML, Koch WM, Capone RB et al. Evidence for a causal association between human papillomavirus and a subset of head and neck cancers. J Natl Cancer Inst 2000; 92: 709–720
11. Byers RM. Squamous cell carcinoma of the oral tongue in patients less than thirty years of age. Am J Surg 1975; 130: 475–478
12. Kuriakose M, Sankaranarayanan M, Nair MK et al. Comparison of oral squamous cell carcinoma in younger and older patients in India. Eur J Cancer B Oral Oncol 1992; 28B: 113–120
13. Franco EL, Dib LL, Pinto DS et al. Race and gender influences on the survival of patients with mouth cancer. J Clin Epidemiol 1993; 46: 37–46
14. Koch BB, Trask DK, Hoffman HT et al. National survey of head and neck verrucous carcinoma: patterns of presentation, care, and outcome. Cancer 2001; 92: 110–120
15. Harrold CC Jr. Management of cancer of the floor of the mouth. Am J Surg 1971; 122: 487–493
16. Panje WR, Smith B, McCabe BF. Epidermoid carcinoma of the floor of the mouth: surgical therapy vs combined therapy vs radiation therapy. Otolaryngol Head Neck Surg 1980; 88: 714–720
17. Nason RW, Sako K, Beecroft WA et al. Surgical management of squamous cell carcinoma of the floor of the mouth. Am J Surg 1989; 158: 292–296
18. Shaha AR, Spiro RH, Shah JP, Strong EW. Squamous carcinoma of the floor of the mouth. Am J Surg 1984; 148: 455–459
19. Fu KK, Lichter A, Galante M. Carcinoma of the floor of the mouth: an analysis of treatment results and the sites and causes of failures. Int J Radiat Oncol Biol Phys 1976; 1: 829–837
20. Pernot M, Hoffstetter S, Peiffert D et al. Role of interstitial brachytherapy in oral and oropharyngeal carcinoma: reflection of a series of 1344 patients treated at the time of initial presentation. Otolaryngol Head Neck Surg 1996; 115: 519–526
21. Memorial–Sloan Kettering Cancer Center. Unpublished data, 2002
22. Callery CD, Spiro RH, Strong EW. Changing trends in the management of squamous carcinoma of the tongue. Am J Surg 1984; 148: 449–454
23. Decroix Y, Ghossein NA. Experience of the Curie Institute in treatment of cancer of the mobile tongue. I. Treatment policies and result. Cancer 1981; 47: 496–502
24. Wallner PE, Hanks GE, Kramer S, McLean CJ. Patterns of Care Study. Analysis of outcome survey data–anterior two-thirds of tongue and floor of mouth. Am J Clin Oncol 1986; 9: 50–57
25. Ildstad ST, Bigelow ME, Remensnyder JP. Squamous cell carcinoma of the mobile tongue. Clinical behavior and results of current therapeutic modalities. Am J Surg 1983; 145: 443–449
26. O'Brien CJ, Lahr CJ, Soong SJ et al. Surgical treatment of early-stage carcinoma of the oral tongue – would adjuvant treatment be beneficial? Head Neck Surg 1986; 8: 401–408

16 Functional outcome and rehabilitation

Snehal G Patel and Jatin P Shah

The tongue and related structures of the oral cavity serve a vital function in mastication, deglutition and articulation of speech. Hence, patients with oral cavity tumors often present with complaints of difficulty in eating and speaking. Treatment of these tumours has the potential to augment any functional impairment that may result from the tumor itself, and the magnitude of these post-treatment functional deficits is related to several factors, including[1–6]:

1. Soft tissue volume loss,
2. Sensory loss,
3. Motor function loss, and
4. Post-treatment limitations in movement secondary to healing and fibrosis.[1–6]

Speech and swallowing in patients with oral cavity tumors are also affected by factors unrelated to the extirpation of the tumor, such as the patient's age, neurologic status, and also non-surgical treatment such as radiation therapy.[7,8] All of these factors should be considered in the rehabilitation of a patient who has been treated for oral cavity cancer.

In order to understand the functional outcomes in patients treated for tumors of the oral cavity, one must first understand the complex and intricate physiologic interplay of the structures in the oral cavity as they relate to normal swallowing and speech. Swallowing has classically been divided into several phases (Table 16.1).[9] While this classification serves as a useful conceptual framework, it is rather artificial and oversimplifies this complex process. Although cancers of the oral cavity can affect all four of these phases, they most commonly and most profoundly impact on the first two: the oral preparatory and oral phases. The oral preparatory phase involves the conversion of solid food into a pulverized bolus that can be easily transported to the posterior aspect of the oral cavity by the tongue. This phase requires the coordinated use and competency of the lips, labiobuccal musculature, jaws, muscles of mastication, tongue, and the hard and soft palate. A lesion that involves any of these structures will have profound effects on the oral preparatory phase of deglutition. For example, loss of a significant amount of the oral tongue will limit the ability to transport the food into position for grinding by the molars. Similarly, if a segment of the mandible is lost, the ability to chew and pulverize the food will be impaired. The treatment of all but the earliest of oral cavity tumors will have profound effects on this stage of deglutition.

The second phase of swallowing is the oral phase. In this phase, the food bolus is transported from the anterior to the posterior region of the oral cavity in the vicinity of the anterior tonsillar pillars. This is the region where the swallowing reflex is initiated and the involuntary, reflexive acts of swallowing begin. This phase is relatively brief, lasting approximately one second, and may also be altered by the treatment of tumors of the oral cavity. The last two phases of swallowing, the pharyngeal phase and esophageal phase, are much less affected by the dynamics of the oral cavity. Adequate rehabilitation requires the determination of which aspects of the normal process are affected by treatment of the oral tumor and then devising methods to minimize or counter these adverse effects.

Table 16.1 Phases of normal deglutition

I:	Oral preparatory phase
II:	Oral phase
III:	Pharyngeal phase
IV:	Esophageal phase

While the majority of the active functions of the oral cavity involve transporting and chewing the food bolus, the sensory components of these activities are also vitally important to deglutition. Consideration, therefore, must be given to any sensory deficits seen after treatment when formulating a rehabilitative plan. Restoration of sensation following surgical excision of oral cavity tumors has become an area of interest with the increasing use of microvascular free flaps. Microneural anastomosis between a sensory nerve supplying a fasciocutaneous flap, e.g. the lateral antebrachial nerve of the radial forearm flap, and a recipient nerve in the vicinity of the surgical defect, e.g. the lingual nerve, is relatively technically simple. However, the practical impact in terms of improved sensation and function after sensate flap reconstruction remains unclear.[10–12] As a general rule, better recovery of sensation may be expected in patients whose lingual and/or inferior alveolar nerves are either intact or have been used for neurorrhaphy compared to other nerves.[13] In addition, because of the innate differences in sensitivity of the oral mucosa and cutaneous surfaces, a considerable degree of sensory re-education may be necessary for useful sensation to return.[14]

The structures of the oral cavity also play a crucial role in the production of speech. Specifically, they are involved in many aspects of articulation as the various components of the oral cavity work to alter the spectral quality of the sound produced by the lungs and larynx. For example, oral competence and the normal function of the lips is critical to the ability to form bilabial phonemes such as /p/ or /b/. Likewise, velopharyngeal competence is critical for the prevention of hypernasal speech.

Functional outcome

One of the major difficulties in reporting functional outcome after treatment of oral cavity tumors is the lack of adequate and standardized measures of oral cavity function. The main problem in creating a comprehensive system that is universally applicable is the vast number of parameters that can be measured to quantify deficits in speech and swallowing. In addition, the interpretations of tests such as videofluoroscopy and some aspects of quality of life measurements are subjective, and prone to variability. Notwithstanding these limitations, several tests have been reported which attempt to measure functional outcome with respect to speech and swallowing. These include videofluoroscopy, scintigraphy, speech tasks, articulation tests, water holding tests, and evaluation of general health, food intake, mastication, and tongue mobility.[5–7,15–17]

Assessment of function and quality of life can be either general or more specific to the disease of interest, e.g. head and neck, or oral cancer. Disease-specific instruments are more relevant to the oral cancer population because they allow comparison of different treatment modalities in defined populations. Table 16.2 lists the salient features of some commonly used head and neck specific instruments. As measurement of quality of life and function is largely indirect and subjective, no particular questionnaire can be expected to be globally useful. Notwithstanding their limitations, instruments that use summary scores, e.g. EORTC QLQ-C30/H&N35, HNQOL or QL-H&N, are practical and have therefore gained common usage. Instruments that are self-administered (EORTC QLQ-C30/H&N35, FACT-H&N, QOL-RTI/H&N, QL-H&N, UW QOL), concise (HNQOL, QLQ, UW QOL), and quick to complete (UW QOL, FACT-H&N) are also likely to be more commonly favored in clinical practice. There are several reports in the literature that have used these instruments to document the functional outcome after surgical treatment of tumors of the oral cavity. Not surprisingly, the postoperative functional deficit is directly proportional to the size of the primary tumor, and hence the magnitude of the surgical defect.[2,4,17] Additionally, the site of the tumor within the oral cavity affects functional outcome. There is a progressive worsening in swallowing function as the site of the index primary changes from anterior to posterior.[4,16] Additionally, resection of the mandible further impairs speech and swallowing postoperatively.[17] From these observations, it can be concluded that the larger and more posterior the primary tumor, the greater the functional impairment postoperatively.

Another factor that has been shown to affect the functional outcome is the method of reconstruction. In one study patients were matched with regard to T stage and volume of tongue resected and then evaluated for functional outcome based on the method of reconstruction. Interestingly, patients who had a primary closure of their surgical defect showed better function then those who had a free flap reconstruction.[16] Obviously, a selection bias exists in this study, with smaller T_3 lesions being more likely to be closed primarily than extensive T_3 lesions, which would be reconstructed with a free flap. In our experience, free flaps are used primarily following major resection and in this setting, the use of free tissue transfer adds tremendously to the functional and esthetic outcome.

The use of adjuvant postoperative radiation therapy can also influence quality of life. Although alterations in speech were reported in one study, patients who received postoperative radiation therapy showed poorer swallowing function than

Table 16.2 Some commonly used quality of life instruments for head and neck cancer

	EORTC-QLQ-C30 HN Module[21]	FACT-HN Module[22]	UWQOL[23]	HNRQ[24]	QOL-RTI/HN[25]
Mode of administration	Self	Self	Self	Interviewer	Self
Number of items	21	11	9	22	12
Internal reliability	Yes	Yes	Not demonstrated	Yes	Yes
Repeat reliability	Not demonstrated	Not demonstrated	Partially demonstrated	Not demonstrated	Yes
Validity	Yes	Yes	Partially demonstrated	Partially demonstrated	Partially demonstrated

EORTC-QLQ, European Organization for Research and Treatment of Cancer – Quality of Life Questionnaire; FACT-HN, Functional Assessment of Cancer Therapy – Head & Neck module; UW QOL, University of Washington Quality of Life questionnaire; HNRQ, Head and Neck Radiotherapy Questionnaire (McMaster University); QOL-RTI/HN, Quality of Life – Radiation Therapy Instrument/Head & Neck module (University of South Florida).

those who did not.[18] Again, the selection bias inherent to such a retrospective study does not allow meaningful interpretation of the data since the patients who need postoperative radiation therapy are more likely to have had larger, more ominous primary tumors.

Finally, in one study, the benefit of rehabilitation treatment in the form of range of motion exercises was evaluated. It was demonstrated that a benefit in swallowing function was seen in those patients who performed range of motion exercises throughout their rehabilitative process.[3] This certainly argues for the routine use of such exercises after treatment of oral cavity tumors.

Rehabilitation

Speech and swallowing rehabilitation of the patient treated for cancer of the oral cavity can be considered in two broad categories: reconstruction of the surgical defect and rehabilitation of the functional defect.

With regard to the reconstruction of the surgical defect, several general principles can be applied. The reconstructive procedure of first choice should be the simplest option likely to provide maximal restoration of form and function. Small defects can be closed primarily without restriction of function. Likewise, if a small defect can be adequately resurfaced with a split-thickness skin graft then the use of free tissue transfer is unwarranted. The second principle in the reconstruction of surgical defects of the oral cavity is to replace like with like. With the evolution of free tissue transfer this aim is much more readily achievable. The variety of donor sites with their unique composition of bone, muscle, skin and even neural innervation allows most defects to be reconstructed with a satisfactory restoration of form and even sensation.[19,20] The challenges that remain in the oral cavity for the reconstructive surgeon include the restoration of the intricate motor function of the resected organ as well as the complex three-dimensional structures of critical regions such as the oral commissure.

It should be realized that the balance in achieving these two overriding principles is often at odds. Striking a balance between the principles of simplicity and sufficiency is governed by the surgical defect, its functional and esthetic implications, and the resources available to the head and neck surgeon. Regardless of the clinical situation, a variety of reconstructive options exist for almost any surgical defect, as outlined in the section on reconstruction.

Once the surgical defect has been adequately reconstructed, rehabilitative efforts are directed toward maximizing the function of the residual and transposed tissue. The initial aspects of this rehabilitation occur shortly after surgery as the operative bed heals and residual sensation and mobility return. Additionally, if innervated free tissue grafts have been utilized, sensation will often return to these tissues with time. During this early postoperative period it is critical for the patient to maintain maximal mobility. Often progressive increase in the movements of the jaws and tongue over time will prevent fibrosis and restriction in movement.

A special note must be made with regard to the preservation of the ability to open the mouth widely and the prevention of trismus. Any patient who undergoes treatment of a lesion in the oral cavity is at risk for the development of trismus. Trismus is much easier to prevent than it is to correct once it has set in. Performing exercises in which the mouth is opened as widely as possible several times a day can prevent trismus. An easy method of actively promoting jaw excursion is to instruct the patient to use fingers to pull the mandible and maxilla in opposite directions as frequently as possible during the post-treatment phase. A stack of wooden tongue depressors may also be used to progressively widen the interincisoral opening over time. Finally, various devices, e.g. TheraBite®, are available to act as aids that facilitate active opening of the mouth. These devices, however, are often cumbersome and difficult to use in all but the most highly motivated patients. The prevention of trismus is obviously critical to all aspects of the rehabilitation of speech and swallowing after treatment of tumors of the oral cavity.

If an anatomical defect persists following surgery, prosthetics can often be used to further restore form and function. One area where great success has been seen with this approach is the use of a palatal obturator in the rehabilitation of the postmaxillectomy defect. The obturator restores velopharyngeal competence, prevents nasal regurgitation, and preserves the esthetic contour of the cheek.

While these aforementioned techniques are all passive methods of rehabilitating the patient with oral cavity cancer, there are also various active techniques that can be utilized. The speech pathologist is a critical player in these efforts. The sophisticated nature and scope of the speech and swallowing evaluation performed by the speech pathologist is beyond the scope of this text. In simple terms, however, an examination of the structural and functional deficits of the patient is obtained. This may include radiographic examination of the swallowing process in the form of a modified barium swallow, as well as functional endoscopic evaluation with sensory testing (FEEST) with the use of a fiberoptic nasolaryngoscope. A treatment plan is formulated which addresses these deficits and uses various exercises and treatments to maximize the function of the remaining structures as well as facilitating the adoption of alternative means to overcome the deficient function. It is important for everyone involved in the patient's care to realize that speech and swallowing rehabilitation is a long process that can often be frustrating. A considerable degree of patience and perseverance is necessary, on the part of both the patient and the caregiver, to achieve the goal of optimal rehabilitation.

Finally, it should be noted that the best postoperative rehabilitation will not overcome the deficits caused by poor surgical planning which does not respect the functional subunits of the oral cavity. A vivid illustration of this fact is the impact on function of the method of closure of the surgical defect after resection of early anterior tongue lesions. When a transverse wedge of tissue is resected which encompasses the tumor and is closed primarily, minimal functional or esthetic deficits result. In contrast, when the same lesion is resected in a longitudinal fashion, resulting in a serpentine elongated tongue, significant effects on speech and swallowing are often seen.

The optimal rehabilitation of patients treated for tumors of the oral cavity therefore requires adequate preoperative planning, optimal reconstruction, postoperative assessment of deficits and limitations, and rehabilitative methods that will allow the patient's quality of life to approximate or return to normal levels.

References

1. Dejonckere PH, Hordijk GJ. Prognostic factors for swallowing after treatment of head and neck cancer. Clin Otolaryngol 1998; 23: 218–223
2. Denk DM, Swoboda H, Schima W, Eibenberger K. Prognostic factors for swallowing rehabilitation following head and neck cancer surgery. Acta Otolaryngol (Stockh) 1997; 117: 769–774
3. Logemann JA, Pauloski BR, Rademaker AW, Colangelo LA. Speech and swallowing rehabilitation for head and neck cancer patients. Oncology (Huntingt) 1997; 11: 651–656; discussion 659
4. McConnel FM, Logemann JA, Rademaker AW et al. Surgical variables affecting postoperative swallowing efficiency in oral cancer patients: a pilot study. Laryngoscope 1994; 104: 87–90
5. Pauloski BR, Logemann JA, Rademaker AW et al. Speech and swallowing function after anterior tongue and floor of mouth resection with distal flap reconstruction. J Speech Hear Res 1993; 36: 267–276
6. Pauloski BR, Logemann JA, Rademaker AW et al. Speech and swallowing function after oral and oropharyngeal resections: one-year follow-up. Head Neck 1994; 16: 313–322
7. Pauloski BR, Rademaker AW, Logemann JA, Colangelo LA. Speech and swallowing in irradiated and

nonirradiated postsurgical oral cancer patients. Otolaryngol Head Neck Surg 1998; 118: 616–624
8. Rademaker AW, Pauloski BR, Colangelo LA, Logemann JA. Age and volume effects on liquid swallowing function in normal women. J Speech Lang Hear Res 1998; 41: 275–284
9. Ardan J, Kemp F. The mechanism of swallowing. Proc R Soc Med 1951; 44: 1038
10. Vriens JP, Acosta R, Soutar DS, Webster MH. Recovery of sensation in the radial forearm free flap in oral reconstruction. Plast Reconstr Surg 1996; 98: 649–656
11. Lvoff G, O'Brien CJ, Cope C, Lee KK. Sensory recovery in noninnervated radial forearm free flaps in oral and oropharyngeal reconstruction. Arch Otolaryngol Head Neck Surg 1998; 124: 1206–1208
12. Netscher D, Armenta AH, Meade RA, Alford EL. Sensory recovery of innervated and non-innervated radial forearm free flaps: functional implications. J Reconstr Microsurg 2000; 16: 179–185
13. Santamaria E, Wei FC, Chen IH, Chuang DC. Sensation recovery on innervated radial forearm flap for hemiglossectomy reconstruction by using different recipient nerves. Plast Reconstr Surg 1999; 103: 450–457
14. Cordeiro PG, Schwartz M, Neves RI, Tuma RA. Comparison of donor and recipient site sensation in free tissue reconstruction of the oral cavity. Ann Plast Surg 1997; 39: 461–468
15. Muz J, Mathog RH, Hamlet SL, Davis LP, King GA. Objective assessment of swallowing function in head and neck cancer patients. Head Neck 1991; 13: 33–39
16. McConnel FM, Pauloski BR, Logemann JA et al. Functional results of primary closure vs flaps in oropharyngeal reconstruction: a prospective study of speech and swallowing. Arch Otolaryngol Head Neck Surg 1988; 124: 625–630
17. Haribhakti VV, Kavarana NM, Tibrewala AN. Oral cavity reconstruction: an objective assessment of function. Head Neck 1993; 15: 119–124
18. Pauloski BR, Rademaker AW, Logemann JA, Colangelo LA. Speech and swallowing in irradiated and non-irradiated postsurgical oral cancer patients. Otolaryngol Head Neck Surg 1998; 118: 616–624
19. Urken ML, Buchbinder D, Weinberg H et al. Functional evaluation following microvascular oromandibular reconstruction of the oral cancer patient: a comparative study of reconstructed and nonreconstructed patients [see comments]. Laryngoscope 1991; 101: 935–950
20. Urken ML. The restoration or preservation of sensation in the oral cavity following ablative surgery. Arch Otolaryngol Head Neck Surg 1995; 121: 607–612
21. Aaronson NK, Ahmedzai S, Bergman B et al. The European Oragnization for Research and Treatment of Cancer QLQ-C30: a quality-of-life instrument for use in international clinical trials in oncology. J Natl Cancer Inst 1993; 85: 365–376
22. D'Antonio LL, Zimmerman GJ, Cella DF, Long SA. Quality of life and functional status measures in patients with head and neck cancer. Arch Otolaryngol Head Neck Surg 1996; 122: 482–487
23. Hassan SJ, Weymuller EA Jr. Assessment of quality of life in head and neck cancer patients. Head Neck 1993; 15: 485–496
24. Browman GP, Levine MN, Hodson DI et al. The Head and Neck Radiotherapy Questionnaire: a morbidity/quality-of-life instrument for clinical trials of radiation therapy in locally advanced head and neck cancer. J Clin Oncol 1993; 11: 863–872
25. Trotti A, Johnson DJ, Gwede C et al. Development of a head and neck companion module for the quality of life – radiation therapy instrument (QOL-RTI). Int J Radiat Oncol Biol Phys 1998; 42: 257–261

17 Prosthetic restoration and rehabilitation of the orofacial cancer patient

Brian F Conroy, Per Ingvar Brånemark and Peter T Blenkinsopp

Introduction

The aim of this chapter is to identify the role of cranio-maxillofacial prosthetic and technological involvement in the management of the patient who presents with malignant disease in the orofacial region and to define essential principles. The origins, objectives, location of prosthetic therapy in the body milieu, clinical foundation criteria and details of modern associated surgical and technical procedures will be described. Our prime intention is to provide proven and relevant information based on wide experience and involvement in this field that leads to optimum restoration and rehabilitation following ablative surgery and the aftermath of radiation therapy. For convenience and brevity the term cranio-maxillofacial prosthetics and technology will hereafter be identified as CMFPT.

This chapter is designed to establish a bridge of understanding between the surgical and clinical oncologist and the CMFPT team. The intention is to identify the essential aims, limitations and the positive possibilities of prosthetic involvement and its potential to make a meaningful contribution to the management of the head and neck cancer patient in general, and in the orofacial area in particular. The other chapters in this book will provide the prosthetist and technologist with a rich and informative overview of the oncologist's aims and objectives, and furthermore an indication of those areas that are problematical and of goals that are difficult to achieve.

It is true to say that modern treatment objectives and the different modalities used in the management of orofacial cancer are tending to move towards synergetic type relationships. Co-operation that transcends the boundaries of surgery, medicine, applied science, engineering, technology and prosthetics is more likely to lead to an end point that is greater than the sum of the individual contributions. The adoption of the team approach in head and neck oncology has been of paramount importance in seeking to offer the patient optimum clinical management and care. CMFPT can contribute much to the team's activities at all stages of the patient's treatment.

Origins and current status

The beginnings of CMFPT are well enshrined in antiquity, there being a plethora of evidence to authenticate that a range of traditional skills and natural materials have been used over several centuries in the construction of prosthetic therapy intended to assist the individual beset by acquired deformity or malfunction.[1] This in the main, however, can be best described as having been essentially the practice of an art and a craft as procedures were very mechanistic and craft orientated (Fig. 17.1). In recent years the more craft orientated stance and mainly artisan approach has given way to a more scientifically based type of service that can now be defined as the practice of an art and a science. This, to a large extent, can be attributed to clinically related procedures having to meet more stringent requirements and the advent of clinical audit. The institution of better training and educational pathways, the deployment of more sophisticated techniques and better understanding of the materials used in modern practice has done much to clinically and scientifically underwrite the role of CMFPT in the management of the orofacial cancer patient.

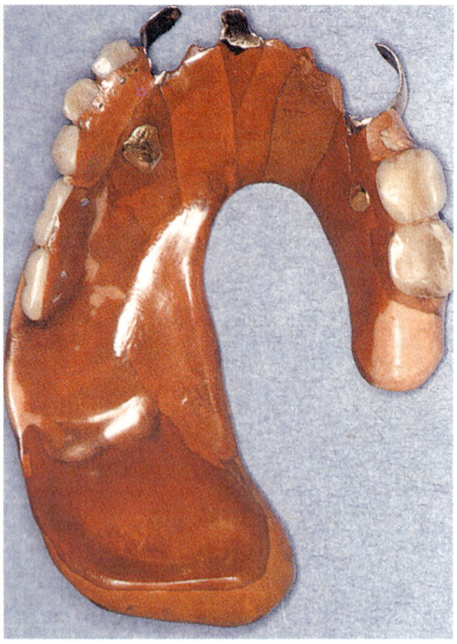

Figure 17.1 A vulcanite obturator prosthesis fabricated circa 1923 for Sigmund Freud, the famous Austrian psychiatrist. Freud underwent a low level posteriorly sited maxillectomy and removal of the coronoid in an attempt to eradicate a malignant lesion said to be a verrucous carcinoma. Freud often referred to his prosthesis as 'his monster' due to the method of retention used and the lack of pre-prosthetic preparation of the defect site.

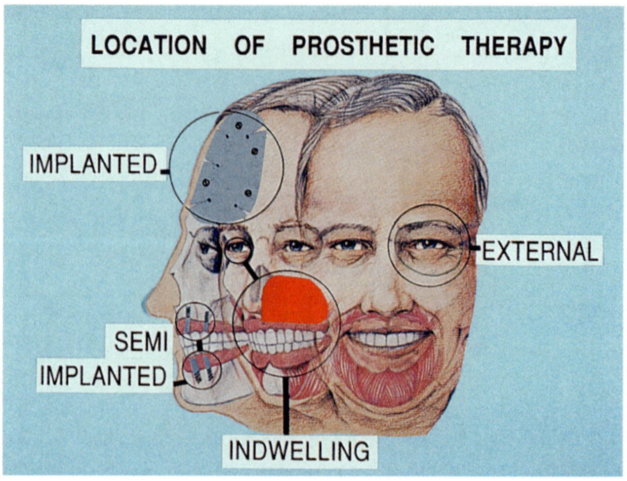

Figure 17.2 The location of prosthetic therapy in the cranio-facial region.

Aims and objectives

The principle aims and objectives of CMFPT are to accomplish the following, when the patients' special needs require prosthetic involvement in their treatment:

1. To facilitate immobilisation and control of compromised structures.
2. To provide protection and support.
3. To aid the elimination of pain and discomfort.
4. To restore or improve functionality.
5. To facilitate therapeutic modalities.
6. To maintain or improve appearance.
7. To lift the spirit and restore morale.

Location and role of prosthetic therapy and devices in the craniomaxillofacial region

The utilisation of prosthetic therapy and the purpose of implanted devices can be identified by the anatomical site they occupy and the service they provide (Fig. 17.2):

1. *The deep buried implant:* devices placed beneath the body exterior and usually sited on or attached to bone in order to maintain skeletal continuity or restore contour (see Fig 17.60).
2. *The semi-implanted device:* this device is essentially in three parts: (1) the fixture, which is sited in bone; (2) the transmucosal or transcutaneous abutment, which projects through the mucosa or skin; (3) the prosthetic abutment, which provides a source of anchorage and a means of load distribution (the key components of osseointegration technology) (see Figs 17.71 and 17.79).
3. *The indwelling prosthesis:* a prosthesis sited in a natural or surgically created body cavity, i.e. the oral or orbital cavity. Its purpose is to maintain the dimensions of the cavity and/or to restore appearance and function (see Figs 17.48 and 17.58).
4. *The external device:* A prothesis sited on the body exterior which serves either to provide protection or to restore a semblance of normality by replicating the colour and form of impaired or absent structures (see Figs 17.70 and 17.80).

Classification of craniomaxillofacial prosthetic therapy services

The service role of prosthetic therapy and the devices deployed in restoration and rehabilitation in the craniofacial region are set out below:

1. *The surgical splint:* the device that facilitates *immobilisation and control* of body structures in order to aid the normal processes of physiological repair. Splintage is generally required

to prevent macro-movement of damaged or surgically modified hard tissue structures or to provide a source of support and protection to soft tissue structures following injury or surgical procedures (see Figs 17.14 and 17.16).

2. *The splint–prosthesis:* the device that provides *basic support and preservation* of form and function where structures are in a compromised state or flux following injury or surgical intervention, especially in the immediate postoperative phase of treatment. This hybrid prosthetic device generally serves in a temporary or intermediate capacity and may also be required to contribute to restoration of appearance (see Figs 17.38 and 17.39).
3. *The functional appliance:* the device that indirectly aids the resolution of *dysfunctionalism* presenting at a site or sites *distant* to the actual location of the appliance. This type of appliance embraces a group of prosthetic devices that provide a means of rest, support or physical activation of distantly located body structures that are impaired, at risk or require to be exercised or activated in order to overcome, for example, trismus becoming more debilitating, or aid speech following a glossectomy (see Fig 17.64).
4. *The therapeutic device:* a device that applies a direct source of *energy or medicament* to a specific site in order to achieve a particular purpose, e.g. stretching, compression, translation, dissipation of body fluids or conveyance of a radiotherapeutic agent or a prophylactic chemical agent (see Fig 17.8).
5. *The definitive prosthesis:* any device that restores or replaces missing or incomplete body structures by artificial means that brings about *restoration of appearance* and/or varying degrees of *functionality* depending on the specific structure involved. For example, a dental obturator prosthesis has the capacity to restore function and appearance, whereas an artificial eye prosthesis will only provide a semblance of normal appearance, but not the patient's vision. While deep buried implanted prostheses are usually expected to serve in a life long capacity, intra- and extra-oral prostheses require to be replaced from time to time, due to changes in the morphology of the supporting body structures, or when wear and tear makes a prosthesis functionally or aesthetically unacceptable (see Figs 17.50–17.72 and 17.80).

Restoration and rehabilitation objectives defined

Replacement or repair of structures that have been lost, modified or impaired following ablative procedures is directed towards the restoration of anatomical form, in other words, return of continuity and cosmesis, whereas rehabilitation is concerned with achieving the return of functionality and psychological well-being. Prosthetic and surgical management should ideally aim to bring about both restoration and rehabilitation. The following identifies some of the residual and functional problems that can arise in the wake of a disease process or following a surgical procedure carried out in or around the oral cavity. They are impairment of:

- the ability to masticate, swallow and control food and liquids
- the ability to maintain full jaw activity
- oral competency
- tongue mobility
- speech performance and
- appearance.

The importance of retaining facial harmony both in relation to colour, texture and form would appear to be an obvious expectation on the part of the patient. However, observations made over many years would seem to indicate that many patients, especially older patients, are more concerned with residual functional problems that are associated with drooling due to loss of oral sphincter performance, the ability to take food and liquid in a controllable manner and moreover, the escape of food and liquid through acquired defects, particularly in the lower third of the external face. Such types of incapacity and impairment are in the main best treated by surgical means, because prosthetic therapy has little to offer in such situations, other than in a palliative or short term role. In the early stages of ablative therapy most patients are more concerned with the inability to speak, eat, drink and swallow than they are about cosmesis. Function is therefore generally perceived as having a higher priority. This is not to say that appearance can be ignored, because the patient's long-term perception of their body image will certainly become a more important aspiration and cause for concern, especially when major changes in facial harmony pertain. Therefore, wherever possible, both restoration and rehabilitation should be the principal objective from the very onset of treatment.

Surgical or prosthetic reconstruction

The decision to use either surgical reconstruction or prosthetic methods to achieve restoration and rehabilitation following ablative surgery is currently very much a matter for debate. Different head and neck cancer units have developed varying views

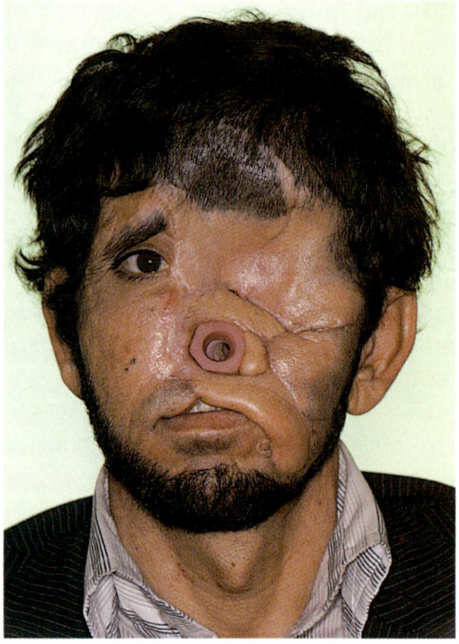

Figure 17.3 Following extensive resection of malignant disease, this patient was managed by a combination of surgical and prosthetic procedures. The former addressed the structures at risk, and the latter, residual dysfunction and appearance. Note the presence of the intra-oral obturator prosthesis already in place.

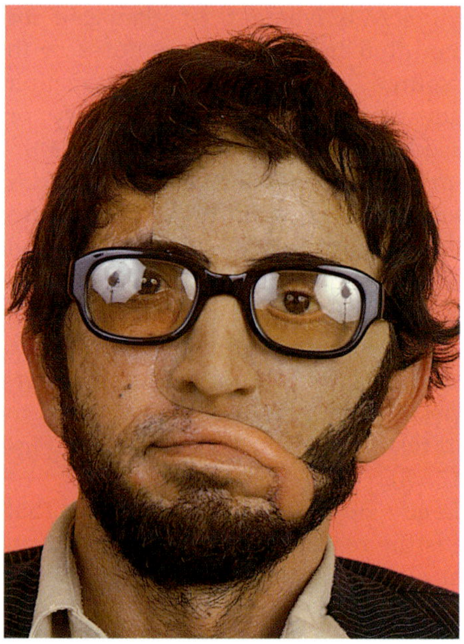

Figure 17.4 The large scalp flap used in this patient's post-resection management covers and protects a massive residual defect site that involves the frontal region, part of the base of skull, the mid face and the dento-alveolar and palatal structures. In order to support the intra-oral obturator during functional activity, the facial prosthesis was designed to extend into the facial defect (on the hollow box principle) to provide a counterforce to resist the upward directed thrusting force exerted against the thin flap by the obturator. The facial prosthesis was purposefully fabricated in hard acrylic to provide strength, stiffness and a lightweight construction. Because of the patient's occupation (a farmer) and the climate in which he lives the facial prosthesis was made in a darker shade bearing in mind that he had been hospitalised for many months. There are many instances when the surgeon and the prosthetist can work together to provide the patient with optimum restoration and rehabilitation.

and, to some extent, the choice of modality has become a controversial issue. Selection of prosthetic or surgical reconstruction requires to be an open and ongoing assessment decision process, in order to serve the patient's best interest. In reality, surgical reconstruction has to be the method of choice, especially where dynamic structures are involved, for example the lips, lower third of the external face and the mandible.

The location and nature of the disease process, especially its propensity to recur, the patient's age, associated medical conditions and the willingness of the patient to undergo additional operative procedures that may leave further evidence of surgical intervention are all important factors that require to be carefully examined and balanced. It also has to be said that, in some institutions, surgeons have no choice but to resort to surgical reconstruction because modern and innovative prosthetic services are not available to them due to lack of locally based, adequately trained and well-motivated staff with appropriate clinical and laboratory facilities.

Surgical or prosthetic rehabilitation should not be allowed to become an issue of competition but used as a thought-provoking process where sound and ethical judgement is applied to each patient's specific clinical, social, functional and psychological needs. Some patients will benefit from a total surgical input, especially where vital structures are at risk and malfunction pertains, and some patients from total prosthetic involvement, and very often from a combination of both modalities (Figs 17.3 and 17.4).

It is important that total adherence to one or other modality does not prevent progress. With all the developments that are being achieved in both fields there is much to be said for joint co-operation and involvement. It should not be overlooked that surgical reconstruction, in some cases, is either not possible, is contra-indicated, or has failed. Prosthetic expertise in this field of activity is the product of considerable experience and long training and, not least, requires the motivation and facilities to provide a viable prosthetic service. In other words, this type of highly skilled and, of necessity, properly resourced service cannot be set in place over night.

It is essential that the maxillofacial prosthetic/ restorative service is seen as an integral part of the oncological team's activities and not a reserve player. Discussion and co-operation from the onset of assessment and treatment planning certainly helps to circumvent any shortfall in the total management of the patient. There are distinct benefits to be accrued if the CMFPT team is fully involved in early assessment and treatment planning because it helps to assure that any special dental, restorative and prosthetic needs are addressed and, furthermore, steps can be taken to provide essential therapy before active treatment begins.

If prosthetic restoration and rehabilitation is to be successful, it is paramount that adequate conditions to achieve retention and stability be in place or steps taken to provide alternative sources of direct and indirect support.[2] This can often be accomplished immediately following resection by utilising preprosthetic surgical procedures or by the placement of osseointegrated implant fixtures at strategic sites in and around the defect.[3] Such procedures need to be discussed and planned well before major surgery is carried out.

Adherence to the team philosophy concept is essential if all the nuances of modern cranio-maxillofacial prosthetic, dental and restorative dentistry are to be fully deployed in the patient's interest. It has to be appreciated that being a member of the oncological team brings with it certain additional responsibilities and duties, not least the requirement to be readily available to serve the patient's special needs as they arise, but also to maintain an ongoing optimistic and sympathetic presence. In addition, there is an obvious need for clinical and technical experience. Satisfactory patient care hinges on the team members having those special social skills that engender confidence and trust. A willingness on the part of the patient to participate in the restorative and/or prosthetic rehabilitation programme, which in all probability has hitherto been a totally unknown field of activity to them, is also a key factor. This aspect of the cranio-maxillofacial prosthetist's work is best described as 'social engineering' because the correct type of approach at the onset can influence the patient's perception of what maxillofacial prosthetics has to offer them.

As already reported, many patients, especially those with acquired major deformity and dysfunction, will also have varying levels of emotional and psychological distress. This places special pressures on the prosthetic team members because they are required to provide not only kind words (which are important) but also a level of prosthetic rehabilitation and restoration which maintains the patient's social and clinical needs. This often takes place in very difficult and demanding clinical circumstances and, not least, from time to time the inability of the prosthetist to match his or her skills or a material's properties to the patient's expectations. This calls for a high level of motivation, innovation and compassion on the part of the prosthetist that must be matched by an equal in-depth understanding of the clinical and technological procedures and the expertise required to provide a viable prosthetic after care service. The true professional will endeavour to make the patient a co-partner in the overall scheme of things and will not promise anything more than he or she can deliver. It is important that the surgical team members do not give the patient an unrealistic idea of what the maxillofacial prosthesis team can provide.

Fundamental oncological treatment protocol

It is imperative that those not directly involved in the surgical and medical management of the cancer patient have an understanding of the clinical treatment protocol and, moreover, its limitations and objectives.

The principal objectives in the management of orofacial malignancy, where circumstances permit, are aimed at the preservation of life. Achievement of this goal may necessitate varying degrees of radicality depending on the type of lesion involved, its specific location and the local extent of the disease and possible general dissemination. Some tumours have an associated poor prognosis, whereas some lesions are more amenable to treatment. Where the prognosis is considered to be unfavourable the procedure of necessity in this type of case is often to offer the patient a less radical form of treatment. This may involve just simple debulking of the tumorous mass to ease the patient from further pain, discomfort and malfunction, which may be carried out in combination with radiotherapy. However, both types of treatment can leave in their wake very varying degrees of disability and morbidity.

Patients with benign lesions may also have to undergo extensive surgical procedures to bring the disease under control and improve functionality. In both situations the consequential aftermath of such ablative procedures has to be addressed if residual deformity and malfunction ensue, in order to achieve optimum restoration of the quality of life.

Essential considerations in surgical and prosthetic management

Clinical considerations

The management of orofacial cancer is all too often considered to be a success if the patient, by the various modalities of treatment available to us, is rendered free of his or her disease for a reasonable period of time. However, our criteria for success should be far more critical than this. Unless the patient is returned to society with a degree of confidence, the ability to communicate with his fellow human beings and the ability to eat and drink in such a way as to gain adequate nourishment there will be a shortfall in maintenance of function. While the doctor may consider this on balance to be a successful outcome, the patient is unlikely to agree.

With the advancement of surgical techniques and improved instrumentation the resection of many tumours today is less destructive than it may have been a decade or so ago. With the ability to replace resected structures with vital hard and soft tissue as autografts, acceptable reconstruction has also become a reality.[4] The morbidity of these reconstruction techniques, however, can be substantial and as many of the patients who develop orofacial cancer may be old or unwell due to alcohol intake and smoking, these advanced surgical techniques of reconstruction may not be appropriate or may have a high risk of failure, for example, in the diabetic and post-radiotherapy patient.

Wherever possible, external structures should be replaced by viable soft tissue taken from a local or distant site but, in doing this, the surgeon, for example, should be aware of the subsequent need to create an adequate cavity to be able to replace a lost eye with a prosthesis and, in the upper jaw, an obturator prosthesis. The need to establish a firm base to resist masticatory forces in a reconstructed maxillary or mandibular site is of prime importance. In the lower jaw structural continuity is highly desirable but, as a compromise, a dental prosthesis can sometimes be managed by the patient even when only half or two-thirds of the mandible remains. Recent advances in osseointegrations technology by van Oort and Reintsema[5] have resulted in great improvement in this area of prosthetic management (Fig 17.5). Insertion of large volumes of soft tissues to fill defects in the oral cavity, without being cognisant of future dental and prosthetic needs, will inevitably end in failure from a total restoration and rehabilitation point of view.

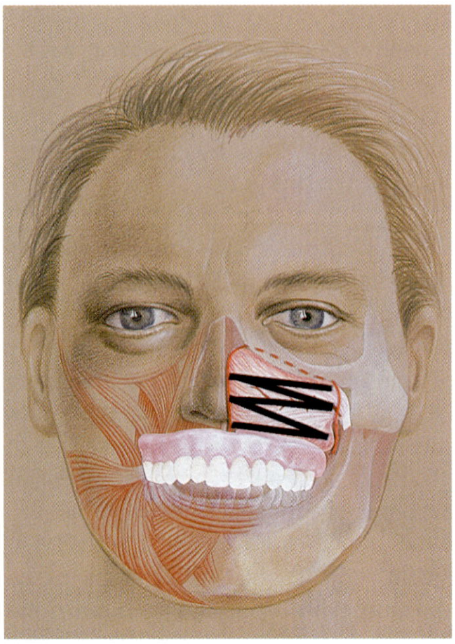

Figure 17.5 Surgical reconstruction of orofacial defects should aim to restore like with like. A mass of soft tissue placed in a mid face defect will provide little support for an intra-oral prosthesis. In this type of surgical reconstruction, the resultant differential stability (due to the lack of a bony framework) will over a period of time result in impairment of the remaining dento-alveolar arch due to shear loading forces.

It is now accepted that the management of the orofacial cancer patient should be planned by the oncologist and surgeon, but the future functional requirements of that patient should also be jointly considered at the initial stages of treatment with the maxillofacial prosthetist, restorative dentist, speech therapist and dietician to ensure that function can be restored as well as elimination of the disease.

The restoration and rehabilitation of the orofacial cancer patient is dependent upon many factors, both general and local, with which the reader will be familiar, but nevertheless are worthy of re-stating. The general health of the patient prior to treatment is of paramount importance and, as already described, many of the patients with this type of disease have been heavy smokers most of their lives and may also have consumed above average amounts of alcohol. Their general metabolism is, therefore, under par, and they may have advanced arterial disease, a factor that can mitigate against successful surgical reconstruction as a good blood supply is crucial for the healing of all tissues.

The diabetic patient and the patient on chemotherapy also present a greater surgical reconstructive risk and, likewise, patients who have had previous radiotherapy will also tend not to heal well and, therefore, will be prone to hard and soft tissue failure due to endarteritis obliterans. Age in itself is not a contra-indication to advanced reconstructive techniques and, in some instances, this may be preferable as tolerance in the older person of a prosthesis may be difficult to achieve.

The site, extension and expected biological progression of the disease are crucial local factors for consideration. Surgical clearance of the tumour may all too often not be possible because of the late presentation of the disease, but surgical palliation is often necessary to prevent the patient developing a debilitating fungating tumour in the orofacial region. In this situation, the patient should not be considered for complicated reconstruction techniques and the emphasis of management be placed on prosthetic rehabilitation.[2]

As already stated, replacement of the external face should, whenever possible, be by soft tissue transfer, as should reconstruction of defects of the floor of mouth, tongue and soft palate. Restoration of the mandible, whenever possible, should be achieved by means of a vascularized bone graft with insertion of dental implants at this time or subsequently when the resection involves the body of the mandible. Restoration of the hard tissue of the upper jaw and mid-face is an area where controversy remains, but reconstruction can only be considered to be successful if full closure of the defect is achieved, to allow swallowing and speech, and the patient is able to masticate and speak. This inevitably implies the necessity to establish a sound bony base to resist the forces conveyed by a dental prosthesis during speech and mastication.

If restoration and rehabilitation are to be realised by surgical reconstruction, the technique most commonly used is a free tissue transfer of bone from the iliac crest using vascular anastomosis of the deep circumflex iliac arteries. This can be a very successful technique as it usually provides an adequate bony base for implants to be inserted, but nevertheless, the morbidity and the time required to carry out surgical reconstruction may preclude its utilisation in many patients.

Prosthetic considerations

Modern obturation of the maxillary defect, especially when using a soft hollow silicone shell/obturator attached to a dental prosthesis, still remains the most satisfactory form of rehabilitation for the majority of patients if sufficient retention and stability is achievable (see Fig. 17.50). However, with the advent of osseointegration implant technology, an alternative source of retention, stability and load distribution is now readily achievable (see Fig. 17.68). It should not be overlooked that successful maxillofacial prosthetic rehabilitation, especially osseointegration technology, has its own demands and a full understanding of the principles associated with these techniques is a prerequisite.[3]

The bony surfaces of a maxillary defect, for example, must be smoothed in all areas and covered by robust mucosa or a skin graft if the obturator prosthesis is not to cause pain when forces are applied to the supporting foundations during mastication and speech. This should be carried out immediately following resection and before skin grafting the defect site.

While certain bony under-cut sites within the maxillary defect can be a valuable source of retention, especially if a soft silicone obturator is to be used, they have the potential to cause pain and ulceration if a hard acrylic obturator is used, particularly during insertion and withdrawal of the prosthesis. The normal dentition, albeit often reduced following resection, is invaluable for the retention of an obturator prosthesis and, therefore, every step should be taken to maintain the patient's natural teeth for as long as possible.

All patients should have an examination by a specialist in restorative dentistry to ascertain what teeth have an extended prognosis and how the dental health may best be restored and preserved. The periodontium supporting the teeth should be brought back to good health, if that is not the case. Daily treatment with fluoride gel in an applicator will reduce any predilection to dental decay. The retention of intra-oral maxillofacial prostheses should be planned at the early assessment stage, noting which teeth can be safely retained and utilised and how the forces generated during mastication and speech will be distributed via the intact remaining maxillary structures. Consideration should always be given as to whether implants can be usefully employed and possibly inserted at the time of primary surgery. Also, at this stage, teeth that are beyond salvage, or those that will have inadequate alveolar bone support due to the margin of the resection having to be extended close to the tooth or teeth, may need to be extracted as their long-term prognosis will be poor. Without supporting alveolar bone, the tooth adjacent to a defect site will soon be lost. It should be anticipated that the alveolus around the tooth socket will need to be cut back and smoothed and then local flaps of mucous membrane placed over these margins to give a comfortable interface between the bony buttress and the prosthesis.

All patients who have undergone a maxillary resection should have a temporary obturator supported by

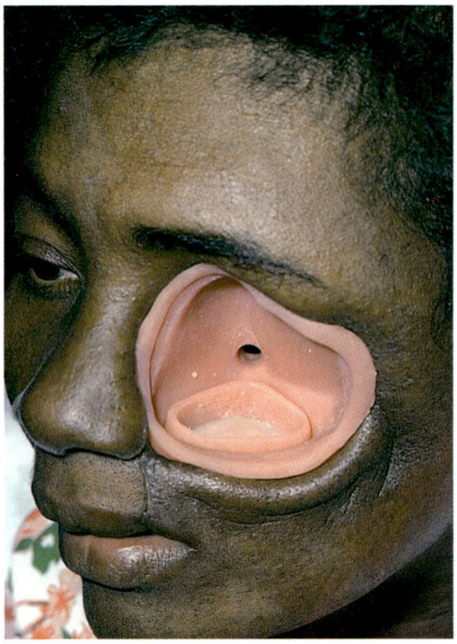

Figure 17.6 All surgically created maxillary defects should be immediately obturated to maintain essential function and, where indicated, external facial contour and appearance.

a surgical splint inserted at the time of the primary surgery to allow a rapid recovery and re-establishment as far as possible of normal nutritional intake and speech (Fig. 17.6). The patient should never be left with a large open intra-oral defect, as this is both demoralising, dysfunctional and inhibits recovery. The raw surfaces at the surgically created defect, especially the inner aspect of the cheek, should be covered with a split skin graft to prevent contraction. (It should be noted that a skin graft will not take on areas of intact respiratory mucosa.) Extra stability and precise location of the skin graft can be achieved by directly suturing its margins to the edges of the surgically created defect. Mucous membrane removed from the bony walls of the nasal cavity, however, will soon become re-epithelialised by local spread of epithelium and therefore does not need to be covered by a split skin graft as contraction at this site will not take place. A split skin graft applied to the mobile cheek tissues, denuded of mucosal cover, will, without doubt, provide a more substantial lining than leaving the raw area to heal by secondary intention. The latter is often friable and does not tolerate the frictional load placed by a prosthesis on the defect site (see Fig. 17.29).

It should be the aim of the surgical team to undertake all preprosthetic surgery at the primary operation. The need to carry out subsequent preprosthetic procedures will only delay prosthetic rehabilitation. Furthermore, healing may be compromised, especially if postsurgical radiotherapy has to be administered (see Figs 17.20–17.22).

Where a tumour directly involves the lower jaw, then clearly that portion of the mandible with an adequate healthy margin of bone has to be resected and, wherever possible, immediate surgical reconstruction undertaken. Various bone grafting techniques are well established, with free tissue transfer providing the optimal results. The aim should not be just to provide bony continuity, but to install an adequate volume of bone to allow the insertion of mucosal penetrating implants to aid the retention of a lower prosthesis (see Fig. 17.73).

It should not be overlooked however, that in certain cases a deep buried mandibular implant prosthesis can effectively restore skeletal continuity and maintain essential function (see Figs 17.60 and 17.61).[6] Restoration of form and function with a deep buried implant prosthesis in this very complex anatomical field is largely dependent on certain important criteria being met. This, to a large extent, is determined by such factors as whether the patient has been in receipt of radiation therapy and the amount given, the site and extent of the defect, the quality and thickness of the overlying soft tissues and the ability to establish mechanical attachment and biomechanics. The latter is perhaps the most important factor because when skeletal continuity is lost deviation of the remaining segment or segments of the mandible will occur. Functional disharmony or imbalance will place the screws retaining the implant-prosthesis, the intact parts of the mandible and the surrounding soft tissues subject to abnormal loading.

Malignant tumours which lie in close proximity to the mandible should, wherever possible, be resected using bone sparing techniques to preserve the continuity of the lower jaw. This may involve the resection of the alveolus leaving the basal bone or, as in tumours of the floor of the mouth, resecting the lingual cortex of the bone along an appropriate length in continuity with the tumour. Resection of the alveolus will often leave adequate basal bone for short implants to be placed in the lower border of the mandible. Additional longer implants can be placed in the remaining intact portions of the alveolar ridge, the number being dictated by the limitations of the anatomy. The long implants will provide anchorage for retention and the short implants will aid stability and load distribution. Experience has shown that, in this situation, it is advisable to make the bar frame work in three separate parts because of the bending moment in the body of the mandible.

The retention of the large maxillary prosthesis has been advanced by the employment of silicone rubber obturator shells which are both comfortable and allow engagement of bony undercut sites which hitherto could not be utilised (see Fig. 17.48).[7] More recently, the development of the osseointegration implant system has revolutionised the prosthetic management of the resectioned patient (see Figs 17.75 and 17.78).[8]

The foregoing has reviewed the essential objectives and has identified those issues that need to be addressed at the early planning stage. Attention will now be turned to outlining the protocol used to gain a systematic assessment of the oral cavity in relation to early and late prosthetic restoration and rehabilitation.

Bioengineering considerations

Research by Conroy[9] and Ghazzawi[10] identifies the importance of biophysical energy in maintaining the integrity and vitality of hard and soft tissue structures. The concept that functional stress is essential to the maintenance of structural form and performance at the macro- and microscopic levels is the basic premise reflected in the design features of the prosthetic therapy promoted in this chapter. Our objective is to apply sound biomechanical engineering principles to the restoration and rehabilitation of the patient with a post-resection defect. This is based on the role played by biophysical energy in maintaining homeostasis. This requires an in-depth understanding of how the human body works and what can impair its integrity, especially following ablative procedures. There is ample evidence that all the musculoskeletal systems work in concert with one another when both systems are intact and operating correctly. The two systems are, in fact, totally dependant on one another, which maintains their integrity and purpose both from a mechanical and biological point of view. Forces generated by the musculature, both at rest and during functional activity, not only result in extrinsic perceived body movement but also in an intrinsic manifestation of forces within the bone, which is not perceivable. These forces functionally stress the bone, both directly and indirectly. The overall situation is one of force and counterforce, since the external and internal forces are of equal magnitude (they are in a *state of balance*). In other words, the human body seems to exhibit all the principles set out in Newton's Third Law of Motion, which states that all forces are met by equal and opposing forces.

In engineering terms, muscles can be identified as being linear motors, exerting either a pulling or squeezing action, but never a pushing action. The muscles are powered by fuel cells which generate the electrical energy that activates the muscle fibres, resulting in contraction. This shows that the human body is essentially dependent upon two elements: (1) a structural framework – bone; (2) a power source – muscle. Study of the former has been described as human engineering, and the latter biomechanics. All of the muscles in the craniofacial area contribute in varying degrees to the realization of functional activity, e.g. mastication and, conjointly, internal stimulation of bone at the cellular level. Both contribute to the maintenance of the stress–strain ratio that dictates vitality, mass, performance, adaptation and optimization of the musculoskeletal system.

In order to determine the service role of the bony structures that make up the craniofacial skeleton, an engineering appraisal has been carried out by Conroy.[11] This research is presented in Fig. 17.7 indicating that the craniofacial skeleton is composed of the following structures: (A) the main load distribution pathways in

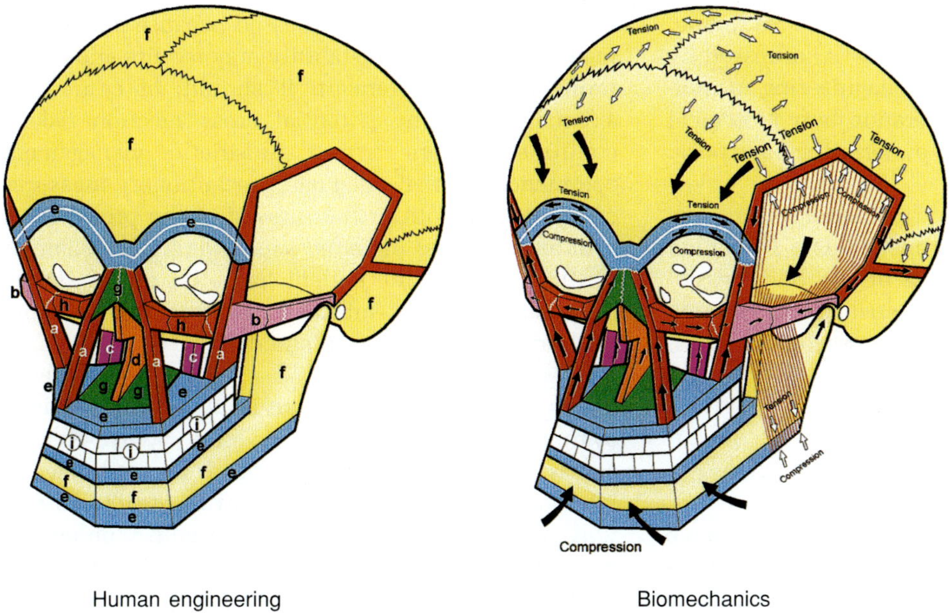

Figure 17.7 An engineering appraisal of the cranio-facial skeleton that identifies the role of the bony framework and the musculature. The former provides support and protection and the latter generates internal and external energy which results in functional activity and internal stimulation of bone.

the mid-facial area, which act as *pillaster buttresses*; (B, C) the zygomatic and pterygoid structures (*horizontal and vertical flying buttresses*, respectively), resisting outward and backward-directed thrusting forces; (D) the vomer (*oblique buttress*), primarily resisting backward and upward-directed forces; (E) the supraorbital ridges, the dentoalveolar ridges and the lower border of the mandible (*arch beams*), resisting forces applied from opposite directions; (F) the corticocancellous structures, i.e. the cranial bones and body and rami of the mandible (*plate buttresses*), responsible for transmitting applied load and resisting bending moments; (G) the hard palate and palatine bone, together with the nasal bones (*tie beams*), preventing outward spread during functional activity; (H) the inferior orbital margins (*joists*), redistributing minor load-bearing forces; and (I) the teeth (*cantilevered beams*).

This research work is based on photoelastic studies and finite element analysis. The sutures that hold the skeletal elements to each other serve as microscopic shock absorbers or dampers and the adjacent bony margins are, in turn, subjected to tensile and comprehensive forces. The periodontal membrane of the teeth also acts as a shockbreaker.

All this would seem to indicate the desirability, wherever possible, of restoring nature's in-built pathways for distributing functional forces, and in maintaining the stress–strain ratio in bone at the microscopic level, because there is ample evidence to confirm that bone that is not functionally stressed or is understressed will undergo adverse change. The important factor is maintaining the optimum magnitude and vector of load distribution within the craniofacial bony structures.[12]

Prosthetic and surgical restoration and rehabilitation should, wherever possible, aim to maintain both essential functional activity and long-term preservation of the structures that form the craniofacial region, at both micro and macro levels. This is addressed by applying sound biomechanical engineering principles, whilst taking into consideration how biological structures are programmed to perform their purpose.

The transmission of bioelectrical energy through bone would appear to be the mechanism by which the brain prevents overloading of the body structures. No doubt, it is also bioelectrical energy sources that play an integral role in osseoperception.

Assessment protocol

The first stage when dealing with patients who have malignant disease in the orofacial region is to establish a good rapport, because this will be the beginning of an ongoing professional relationship. It is essential that the patient is made aware of what the CMFPT team can bring to their treatment, both during the early ablative phase and, moreover, in the long term. Of prime importance at this stage is to offer the patient and other family members reassurance and confirmation that prosthetic therapy will be commenced at the operative stage (if the treatment requires it), and continue on an ongoing basis. Interestingly, patients often state, years after their surgery, that it was the commitment to provide prosthetic after-care and the sympathetic support they received initially, that gave them the strength and motivation to undergo ablative surgery. One should endeavour to create a sense of trust. The fact that someone has made a commitment to achieve their optimum restoration and rehabilitation, helping to assure their place in society, will provide the patient with hope for the future.[2,13]

At the first assessment it is necessary to determine the patient's general status including mental state, followed by assessment of the oral cavity. This should be carried out systematically starting with a series of pertinent questions that help to clarify the patient's general medical condition, especially any problems that might affect or compromise prosthetic management, such as arthritis, especially in the hand, or limited sight. These two factors alone can often mitigate against using a complicated device which involves intricate manual dexterity to locate and remove it. It should not be overlooked that poor eye sight can also impair the patient's ability to maintain good oral hygiene, which may be a contraindication to using crown and bridgework, or even osseointegrated implants unless other family members can fulfil this requirement.

It should not be forgotten that the patient may have other medical conditions that can affect their general well-being and mental stability. The patient's general mental state needs to be assessed because long-standing and deep-seated instability may require additional professional management. It should, of course, be axiomatic that any potential cross-infection risk is confirmed before active prosthetic management commences so that adequate precautionary measures can be taken, both in the interest of the professional staff and of other patients. It is strongly advisable to confirm whether the patient has a history of allergy or sensitivity to any substance, especially if a custom made device is to be implanted.

In the first instance, it is advisable, when about to evaluate the condition of the oral cavity, first to assess what is not compromised by the disease. Ultimately, it is the intact remaining structures that will afford retention and stability for prosthetic reconstruction. Examination should be carried out in the order shown in Table 17.1.

Table 17.1 Order in which examination for prosthetic therapy should be carried out

1. Assess the state and mobility of the oral stoma. Previous surgery may have left in its wake residual scarring and limited opening of the mouth.
2. Examine the buccal sulci for signs of scarring, fibrosis, lack of sulcus depth and restricted mobility.
3. Examine the floor of the mouth and the tongue, especially in relation to limitation of functional activity, i.e. tethering, and signs of possible traumatic injury to the tongue by adjacent teeth or prostheses.
4. Examine the hard palate for abnormal morphology, i.e. an excessively large maxillary torus or fistuli.
5. Attempt to quantify the functional status of the soft palate and note if any residual scarring or any other abnormality is present, i.e. swallowing difficulties.
6. Examine the remaining natural teeth and their supporting structures on an individual basis and quantify their status in relation to:
   (a) Oral hygiene
   (b) Periodontal disease and especially signs of furcation involvement compromising the molar teeth
   (c) Grossly carious and broken down teeth
   (d) Teeth with symptomatic evidence of irreversible pulpitis
   (e) Periapical infection
   (f) Overerupted and unopposed teeth
   (g) Grossly malpositioned individual and quadrants of teeth
   (h) Teeth with razor sharp edges
   (i) Malocclusion or lack of adequate occlusal stability
   (j) Condition of any crown and bridge restorative work
7. Assess the quality of any removable dental prosthesis and its potential use in future operative or dental restorative procedures.
8. Determine and record the maximum amount of jaw opening the patient can accomplish.
9. Assess any possibility of neuromuscular impairment, for example facial palsy, or swallowing difficulties.

Information gathering

The foregoing primary clinical assessment requires to be substantiated by radiographic evidence. This should include facial, intra-oral and panoral radiographs. It is advisable also to obtain intra-oral and facial photographs of the patient. Of principal importance is the taking of upper and lower impressions which should include as much as possible of the lesion and its surrounding structures. The centric jaw relationship should be recorded and the study models mounted on an articulator. If a surgical splint or immediate obturator is to be constructed it is advisable also to take the shade of the patient's teeth (see Fig. 17.30). It is also advisable at this stage to measure how far the patient can open the lower jaw and whether any degree of deviation occurs.

Dental study models will provide useful information and help in forming both the surgical and prosthetic treatment plan and, furthermore, allow the surgical splint and any other therapeutic appliance that may be required to be fabricated on a duplicate model (see Fig 17.12). Mounted study models will allow for an immediate obturator to be constructed and fitted following a maxillary resection.

It is only on the basis of assessing the patient's general medical and oral status, coupled with an understanding of the histological and radiographic evidence and the principles of prosthetic management, that an informed assessment and choice of the optimum type and level of prosthetic management can be made.

Implementation of urgent dental and restorative procedures

When a benign or malignant lesion presents in the oral cavity and where surgical intervention or radiotherapy is envisaged in the dentate patient, a course of oral hygiene and any urgent need for restorative dentistry should be implemented immediately. The patient with a high level of oral hygiene and teeth in good condition will certainly tolerate the ablative procedures, from a dental point of view, better than those with a poor standard of care. The following sets out the principal investigative and treatment measures that should be taken.

1. Establish the status and prognosis of individual teeth and their supporting structures and carry out essential restorative repair.
2. Identify those teeth immediately adjacent to a malignancy, especially those involving the tongue, floor of mouth and cheeks, as this may be a strong indication for extracting such teeth in order to facilitate the following:
   (a) Achievement of a tension-free flap from the tongue or cheek
   (b) Avoidance of postoperative traumatisation of irradiated soft tissues and ulceration of locally diverted flaps
   (c) Circumvent the possibility of radiation-induced caries at the site of maximum dosage

(d) Avoid the need for late extraction of teeth with a poor prognosis leading to osseoradionecrosis.

Post-radiation induced complications

It is well understood that the orofacial hard and soft tissue structures undergo adverse degenerative changes following radiotherapy that can influence and, on occasion, complicate or delay prosthetic management. Experience has shown that radiation will result in epithelial structures undergoing atrophy, and connective tissues becoming fibrosed and less vascular. The bone, especially the marrow, can be expected to change in character, as it will become avascular with associated ongoing fatty and fibrous degeneration.

A decreased rate of salivary flow with an increase in viscosity should also be anticipated, especially if the parotid gland is involved in the field of irradiation. All these factors can influence prosthetic management, especially in the early stages of treatment, but will rarely preclude long-term prosthetic care. It used to be advocated that patients should be advised not to wear their prosthesis for at least 2 to 3 years following receipt of radiation. However, current clinical practice would indicate that, when the mucosal structures are healed, there is no good reason to prevent patients from using their prostheses as they will in fact provide functional stimulation of the underlying hard and soft tissue structures. A requirement, however, is to make the prosthesis atraumatic by removing any irregular areas, i.e. sharp cusps and making the fitting surfaces as smooth as possible.

It is our experience in the lower jaw that, following radiotherapy, healing is much slower than in the upper jaw, and furthermore, that osseointegrated implants placed in the irradiated mandible do less well than those placed in the maxilla. This can, no doubt, be attributed to the fundamental differences relating to the blood supply in the lower more dense mandibular bone as compared to the more vascular maxillary structures. This leads to an overall impairment in osteoblastic and osteoclastic activity. There may in fact be some merit in placing implants in the irradiated bone, especially the mandible, at an early stage before the endarteritis obliterans becomes established, as they may reduce this adverse change by enhancing functional stimulation.

Extractions should be carried out atraumatically at least 14 days prior to the commencement of radiotherapy or at the time of surgery under antibiotic cover. A local alveolectomy should be performed to hasten bony remodelling and aid epithelial healing over the site, which otherwise will be impaired. Primary closure without tension between the flaps is essential. Experience has shown that if sharp projecting bony spurs are not removed they have the potential to cause necrosis and ulceration of the overlying mucosa.

The delivery of radiation may be interstitial or external beam. A common aftermath of such treatment is the onset of xerostomia, which is dose related, especially if the parotid gland is in the radiation field. Xerostomia is directly related to the reduction of the volume of saliva and changes in its viscosity and pH. The symptoms of this debilitating and miserable condition are impaired speech and mastication, difficulty in swallowing, lack of taste and appetite and general discomfort. Furthermore, many patients find it impossible to wear their prosthesis and any remaining natural teeth can quickly develop extreme sensitivity to hot and cold associated with rapid onset of rampant caries, especially at the cervical margins.

The use of artificial saliva substitutes, usually delivered in a carrier, brings a degree of respite and relief (Fig. 17.8). The use of pilocarpine hydrochloride may help to induce improved secretory activity in some patients. Dosage is up to 30 mg per day.

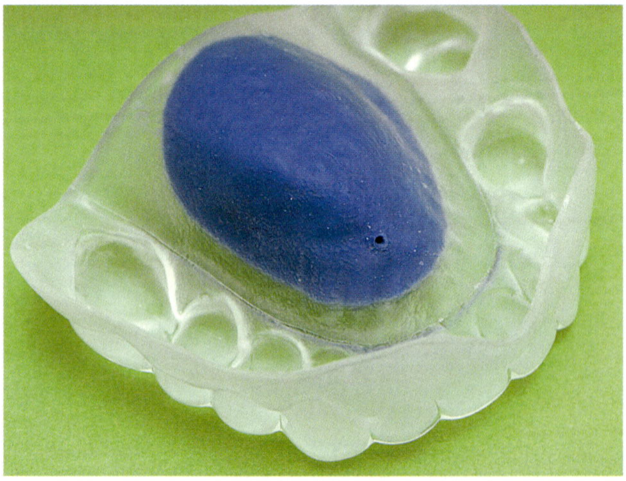

Figure 17.8 This therapeutic appliance delivers a supply of artificial saliva when a palatal soft membrane is compressed by the patient's tongue. The holding chamber above the membrane is filled with artificial saliva through a small hole on the superior fitting surface of the device. When the membrane is activated by the patient the viscous fluid is expressed via the aperture and filters out from the under surface of the device.

Mucositis

This condition usually begins some 2 to 3 weeks into radiation and continues to the completion of this modality. The signs of mucositis are the presence of mucosal erosions and oedema coupled with ulceration and pain, with associated difficulty in maintaining oral hygiene and eating. The optimum treatment is to irrigate or swab the mouth with 0.2% chlorhexide gluconate (for plaque control) and to use a 0.2% benzydanine HCI (Difflam) analgesic mouthwash. Topical or systemic corticosteroids are also useful when the condition is acute. Candida overgrowth can be treated with miconazole gel, or any other antifungal agents. When mucositis is very severe and the patient has intractable pain, and nutritional input is severely compromised, the insertion of a PEG may be indicated to keep the oral cavity clean and maintain nourishment.

Osteoradionecrosis

Bony structures of high density (particularly the mandible) tend to absorb a greater amount of radiation. Occasionally this is manifested as ischaemic necrosis combined with superficial contamination of exposed bone, which usually does not sequestrate due to failure of osteoclastic activity. This very incapacitating condition is one of the serious complications that can arise following extraction of teeth in patients who have undergone a course of radiotherapy. This situation can also occur spontaneously in the presence of periodontal or periapical disease or following mucosal ulceration and the local removal of exposed bone. Severe examples may be associated with an acute infection or pathological jaw fracture. Treatment necessitates the atraumatic removal of any involved teeth and utilisation of metronidazole 400 mg 8 hourly, for soft tissue control. Ultrasound has been used at a dose of 1 watt/cm^2, 3 megahertz, pulsed 1 in 4 to the mucosa overlying the site of radionecrosis for 15 minutes daily for up to 25–50 treatments. Hyperbaric oxygen therapy may, however, be the treatment of choice. Severe cases in the lower jaw may eventually need a partial mandibulectomy.[14]

All patients who have to undergo orofacial radiation are potentially at risk from dental caries and as a prophylactic measure rigorous pretreatment is essential. The most effective preventative regime is to use fluoride gel rather than toothpaste which is an irritant, especially in the inflamed mouth. Sodium fluoride thixotropic gel 1% is placed in an applicator which is worn over night. Patients should be advised to avoid high sugar content foods and drinks. Promotion of chewing to encourage saliva stimulation should be recommended. This group of patients will require ongoing specialist management of their dental needs for at least 5 years following their course of radiotherapy.

Design and construction of splintage and therapeutic appliance therapy devices

Maxillary considerations

Where the integrity of the maxillary structures are to be changed following resection, resulting in skeletal discontinuity with associated loss of oral competence, a surgical splint and obturator mould will be required (Fig 17.9). The role of the surgical splint and obturator mould is defined in Table 17.2.

The design features of surgical splints that are to be employed in the maxillary region will vary depending on the type of resection to be carried out, location of the defect and its magnitude. The surgical splint should meet the criteria listed in Table 17.3.

A simple classification of maxillary resections is shown in Fig. 17.10.

Armed with the information of the location of the lesion and the provisional plan of the resection

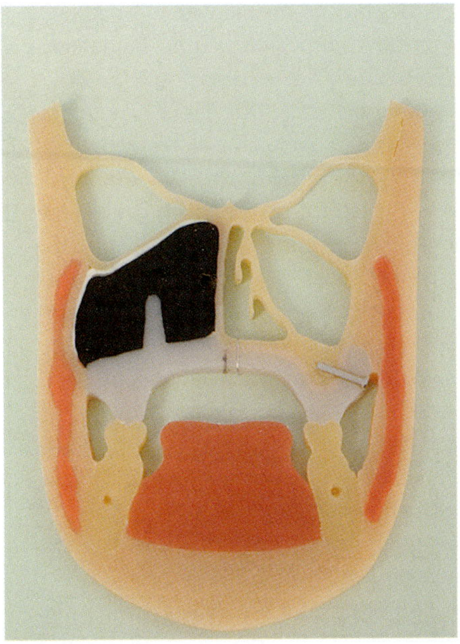

Figure 17.9 The role of the split-plate and the obturator mould. Note the method of fixation used to retain the surgical splint and the mechanical means of securing the obturator mould, i.e. the tapered vertical post.

Table 17.2 Role of the surgical splint

1. Seal off the defect site from the oral cavity in order to prevent escape of air, food and liquid.
2. Maintain the volume of the surgically created defect in order to prevent contractual shrinkage of the surrounding non-bony supported soft tissues structures, i.e. the cheeks and lips.
3. Maintain an oral seal to permit normal speech.
4. Allow mastication and swallowing.
5. Facilitate the close adaptation of a skin graft to areas that are denuded of mucosal cover within the defect site, especially the inner aspects of the cheeks and lip.
6. Maintain the patient's vertical intermaxillary dimension.
7. Prevent the condylar head being drawn upward into the glenoid fossa by contractual forces causing pain in the joint and the ear.
8. Maintain a semblance of normal appearance (dental and facial)
9. Maintain the patient's morale.

Table 17.3 Criteria for the surgical splint

1. Provide mechanical support for the obturator mould.
2. Be sufficiently well retained by direct or indirect fixation in order to resist displacement by functional forces that will be applied against it and prevent movement of the obturator mould within the defect.
3. Allow postoperative inspection in the immediate post-resection phase of the defect site without having to remove the source of direct or indirect fixation, e.g. transnasal or per-alveolar wiring or bone screws. This is achieved by making the surgical splint a two-part device, i.e. a fixed element and a removable element.)
4. Allow the surgical splint to be used, even if the operative procedure requires to be more extensive than originally planned by providing a facility for local extension or an alternative method of fixation.
5. Maintain speech, mastication, and swallowing in the immediate postoperative phase.
6. Cause no hindrance or discomfort during tongue activity, mastication and swallowing.
7. Maintain external facial contour where skeletal support has been lost.
8. Ensure that the device does not damage teeth and soft tissue structures.
9. Allow the surgical splint, at the completion of treatment, to be removed with minimum inconvenience or discomfort to the patient.

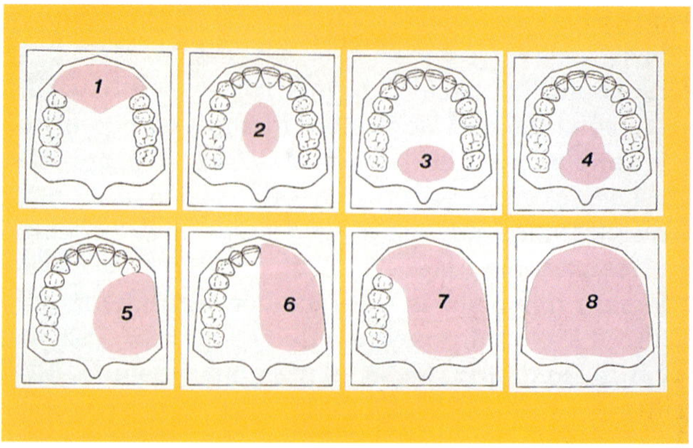

Figure 17.10 A classification of standard maxillary resection procedures. Please note, the precise delineation of each maxillary defect can vary to some degree, depending on the location and the size of the lesion.

procedure to be carried out, steps can then be taken to design and fabricate the surgical splint.[15] If maxillofacial laboratory facilities are not to hand, it may be possible to convert an existing denture into a surgical splint. While this is not the ideal method circumstances will prompt the need for innovation and compromise. In a hemi-maxillectomy case, for example, the patient's full upper denture can be modified by cutting back the labial and buccal flanges and creating a flat platform in the area of the proposed resection. In a posteriorly extended resection case it may also be necessary to extend the back edge of the dental prosthesis with auto-polymerising acrylic. Using the same material, a vertical location post can also be fabricated on the fitting surfaces of the modified denture in the anticipated area of the resection, siting the post in the centre of the platform.

In large resection cases, a vertically orientated location post/s has the distinct advantage of allowing the modified denture and, moreover, any type of maxillary sited surgical splint to be removed independently from the surgical mould, in its own dictated pathway, and the obturator mould in a different pathway as dictated by the shape and orientation of the defect site (Fig. 17.9). This applies to all maxillary defect sites, with the exception of defects 2, 3 and 4 in the maxillary resection classification (Fig. 17.10). Surgical obturation in these cases is primarily concerned with providing local support for the resection margins and maintenance of the oronasal/antral seal. Defects in the posterior maxillae and, more especially, in the soft palate area are better managed with a one-piece surgical splint or a mechanically retained extension to which the surgical mould is firmly bonded because it is easier to insert and remove such devices (Fig. 17.11; see Fig. 17.16). To prevent accidental inhalation of the

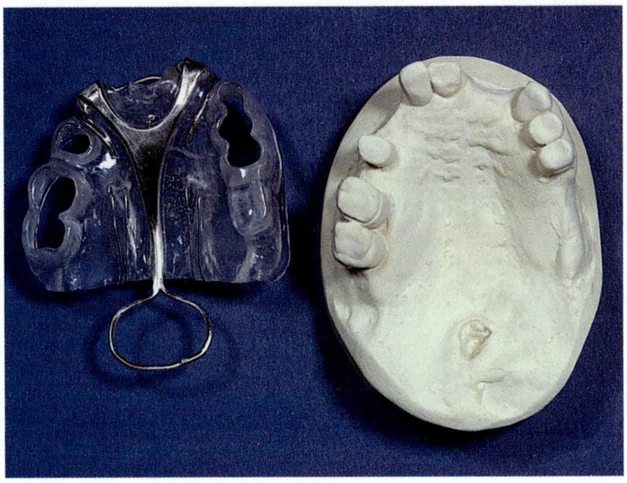

Figure 17.11 An example of a two-part splint that establishes a source of positive fixation (when wired in position) and provision of a detachable unit, which allows withdrawal of the obturator section, without having to remove the fixed element. This type of splint allows the obturator unit to be removed in the immediate postoperative phase when the patient is conscious and capable of functionally determining the shape of the surgical mould.

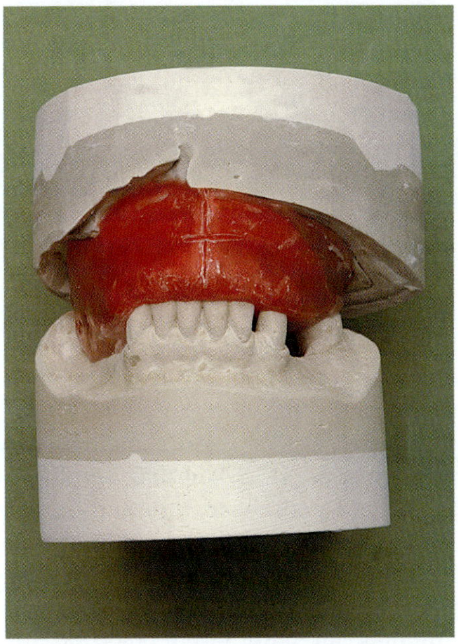

Figure 17.12 The articulated study models allow the surgical splint to be constructed and facilitate the fabrication of an immediate obturator prosthesis, when this is required.

obturator section it is safer to have the mould as an integral part of the surgical splint when obturating posteriorly sited defects. This can be a wire loop processed into the acrylic splint or a mechanically linked extension based on the sliding pair method of attachment, i.e. a double rod and tube system or screw retained device (Fig. 17.11).

Many surgeons still, however, use a wire loop around which the obturator mould is formed in maxillary resection cases 4–8. This technique has the disadvantage in large maxillary defect cases of the surgical mould and the attached surgical splint having to be removed as one element and in one path of insertion. This will involve the patient having to overextend their jaw opening when removing the splint and mould, which can be very difficult and painful, especially in the immediate postoperative stage. The need to remove the maxillary surgical splint and the surgical mould as one unit can also lead to skin grafted surfaces within the defect being damaged during withdrawal of the surgical mould. (Please note: the aforegoing does not apply to maxillary defects type 2, 3 and 4, where a one-piece device with facility to mechanically bond the obturator mould to the surgical splint is a better option.)

For optimum results, the surgical splint should be fabricated on a new model that represents the current state of any remaining teeth and the dento-alveolar and palatal structures. Using the patient's current denture as a source of obtaining a model on which to fabricate the surgical splint is not always advisable, as the prosthesis may not be well-fitting and, moreover, may have a poor occlusal relationship with the opposing lower dentition or denture. The upper and lower models should always be articulated, especially if the patient is edentulous, with the aid of a jaw registration block in order to assure maintenance of the correct vertical dimension and jaw relationship. It is essential if a Roehampton type immediate obturator prosthesis is to be fabricated to place the arm of the plane line articulator over what is considered to be the tumour free part of the maxilla (Fig. 17.12; see Fig. 17.35).

The design of the surgical splint will vary according to the following circumstances:

- If the patient is dentate and will have a sufficient number of sound teeth spread over two quadrants following the resection procedure.
- The location and magnitude of the resection site.
- If the patient is, or will be edentulous following the resection procedure.

If the patient has an adequate number and distribution of sound teeth and the operative procedure will fall into types 1, 2, 3 and 4 of the maxillary resection classification or involve operative procedures in the soft palate region, then a surgical splint fabricated in acrylic incorporating wrought metal clasps will usually provide adequate control of the surgical mould.

If the patient is, or will become edentulous following the resection, in the maxillary region or the soft palate or both, the surgical splint (either a one-piece or a two-piece device) can be retained by screw fixation or wire suspension. All edentulous patients will require some form of internal fixation and defects 4–7 will usually also benefit from a two-part surgical splint system (see Fig 17.14).

Traditionally, the surgical splint and the method of fixation for the edentulous patient and, on some occasions, patients with a poor dentition has been to use a one-piece base plate that is retained by either circum-zygomatic suspension or per-alveolar wiring and, more recently, bone screws. The disadvantages of this type of splint and, moreover, the methods of fixation used are that it is not possible to gain access easily to the defect site for inspection and cleaning purposes without removing the means of fixation. This has precipitated an alternative method of fixation using the trans-nasal wiring technique and the development of the sectional splint or split-plate technique (see Figs 17.9 and 17.14).

Our approach has not only been directed to the immediate requirement to provide a surgical obturator, but also to maintain the well-being of the remaining hard and soft tissues that are involved in load distribution and providing retention. This helps to maintain functionality and aid patient comfort throughout the postoperative phase and, from a prosthetic point of view, addresses the need to be able to prefabricate during the postoperative period an intermediate splint-prosthesis that can be inserted at the time that the surgical splint and surgical mould are removed (see Figs 17.36–17.40). The latter is dependent on the specific design features of the surgical splint.

The surgical splint basic laboratory construction techniques

Table 17.4 identifies the basic laboratory procedures that are common to all the various types of surgical splints that will be described in this section.

If the Roehampton immediate obturator technique is to be used (appropriate in maxillary resections 5, 6 and 7), it is necessary to make a duplicate of the surgical splint (see Fig. 17.33). This replica serves as a transfer jig, allowing the unknown, i.e. the shape of the surgically-created defect, to be married to the known, i.e. the intact dentoalveolar and palatal structures (see Fig. 17.34).

Table 17.4 The basic laboratory procedure relating to the design and construction of the surgical splint

1. Articulate the upper and lower models in centric occlusion (Fig. 17.12).
2. Discuss with the surgeon the extent of the proposed resection and indicate on the model (Fig. 17.13).
3. Reduce the plaster model where the tumour has caused enlargement, including involved teeth, and establish a flat platform over the proposed resection site (Fig. 17.13).
4. In dentate cases, survey the model and block out unusable dentoalveolar under-cuts, other than those sites on the labial/buccal surfaces of the teeth, that will be required for retentive purposes, i.e. placement of clasps.
5. Drill one or more 1 cm diameter holes in the plaster model at the centre of the anticipated resection area to facilitate provision of location post/s. (The number of holes it will be necessary to drill in the model will depend on the magnitude of the defect.) In the dentate case, the holes for the retention post should be in the same path of insertion as it is proposed the surgical splint will follow, so to establish a common alignment between the teeth and the surgical mould. In maxillary resections type 3 and 4 it is advisable to use a wire loop or other means of positive attachment for the surgical mould.
6. When a two-part surgical splint is indicated, the mechanical means of linking the two sections together is then constructed, i.e. the sliding rod and tube system (Fig. 17.13). This device is then located on the model close to the anticipated margin of the planned defect. One half of the linking sytem is located in the fixed element and the other in the removable element. The two sections are processed separately (Fig. 17.14).
7. Remove the upper model from its mounting assembly and duplicate it, to provide a second model on which to fabricate the surgical splint. This will allow the wax prototype surgical splint to be assembled on the master model in relation to occlusion, etc., and then transferred to the duplicate model for processing.
8. Following processing, the surgical splint is fitted back to the master model in order to confirm the fit and that the occlusion has been maintained.
9. The sides of the locating post are made flat to prevent rotation of the surgical mould within the defect site (Fig. 17.15). (When a wire loop is used, this should be checked for alignment and length in relation to the anticipated shape of the defect.)

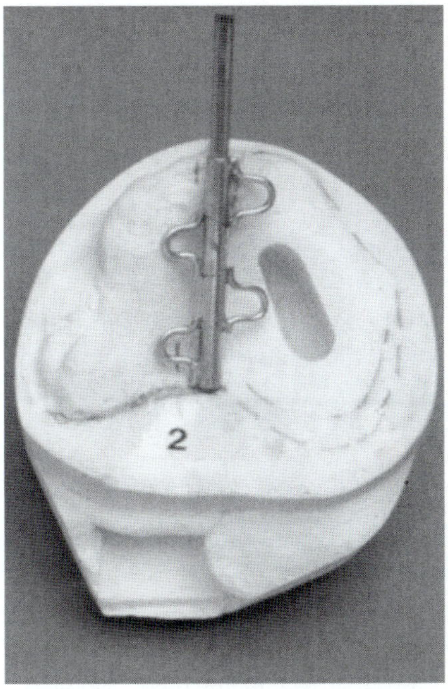

Figure 17.13 The proposed resection drawn on the model and the linking mechanism positioned adjacent to the planned operative site prior to fabricating the two-part surgical splint. Note the retention tags soldered to the oval tubing.

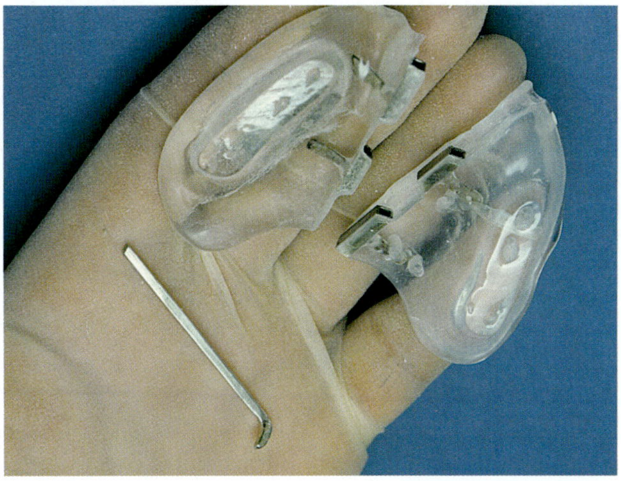

Figure 17.14 The two-part surgical splint after conversion to acrylic.

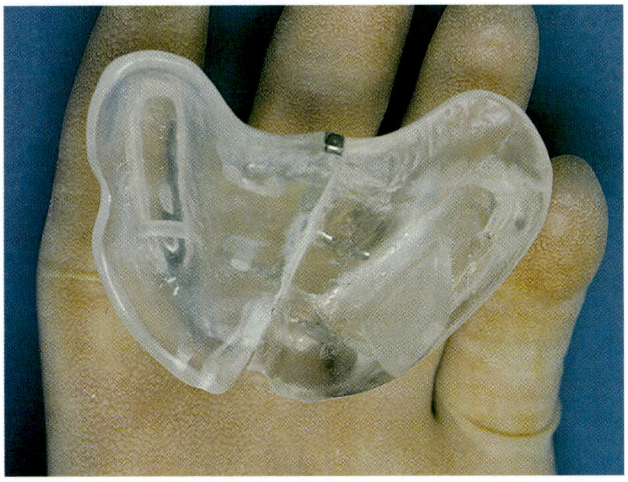

Figure 17.15 The two halves of the split-plate joined together with the linking pin. Note the small holes sited in the posterior aspect of the fixed element to provide a point of attachment for the transnasal wire. The double strand of 0.4 mm soft stainless steel wire is passed from the fitting surface of the acrylic plate so that the wires rest on the back edge of the splint.

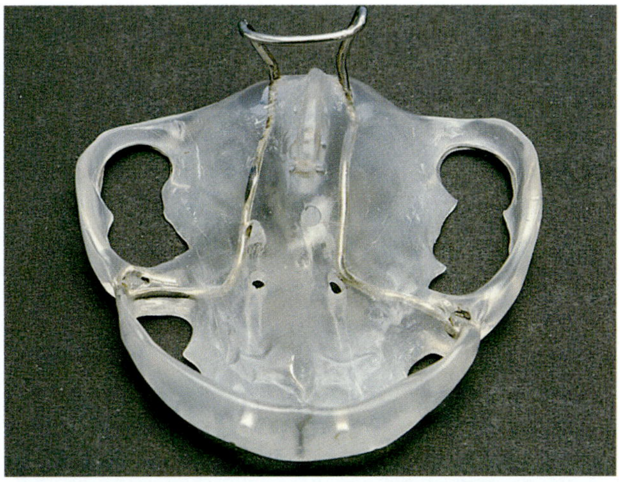

Figure 17.16 A surgical splint designed to retain an obturator mould following resection of a lesion involving the hard and soft palate structures. In this situation it is advisable to use some means of wire fixation or suspension, unless the patient has a good complement of sound teeth distributed in all four quadrants.

Soft palate resections

Loss of part or the whole of the soft palate, following ablative procedures, requires special consideration as it is a dynamic structure, that is to say, it is constantly changing in shape and orientation during functional activity. A surgical mould formed around a wire extension projecting out of the posterior aspect of a surgical splint (Fig. 17.16), at the time of surgery (when of course, the patient is under anaesthetic) is rarely a true facsimile or correctly physiologically shaped during the operative procedure with the exception of a sub- or total resection of the soft palate. The latter can be attributed to the fact that very little tactile soft tissue is left following these types of resection. Remoulding is easily accomplished if black gutta percha is used (which is a thermoplastic material) or by application of a denture conditioning paste. During the postoperative obturator moulding process the patient is instructed to swallow and speak in order to adapt the surfaces of the mould to a shape which is both comfortable, improves speech and establishes a functional seal.

If the wire framework is fabricated as a detachable unit from the surgical splint (Fig. 17.11), it will be possible at a later date to convert the moulding separately to acrylic, thus preventing distortion of the retaining plate on recuring. This technique allows a temporary obturator mould to be formed (if a second wire framework is available) that maintains function during conversion of the surgical mould to a more durable material. Following the processing of the acrylic extension, it is returned to the acrylic plate and luted in position with a mixture of quick-curing resin.

If the patient is edentulous or has a limited number of sound teeth it is advisable, if not axiomatic, to make the surgical splint a fixed component, that is to say, use trans-nasal suspension, per-alveolar wiring or bone screws. Failure to establish a means of direct fixation will almost certainly result in the edentulous case in the surgical splint and the obturator mould being displaced by applied functional forces and gravity.

Mandibular defects

Resections involving the mandible may be (1) marginal (both in the horizontal and vertical planes), (2) partial (mandibulectomy with loss of continuity) or (3) total mandibulectomy. In situation (1) it may be advisable to use some type of splint fixation in order to prevent a possible fracture of the weakened remaining lower border of the mandible during the postoperative period or in situation 2, to control the remaining fragment or fragments. Partial loss of the anterior dento-alveolar ridge can result in inward rotatory re-alignment of the posterior quadrants due to remodelling of the remaining strut of basal bone. Lingual inclination of the posterior dental quadrants can compromise the fitting of a lower partial dental prosthesis. Splint fixation will help to prevent inward rotation of the posterior quadrants (Fig. 17.17).

Where gross inclination of the posterior quadrants of the horizontal body of the mandible is long standing, this is often an indication to use a two-part prosthesis that engages the lingual under-cuts of the posterior teeth, thus gaining both retention and providing a form of splintage to prevent further inward deviation (see Figs 17.53 and 17.54).

When there is loss of bony continuity, a surgical splint with a detachable training flange can often be of great assistance, as it will help to prevent lateral and rotatory deviation of the major fragment (Fig. 17.18). This device also helps prevent the muscles undergoing contracture owing to loss of force and

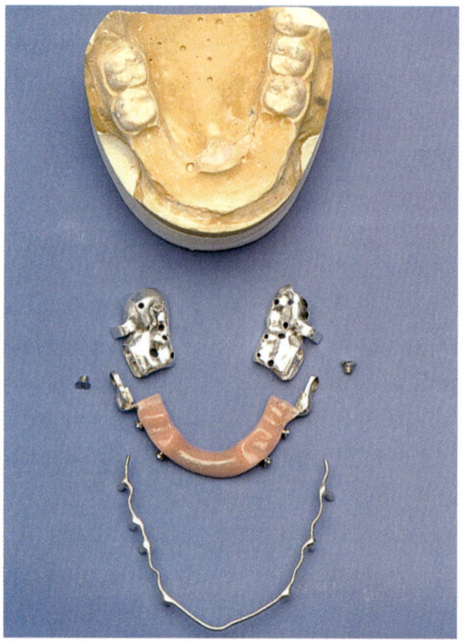

Figure 17.17 The use of cast metal cap splints and a localising block which incorporates locking plates to immobilise the posterior fragments. The arch bar allows intermaxillary fixation to be established during the immediate postoperative phase.

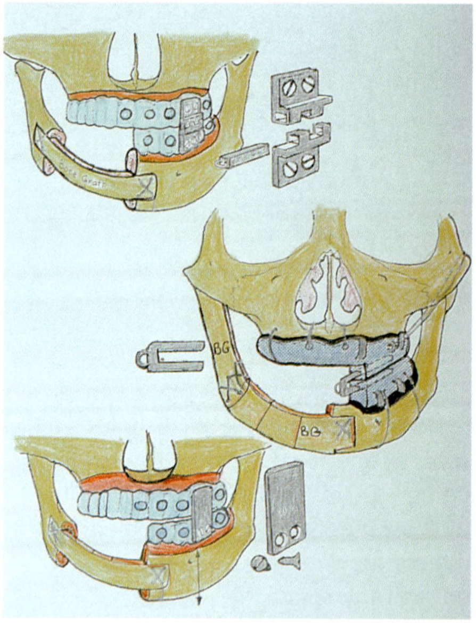

Figure 17.18 A method of immobilising the main mandibular fragment following resection in a dentate patient's treatment. The top illustration shows the lower fragment localised to the upper jaw utilising a removable plate secured with four screws. The mid illustration shows the use of Gunning type splints with a double pin localising device. The lower illustration shows how the splint system described in the upper illustration can be modified to allow the patient to open and close the lower jaw without the fragment being laterally displaced.

Table 17.5 Essential design objectives of the mandibular located splint

1. To provide adequate control and stabilisation of the mandibular fragment or fragments during the postoperative phase.
2. To provide temporary stress shielding for a bone grafted area in the immediate postoperative period (this should be discontinued after approximately 6 weeks) (Fig. 17.18).
3. The design concept should have sufficient latitude in case the resection has to be more extensive than originally planned to allow it to fulfil its proposed role.
4. The surgical splint should not interfere with normal occlusion or local functional activity.
5. Where required, the surgical splint should have an in-built facility to prevent lateral deviation of the major fragment.
6. To facilitate easy removal of the splint at the completion of treatment.

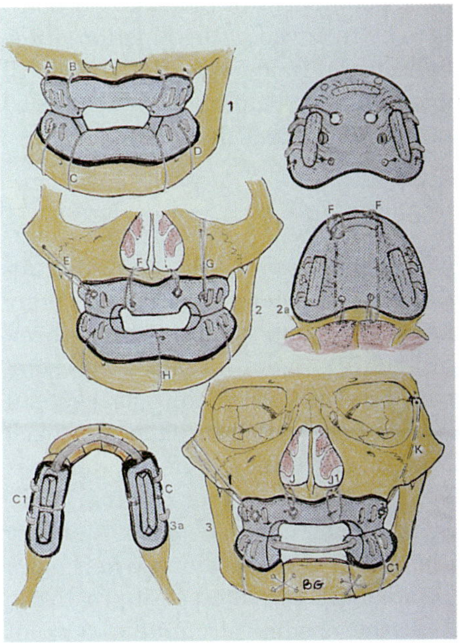

Figure 17.19 Methods of splint fixation used in the treatment of edentulous patients.

counterforce, and to overcome the forces exerted by the formation of scar tissue being an additional debilitating factor. When contemplating bone grafting, a training flange should also be considered, because it can assist in preventing harmful bending forces being placed on the bone graft itself and, more especially, on the retaining screws or wire fixation, in the immediate postoperative phase. The possibility exists for bone grafts to become disattached due to bone plates or screws either fracturing or being loosened due to stressing the means of fixation beyond the material's proportional limit and, moreover, the bone in which the screws are located.

The essential design objectives of the mandibular located splint are set out in Table 17.5.

Custom made splintage is usually in the form of a laboratory constructed fitted arch bar, metal and acrylic devices and Gunning type splints. Cast metal rings or cap splints in some cases still have a role to play in this type of reconstructive surgery if laboratory personnel with appropriate skills are available. Increasing use is being made of bonded orthodontic brackets and arch wires to obtain a means of intermaxillary fixation and stabilisation. Methods of retaining different type of custom made surgical splints as used in the edentulous patient are demonstrated in Fig. 17.19).[15]

Preprosthetic surgical considerations

The need to carry out secondary preprosthetic surgery should be avoided if at all possible and the surgical defect adequately prepared for prosthetic restoration at the time of the primary surgery.

Common problems following resection are:

1. Areas of exposed non-vital bone following radiotherapy either in the upper or lower jaw.
2. Loose fragments of bone causing pain and soft tissue inflammation.
3. Retained turbinates in the defect site.
4. Bands of scar tissue.
5. Excess flabby and compressible tissue that interferes with prosthesis stability.

Exposed non-vital bone should be trimmed back using a rotating burr with copious water coolant until, if possible, underlying vital bone becomes exposed. If this is the case, then a skin graft can be placed over the larger defect site, but minor soft tissue defects may be left ungrafted and allowed to re-epithelialise spontaneously. Very often, vital bone cannot be found following radiotherapy, in which case the bone should be cut back to a level beneath the surrounding soft tissue and left to re-epithelialise. Any sharp projections of bone should be cut back until a smooth flat surface is achieved. Bare areas of bone may be covered by local flaps, but the risk is always that the donor area may then become non-vital and a process of re-epithelialisation may be more satisfactory (Fig. 17.20).

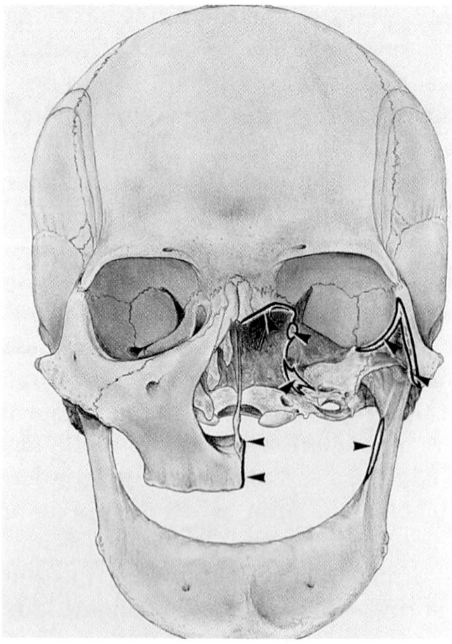

Figure 17.20 The principle sites where pre-prosthetic surgery following resection can improve the bony foundation and aid subsequent prosthetic rehabilitation and reconstruction. Note that a coronoidectomy has been carried out following a posteriorly extended maxillectomy.

Soft tissue contractures within the oral cavity following surgical intervention may abolish the normal sulci between the alveolus and the cheeks or between the alveolus and the tongue, which are important sites for prosthesis retention. Minor contractures may be relieved by Z-plasty techniques or local flaps but, generally speaking, the procedure of sulcoplasty with the insertion of a split-skin graft is the most satisfactory. The split-skin graft needs to be retained by a surgical splint that is firmly fixed in position for a period of several weeks, not only to facilitate the close apposition of the skin graft to the raw surface, but also to prevent further contraction during the healing phase. The technique of sulcoplasty may be especially valuable in the patient who has had a resection involving the floor of mouth where the operative procedure results in the tongue becoming fixed to the alveolus or cheek. This occurs either following direct repair of the remaining tissues following the resection or after insertion of soft tissue from a distant site. It should, however, be remembered that while the creation of a sulcus may assist the insertion of a prosthesis, any extra mobility of the tongue, so achieved, will be dependent upon the amount of innovated muscle still remaining.[16]

Soft palate resections

A posteriorly extended maxillectomy which involves resection of the hamulus may interfere with soft palate function. This is due to loss of tension in the soft palate, resulting from the tensor veli palatinus losing its attachment. This important structure can be relocated to the lateral pharyngeal vault, which often helps to preserve some function and, moreover, circumvents nasal regurgitation. It is also advantageous to suture the oral mucosa to the nasal mucosa following a resection that involves the soft palate structures, as this will encourage rapid healing and, moreover, permit early prosthetic restoration and rehabilitation to be instituted.

Alveolar buttresses

Following operative procedures that involve the continuity of the alveolar arch, the cut bony ends should be assessed in relation to their orientation and, where gross under-cuts are present, the overhanging bone should be reshaped to establish a common path of insertion for a prosthesis (Fig. 17.20). Failure to do so will reduce the opportunity to gain full access to the site, thus forfeiting useful stability and retention. Sharp cortical bony margins should be rounded off and, if sufficient mucoperiosteal tissue is not locally available, a flap from the cheek or buccal sulcus advanced to provide good cover of the exposed bone. When a tooth has to be removed at the junction of the defect, sufficient additional mucoperiosteal cover will be readily available following trimming back the bone tissues that previously supported the tooth.

Palatal structures

In palatal and maxillary resections, it is counterproductive to leave a large unilateral overhang of bony palate when the vomer and septum have been removed because it will prevent a seal being established between the prosthesis and the nasal lateral wall of the defect site (Fig. 17.21). This approach also applies in type 2 resections when the defect is centrally sited, i.e. mid-palate, where residual bilateral bony shelves have been created by the operative procedure. This is one of the occasions when extra bone should be removed in the interest of prosthetic rehabilitation. A further benefit from this type of approach is that the extra mucoperiosteal length will allow a cushion of soft tissue to be placed around the cut bony edges which will enhance comfort and improve oral seal and prosthesis stability. Unsupported bony shelves will, in time, atrophy due to cantilevered loading, resulting in the bone being replaced by a mobile and fibrotic mass (Fig. 17.21). If a type 5 resection has been carried out, the bony margins of the hard palate should be rounded off leaving about a 2 mm projection as this will aid retention. If it has been possible to preserve a palatal mucosal flap, this is then wrapped around the margin of the bony palate and sutured to the nasal mucosa (Fig. 17.22). If the latter is very friable, it

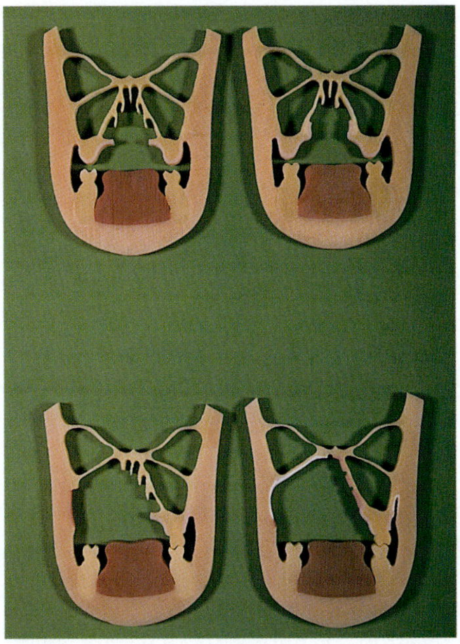

Figure 17.21 Pre-prosthetic preparation in maxillary defects 2 and 7. Upper models: trimming the residual palatal shelf and removal of the turbinates will allow access to the vertical bony supported wall of the defect site. Lower models: the recommended surgical procedure in the laterally extended maxillary resection will facilitate utilisation of the vertical wall of the defect in order to achieve maximum indirect retention and stability.

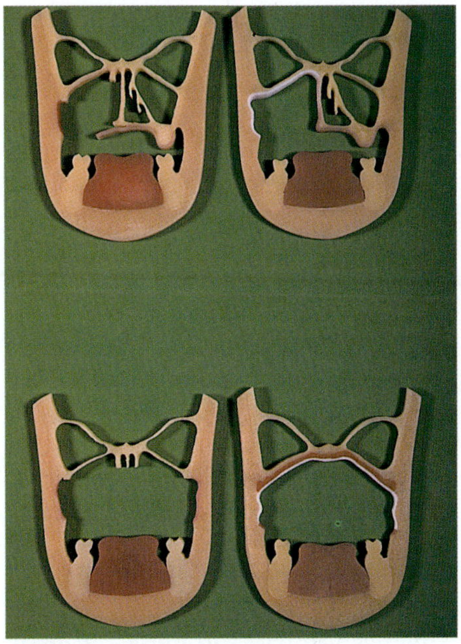

Figure 17.22 Pre-prosthetic preparation in maxillary defects 6 and 8. Upper models: reshaping the cut margin of the palatal shelf and resiting the palatal mucosa to provide a cuff of soft tissue over the bony surfaces. If the edge of the bone is left 2 mm in length this will provide a degree of biomechanical retention. Lower models: removal of projecting bony structures in the roof of the defect in the total maxillectomy case and angulating the margins of the cuts made in the zygomatic complex will aid prosthetic management.

may be necessary to drill a series of fine holes through the edges of the bony palatal shelf and secure the palatal flap with a continuous suture.

Flabby ridges

The presence of a fibrous tissue mass sited over the crest of the residual ridge, which is excessively mobile, will interfere with stability of a prosthesis. Therefore it is advisable to make an incision along the crest of the ridge and carefully dissect out sufficient fibrous tissue to allow a layer of firm mucoperiosteum to be relocated over the bony alveolus.

Sharp bony alveolar ridges

It is quite a simple task to expose such areas at the time of surgery and eliminate any sharp bony structures with a cross-cut dental burr, and then resuture the mucosa.

Orbital floor

If it has been necessary to resect the orbital floor, the function of the associated eye should be carefully assessed, as there is little point in retaining, in this situation, a globe with no vision. Adequate support for a globe that has vision needs to be established. Ideally, the orbital floor should be reconstructed with a bone graft, preferably based on the temporalis muscle. Alternatively, the buccal fat pad can be used on some occasions as a rotation flap, when not tumour involved, to provide a sling. The buccal fat pad will tend to fibrose and, in time, will provide adequate support for the orbital contents.

Zygomatic buttress

In maxillary resections, especially types 4–8, it is extremely beneficial from a prosthetic point of view if the orientation of the bony division at the zygomatic buttress is made as oblique as possible. This creates a small area of lateral bony support for the obturator and helps to distribute functional load via the lateral margin of the orbit and along the zygomatic arch to the base of the skull (Figs 17.22 and 17.23). Changing a vertical cut surface to a slightly angulated plane of orientation will improve access to place zygomatic-sited implants.

Mandibular resections

Resections of the mandible should always be carried out in such a way so as to provide a steped surface at the cut bony margins. This allows the soft tissue reconstruction to be supported by the residual basal bone, producing less stress at the suture margin between the flap and the mucous membrane, thus reducing the risk of breakdown. All bone margins should be left smooth and rounded.

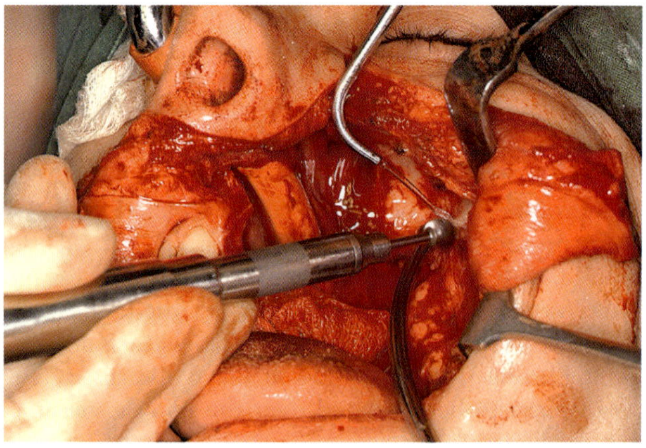

Figure 17.23 Removing sharp irregularities and reshaping the angulation of the bony surfaces of the zygomatic structures with a barrel-shaped cutting burr. Note the use of a cooling medium to prevent overheating of the bone.

Modification of the leading edge of the ascending ramus and coronoid process

The leading edge of the ascending ramus normally advances on opening the lower jaw into the upper posterior buccal sulcus, but in the posteriorly extended maxillary resection patient this area requires to be closed by the back edge of the obturator prosthesis to establish a seal. The coronoid process, if not surgically modified, will impinge upon the obturator prosthesis during functional activity causing either pain, an inability to open the jaw or dislodgement of the obturator. At the time of primary surgery, therefore, a cut should be made from the sigmoid notch to the retromolar area of the mandible to remove the coronoid and the anterior portion of the ascending ramus of the mandible (Fig. 17.23).

Establishing the optimum conditions for prosthetic restoration is not unlike building a house. Both require to be underpinned by a sound foundation.

Fitting the surgical splint and construction of the obturator mould

Maxillary defects

Following the resection procedure and preprosthetic preparation of the defect, attention can be turned to fitting the surgical splint. If a simple type of splint is to be used, that is to say retention will be obtained by clasping the remaining teeth, the splint should be placed in position and checked for stability and retention. This should be done prior to luting any additional material, i.e. silicone putty, gutta percha, Stents composition, to the splint. In many instances it should be noted that the surgical splint will, at this stage, be fitted for the first time. This is often due to the need to modify the shape of the model pre-operatively, particularly to eliminate tumour bulk or teeth where it is known there will be a need for their extraction, which makes it impossible to try-in the surgical splint prior to surgery. It may be necessary to make minor adjustment to the tension on the clasps to achieve adequate retention. It is imperative, however, that excessive pressure is not placed on the teeth by overadjustment of the clasps at the time of surgery when fitting the splint as this can led to pain and compromise the teeth. It should be remembered that it will be necessary to remove the splint at a later stage, usually when the patient is not anaesthetised.

In order to prevent ingress of food and other debris becoming trapped under the plate, attention must be paid, at the construction stage, to site the margins of the acrylic plate, especially around the teeth, to lie above the survey line. Where this has not been accomplished, a thin wash of denture conditioning paste can be applied to obtain a better seal.

Gutta percha, or a denture conditioning paste such as Viscogel or Co-Comfort, can be used to obturate minor defect sites, especially in types 2, 3 and 4 defects. It should be appreciated that it will be necessary in these types of defects to make only minimal extension into the vestibule of the defect, sufficient to establish a seal. In such defects it is advisable to pack the under-cut areas within the defect site with ribbon gauze or tulle gras prior to introducing the gutta percha or denture conditioning material. Totally filling such bony defect sites with a surgical mould is both contraindicated and unnecessary as often the entrance is smaller than the defect itself and it will be difficult, if not impossible, to remove the splint and the obturator extension in one piece. At the moulding stage it is advisable, after the material has reached a non-distortable state, to remove the plate and the surgical mould and trim off any extraneous extensions that will prevent easy re-insertion and removal. Most materials will become less compliant with time and, therefore, more difficult to remove. It should not be necessary to skin graft nasal defects types 2, 3 and 4, but it is advisable to suture the oral mucosa to the nasal mucosa at the entrance to the defect site (Figs 17.21 and 17.22). Remember to remove any packing used to pack-off unusable areas within the defect site, as this may be subsequently inhaled or swallowed by the patient.

In other larger type defects, and where retention cannot be adequately obtained from the dentition, it will be necessary to effect some means of direct fixation or suspension. The methods that can be utilised to provide anchorage or suspension in the maxillary region are set out below.

Methods of fixation and suspension

1. Per-alveolar wiring
2. Screw fixation
3. Transnasal suspension
4. Piriform fossa suspension
5. Circum-zygomatic and orbital suspension
6. Circum-vomer suspension

In our practice, the use of circum-zygomatic suspension has been superseded by the transnasal wiring technique, because this method of fixation involves minimal passage through soft tissue structures and provides central support for the surgical splint. A transnasal wire can be supplemented, where necessary, by either a per-alveolar wire or an appropriately sited bone screw in order to effect maximum stability (Fig. 17.9). If a bone screw is used it should be sited horizontally in the alveolar ridge and not in the palate. The hard palate is a very thin structure and will not permit many threads to be engaged in bone and can leave in its wake a defect in the palate. Figure 17.28 shows the optimum alignment of the bone screw. If the patient is dentate, due attention should be paid to the roots of the teeth.

First, the fixed element of the split-plate is tried in and checked for possible overextension, especially into the buccal sulci or adjacent to the tuberosities. The point where the transnasal wire will emerge through the soft tissues, at the junction of the hard and soft palate, is marked on the mucosa using the back edge of the surgical splint as a guide (Fig. 17.24). A curved awl is then passed into the contralateral nasal cavity and, after transversing the nasal floor lateral to the nasal septum and vomer, is driven through the soft palate immediately behind the palatine bony margin (Fig. 17.24). Placing a finger on the oral surface of the palate will help to guide the precise entry of the tip of the awl into the oral cavity. Soft 0.04 prestretched (10%) stainless steel wire is then threaded through the holes drilled in the back edge of the fixed element of the surgical splint to form a double loop. The wires are inserted from the fitting surface of the splint so that the wire rests on the back edge of the acrylic plate, thus placing the load on the splint rather than the soft tissues (Fig. 17.25). The ends of the wire are then threaded through the vent in the tip of the awl, making sure that they are well secured and bent back on themselves. The awl and the attached wires are then carefully withdrawn in a forward direction and immediately above the anterior aspect of the buccal sulcus it is redirected into the mouth. At this point the two strands of wire are pulled tightly so that they lie close to the nasal floor. The awl is then disattached from the two strands of wire and the free ends are passed around an anteriorly sited bollard or through a hole drilled in the buccal flange of the surgical splint (Fig. 17.25).[16]

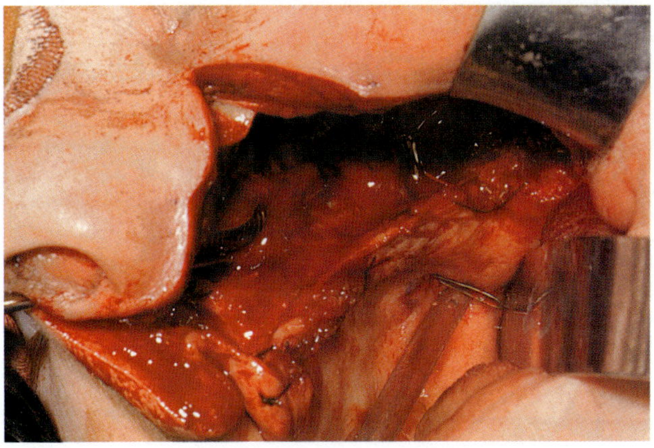

Figure 17.24 Fitting of a two-part surgical splint following a modified type 7 maxillary resection (the anterior maxillary quadrant and a strip of the bony palate were retained in this case), making it possible to use transnasal fixation. It is advisable to cut a notch in the back edge of the palatine bone to prevent the retaining wire from slipping. This illustration shows the insertion of a curved awl through the nasal aperture and penetration of the soft palate immediately behind the remaining sectioned segment of the palatine bone on the non-defect side. The two strands of soft stainless steel wire are threaded through the hole in the tip of the awl. The awl is then withdrawn through the nasal cavity and the instrument and the wires reintroduced into the anterior buccal sulcus. The wires previously threaded through holes in the fixed element of the split-plate are then drawn tightly and twisted around the bollard sited on the anterior surfaces of the acrylic plate. This method of fixation will usually be sufficient to provide stability, but when this is not the case a bone screw can be passed through the buccal flange in a horizontal alignment to engage the bony alveolus (see Fig. 17.9).

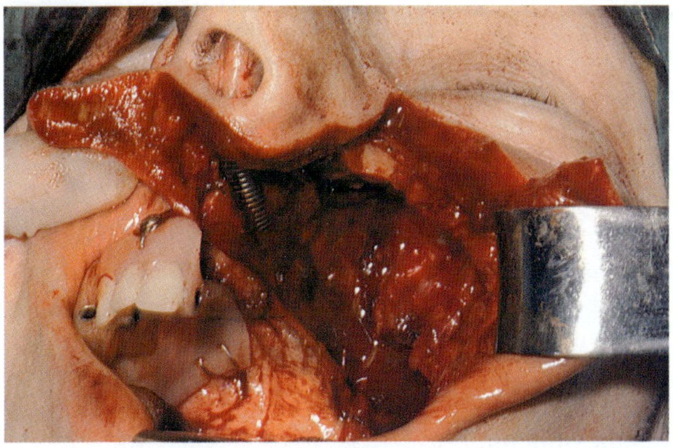

Figure 17.25 The fixed element in situ. Note the position of the double strand of wire resting on the back edge of the splint. This method of fixation involves minimal penetration of the soft tissues and, therefore, does not cause discomfort. More to the point, it is not a potential focus for tracking infection, which can occur when using circum zygomatic suspension fixation.

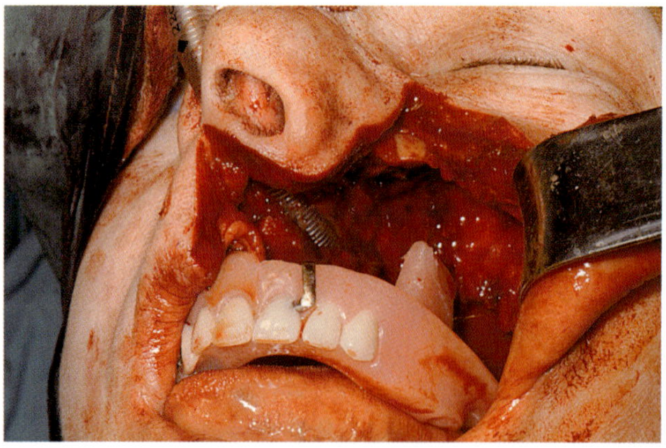

Figure 17.26 The removable element joined to the fixed element by means of the linking pin. Note the location of the vertical post within the defect site that will secure the obturator mould during the postoperative healing phase.

This completes the fitting and anchorage of the fixed element. The removable section is then joined to the fixed element with the pin or pins depending on the design freatures of the surgical splint (Fig. 17.26; and see Fig. 17.30 for an alternative method of linkage). In this case, two rods and tubes have been used. Using a single round rod and tube system will create a hinge device which is contraindicated.

Construction of the surgical mould or obturator

When subsidiary minor defects lead off the principal defect, it is advisable to pack such areas with ribbon gauze or tulle gras to prevent ingress of the compliant obturator material during the moulding procedure and thus becoming trapped in these inaccessible sites. The defect site should also be carefully assessed in order to identify the static and dynamic zones and the possibility of potential difficulty in removing the obturator mould where conflicting under-cut sites are present. When the shape of the defect is very large and there are conflicting under-cut areas it is necessary to make the surgical mould in two or more sections (see Fig. 17.32). This illustration also shows the second half of the room temperature vulcanising (RTV) silicone mould being physiologically shaped, i.e. in the ramus and buccal pad area. It is essential to lubricate the surface of each section of the obturator to prevent bonding, which would make removal of the surgical mould difficult.

The use of RTV silicone foam or ribbon gauze as a surgical pack or temporary obturator should be discouraged because such materials tend to become reservoirs of infection and require frequent replacement. A further disadvantage is that these materials cannot be selectively shaped and lack form stability.

If a pack has to be used it is advisable to soak the ribbon gauze in BIP solution, which is an antibacterial agent. BIP also helps to give the pack a firmer consistency. Overpacking when using this technique can result in the patient postoperatively being unable to open his other lower jaw due to mechanical obstruction.

In all large maxillary defects, especially where conflicting under-cut areas are present, it is necessary to use a sectional moulding technique, otherwise it will be extremely difficult to remove the surgical mould and/or the impression of the defect as used in the construction of the immediate obturator prosthesis (see Fig. 17.32). During the fabrication of the facsimile of the defect site a physiological or functional moulding technique should be used. The aim of this procedure is to establish a shape that is a response to dynamic activity within the confines of the defect site, i.e. the shape of the soft tissues over the modified ascending rami, the soft tissues of the face overlying the defect and the soft palate during function (see Fig. 17.32).

This is achieved by manually opening and closing the lower jaw and repositioning the facial flap while the mould material is still in a compliant state. Make sure that a sufficient mass of material has been used in order to fill the defect and restore external facial contour.

The main purpose of the functional moulding technique is to produce a form that will allow full jaw opening without mechanical obstruction by impingement on the surgical obturator mould or the semi-definitive obturator prosthesis and to create a defect cavity that will, in the long term, aid retention rather than reject the prosthesis. A further objective of the functional moulding technique is to restore a semblance of normal external facial contour and produce a shape that is narrower at the entrance to the defect than in the main bulk of the obturator.

When the resection is carried out in conjunction with a facial flap, i.e. Weber Ferguson approach, the construction and shaping of the surgical obturator and the impression moulding of the defect are carried out with the removable element of the surgical splint in situ (Fig. 17.27). This will provide a platform on which to place the compliant material and also help to contain it within the defect site during the moulding procedure.

Gutta percha, being a thermoplastic material, is softened by placing it in hot water approximately at 80°C where it will become readily compliant and mouldable. When RTV silicone putty is selected appropriate amounts of the putty are catalysed and mixed together. Prior to catalysation a small amount of Vaseline can be added to the mix which will

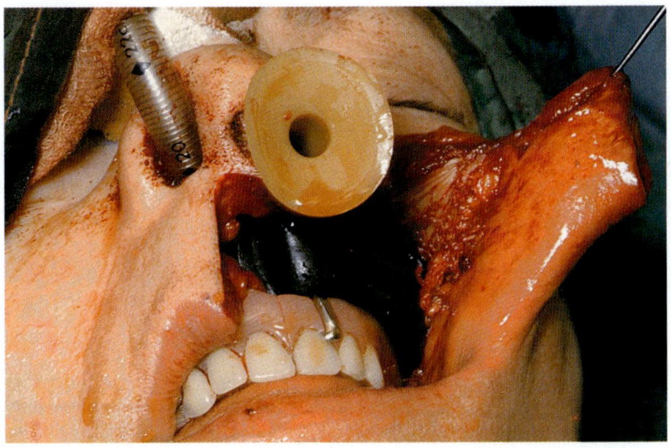

Figure 17.27 The gutta percha surgical mould physiologically shaped to obturate the defect and give support to the overlying soft tissues of the face. Note the nasal airway that passes through the surgical mould. When the mould material has become firm, the lubricated plastic airway is withdrawn through the nose, leaving a channel in the obturator.

extend the working time. Irrespective of the mould material used, it is essential when a sectional mould is indicated that each section or layer is wiped with Vaseline before introducing the next section, otherwise all the segments of the mould will become bonded to one another, thus making retrieval extremely difficult, especially where large undercuts exist.

It is advantageous to both the patient and the medical team if an airway is incorporated into the surgical mould, especially in maxillary resections 5, 6, 7 and 8 (Fig. 17.27). This is accomplished by introducing a well-vaselined paediatric anaesthetic tube through the ipsilateral nasal cavity in maxillary resections 5, 6, 7 and 8 and locating the end of the tube or naso-pharyngeal airway over the soft palate (in defects 7 and 8 the airway can be formed bilaterally). The surgical mould is then fashioned around the tubing/s and when the material is set or firm the tube is withdrawn from the nose, which will allow the obturator mould to be removed via its own path of insertion through the mouth. This small additional task has proved very worthwhile, in as much that the patient can breathe normally after surgery and the anaesthetist can easily suck out any blood or other debris in the postoperative recovery phase (Fig. 17.27).

Having constructed the obturator mould, when using the sectional splint method, the pin or pins are withdrawn, thus allowing the removable element to be separated from the fixed element. The removable element and the surgical mould are then carefully separated in situ and individually eased out of the defect site. The obturator mould is examined and any sharp edges or extraneous extensions, which will complicate subsequent reinsertion of the obturator, are removed. This completes the fabrication of the surgical mould.

If it is intended to construct an immediate Roehampton maxillary obturator prosthesis, the moulding procedure is repeated, again using the second half of the splint as a platform and the vertical post as a location point. It may be necessary to use the sectional impression moulding technique (Fig. 17.28; see immediate Obturator Technique). The next stage is to harvest a split-skin graft and suture this at its margins to the edges of the defect covering the cheek and the roof of the defect with the skin graft (Fig. 17.29). An alternative is to drape the skin graft over the surgical mould, having previously painted it with an adhesive. This technique

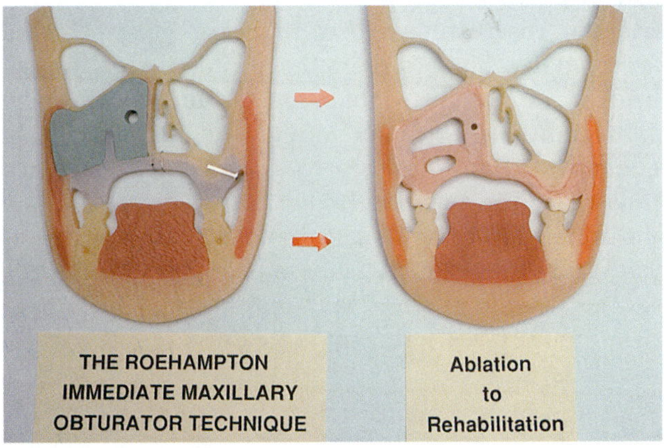

Figure 17.28 Immediately following construction of the surgical mould that will support the skin graft and, in turn, the overlying facial structures, a second mould is made of the defect in RTV silicone rubber to permit at a later stage fabrication of an immediate obturator prosthesis. This technique allows for continuous obturation to be achieved.

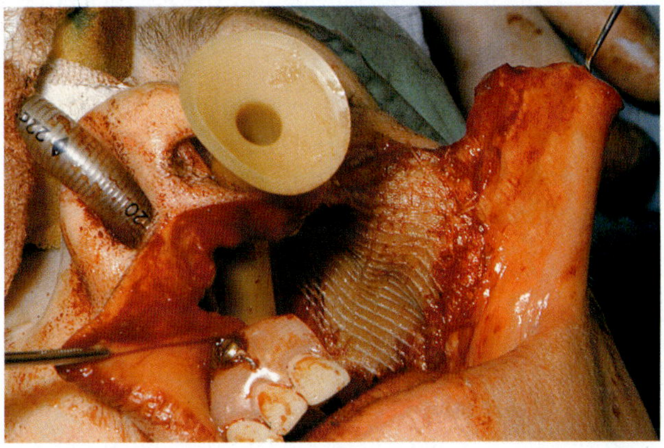

Figure 17.29 The split-skin graft in place. Note that it is secured at its margins with sutures and protected with tulle-gras prior to reinsertion of the previously described surgical mould.

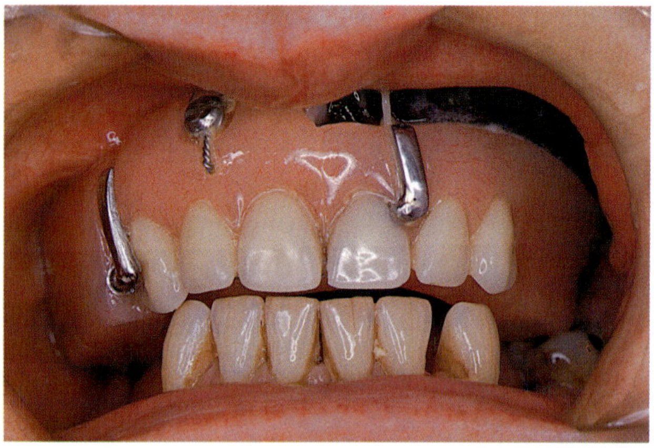

Figure 17.30 The split-plate securely supporting the surgical mould and restoring palatal continuity, thus maintaining the patient's ability to speak and control food and liquid.

has the disadvantage that the skin graft may be accidentally dislodged in the postoperative phase, leading to possible inhalation. After securing the skin graft, the obturator mould and the removable element of the splint are relocated and the pin or pins placed in position (Fig. 17.30). This will allow the facial flap to be replaced and the cut margins of the Weber Ferguson incision to be repaired in layers, i.e. at both the mucosal and skin layers. One or two deep gut sutures will provide extra support for the facial flaps.

When it is necessary to carry out a superiorly extended maxillectomy, that is to say, involving the orbital floor and contents, the surgical mould will require to be in two or more sections to allow removal either via the orbit or through the mouth.

The foregoing describes the basic steps in installing the two-part surgical splint, constructing the surgical mould and making a duplicate impression of the defect to facilitate the fabrication of the immediate resection prosthesis.

With the advent of extended delivery of medicaments, evaluation is currently being given to using the obturator mould, especially RTV silicone rubber, as a vehicle for the slow discharge of suitable topical agents, for example antibacterial preparations to keep the operative site as healthy as possible.

The optimum period to maintain the surgical obturation will depend on the site and size of the defect, and may be influenced by the type of suspension or fixation used. Where skin grafting has been carried out, it should be appreciated that approximately 16 days are required for the graft to take. It is our practice, especially in large defect cases, to maintain the surgical splint and mould for at least 6 to 8 weeks. This is often indicated in resections 6, 7 and 8 (see maxillary resection classification; Fig. 17.10). The transnasal wiring technique and two-part splint system have allowed in some cases for the surgical splint and mould to be retained for up to 14 weeks, when special circumstances have indicated the need for prolonged positive splintage, i.e. gross contracture (Fig. 17.24).

Mandibular resections

As already pointed out, resection procedures involving the mandible or in close proximity to the lower jaw will usually involve loss of bone and overlying soft tissue, or result in loss of skeletal continuity. In both situations a prosthetic input may be required to restore form and function or maintain structural integrity.

Loss of dento-alveolar structures

Where substantial loss of alveolar bone has taken place, leaving only a thin strut of the lower border of the mandible intact, splint fixation may be necessary to prevent a pathological or accidental fracture occurring. A prefabricated arch bar or cast metal cap splint, depending on the number of teeth remaining following resection, may be indicated. Where a limited number of teeth are retained following resection, an arch bar with supplementary augmentation of a light cured acrylic strut can also help to bring additional stabilisation and control of the remaining quadrants (Fig. 17.17).

Loss of skeletal continuity

Splint fixation can play an important role in preventing displacement of the remaining fragment or fragments, especially if a reasonable complement of sound teeth are retained following the surgical procedure. Again, some form of prefabricated sectional splint should be prepared and located immediately before or after resection (Fig. 17.17). In the edentulous patient, a modified Gunning type splint will offer an element of control and stabilisation, especially if the remaining alveolar ridge or ridges are of a reasonable shape and size. For such splints to provide adequate stability, they require to be firmly located to the body of the mandible with either a circumferential wire or by the insertion of bone screws (Fig. 17.19).

In anticipation of deviation of the remaining fragment, a training flange which is attached to a lower splint should be considered. The degree of success in preventing inward and upward deviation of the fragment will depend on the number of sound teeth that are present to provide anchorage for the prosthetic device. An example of the role that a functional appliance can play in this situation is presented in Fig. 17.18, where the prosthetic device provides both a source of immobilisation and the facility of a training flange by using interchangeable components. It will be noted that in addition to the lower splint it will also be necessary to fit some type of upper appliance to prevent the forces generated by the musculature from traumatising the upper dentition and buccal mucosa (Fig. 17.18; see Fig. 17.56).

Soft tissue repair and restoration of sulci

Where sulcus depth has been lost and this interferes with form and function, it is necessary to recreate lingual and buccal sulci and to line the operative site with either a local flap or a skin graft. An integral part of this procedure is the use of a surgical splint which will retain a flap (which should be as thin as possible) or a skin or mucosal graft in order to maintain the shape and depth of the surgically established pocket. The splint and mould will also provide protection to the graft area. The mucosal covering of the turbinate is very useful for this purpose as it offers a very robust surface layer. A correctly designed surgical splint and component elements will allow gentle pressure to be applied to a grafted area and, moreover, will help to prevent oral fluids collecting under the graft.

The dynamic state of the surgically modified soft tissues in the lingual and buccal vestibules makes them very prone to undergo major contracture, often resulting in total loss of the sulcus depth, if not splinted during the contractile healing phase. In such cases it is necessary to fashion a surgical mould from either gutta percha, Stents composition or RTV silicone rubber, which is retained by an extension from a well-retained splint. Such devices play an important role, especially when the defect site is extensive. Failure to restore full sulcus depth, especially the lingual sulcus area, will result in impaired function due to contracture and tethering, which can interfere with tongue mobility and the eventual placement of a prosthesis. Loss of the buccal sulcus will also interfere with functional activity and may also compromise external facial appearance due to internal contracture of the oral surfaces of the cheeks. The presence of bands of scar tissue and lack of compliance, especially around the oral stoma, can also be a major complication when attempting to fit a prosthetic device.

For such procedures to achieve their full potential, it is essential that the defect site is supported and, in turn, the graft is compressed for several weeks to resist the forces of contracture and, in turn, prevent fluid collecting under the graft. After approximately 16 days the surgical mould can be temporarily removed to allow the operative site to be irrigated. Hydrogen peroxide is highly recommended for this procedure. At this stage, that is to say when the skin graft has taken, it may be possible to modify the shape of the surgical mould, which is often used initially oversized in anticipation of contractional activity.

Immediate postoperative care

As already stated, it is important to keep the oral cavity and the adjacent structures, especially the commissures of the lips, clean and free of fungal or other infections. Cleaning of the nasal passages with the intention of removing remnants of dried blood or other debris will also make the patient more comfortable and make breathing through the nose possible, especially if a nasal airway has been created in the obturator mould (Fig. 17.27).

Early and ongoing oral hygiene is essential and should include instruction on mouth care and use of topical fluoride agents, especially when the patient is still in possession of natural teeth. Immediately following surgery it is important to keep the oral cavity clean and moist by gentle irrigation or swabbing with a solution of 0.2% chlorhexidene or normal saline. The modern practice of nasogastric or direct feeding into the stomach using the technique of percutaneous endoscopic gastrostomy has also brought about an associated improvement in mouth care and healing of the oral tissues in resection cases.

Ideally, the oral cavity should be irrigated daily by an oral hygienist, or by the patient after taking food and drink. It should be noted that vigorous irrigation of the defect site should be avoided for at least 16 days after surgery if the defect has been skin grafted, as this may result in separation of the graft from the host structures (Fig. 17.29). It is important that the patient is fully instructed on how to keep the oral cavity clean and free of debris, especially when they leave hospital care. Maintenance of dietary input should also be monitored and guidance given to the patient in the form of written instructions as what constitutes an optimum nutritious diet. Immediately after surgery the lips should be examined for signs of trauma, and hydrocortisone cream applied where necessary.

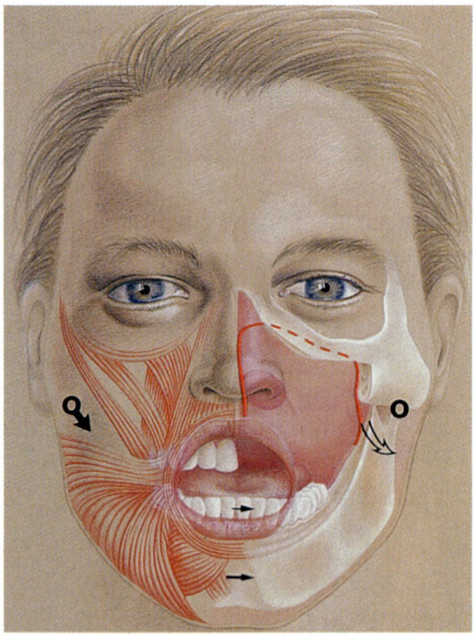

Figure 17.31 Following a posteriorly extended maxillectomy the patient will have acquired TMJ dysfunction, in as much as the joint on the defect side will be restricted to a hinge movement and no forward glide, whereas on the contralateral side there will be increased rotation and forward glide. This often results in lateral deviation of the lower jaw on opening and reduction of the posterior buccal sulcus, especially around the tuberosity on the non-defect site.

In certain types of maxillary resections, lateral deviation of the mandible on opening may occur, due to unilateral loss of pterygoid muscle attachment (Fig. 17.31).

The need to move to a definitive obturator is today not as pressing as it was in the past, due to improved methods of fixation, i.e. the transnasal wire, bone screws and better splint design (Fig. 17.25). It is our basic objective to allow tissue changes which are an inevitable consequence of surgical intervention and radiotherapy in this area to take place around a well supported and retained splint and mould and not a poorly and inadequately retained removable definitive prosthesis subjected to contractual forces that will ensue for some time after surgical intervention. Attendance at the maxillofacial surgical/prosthetic department for treatment during the healing phase should also be utilised to furnish information regarding future prosthetic restoration and rehabilitation and to provide sympathetic support and guidance.

When the defect site is fully healed and contracture has abated steps can be taken to remove the surgical splint and obturator mould. The following text will describe a new technique that allows immediate obturation of the defect and the fitting of a dental prosthesis (see Fig. 17.28).

Construction of the immediate obturator prosthesis

A major advancement in the management of the maxillary resection patient, as already stated, has been the development of the Roehampton Immediate Obturator Technique, which can be applied to both maxillary and soft palate resection cases. This technique has been specifically developed to be used in dentate and endentulous maxillary resection cases and 3–7 (Fig. 17.28). As already stated earlier in this chapter, this technique is based on the utilisation of information obtained prior to and during the surgical procedure. This, in the main, relates to having articulated master models (Fig. 17.12) (which identify the patient's jaw relationship and vertical dimension) and an impression of the defect site (Fig. 17.32). With the aid of a facsimile of the surgical splint (Fig. 17.33), which acts as a transfer jig, and the impression moulding made immediately following the resection, it is possible to marry the shape and orientation of the defect to the intact maxillary structures present in the master model (Fig. 17.34).

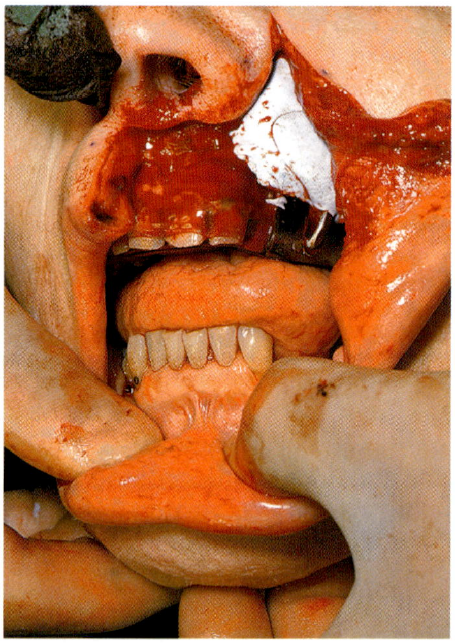

Figure 17.32 When shaping the surgical mould and the impression of the defect for the construction of the immediate obturator prosthesis, it is advisable to manually open and close the lower jaw whilst the material is still in a plastic state. This will produce a dynamically shaped replication of the defect site and, more especially, of those structures that will change shape during functional activity. Failure to carry out physiological moulding of the obturator and the impression will result in discomfort and possible displacement of the obturator at a later stage.

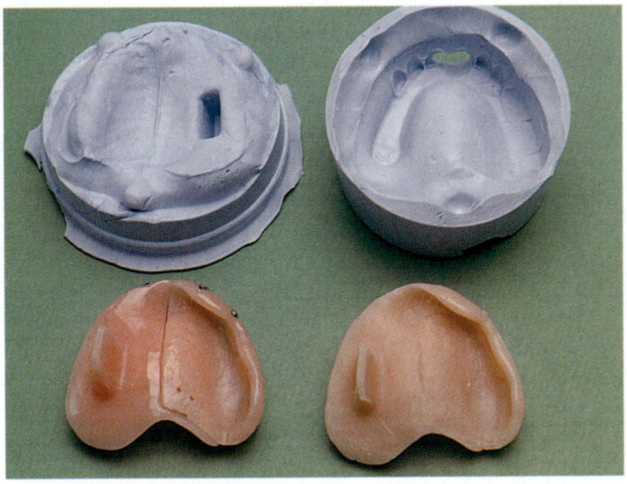

Figure 17.33 Prior to surgery, the surgical splint is duplicated in order to produce a replica or facsimile of the device. This acts as the transfer jig in the immediate obturator technique.

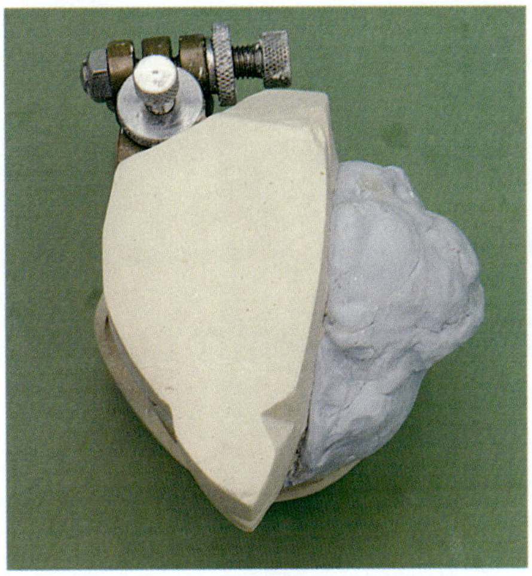

Figure 17.35 The impression of the defect mounted on the replica splint is then married to the cut model with a plaster matrix. The outer wall of the model is fabricated as a separate unit.

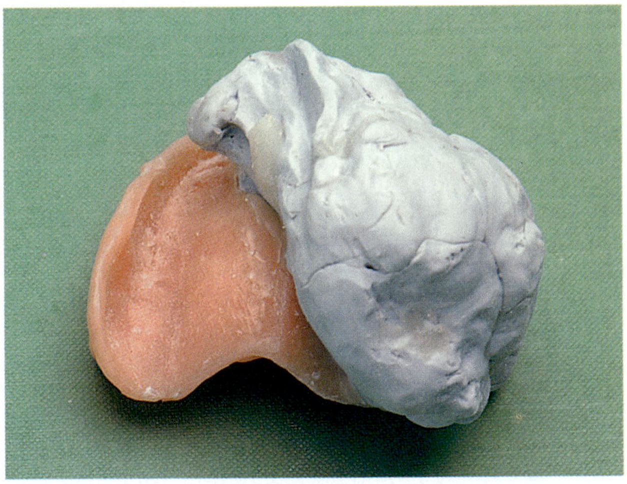

Figure 17.34 Following the resection, the impression moulding of the defect (after cleaning) is located on the transfer jig using the vertical post as a point of reference. This assembly of information provides a precise representation of the known and the previously unknown data i.e. the shape of the surgically created defect and its relationship to the intact dento-alveolar and palatal structures.

Step 1 The upper model and its mounting assembly (on which the surgical splint was constructed) are sectioned close to the inner aspect of the surgically created defect. The RTV silicone rubber impression of the defect is then located on the superior surface of the transfer jig (the facsimile of the acrylic surgical splint), using the vertical posts as a means of precise orientation.

Step 2 The transfer jig and the silicone rubber moulding of the defect (Fig. 17.34) are then offered up to the dentoalveolar structures of the sectioned model with the intention of locating the fitting surfaces of the replica of the surgical splint back to the modified master model and mounting assembly (Fig. 17.35). It may be necessary to carry out further trimming of the plaster surfaces of the sectioned model and its mounting assembly in order to accommodate the silicone moulding and locate the transfer jig on the dento-alveolar ridge. When the latter has been achieved the replica of the splint is sealed at its margins to the modified model to allow a plaster matrix to be poured around the silicone rubber moulding to make it integral with the mounting assembly. It is advisable to make this in two parts to facilitate access to the simulated defect site within the modified articulated model (Fig. 17.36). Note the use of locating vents to precisely relate to two halves of the extended model. Having married the 'unknown' to the 'known' it is now possible to proceed with the design and construction of the immediate obturator prosthesis (Figs. 17.36 and 17.37).

Step 3 Any minor surface roughness within the model of the replicated defect site is made smooth with fine sandpaper. A wax shell is then adapted to the walls and roof of the defect site terminating at the entrance of the resection cavity. The halves of the master model are separated to allow the wax shell to be removed. The wax pattern is then invested in a two-part plaster mould. When the stone plaster is sufficiently hard, the two halves of the flask are heated to allow separation and elimination of the wax with boiling water. After sealing the surfaces of the stone plaster mould, the mould cavity is packed with Molloplast B silicone rubber and the two halves of the flask closed under

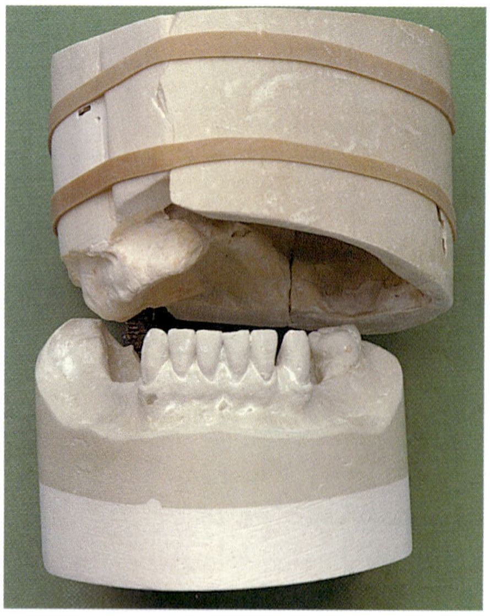

Figure 17.36 The working model of the defect and the intact structures following removal of the acrylic resin transfer jig and silicone moulding of the defect site.

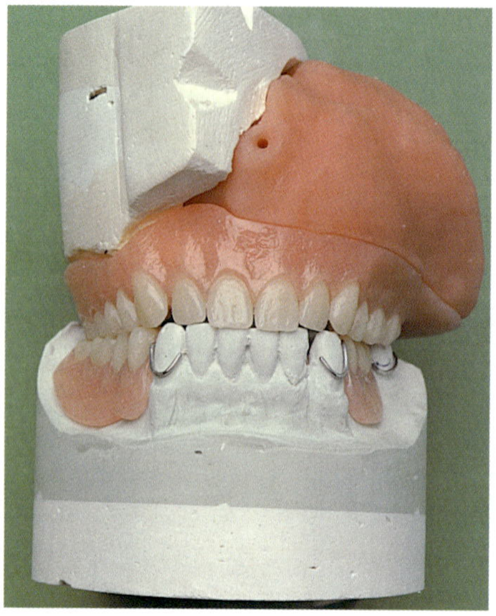

Figure 17.37 Having a split cast it is possible to fabricate a wax shell that utilises the full extend of the defect site. The wax pattern is then removed from the model assembly and converted to a Molloplast B silicone rubber obturator. The silicone obturator has an inbuilt circumferentially-sited groove situated approximately 1 cm from the entrance to the shell. This provides mechanical linkage between the compliant obturator and the rigid extension from the dental prosthesis which engages the inner aspect of the obturator. Subsequently the dental prosthesis is fabricated on a duplicate plaster model that records the margins of the silicone obturator shell and the intact dento-alveolar and palatal structures.

pressure making sure that excess material is seen. The clamped flask and contents are then processed at 100°C for at least 3 hours. The cured shell is removed from the mould and the excess trimmed from the margins.

Step 4 The cured silicone rubber obturator shell is fitted back to the two-part master model and examined for close adaptation at its margin. Any excess material is trimmed back in order to establish a smooth junction between the silicone shell and the intact palate. An acrylic shell is then made of the inner surfaces of the silicone obturator. This engages a groove sited in the walls of the silicone obturator which provides a means of mechanical purchase between the obturator and the denture.

Step 5 At this stage it is advisable to duplicate the upper model with the silicone shell and the acrylic insert in situ. The duplicated upper model is subsequently re-articulated to the lower master model and assembly, using a jaw registration block to record the patient's centric relationship and vertical dimension. (This information is obtained from the articulated master models.) By processing the denture component on the duplicate model, it is possible to relocate it on the two-part master model, thus allowing the occlusion to be checked and, where necessary, corrected. This procedure also facilitates monitoring the precise relationship of the silicone obturator to the denture.

Step 6 The construction of the acrylic denture follows conventional lines, except that it will partially extend into the vestibule of the silicone shell to allow attachment with the acrylic shell. When the patient is dentate, it is essential that every endeavour is made to distribute load as widely as possible and to use wrought clasps that have optimum resilience. The prosthesis is processed in the usual manner and subsequently fitted back to the master model, making sure that the interface between the retaining part of the dental prosthesis and the silicone shell is satisfactory. The acrylic thin-walled shell is bonded to the denture with cyanoacrylate adhesive (Fig. 17.37). Please note: the second moulding procedure to allow the obturator prosthesis to be constructed is carried out immediately following fabrication of the surgical mould, i.e. at the time of resection (Fig. 17.32). If a surgical mould change is planned some two or three weeks after the surgery, the impression procedure can be carried out at this stage if necessary.

Removal of the surgical splint and mould and fitting of the immediate obturator prosthesis

At the time of finally removing the surgical splint and surgical mould, the immediate obturator denture

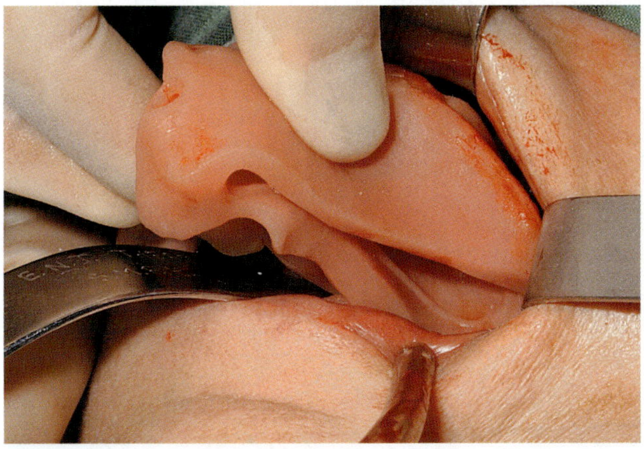

Figure 17.38 When the soft tissues within the defect are healed and major contracture has ceased, the surgical splint and mould are removed and the defect cleaned of any residual debris. The immediate obturator shell is then inserted into the defect. This procedure should be carried out as quickly as possible, as there will still be the tendency for the defect to undergo contracture.

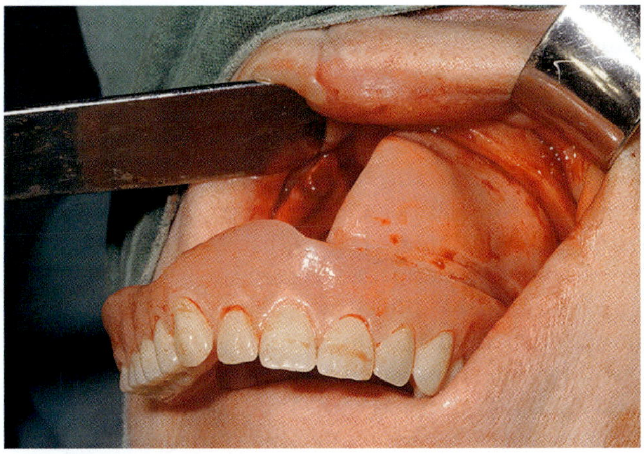

Figure 17.39 The dental prosthesis being inserted to engage the retentive groove within the inner aspect of the silicone shell.

is taken to the operating theatre and placed in a suitable disinfecting fluid. *Do not attempt to autoclave the denture as this will result in distortion.* The silicone rubber shell can, however, be autoclaved without fear of structural modification or damage. The surgical splint and surgical mould are then removed and the defect site profusely irrigated with hydrogen peroxide. The silicone shell obturator is immediately inserted into the defect and the dental prosthesis fitted as a separate unit (Figs 17.38 and 17.39). This procedure should be carried out as quickly as possible as contracture will soon ensue. It is contraindicated to attempt to carry out any occlusal equilibration while the patient is under a general anaesthetic as the muscles that control the mandible are not under dynamic control and the occlusion may be quite different when the patient is conscious.

It is also inadvisable to attempt to remove the prosthesis for approximately 24 hours as the surrounding soft tissues will be in a state of adaptation and may not yet have reached a state of balance in relationship to the obturator. The object is to allow the facial structures to contract down on to the obturator. The patient should be instructed that in the early stages when the prosthesis and obturator are removed for cleaning purposes they should be returned as quickly as possible. This type of immediate obturator will usually remain satisfactory for approximately 6 months after its primary insertion.

It has to be recognised that failure from the onset to provide a form of immediate obturation will almost certainly result in concomitant contracture of the defect site, with associated impairment of the patient's morale. The maxillary obturator is essentially at this stage a space maintainer, but a major step in the patient's rehabilitation (Fig. 17.40).

When the obturator fully occupies the defect site (in resections 1 and 5–8) and the upper surfaces of the prosthesis occlude with the roof of the defect, the first stage of conditioning the soft tissues that line the defect to accept functional load begins to take place. In addition, the underlying bony structures, if suitably shaped, also take on the task of being a load-bearing foundation. This re-establishes internal stimulation of the bony structures. The foregoing is in keeping with Wolff's Law, which states that bone requires to be constantly subjected to functional loading in order to maintain its viability.[12] Experience has shown that respiratory type mucosa will change histologically and will take on the characteristics of the tissues that are normally

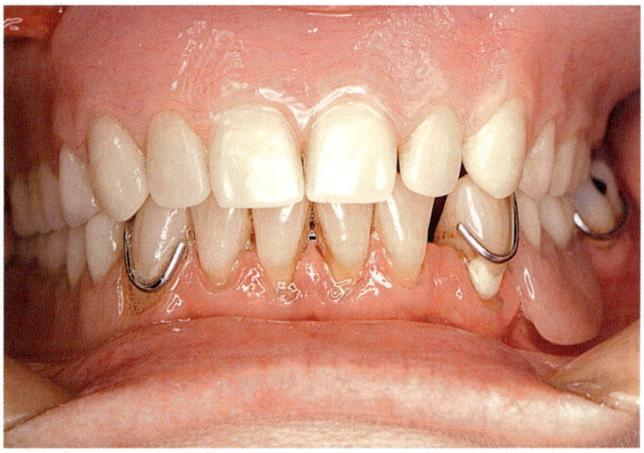

Figure 17.40 The obturator shell and attached dental prosthesis in situ some two days after insertion.

required to function in a more robust role when subjected to functional loading by the obturator shell and denture.

Implementation of definitive maxillofacial prosthetic restorative procedures: maxillary, mandibular and tongue

When the intra-oral structures have healed and contractual forces have abated, attention can be turned to providing some form of more permanent prosthetic restoration and rehabilitation. It is, however, important to appreciate that the provision of the so-called 'definitive prosthesis' is but a step along what is often a lifelong commitment, both on the part of the patient and the CMFPT team. Nothing is permanent in maxillofacial prosthetics, other than deep buried implants that are usually required to serve in a lifetime capacity. Indwelling and externally prosthetic devices have a finite lifespan due to deterioration and wear. The body tissues will also undergo changes, due to the ageing processes and, moreover, the additional load bearing forces that the prosthetic therapy will impose on the intact body structures. This is amplified when functional load is, of necessity, placed on a reduced foundation and in a different plane of orientation from the norm.

The biomechanical engineering implications when dealing with patients who have suffered major loss of hard and soft tissue structures in an around the oral cavity are far more complex and demanding than seen in conventional dental prosthetics. The forces involved are greater and the vector of application is usually different. The patient's reliance also on maxillofacial prosthetic restoration and rehabilitation ceases to be a matter of choice, but more of a necessity, if an acceptable quality of life is to be maintained.[17]

At the early assessment stage it is necessary to identify the potential to achieve optimum load distribution and to obtain a viable source of retention. Figure 17.41 demonstrates the static structures in a maxillary resection case that can be utilised for direct and indirect retention and, moreover, distribution of load bearing forces. The teeth and bony based areas which are static structures are shown in white and yellow. The pink and dark red areas signify those structures that are subject to dynamic activity. (The white area within the defect site identifies a skin grafted area which is also under the influence of dynamic activity.) The two blue zones denote further areas that will undergo dynamic change during functional activity (Fig. 17.41).

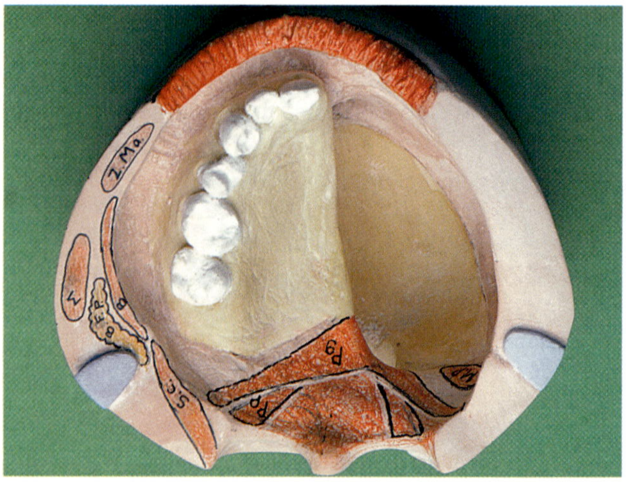

Figure 17.41 The design of prosthetic therapy should be based on careful assessment of the static structures (the white and yellow zones) and the dynamic structures (the red and blue zones) and the degree of direct and indirect retention that can be derived from both the defect and the intact dento-alveolar and palatal components.

Our philosophy in approaching the prosthetic management of the intra-oral post-resection patient has been to endeavour to achieve maximum return of form and function without, if possible, impairing the integrity of the remaining structures. These objectives have in some instances taken us away from conventional or traditional methods of prosthetic treatment. For example, to expect one quadrant of the intact maxillary arch in a post-resection patient to provide the total retention and stability for a prosthesis is to expect nature to accommodate applied forces for which these structures were never intended to cope with. Traditionally, in this situation, it has been common practice in many centres to make minimal extension into a unilaterally sited defect for retentive purposes and to expect the remaining dentoalveolar structures to withstand applied transverse loading. Experience has shown, when observing such patients over a period of time, that the long term sequelae are often the loss of the remaining teeth, and subsequently, rapid alveolar bone resorption and traumatisation of the margins of the defect.

Our modus operandi over the last 20 years has been to apply sound biomechanical engineering principles to design concepts that are based on an understanding of human engineering and biomechanics, and attempting to restore load distribution pathways (Fig. 17.7). In other words, this has led us to attempt to replace 'like with like' in broad mechanical terms. This, in some instances, has led to a major shift in technique, which has been to move away from hard acrylic hollow-box obturators in favour of obturators fabricated in a compliant material such as Molloplast

B silicone rubber, to use wrought metal clasps rather than cast clasps and not to use rigid metal frameworks. The advent of osseointegration has played a major role in our ability to advance the frontiers of CMFPT and bring great benefit to the post-resection patient.

Clinical assessment criteria

The clinical assessment should address the following factors in order to determine the level and severity of acquired deformity and disability (Table 17.6).

The basic principles of prosthetic management

The essential objectives are set out in Table 17.7.

Basic design objective

The paramount objective should always be to achieve maximum restoration of form and function without placing the remaining hard and soft tissues at risk. This, in the main, relates to accomplishing wide distribution of load, ideally three-dimensionally. In the dentate case, this involves distributing the applied load over the maximum number of natural teeth as possible, to obtain direct retention from the remaining intact structures and also from within the defect site itself (Fig. 17.42). Maximum usage of indirect retention should also be implemented to resist lateral and rotatory forces. The bony supported walls within the defect can often be used to improve stability, thus preventing or reducing harmful forces being placed on the dento-alveolar structures. The viability of using the surgically exposed vomer, or the lateral wall/s of the nasal

Table 17.6 Clinical assessment criteria

1. Review of the efficacy of the patient's stoma opening and oral seal competency.
2. Determine the ability to achieve full jaw opening and whether mandibular deviation occurs with consequent disturbance of normal functional activity, especially the following: (a) impingement of the leading edge of the ascending ramus on the lateral wall of the maxilla in the tuberosity region on the non-operated side; (b) the potential displacement of a posteriorly extended maxillary obturator due to advancement of the coronoid process into the confines of the maxillary defect.
3. Determine the site and size of the defect and other possible sources of disability.
4. Examine the state of the remaining soft tissue structures and identify any compromised areas, i.e. bands of scar tissue, loss of sulcus depth, presence of flaps in relation to bulk, compressibility, mobility and interference with functional activity and signs of ongoing traumatic injury.
5. Examine by palpation the underlying bony foundations both within the confines of the defect site and the intact dentoalveolar quadrants for sharp or irregular structures that will complicate insertion of the prosthesis, load distribution and interfere with comfort.
6. Examine the condition of the remaining teeth and the associated structures in order to identify the following:
   (a) The number, orientation and distribution of teeth in both arches. Please note that each dental arch is divided into four quadrants and 16 units.
   (b) Their individual status and the need for restorative procedures to be carried out.
   (c) The occlusal relationship with opposing teeth.
   (d) The degree and quality of bony support.
   (e) The possible need for minor tooth modification to establish (i) guide planes, (ii) retention, (iii) improved occlusion and (iv) channels over the occlusal surfaces to permit siting of clasp arms that do not interfere with occlusion. (The latter will require careful reference to diagnostic study models.)
   (f) Examine the oral cavity and lips for signs of injury, infection or disease, and refer for appropriate treatment.
   (g) Assess the defect site in relation to shape, size, orientation and quantitate the potential for gaining retention from this source.
   (h) Identify the potential foundations available to obtain support and retention from the intact structures.
   (i) Examine the tongue, especially in patients who have undergone ablative procedures in this area, to assess whether the provision of a prosthetic device will improve speech and control of food.
   (j) Assess the patient generally in relation to their ability to insert and remove a prosthetic appliance, and also identify any concomitant disabilities such as impaired intellect, eyesight and arthritic conditions, particularly afflicting the hands. These factors may complicate their day to day management, e.g. oral hygiene and maintenance of their prosthetic appliance.

Table 17.7 Basic principles of prosthetic management

1. To obtain maximum restoration of form and function.
2. To facilitate maximum long-term preservation of the remaining hard and soft tissue foundations that will provide retention and support.
3. To apply simplicity to the design concept where-ever possible.
4. To apply sound applied biomechanical engineering principles to the design concept.
5. To select a method of retaining the prosthesis or device that does not impair the long-term integrity of remaining hard and soft-tssie structures that are required to provide anchorage and stabilization.
6. To provide a prosthetic service that realistically and ethically reflects the true cost implications which ideally should be at a level that the user of the service can afford.
7. To provide ongoing monitored aftercare, which should include encouragement, support and maintenance of any prosthetic appliance supplied.
8. To keep the wider team fully acquainted of the patient's prosthetic progress and, moreover, to report any reason for concern, especially changes in medical, psychological and social status and, most importantly, any evidence of recurrence.

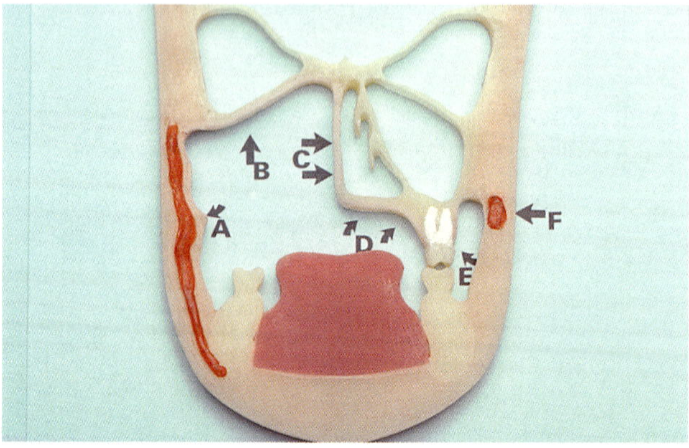

Figure 17.42 The potential sites in a type 6 maxillary resection defect that can offer a source of retention and indirect stability for prosthetic rehabilitation and restoration are: (a) creation of a scarband at the vestible of the defect (a non grafted area); (b) the bony roof of the defect, which offers a source of resistance against upward displacement of the prosthesis; (c) the vertical bony structures, i.e. the vomer and nasal septum, which offer indirect support; (d) the hard palate, which when used in combination with (c) provides resistance to rotatory directed forces; (e) the teeth, which provide a source of direct and indirect retention and resistance against vertical displacement of the prosthesis under load; (f) the presence of a dynamic strap i.e. the buccinator muscle, which provides resistance to downward directed displacing forces exerted by the soft tissues of the face during functional activity on the obturator.

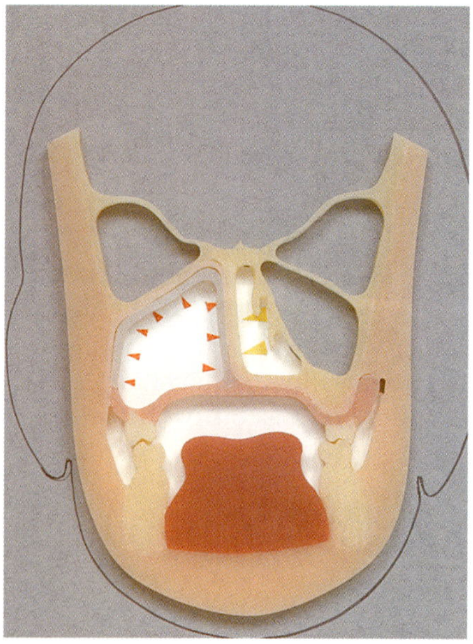

Figure 17.43 The acrylic hollow-box obturator is a lightweight construction and offers the potential to gain a limited amount of physical retention i.e. adhesion, cohesion and atmospheric pressure if a seal can be effected around the margins of the obturator prosthesis.

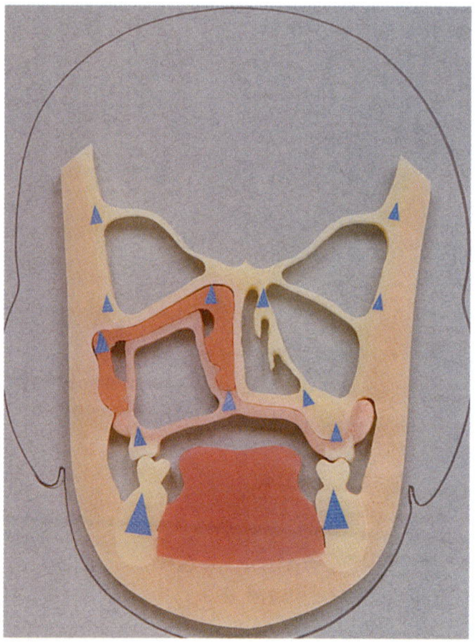

Figure 17.44 The silicone rubber shell and attached dental prosthesis provide opportunity to gain biomechanical retention from within the defect, especially when undercut bony supported areas are present. In turn, the soft silicone shell acts as a stress breaker during mastication and conveys functional stimulation to both hard and soft tissues within the defect site.

cavity, will depend on the thoroughness of previous preprosthetic surgery having been carried out (Figs 17.41 and 17.42). All static bony supported structures that are exposed to the oral cavity, particularly within the defect, have the potential to offer indirect retention and support (Figs 17.41).

Table 17.8 Advantages and disadvantages of the hard acrylic hollow-box obturator prosthesis and the soft silicone rubber shell and dental prosthesis

Hard acrylic hollow-box obturator prosthesis technique (Fig. 17.42)	Soft silicone rubber shell and dental prosthesis technique (Fig. 17.43)
Advantages	**Advantages**
More applicable in a non-retentive defect More appropriate in the presence of reduced manual dexterity in the older patient A more light-weight construction A better option in small palatal defects Easier to clean Less labour intensive to construct Materials used are relatively inexpensive The surfaces of the obturator element can be polished to a high degree of smoothness	Can utilise the maximum potential for gaining retention from within the defect Compliant and easy to insert and remove More compatible to soft tissue structures Permits functional stimulation of the tissues Allows sites within the defect to be more fully obturated thus preventing collection of debris Allows maximum indirect retention to be achieved from within the defect Allows selective use of stiff or rigid sections in the obturator element Allows the silicone rubber obturator to be replicated independently of the denture element Allows areas of the obturator to be modified in relation to establishing different surface energy characteristics Can aid the stability and retention of the attached dental prosthesis Permits a good seal to be established in dynamic areas
Disadvantages	**Disadvantages**
Hard and unyielding Prone to damage The hollow-box is prone to leakage Not form stable on reprocessing Requires total replacement Less comfortable The amount of potential extension into retentive areas within the defect is reduced A functional seal is more difficult to achieve	Is more labour intensive to construct Materials used are more expensive The silicone shell is more difficult to keep clean The silicone rubber obturator is more susceptible to fluid uptake

As already mentioned, it is our practice to make full use of the roof and walls of the defect, especially in maxillary resection defects 1 and 5–8, for load transference, retention and to facilitate restoration of the external facial contour by using the obturator section as a substitute for the lost bony framework. Because of the shape of most maxillary defects we prefer to use a compliant, shell-like obturator which permits full extension into under-cut areas with relative ease, thus improving retention, maximum stimulation of the tissues within the defect surfaces, optimum load transmission and, moreover, preventing the collection of food and other debris in inaccessible areas. A facility is built into the obturator design concept to allow the obturator shell and the supporting denture to be mechanically linked to one another and for the two components to collectively engage the maximum extent of the usable retentive sites that are present, both in the defect site and in the intact dental arch (Figs 17.39 and 17.44).

In our practice we tend to deploy the two-part silicone rubber shell and obturator denture technique in the majority of our patients, especially in large defects where it is possible to gain bio-mechanical retention. However, there are occasions when it is advisable to use a hard acrylic hollow-obturator type denture either as a one-piece device or in two parts. The latter is usually determined by the patient's ability to introduce a large prosthesis into the oral cavity. However, the hollow-box technique is usually the ideal method when used in conjunction with an osseointegration supported framework (see Fig. 17.77).

The relative indications for using either a soft silicone rubber shell and detachable dental prosthesis or a hard acrylic resin hollow-box obturator prosthesis are set out in Table 17.8.

Maxillary resection: case reports

Case 1: hard and soft palate resection

This patient presented with a large lesion sited in both the antrum and in the lateral aspect of the soft palate. The patient was partially endentulous in the upper arch and there was considerable wear abrasion of the remaining teeth, especially the anterior teeth. The remaining posterior teeth were quite sound and adequate to provide retention for a clasp supported surgical splint and wire extension. An extended fenestration was carried out involving the lateral hard palate and the soft palate (Fig. 17.45). Temporary obturation of the linked defects was achieved by luting gutta percha to a wire staple processed into the fitting surfaces of an acrylic splint. After approximately 4 weeks the splint and surgical mould were removed from the defect and the obturator section converted to heat cured acrylic resin utilising the immediate obturator technique. When the tissues in and around the defect had totally healed and contraction had ceased the patient's own dental practitioner carried out a planned programme of restorative dentistry. This involved crowning and lengthening of the anterior teeth to increase the vertical dimension and the placement of precision attachments in the anterior bridgework and in the remaining crowned posterior teeth. During this phase the changes around the crowned teeth were made-up by extending the prosthesis with a light cured acrylic resin.

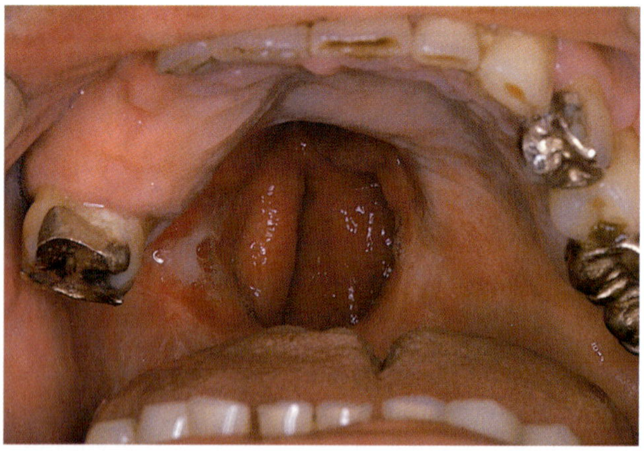

Figure 17.45 A laterally-sited communicating hard and soft palate defect involving a combination of static and dynamic structures. The remaining natural teeth were restored with fixed bridge work that incorporates precision attachments. Two non-saveable posterior teeth on the contralateral quadrant to the defect had to be extracted.

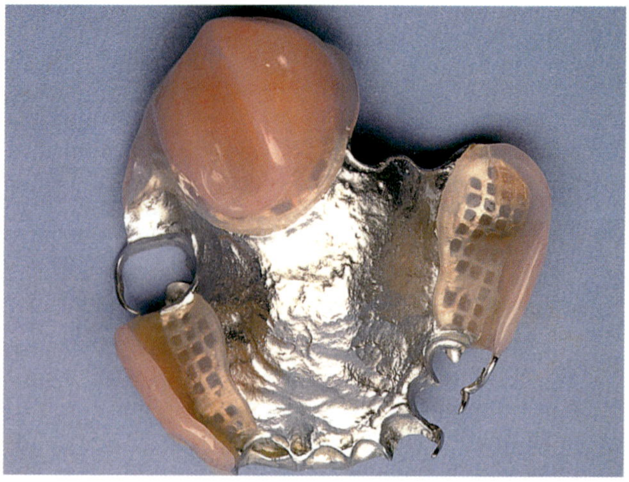

Figure 17.46 The obturator extension was physiologically shaped during functional activity accommodate the dynamic changes in the soft palate during speech and swallowing in order to prevent shear loading forces being placed on the supporting teeth during function by the prosthesis.

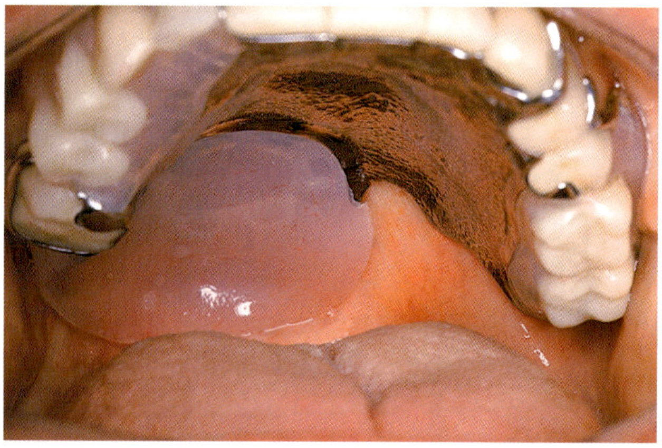

Figure 17.47 The metallic and acrylic prosthesis in situ. Note the shape of the obturator extension that covers the margins of the soft palate defect.

Finally, a cast metal framework was made and the obturator extension that closes off the defect in both the hard and soft palate was physiologically shaped to obtain optimum speech and control of food and liquid (Fig. 17.46). Subsequently teeth were added to the metal plate and the obturator section converted to acrylic. This case demonstrates the advantages to be accrued when there is both a maxillofacial prosthetic and restorative dentistry input focusing on a patient's restorative and rehabilitation needs (Fig. 17.47).

Case 2: posteriorly extended maxillary resection

This maxillary resection case (type 5 in the classification) demonstrates the benefit of retaining the ipsilateral central incisor in order to increase the potential for support and load distribution. Following resection and preprosthetic preparation of the defect site (which also included planned removal of the coronoid process and the leading edge of the ascending ramus), provision was made at the resection to fabricate a two-part mould of the defect to permit the subsequent fitting of an immediate maxillary obturator prosthesis. The defect was skin grafted and the resection site obturated with a two-part silicone rubber putty surgical mould. This was retained by a two-part surgical splint.

Some 8 weeks after the primary surgery the splint and obturator mould were removed and an immediate obturator prosthesis fitted. This consisted of a silicone rubber obturator shell that fully engaged the very retentive defect, gaining additional support for the overall prosthetic restoration and, more importantly, full restoration of external facial contour. The silicone obturator was supported in the late postoperative phase by a clasp retained dental prosthesis.

A more definitive two-part obturator prosthesis was constructed and fitted some 6 months later. Retention and stability for the prosthesis was achieved by the strategic placement of wrought metal clasps and by the use, wherever possible, of occlusal rests. It will be noted from Fig. 17.48 that this prosthesis incorporates a buccal acrylic extension that helps to resist applied lateral and rotatory load bearing forces and distributes load to the zygomatic buttress. In order to provide a counter force to resist the anteroposterior load placed on the palatal surfaces of the last tooth in the intact anterior dental arch a modified Roach clasp was used. The long double arm connecting element of the clasp (approximately 1 cm in length) facilitated maximum stress breaking and utilisation of a relatively deep under-cut surface on the labial surface of the tooth. Placement of a clasp arm on the buccal surfaces of the tooth invokes Newton's Third Law of Motion – force and counterforce. The clasp is incorporated into the vertical margin of the acrylic gum work where it is less obtrusive and hidden by the upper lip. The clasps are fabricated in a heat-treated type of wire (Figs 17.49 and 17.50).

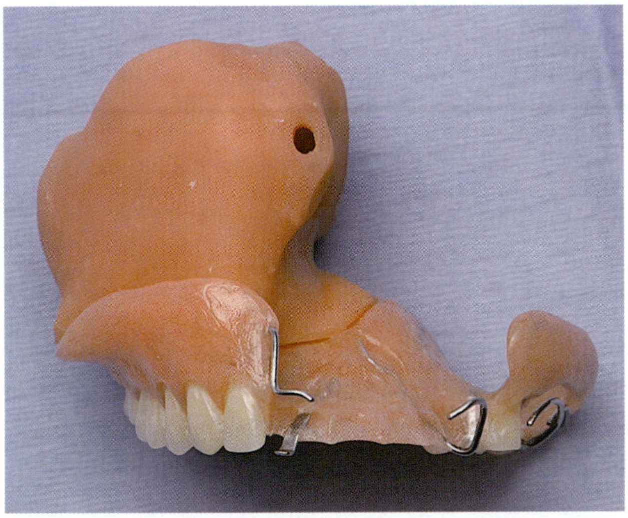

Figure 17.48 A two-part silicone shell obturator and denture which illustrates the following: (a) the viability of using opposing undercut sites; (b) the presence of a built-in airway in the silicone rubber obturator; (c) wide distribution of clasps and occlusal rests; (d) the use of a buccal extension from the dental prosthesis to improve load distribution and resist forces applied during opening of the mouth.

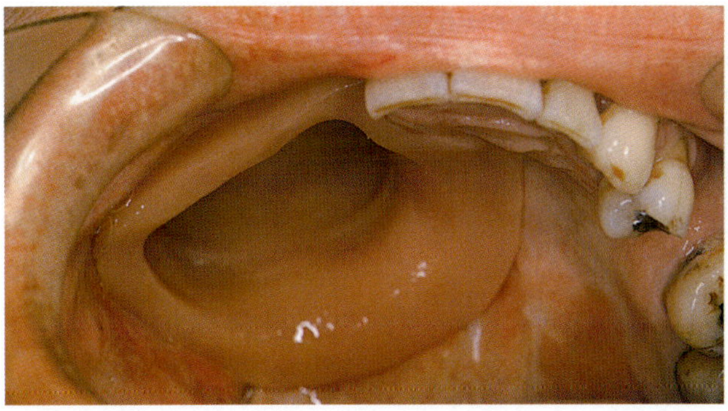

Figure 17.49 The silicone shell in situ demonstrating that it is self-retentive by occupying areas within the defect that permit biomechanical retention to be realised, which is further enhanced when the dental prosthesis is engaged.

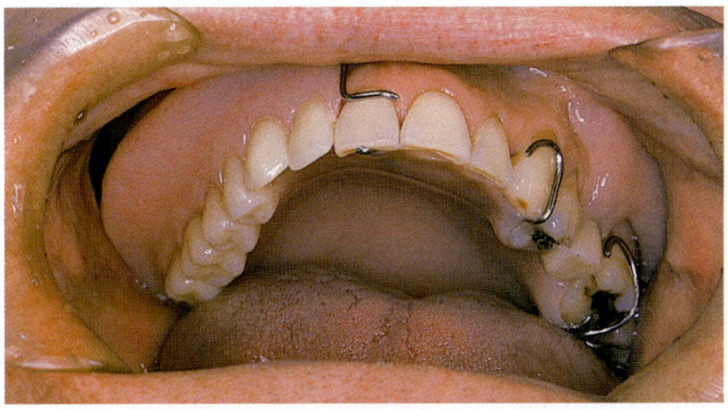

Figure 17.50 Obturation of the maxillary defect and restoration of the dento-alveolar structures. Note (a) the distribution of clasp arms and rests invoking the principles of force and counterforce, (b) the buccal extension which improves stability and performance (the latter does not compress the soft tissues overlying the dento-alveolar ridge as this would cause bony resorption). This component, if optimally shaped, is tightly gripped by the bucconator muscle during functional activity, especially on jaw opening.

This two-part prosthetic device is designed to aid bilateral distribution of functional load and maintenance of appearance, oral seal and speech. This patient retains his full professional role in a busy executive position and, moreover, leads a full social life some 15 years after his primary surgery.

Case 3: maxillary resection (paediatric patient)

Maxillary resection in children is relatively rare. However, when it is necessary the aftermath of removing bone and soft tissue in the growing child invariably has serious consequential ramifications. The need to use adjuvant radiotherapy will also contribute to residual long-term deformity and malfunction.

Development and growth of orofacial structures will usually be modified as a result of impairment of the growth centres initiated by the ablative intervention. As in common with adults who undergo such procedures, mastication and speech can be compromised. In the child, however, there may also be associated psychological implications. Prosthetic management is invariably complicated by the lack of teeth with appropriately sized and shaped clinical crowns and, moreover, the need not to hinder or compromise any residual potential for growth (Fig. 17.51).

The treatment of a young child that came under our care is presented to demonstrate how the above objectives can be efficaciously met and a reasonable level of rehabilitation and restoration be achieved. The design concept adopted in this patient's treatment was aimed at restoring essential form and function by supplying what is essentially a full upper hollow-box obturator prosthesis. The aim was to realise maximum biophysical retention, restore occlusion (hence stimulation of the remaining hard and soft tissue structures) and allow the remaining teeth to erupt and descend through the prosthesis. The collets of the prosthesis around the remaining posterior natural teeth were fabricated in a compliant material to provide a degree of latitude for potential growth (Fig. 17.52).

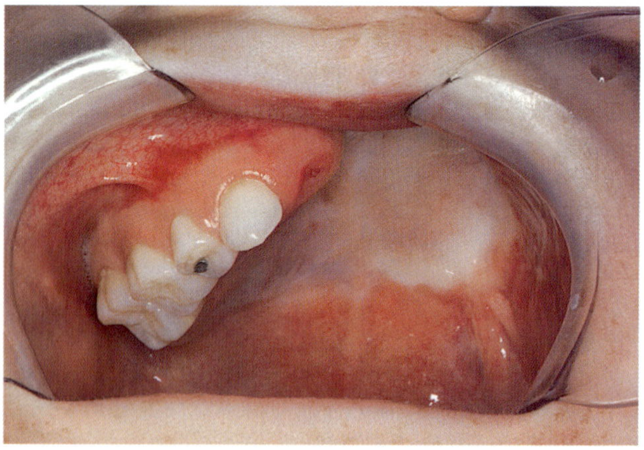

Figure 17.51 A maxillary defect in a eight-year old child following a resection carried out three years previously. Note the collapse of the dental arch and lack of forward development of the upper jaw. The crowns of the few remaining teeth and the shape of the defect provided little or no potential for retention.

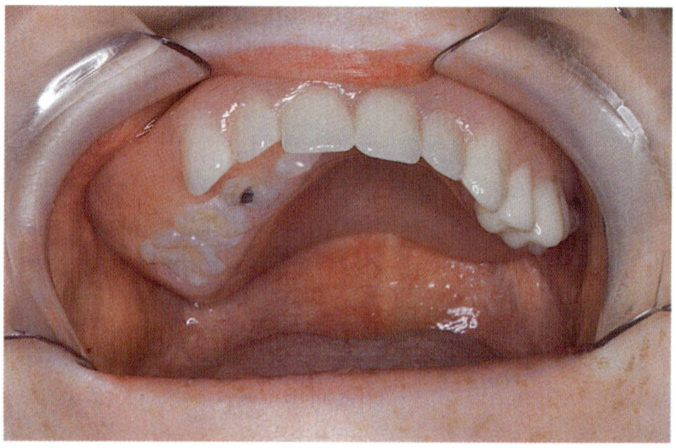

Figure 17.52 The acrylic hollow-box obturator in clinical use. Note that full use of the buccal sulcus on the contralateral side has been utilised in order to use the zygomatic buttress for additional support. The prosthesis; where it encompasses the natural teeth, has an integral soft plastic insert which acts as stress breaker and facilitates a degree of viscoelastic-derived retention, and also allows the teeth to undergo further eruption.

The prosthetic input into this young girl's restoration and rehabilitation was focused to recognise that a young patient is still growing and that a prosthesis can provide the biophysical stimulus to facilitate hard and soft tissue development and growth.

Mandibular defects:

This section discusses the prosthetic management of surgically acquired dento-alveolar and mandibular ridge resections. The former type of defect is usually central, posterior, unilateral or bilateral. However, minor variations will be encountered when less or more dental units are involved. However, the same basic principles of prosthetic management pertain. When mandibular continuity is lost the resulting defect can vary from a minor resection to total removal of the mandible.

Important treatment objectives are:

1. Maximum distribution of applied load over the intact structures.

2. Establishment of a smooth and ideally broad-based bony foundation.
3. Establishment of soft tissue coverage over the bony defect site with minimal differential compressibility.
4. Occlusal stability and maximum contact between opposing natural or artificial teeth.
5. Elimination of unyielding scar bands and bulky flaps that encroach upon the denture-bearing area or complicate insertion of the prosthesis.

The main factors that complicate prosthetic restoration are:

1. The lack of an adequate number of sound teeth that are aligned in a path of common orientation and which allow access and provision of support and retention for a prosthesis.
2. The absence of lingual and buccal sulci of adequate depth to obtain resistance against laterally applied forces.
3. Lack of dento-alveolar structures to provide direct and indirect support for a prosthesis.
4. Bulky flaps of variable compressibility.
5. Limitation of access due to reduction of jaw opening potential; reduced stoma due to residual scar.
6. Lack of neuromuscular input and associated impairment of perception.
7. Malocclusion following loss of skeletal continuity.

The following will identify some of the relevant problems and objectives associated with the management of the dento-alveolar case.

Dento-alveolar resection defects

Loss of the anterior quadrants and associate supporting bony structures will often bring about collapse of the posterior dental quadrants due to remodelling of the remaining bony ridge which forms the lower border of the mandible. This, in the dentate case, will usually result in the posterior teeth and also the alveolar structures undergoing varying degrees of lingual rotation.

The common method of overcoming this prosthetic problem is to block out the under-cut areas on the lingual aspect of the dento-alveolar structures and fit a prosthesis that has minimal physical contact with the lingual aspect of the teeth and mucosa. Unfortunately this usually results in accumulation of food in that area which can mean that the remaining teeth have a poor prognosis due to lingual caries.

Our approach to this situation, as reported earlier, has been to endeavour to prevent the deviation of the posterior quadrants at the time of surgery by fitting an appropriate splint prosthesis at the time of surgery. However, when adverse remodelling of the remaining bone has occurred, prosthetic management is, in our practice, by the use of a two-part prosthesis technique. The design concept of the two-part or sectional partial prosthesis as used in the first case is that it allows the component elements to be located from two paths of insertion (Fig. 17.53). This facilitates full engagement of both lingual under-cut surfaces of the remaining posterior teeth, thus eliminating the potential for food and other debris to accumulate under the prosthesis. When the two sections of the cast metal framework are located in their respective quadrants, a locking mechanism is activated which mechanically prevents the joined prosthesis from being withdrawn (Fig. 17.54). Many designs have been advocated, but each case will need to be treated on an individual basis. The design concept should meet the following criteria:

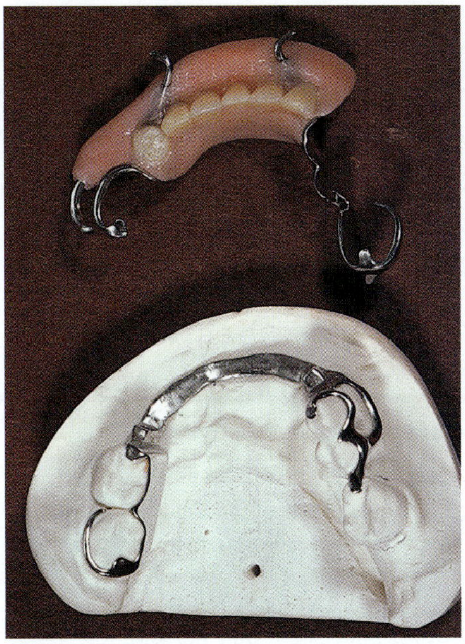

Figure 17.53 A two-part cast metal framework and denture designed to overcome lingual inclination of the remaining posterior teeth following earlier resection of the anterior dento-alveolar ridge and the underlying body of the mandible, leaving a thin strip of lower border. Each section of the prosthesis is located from its own path of insertion thus fully occupying all the lingual surfaces of the remaining posterior teeth.

1. Spread the functional load over the maximum number of teeth.
2. Address the need that every force requires to be met by an equal and opposite force (failure to meet this requirement will cause the appliance therapy to take on the role of an orthodontic-like

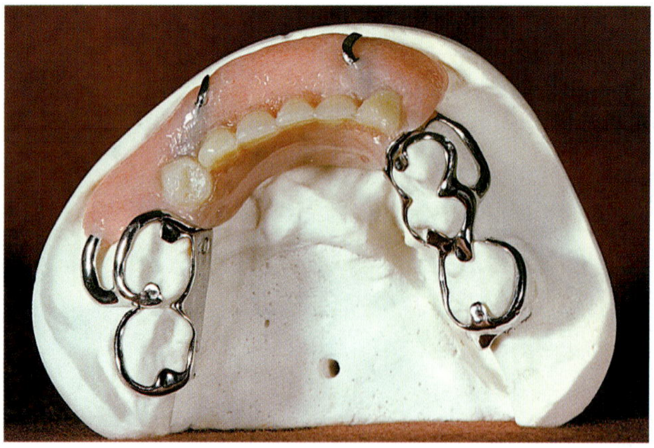

Figure 17.54 The two halves of the prosthesis locked together following activation of the two Pullen–Warner bolts. Note that the design of such cases should reflect the need for force and counterforce to be employed, i.e. all forces must be met by equal and opposite forces (albeit static), otherwise the device will become an orthodontic appliance resulting in tooth movement and possible bone loss.

appliance, resulting in subsequent tooth movement with associated loss of supporting alveolar bone).

3. Allow relatively easy access to the locking mechanism

Case presentations

This patient underwent an anterior resection some 45 years ago to remove a tumour which involved the lower anterior dento-alveolar quadrants. Fortunately, the cut ends of the alveolar ridge at the resection site were ideally shaped to provide a common path of insertion. The superior surface of the lower border of the mandible was also suitably shaped and covered with a relatively thin layer of mucosal tissue.

Because of the gross lingual rotation of the posterior quadrants, almost certainly attributable to the lack of splintage during the early postoperative phase, it was necessary to construct a two-part cast metal prosthesis for this patient. The two halves of the prosthesis were mechanically locked to one another by means of two Pullen–Warner locking bolts (Figs 17.53 and 17.54).

Over the last 45 years the patient has been supplied with two sectional or two-part prostheses. The second prosthesis was necessary only because the lower anterior acrylic teeth had become grossly foreshortened due to wear abrasion, otherwise the metal framework maintained its original precise contact with the remaining teeth. During the 45-year period the patient has worn his lower two-part prosthesis he has lost only one of his natural teeth. The remaining natural teeth are surprisingly firm and in good condition. The patient still uses this type of prosthesis some 45 years after surgery and even in his late 80s he has little difficulty in activating the locking devices.

Intra-oral prosthetic management of the mandibular discontinuity patient

The role of intra-oral prosthetic therapy in the management of the mandibular discontinuity patient is primarily to accomplish the following objectives:

1. To maintain the patient's vertical dimension.
2. To preserve functional activity, i.e. mastication and swallowing.
3. To restrict uncontrolled lateral deviation of mandibular fragments or fragment.
4. To maintain symmetry in the lower third of the face.
5. To maintain the musculature in its original functional state, i.e. to prevent contracture due to an imbalance between the muscles that are responsible for jaw activity.
6. To aid the preservation of speech.

As already stated, varying degrees of mandibular dysfunction following loss of mandibular continuity will pertain where it has not been possible to bridge the surgically created defect, with either a bone graft or a deep buried implant prosthesis. The latter may be of short-term duration, while staged surgical reconstruction is awaited, or it can be of a permanent nature when surgical reconstruction is contraindicated for medical reasons, or has been declined by the patient.

The ability to restore a degree of functional activity and, moreover, restore facial harmony where a discontinuity type defect pertains by means of intra-orally sited prosthetic devices is, to a large extent, determined by the number of teeth that are present in both arches. A reasonable number of well supported teeth in both jaws will allow the use of a training flange. This device consists essentially of a plate or wire frame that mechanically allows vertical jaw opening, but restricts lateral deviation of the intact mandibular fragment (Figs 17.55 and 17.56).

When the patient is edentulous, full restoration of form and function by prosthetic therapeutic means is less successful. The displacing forces placed on

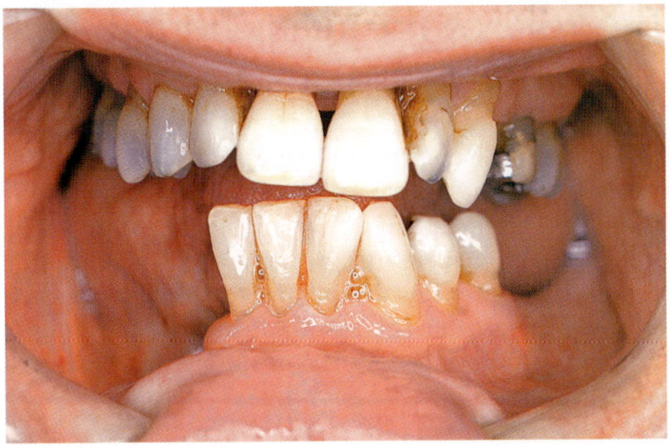

Figure 17.55 Fragment instability following an almost hemimandibulectomy owing to loss of muscular equilibrium in the floor of the mouth, resulting in lateral and upward deviation.

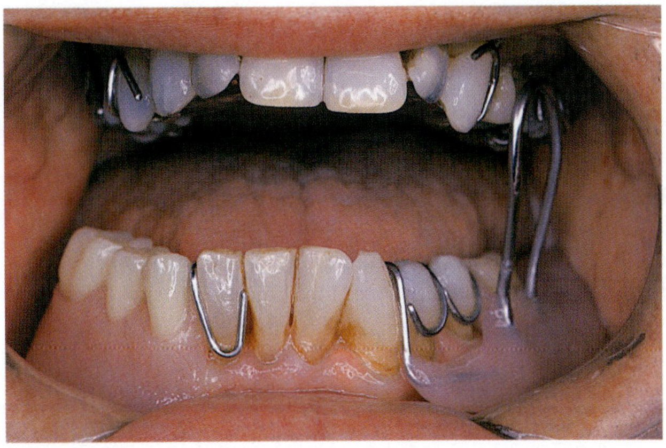

Figure 17.56 The wire framework processed as a integral part of the clasp retained lower prosthesis abuts against an acrylic platform, which is part of the clasp retained upper acrylic plate. This appliance allows vertical opening of the jaw but prevents lateral deviation of the sectioned mandibular fragment.

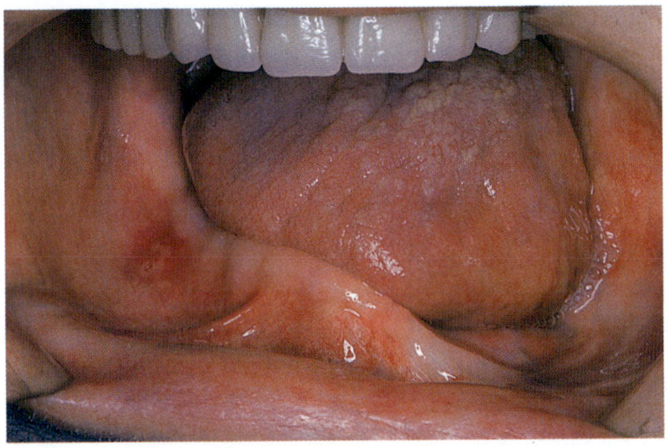

Figure 17.57 Hemimandibulectomy in the edentulous patient presents a substantial challenge in relation to achieving satisfactory prosthetic management. This is further compromised if the remaining alveolar ridge and sulci do not offer some physical resistance against functional displacement of the prosthesis. Fortunately, in this case sufficient ridge height and sulcus depth pertained to make a prosthetic input to the patient's treatment a viable proposition. The occlusal platforms of both the upper and lower teeth were widened and the occlusal plane canted to encourage the fragment to be returned to its correct position on closure of the jaw.

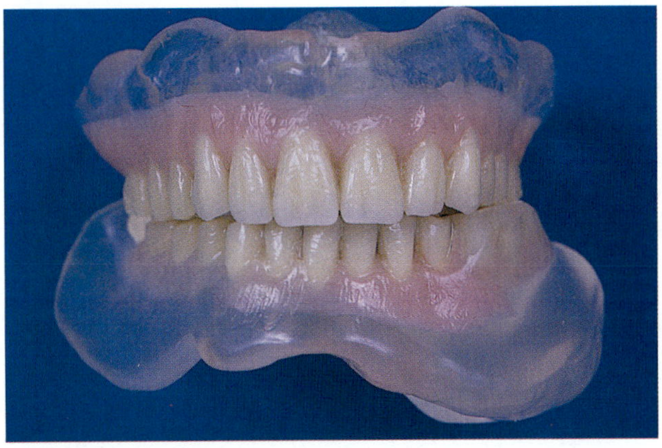

Figure 17.58 The upper and lower prostheses in occlusion. Note the full peripheral extension of both prostheses to achieve maximum physical retention and stability.

the edentulous prosthetic device are often much greater than the level of physical retention that can be achieved at the prosthesis/tissue interface.

Experience has shown, in the mandibular discontinuity cases, that it is possible to use intra-orally sited devices in order to effect improvement of function and appearance. Prosthetic therapy can help to improve masticatory performance and in some instances also cosmesis. The overall governing factor is how stable the intra-oral prosthetic device can be made, if the stated objectives are to be achieved. The presence of teeth in both jaws is essential if the forces that cause mandibular deviation are to be resisted.

Prosthetic rehabilitation in the edentulous patient is essentially directed to establishing a means of occlusal contact. This is accomplished by extending the occlusal platform in the upper prosthesis towards the palatal mid-line. By creating a slight cant in the occlusal plane of the bite platform it is sometimes possible to reduce the amount of deviation that actually takes place and, at the same time, maintain a degree of occlusal contact. The presence of lingual and labial vestibular sulci of adequate depth will influence the prosthetist's ability to establish prosthesis stability (Figs 17.57 and 17.58).

Case 1: mandibular resection: dentate patient

This patient's treatment demonstrates the use of a guide system in a dentate patient where the remaining sound natural teeth provided adequate anchorage to prevent the prosthesis being displaced during functional activity. The wire extension was fabricated from 1.5 mm diameter hard stainless steel wire and is joined to the lower prosthesis in the first and second premolar region contralateral to the defect site (Fig. 17.55).

The intention was to clasp as many teeth as possible and use occlusal rests in order to distribute the incurred loading widely over the dental arches. When first seen, this patient's jaw relationship following the resection was being exacerbated and the overall displacement was made considerably worse as the lower dental arch had taken up a position within the palatal vault. In fact, the palatal mucosa was acting as an inclined plane, thus adding to the overall displacement of the jaw fragment. The sequela of this was that a considerable amount of rotation was taking place in the remaining temporomandibular articulation with accompanying discomfort. The lower teeth had also caused considerable laceration to the palatal mucosa. A further complication was that the remaining musculature in the floor of the mouth had undergone severe contracture, which added to the displacement of the mandibular fragment.

This type of device is very useful in a 'holding position', which aptly describes its purpose when surgical reconstruction is planned at a later stage. Any improvement in the relationship of the remaining mandibular arch to the maxilla and prevention of further contracture of the musculature will help to prevent harmful contractual forces being placed on the bone graft (Fig. 17.56).

Case 2: mandibular resection: edentulous patient

This patient's prosthetic management facilitated considerable improvement in both masticatory performance and extra-oral appearance. Careful attention to physiological moulding of the base of the lower prosthesis and its extension into part of the defect space did much to improve overall stability and the restoration of function. Minimal increase in the width of the occlusal platform was sufficient to maintain masticatory performance and prosthesis stability. It is mainly the bulk extension of the lower prosthesis into the defect site that prevents the main fragment being drawn in a lateral direction by the remaining musculature and the presence of scar tissue (Figs 17.57 and 17.58).

The role of the deep buried mandibular implant

Mandibular discontinuity type defects following resection can vary in length, site and magnitude. The level of incapacity that arises following such procedures also varies according to the type of resection carried out. The further the resection procedure extends, the greater the resultant incapacitation and the more pronounced is the resultant facial deformity.

Normal mandibular functional activity is dependent on skeletal continuity, the presence of teeth and an intact and co-ordinated muscular system. When one or both of the temporomandibular articulations is compromised, the remaining mandibular element or elements are placed in a state of imbalance. This, in the main, is due to the loss of the equilibrium that normally exists in the musculature that is responsible for mandibular activity being disturbed. As the extent of the ablative procedure increases, the level of malfunction and skeletal deviation also increases. Bony fragments, following loss of continuity, undergo varying patterns of medial, rotational and superior deviation.

This sequence of events has the potential to compromise the patient's ability to masticate, swallow and articulate, and can also interfere with respiration when gross deviation occurs. A degree of cosmetic impairment can also be anticipated depending on the severity and location of the defect site. Wherever possible, the prime objective is to attempt to restore mandibular skeletal continuity with either a bone graft or by the placement of a deep buried implant prosthesis.

The cardinal rule in both the surgical and prosthetic management of the patient with a mandibular discontinuity defect is not to perceive this type of deformity as being primarily a structural problem. The aftermath of this type of resection has to be seen as also constituting a biomechanical problem, as the musculature that controls mandibular activity can no longer function as a co-ordinated and controlled entity. Unless both skeletal continuity and muscular control are fully addressed, the end result is highly likely to be less than satisfactory. The roles of human engineering and biomechanics in this situation should always be viewed as having equal importance. In certain situations, especially when the patient is reluctant to allow a secondary procedure to obtain a bone graft or where the medical condition is a contra-indication, consideration has to be given to prosthetic replacement to achieve skeletal continuity. Experience has shown that certain types of mandibular defects are more amenable to prosthetic management than others. Success is usually determined by the quality and thickness of the surrounding soft tissue envelope. Irradiated structures can also influence the viability of the host structures and be a contra-indication for prosthetic involvement. It is interesting to note that radiotherapy can be safely delivered in the presence of a titanium implant prosthesis due to the special physical characteristics of this material.

The component parts required to replace the missing sections of the mandible can be hand made in the maxillofacial laboratory if suitable equipment and titanium of the correct grade and shape are available. Again, our experience has shown that titanium is the metallic material of choice for replacement of the mandible. It is well tolerated by the body and, moreover, has the optimum physical and mechanical properties to make it suitable for implantation in this anatomical site.

Case presentation

This patient presented with a tumour at the angle of the mandible, which fortunately had not eroded through the overlying soft tissues (Fig. 17.59). Unfortunately, the patient's general health

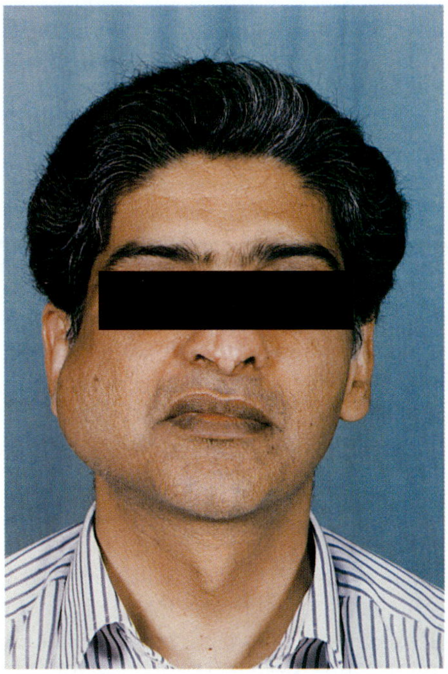

Figure 17.59 The presence of a malignant tumour involving the angle and horizontal body of the mandible (but not the overlying soft tissues) indicated the need for surgical intervention. The patient's health and disinclination to embark on surgical reconstruction prompted the decision to maintain mandibular continuity by using a custom-made deep buried implant prosthesis.

precluded the possibility of immediate surgical reconstruction following the resection procedure. In anticipation of this, a two-part titanium prosthesis was fabricated using radiographs to determine the dimensions of the device. The device consists of the following components:

1. A ramus section;
2. A pre-angulated body section;
3. Two screw bolts;
4. Two retaining devices.

Both the fixing plates at the ends of the body section have a long slot rather than individual holes to accommodate the bone screws or nut and bolt retaining mechanism. The purpose of the vents is to allow the vertical alignment of the ramus section to be determined at the time of surgery, and also to permit more latitude for locating the fixing plates to the buccal wall of the sectioned mandible.

The ramus section, fabricated in T160, is relatively hard and unyielding and offers the best mechanical conditions in which to create a screw thread, whereas the angulated body section was fabricated in T115, which is relatively ductile and malleable. Both types of titanium are compatible with one another and can be safely used in combination without electrolytic action taking place. The use of T115 allows cold bending to be carried out in the operating theatre at the time of contouring and fitting the prosthesis. Following attachment of the preangulated body section to the remaining bony fragment, the ramus section was adjusted to take up a passive relationship within the glenoid fossa. (If necessary, the orientation of the ascending ramus section can be adjusted with a special bar bending tool.) The contour of the horizontal bar of the body section was fashioned to establish a passive relationship with both the internal and external soft tissue structures.

For many years we have placed a perforated silicone rubber sleeve over the contoured implant (Fig. 17.60). This aids soft tissue in-growth and helps to form a cushion over the metal framework, thus preventing stress points being created in the overlying soft tissue structures. (A narrow bar abutting against a tight soft tissue surface creates a 'stiletto heel' effect.) The advantage of the silicone tubing is that it increases the volume of the implanted device without adding to the weight of the metallic structure and, in addition, creates a pseudo-periosteal sheath which aids tissue attachment.

Finally, to address biomechanical requirements, the anterior part of the temporal muscle was relocated to act as a static sling and to provide upward lift and full-thickness cover over the angle of the prosthesis.

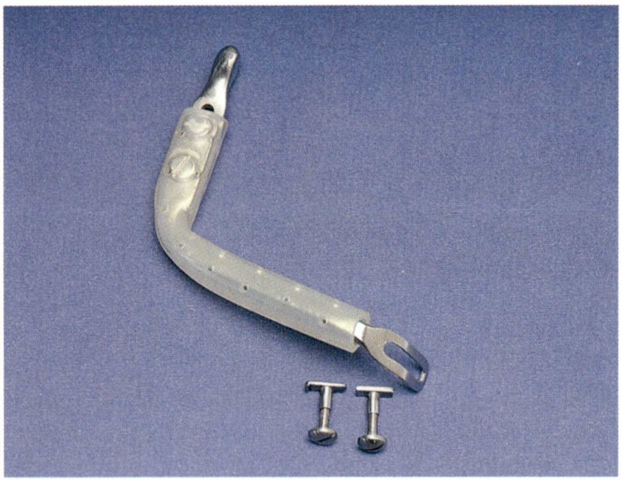

Figure 17.60 The two-part titanium implant (which has an in-built capacity to allow vertical adjustment) of the ramus height and orientation of the condylar head, bolted together and covered with a thick walled perforated medical grade silicone tube, immediately before placement in the body.

This manoeuvre brings in additional cover and bulk which helps to reduce lateral deviation of the mandible. This important additional input is of great importance in addressing the problem of restoring biomechanical control and support. This prosthetic device is still in full functional use some 10 years after it was installed and the patient has declined further reconstructive surgery (Fig. 17.61). This patient's treatment was carried out under the management of Mr Daniel Archer FRCS, Consultant Maxillofacial Surgeon at the Royal Marsden Hospital, London.

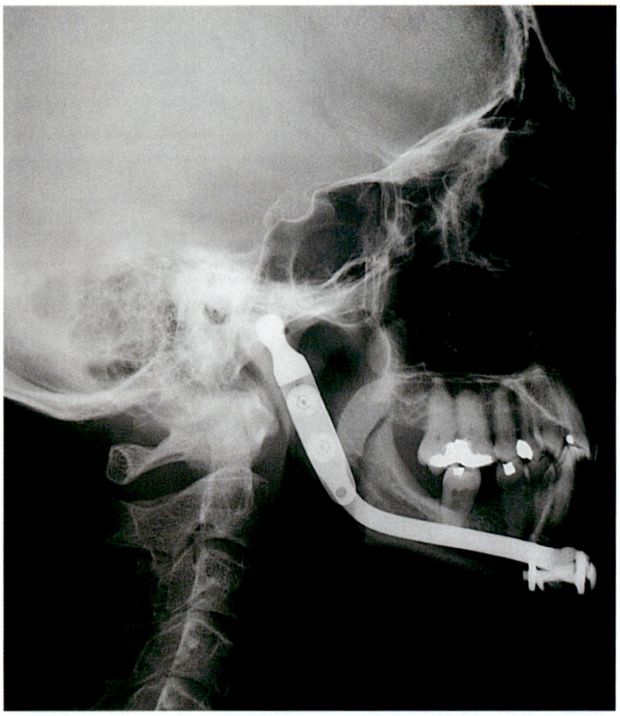

Figure 17.61 An x-ray showing the internal location of the implant and the presence of the two retaining devices which attach the implant to the remaining bony fragment in the symphesis region. A turned-down portion of the anterior fibres of the temporal muscle was attached to the angle of the implant to provide a static sling.

Prosthetic management of the glossectomy patient

Patients that have undergone a partial or total glossectomy will have varying degrees of disability depending on the extent of the resection procedure carried out. In the main, dysfunction is manifested by speech impairment and lack of control of food and saliva and often the ability to swallow.

Interference in articulation is usually proportional to the volume of the tongue mass that has been lost. Minimal loss of tongue volume will usually cause only slight interference in speech intelligibility. Patients with partial resection of the tongue tend to use the residual remnant to simulate adaptive normal articulatory functional movements.

The location of the resection site is also of considerable importance as loss of the tip of the tongue, for example, will result in greater impairment of speech as compared with a hemi-glossectomy. This relates to the patient's ability to maintain physical contact between the tongue and the palate. Obviously, after total glossectomy, the patient is unable to articulate.

To have a better understanding of this type of surgical deformity it is essential to have some basic understanding of the mechanism of speech. Essentially, human speech is created by a projected air stream that is directed through a vibrating mechanism, which consists of a resonating area and a patent oral cavity. These component parts make up the so called vocal tract.

Various authors have reported their findings in relation to the provision of prosthetic appliance therapy designed to improve speech and control of food and oral fluids for the post-resection patient. It is true to say that the prosthetic management of such patients is complex and demanding and calls for close interdisciplinary co-operation between the speech therapist and the CMFPT team. In the main, most experts in this field seem to agree that partial glossectomy patients are best treated by lowering the palatal vault by prosthetic means. This enables the patient to maintain a degree of physical contact between the tongue and the palatal surfaces.

However, patients who have undergone a total glossectomy can also benefit from a prosthesis that simulates the volume of the tongue mass that has been lost. The missing structure is replaced with an appropriately shaped facsimile that fills the floor of the mouth. Most of the devices that have been described in the literature have been essentially static structures other than the facility for minor flexibility due to the intrinsic compliance of devices when constructed in materials such as silicone rubber.

The tongue is a dynamic structure that changes its position within the oral cavity, but maintains a semblance of contact with the palate and the walls of the teeth in certain speech forms. The foregoing criteria have prompted one of the authors (BC) to design and construct a new type of artificial tongue prosthesis that is a dynamic component, in an attempt to replicate the basic function of the tongue, in the hope of restoring some semblance of speech.

Case report

This edentulous patient presented with a large malignant tumour that involved the tongue, floor of the mouth and the alveolar ridge. Because of the type of tumour and its spread, it was decided that it would be necessary to carry out a total glossectomy and, moreover, resection of the lower alveolus. A free flap was used to repair the resultant soft tissue defect in the floor of the mouth and to provide cover for the remaining strut of basal bone that constituted the lower border of the mandible. The flap was shaped posteriorly to provide bulk with the intention of simulating the tongue so that this would improve speech performance. Unfortunately this objective was not realised. A further impediment that caused the patient great concern was that the lower lip, having lost its underlying bony support, collapsed into the floor of the mouth. This resulted in the escape of oral fluids and food and was also contributory to his speech problems (Fig. 17.62).

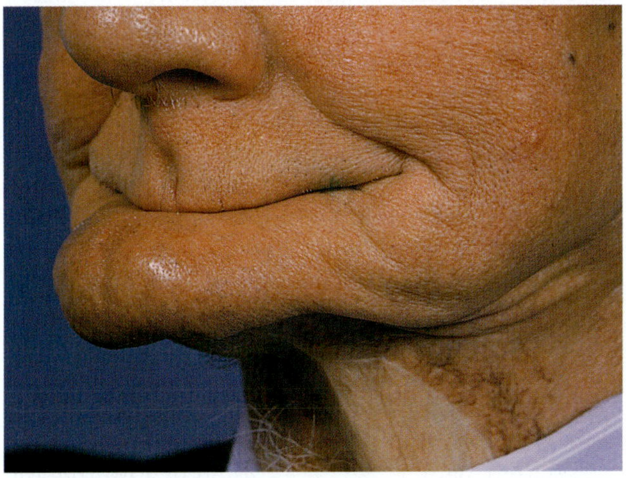

Figure 17.62 Collapse of the lower facial structures and associated dysfunction following resection of the lower alveolar ridge and the tongue.

The first priority from a prosthetic point of view was to restore the patient's vertical dimension and to provide support for the lower lip. Upper and lower dentures were therefore constructed using the residual basal bone as a pseudo-dental alveolar base. The almost flat floor of the mouth offered little or no resistance to counteract the powerful backward-directed contracting force exerted by the lower lip. In an attempt to oppose this, the lower prosthesis was extended to engage the vertical surfaces of the ascending rami. Once the patient's vertical relationship had been restored and support provided for the lower lip, a state of equilibrium was established.

The next stage in the prosthetic management involved extending the lower denture to cover the reconstructed floor of the mouth with a view to improving overall stability and to provide a foundation for the artificial tongue. When the patient became accustomed to this, which took approximately 2 weeks, steps were taken to design and construct the artificial tongue.

The design concept attempted to address the need for establishing a 'vibrating' component and to replace the volume previously occupied by the tongue within the oral cavity. This was achieved by a trial and error process by building up a form in wax and bonding it to the lower prosthesis and then modifying the shape until some improvement in the patient's speech could be discerned. The next stage involved the construction of a hinged linking system that allows the artificial tongue to be joined to the most posterior aspect of the base plate. The wax form of the artificial tongue, in which one half of the linking mechanism (i.e. two lengths of 2 mm internal diameter stainless steel tubing) are housed, was subsequently converted to hard acrylic (Fig. 17.63).

To introduce a means of creating the vibrating action, two magnets were located at the anterior tip of the under surface of the artificial tongue and directly below, in the base plate. The magnets were arranged in a repulsion relationship, separated by approximately 1 cm (Fig 17.63). At this distance the magnetic forces were in a 'making and breaking' state. The actual mobility of the artificial tongue is created by movement of the head, which influences the delicate balance between the opposing magnets to change. Closure of the lower jaw also results in the tongue being rotated at the hinge. On opening the jaw the tongue tip is again activated by the action of the repelling force of the

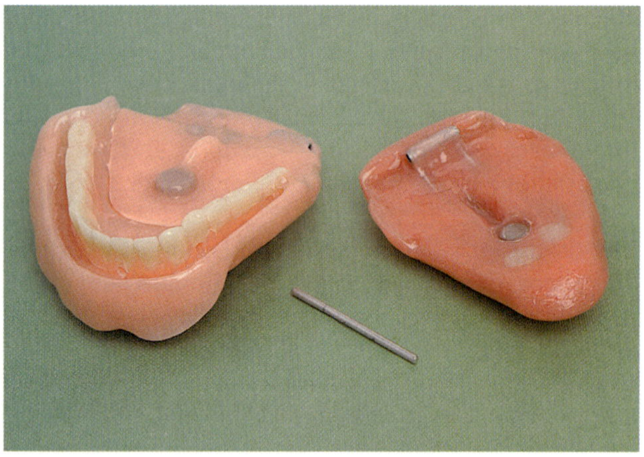

Figure 17.63 The intra-oral prosthesis (which totally covers the floor of the mouth and relies on the cut margin of the lower border of the mandible for support), together with the detachable artificial tongue. The two darker areas under the tongue and in the anterior part of the base plate immediately behind the anterior teeth indicate the location of the rare earth magnets that are encompassed within the acrylic. The magnets are arranged to be in a state of repulsion and are approximately 1 mm apart when the tip of the tongue is in its most superior position.

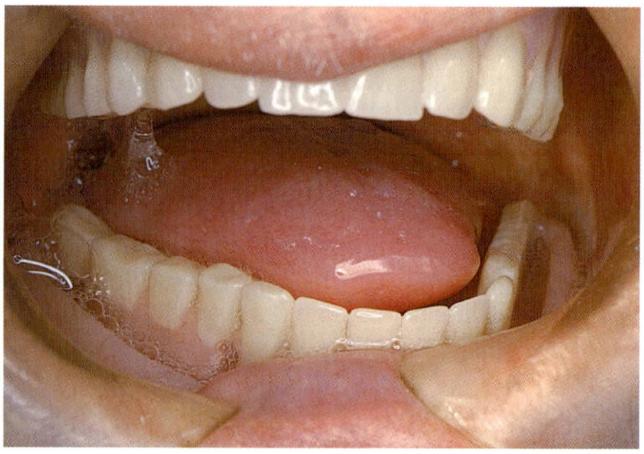

Figure 17.64 The artificial tongue hinged to the lower dental prosthesis. The lowered palatal vault of the upper denture depresses the tip of the artificial tongue around the axis of the hinge, thus bringing the magnets together. When the jaw is opened the action of the opposing magnets is then activated, which sets the tongue in a state of oscillation. The volume of the tongue in the floor of the mouth, the lowered palate and the changing position of the hinged tongue assists the patient to form speech sounds.

magnets. In order to fill the intervening space between the upper surface of the artificial tongue and the palate of the upper denture, the latter was lowered to create a point of contact when the dental prostheses are in occlusion. When the teeth are in contact the tip of the artificial tongue is depressed by contact with the palatal surfaces of the upper denture, thus overcoming the repulsive forces between the opposing magnets. On opening the jaw, the opposing magnets come into play and the tongue enters into a state of temporary vibration (Fig. 17.64).

The patient has learnt by practice to adopt different head positions and different degrees of occlusal contact to produce the conditions for a level of intelligibility. If the patient speaks slowly to allow the saliva which tends to collect in the anterior part of the mouth to dissipate, a reasonable semblance of speech can be produced. Special channels were made in the buccal surfaces of the lower prosthesis to aid the flow of the excess saliva to the posterior aspect of the mouth (Fig. 17.63).

The artificial tongue almost fills the space between the anterior and posterior artificial teeth, leaving just enough latitude for free movement in the vertical direction to take place. The tongue element also helps to project the bolus of food in a posterior direction. The patient can withdraw the locating pin that links the artificial tongue to the lower denture to simplify cleaning.

The developing role of osseointegration technology in orofacial prosthetic restoration and rehabilitation

Few would disagree, especially among those who are charged with providing a prosthetic solution for patients with varying degrees of disability and deformity in different parts of the body, that the ability to 'forge a biophysical bond' with living bone to be the most important single advancement in prosthetics. For many decades the means of gaining attachment to the body has remained unchanged. In the main, the traditional techniques used to establish a means of attachment between the body tissues and prosthetic devices can be described as constituting 'socket-type retention', with dentures, obturators, artificial eyes, finger and limb prostheses all being examples of this methodology. It is true to say, that in certain areas of maxillofacial prosthetic management many of the conventional methods of retention are not suitable, or cannot be deployed because of the severity of the deformity, especially in relation to the sparsity and quality of the remaining structures.

With one gigantic leap however, some three decades ago a new dimension entered the field of prosthetic restoration and rehabilitation that has become known as osseointegration technology. Scientific and clinical examination have since demonstrated that this technology can offer, in certain circumstances, a dependable and safe system which allows direct mechanical attachment of prosthetic devices to the human body, if certain basic principles are adhered to.[18,19]

The ability to mechanically link prosthetic devices to the bony skeleton not only overcomes many of the problems of gaining retention, but also offers a means of functionally stimulating the body tissues. This maintains the vitality of the body structures in and around the affected defect site and, moreover, the facility to restore in part tactile perception. These three factors, in the maxillofacial region, are of seminal importance because:

1. Without adequate retention and stability, essential functions such as speech, mastication and control of food and liquids are disturbed. In addition a prosthesis that is poorly retained can cause traumatic injury and in the long-term contribute to the loss of natural teeth.
2. Without functional stimulus, the body structures, especially bone, soon undergo resorption, becoming less dense and weaker as a result and, thus, less able to perform their intended role.[20]

Disuse atrophy is well recognised in the management of the amputee patient and the heavily resorbed edentulous jaw is also a good example of the role played by natural teeth in delivering a source of functional stress to the alveolar bone. It is well recognised that bone, when exposed to less than normal functional activity, and when the vector of applied load is changed, can exhibit adverse structural modification, due to loss of equilibrium in the stress–strain ratio.

The sequelae of this phenomenon can be readily observed in many post-resection maxillofacial patients where excessive dentoalveolar bone resorption and loss of vitality in the overlying soft tissues have occurred. This is brought about because the prosthetist has to rely on a reducing bony foundation for support and retention often due to adverse loading, that is further compounded by the inevitable ageing process. An example of this is the long-standing practice in maxillofacial prosthetics of expecting a few remaining teeth and their supporting structures to retain a large obturator prosthesis indefinitely, when the skeletal foundation has been reduced. This reflects the importance of applying sound and defensible biomechanical engineering principles to the management of the resection patient's post-prosthetic treatment. This failing, in part, is often due to a lack of understanding of human engineering and an ability to establish alternative methods of gaining retention and load distribution.

Fortunately, with the advent of osseointegration and its successful impact in dentistry, new technology now exists in maxillofacial prosthetics to improve the prosthetic management of the orofacial amputee patient. Osseointegration represents the very interface of biology and engineering, surgery and prosthetics and the marriage of living and non-living materials to create a link between the human body and prosthetic therapy.[21] There is also growing evidence that a degree of osseoperception exists following the placement of implants into bone. This increases the patient's awareness of local conditions during functional activity, thus improving performance and control of the prosthetic devices.

It would be wrong to imply that this scientific and technical advancement relating to the development of osseointegration took place over a short period of time, when in fact this concept is the result of painstaking research spread over at least four decades. Early research relating to osseointegration has shown that bone and marrow act as a functional unit and that the microcirculation, tissue injury and its repair are integral elements in understanding tissue integration phenomena. Examination of a host of metallic materials, especially titanium, at the microscopic and macroscopic levels, demonstrates that this element, in certain circumstances, forms a biophysical bond with bone (Fig. 17.65).

It has been well recognised in surgery that certain metallic materials have special intrinsic characteristics, particularly their non-corrosive qualities, which

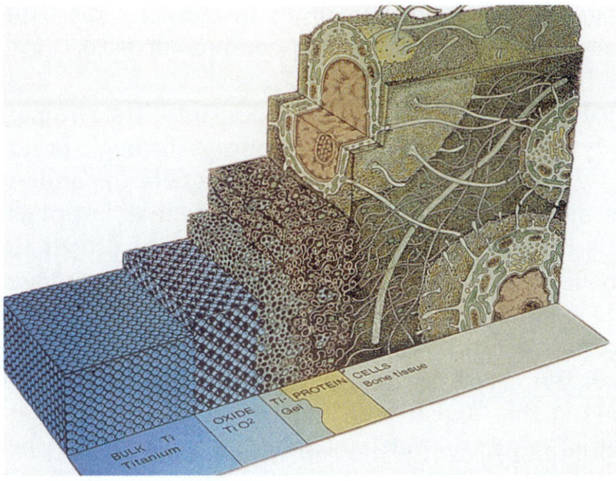

Figure 17.65 A precise explanation of the scientific basis of the phenomenon of osseintegration is currently not available. However, the essential structures that would seem to influence the establishment of a biophysical and biochemical bond between metal and bone are graphically presented in the above illustration. Reprinted with permission from International Workshop on Osseointegration in Skeletal Reconstruction and Joint Repair. Gothenburg, Sweden: Institute for Applied Technology, 1991.

to a large extent can be attributed to a tenacious outer oxide layer. It was, however, not fully appreciated that it is the outer coating and, in turn, the irregular surface morphology of the element titanium that are the integral and essential factors in establishing a biophysical bond between metal and bone. The outer surface of titanium is, in fact, a ceramic substance which is rich in oxide. What, hitherto, had also not been fully appreciated is that a special substance is also present over the oxide coating of titanium, that is called titanium per-oxy gel (Fig. 17.65). This gel or 'flux' not only appears to annul the body's defence mechanism and ability to mount an immune attack on substances it does not recognise, but also seems to have the facility to inhibit any inflammatory response around implanted titanium devices (Fig. 17.65).

There is now evidence to show that external and internal functional loading of bone plays an integral role in maintaining hard tissue volume and vitality which, in turn, influences the phenomenon of osseointegration.

Engineering technology has played no small part in developing a range of implants and component parts that offer, respectively, a means of intra-oral anchorage and extra-oral attachment of prosthetic devices. The design features of the implant fixture and its component elements are essentially based on the 'matching pair concept' invoking the engineering principles of locating and screw pairs. These devices require to be manufactured to the highest level of precision in order to allow the various components to be used in many different combinations. Furthermore, it has been necessary to develop a range of instruments in order to correctly drill the bone and install the various component parts.

Introducing implantable devices into the human body is not unlike making a journey through previously uncharted terrain and being totally dependent on mechanical equipment and essential supplies. This can be compared to the delivery of prosthetic rehabilitation based on osseointegration technology. It is axiomatic that the equipment used should meet rigorous scrutiny and be designed ergonomically to meet the needs of the task involved. The individual making the 'expedition' requires to have the intellectual capacity and knowledge of the terrain, plus the technical skills to achieve the requisite end result efficaciously without putting themselves or others at risk. In other words, it is necessary to acquire the correct education and training on how to manage the osseointegration patient appropriately, and to use the components and associated equipment that have been specifically designed for the task correctly.[8]

Some clinical colleagues are of the opinion that the loss of implants in patients who have undergone conjunctive radiotherapy and surgical ablative procedures is due primarily to being irradiated. There can be little doubt that where irradiation and, more especially, high dosage are involved that vascularisation will be impaired, with an associated reduction in osseoblastic and osseoclastic activity. We, however, are equally of the opinion that one must not overlook other potential contributory factors for the loss of implants, especially adverse biomechanical loading. It is well recognised in dentistry that when teeth are exposed to shear or tortional applied forces this produces adverse loading and bending moments. This compromises the long-term preservation of teeth, or more to the point, the supporting bone. It has to be recognised too that, in engineering terms, teeth and soft tissue penetrating implants are both classified as cantilevered beams. Therefore, both become vulnerable when shear, transverse or bending type forces are imposed upon them, especially on exceeding certain limits. The rigidity of teeth and implants at their interfacial relationship with bone is also determined, in part, by the surface area of the roots of the teeth that are encapsulated in bone and, in the case of the implant, the surface area that is biophysically bonded in healthy bone.

Granstrom has advocated the use of hyperbatic oxygen therapy to improve the success rate in the post-irradiated patient.[14]

There is ample evidence to demonstrate that the craniofacial skeleton per se is not a rigid structure, but rather a collection of linked independent units that function as a structural entity. This allows a degree of micromovement between the different bony elements, where they are joined together at the sutures (see Fig. 17.7). This facility needs to be introduced into the design concept of bar frameworks as used in large maxillary resection cases. This has been achieved in many of our patients, for example by extending the bar framework across the palate and, where necessary, into the defect site. The extra length of the super structure (it is often angulated where it enters the defect) and its shape allows greater potential for stress breaking under load. The vertical orientation of the bar framework also helps to prevent lateral movement of the attached prosthesis (Fig. 17.66). The bar framework, where it crosses the palate or the roof of a defect, acts as a tie beam (see Figs 17.65 and 17.76).

We also endeavour, wherever possible, to distribute applied functional load three-dimensionally by the strategic placement of implants. On some occasions this necessitates creating an adequate bony foundation in which to place an implant by utilising grafting procedures where there is a deficiency of bone.

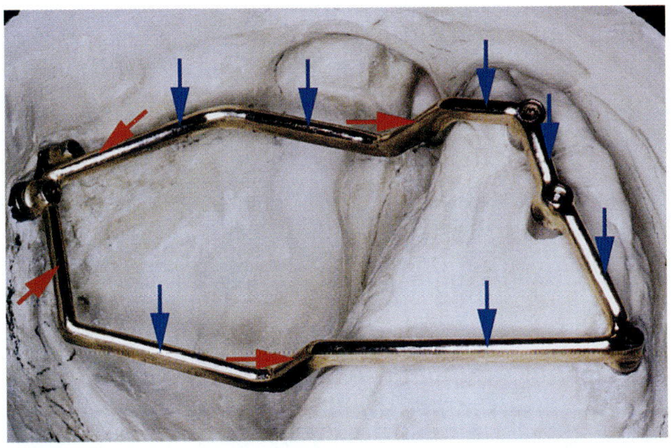

Figure 17.66 The location of implant fixtures in the post-resection defect and the design of the bar framework should be based on sound biomechanical engineering principles. In the above case attention has been paid to achieving the following: (a) bilateral distribution of load to structures capable of absorbing and retransmitting load; (b) to provide a tie beam system; (c) to address antro posterior loading; (d) to distribute vertical load (blue); (e) to resist lateral displacing forces (red); (f) to facilitate stress breaking in the bar framework. Short angulated zygomatic implants have been used in the defect.

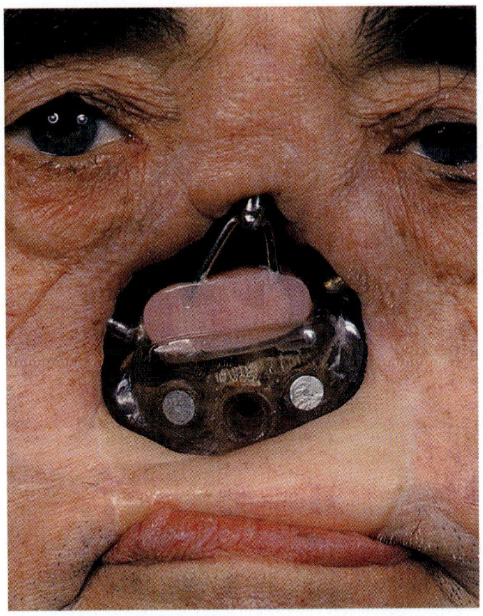

Figure 17.68 Because of the orientation of the implants it was necessary to use a three-part framework system that resembles a tripod, thus achieving a three-dimensional distribution of applied load. A sectional acrylic platform was processed around the terminal ends of the bar framework to establish a pseudo alveolus and palate. The three plastic sections contain rare earth magnets which, when in contact with magnets sited in the superior surfaces of the hollow-box obturator, provide retention. The male and female relationship between the acrylic platform and the upper surface of the obturator firmly holds the three components together yet allows a degree of stress breaking, thus protecting the implants and the supporting bone from being exposed to torque.

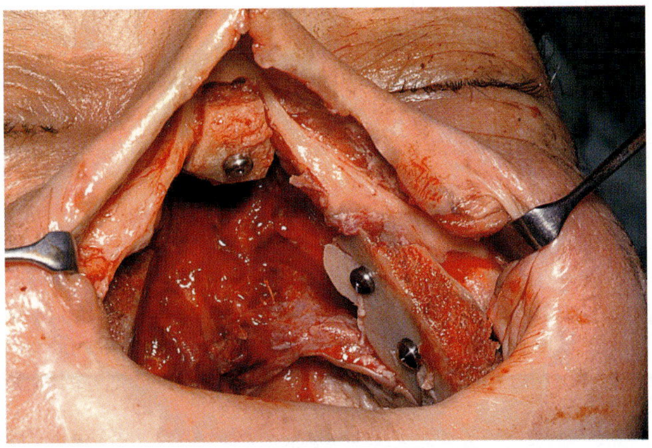

Figure 17.67 This patient underwent a total maxillectomy and removal of the nose and upper lip. The latter was surgically repaired by rotation of bilateral facial flaps. Due to lack of adequate bone it was necessary to place bone grafts at strategic sites within the defect. The implants were also used to secure the bone grafts in place. Soft tissue was advanced from the surrounding mid face to cover the exposed bone and the implants.

The sites where implants can be placed in post-resection cases that have been found to be useful are the anterior maxillary alveolus, the tuberosity and the bony area between these two points, if adequate bone is present or when bone grafted. The inferior orbital margin (when augmented with bone), the lateral orbital margin, the zygomatic buttress, the base of the skull at the root of the pterygoid plates (following resection), the supra-orbital ridge and the nasal bridge following bone grafting are additional areas that can be utilised for implant placement (Figs 17.66–17.68; see Figs 17.76 and 17.79). In the case of the mandible, as much of the alveolar ridge as circumstances permit should be used, avoiding the neurovascular bundle. The siting of implants in the retromolar region and linking them rigidly to anteriorly sited implants has proven to be problematic in certain cases. This can be attributable to the inevitable internal bending action that takes place in the horizontal body of the mandible whenever the lower jaw is subjected to functional activity during mastication. A sectional bar system is advocated in this situation. Masticatory muscle activity produces a bending moment at the midline of the mandible with inward rotation of the posterior horizontal body of the mandible and similar deviation of the ascending rami. This problem may be overcome by incorporating a facility for the linked bar system to have a degree of flexibility as a means of stress breaking between the anteriorly and posteriorly sited implants or as stated above a sectional framework.

Planning

As already stated, a full radiographic and clinical survey is essential, as this forms the very basis on which to conduct planning. This information, in conjunction with the mounted study models, is invaluable. We always begin the assessment procedure by making a two-dimensional drawing of where the implants ideally should be sited and the general alignment of the bar framework. This serves as a provisional indication of what is considered to be a possible surgical and prosthetic option (Fig. 17.69). Such drawings have proven to be extremely useful in giving the patient some idea of what is planned. This information is correlated with the radiographic and clinical evidence, e.g. bone density studies, and on the basis of this a three-dimensional representation or model planning system is constructed. It is important to relate this model to the opposing dental arch in order to assess the intermaxillary relationship to circumvent where possible high torque forces being placed on the implants. The purpose of the model planning system is to provide a three-dimensional representation of both the defect site and the intact structures with simulation of the optimum alignment of the implants and the bar framework. The implants are replicated by incorporating engineering type screw bolts into the study model and simulating the proposed alignment and cross-sectional shape of the bar framework with preformed wax strips. This type of planning model demonstrates to the surgical team, especially in the operating theatre, what will provide the prosthetic team with the ideal distribution of implants in which to carry out bar construction and the best way to gain optimum retention and load distribution. It should be noted that the correct spacing, alignment and the number of implants used can do much to influence the realisation of a satisfactory end result. This type of planning aid is extremely simple to construct and is inexpensive in relation to the materials used and the time taken to fabricate the model system. This completes the definitive planning.

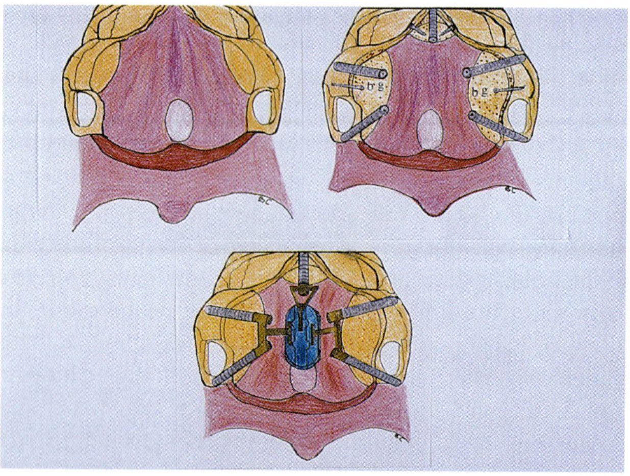

Figure 17.69 A simple two-dimensional planning aid that identifies: (a) the bony margins of the intra-oral and facial defect; (b) the proposed location of the bone grafts and the implants; (c) the design of the three-part bar framework and sectional acrylic platform (this planning aid relates to the treatment of the patient presented in Figs 17.67–17.68 and 17.70). A drawing of this type is made for all osseointegration cases by the CMFPT team prior to surgery.

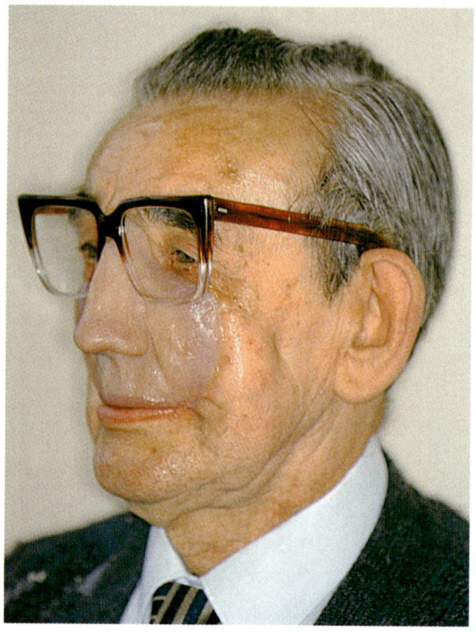

Figure 17.70 The external facial prosthesis is retained by a combination of gold clips that engage the vertical bar framework and strategically-sited platinum–cobalt magnets in the obturator. The facial prosthesis simulates the vermillion border of the upper lip and provides contact for the lower lip.

Insertion of implants

As already stated, the most appropriate sites in which to place implants must be investigated pre-operatively by a radiographic survey of the structures adjacent to the defect site to ascertain the quantity and quality of bone present, and especially its density to see if such areas can be utilised. The preparation of the bone to receive the implant and its eventual insertion should be carried out as atraumatically as possible. The operative site should be kept as cool as possible, to prevent thermal injury during drilling and the implant insertion procedure. The location and number of implants should reflect the degree of loading that will be placed on the source of retention and, moreover, to the location and quality of the bony foundations that can be utilised (see Fig. 17.74).

Operative criteria

The successful realisation of satisfactory prosthetic rehabilitation based on osseointegration is determined by biological and biomechanical engineering criteria, as set out in Table 17.9.

Table 17.9 Operative criteria

1. The quality and quantity of suitable bone that is available or can be established by bone grafting.
2. The length of implant that can be used.
3. The surface area of the implant that actually forms a biophysical bond with the surrounding bone.
4. The ability to address both anteroposterior and bilateral load-bearing forces (see Fig. 17.76).
5. The number of implants it is possible to place.
6. The distribution and orientation of the implants and their individual relationships to one another.
7. Achievement of a satisfactory emergence of the transmucosal abutment through the oral mucosa into the oral cavity (see Fig. 17.75).
8. The dynamic state of the soft tissue structures adjacent to the transcutaneous or transmucosal abutment.
9. The ideal placement of the retaining clips to distribute the forces created during insertion and withdrawal of the prosthesis and during functional activity. Ideally the applied load should be directed as close as possible to the source of bony support (see Fig. 17.77).
10. The achievement of satisfactory hygiene around the implants where they perforate the mucosa and also under the framework.
11. Optimum linkage between the implanted elements to distribute applied load three-dimensionally and to provide cross-bracing between distant sited implant fixtures. The need for stress breaking should also be considered in the design of the framework. This is required so as to prevent differential areas of tension and compression being created at the bone/implant interface (Fig. 17.66; see Fig. 17.77).
12. The ability to locate the various component parts safely, i.e. prosthetic abutments, screws and the bar framework, in the oral cavity.
13. The facility to locate and accommodate the dental prosthesis over the bar framework without interfering with the freeway space and allow an accessible path of insertion.
14. The facility to establish a functional seal around the margins of the removable prosthesis (see Fig. 17.77).

Design and construction of the bar framework

In the resection patient, as already pointed out, the distribution of applied load requires to be carefully balanced and distributed to those structures that can absorb and, in turn, retransmit load. Anteroposterior and bilaterally applied forces should be identified and addressed. Likewise, the bending moment in the mandible should be noted.

Because of the topography of many defect sites, especially in the maxillae, the alignment of the bar framework is of great importance, especially when using square or oblong bars as compared to round bar systems. Correct alignment of the bar framework can only be assured by using a paralleling instrument. This piece of equipment must be as accurate as possible, especially in relation to the articulated arm, as side play within the joint mechanism will introduce a discrepancy. Paralleling machines used in crown and bridge techniques, which also have facility for drilling and milling, are highly recommended for ensuring accurate alignment of the bar system. The complex shape of some defects and, moreover, the morphology and orientation of the dentoalveolar quadrants can on occasion involve the need for multiple sectioning of the prefabricated gold bar in order to establish a framework that follows the contours of the arch, palate and the defect. In some of our cases, in order to achieve the required configuration of the bar framework, it has been necessary to make over 25 separate soldered joints. This requires careful planning and a precise soldering technique in order to achieve close adaptation to maintain parallelism and prevention of distortion of the bar system during its construction (see Fig. 17.76).

In our experience the Dolder square sectioned bar and matching clips have proven to be more satisfactory than the conventional round bar and clip system. Without doubt the latter, while more universal in its application and easier to use, often has the disadvantage that the gold clips soon become bent or fractured when used in the very demanding intraoral post-resection patients' treatment.

Circumstances, will, on some occasions, indicate the need to use separate frameworks with the incorporation of a mechanical linkage between the different elements (see Fig. 17.76). This will be dictated by the orientation of the individually sited implants or groups of implants. While the new angulated implant and angulated abutments provide greater flexibility to overcome the problems of establishing a common alignment, this cannot always be fully realised, even when using transmucosal abutments with 30° or 45° potential for realignment. This is very often the case when zygomatic type implants are used in defect cases (Fig. 17.68).

When it is necessary to link the different bar elements mechanically, a special two-screw locating plate is used. Two lengths of Dolder bar soldered together will provide the dimensions and the type of gold in which to place a thread. We use the standard gold or titanium screws as supplied with the Branemark implant system. The use of locating devices involves miniature engineering skills and access to precise drilling and thread-making equipment (see Fig. 17.76). With the advent of the laser welder it is now possible to use an all-titanium assembly of implants, abutments, prosthetic abutments, screws, bars and clips.

Once the bar framework has been constructed it is tried in, to ensure that is marries up accurately with the matching interfaces of the transmucosal abutments. We have found it advisable to make a duplicate model of the bar framework while it is sited on the master model (see Fig. 17.76). This allows the gold framework to be left in situ and the denture prosthesis to be fabricated on the duplicate model. It is, however, necessary to block out the undersurfaces of the bar framework with wax and trim the lateral surfaces of the wax infill using the gold framework as an indication of the overall vertical alignment. This can only be accurately achieved by using a model surveyor and the appropriate shaping tool. The latter procedure should be carried out prior to pouring the RTV silicone rubber duplicating material. Failure to eliminate the spaces under the bar framework will prevent removal of the master model and attached gold framework from the silicone rubber duplicate mould. To ensure that the duplicate plaster model has maximum surface hardness and is dimensionally accurate, it is advisable to use a crown and bridge die stone type of plaster (see Fig. 17.76).

Leaving the bar framework in situ will simplify the bite registration and try-in procedures. Removing and re-inserting the framework at the various clinical stages in large orofacial resection cases is both time-consuming and increases the possibility of the patient accidentally swallowing the minute gold screws or other components.

The following stages of prosthesis construction largely follow conventional laboratory procedure. However, it is advisable to tin foil the fitting surfaces of the duplicate model, covering the entire dental arch, palate and the prosthetic abutments plus those parts of the bar system that will not be used for placement of the gold clips. Experience has shown that the placement of a thin layer of tin foil at the prosthesis/model interface helps to compensate for the inevitable contractual changes that occur in all acrylic prostheses during curing. The tin foil layer can be bonded to the stone plaster surfaces by use of an acrylic cement.

When the prosthesis has been processed, deflasked, trimmed and polished it is fitted back to a second duplicate model in order to ascertain that the denture satisfactorily fits the model and the replicated gold framework (see Fig. 17.77).

The lower jaw

It is advantageous to place implants in a bone grafted mandible as this can provide both support and retention for the prosthesis, which in turn functionally stimulates the grafted area. Such reconstructive procedures usually involve the use of a composite graft of bone, attached muscle, fat and skin. The soft tissue covering of this type of flap is usually thick and bulky. Where the flap is bulky and accordingly mobile and compressible it will be necessary before prosthetic restoration to thin out the flap and establish an attachment of the skin to the underlying bone. (This should be carried out when the implants are inserted and further adjusted, if necessary, at the second stage when the abutments are fitted.) Failure to do so will allow movement of the soft tissues over the underlying bony surfaces and around the abutments. This will result in the failure to ‘establish a satisfactory relationship’ between the soft tissues and the transmucosal abutments. Ideally, the soft tissue over the mandible and around the transmucosal abutments should consist primarily of epithelium and little else.

In non-reconstructed cases, Reintsema, van Oort and Schoen in The Netherlands have had considerable success in placing implants in the remaining alveolar ridge of the mandibular fragment following hemimandibulectomy (Figs 17.71 and 17.72).

The previous description is intended to present an overview of the role that osseointegration technology can play in intra-oral prosthetic restoration and rehabilitation to illustrate the salient factors that influence the realisation of a satisfactory level of treatment. The following case reports are presented to illustrate how certain defect cases have been managed successfully.

Case 1: dento-alveolar resection

This patient’s treatment demonstrates the advantages to be gained by carrying out immediate surgical reconstruction of the defect coupled with the insertion of implants into the bone graft. Following resection of a lesion presenting in the dentoalveolar region, a substantial block of bone from the iliac crest was introduced into the defect site. Two 22 mm long Branemark implants were inserted through the bone graft and into the remaining strut

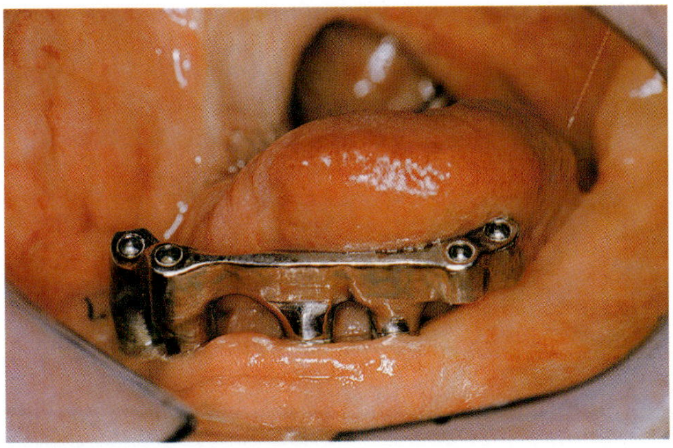

Figure 17.71 An implant-supported milled bar framework used in the treatment of a patient with a major mandibular discontinuity defect. The bar framework incorporates precision attachments.

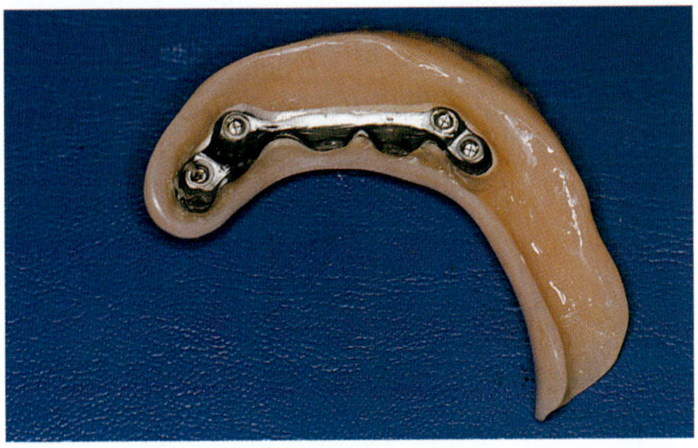

Figure 17.72 The male part of the retaining mechanism is encompassed within the lower prosthesis. Note that this prosthesis terminates close to the end of the sectioned mandibular arch to prevent shear loading forces being applied. This case is presented courtesy of Drs R van Oort, H Reintsema and P Schoen based at the Academische Zickhuis, Groningen in The Netherlands.

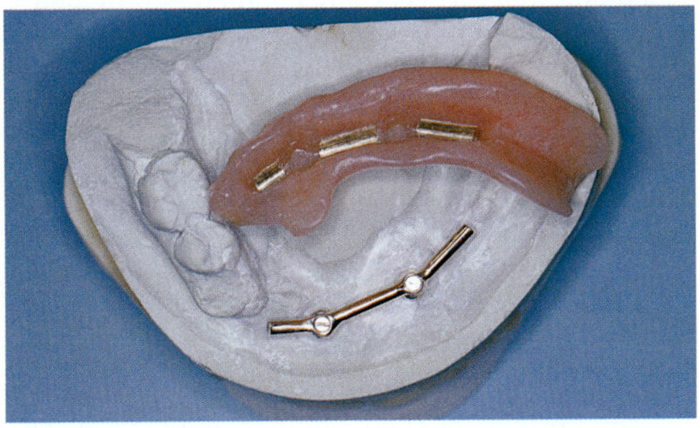

Figure 17.73 Implant fixtures were used in this case to retain both a bone graft placed in a large defect in the anterior dento-alveolar and body of the mandible, and to provide retention for a lower prosthesis. The 22 mm implants engage both the graft and the lower border of the mandible.

of the mandible (Fig. 17.73). The intended objectives of this were:

1. Immobilisation of the bone graft in the host site.
2. To provide a source of functional stimulation to the bone graft.
3. To augment the retention and stability of a lower prosthesis.

Some 4 months after surgery, the soft tissue bulk over the bone graft was thinned and 7 mm trans-mucosal abutments inserted. It was subsequently necessary to remove areas of granulation that had formed around the abutments and replace the loss of cover with thin mucosal grafts. This helped to prevent further build-up of granulation tissue in these areas. A gold bar was fitted to link the two implants and subsequently a removable lower prosthesis was inserted which was retained by gold clips. The early physical stimulation of the grafted area in this case, and the fitting of an implant-retained prosthesis, has contributed considerably to the viability of the bone graft and the overall stability of the mandibular arch.

Case 2: partial maxillary resection

This patient originally presented with a sarcoma in the upper jaw. Treatment necessitated an extensive resection of the anterior dentoalveolar quadrants and variable amounts of alveolar bone in the right and left posterior quadrants plus most of the hard palate. The support for the nose was also lost. A full course of radiotherapy was given, resulting in extensive contracture of the external face, especially the upper lip. Sometime later there was a recurrence of the disease and further radiotherapy was administered.

Prosthetic rehabilitation proved to be difficult because of the sensitivity of the irradiated soft tissues, which were extremely friable, and the lack of a bony foundation that could be used within the defect for load distribution. A further complication was that the patient had a mandibular protrusive dental relationship. While it is true to say that the patient managed to control his prosthesis, the level of rehabilitation achieved was inadequate by our standards. Retrospectively, it also has to be recognised that this removable prosthesis caused rotational forces to be placed on the remaining alveolar and palatal structures. Over a period of time this contributed to the remaining alveolar ridges undergoing considerable resorption. In May 1989 it was decided to insert Branemark type implants in an attempt to improve his functional activity. Exposure of the residual alveolar bony foundations showed that the previous use of per-alveolar wiring to retain surgical splints during three earlier operative procedures had left in their wake a honeycomb appearance in the bone. This, of course, could also be attributed to the high levels of radiation that had been given.

This prompted the decision to place bone grafts in the remaining antral vaults and to use implants to retain these grafts. Three other implants approximately 11 mm in length were placed in both tuberosities and in a small remaining extension of the canine eminence to engage the anterior pillaster buttress. Some 6 months later the implants were exposed. The bone around some implants, especially those that had been placed in the bone grafted sites, were found to have undergone a certain amount of resorption. Approximately 2 mm of thread was exposed but, otherwise, the implants were firmly osseointegrated. A one-piece bar framework of round cross-sectional specification was subsequently constructed and fitted. Reference to Fig. 17.74 will show that this was an open-ended bar system connected anteriorly by a linking strut that extended into and across the roof of the defect. Within the defect site an acrylic pad that housed a rare earth magnet was processed around the connecting bar in order to provide a site of additional stability and retention.

This prosthetic device functioned quite well for approximately 8 years, after which time increasing problems presented around those implants that had been placed in the irradiated bone rather than in the bone grafted sites. One can only postulate on whether the aftermath of irradiation or the design features of the bar system, including the use of a round bar, were the *raison d'être* for these implants becoming compromised. In all probability it was the result of a combination of both factors. In hindsight, the placement of a second tie bar across the intact palatine bone would have provided additional stability to the framework during functional activity, thus reducing torque on the posteriorly sited implants and, in turn, the supporting bone.

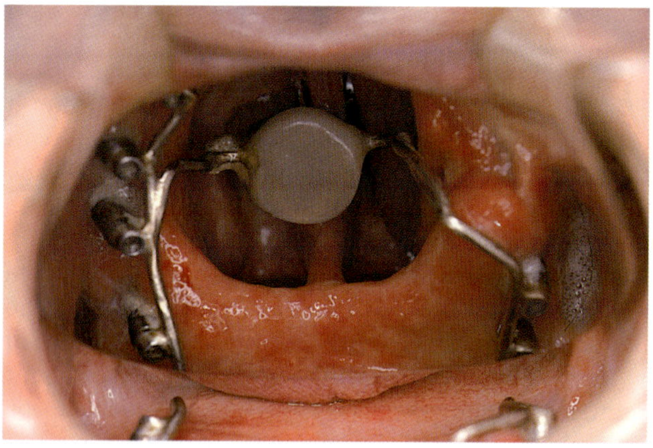

Figure 17.74 A one-piece bar framework which incorporates an integral acrylic platform in the anterior part of the large maxillary defect. The acrylic platform encompasses a rare earth magnet. The posterior margin of the defect is essentially the sectioned palatine bone and the tuberosities. The round bar framework is of a U-shaped configuration in both the horizontal and vertical planes.

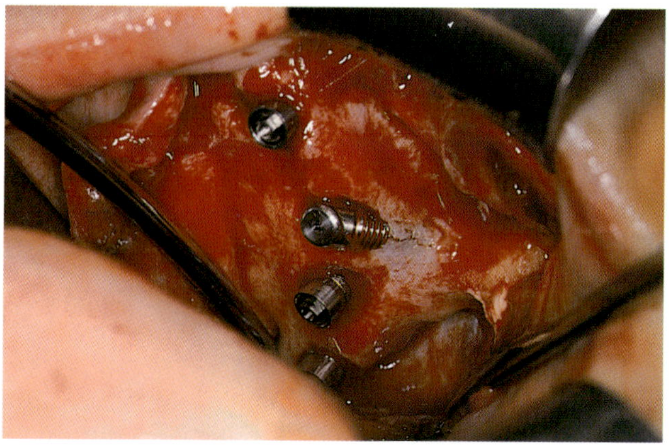

Figure 17.75 The placement of the zygomatic implants in the same patient as shown in Fig. 17.74 some eight years later. Note the necessity to locate the implants in different alignments owing to the sparsity of bony foundation around the defect site.

The loose implants were subsequently removed and, at the same time, four new transzygomatic implants of length 35 mm and 40 mm, respectively, were installed. Two additional implants approximately 20 mm in length were placed in both the tuberosities and pterygoid plates (Fig. 17.75). This new configuration and the introduction of longer and more appropriately sited implants provided a more even distribution of applied load in both the sagittal and coronal planes. Because of the unfavourable orientation of two of the anterior sited transzygomatic implants it was necessary to construct the bar framework in two sections and link them together with a locating plate (Figs 17.76 and 17.77). A very satisfactory level of prosthetic restoration has been achieved in this patient's rehabilitation. This reflects the positive attributes to be gained from wide distribution of load, made possible by the new long transzygomatic implants and the posteriorly sited standard implants placed in the tuberosity and pterygoid regions. The new short angulated zygomatic implants have been found to be advantageous when placed in the sectioned zygoma. Square Dolder bar was used in the fabrication of the two-part framework (note the distribution of gold clips). Subsequently, soft tissue

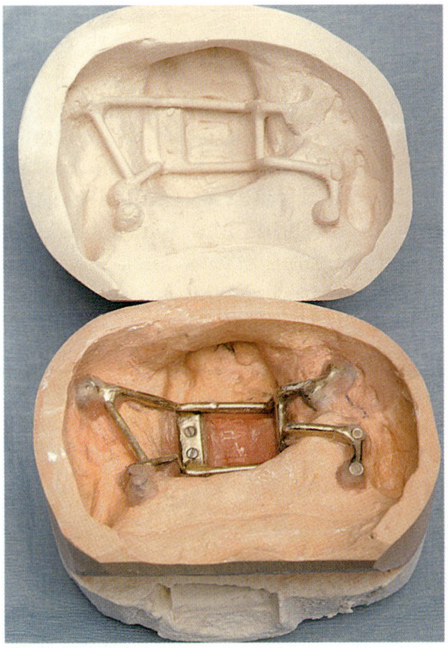

Figure 17.76 Owing to the orientation of the implant fixtures it was necessary to fabricate a two-part gold framework (using a Dolder bar). Note the use of a box frame system to provide both anterior- and posterior-sited tie beams and a two-screw locating plate that links the two frameworks together. The duplicate of the working model and bar framework is shown above and it is on this model that the hollow-box acrylic obturator was processed.

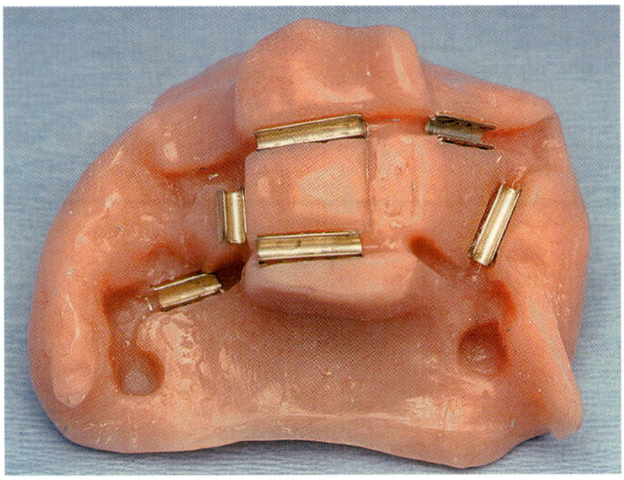

Figure 17.77 The large hollow-box obturator showing the placement of the retaining clips that are sited to resist both antro-posterior and laterally directed forces.

reconstruction and modification was carried out in this patient to lift the tip of the nose and to introduce greater length in the upper lip (Fig. 17.78). With the aid of osseointegration technology this patient is currently well-rehabilitated in terms of speech, mastication, control of food and liquid and facial appearance, despite having little or no maxillea.

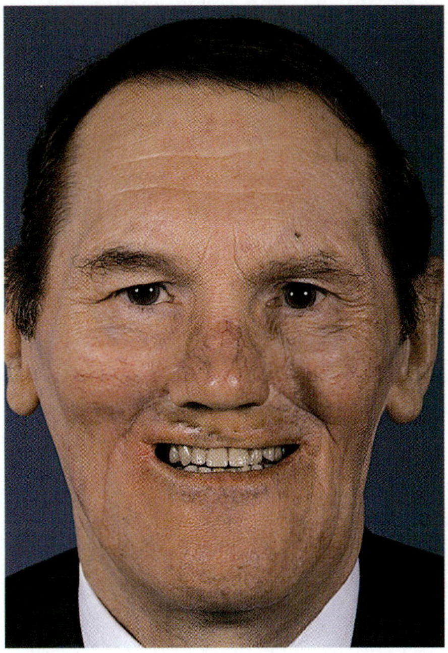

Figure 17.78 The patient's appearance (following lengthening of the upper lip) with the obturator in situ.

Case 3

This patient underwent a major resection some 25 years ago, leaving a large residual orofacial defect. The bony palate and the remnants of the alveolar ridge in the defect area (which had become a cantilever structure after the ablative procedure) soon lost vitality and rigid status due to the adverse shear loading forces applied by the intra-oral prosthesis. Some 15 years ago osseointegrated implant fixtures were placed in the supra-orbital ridge (with the intention of using this bony structure as a pseudo dento-alveolar ridge) and the stump of the pterygoid process. This arrangement of implant fixtures allowed a tripoidal bar framework to be installed, creating a pseudo facial skeleton. Owing to the presence of three small defects in the soft tissues overlying the oral cavity, it was possible to provide direct stability and retention for the intra-oral dental prosthesis (Fig. 17.79).

The bar framework also provides a source of retention for the large facial prosthesis. This was fabricated in Cosmesil silicone rubber (Cosmedica Ltd, Cardiff, United Kingdom), which is a soft compliant material. The facial restoration was processed over and bonded to a thin lightweight acrylic base plate in which the retentive gold clips are sited. This prosthetic restoration

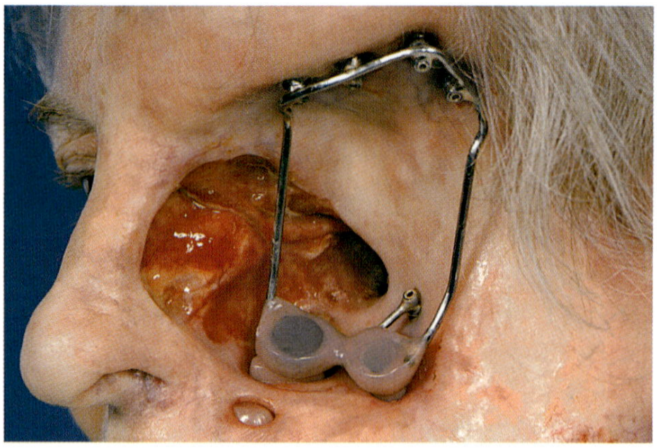

Figure 17.79 Strategic placement of fixtures and the arrangement of the bar framework to create a pseudo facial skeleton. Note the use of magnets within the acrylic pads that are located over minor defects in the residual palate (which is devoid of bone) that transmit vertically directed forces from the intra-oral prosthesis via the framework to the super-orbital ridge and the root of the pterygoid plates.

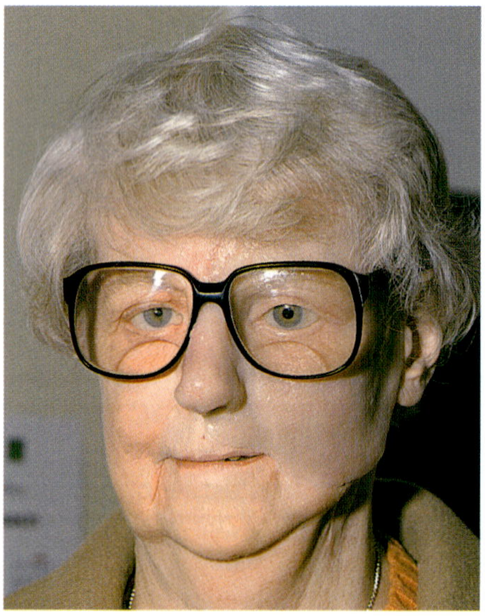

Figure 17.80 The patient's appearance following fitting of a large silicone rubber facial prosthesis which was processed over a thin acrylic base plate in which the gold clips are housed.

and bar framework has been in clinical use for almost 15 years, and the patient maintains a full family and social life (Fig. 17.80). This case demonstrates that when the disease process has compromised the facial structures, the resection procedure often involves the sacrifice of large areas of bone and soft tissue, including the orbital structures, that prosthetic restoration and rehabilitation can play a meaningful role. Surgical reconstruction in this patient's management was considered inadvisable due to previous extensive radiotherapy.

Summary

It should not be assumed that osseointegration technology is the total panacea for all patients needing prosthetic restoration. It has to be recognised that some resection patients can be treated adequately by simpler methods and that some will benefit from osseointegration. It has been standard practice, when placing osseointegrated implants in the craniofacial region, to wait approximately 6 months before bringing them into service. This has become known as the osseointegrating or healing period. Current research and clinical experience, however, would seem to indicate in some situations that a shorter period sufficient to allow repair at the implant/bone interface may be a viable option. This has special implications for the resection patient because it opens up the possibility of the immediate insertion of implants at the time of resection, allowing their early exposure and utilisation. The period for postoperative healing and the control of contracture within the defect site may in fact coincide with the time required for a sufficient level of osseointegration to take place. This of course has to be balanced with the need to administer postoperative radiotherapy in some cases.

Our current knowledge of osseointegration and its application in the treatment of the tumour patient is still at an early stage. The international pooling of clinical findings and scientific research will, without doubt, make for greater understanding of the most efficacious use of osseointegration procedures in the treatment of the compromised patient.

Concluding remarks

If the provision of prosthetic restoration and rehabilitation of all parts of the body is to meet patients' expectations and their clinical needs and, moreover, keep pace with advancements made in other fields, this requires an input of surgical, scientific, bioengineering and technological expertise. To a large extent, this has in recent years been realised in the craniofacial region following the introduction of new techniques such as osseointegration technology, improved materials and equipment and, importantly, better understanding of the clinical, scientific and artistic foundations that underpin CMFPT.

The foregoing helps to prompt the 'notion that man is endeavouring to extend and improve his ability to repair and, where necessary, rebuild man' by the skilful deployment of surgical and engineering procedures coupled with the application of materials science. The practice of CMFPT today requires the prosthetist/technologist to be a combination of clinician, technologist, prosthetist, bioengineer and artist. The skills from each of the above-mentioned disciplines play an integral part in the delivery of prosthetic management in the craniofacial region. It is no doubt because of this remit that the members of the CMFPT team are often seen as the 'bridge' between surgery and engineering because they have, so to speak, a foot in both camps.

Experience over many years has shown that a close working relationship between the surgeon and the prosthetist/technologist is essential to achieve optimum results.

The treatment of oral cancer can produce many levels of residual deformity and disharmony which requires the involvement of those who have the requisite knowledge, motivation and skill, together with ingenuity and compassion, to meet this challenge. The force to deliver and extend one's personal service to mankind over many decades, especially to the orofacial cancer patient, along with the ability to innovate can be developed and strengthened; the feeling of compassion for others, however, comes from within.

Ex Hypothesi – Experientia Docet – Omnia Vincit Amor (From the facts advanced – Experience teaches – Love conquers all difficulties)

References

1. Conroy BF. A brief sortie into the history of cranio-oculofacial prosthetics. Facial Plast Surg 1993; 9: 89–115
2. Bowerman JE, Conroy BF. Maxillofacial prosthetics: general principles. In: Wilson JSB (ed). Operative Surgery: Head and Neck, 3rd edn. London: Butterworth, 1981
3. van Oort R, Roodenburg JL, van Dijk G, Reintsema H, Raghoebar GM. Prosthetische reconstructie na oncologische ingrepen in het hoofd-halsgebied. Oncology in the dental profession. Ned Tijdschr Tandheelkd 1996; 103: 365–368
4. Wilson JSP. General principles of reconstruction. In: Wilson JSB (ed). Operative Surgery: Head and Neck, 3rd edn. London: Butterworth, 1981
5. van Oort R, Raghoebar GM, Schoon PJ. Implant retained mandibular prosthesis following continuity resection of the mandible prosthodontic considerations. Unpublished data.
6. Conroy BF, Bowerman JE, Harrisson JM. Restoration of the mandible by implant prosthesis. In: Williams DF (ed). Biocompatibility in Clinical Practice, vol 11. Bocca Raton, USA: CRC Press, 1982
7. Conroy BF. Maxillofacial prosthetics. In: Rowe NL, Williams JL. Maxillofacial Injuries. London: Churchill Livingstone, 1986
8. Worthington P, Branemark PI. Advanced Osseointegration Surgery: Applications in the Maxillofacial Region. Chicago: Quintessence, 1992
9. Conroy BF. The modern role of implanted devices in the craniofacial region. Dent Tech 2002; 55: 4–7
10. Ghazzawi Z. Modelling of the craniofacial skeleton: an investigation of bone functional adaptation. MSc thesis submission, University of Surrey Library, Guildford, Surrey 1999
11. Conroy BF. An engineering appraisal of the craniofacial skeleton. 2002, unpublished data
12. Lenihan J. Human Engineering. London: Weidenfield and Nicholson, 1974
13. Blenkinsopp PT. Clinical considerations relating to the prosthetic management of orofacial defects. In: Conroy (ed). The proceedings of the IMFT international congress on maxillofacial prosthetics and technology. Southampton: Millbrook Press, 1986; 164–171
14. Granstrom G, Tjellstrom A, Albrektsson T. Postimplantation irradiation cancer treatment. Int J Oral Maxillofac Implants 1993: 8; 495–501
15. Conroy BF, Bowerman JE. Maxillofacial prosthetics: maxilla and orofacial resections. In: Wilson JSB (ed). Operative Surgery: Head and Neck, 3rd edn. London: Butterworth, 1981
16. Bowerman JE, Conroy BF. Maxillofacial prosthetics: general principles. In: Operative Surgery: Head and Neck, 3rd edn. London: Butterworth, 1981
17. Conroy BF. Recent advances in the prosthetic management of large orofacial defects following ablative surgery. In: Conroy (ed). The proceedings of the IMFT international congress on maxillofacial prosthetics and technology. Southampton: Millbrook Press.
18. Branemark PI. Introduction to osseointegration. In: Branemark PI, Zarb G, Albrektsson T (eds). Integrated Prosthesis. Osseointegration in Clinical Dentistry. Chicago: Quintessence, 1985
19. Williams E. A Matter of Balance. Gothenberg, Sweden: Ab Akademiforlaget, 1992
20. Branemark PI. Intravascular anatomy of blood cells in man. Monograph. Basel: S Karger, 1971
21. Branemark PI. Osseointegration: biotechnological perspective and clinical modality. In: Branemark PI, Rydevik BL, Skalak R (eds). Osseointegration in Skeletal Reconstruction and Joint Replacement. Chicago: Quintessence, 1997

18 Prevention of oral cancer

Newell W Johnson

Some definitions

Approaches to disease prevention are often classified at three levels:

- *Primary prevention* is the approach which concentrates on removing risk factors from the community with the intention of minimizing the number of cases of the disease which arise in that community, namely reducing the incidence of disease. If effective at an affordable cost, this is clearly the best approach in terms of both public and personal health gain.
- *Secondary prevention* refers to the detection of cases of the disease in question at an early stage in its natural history at which intervention is likely to lead to cure, or to minimize morbidity and reduce eventual mortality. This is the category which encompasses *screening*. It is a complex area of science and the risks and benefits need careful evaluation in every situation.
- *Tertiary prevention* refers to interventions designed to reduce recurrence of disease after treatment or to minimize the morbidity arising from treatment.

Primary prevention of oral cancer

The major risk factors for oral cancer are well understood and are exhaustively analysed in Chapter 2. Taken together, the effects of tobacco use, heavy alcohol consumption and poor diet probably explain over 90% of cases. The preventive approach is therefore clear and all health care professionals have an obligation and excellent opportunities to contribute.[1] Major international and national agencies are currently very active in this area.[2–4] Many of these documents can be downloaded from the Internet (Table 18.1).

Disease prevention or health promotion messages can be directed at whole communities, targeted at sectors of the population such as youth, prepared specifically for defined populations such as employees of a business or factory or delivered to individual 'clients' such as dental patients or those attending a health centre, antenatal clinic, physician's office, etc. There will be much common ground in the material suitable for these approaches. Dentists and doctors can obtain literature suitable for use in their offices or hospitals from many sources including, in many cases, national medical and dental associations and national health promotion and cancer prevention agencies. Much excellent material is available on the Internet, by inserting simple terms like 'oral cancer', 'tobacco control' or 'alcoholism' into one of the common search engines. A number of suggestions are given in Table 18.1.

Deaths through tobacco use

One of the most valuable critical but concise analyses of the role of tobacco in health and disease, and of the approaches to prevention, is that produced by the Department of Health for England.[5] Every 10 seconds another person dies somewhere in the world as a result of tobacco use. In developed countries as a whole tobacco is responsible for 24% of all male deaths and 7% of female deaths, rising to over 40% for men in some of the former socialist countries and 17% for women in the USA. This has been calculated to represent an average loss of life for all cigarette smokers of 8 years and, for those whose deaths are directly attributed to tobacco, of 16 years:[6]

> for every 1000 20-year-old smokers it is estimated that one will be murdered, six will die in road accidents and 250 will die in middle age from smoking

The proportions of cancer deaths attributed to smoking in developing countries as a whole are lower, being about 21% for men and only 4% for women. However these figures are rising, the fall in global tobacco consumption in the West being matched by growth in developing countries. Indeed of the vast

Table 18.1 Souces of information on tobacco cessation programmes

- Action on Smoking and Health (ASH)
  www.ash.org
- Agency for Healthcare Research and Quality, Clinical Practice Guideline: *Treating Tobacco Use and Dependence* and supplements
  www.surgeongeneral.gov/tobacco.default.htm
  www.guideline.gov
- American Cancer Society
  www.cancer.org/tobacco/
- American Dental Association
  www.ada.org
- American Dental Schools Association
  www.adsa.jhu.edu
- American Heart Association
  www.americanheart.org/CATALOGUIE/Health_catpage 14.html
- American Lung Association
  www.lungusa.org/tobacco/index.html
  www.smokesignals.org
- American Medical Association – Archives of Family Medicine, clinical review
  http://archfami.ama-assn.org/issues/v9n3/full/fcr9009.html
- Breed's Tobacco Activism Guide
  www.tobacco.org/resources/lbguide.html
- British Dental Association
  www.bda-dentistry.org.uk
- Campaign for Tobacco-Free Kids
  www.tobaccofreekids.org/home.cfm
  Global issues
  http://tobaccofreekids.org.campaign/global
- Canadian Council for Tobacco Control
  www.cctc.ca
- FCA leaflet – Tobacco in Developing Countries
  www.fctc.org/ldc.shtml
  www.fctc.otg/ldcf.shtml
- FDI World Dental Federation
  www.worlddental.org
- Food and Drug Administration: children and tobacco page
  www.fda.gov/opacom/campaigns/tobacco.html
- Framework Convention on Tobacco Control Alliance (FCA)
  English www.fctc/org/statement.shtml
  French www.fctc/org/statementf.shtml
  German www.fctc/org/statementg.shtml
  Indonesian www.fctc/org/statementin.shtml
  Italian www.fctc/org/statementi.shtml
  Vietnamese www.fctc/org/statementv.shtml
  Urdu www.fctc/org/statementu.pdf
  Chinese www.fctc/org/statementC1.pdf
  www.fctc/org/statementC2.shtml
- For reference to tobacco control organizations within a specific country, contact Belinda:
  www.fctcalliance@inet.co.th
- Guide to internet resources for cancer
  www.fctc.otg/ldcf.shtml
- Health and Behaviour Alliance – 26 professional research organizations
  www.cfah.org/alliance/main.htm
- International Union for Cancer Control (UICC)
  www.globalink.org
  UICC factsheets
  http://copies.uicc.org/extranet/cancerinformation/tobaccorelatedcancers.shtm
- Journal of Tobacco Control
  www.tobaccocontrol.com
- Master Anti-Smoking Page – anti-smoking web resources
  www.autonomy.com/smoke.htm
- National Cancer Institute
  www.cancer.gov
- National Cancer Institute
  Publications locator
  www.cancer.gov/publications/
  Soccer website
  www.smokefree.gov
- National Center for Tobacco-Free Kids
  www.tobaccofreekids.org
- National Center for Tobacco-Free Older Persons
  www.tesg.org/tobacco.htm
- National Institute of Drug Abuse
  www.drugabuse.gov
  Strategic plan
  www.nida.nih.gov/strategicplan/plan.html
- National Oral Health Clearing house: spit tobacco, oral cancer
  www.aerie.com/nohicweb
- National Spit Tobacco Education Program (NSTEP)
  www.nstep.org
- Not-On-Tobacco
  www.lungusa.org/tobacco.not
- Office on Smoking and Health, CDC
  www.cdc.gov/tobacco/industrydocs/index.htm
  Reports
  www.cdc.gov/tobacco
- Oral Health America Foundation
  www.oralhealthamerica.org
- Program Against Teen Chewing
  www.patchproject.org
- Research protocol evaluation – Cochrane Collaboration
  Australia http://som.flinders.edu.au/fusa/cochran
  Canada http://hiru.mcmaster.ca/cochrane
  Denmark www.cochrane.dk/default.html
  Germany www.cochrane.de
  Japan www.nihs.go.jp/acc/default.html
  Spain www.cspt.es/cochrane/cochrane/default.html
  UK www.update-software.com/ccweb/default.html
  USA www.cochrane.org
- Society for Research on Nicotine and Tobacco
  www.srnt.org
- Surgeon General's report, 1989, Chapter 2
  www.cdc.gov/tobacco/sgr/sgr_1989/1989SGRChapter2.pdf
- Tar Wars – a partnership in youth education
  www.tarwars.org
- Tobacco and the elderly
  www.tesg.org/tobacco.htm
- Tobacco Control Research Branch
  www.dccps.nci.gov/tcrb
- Tobacco Control Resource Center
  www.tobacco.neu.edu
- Tobacco marketing and kids – assessing company strategies
  www.tobaccofreezone/marketing.htm
- Tobacco News
  http://tobacco-control.org
- Tobacco Week
  www.tobaccoweek.com
- Try to Stop Org
  www.trytostop.org
- UK government report
  www.official-documents.co.uk/document/doh/tobacco/part-1.htm#1.31
- US national tobacco objectives. In: *Healthy People 2010*
  www.health.gov/healthypeople
- World Health Organization, Tobacco or Health Programme
  www.who.int/toh
  Programs and publications
  www.who.ch/programmes/psa/psahome.htm
  www.ahrq.gov/clinic/
- Youth Media Network
  www.ymn.org

majority of the estimated 1100 million smokers in the world, some 800 million are in developing countries, 300 million in China alone! Globally some 3 million deaths a year have been estimated to be attributable to smoking, rising to 10 million a year in 30–40 years time when some 7 million will be in developing countries.[7,8] When the use of oral smokeless tobacco is added to these figures, and the deaths it contributes through oral, pharyngeal and oesophageal cancer, the seriousness of the global epidemic of tobacco-related diseases is even more staggering. We all share a responsibility to help quell this epidemic.

According to Doll et al.,[9] who used data from the long-term study on male British doctors, about half of all regular smokers will be killed by their habit. The major causes of such deaths are listed in Table 18.2.

Among men in industrialized countries, smoking is estimated to be the cause of 40–45% of all cancer deaths, 90–95% of lung cancer deaths, over 85% of oral cancer deaths, 75% of chronic obstructive lung disease deaths and 35% of cardiovascular disease deaths in those aged 35–69 years. Thus, while oral and pharyngeal cancer figure prominently, prevention of lung cancer, other pulmonary diseases and cardiovascular diseases should be the starting point for anti-tobacco counselling.

The World Health Organization supplies data which rank smoking prevalence around the globe. The top 20 nations are listed in Table 18.3. Thus, while considerable success has been achieved in many Western industrialized countries, notably in North America, in the last decade, where adult smoking prevalences are now below 30%, many countries have very serious challenges ahead to reach these levels. In the UK the decline in smoking prevalence has plateaued (Fig. 18.1). Indeed, even in those countries which have been relatively successful there are well-documented increases in the proportion of teenagers taking up smoking habits, particularly females (Fig. 18.2). This is of great concern for the future, because many of these will go on to smoke all their lives. Furthermore it has recently been reported that females are at greater risk than male smokers of developing the most lethal form of bronchogenic carcinoma—small cell lung cancer.

There is a good deal of scientific evidence on the cost-effectiveness of approaches to tobacco (principally smoking) prevention/intervention. Table 18.4 ranks these: individual action by doctors and dentists is clearly important. The effectiveness of brief individual action by doctors and dentists is strikingly shown in the study from the UK Centre for Health Economics (Table 18.5).[11]

Table 18.2 Major causes of death from smoking tobacco

- Cancers: of the lung, bladder, pancreas, mouth, oesophagus, pharynx and larynx
- Chronic obstructive pulmonary and other respiratory diseases
- Vascular diseases, including coronary artery and peripheral arterial diseases
- Peptic ulceration

Table 18.3 Estimated smoking prevalence among men and women, 15 years of age and over, by country. (Source: WHO[8])

	Men	Women
Republic of Korea	68.2	6.7
Latvia	67.0	12.0
Russian Federation	67.0	30.0
Dominican Republic	66.3	13.6
Tonga	65.0	14.0
Turkey	63.0	24.0
China	61.0	7.0
Bangladesh	60.0	15.0
Fiji	59.3	30.6
Japan	59.0	18.4
Sri Lanka	54.8	0.8
Algeria	53.0	10.0
Indonesia	53.0	4.0
Samoa	53.0	18.6
Saudi Arabia	52.7	N/a
Estonia	52.0	24.0
Kuwait	52.0	12.0
Lithuania	52.0	10.0
South Africa	52.0	17.0
Poland	51.0	29.0

Table 18.4 A hierarchy of the cost-effectiveness of approaches to smoking cessation[10]

- Imposition/raising of taxes
- Legislation against advertising and sponsorship
- Legislation for smoke-free areas in public places, transport, etc.
- Medical action: advice/intervention by health care professionals
- Education/health promotion at following levels:
  - national
  - state
  - school
  - workplace, etc.
- Dedicated quitting group activities
- Dedicated individual quitting activities

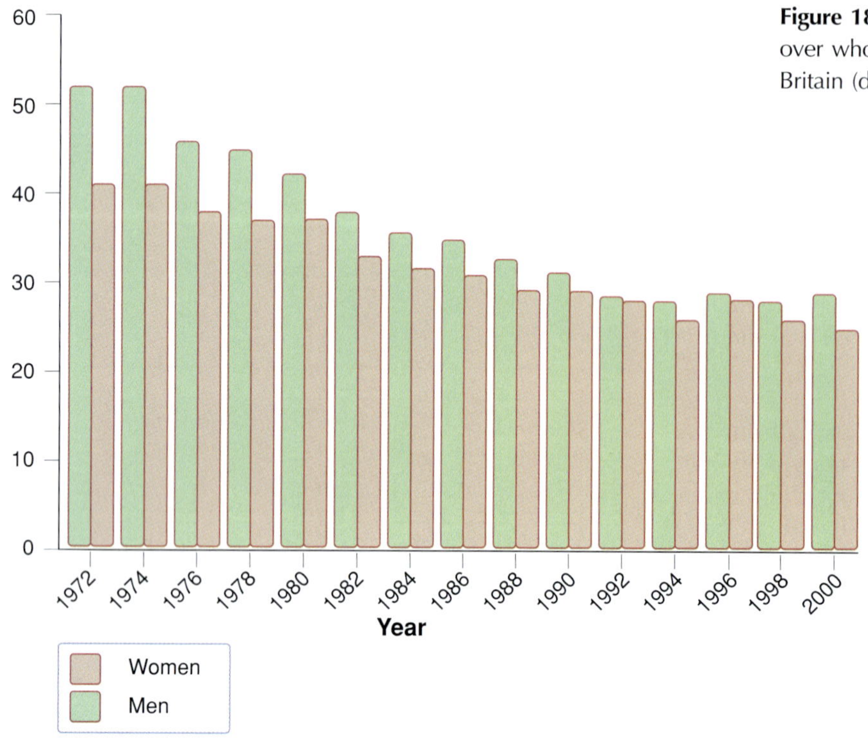

Figure 18.1 Percentage of adults aged 16 and over who smoke cigarettes, 1972–2000, Great Britain (data from www.ash.org.uk/html/factsheets).

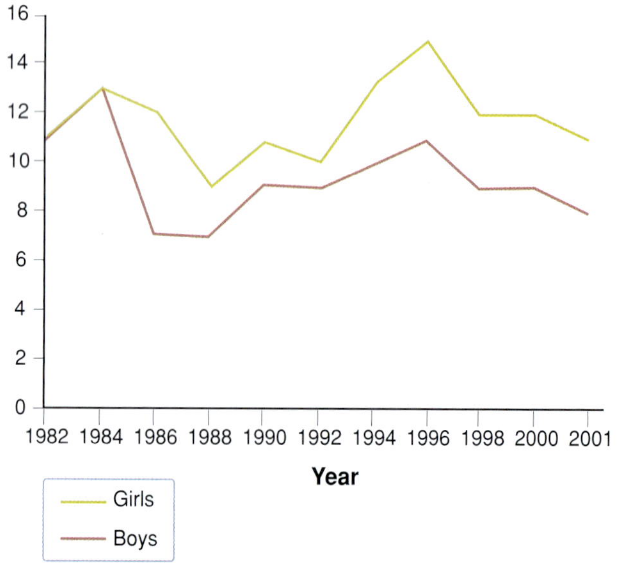

Figure 18.2 Percentage of children aged 11–16 who smoke regularly, 1982–1996, England (data from www.ash.org.uk/html/factsheets).

Adolescent smoking is a particular concern. A comprehensive review of the world literature concludes that there is no single cause, and that personal, socio-cultural and environmental factors all encourage smoking uptake. All three types of influence need to be addressed and there is evidence for modest success for interventions via schools, mass media, community-based programmes and environmental measures covering controls on advertising, packaging, pricing, retailing and smoking policies.

Clinicians and tobacco control

Members of the health professions can be active in influencing politicians and community leaders to adopt appropriate legislative approaches. All professional associations are urged to adopt a policy on tobacco and health, and many have done so. That produced by the FDI World Dental Federation might serve as a model (Table 18.6).[12]

Health care professionals can work within their clinical environment to great effect. There is ample evidence that general medical practitioner advice to quit tobacco use is respected by the majority of patients, and several recent studies show that dentists can be equally effective (Table 18.7). This is achieved by following the simple scheme of the 4As (expanded in Table 18.8 to the 5As), widely used around the world.

Dentists, and all clinicians involved in oral health care,[13,14] have a natural entrée to discussion of tobacco-related diseases with their patients because of the oral signs of tobacco use and its influence on many oral diseases and conditions.[15] Many of these are covered in detail elsewhere in this book; they are summarized in Table 18.9. The malignant and potentially malignant lesions and conditions are of obvious importance: realistically, however, they are not common and do not give rise to opportunities for true primary prevention. The socially important changes—bad breath and tooth staining—are often sufficient to focus clinicians and patients alike on the desirability of quitting. Because periodontal diseases

Table 18.5 Life years gained over age 45 for a Western population of about 500 000, smoking at a 27% prevalence, and estimated costs per life year gained[10]

Intervention	Effectiveness (%)	Population reached (%)	Life years gained	Cost per life year (undiscounted) (£)
Primary health care interventions				
Brief advice	2	80	3034	94
Additional gains and costs on top of brief advice from:				
brief counselling	2	70	2665	545
nicotine gum	8	50	7601	463
Community interventions				
Local 'no smoking' days	0.15	90	284	21
Broader community-wide programmes	0.50	100	948	54
	0.10	100	190	271
	0.05	100	95	541

Table 18.6 FDI policy statement on tobacco

Tobacco in daily practice

The use of tobacco is harmful to general health, as it is a common cause of addiction, preventable illness, disability and death. The use of tobacco also causes an increased risk for oral cancer, periodontal disease and other deleterious oral conditions and it adversely affects the outcome of oral health care.

The FDI urges its Member Associations and all oral health professionals to take decisive actions to reduce tobacco use and nicotine addiction among the general public.

The FDI also urges all oral health professionals to integrate tobacco use prevention and cessation services into their routine and daily practice.

Tobacco in all education

Brief interactions, for example by identifying tobacco users, giving direct advice, supportive material and follow-up, all have a significant impact on the patients' use of tobacco products.

The FDI urges all oral health institutions and all continuing education providers to integrate tobacco-related subjects into their programmes.

Protect the children

The adverse consequences of environmental tobacco smoke are particularly severe for children—and lifelong.

The FDI strongly endorses and promotes public and professional education and policies that prevent and/or reduce the exposure to tobacco smoke for infants, children and young people.

Prevent the initiation

More than 80% of adults who use tobacco started their use of tobacco before the age of 18. Use of tobacco among children and youths easily produces a nicotine dependency, the risk of which is vastly underestimated by the young people themselves.

The FDI vigorously supports all measures that endeavour to prevent the initiation of tobacco use.

are common in all populations, increased severity and extent of disease, and limitations in response to periodontal treatment, can be an important 'hook' for involving an affected patient in tobacco control. Knowledge in this area is growing rapidly and has been summarized in a position paper from the American Academy of Periodontology.[22] The scientific evidence on the harm to general and oral health of tobacco use, with special emphasis on oral cancer and precancer, oral candidiasis, other mucosal

Table 18.7 A selection of smoking cessation trials in primary care

Reference	Country	Year	Setting	*n*	Method	Period	Quit rate (%)
Cohen et al.[16]	USA	1989	Private dentists	374	Dentist training + brief advice (a)	1 year	7.7
					(a) + nicotine gum	1 year	16.3
					(a) + reminders on notes	1 year	8.6
					(a) + gum and reminders	1 year	16.9
Segnan et al.[17]	Italy	1991	GMP	923	Minimal intervention	1 year	4.8
					Repeated counselling	1 year	5.3
					Counselling + gum	1 year	7.5
					Counselling + spirometry	1 year	6.5
Russell et al.[18]	UK	1993	GMP	400	Brief advice + nicotine pratches	1 year	9.3
			GMP	200	Brief advice + placebo patches	1 year	5.0
Stapleton et al.[19]	UK	1995	GMP	800	Nicotine patches	1 year	9.6
				400	Placebo patches	1 year	4.8
Macgregor[20]	UK	1996	Hospital periodontal	98	Dental health education + advice against smoking	3–6 months	13.3
			clinic	98	Dental health education only	3–6 months	5.3
Smith et al.[21]	UK	1997	GDP	154	Brief advice + optional nicotine patches	9 months	11.0

Table 18.8 The five As

- Ask patients about their tobacco habits
- Advise them on the importance of quitting
- Agree with them a quit date
- Assist them in achieving this
- Arrange follow-up

Table 18.9 Tobacco-induced and associated conditions. (Source: Mecklenburg et al.[25])

Oral cancer

Leukoplakia
- Homogenous leukoplakia
- Non-homogeneous leukoplakia (precancer)
  - verrucous leukoplakia
  - nodular leukoplakia
  - erythroleukoplakia

Other tobacco-induced oral mucosal conditions
- Snuff dipper's lesion
- Smoker's palate (nicotine stomatitis)
- Smoker's melanosis

Tobacco-associated effects on the teeth and supporting tissues
- Tooth loss (premature mortality)
- Staining
- Abrasion
- Periodontal diseases
  - destructive periodontitis
  - focal recession
  - acute necrotizing ulcerative gingivitis

Other tobacco-aassociated oral conditions
- Gingival bleeding
- Calculus
- Halitosis
- Leukoedema
- Chronic hyperplastic candidiasis (candial leukoplakia)
- Median rhomboid glossitis
- Hairy tongue

Possible association with tobacco
- Oral clefts
- Dental caries
- Dental plaque
- Lichen planus
- Salivary changes
- Taste and smell

Table 18.10 Constraints felt by dental practitioners in the UK towards giving clients advice against tobacco use

	Those who feel dentists should give advice (71%) (%)	Those who feel dentists should not give advice (29%) (%)
It is frustrating	26	15
It is not important	3	6
It is not effective	9	22
It is not cost effective	24	21
We are not trained	28	21
Other reasons	10	14

diseases, periodontal diseases, salivary flow rate and composition, susceptibility to dental caries, impact on wound healing and the success or failure of dental implants is summarized in a report of the EU Working Group on Tobacco and Oral Health 1998.[23,24]

In the USA the National Cancer Institute, the American Medical Association and the American Dental Association have produced extensive literature to help train physicians, dentists and their teams in anti-tobacco counselling, as have a number of other countries.[25] Almost all countries in the world have educational material designed for professionals and health promotion material designed for the public: these should be easily accessed by approaching the appropriate agencies, some of whom have been listed in Table 18.1. The FDI head office is in the process of cataloguing such materials. Most of these agencies can, of course, be accessed on the World Wide Web, and much of the information can be downloaded.

Even in the absence of oral stigmata of tobacco use, dentists should *ask and advise* in order to detect new tobacco addicts, and engage in early preventive activities. This is a particular challenge with young people. Surveys of dental practitioner knowledge, attitudes and behaviour towards tobacco control have been conducted in a number of countries with, unsurprisingly, variable results. Encouragingly, a recent US national survey showed that a quarter of tobacco users had been advised to quit by their dentist.[27] However, even in Northern Europe and North America, a substantial proportion, usually a majority, of colleagues are inhibited from asking, and reluctant to advise. A large questionnaire survey of UK dentists found that half of the respondents did not routinely enquire about risk habits related to oral cancer; 30% inquired of their patients regarding smoking habits and 19% questioned on both smoking and alcohol use. (However, this sample is unrepresentative, as out of 2532 dentists addressed, only 16% responded.) Of those enquiring into these risk habits, only 19.5% made appropriate notes in patients' records. Only 30% of dentists who inquired into smoking habits provided brief advice routinely to patients and a further 31% only to patients they regarded as being at high risk of oral cancer or another serious disease. A much smaller proportion (20%) of dentists in this study attempted to provide advice on alcohol moderation when patient histories suggested excess consumption. Dentists who were regular smokers themselves were less likely to inquire about the risk habits of their patients compared to those professionals who had either never smoked or were ex smokers ($p < 0.05$). When asked whether dental practitioners should be involved in giving advice against tobacco use, 71% of respondents agreed that this was desirable, but many constraints were perceived, listed in Table 18.10. Understandably, dentists not already providing such advice felt constrained by a wider range of these items.[28] Knowledge, attitudes and behaviour surveys of US dentists indicate similar gaps.[29,30]

These results are similar to those reported from Texas.[31] Educational efforts are thus required for both the public and for the profession in the hope of developing a growing awareness of the appropriateness of dentists addressing these issues. At present it is likely that many practitioners will opt to refer interested dental patients to an individual specialist or group: the AA-R approach (Ask, Advise, Refer) rather than the AAAAA approach. Advice leaflets, which include telephone numbers and addresses of such resources, should be available in every health care setting.

Increasingly, dentists and other clinicians are willing to receive training in tobacco control methods, via the many sources listed above. This may involve advice to clients on the use of nicotine replacement to help over the period of withdrawal.

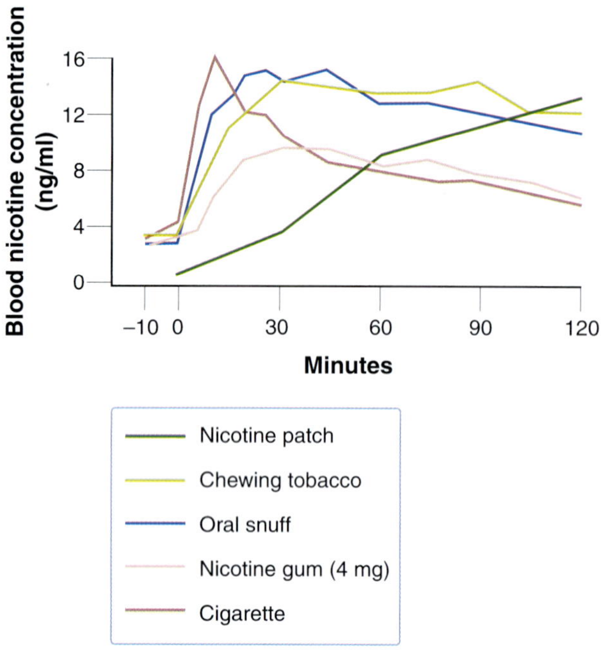

Figure 18.3 Blood nicotine concentration over time by method of administration.

As an active substance, nicotine, on a milligramme for milligramme basis, is ten times more potent than heroin.[32] An important study in the UK has shown that the use of nicotine skin patches can double the rate of smoking cessation handled through a medical practitioner, from around 5% to around 10% of recruits.[33] This played a role in the comparable 11% quit rate we have demonstrated as possible in dental practice.[21] The California tobacco survey shows that such patches are significantly important aids to smokers who want to quit when used as an adjuvant to other forms of assistance.[34] Nicotine replacement is available as skin patches, chewing gums, nasal sprays or as an inhaler fashioned like a cigarette (which then helps with the oral and tactile stimulation which is part of smoking addiction). All have a role to play in appropriate circumstances.[35] These devices deliver nicotine with different pharmacokinetic consequences, as shown in Fig. 18.3. Advice on their appropriate use, including dosages and contraindications, is included in the training literature referred to above, and from the manufacturers. In some countries these products are available over the counter, with detailed instructions: pharmacists/drug stores can also be consulted by doctor, dentist or patient for advice.

Oral smokeless tobacco

As shown in Chapter 2, there is no doubt that the addition of tobacco to areca nut (betel) quids, consumed by millions in south and south east Asia, confers a major increase in their carcinogenicity[36] and habitués must be encouraged to quit; indeed the benefits of doing so are clear.[37] Omitting tobacco from quids, and washing the mouth well after use, may be helpful intermediate steps. We have seen that the tobaccos used in mixtures such as *nass*, *niswar* or *toombak* in North Africa, the middle East or northern parts of the Indian subcontinent also contain high levels of nitrosamines and are dangerous.[38] A clear summary of the evidence for oral cancer associated with the various forms of tobacco use around the world is provided by Gupta et al.[39]

Controversy exists, however, as to the danger of moist loose or portion-bag-packed snuff in the west, notably Scandinavia and the USA. It appears that the risk of oral cancer is low with these products,[40] and the chemical, behavioural and risk differences associated with Swedish *snus* and Sudanese *toombak* have been compared in detail by Idris et al.[41] There is even the suggestion that smokers should be encouraged to take up oral smokeless tobacco as a less dangerous means of coping with nicotine addiction.[42] However, this is an unproven and potentially dangerous approach; there are safer

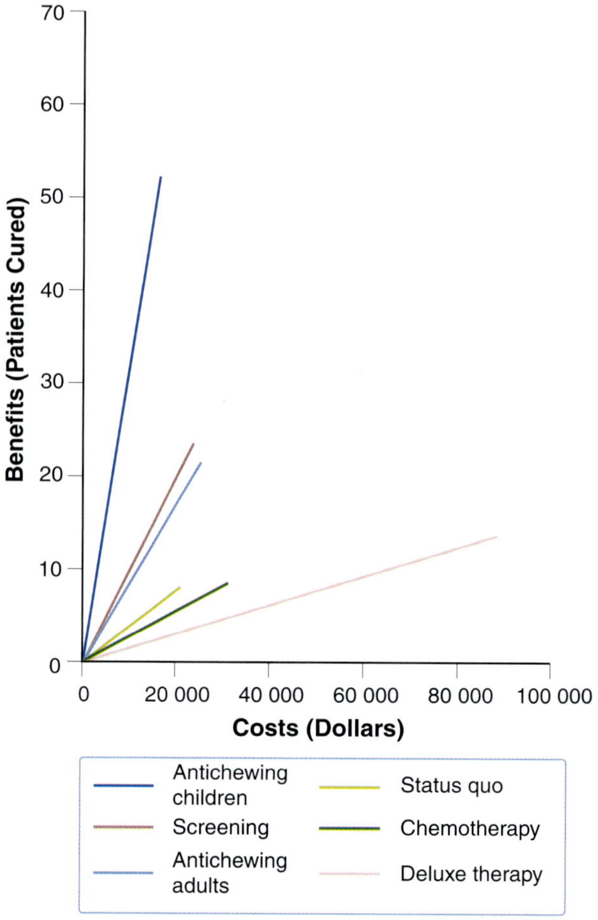

Figure 18.4 Cost-benefit analysis of oral cancer in Sri Lanka.

forms of nicotine replacement available and the cardiovascular effects and risks of cancer at other sites have not been fully evaluated.

There is no doubt that primary prevention by habit intervention is the most cost-effective approach to the management of oral cancer. This is strikingly demonstrated in a model of the situation in Sri Lanka (Fig. 18.4) (Stjernsward J, WHO, personal communication).

Passive smoking

Two recent critical meta-analyses of the world literature from the Wolfson Institute of Preventive Medicine in London[43,44] and reviews from the California Environmental Protection Agency[45] and the US Environmental Protection Agency[46] show conclusively that exposure to environmental tobacco smoke is a major cause of serious illness. In the US alone it is calculated to be responsible for 3000 deaths from lung cancer each year, 35 000–62 000 deaths from ischaemic heart disease (tobacco smoke has a marked effect on platelet biology, even at low doses), 150 000–300 000 cases of bronchitis or pneumonia in infants and children up to 18 months of age (of whom a proportion die), 8000–26 000 new cases of asthma and exacerbation of asthma in up to a million children, 9700–18 600 cases of low birth weight and 1900–2700 sudden infant deaths.[47] All health professionals should set an example by not smoking (seeking help if we are current smokers) and by ensuring that the whole work environment is smoke free.

Clinicians and the management of heavy alcohol consumption

Excessive alcohol consumption is a major cause of individual morbidity and mortality and contributes much damage to society. In the USA it is estimated that alcohol-related diseases contribute 100 000 excess deaths each year. In this respect tobacco and alcohol abuse are much more significant than hard drugs, when measured by outcomes such as person years of life lost or bed days occupied in hospital. Figure 18.5 shows data from Australia, which illustrate this dramatically. All health care clinicians have a responsibility, therefore, to help their clients (patients, colleagues and students) use alcohol sensibly. This is especially true in teaching and training centres, because students and staff in medical institutions are amongst the highest risk groups for dangerous drinking.[48]

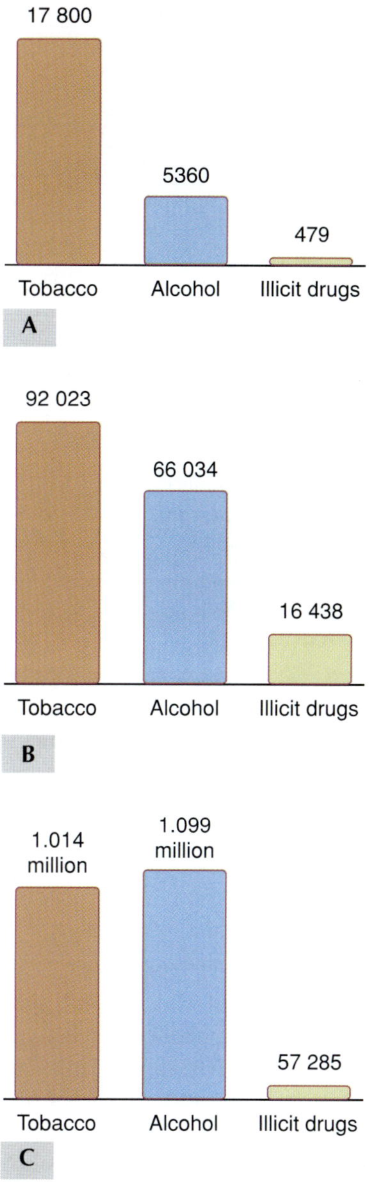

Figure 18.5 (A) deaths (0–69) due to tobacco, alcohol and illicit drugs, Australia 1996. (B) Person years lost (0–69) due to tobacco, alcohol and illicit drugs, Australia 1996. (C) Bed days (0–69) due to tobacco, alcohol and illicit drugs, Australia 1996. (Courtesy of Dr Nigel Gray, UICC and Anticancer Council of Victoria.)

Many primary care clinicians are inhibited from taking alcohol histories from their patients, but all should, with tact, be able to help their patients see that such questioning is directed at genuine concerns for their general health and that this is relevant to their oral health. Oral and other upper aerodigestive tract cancers, and potentially malignant lesions, are perhaps our major concerns as clinicians interested in diseases of the head and neck. As explained earlier, many epidemiologists believe that the rise in both incidence and mortality of these cancers seen in a number of countries, particularly in Europe, is related to rising alcohol consumption over recent years. Differences in

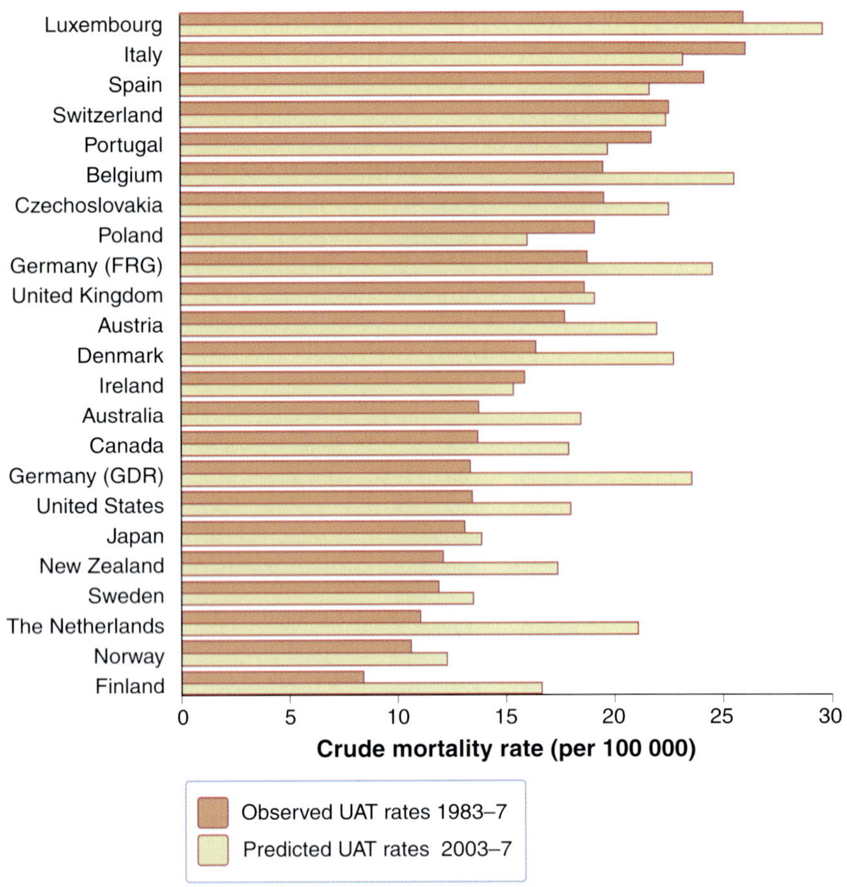

Figure 18.6 Current and future mortality from upper aerodigestive tract (UAT) cancers in males.

alcohol consumption (particularly amongst those who also smoke) explain most of the increasingly higher rates of oral cancer amongst Blacks, as compared to Whites in the USA.[49] Projections of disease levels based on trends in alcohol consumption lead to disturbing predictions of future cancers at these sites (Fig. 18.6).[50] In addition, alcohol contributes to dental and maxillofacial injuries, and by secondary effects following liver damage and, often, undernutrition, compromises periodontal health, wound healing and resistance to infection.[51]

All clinicians can see these facial and intra-oral signs in their patients, and suspicion may be aroused because of patient behaviour. There are a number of well-established tools for the estimation of problem drinking in our patients. These include the so-called CAGE and AUDIT (Alcohol Use Disorders Identification Test) questionnaires, of which a recent study showed the AUDIT to be marginally superior.[52] We have validated the AUDIT questionnaire, as developed by the World Health Organization.[53] In a study of 107 south London misusers, over half of whom consumed more than 200 units of alcohol per week, and 80% of whom also smoked, eight subjects had oral mucosal lesions, including two previously treated carcinomas in one individual. Dental caries experience did not differ from an age-matched national sample, but periodontal disease was more severe, and was related to both smoking and undernutrition as recorded by body mass index and mid-arm muscle circumference measurements. Clearly such individuals, to be found in most societies worldwide, are a priority group for preventative counselling.[54] A policy of *Ask, Advise* ought then to be followed, accepting that *Referral* is probably wise for patients with a suspected alcohol problem, given the complexity of the addictive process and the therapeutic challenges in this demanding, specialized field. A wide variety of dedicated groups, agencies and clinics exist in most countries, and practitioners are advised to be aware of what networks exist locally. Serious alcohol dependence often requires inpatient and/or day stay treatment, which is both demanding and expensive.[55] Again, the Internet is a source of much professonal advice and access to self-help and support groups for individuals with alcohol problems and their families.

It is clear that specific training can enhance the effectiveness of primary care physicians in detecting and managing hazardous drinking in their patients, and that direct contact with trainers, face to face or on the telephone, is more effective than mailed training kits.[56] In a study in Sydney, Australia, 36 trained general medical practitioners recruited 179 patients with an alcohol problem over 3 months,

Table 18.11 Major causes of drink-related death

- Stroke
- Cardiomyopathy
- Cancer (several sites)
- Liver cirrhosis
- Pancreatitis
- Accidents
- Suicide
- Homicide

32% of whom reported reduced drinking to the researchers.[57] As with tobacco control, education and health promotion interventions need to be taken at all levels of society, and many governments around the world are working to improve their effectiveness and cost effectiveness.[58]

Moderate alcohol consumption is not harmful, and may even be beneficial, particularly in reducing the risk of cardiovascular diseases. The so-called J-shaped curve relation between alcohol consumption and total mortality has been established for some years.[59] The lowest mortality occurs in those who consume one or two drinks per day. In teetotallers or very occasional drinkers the mortality rate is higher than those who take one or two drinks per day. Importantly, in those who take three or more drinks per day, mortality rises rapidly in a dose-dependent manner. The major causes of death are shown in Table 18.11.

The protection against coronary heart disease provided by one or two drinks per day is of the order of 30–50%,[60] and there is demonstrably less atherosclerosis in such moderate drinkers, visible at catheterization or at autopsy. This effect seems to be independent of possible confounders such as smoking and poor diet. It is generally considered[61] that about half of the protective effect is mediated through increased levels of HDL-cholesterol, which carries cholesterol from arterial walls back to the liver.[62] Other beneficial effects are mediated through reduction in clotting factor and platelet activity and/or clot lysis.[63,64]

Other protective substances have been identified in several beverages, such as the antioxidants in wine derived from grape skins[65] and in dark beer. However the available epidemiological evidence does not show any particular type of beverage to be consistently more effective in reducing coronary heart disease, perhaps because of considerable variability on confounding factors such as smoking, diet and age in the various studies.[66] The frequency of alcohol consumption is also critically important: Studies in eastern Europe, where patterns of alcohol use and heart disease are different from the west, show binge drinking to be dangerous, without the raised HDLs, indeed with raised LDLs, and with a tendency to increased thrombosis after cessation of drinking.[67]

What, therefore, constitutes potentially unhealthy levels of alcohol consumption? Many governments and agencies suggest a healthy limit of 21 units of alcohol a week for men and 14 for women, with at least two alcohol-free days per week. A unit of alcohol is taken to be a single glass (approximately 284 ml) of average strength beer or lager, a single measure (approximately 25 ml) of spirits or a single standard (approximately 113 ml) glass of wine or aperitif (50 ml).[68]

It is clear that national policies are needed to prevent tobacco use and to limit alcohol consumption in the young, to reduce future morbidity and mortality from UADT cancers.[69] A recent study in Switzerland, however, suggests that it takes some years for alcohol cessation to have an effect on cancer risk.[70] And public recognition of the importance of alcohol as a risk factor for cancer, especially oral cancer, is poor.[71,72]

Healthy eating in the prevention of oral cancer

Clinicians, it is hoped, routinely enquire about the dietary habits of their patients, usually because they are interested in their likely adverse effects on cardiovascular health or—particularly for dentists—in their possible carcinogenicity. Adequate (neither under- nor over-) nutrition is essential to host resistance against all diseases and this is strongly true of cancer. Table 18.12 summarizes dietary measures suggested for the prevention of cancer, based on a critical review by Sir Richard Doll, the epidemiologist who has made perhaps the biggest single contribution to knowledge of causes and prevention of cancer this century.[73] He believes that the risk of cancer overall can be reduced by a third or more by modification of diet in a way that has already proved acceptable to many.

The protective role of diets adequate in trace elements, minerals and vitamins (particularly the antioxidant or free-radical scavenging vitamins A, C and E) has been emphasized in Chapter 2. An extensive literature in relation to head and neck cancer has been reviewed by La Vecchia et al. 1997.[74] Two recent publications, produced with characteristic thoroughness, by the International Agency for Research on Cancer, are strongly recommended.[75,76] The benefits are apparent even in the case of such high-risk habits as reverse smoking.[77]

Many studies have shown that intake of protective nutrients is more effective when these are derived from natural foodstuffs rather than from synthetic

Table 18.12 Dietary measures suggested for the prevention of cancer. (Modified from Doll[73])

Measure	Type of cancer affected
Reduce:	
Calories (avoid obesity)	Gallbladder, body of uterus, possibly breast
Fat	Breast, colon and rectum, prostate and endometrium
Smoked and grilled food	Stomach, perhaps others
Salt cured food	Stomach
Nitrates	Stomach, possibly others
Saccharin	Possibly bladder
Increase:	
Fibre	Colon and rectum
Vegetables	Colon and rectum; many sites, including head and neck
Fruit	Colon and rectum; many sites, including head and neck
Vitamins A, C, E	Many sites, including head and neck
Beta-carotene	Many sites, including head and neck
Selenium	Many sites, including head and neck

Table 18.13 American Cancer Society guidelines on diet, nutrition and cancer prevention[80]

1. Choose most of the foods you eat from plant sources.
   - Eat five or more servings of fruits and vegetables every day.
   - Eat other foods from plant sources, such as breads, cereals, grain products, rice, pasta or beans several times each day.
2. Limit your intake of high-fat foods, particularly from animal sources.
   - Choose foods low in fat.
   - Limit consumption of meats, especially high-fat meats.
3. Be physically active: achieve and maintain a healthy weight.
   - Be at least moderately active for 30 minutes or more on most days of the week.
   - Stay within your healthy weight range.
4. Limit consumption of alcoholic beverages, if you drink at all.
5. Do not smoke.
6. Avoid sexually transmitted infections.

food supplements.[78] This is particularly important in smokers and drinkers.[79] Thus, the advice which we should give to our patients, which is part of every nation's health promotion guidelines, is summarized in Table 18.13, developed from the 1997 version of the American Cancer Society.[80]

Secondary prevention: screening for oral cancer and potentially malignant lesions

Screening for disease is a very precise science[81] and must follow established principles (Table 18.14).[82] Oral cancer meets some, but not all, of these criteria and, although there are clear potential advantages (Table 18.15), there are also potential disadvantages (Table 18.16).

The rationale for screening for oral cancer is based on the fact that these malignancies are asymptomatic and localized for a period of their natural history and are often preceded by potentially malignant lesions and conditions such as leukoplakia, erythroplakia and submucous fibrosis, when they can be detected by simple systematic oral examinations.

Table 18.14 Screening for disease. (Source: Wilson and Junger[82])

The basic principles concerning are:

- The condition should be an important health problem, whose natural history is understood.
- There should be an accepted and proven intervention.
- There should be a suitable and accepted diagnostic test.
- The cost of screening should be balanced in relation to other health care expenditure.

Table 18.15 Potential advantages of screening for oral cancer and precancer

- Reduced mortality
- Reduced incidence of invasive cancers
- Improved prognosis for individual patients
- Reduced morbidity for cases treated at early stages
- Identification of high-risk groups and opportunities for intervention
- Reassurance for those screened negative
- Cost savings

Table 18.16 Potential disadvantages of screening for oral cancer and precancer

- Detection of cases already incurable may increase morbidity for some patients
- Unnecessary treatment of those potentially malignant lesions which may not have progressed
- Psychological trauma for those with a false positive screen
- Reinforcement of bad habits among some individuals screened negative
- Costs

This is important because habit intervention,[83] dietary intervention[84] and surgical treatment[85,86] can result in their resolution or elimination.

However, *population screening* for oral cancer cannot be recommended,[87,88] because there is inadequate understanding of its natural history[89] and there is insufficient evidence for its utility[90] or cost-effectiveness. Oral cancer screening programmes have been carried out on several hundreds of thousands of individuals in developing countries (mostly Sri Lanka, India and Cuba) and several thousands in developed countries (mostly the USA, UK and Italy) and the evidence from these is reviewed by Warnakulasuriya and Johnson[91] (from which Table 18.17 is derived) and by Franceschi et al.[89] A meta-analysis of these studies has just been published.[92] In the high incidence parts of the world a substantial proportion of suspicious lesions has been found (ranging from 2 to 16% in south Asia), but compliance of patients to attend follow-up was poor. In the west the yield is substantially lower. For example, the largest study group was in Minnesota and consisted of over 23 000 adults, over age 30, whose mouths were examined by dentists between 1957 and 1972. Although more than 10% of those screened had an oral lesion these were mostly benign; 'precancer' was encountered in 2.9% and cancer in less than 0.1%. A very large, community-based, controlled oral cancer screening trial is currently underway in Kerala, with encouraging early results.[93]

Logically, a stronger case can be made for *targeting screening* to at-risk populations—in the context of oral cancer perhaps to smokers and heavy drinkers over the age of, say, 40. Such individuals can be identified from the records of family medical practitioners or occupational health records. Even so, studies of this kind conducted in the UK[94] and in Japan[95,96] have shown high non-attendance rates for the initial oral examination. This, together with the still low prevalence of lesions, makes even this type

Table 18.17 Results of oral cancer/precancer[a] screening programmes. (Source: Warnakulasuriya and Johnson[91])

Investigators[b]	Year	Country	Sample	Cancer		Precancer	
				No.	#[c]	No.	%[d]
Ross and Gross	1971	USA	12 868	1	(8)	339	(2.6)
Folsom et al.	1972	USA	158 996	120	(75)	802	(0.5)
Axell et al.	1976	Sweden	20 333	1	(5)	732	(3.6)
Mehta et al.	1969	India	50 915	26	(51)	881	(1.7)
Warnakulasuriya et al.	1983	Sri Lanka	28 295	4	(14)	1220	(4.2)
Bouquot and Gorlin	1986	USA	23 616	22	(93)	682	(2.9)
Ikeda et al.	1991	Japan	3 131	None		77	(2.5)
Banoczy et al.	1991	Hungary	7 820	1	(13)	104	(1.3)

[a]Includes benign keratoses in some surveys.
[b]See Warnakulasuriya and Johnson[78]
[c]Rate per 100 000.
[d]Rate as percentage.

Table 18.18 Screening for oral cancer and potentially malignant lesions. Based on clinical and digital examination of the oral mucosa by dentists, with confirmation by an oral medicine specialist. The first three studies provided the data for training the neural network

Location	*n*	Lesion prevalence (%)	Sensitivity	Specificity
Dental hospital	1042	3.00	0.81	0.99
Medical practice	985	2.22	0.64	0.99
Company headquarters	309	5.50	0.71	0.99
Neural network	365	2.74	0.80	0.77

of screening of dubious utility. In a series of studies conducted by ENT specialists in Northern Italy between 1994 and 1998 the yield was substantially increased by adding inspections of the pharynx and larynx (with appropriate instrumentation), and aiming the programme at smokers and/or heavy drinkers, relying on general practitioners for the identification of these high-risk groups. Even so, only 1564 out of 4419 (35%) individuals complied with the examination. This yielded 152 (9.7%) 'precancerous' lesions (mostly low-risk flat leukoplakias) and 20 (1.3%) cancers at any of these upper aerodigestive sites. A better participation rate can be obtained when oral screening is part of general health screening.[97]

The Oral Cancer Screening Group at the Eastman Dental Institute, London, has carried out an outstanding series of investigations in recent years. They have shown that the sensitivity and specificity of lesion detection is comparable to that of oral examination by the use of artificial intelligence systems to compute all known risk factors for oral cancer (Table 18.18).[98] This is an exciting way forward for the future, but bringing these individuals to early treatment will remain a problem.

In a simulation model, estimates of quality adjusted life years (QALYs) and of lives gained from screening were obtained, compared with the status quo of no screening. Participants were a notional population of 100 000 adults of average age 55 years and 20 years' life expectancy. The basic assumptions were a 50% attendance of the eligible population, a prevalence of oral cancer of 0.098% and of precancer 2.57%, a positive predictive value of the screening test of 0.67 and a negative predictive value of 0.99. The cancers were assumed to be 40% stage 1, 60% stage 2+ without screening and 60% stage 1 and 40% stage 2+ with screening. Patients with oral precancer were assumed to have a survival of 19.2 years, with stage 1 cancer 14.6 years and stage 2+ cancer 10.8 years. The public's perceived utilities were 0.92 for precancer and 0.88 and 0.68 for stage 1 and stage 2+ cancer, respectively, compared to a utility of 1.0 for health. One cycle of the programme was modelled over one year in a dental practice setting. Under these circumstances the cost benefits obtained are shown in Table 18.19.

This estimate of a cost per life saved by screening a high-risk population for oral cancer, £8333, compares very favourably with costs estimated for other, more common, cancers, for which population screening programmes already exist in many countries (Table 18.20). Indeed the longest established cancer screening programmes in the world, those for cancer of the uterine cervix, are extremely expensive and controversial. They have never been evaluated by means of a randomized controlled trial and, although changes in incidence make it difficult to estimate the effect of a screening programme

Table 18.19 Hypothetical cost-benefits of oral cancer screening programmes (assuming the cost of a screening examination to be £5)

Screening of whole population
- Cost of screening 100 000 = £500 000
- Lives saved = 5.6
- Cost per life saved = £89 286

Screening a high-risk population
- Cost of screening 25 000 = £125 000
- Lives saved = 15
- Cost per life saved = £8333

Table 18.20 Costs per life saved for cancer screening programmes (Source: Roberts et al.[99])

Breast cancer	£80 000
Cervical cancer	£300 000
Colon cancer	£6500
Oral cancer (high-risk)	£8883

quantitatively, the impact on this disease is less than that which might be thought feasible.

Opportunistic screening, namely offering a screening test for an unsuspected disorder at a time when a person presents to a doctor—or a dentist or any other suitably trained primary health care professional[100]—for another reason, is rational and cost-effective. This is the basis of the screening examination of the oral soft tissues recommended at every dental visit, perhaps also at periodic visits to a family physician. We have the manpower available—ourselves as trained specialists in what constitutes normal and abnormal tissues—and it need take only approximately 3 minutes for the month at least. This we have a duty to perform. The clinical identification of suspect lesions by visual observation and manual palpation is a skill which can be taught to any primary health care worker, even those with quite basic training such as the medical auxiliaries found in some developing countries.[101] The most encouraging outcome of such studies so far published comes from the Oral Cancer Case Finding Programme in Cuba. Between 1983 and 1990, 10 167 999 patients were examined nationwide when they attended stomatological clinics: only 8259 out of 30 478 patients (27%) with suspect lesions complied with referral and of these there were 3220 potentially malignant lesions, 581 squamous cell carcinomas and 127 other malignancies. However, although no doubt at considerable cost, the programme was shown to be effective because there was 'downstaging' of the cancers seen: stage I lesions rising from 22.8% to 48.2% and stages II, III and IV lesions falling from 77.2% to 51.8%.[102] This study used specially trained stomatologists. In spite of their lower cost and comparable accuracy to dentists, use of auxiliaries for population screening still cannot be recommended because there is no evidence yet available of the efficacy of such an approach in reducing the incidence and mortality of oral cancer.

Toluidine blue

The use of toluidine blue (tolonium chloride) dye as a mouthwash or topical application is currently receiving much attention as an aid to the diagnosis of oral cancer and potentially malignant lesions. It certainly has a place, with appropriate training, in screening of high-risk subjects and in helping to define the site for biopsy. There have been a number of clinical trials using toluidine blue and these are summarized in Table 18.21.[103] The table shows that the method has good sensitivity, with a very low false negative rate. However, it is important to realize that most of these studies have taken both overtly invasive carcinomas and severe (or even moderate) dysplasia as true positive lesions under the umbrella 'oral cancer'. Although 100% of invasive lesions will stain, most studies show that only 50% or less of dysplasias are detected. The false positive rate is likely to be very low in patients presenting with perfectly healthy mucosae, but areas of inflammation, ulceration or erosion stain positively whatever their cause. False positives may be as high as 48% following a single application. Repeating the stain 10 to 14 days later to allow for the healing of acute ulcerative or traumatic lesions has been shown to reduce the false positive rate to 11%. The dorsum of the tongue always stains positively, due to retention of dye in crevices between the papillae, making it of limited value for studying lesions at this site, unless the lesion arises out of an atrophic area. Likewise, crevices and cracks within thick keratotic plaques retain dye and produce a false positive result.

Thus good clinical judgement, training and experience in the use of toluidine blue ensure rational use of this diagnostic aid. Biopsy remains the gold standard for the diagnosis of oral cancer and potentially malignant lesions. False positives are of less concern than false negatives. All positive stain reactions require biopsy, as do any suspicious lesions which do not stain.

Figure 18.7 shows a speckled leukoplakia at the commissure heavily stained. Fig. 18.8 shows an area of

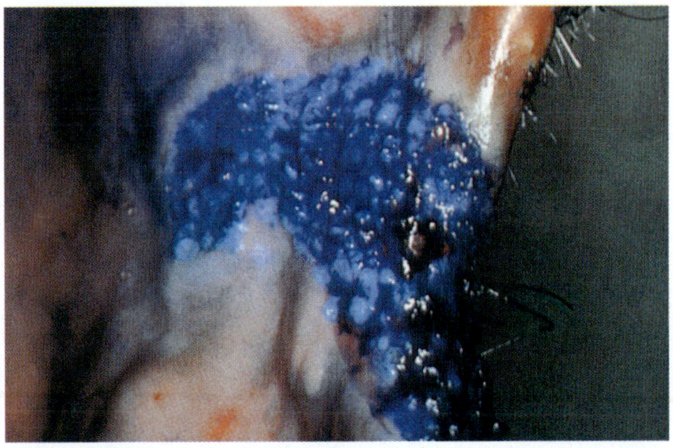

Figure 18.7 Speckled leukoplakia at the commissure—heavily stained.

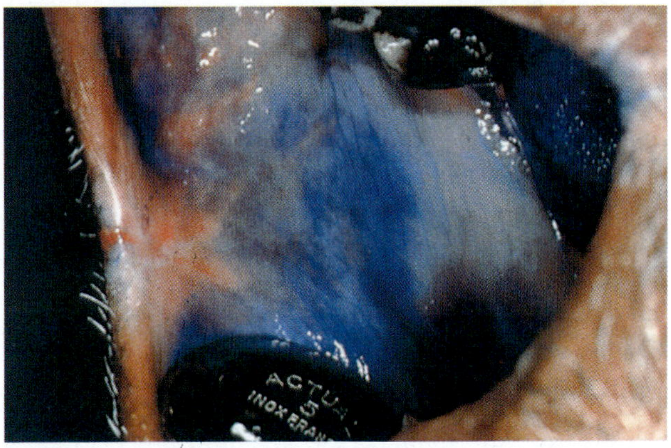

Figure 18.8 Stained area of atrophic mucosa, which on biopsy proved to be epithelial dysplasia.

Table 18.21 Evaluation of toluidine blue staining as a screen for oral cancer

Study	Number of reported evaluations	Sensitivity (%)	Specificity (%)	False positives	False negatives
(a) Trials involving a single application of stain					
Nibel and Chomet 1964	11[a] (20 patients)	100	NR	NR	0/11
Shedd et al. 1965	44[b] (50 patients)	100	85	2/13	0/31
Shedd et al. 1967	62 (23 volunteers)	100	(a) 85[c] (b) 94	3/20 0/23	0/42
Myers 1970	71	98	100	0/19	1/52
	100L[d]	NR	75	18/71	NR
Srivastava and Mathus 1971	100P	NR	94	6/97	NR
	(Combined)	NR	86	24/168	NR
Rosen et al. 1971	45	50	50	20/39	3/6
Vahidy et al. 1972	1030 (+ 160 cases[e] excluded)	86	76	131/549 (+106 doubtful)	66/481 (+54 doubtful)
Reddy et al. 1973	490	99	83	6/37	2/453
Sigurdson and Willen 1975	54	100	87	2/23	0/31
Barrellier et al. 1982	115 (111 patients)	100	93	7/105	0/6
Silverman et al. 1984	132	98	70	10/33	2/99
Epstein and Scully 1992	59	93	63	7/19	3/40
Barellier et al. 1993	235	95.7	85.9	30/212	1/23
Warnakulasuriya and Johnson 1996	86 (102 patients)	100	62	11/29[8]	0/18
Portugal et al. 1996	50	100	86	6/44	0/6
Epstein et al. 1997	81 (46 patients)[7]	100	52[6]	26/53	0/28
Total	**2948**				
(b) Trials involving a second application of stain or a period for resolution of transient inflammatory lesions					
Pizer and Dubois 1979	255	NR	99	3/248	0/7
Mashberg 1980	235	93	92	11/130	7/105
Mashberg 1981, 1983[9]	179 (a) rinse	89	91	9/98	9/81
	179 (b) direct application	98	88	12/98	2/81
Moyer et al. 1986	76 (75 patients)	NR	92	7/76	NA
Total	**924**				

[a]Malignant lesions only reported on.
[b]Results from 44 patients given.
[c](a) Specificity with respect to negatively staining patients; (b) specificity including volunteers.
[d]100 patients with lesions (L); 100 randomly selected patients (P).
[e]Excluded as stain reading doubtful.
6. Benign and all levels of dysplasia regarded as negative.
7. Treated patients with a 33% prevalence of new lesions.
8. This includes precancer.
9. Figures counted twice as two evaluations per patient were carried out.
NR: not reported, NA: not applicable

atrophic mucosa without a distinctive lesion which took up the dye and which proved, on biopsy, to show epithelial dysplasia, indicating an increased risk of progressing to malignancy if untreated. Figures 18.9–18.11 show pre- and post-stain results for an overt cancer, a severe dysplasia and a benign keratosis.

The FDI Commission, through its project on oral cancer, has recently agreed a statement on the use of toluidine blue, supporting its use in appropriately experienced hands and urging further research on its clinical utility in primary care settings. This states that the use of toluidine blue,

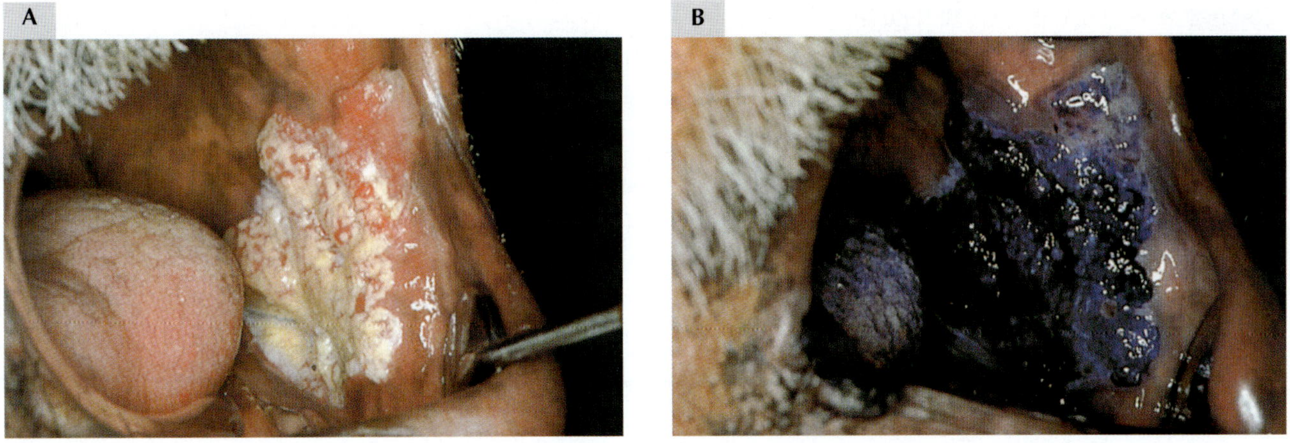

Figure 18.9 (A) A large exophytic tumour with a partly red, partly white surface. Clinically, this is almost certainly a carcinoma of the oral mucosa which, nevertheless, requires diagnostic confirmation by biopsy. Several biopsies from the junction between clinically normal and tumour tissue, including the deep invasive front, are desirable to provide details for treatment planning. (B) The tumour mass is stained a deep royal blue, with clearly defined borders. In this example, toluidine blue has not contributed to the diagnosis because the lesion is so clinically obvious. It may help delineate the margins and thus indicate appropriate sites for biopsy.

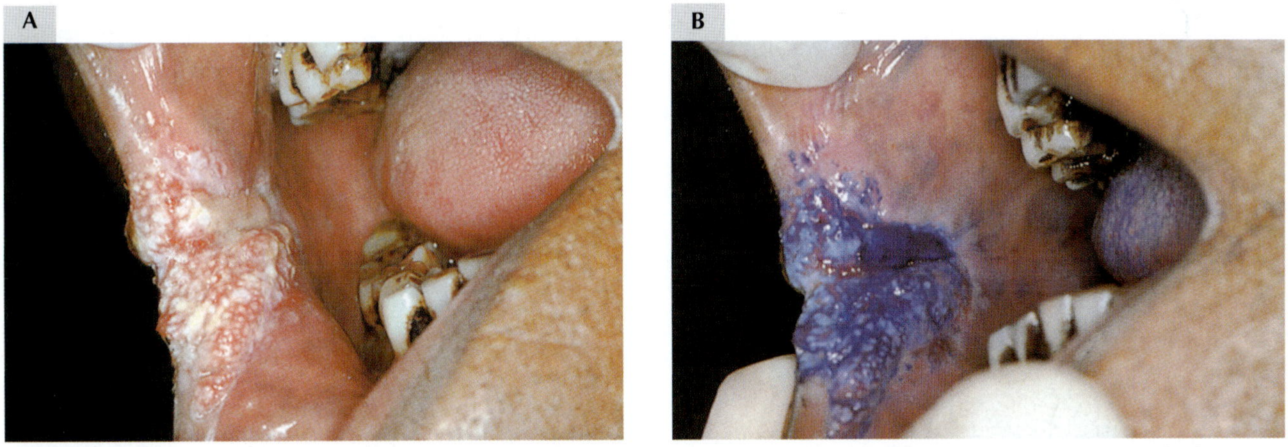

Figure 18.10 (A) A mixed nodular leukoplakia and erythroplakia at the commissure. (B) This also shows clearly demarcated, intense staining, including an area of ulceration in the upper posterior part of the lesion. Once again, biopsy would have been mandatory on the basis of clinical appearance alone. In this case, histology demonstrated severe epithelial dysplasia, short of overtly invasive carcinoma.

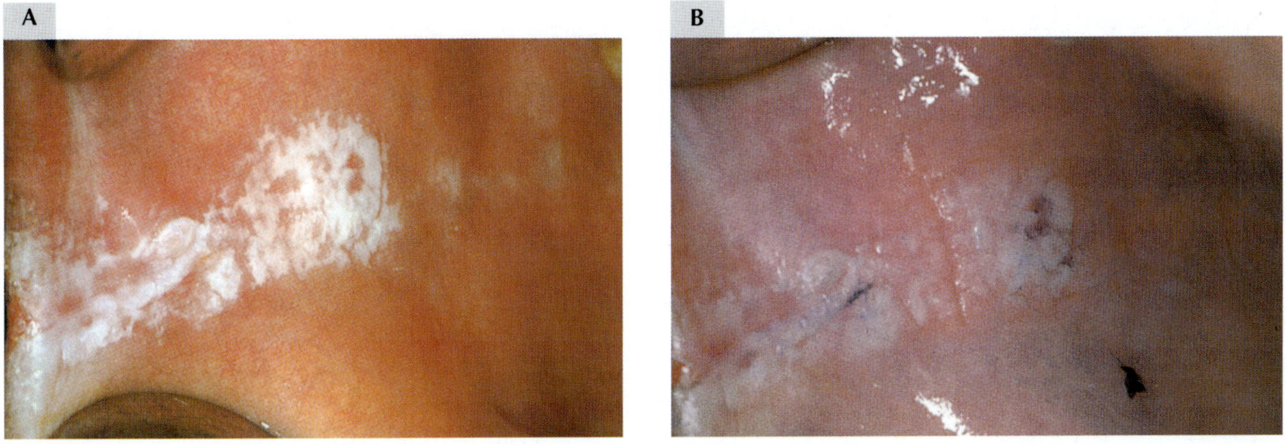

Figure 18.11 (A) A homogenous leukoplakia on the right commissure, with intervening areas of more normal mucosa. This appearance does not suggest a high risk lesion. (B) Apart from retention of a little dye in creases in the surface keratin, this lesion is toluidine blue negative. Nevertheless, biopsy is still required, on the basis of the initial clinical observations alone.

in expert and experienced hands, is recommended for:

- Monitoring of suspicious lesions over time.
- Screening for oral mucosal malignancy and premalignancy in high-risk individuals and population groups.
- Follow-up of patients already treated for upper aerodigestive tract cancer.[104]
- Helping to determine an optimal site for biopsy when a suspicious lesion or condition is present.
- Intra-operative use during surgery for upper aerodigestive tract malignancy as an application to help judge the borders of the neoplasm.[105]

Other fluorescent dyes,[24,106,107] direct microscopy[108,109] and image analysis of brush biopsies[110] are currently under study.

Molecular screening

It is possible to analyse tissue, and indeed a variety of body fluids, increasingly including saliva, for markers of aberrations in oncogenes or tumour suppressor genes or their protein products. It is also possible to screen chromosomes from oral epithelial cells in health, from potentially malignant lesions and from overt cancers and to record abnormalities such as loss, amplification or transposition of parts of the genome thought to be important in carcinogenesis. Existing knowledge in the rapidly developing field is given in Chapter 5.

It is not known precisely how many 'hits' or aberrations are necessary to render a clone of cells malignant, although a figure of around six is often quoted. Recent research of the above kind has led to models for the development of head and neck cancer (Fig. 18.12). Such models should not be taken to imply that precisely this series of abnormalities, in precisely that order, are necessary or sufficient for a cancer to develop: the number, type and order may differ from patient to patient. Nevertheless, the accumulation of such changes indicates an increasing risk of malignant transformation and this information will, in the future, be put to use in:

- Screening clinically normal patients, who are heavy smokers and drinkers, to determine their risk of a future cancer.
- Screening potentially malignant lesions and conditions in order to assess how far along the path to malignancy has been reached, and thus to focus intervention for the individual patient.
- Determining completeness of excision/killing by radiotherapy/chemotherapy, by sampling tissue in situ after treatment for an overt cancer, in order to assess the risk of recurrence or second primary. This encompasses the concepts of 'field change' and of 'residual disease'.
- Screening peripheral blood or bone marrow for malignant cells disseminated from the primary lesion.
- Screening blood or saliva,[111] or scrapings/washing[112–114] for the presence of a marker indicative of the presence of neoplasm—residual or recurrent primary, new primary or metastatic disease.[115]

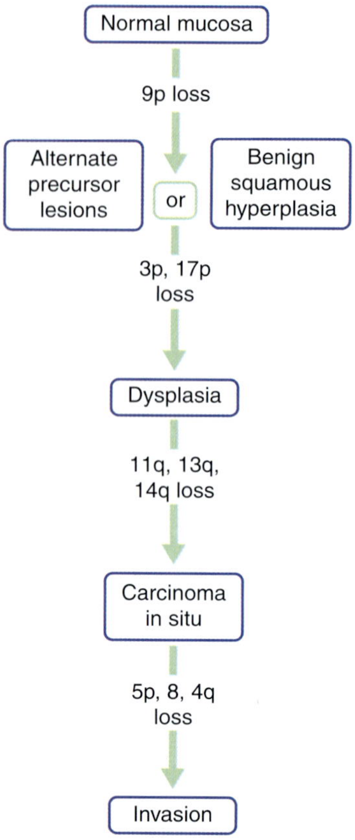

Figure 18.12 Genetic progression model for head and neck cancer: implications for field cancerization (adapted from Califano et al.[116]).

Tertiary prevention: preventing recurrence or further primary cancers and minimizing morbidity

When a patient treated for an oral cancer develops further cancer in the mouth, months or years after apparently successful treatment, it is often not clear whether the new lesion is a recurrence, arising because of incomplete removal of the primary lesion, or a second primary lesion, arising in a field of altered mucosa. The concept of *field cancerization* is that the patient's genetic predisposition, plus the lifelong accumulation of potentially carcinogenic insults from known and unknown risk factors renders the patient, and the anatomical area most affected, at increased

Table 18.22 Selected chemoprevention trials in oral premalignancy. (Source: Khuri et al.[117])

Reference	Year	Agent(s)	No. of patients	Results
Hong et al.[118]	1986	13cRA at 1–2 mg/kg per day for months versus placebo	44	67% response (13cRA) versus 10% response (placebo) (p = 0.0002)
Stich et al.[119]	1988	β-carotene + retinol (100 000 IU/week) (180 mg/week) versus placebo	103	27.5% versus 14.8% versus 3.0% ($p < 0.001$)
Stich et al.[120]	1988	Vitamin A (200 000 IU/week) orally for 6 months versus placebo	64	57.1% complete remission (vitamin A) versus 30% (controls) ($p < 0.01$)
Han et al.[121]	1990	4-HCR (40 mg/day) versus placebo	61	87% complete remission versus 17% ($p < 0.01$)
Lippman et al.[122]	1993	13cRA (1–5 mg/kg per day) for 3 months followed by 13cRA (0.5 mg/kg per day) for 9 months versus β-carotene (30 mg/day) for 9 months	70	Initial response 55% to high dose 13cRA; continued response or stable disease 92% in 13cRA maintenance versus 45% in β-carotene ($p < 0.001$)
Chiesa et al.[123], Costa et al.[124]	1993, 1994	4-HPR (200 mg/day) for 52 weeks versus placebo	153	Failure in 6% (4-HPR) versus 30% (placebo) ($p < 0.05$)

13cRA: 13-*cis*-retinoic acid; 4-HCR: 4-(hydroxycarbophenyl)retinamide; 4-HPR: 4-*N*.

risk of cancer. This applies whether the second cancer is synchronous with the first or arises later (metachronous). An alternative view is that a clone of genetically damaged and therefore 'premalignant' cells migrates in the anatomical area and may give rise to second tumours.[125] Either way, it is clear that with oral cancer the whole of the upper aerodigestive tract can be regarded as the susceptible field.[126] Unsurprisingly, therefore, the risk of a further cancer is high once a patient has been treated for oral cancer, amounting to some 20% of patients over a 5-year period. This is especially so if the tobacco, alcohol and dietary risk factors continue to be present. All of the above primary prevention approaches are, therefore, especially important at this stage, including supplementation with antioxidants such as vitamin A[127] or retinoids.[128,129]

Chemoprevention of malignant transformation of oral precancerous lesions (leukoplakia has been most extensively investigated, as it is the commonest, even if variably and loosely defined) and conditions by dietary supplementation is another exciting field under active investigation. Data from some selected trials are summarized in Table 18.22. Synthetic retinoids[130] and curcumin[131] are currently attracting interest.

The current position was thoroughly evaluated by Sankaranarayanan et al.,[132] from which the following summary is partly derived. Both the experimental animal evidence and the then published clinical trials were thoroughly analysed by Tanaka in 1995.[133] Many of the field studies have been conducted in India on pan or other smokeless tobacco-associated lesions, with or without beedi smoking and alcohol as cofactors. Those from the West relate to smoking and alcohol related cancers. The essential conclusions are:

- In the *primary prevention* of oral and other epithelial cancers, as discussed earlier, a substantial reduction in risk can be obtained by increasing fruit and vegetable consumption.[134,135] This is quite distinct from the use of nutritional supplements in *secondary and tertiary prevention.*
- Retinoids and β-carotene have been shown to result in the regression of oral leukoplakia, but the lesions soon recur after the chemopreventive agents are stopped.[136]
- Lower frequencies of malignant transformation have been observed in a small number of subjects with leukoplakia receiving retinoids compared to subjects receiving β-carotene.[122]
- Supplementation has not been shown to reduce the risk of locoregional recurrence in treated head and neck cancer patients.
- A reduction in the frequency of second primaries has been observed with 13-*cis*-retinoic acid,[137] but not with etretinate.[138]

- Although retinoids seem to be effective in inhibiting head and neck carcinogenesis, compared with β-carotene, the synthetic retinoids are quite toxic, which limits their usefulness.[122]
- Retinoids have the potential to enhance carcinogenesis under certain conditions, perhaps due to an angiogenic effect, so their use cannot yet be justified outside of clinical trials.[139]
- There is insufficient evidence to evaluate the chemopreventive effects of vitamin E or of selenium in head and neck cancer. Some early results on combinations of vitamin E and β-carotene are encouraging.[140]
- None of the potential intermediate biomarkers studied for the effect of chemopreventive regimes have yet been fully validated. Amongst these micronucleated epithelial cells have received the most attention,[141] and Sankaranarayanan et al.[132] concluded that this method has value in monitoring compliance amongst patients.
- Many other potential biomarkers, discussed in Chapter 5, are under investigation. These include DNA adducts,[141] cell proliferation markers such as Ki67 and PCNA, EGFR and erbB expression, aberrations of the p53 gene or its protein and HPV gene expression or integration. In respect of studies on retinoid chemoprevention it may be possible to use nuclear retinoic acid receptors for this purpose.[142]
- Attempts at chemoprevention of head and neck cancer should only be made in the context of well-planned, preferably multicentre, clinical trials. Many of these are ongoing.

Further secondary prevention (by screening) is also especially important. Treated patients should be monitored regularly in order to ensure that their mastication, swallowing, speaking, smiling and other functions, their physical appearance and their social integration are as good as the cancer care team can manage, and to screen for the possibility of new lesions. In this latter respect toluidine blue application may have particular utility. The cost-effectiveness of regular upper aerodigestive tract endoscopy has yet to be established.

Nowhere is teamwork in cancer care more important than with treated patients, in order to maximize the quality of life for those afflicted and to ensure the best possible quality of death.

References

1. Alfano MC, Horowitz AM. Professional and community efforts to prevent morbidity and mortality from oral cancer. J Am Dent Assoc 2001; 132: 24S-29S
2. WHO. Tobacco control initiative: rationale, update and progress. Geneva: World Health Organization, 1998
3. Centres for Disease Control and Prevention. Preventing and controlling oral and pharyngeal cancer, MMWR 1998; Vol 47, No RR-14. Washington DC: US Department of Health and Human Services
4. Smoking kills: a white paper on tobacco. London: The Stationery Office, 1998
5. Department of Health. Report of the Scientific Committee on Tobacco and Health. London: HMSO, 1998
6. Peto R, Lopez AD, Boreham J et al. Imperial Cancer Research Fund and World Health Organization. Mortality from smoking in developing countries 1950–2000. Oxford: Oxford University Press, 1994
7. Peto R, Lopez AD, Boreham J, Thun M, Heath C Jr, Doll R. Mortality from smoking worldwide. Br Med Bull 1996; 52: 12–21
8. WHO. Tobacco or health: a global status report. Geneva: World Health Organization, 1997
9. Doll R, Peto R, Wheatley K et al. Mortality in relation to smoking: 40 years' observations on male British doctors. Br Med J 1994; 309: 901–911
10. Cost effectiveness of smoking cessation interventions. London: Centre for Health Economics, University of York and Health Education Authority, 1997
11. Stead M, Hastings G, Tudor-Smith C. Preventing adolescent smoking: a review of options. Health Educ J 1996; 55: 31–54
12. FDI World Dental Federation. Position statement on tobacco. FDI World 1996; 6: 9
13. Watt RG, Johnson NW, Warnakulasuriya KA. Action on smoking – opportunities for the dental team. Br Dent J 2001; 190: 227
14. Tomar SL. Dentistry's role in tobacco control. J Am Dent Assoc 2001; 132: 30S-35S
15. Johnson NW, Bain CA. Tobacco and oral disease. EU-Working Group on Tobacco and Oral Health. Br Dent J 2000; 189: 200–206
16. Cohen SJ, Stookey GK, Katz BP et al. Helping smokers quit: a randomised controlled trial with private practice dentists. J Am Dent Assoc 1989; 118: 41–45
17. Segnan N, Ponti A, Battista RN et al. A randomised trial of smoking cessation interventions in general practice in Italy. Cancer Causes Contr 1991; 2: 239–246
18. Russell MA, Stapleton JA, Feyeraband C et al. Targeting heavy smokers in general practice: randomised controlled trial of transdermal nicotine patches. Br Med J 1993; 306: 1308–1312
19. Stapleton JA, Russell MAH, Feyerabend C et al. Dose effects and predictors of outcome in a randomised trial of transdermal nicotine patches in general practice. Addiction 1995; 90: 31–42
20. Macgregor IDM. Efficacy of dental health advice as an aid to reducing cigarette smoking. Br Dent J 1996; 180: 292–296
21. Smith SE, Warnakulasuriya KAAS, Feyerabend C, Belcher M, Cooper DJ, Johnson NW. A smoking cessation programme conducted through dental practices in the UK. Br Dent J 1998; 185: 299–303

22. Tobacco use and the periodontal patient. J Periodontol 1996; 67: 51–56
23. EU Working Group on Tobacco and Oral Health Consensus Meeting. Copenhagen, 23–26 October 1997. Oral Diseases 1998; 4: 48–67
24. van Staveren HJ, van Veen RL, Speelman OC, Witjes MJ, Star WM, Roodenburg JL. Classification of clinical autofluorescence spectra of oral leukoplakia using an artificial neural network: a pilot study. Oral Oncol 2000; 36; 286–293
25. Reibel J, Stoltze K, Pindborg JJ. Tobakkens skadelige virkninger i mundhulen. Copenhagen: Danish Dental Association
26. Mecklenburg RE, Greenspan D, Kleinman DV et al. Tobacco effects in the mouth. NIH Publication No 96-3330. Washington DC: US Dept of Health and Human Services
27. Martin LM, Bouquot JE, Wingo PA, Heath CW Jr. Cancer prevention in the dental practice: oral cancer screening and tobacco cessation advice. J Public Health Dent 1996; 56: 336–340
28. Warnakulasuriya KAAS, Johnson NW. Dentists and oral cancer prevention in the UK: opinions, attitudes and practices to screening for mucosal lesions and to counselling patients on tobacco and alcohol use. Baseline data from 1991. Oral Dis 1999; 5: 10–14
29. Horowitz AM, Drury TF, Goodman HS, Yellowitz JA. Oral pharyngeal cancer prevention and early detection. Dentist's opinions and practices. J Am Dent Assoc 2000; 131: 453–462
30. Yellowitz JA, Horowitz AM, Drury TF, Goodman HS. Survey of US dentists' knowledge and opinions about oral pharyngeal cancer. J Am Dent Assoc 2000; 131: 653–661
31. Dodds AP, Rankin KV, Jones DL, Seals RR. What are you doing about oral cancer? Report of a survey of Texas dentists. Texas Dent J 1994; 114: 39–41
32. Sachs DPL. Advances in smoking cessation treatment. In: Simmons DH (ed). Current pulmonology, Vol 12. Chicago: Year Book Publishers, 1991: 139–198
33. Russell MA. Targeting heavy smokers in general practice: randomised controlled trial of transdermal nicotine patches. Br Med J 1993; 306: 1308–1312
34. Pierce JP, Gilpin E, Farkas AJ. Nicotine patch use in the general population: results from the 1993 California Tobacco Survey. JNCI 1995; 87: 87–93
35. Silagy C, Mant D, Fowler G, Lodge M. Meta-analysis on efficacy of nicotine replacement therapies in smoking cessation. Lancet 1994; 343: 139–142
36. Johnson NW. A global view of the epidemiology of oral cancer. In: Johnson NW (ed.). Risk markers for oral diseases, Vol 2. Oral cancer: detection of patients and lesions at risk. Cambridge: Cambridge University Press, 3–26
37. Gupta PC, Murti PR, Bhonsle RB et al. Effect of cessation of tobacco use on the incidence of oral mucosal lesions in a ten year follow up study of 12 212 users. Oral Dis 1995; 1: 54–58
38. Idris AM, Warnakulasuriya, KAAS, Ibrahim YE et al. Toombak-associated oral mucosal lesions in Sudanese show a low prevalence of epithelial dysplasia. J Oral Pathol Med 1996; 25: 239–244
39. Gupta PC, Murti PR, Bhonsle RB. Epidemiology of cancer by tobacco products and the significance of TSNA. Crit Rev Toxicol 1996; 26: 183–198
40. Lewin F, Norell SE, Johansson H et al. Smoking tobacco, oral snuff and alcohol in the aetiology of squamous cell carcinoma of the head and neck. A population based case-referent study in Sweden. Cancer 1998; 83: 1367–1375
41. Idris AM, Ibrahim SO, Vasstrand EN et al. The Swedish *snus* and the Sudanese *Toombak*: are they different? Oral Oncol 1998; 34: 558–566
42. Rodu B. For smokers only: how smokeless tobacco can save your life. New York: Sulzberger and Graham, 1995: 190
43. Hackshaw AK, Law MR, Wald NJ. The accumulated evidence on lung cancer and environmental tobacco smoke. Br Med J 1997; 315: 980–988
44. Law MR, Morris JK, Wald NJ. Environmental tobacco smoke exposure and ischaemic heart disease: an evaluation of the evidence. Br Med J; 315: 973–980
45. California Environmental Protection Agency, Office of Environmental Health Hazard Assessment. Health effects of environmental exposure to tobacco smoke. http://www.calepa.cahwnet.gov/oehha/docs/finalets.htm
46. US Environmental Protection Agency. Respiratory health effects of passive smoking: lung cancer and other disorders. Publication EPA/600/6–90/006F. Washington DC: US Environmental Protection Agency, 1992
47. McGinnis JM, Foege WH. Actual causes of death in the United States. JAMA 1993; 270: 2207–2212
48. Gray JD, Bhopal RS, White M. Developing a medical school alcohol policy. Med Educ 1998; 32: 138–142
49. Day GL, Blot WJ, Austin DF et al. Racial differences in risk of oral and pharyngeal cancer: alcohol, tobacco and other determinants. J Natl Cancer Inst 1993; 85: 465–473
50. Macfarlane GJ, Macfarlane TV, Lowenfels AB. The influence of alcohol consumption on world wide trends in mortality from upper aerodigestive tract cancers in males. J Epidemiol Comm Health 1996; 50: 636–639
51. Harris CK, Warnakulasuriya KAAS, Johnson NW, Gelbier S, Peters TJ. Oral health in alcohol misusers. Comm Dent Health 1996; 13: 199–203
52. Bradley KA, Bush KR, McDonell MB, Malone T, Fihn SD. Screening for problem drinking: comparison of CAGE and AUDIT. Ambulatory care quality improvement project (ACQUIP). Alcohol use disorders identification test. J Gen Intern Med 1998; 13: 379–388
53. Saunders JB, Aasland OG, Babor TF, De La Fuente JR, Grant M. Development of alcohol use disorders identification test (AUDIT): WHO collaborative project on early detection of persons with harmful alcohol consumption – 11. Addiction 1993; 88: 791–804
54. Harris C, Warnakulasuriya KAAS, Gelbier S, Johnson NW, Peters TJ. Oral and dental health in alcohol misusing patients. Alcohol Clin Exp Res 1997; 21: 1707–1709

55. Long CG, Williams M, Hollin CR. Treating alcohol problems: a study of programme effectiveness and cost effectiveness according to length and delivery of treatment. Addiction 1998; 93: 561–571
56. Gomel MK, Wutzke SE, Hardcastle DM, Lapsley H, Reznik RB. Cost-effectiveness of strategies to market and train primary health care physicians in brief intervention techniques for hazardous alcohol use. Soc Sci Med 1998; 47: 203–211
57. Richmond RL, Novak K, Kehoe L, Calfas G, Mendelsohn CP, Wodak A. Effect of training on general practitioners' use of brief intervention for excessive drinkers. Aust NZ J Public Health 1998; 22: 206–209
58. Subcommittee on Health Services Research, National Advisory Council on Alcohol Abuse and Alcoholism. Improving the delivery of alcohol treatment and prevention services: executive summary. NIH Publication No 4224. Bethesda MD: National Institute on Alcohol Abuse and Alcoholism, National Institutes of Health, Department of Health and Human Services, 1997
59. Klatsky AL, Armstrong MA, Friedman GD. Alcohol and mortality. Ann Intern Med 1992; 117: 646–654
60. Gazioano JM, Buring JE, Breslow JL et al. Moderate alcohol intake, increased levels of high-density lipoprotein and its sub-fractions, and decreased risk of myocardial infarction. N Engl J Med 1993; 329: 1829–1834
61. Pearson TA. Alcohol and heart disease. Circulation 1995; 94: 3023–3025
62. Suh I, Shaten BJ, Cutler JA, Kuller LH for the Mutiple Risk Factor Intervention Trial research group. Alcohol use and mortality from coronary heart disease: the role of high-density lipoprotein cholesterol. Ann Int Med 1993; 116: 881–887
63. Ridker PM, Vaughan DE, Stampfer MJ, Glynn RJ, Hennekens CH. Association of moderate alcohol consumption and plasma concentration of endogenous tissue-type plasminogen activator. JAMA 1994; 272: 929–933
64. Renaud S, de Lorgeril M. Wine, alcohol, platelets, and the French paradox for coronary heart disease. Lancet 1992; 339: 1523–1526
65. Jang M, Cai L, Udeani GO et al. Cancer chemopreventive effect of resveratrol, a natural product derived from grapes. Science 1997; 275: 218–220
66. Rimm EB, Klatsky A, Grobbee D, Stampfer MJ. Review of moderate alcohol consumption and reduced risk of coronary heart disease: is the effect due to beer, wine or spirits. Br Med J 1996; 312: 731–736
67. McKee M, Britton A. The positive relationship between alcohol and heart disease in eastern Europe: potential physiological mechanisms. J R Soc Med 1998; 91: 402–407
68. UK Health Education Authority. That's the limit – a guide to sensible drinking. London: HEA
69. Bray I, Brennan P, Boffetta P. Projections of alcohol- and tobocco-related cancer mortality in Central Europe. Int J Cancer 2000; 87: 122–128
70. Franceschi S, Levi F, Dal Maso L et al. Cessation of alcohol drinking and risk of cancer of the oral cavity and pharynx. Int J Cancer 2000; 85: 787–790
71. Warnakulasuriya KA, Harris CK, Scarrott DM et al. An alarming lack of public awareness towards oral cancer. Br Dent J 1999; 187:319–322
72. Hay JL, Ostroff JS, Cruz GD, LeGeros RZ, Kenigsberg H, Franklin DM. Oral cancer risk perception among participants in an oral cancer screening program. Cancer Epidemiol Biomarkers Prev 2002; 11: 155–158
73. Doll R. The prevention of cancer: opportunities and challenges. In: Heller T, Davey B, Bailey L (eds). Reducing the risk of cancers. London: Hodder and Stoughton, 1989
74. La Vecchia C, Tavani A, Franceschi S et al. Epidemiology and prevention of oral cancer. Oral Oncol 1997; 33: 303–312
75. Hakama M, Beral V, Buiatti E, Faivre J, Parkin DM (eds). Chemoprevention in Cancer Control. IARC Scientific Publication No 136, Lyon: IARC, 1996
76. Stewart BW, McGregor D, Kleihues P (eds). Principles of chemoprevention. IARC Scientific Publication No 139, Lyon: IARC, 1996
77. Hebert JR, Gupta PC, Bhonsle RB et al. Dietary exposures and oral precancerous lesions in Srikakulam District, Andhra Pradesh, India. Public Health Nutr 2002; 5: 303–312
78. Negri E, Franceshi S, Bosetti C et al. Selected micronutrients and oral and pharyngeal cancer. Int J Cancer 2000; 86: 122–127
79. Morse DE, Pendrys DG, Katz RV et al. Food group intake and the risk of oral epithelial dysplasia in a United States population. Cancer Causes Control 2000; 11: 713–720
80. American Cancer Society. Advisory Committee on Diet, Nutrition and Cancer Prevention; guidelines in diet, nutrition and cancer prevention: reducing the risk of cancer with healthy food choices and physical activity. CA – A Cancer Journal for Clinicians 1996; 46: 325–341
81. Chamberlain J, Moss S. Focus on cancer: evaluation of cancer screening. London: Springer, 1996
82. Wilson JMG, Jungner G. Principles and practice of screening for disease. Public Health Paper No 34. Geneva: WHO, 1968
83. Gupta PC, Murti PR, Bhonsle RB et al. Effect of cessation of tobacco use on the incidence of oral lesions in a ten year follow up study of 12,212 users. Oral Dis 1995; 1: 54–58
84. Sankaranarayanan R, Matthew B, Varghese PR et al. Chemoprevention of oral leukoplakia with vitamin A and beta carotene: an assessment. Oral Oncol 1977; 33: 231–236
85. van der Waal I, Schepman KP, van der Meij EH et al. Oral leukoplakia: a clinicopathological review. Oral Oncol 1997; 33: 291–301
86. Tradati N, Grigolat R, Calabrese L et al. Oral leukoplakias: to treat or not? Oral Oncol 1997; 33: 317–321

87. Speight PM, Downer MC, Zakrzewska JM (eds). Screening for oral cancer and precancer: report of a UK working group. Comm Dent Health 1993; 10: (Suppl 1): 1–89
88. Rodrigues VC, Moss SM, Tuomainen H. Oral cancer in the UK: to screen or not to screen. Oral Oncol 1998; 34: 454–465
89. Franceschi S, Barzan L, Talamini R. Screening for cancer of the head and neck: if not now, when? Oral Oncol 1997; 33: 313–316
90. Downer MC, Jullien JA, Speight PM. An interim determination of health gain from oral cancer and precancer screening: 1. Obtaining health state utilities. Comm Dent Health 1997; 14: 139–142
91. Warnakulasuriya KAAS, Johnson NW. Strengths and weaknesses of screening programmes for oral malignancies and potentially malignant lesions. Eur J Cancer Prev 1996; 5: 93–98
92. Moles DR, Downer MC, Speight PM. Meta-analysis of measures of performance reported in oral cancer and precancer screening studies. Br Dent J 2002; 192: 340–344
93. Sankaranarayanan R, Mathew B, Jacob BJ et al. Early findings from a community-based, cluster-randomized, controlled oral cancer screening trial in Keral, India. The Trivandrum Oral Cancer Screening Study Group. Cancer 2000; 88: 664–673
94. Jullien JA, Zakrzewska JM, Downer MC et al. Attendance and compliance at an oral cancer screening programme in a general medical practice. Oral Oncol, Eur J Cancer 1995; 31B: 202–206
95. Ikeda N, Downer MC, Ozowa Y et al. Characteristics of of participants and non-participants in annual mass screening for oral cancer in 60 year old residents of Tokoname city, Japan. Comm Dent Health 1995; 12: 83–88
96. Nagao T, Ikeda N, Fukano H, Miyazaki H, Yano M, Warnakulasuriya S. Outcome following a population screening programme for oral cancer and precancer in Japan. Oral Oncol 2000; 36: 340–346
97. Nagao T, Warnakulasuriya S, Ikeda N, Fukano H, Fujiwara K, Miyazaki H. Oral cancer screening as an integral part of general health screening in Tokoname City, Japan. J Med Screen 2000; 7: 203–208
98. Speight PM, Elliott AE, Jullien JA et al. The use of artificial intelligence to identify people at risk of oral cancer and precancer. Br Dent J 1995; 179: 382–387
99. Roberts CJ, Farrow SC, Charny MC. How much can the NHS afford to spend to save a life or avoid a severe disability? Lancet 1985; i: 89–91
100. Sankaranarayanan R. Health care auxiliaries in the detection and prevention of oral cancer. Oral Oncol 1997; 33: 149–154
101. Warnakulasuriya KAAS, Pindborg JJ. Reliability of oral precancer screening by primary health care workers in Sri Lanka. Comm Dent Health 1990; 7: 73–79
102. Santana JC, Delgado L, Miranda J et al. Oral cancer case finding programme (OCCFP). Oral Oncol 1997; 33: 10–12
103. Onofre MA, Sposto MR, Navarro CM. Reliability of toluidine blue application in the detection of oral epithelial dysplasia and in situ and invasive squamous cell carcinomas. Oral Surg Oral Med Oral Pathol Oral Radiol Endod 2001; 91: 535–540
104. Guo Z, Yamaguchi K, Sanchez-Cespedes M, Westra WH, Koch WM, Sidransky D. Allelic losses in OraTest-directed biopsies of patients with prior upper aerodigestive tract malignancy. Clin Cancer Res 2001; 7: 1963–1968
105. Kerawala CJ, Beale V, Reed M, Martin IC. The role of vital tissue staining in the marginal control of oral squamous cell carcinoma. Int J Oral Maxillofac Surg 2000; 29: 32–35
106. Leunig A, Mehlmann M, Betz C et al. Fluorescence staining of oral cancer using a topical application of 5-aminolevulinic acid: fluorescence microscopic studies. J Photochem Photobiol B 2001; 60: 44–49
107. Leunig A, Betz CS, Mehlmann M et al. Detection of squamous cell carcinoma of the oral cavity by imaging 5-aminolevulinic acid-induced protoporphyrin IX fluorescence. Laryngoscope 2000; 110: 78–83
108. Suhr MA, Hopper C, Jones L, George JG, Bown SG, MacRobert AJ. Optical biopsy systems for the diagnosis and monitoring of superficial cancer and precancer. Int J Oral Maxillofac Surg 2000; 29: 453–457
109. Gynther GW, Rozell B, Heimdahl A. Direct oral microscopy and its value in diagnosing mucosal lesions: a pilot study. Oral Surg Oral Med Oral Pathol Oral Radiol Endod 2000; 90: 164–170
110. Christian DC. Computer-assisted analysis of oral brush biopsies at an oral cancer screening program. J Am Dent Assoc 2002; 133: 357–362
111. Warnakulasuriya S, Soussi T, Maher R, Johnson N, Tavassoli M. Expression of p53 in oral squamous cell carcinoma is associated with the presence of IgG and IgA p53 autoantibodies in sera and saliva of the patients. J Pathol 2000; 192: 52–57
112. Califano J, Ahrendt SA, Meininger G et al. Detection of telomerase activity in oral rinses from head and neck squamous cell carcinoma patients. Cancer Res 1996; 56: 5720–5722
113. Nunes DN, Kowalski LP, Simpson AJ. Detection of oral and oropharyngeal cancer by microsatellite analysis in mouth washes and lesion brushings. Oral Oncol 2000; 36: 525–528
114. Spafford MF, Koch WM, Reed AL et al. Detection of head and neck squamous cell carcinoma among exfoliated oral mucosal cells by microsatellite analysis. Clin Cancer Res 2001; 7: 607–612
115. Forastiere A, Koch W, Trotti A, Sidransky D. Head and neck cancer. N Eng J Med 2001; 345: 1890–1900
116. Califano J, van der Riet P, Westra W et al. Genetic progression model for head and neck cancer; implications for field cancerization. Cancer Res 1996; 56: 2488–2492
117. Khuri FR, Lippman SM, Spitz MR, Lotan R, Hong WK. Molecular epidemiology and chemoprevention of head and neck cancer. J Natl Cancer Inst 1997; 89: 199–211

118. Hong W, Endicott J, Itri LM et al. 13-*cis* retinoic acid in the treatment of oral leukoplakia. N Engl J Med 1986; 315: 1501–1505
119. Stich HF, Hornby AP, Mathew B, Sankaranarayanan R, Nair MK. Response of oral leukoplakias to the administration of vitamin A. Cancer Lett 1988; 40: 93–101
120. Stich HF, Rosin MP, Hornby P, Mathew B, Sankaranarayanan R, Nair MK. Remission of oral leukoplakias and micronuclei in tobacco/betel quid chewers treated with β-carotene and with β-carotene plus vitamin A. Int J Cancer 1998; 42: 195–199
121. Han J, Jiao L, Lu Y, Sun Z, Gu QM, Scanlon KJ. Evaluation of *N*-4-(hydroxycarbophenyl) retinamide as a cancer prevention agent and as a cancer chemotherapeutic agent. In Vivo 1990; 4: 153–160
122. Lippman SM, Batsakis JG, Toth BB et al. Comparison of low dose isotretinoin with beta carotene to prevent oral carcinogenesis. N Engl J Med 1993; 328: 15–20
123. Chiesa F, Tradati N, Marazza M et al. Fenretinide (4–HPR) in chemoprevention of oral leukoplakia. J Cell Biochem Suppl 1993; 17F: 255–261
124. Costa A, Formelli F, Chiesa F, Decensi A, De Palo G, Veronesi U. Prospects of chemoprevention of human cancers with the synthetc retinoid fenretinide. Cancer Res 1994; 54 (Suppl): 2023s–2037s
125. Partridge M, Emilion G, Pateromichelakis S et al. Field cancerization of the oral cavity: comparison of the spectrum of molecular alterations in cases presenting with both dysplastic and malignant lesions. Oral Oncol 1997; 33: 332–337
126. Ogden GR. Field cancerization in the head and neck. Oral Dis 1998; 4: 1–3
127. Jyothirmayi R, Ramadas K, Varghese C et al. Efficacy of vitamin A in the prevention of loco-regional recurrence and second primaries in head and neck cancer. Oral Oncol, Eur J Cancer 1996; 32B: 373–376
128. Lippmann SM, Spitz MR, Huber MH et al. Strategies for chemoprevention study of premalignancy and second primary tumours in the head and neck. Curr Opin Oncol 1995; 7: 234–241
129. Anderson WF, Hawk E, Berg CD. Secondary chemoprevention of upper aerodigestive tract tumors. Semin Oncol 2001; 28: 106–120
130. Femiano F, Gombos F, Scully C, Battista C, Belnome G, Esposito V. Oral leukoplaskia: open trial of topical therapy with calcipotriol compared with tretinoin. Int J Oral Maxillofac Surg 2001; 30: 402–406
131. Cheng AL, Hsu CH, Lin JK et al. Phase I clinical trial of curcumin, a chemopreventive agent, in patients with high-risk or pre-malignant lesions. Anticancer Res 2001; 21: 2895–2900
132. Sankaranarayanan R, Mathew B, Nair PP et al. Chemoprevention of cancers of the oral cavity and the head and neck. In: Stewart BW, McGregor D, Kleihues P (eds). Principles of chemoprevention. IARC Scientific Publication No 139. Lyon: IARC, 1996
133. Tanaka T. Chemoprevention of oral carcinogenesis. Oral Oncol 1995; 31B: 3–15
134. La Vecchia C, Tavani A. Fruit and vegetables and human cancer. Eur J Cancer Prev 1998; 7: 3–8
135. De Stefani E, Deneo-Pelligrini H, Mendilaharsu M, Ronco A. Diet and risk of cancer of the upper aerodigestive tract – I. Foods; II. oral. Oncology 1999; 35: 17–21
136. Stich HF, Mathew B, Sankaranarayanan R, Krishnan Nair M. Remission of oral precancerous lesions of tobacco/areca nut chewers following administration of β-carotene or vitamin A, and maintenance of the protective effect. Cancer Detect Prev 1991; 15: 93–98
137. Benner SE, Pajak TF, Lippman SSM, Earley C, Hong WK. Prevention of second primary tumours with isoretinoin in patients with squamous cell carcinoma of the head and neck: long-term follow up. J Natl Cancer Inst 1994; 86: 140–141
138. Bolla M, Lefur R, Ton Van J et al. Prevention of second primary tumours with etretinate in squamous cell carcinoma of the oral cavity and oropharynx. Results of a multicentric double blind randomised study. Eur J Cancer 1994; 30A: 767–772
139. Schwartz JL, Shklar G. Retinoid and carotenoid angiogenesis: a possible explanation for enhanced oral carcinogenesis. Nutr Cancer 1997; 27: 192–199
140. Garewal H. Antioxidants in oral cancer prevention. Am J Clin Nutr 1995; 62 (Suppl): 1410s–1416s
141. Prasad MPR, Mukundan MA, Krishnaswamy K. Micronuclei and carcinogen DNA adducts as intermediate end points in nutrient intervention trial of precancerous lesions in the oral cavity. Oral Oncol 1995; 31B: 155–159
142. Khuri FR, Lippman SSM, Spitz MR, Lotan R, Hong WK. Molecular epidemiology and chemoprevention of head and neck cancer. J Natl Cancer Inst 1997; 39: 199–211

Index

Numbers in italics indicate *tables* or *figures*.